Textbook of

HISTOLOGY

Textbook of

HISTOLOGY

FIFTH EDITION

Leslie P. Gartner, PhD
Professor of Anatomy (Ret.)
Department of Biomedical Sciences
Baltimore College of Dental Surgery
Dental School
University of Maryland
Baltimore, Maryland

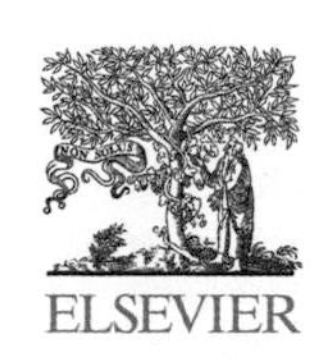

1600 John F. Kennedy Blvd.
Ste 1600
Philadelphia, PA 19103-2899

TEXTBOOK OF HISTOLOGY, FIFTH EDITION ISBN: 978-0-323-67272-6

Content Strategist: Alexandra Mortimer
Content Development Manager: Meghan Andress
Publishing Services Manager: Deepthi Unni
Project Manager: Haritha Dharmarajan/Aparna Venkatachalam
Design: Bridget Hoette

Printed in Canada

Last digit is the print number: 9 8 7 6 5 4 3 2 1

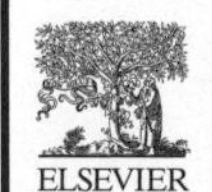

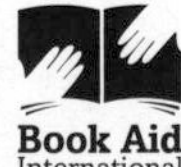

To my wife Roseann,
my daughter Jen,
and my mother Mary.
L.P.G.

PREFACE

Once again, I am gratified to release a new edition of a histology textbook that has become well established not only in its original language but also in seven other languages into which it has been translated: Italian, Portuguese, Indonesian, Korean, Spanish, Greek, and Turkish. The place of histology has altered as the biological sciences have progressed in the last half a century. It evolved from the purely descriptive science of microscopic anatomy to its current position as the linchpin that connects functional anatomy, molecular and cell biology, physiology, and histopathology.

The current edition has been thoroughly revised to be consistent with new information in cell and molecular biology that pertains to the subject matter of histology. While incorporating new material, the author was mindful of the time constraints that students face in an ever-expanding curriculum and an exponentially increasing information glut. Therefore, the goal was to maintain the brevity while at the same time retaining the readability of the textual material.

I have added numerous new clinical considerations, several new drawings, 16 new tables, and over 170 new photomicrographs created specifically for this edition of the *Textbook of Histology*. The most visible change is the addition of a segment called "Histology Laboratory Instructions" for Chapters 5 through 22. These instructions are designed to be photocopied (or downloaded from the website for this textbook on Elsevier's studentconsult.com) and to be used as a histology laboratory manual, referring back to the photomicrographs illustrating this textbook. I decided to write the histology manual because, in many schools, the laboratory component of the histology course had to be partially sacrificed due to the loss of instruction time with the drastic reduction in the basic science elements of the medical curriculum.

As with all of my textbooks, this *Textbook of Histology* has been written with the student in mind. Thus, the material presented is complete but not esoteric. It is not meant to train the reader to be a histologist but rather to provide the necessary basis for the understanding of the microscopic structure of the human body and to lay a foundation for the student's progress through the biomedical sciences.

Although I have attempted to be accurate and complete, I realize that errors and omissions may have escaped my attention. Therefore, I welcome criticisms, suggestions, and comments that would help improve this textbook. Please address them to LPG21136@yahoo.com.

Leslie P. Gartner

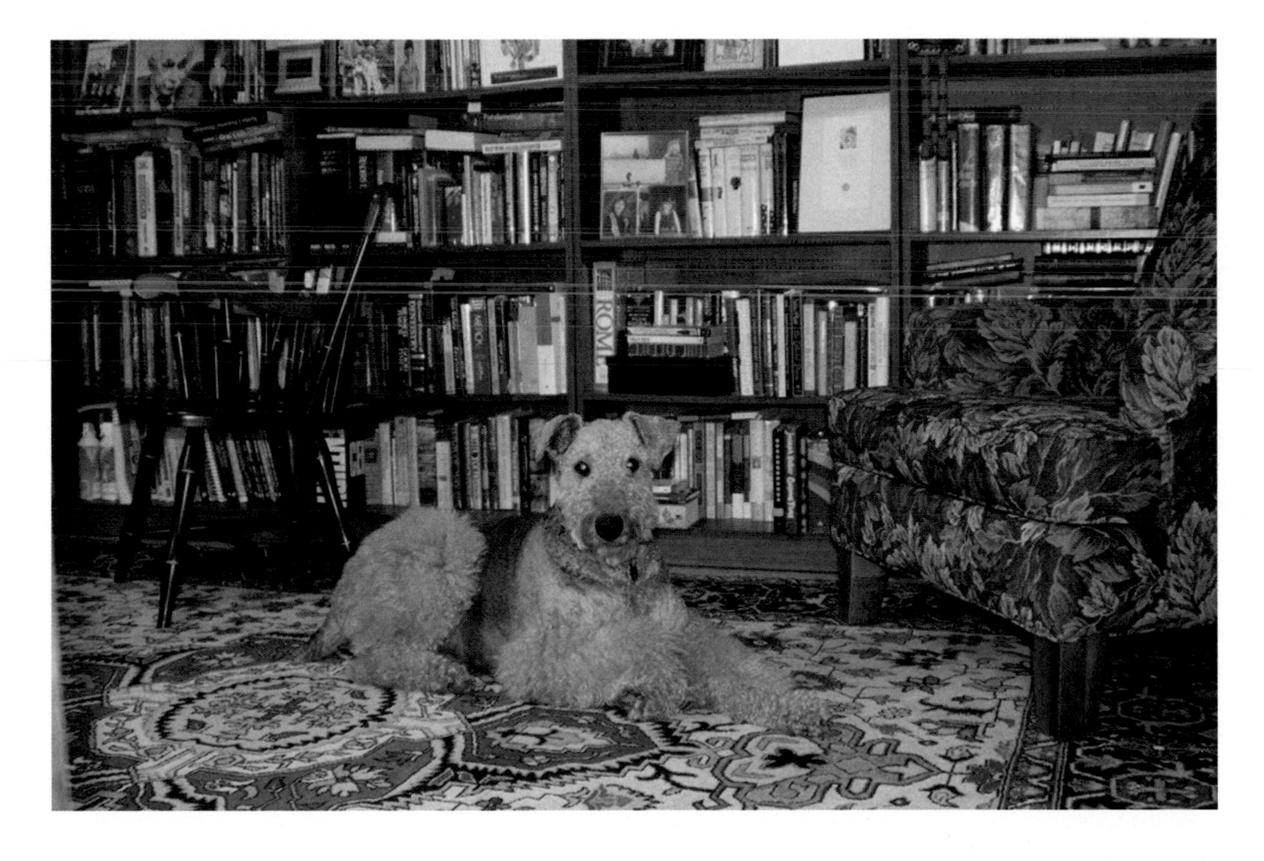

Although it has been stated that writing is a lonely profession, I have been very fortunate in having the company of my faithful Airedale Terrier, Skye, who, as is evident in the accompanying photograph, kept me company as I was sitting at my computer.

ACKNOWLEDGMENTS

I would like to thank the following individuals for the help and support that they have provided in the preparation of this book.

Because histology is a visual subject, it is imperative to have excellent graphic illustrations. For that, I am indebted to Todd Smith for his careful attention to detail in revising the illustrations from the previous editions and for the creation of new figures. I also thank my many colleagues from around the world and their publishers who generously permitted me to borrow illustrative materials from their publications.

Finally, my thanks go to the project team at Elsevier for all their help, namely Alexandra Mortimer, Content Strategist, who was instrumental in initiating and bringing to fruition the possibility of this new edition; and Humayra R. Khan and Meghan B. Andress, Content Development Specialists, who worked tirelessly in ensuring that the "i's" were dotted and the "t's" were crossed, with special thanks to Meghan, who was always available to help solve all of the problems that arose doing the revision. Finally, I would like to thank Haritha Dharmarajan, Project Manager, for her great help in orchestrating the corrections of the page proofs.

CONTENTS

1 Introduction to Histology and Basic Histological Techniques

Although **histology** is the microscopic study of tissues of living organisms, be they animals or plants, this textbook discusses only mammalian—more specifically, human—tissues. However, the term has evolved to have a broader concept, named **microscopic anatomy**, because its subject matter encompasses not only the microscopic structure of tissues but also those of the cell, organs, and organ systems.

The body is composed of cells, extracellular matrix, and a fluid substance, the extracellular fluid (tissue fluid), which bathes these components. Extracellular fluid, which is derived from plasma of blood, carries nutrients, oxygen, and signaling molecules to cells of the body. Conversely, waste products, carbon dioxide, signaling molecules, and additional products released by cells of the body reach blood and lymph vessels by way of the extracellular fluid. Extracellular fluid and much of the extracellular matrix are not visible in routine histological preparations, yet their invisible presence must be appreciated by the student of histology.

Moreover, the subject of histology encompasses more than just the microscopic structure of the body; it is also concerned with the body's function. In fact, histology has a direct relationship to other disciplines and is essential for their understanding. This textbook intertwines the disciplines of cell biology, biochemistry, physiology, embryology, gross anatomy, and, as appropriate, pathology. Students will recognize the importance of this subject as they refer to the text later in their careers. An excellent example of this relationship should be evident when the reader learns about the histology of the kidney and realizes that it is the intricate and almost sublime structure of that organ (down to the molecular level) that is responsible for the kidney's ability to perform its function. Alterations of the kidney's structure are responsible for a great number of life-threatening conditions. Another example is the microscopic—indeed, molecular—structure of muscle cells. The ability to contract is intimately dependent on the microscopic, submicroscopic, and molecular organization of the various components of the muscle cell.

The remainder of this chapter discusses the methods used by histologists to study the microscopic anatomy of the body.

Light Microscopy

TISSUE PREPARATION

The steps required in preparing tissues for light microscopy are (1) fixation, (2) dehydration and clearing, (3) embedding, (4) sectioning, and (5) mounting and staining the sections.

Numerous techniques have been developed to prepare tissues for study so that they closely resemble their natural living state. These include **fixation**, **dehydration** and **clearing**, **embedding** in a suitable medium, **sectioning** into thin slices to permit viewing by transillumination, **mounting** onto a surface for ease of handling, and **staining** so that tissue and cell components may be differentiated.

Fixation

Fixation not only retards the alterations of the tissue subsequent to removal from the body but also maintains its normal architecture. The most common fixative agents used in light microscopy are neutral buffered **formalin** and **Bouin's fluid**. Fixatives cross-link proteins, thus preventing them from altering their position, which preserves a lifelike image of the tissue.

Dehydration and Clearing

Alcohol baths, beginning with 50% alcohol and progressing in graded steps to 100% alcohol, are used to remove the water (**dehydration**) from the tissue, which is then treated with xylene, a chemical that is miscible both with alcohol and melted paraffin. This process is known as **clearing**, since xylene causes the tissue to become transparent.

Embedding

Tissues are **embedded** in a proper medium and then sliced into thin sections. For light microscopy, the usual embedding medium is paraffin. The tissue is placed into melted paraffin until it is completely **infiltrated** and then placed into a small receptacle, covered with melted paraffin, and allowed to harden, forming a paraffin block containing the tissue.

Sectioning

The hardened blocks of tissue are trimmed of excess embedding material and are mounted for **sectioning** on a microtome, where thin slices are removed from the block. For light microscopy, the thickness of each section is about 5 to 10 μm and each section or a series of sections are mounted (placed) on glass slides.

Sectioning can also be performed on specimens frozen either in liquid nitrogen or on the rapid-freeze bar of a cryostat. These sections are mounted by the use of a quick-freezing mounting medium and sectioned at subzero temperatures by means of a precooled steel blade. The sections are placed on precooled glass slides, permitted to come to room temperature, and stained with specific dyes (or treated for histochemical or immunocytochemical studies).

Mounting and Staining

Paraffin sections are mounted (placed) on glass slides and then stained by water-soluble stains that permit differentiation of the various cellular components.

The sections for conventional light microscopy are **mounted** on adhesive-coated glass slides. Because many tissue constituents have approximately the same optical densities, they must be **stained** for light microscopy, mostly with water-soluble stains.

Therefore, the paraffin must first be removed from the mounted sections, after which the tissue is rehydrated and stained. After staining, the section is again dehydrated so that the coverslip may be permanently affixed by the use of a suitable mounting medium. The coverslip not only protects the tissue from damage and drying but also is necessary for viewing the section with the microscope.

Stains are grouped into three classes:

- Those that differentiate between acidic and basic components of the cell
- Specialized stains that differentiate the fibrous components of the extracellular matrix
- Metallic salts that form a metal deposit on tissues

The most commonly used stains in histology are **hematoxylin** and **eosin (H & E).** Hematoxylin is a base that preferentially binds to the acidic components of the cell, such as deoxyribonucleic acid (DNA) and ribonucleic acid (RNA), staining them blue; these components of the cell are referred to as **basophilic**. Eosin is an acid that binds to cytoplasmic constituents that have a basic pH, staining them pink; these elements of the cell are said to be **acidophilic**. Many other stains have been developed for histological study (Table 1.1).

Molecules of some stains, such as **toluidine blue**, polymerize with each other when exposed to high concentrations of polyanions in tissue. This stain dyes tissues blue, except for those tissues that are rich in polyanions (e.g., cartilage matrix and granules of mast cells), which are stained purple. A tissue or cell component that stains purple with this stain is said to be **metachromatic**, and toluidine blue is said to exhibit **metachromasia**. Examples of tissues stained with common histological stains are presented at the end of this chapter (Figs. 1.11 to 1.17).

LIGHT MICROSCOPE

Compound microscopes are composed of a specific arrangement of lenses that permit a high magnification and good resolution of the tissues being viewed.

Because current light microscopes employ specific arrays of **lenses** in magnifying an image (Fig. 1.1), they are known as **compound microscopes**. The light source is an electric bulb with a tungsten filament whose light is gathered into a focused beam by the **condenser lens**.

TABLE 1.1 Common Histological Stains and Reactions

Reagent	Result
Hematoxylin	*Blue:* Nucleus, acidic regions of the cytoplasm, cartilage matrix
Eosin	*Pink:* Basic regions of the cytoplasm, collagen fibers
Masson's trichrome	*Dark blue:* Nuclei. *Red:* Muscle, keratin, cytoplasm
	Light blue: Mucinogen, collagen
Weigert's elastic stain	*Blue:* Elastic fibers
Silver stain	*Black:* Reticular fibers
Iron hematoxylin	*Black:* Striations of muscle, nuclei, erythrocytes
Periodic acid–Schiff	*Magenta:* Glycogen- and carbohydrate-rich molecules
Wright and Giemsa stains	Used for differential staining of blood cells
	Pink: Erythrocytes, eosinophil granules
	Purple: Leukocyte nuclei, basophil granules
	Blue: Cytoplasm of monocytes and lymphocytes

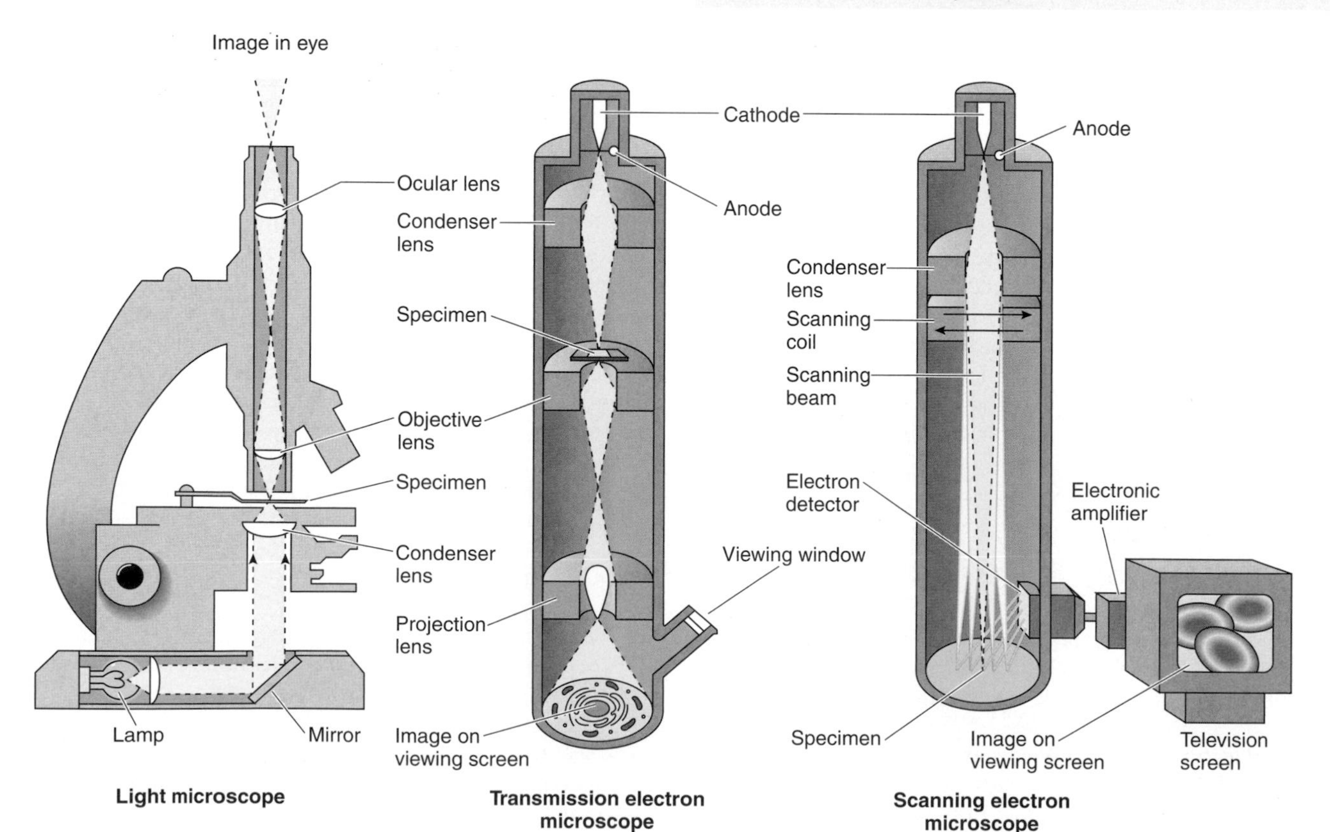

Fig. 1.1 Comparison of light, transmission, and scanning electron microscopes.

Light passing through the stained specimen from below enters one of the usually four objective lenses attached to a movable turret positioned above the specimen. Generally, in most microscopes, the first 3 lenses magnify 4, 10, and 40 times, respectively, and are used without oil; the oil lens magnifies the image 100 times.

The image from the objective lens is gathered and further magnified by the ocular lens of the eyepiece. This lens usually magnifies the image by a factor of 10—for total magnifications of 40, 100, 400, and 1000—and focuses the resulting image on the retina of the eye (or on the film of a film camera or on the sensor of a digital camera).

The image is focused by moving the objective lenses up or down above the specimen. It is interesting to note that the image projected on the retina (or film or sensor) is reversed from right to left and is upside down.

Image quality is a function of the ability of a lens to magnify and its **resolution**—the ability of the lens to show that two distinct objects are separated by a distance. Due to the wavelength of visible light, the theoretical limit of resolution is 0.25 μm and the quality of a lens is judged by how closely the lens can approach that limit.

There are several types of light microscopes, distinguished by the type of light used as a light source and the manner in which they use the light source. However, most students of histology are required to recognize only images obtained from compound light microscopy, transmission electron microscopy, and scanning electron microscopy. Therefore, the other types of microscopy are not discussed.

Digital Imaging Techniques

Digital imaging techniques use computer technology to capture and manipulate histological images.

Computer technology permits the capture of images digitally, replacing the use of film, providing results as good as, if not better than, that afforded by film technology.

In addition, because these images are stored in a digital format, thousands may be archived on removable-disk technology and their retrieval is almost instantaneous. Finally, their digital format permits the electronic transmission of these images via the Internet without risking the loss of the original files.

Interpretation of Microscopic Sections

One of the most difficult and frustrating skills needed in histology is learning to interpret what a two-dimensional section looks like in three dimensions. If one imagines a garden hose coiled, as in Fig. 1.2, and then takes the indicated thin sections from that hose, it becomes clear that the three-dimensional object usually cannot be discerned from any *one* of the two-dimensional depictions. However, by viewing many of the sections drawn from the coiled tube, one can mentally reconstruct the correct three-dimensional image.

ADVANCED VISUALIZATION PROCEDURES

Histochemistry

Histochemistry is a method of staining tissue that provides information concerning the presence and location of intracellular and extracellular macromolecules.

Specific chemical constituents of tissues and cells can be localized by the method of **histochemistry** and **cytochemistry**. These methods capitalize on enzymatic activity, chemical reactivity,

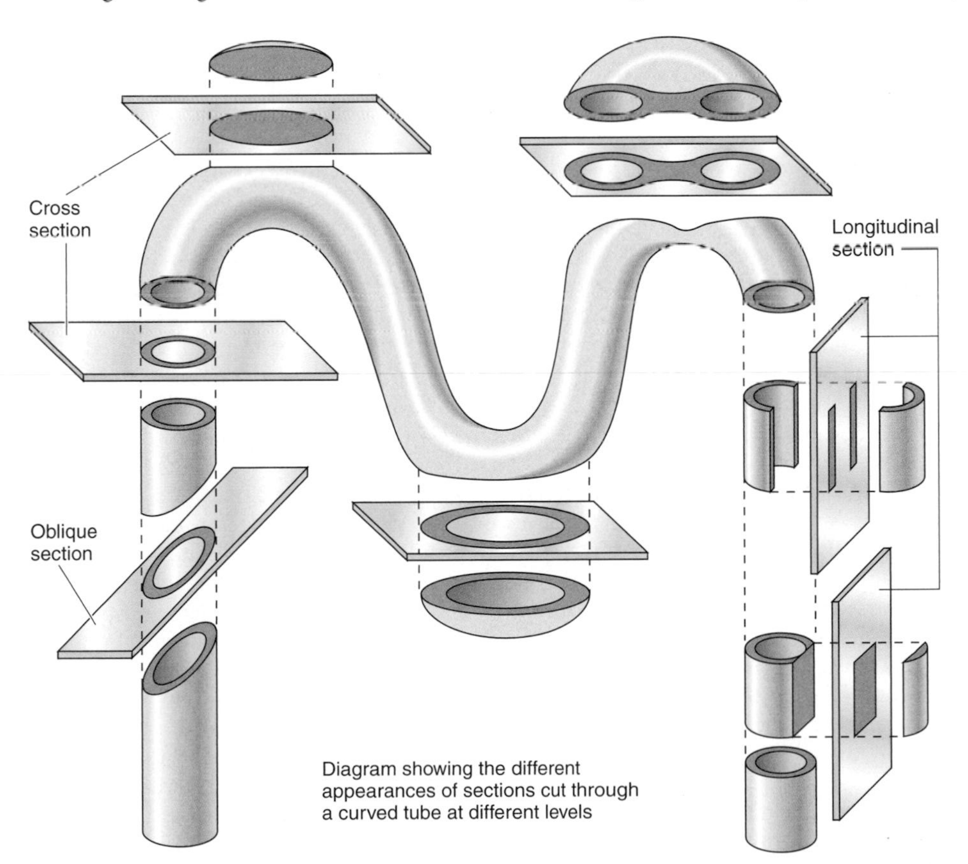

Fig. 1.2 Histology requires a mental reconstruction of two-dimensional images into the three-dimensional solid from which they were sectioned. In this diagram, a curved tube is sectioned in various planes to illustrate the relationship between a series of two-dimensional sections and the three-dimensional structure.

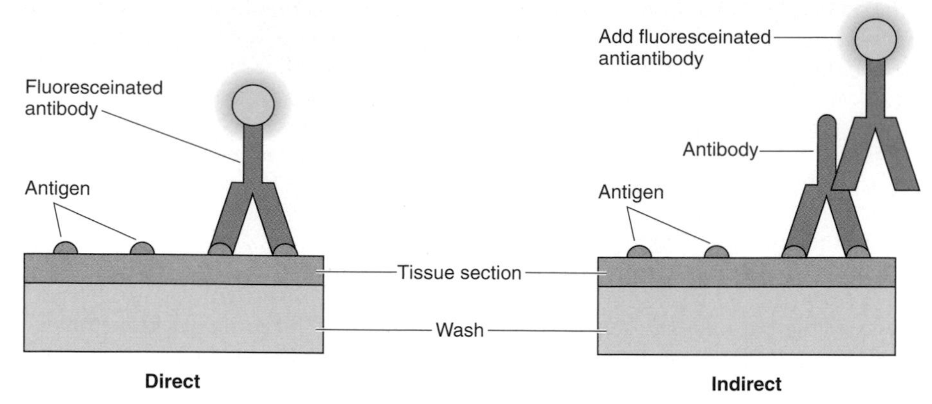

Fig. 1.3 Direct and indirect methods of immunocytochemistry. *Left:* An antibody against the antigen was labeled with a fluorescent dye and viewed with a fluorescent microscope. The fluorescence occurs only over the location of the antibody. *Right:* Fluorescent-labeled antibodies are prepared against an antibody that reacts with a particular antigen. When viewed with fluorescent microscopy, the region of fluorescence represents the location of the antibody.

or other physicochemical phenomena associated with the substance of interest. Particular chemical reactions are monitored by the formation of insoluble precipitates that take on a certain color. Frequently, histochemistry is performed on frozen tissues and can be applied to both light and electron microscopy.

One of the most common histochemical reactions uses the periodic acid–Schiff (PAS) reagent, which forms a magenta-colored precipitate with molecules rich in glycogen and carbohydrates. Consecutive sections are treated with amylase prior to applying the PAS reagent to ensure that the reaction is specific for glycogen. Thus, sections not treated with amylase display a magenta deposit, whereas amylase-treated sections display a lack of staining in the same region.

Although enzymes can be localized by histochemical procedures, the product of enzymatic reaction, rather than the enzyme itself, is visualized. The reagent is designed so that the product precipitates at the site of the reaction and is visible either as a metallic or colored deposit.

Immunocytochemistry

Immunocytochemistry uses fluoresceinated antibodies and antiantibodies to provide more precise intracellular and extracellular localization of macromolecules than is possible with histochemistry.

Although histochemical procedures permit relatively good localization of some enzymes and macromolecules in cells and tissues, more precise localization can be achieved by the use of **immunocytochemistry**. This procedure requires the development of an antibody against the particular macromolecule to be localized and labeling the antibody with a fluorescent dye, such as fluorescein or rhodamine.

There are two common methods of antibody labeling: **direct** and **indirect**. In the direct method (Fig. 1.3), the antibody against the macromolecule is labeled with a fluorescent dye. The antibody is then permitted to react with the macromolecule, and the resultant complex may be viewed with a fluorescent microscope (Fig. 1.4).

In the indirect method (see Fig. 1.3), a fluorescent-labeled antibody is prepared against the primary antibody specific for the macromolecule of interest. Once the primary antibody has reacted with the antigen, the preparation is washed to remove unbound primary antibody. The labeled antibody is then added and reacts with the original antigen-antibody complex, forming a secondary complex visible by fluorescent microscopy (Fig. 1.5). The indirect method is more sensitive than the direct method because numerous labeled antiantibodies bind to the primary antibody, making them easier to visualize. In addition, the indirect method does not require labeling of the primary antibody, which often is available only in limited quantities.

Immunocytochemistry can be used with specimens for electron microscopy by labeling the antibody with ferritin, an electron-dense molecule, instead of with a fluorescent dye. Ferritin labeling can be applied to both the direct and indirect methods.

Autoradiography

Autoradiography is a method that uses the incorporation of radioactive isotopes into macromolecules, which are then visualized by the use of an overlay of film emulsion.

Autoradiography (radioautography) is a particularly useful method for localizing and investigating a specific temporal sequence of events. The method requires incorporation of a radioactive isotope—most commonly tritium (^3H)—into the compound being studied (Fig. 1.6). An example would be the use of tritiated amino acid to follow the synthesis and packaging of proteins. After the radiolabeled compound is injected into an animal, tissue specimens are taken at selected time intervals. The tissue is processed as usual and placed on a glass slide. However, instead of the tissue being sealed with a coverslip, a thin layer of photographic emulsion is placed over it. The tissue is placed in a dark box for a few days or weeks, during which time particles emitted from the radioactive isotope expose the emulsion over the cell sites where the isotope is located. The emulsion is developed and fixed by means of photographic techniques, and small silver grains are left over the exposed portions of the emulsion. The specimen then is sealed with a coverslip and viewed with a light microscope. The silver grains are positioned over the regions of the specimen that incorporated the radioactive compound.

Autoradiography has been used to follow the time course of incorporation of tritiated proline into the basement membrane underlying endodermal cells of the yolk sac (see Fig. 1.6). An adaptation of the autoradiography method of electron microscopy has been used to show that the tritiated proline first appears in the cytosol of the endodermal cells, then travels to the rough endoplasmic reticulum, then to the Golgi apparatus, then into

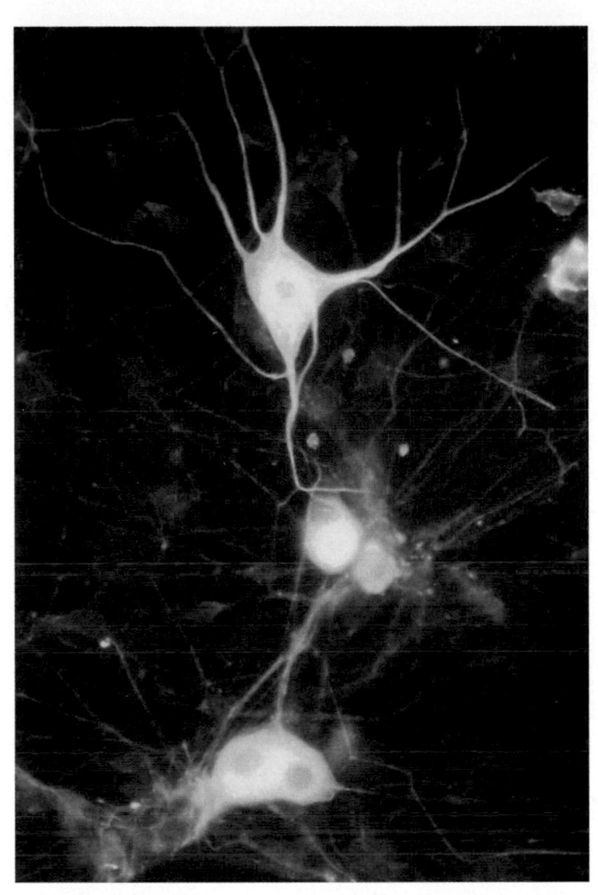

Fig. 1.4 Example of direct immunocytochemistry. Cultured neurons from rat superior cervical ganglion were immunostained with fluorescent-labeled antibody specific for the insulin receptor. The bright areas correspond to sites where the antibody has bound to insulin receptors. The staining pattern indicates that receptors are located throughout the cytoplasm of the soma and processes, but are missing from the nucleus. (From James S, Patel N, Thomas P, Burnstock G. Immunocytochemical localisation of insulin receptors on rat superior cervical ganglion neurons in dissociated cell culture. J Anat. 1993;182:95–100.)

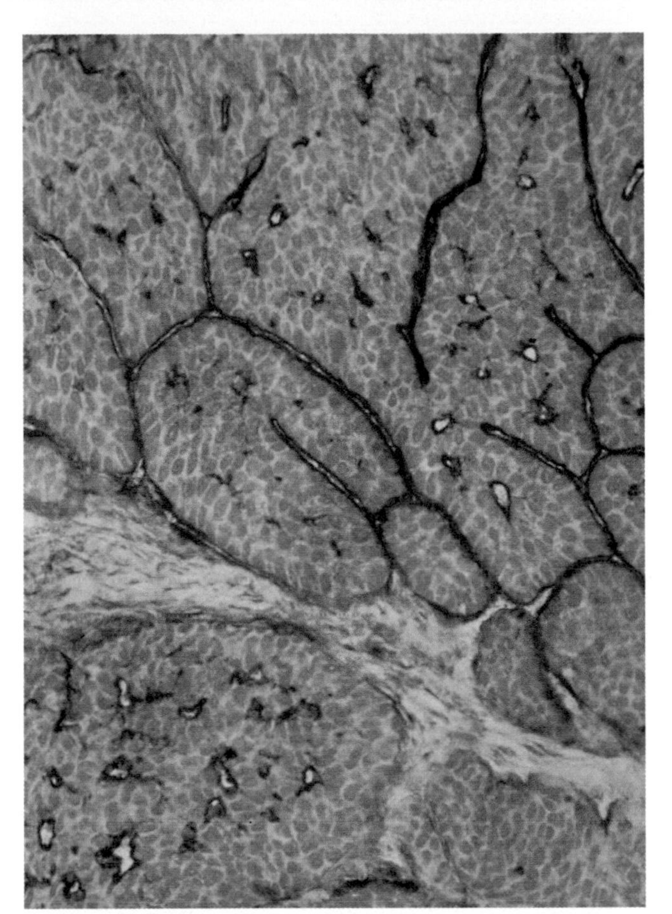

Fig. 1.5 Indirect immunocytochemistry. Fluorescent antibodies were prepared against primary antibodies against type IV collagen to demonstrate the presence of a continuous basal lamina at the interface between malignant clusters of cells and the surrounding connective tissue. (From Kopf-Maier P, Schroter-Kermani C. Distribution of type VII collagen in xenografted human carcinomas. *Cell Tissue Res.* 1993;272:395–405, 1993.)

vesicles, and, finally, into the extracellular matrix (Fig. 1.7). In this manner, the sequence of events leading to the synthesis of type IV collagen—the main protein in the lamina densa of the basal lamina—was visually demonstrated.

CONFOCAL MICROSCOPY AND CONFOCAL LASER ENDOMICROSCOPY

Confocal microscopy relies on a laser beam for the light source and a pinhole screen to eliminate undesirable reflected light from being observed. Thus, the only light that can be observed is what is located at the focal point of the objective lens, making the pinhole conjugate of the focal point. Confocal laser endomicroscopy gathers real-time representations of the mucosa at the microscopic level during endoscopy.

In confocal microscopy, a laser beam passes through a dichroic mirror to be focused on the specimen by two motorized mirrors, whose movements are computer controlled to scan the beam along the sample. Since the sample is treated with fluorescent dyes, the impinging laser beam causes the emission of light from the dyes. The emitted light follows the same path taken by the laser beam but in the opposite direction, and the dichroic mirror focuses this emitted light on a pinhole in a plate. A photomultiplier tube collects the emitted light passing through the pinhole, while the plate containing the pinhole blocks all of the extraneous light that would create a fuzzy image. It must be remembered that the light emerging from the pinhole at any particular moment in time represents a single point in the sample and, as the laser beam scans across the sample additional individual points are collected by the photomultiplier tube. All of these points gathered by the photomultiplier tube are then compiled by a computer, forming a composite image, one pixel at a time. Since the depth of field is very small (i.e., only a thin layer of the sample is observed at any one scan), the scanning may be repeated at increasingly deeper levels in the sample, providing the capability of compiling a very good three-dimensional image (Fig. 1.8).

A variation of confocal microscopy, known as confocal laser endomicroscopy (CLE), is designed to gather real-time representations of the mucosa at the microscopic level during endoscopy. Basically, CLE is capable of providing the physician with a *virtual biopsy* of the structure being examined. In order to use this ability of CLE, a fluorescent dye is administered intravenously or topically. The fluorescent light that is produced in response to the incident laser beam is captured by a photodetector, which converts the light signals into electrical signals that can be computerized. The same process is also available for examining tissues that were quick frozen after removal from the body by probe-based CLE (pCLE). Using these techniques, previously unknown microscopic tissue spaces were discovered in dense irregular collagenous connective tissue (Fig. 1.9). These fluid-filled **interstitial spaces**, bolstered by bundles of collagen fibers, appear to be lined by highly attenuated cells bearing

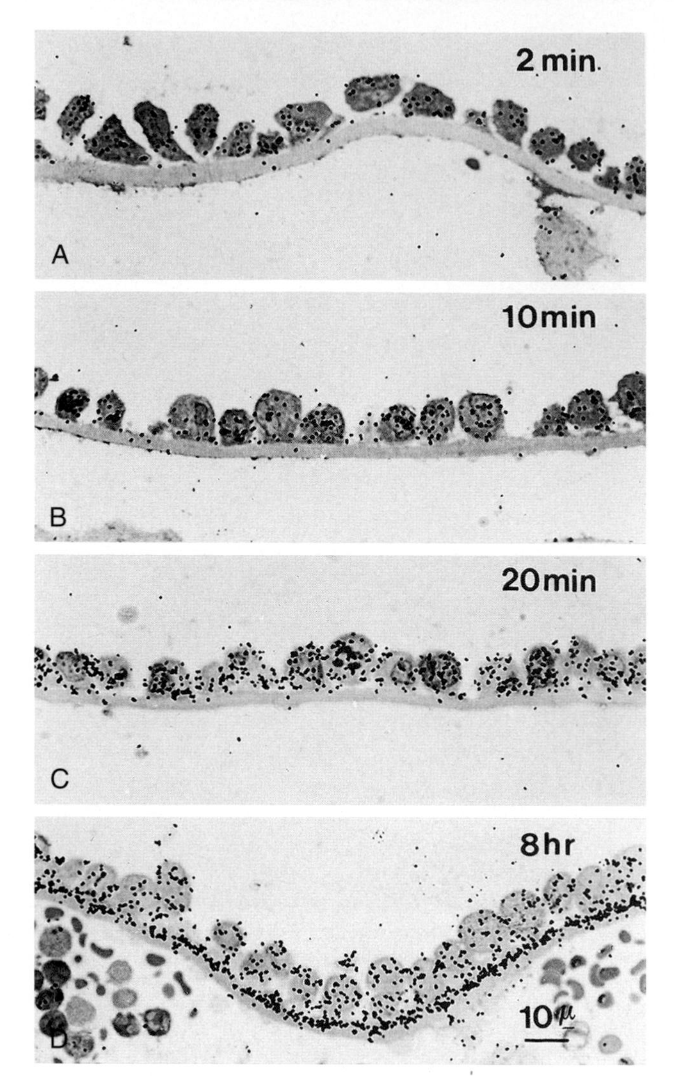

Fig. 1.6 Autoradiography. Light microscopic examination of tritiated proline incorporation into the basement membrane as a function of time subsequent to tritiated proline injection. In photomicrographs (A) to (C), the silver grains *(black dots)* are localized mostly in the endodermal cells. After 8 hours (D), however, the silver grains are also localized in the basement membrane. The presence of silver grains indicates the location of tritiated proline. (From Mazariegos MR, Leblond CP, van der Rest M. Radioautographic tracing of 3H-proline in endodermal cells of the parietal yolk sac as an indicator of the biogenesis of basement membrane components. *Am J Anat.* 1987;179:79–93.)

CD34 molecules on their cell membranes. The fluid contained in these spaces is believed to be prelymphatic fluid that probably makes its way to lymph nodes. It is postulated that this tissue compartment has not been observed because the fluid is drained from the tissues during excision and the tissue collapses onto itself during routine histological preparation. In the living organism, these prelymphatic fluid-filled interstitial spaces act as "shock absorbers" that counter forces of compression.

Electron Microscopy

The use of electrons as a light source in electron microscopy permits the achievement of much greater magnification and resolution than that realized by light microscopy.

In light microscopes, optical lenses focus visible light (a beam of photons). In electron microscopes, electromagnets focus a beam of electrons. Because the wavelength of an electron beam is much shorter than that of visible light, electron microscopes theoretically are capable of resolving two objects separated by 0.005 nm. In practice, however, the resolution of the **transmission electron microscope (TEM)** is about 0.2 nm, still more than a thousand-fold greater than the resolution of the compound light microscope. The resolution of the **scanning electron microscope (SEM)** is about 10 nm, considerably less than that of TEMs. Moreover, modern electron microscopes can magnify an object as much as 150,000 times; this magnification is powerful enough to see individual macromolecules, such as DNA and myosin.

TRANSMISSION ELECTRON MICROSCOPY

Transmission electron microscopy uses much thinner sections compared with light microscopy and requires heavy metal precipitation techniques rather than water-soluble stains to stain tissues.

Preparation of tissue specimens for transmission electron microscopy involves the same initial basic steps as in light microscopy. Special fixatives had to be developed for use with transmission light microscopy, since the greater resolving power of the electron microscope requires much smaller end products and more specific cross-linking of proteins. These fixatives, which include buffered solutions of **glutaraldehyde**, **paraformaldehyde**, **osmium tetroxide**, and **potassium permanganate**, preserve fine structural details and act as electron-dense stains, which permit observation of the tissue with the electron beam.

Because the ability of these fixatives to penetrate fresh tissues is much less than that for light microscopy, relatively small pieces of tissues have to be infiltrated in large volumes of fixatives. Tissue blocks for transmission electron microscopy are usually no larger than 1 mm^3. Suitable embedding media have been developed, such as epoxy resin, so that plastic-embedded tissues may be cut into extremely thin (ultrathin) sections (25–100 nm) that absorb only a small fraction of the impinging beam of electrons.

Electron beams are produced in an evacuated chamber by heating a tungsten filament, the **cathode**. The electrons then are attracted to the positively charged **anode**, a donut-shaped metal plate with a central hole. With a charge differential of about 60,000 volts placed between the cathode and anode, the electrons that pass through the hole in the anode have high kinetic energy.

The electron beam is focused on the specimen by the use of electromagnets, which are analogous to the condenser lens of a light microscope (see Fig. 1.1). Because the tissue is stained with heavy metals that precipitate preferentially on lipid membranes, the electrons lose some of their kinetic energy as they interact with the tissue. The heavier the metal concentration that is encountered by an electron, the less energy the electron will retain.

The electrons leaving the specimen are subjected to the electromagnetic fields of several additional electromagnets, which focus the beam on a fluorescent plate. As the electrons hit the fluorescent plate, their kinetic energy is converted into points of light whose intensity is a direct function of the electron's kinetic energy. One may make a permanent record of the resultant image by substituting an electron-sensitive film in place of the fluorescent plate and by producing a negative from which a black-and-white photomicrograph can be printed. Recently, digital electron microscopy has been introduced in which the photographic film is replaced by charge-coupled device technology to capture the image produced by the electrons.

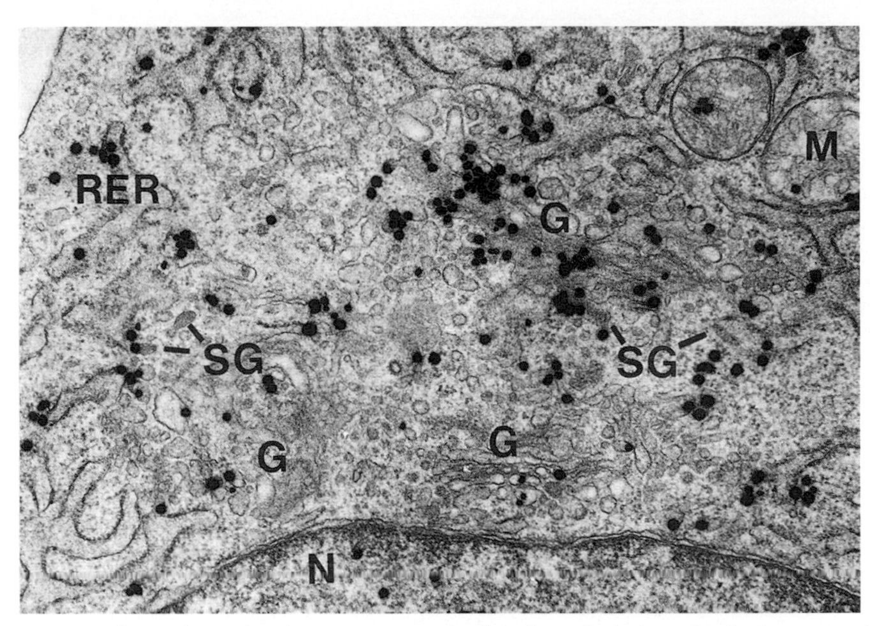

Fig. 1.7 Autoradiography. In this electron micrograph of a yolk sac endodermal cell, silver grains (similar to those in Fig. 1.6) representing the presence of tritiated proline are evident overlying the rough endoplasmic reticulum (rER), Golgi apparatus (G), and secretory granules (SG). Type IV collagen, which is rich in proline, is synthesized in endodermal cells and released into the basement membrane. The tritiated proline is most concentrated in organelles involved in protein synthesis. (From Mazariegos MR, Leblond CP, van der Rest M. Radioautographic tracing of 3H-proline in endodermal cells of the parietal yolk sac as an indicator of the biogenesis of basement membrane components. *Am J Anat.* 1987;179:79–93.)

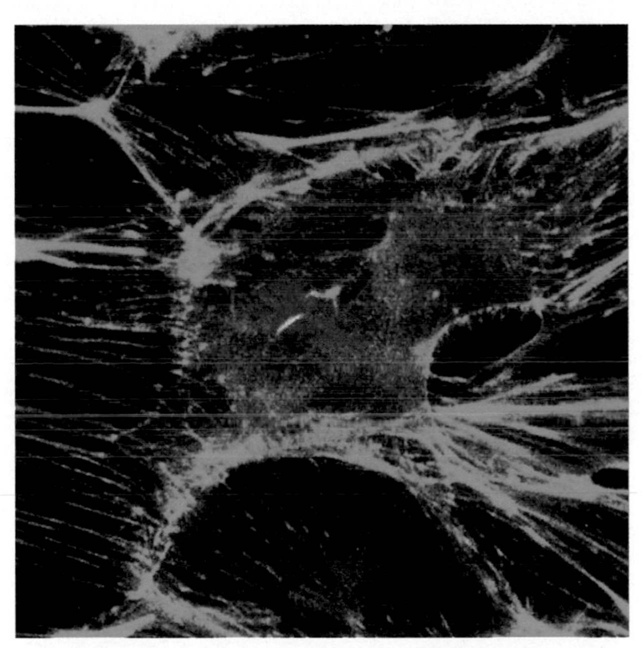

Fig. 1.8 Confocal image of a metaphase rat kangaroo cell (PtK2) stained with FITC-phalloidin for F-actin *(green)* and propidium iodide for chromosomes *(red)*. (Courtesy Dr. Matthew Schibler, UCLA Brain Research Institute.)

SCANNING ELECTRON MICROSCOPY

Scanning electron microscopy provides a three-dimensional image of the specimen.

Unlike transmission electron microscopy, scanning electron microscopy is used to view the surface of a solid specimen. Using this technique, one can view a three-dimensional image of the object. Usually, the object to be viewed is prepared in a special manner that permits a thin layer of heavy metal, such as gold or palladium, to be deposited on the specimen's surface.

As a beam of electrons scans the surface of the object, some (backscatter electrons) are reflected and others (secondary electrons) are ejected from the heavy metal coat. The backscatter and secondary electrons are captured by electron detectors that are interpreted, collated, and displayed on a monitor as a three-dimensional image (see Fig. 1.1). One may make the image permanent either by photographing it or digitizing it for storage in a computer.

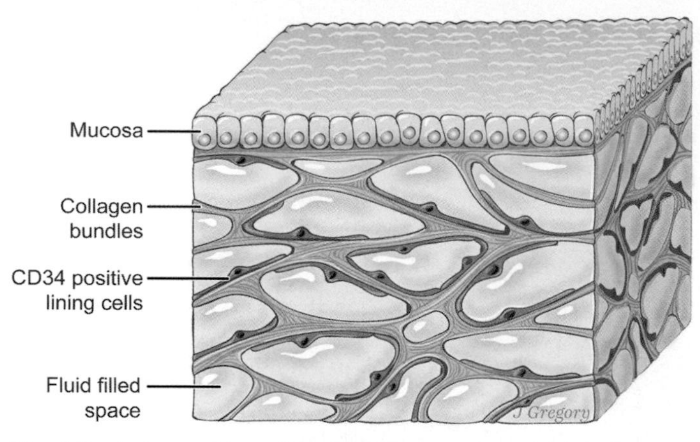

Fig. 1.9 Artist rendition of the fluid-filled spaces in the bile duct connective tissue as visualized by probe-based confocal laser endomicroscopy (pCLE). Using regular histological preparation of connective tissue proper, the collagen fiber bundles are pressed against each other, obscuring the fluid-filled spaces revealed by pCLE. These spaces are lined by CD34-positive lining cells. (Illustration by Jill K. Gregory, CMI. Printed with permission from Mount Sinai Health System.)

FREEZE-FRACTURE TECHNIQUE

The macromolecular structure of the internal aspects of membranes is revealed by the method of **freeze fracture** (Fig. 1.10). Quick-frozen specimens that have been treated with cryopreservatives do not develop ice crystals during the freezing process; hence, the tissue does not suffer mechanical damage. As the frozen specimen is hit by a supercooled razor blade, it fractures along cleavage planes, which are regions of least molecular bonding. In cells, fracture frequently occurs between the inner and outer leaflets of membranes.

The fracture face is coated at an angle by evaporated platinum and carbon, forming accumulations of platinum on one side of a projection and no accumulation on the opposite side next to the projection, thus, generating a replica of the surface. The tissue is then digested away and the replica is examined by transmission electron microscopy. This method enables the transmembrane proteins of cellular membranes to be displayed.

Figs. 1.11 to 1.17 show examples of tissues stained with common histological stains.

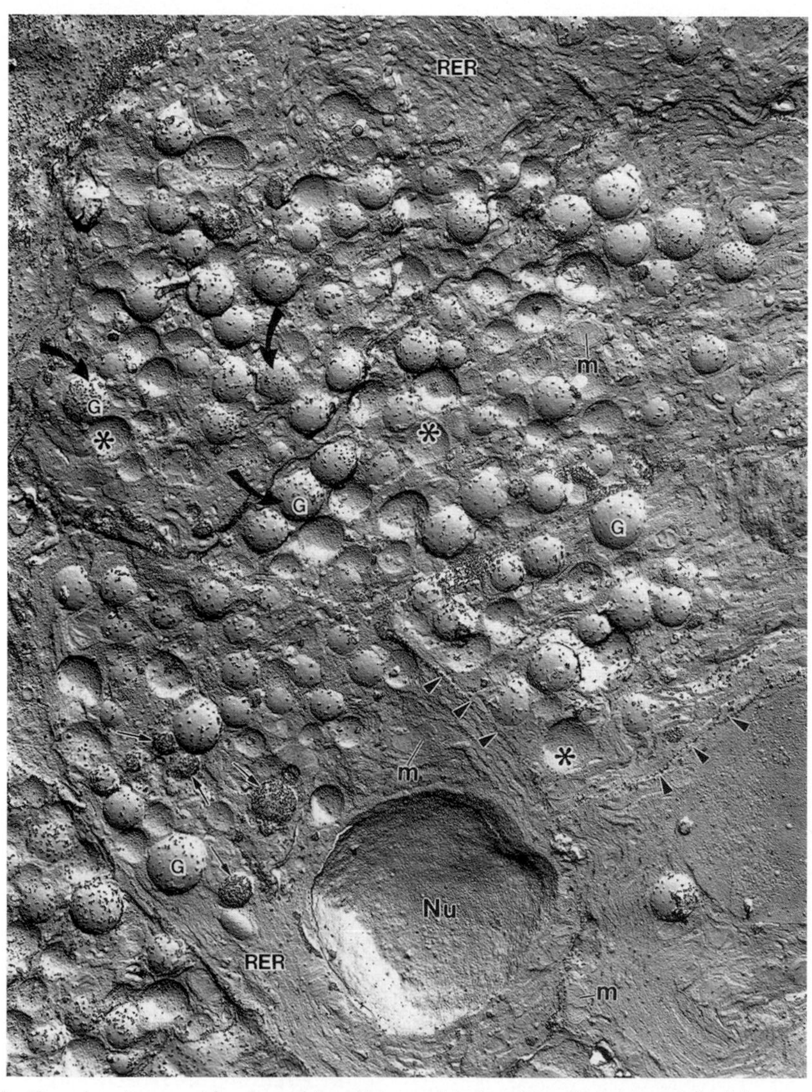

Fig. 1.10 Cytochemistry and freeze etching. Fracture-label replica of an acinar cell of the rat pancreas. *N*-acetyl-*d*-galactosamine residues were localized by the use of *Helix pomatia* lectin-gold complex, which appears as black dots in the image. The nucleus (Nu) appears as a depression, the rough endoplasmic reticulum (rER) as parallel lines, and secretory granules (G) as small elevations or depressions. The elevations (IG) represent the E-face half and the depressions *(asterisk)* represent the P-face of the membrane of the secretory granule. (From Kan FWK, Bendayan M. Topographical and planar distribution of *Helix pomatia* lectin-binding glycoconjugates in secretory granules and plasma membrane of pancreatic acinar cells of the rat: Demonstration of membrane heterogeneity. *Am J Anat.* 1989;185:165–176.)

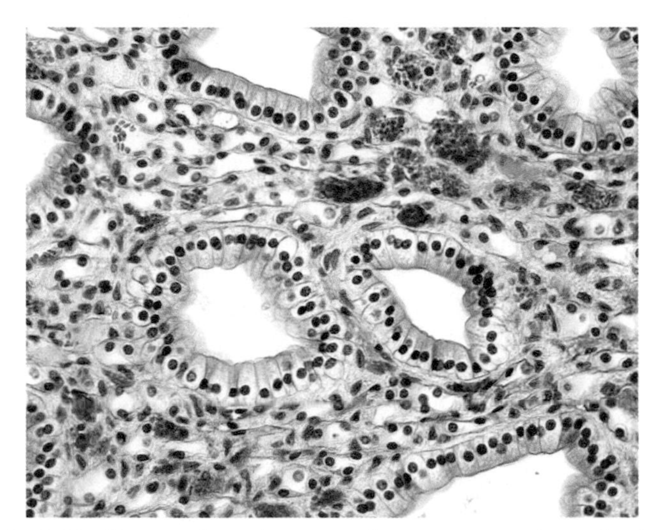

Fig. 1.11 Hematoxylin and eosin are the most commonly used stains. Hematoxylin stains acids blue. Nuclei are rich in deoxyribonucleic acids and consequently they stain blue. Basic regions of the cytoplasm stain pinkish-red with eosin.

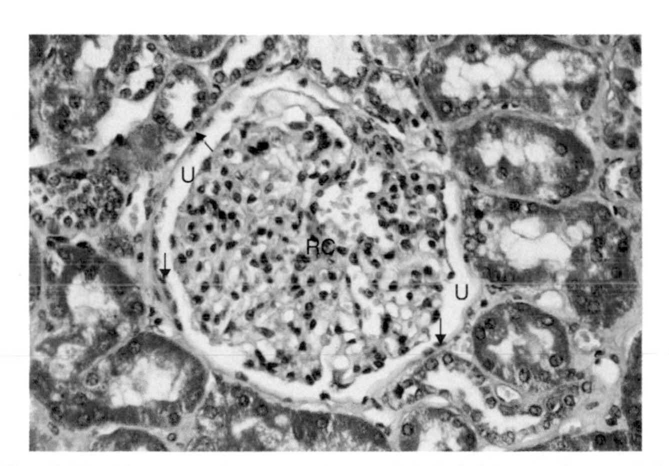

Fig. 1.12 Masson-trichrome stains nuclei dark blue, collagen light blue, and cytoplasm pink to red. (From Standring, S. *Gray's Anatomy*. 40th ed. Philadelphia: Elsevier; 2008.)

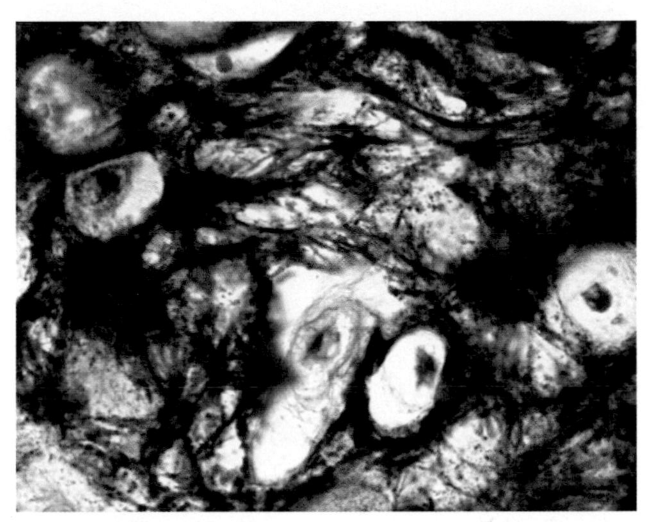

Fig. 1.13 Weigert's elastic stain stains elastic fibers blue.

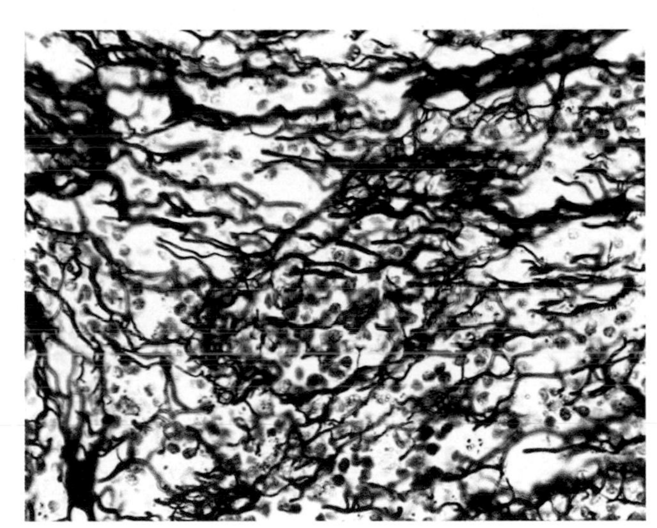

Fig. 1.14 Silver stain stains reticular fibers (type III collagen fibers) black.

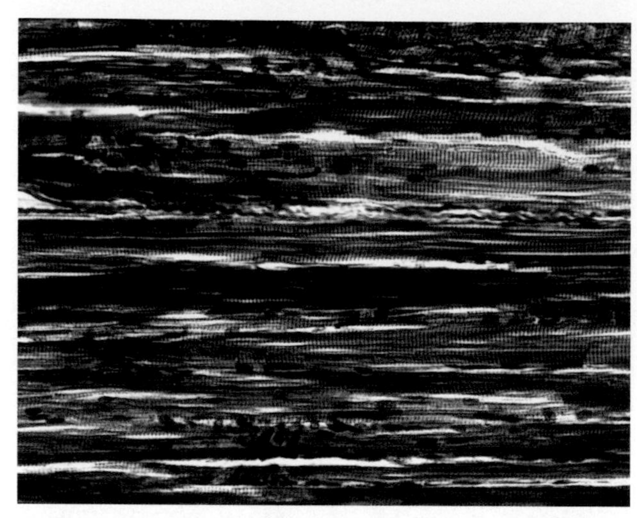

Fig. 1.15 Iron hematoxylin stains cross striations and nuclei of striated muscle cells as well as red blood cells black.

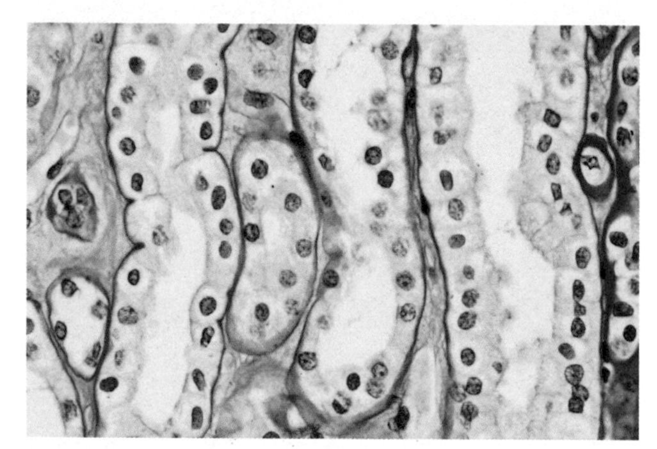

Fig. 1.16 Periodic acid Schiff (PAS stain) reagent stains glycogen and carbohydrate-rich molecules a magenta color. (From Standring S. *Gray's Anatomy*. 40th ed. Philadelphia: Elsevier; 2008.)

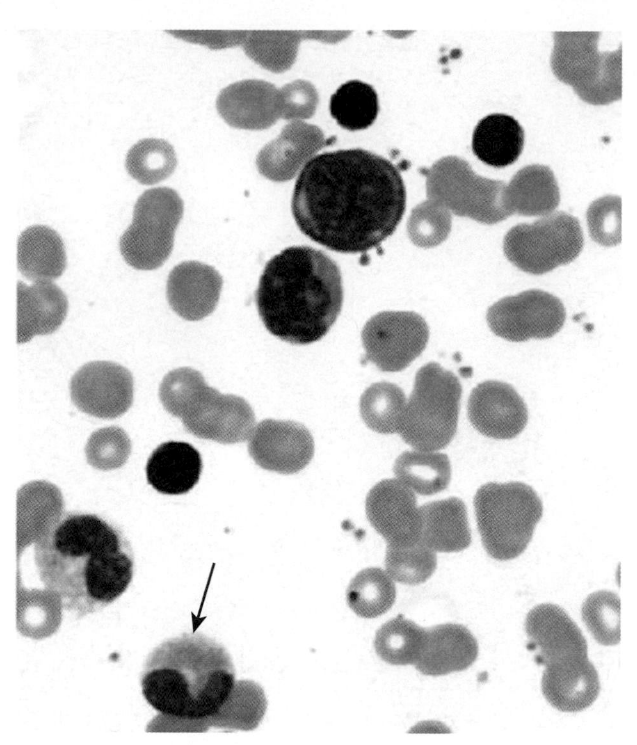

Fig. 1.17 Wright and Giemsa stains are used for differential staining of blood cells. Erythrocytes and eosinophilic granules stain pink, white blood cell (arrow) nuclei and basophilic granules stain purple, and monocyte and lymphocyte cytoplasms stain blue.

2 Cytoplasm

The basic functional unit of complex organisms is the cell. Cells that have or serve a common purpose congregate to form tissues, which, in animals—specifically, mammals—are placed in four categories (epithelium, connective tissue, muscle, and nervous tissue). These tissues assemble to form organs, which, in turn, are collected into the various organ systems of the body. Each organ system performs a collection of associated functions, such as digestion, reproduction, and respiration.

Although there are more than 200 different types of cells that comprise the body, each having a different function, they all possess certain unifying characteristics and, thus, can be described in general terms (Figs. 2.1 to 2.4). Every cell is surrounded by a plasma membrane, possesses organelles that permit it to discharge its functions, synthesizes macromolecules for its own use or for export, produces energy, and is capable of communicating with other cells. The number and disposition of the organelles varies not only with the cell in question but also with the particular stage in life cycle of that cell.

Protoplasm, the living substance of the cell, is subdivided into two compartments: the **cytoplasm**, extending from the plasma membrane to the nuclear envelope, and the **karyoplasm**, the material forming the contents of the nucleus. The cytoplasm is detailed in this chapter; the nucleus is discussed in Chapter 3.

The cytoplasm is composed mostly of **water**, in which various inorganic and organic chemicals are dissolved and/or suspended. This fluid suspension is called the **cytosol** (**intracellular fluid**), and it is that portion of the cytoplasm that is left after all organelles, the cytoskeleton, and inclusions are removed from the cytoplasm. **Organelles** are metabolically active structures that perform distinctive functions (Figs. 2.5 and 2.6). The **cytoskeleton**, a system of tubules and filaments, maintains the shapes of cells and enables them to move and form the intracellular pathways within cells. **Inclusions** consist of metabolic by-products, storage forms of various nutrients, or inert crystals and pigments.

Organelles

Organelles are metabolically active cellular structures that execute specific functions.

Although some organelles were discovered by light microscopists, their structure and function were not elucidated until the advent of electron microscopy, separation techniques, and sensitive biochemical and histochemical procedures. As a result of the application of these methods, it is now known that the membranes of organelles are composed of a **phospholipid bilayer**, which not only partitions the cell into compartments but also provides large surface areas for the biochemical reactions essential for the maintenance of life.

CELL MEMBRANE

The cell membrane forms a selectively permeable barrier between the cytoplasm and the external milieu.

Each cell is bounded by a cell membrane (plasma membrane; plasmalemma) that

- Maintains the structural integrity of the cell
- Controls movements of substances in and out of the cell (selective permeability)
- Regulates cell–cell interactions
- Recognizes, via receptors, antigens and foreign cells, as well as altered cells
- Acts as an interface between the cytoplasm and the external milieu
- Establishes transport systems for specific molecules
- Sustains a potential difference between the intracellular and extracellular aspects of the membrane
- Transduces extracellular physical or chemical signals into intracellular events

Cell membranes are not visible with the light microscope. In electron micrographs, the plasmalemma is about 7.5 nm thick and appears as a trilaminar structure of two thin, dense lines with an intervening light area. Each layer is about 2.5 nm in width, and the entire structure is known as the **unit membrane** (Fig. 2.7). The inner (cytoplasmic) dense line is its **inner leaflet**; the outer dense line is its **outer leaflet**.

MOLECULAR COMPOSITION

The plasmalemma is composed of a phospholipid bilayer and associated integral and peripheral proteins.

Each leaflet is composed of a single layer of **phospholipids** and associated **proteins**, usually in a 1:1 proportion by weight. In certain cases, such as myelin sheaths, however, the lipid component outweighs the protein component by a ratio of 4:1. The two leaflets, the **phospholipid bilayer** with associated **proteins**, form the basic structure of all membranes of the cell (Fig. 2.8). Although the two leaflets appear indistinguishable from each other, their phospholipid compositions are different, making the two leaflets *asymmetrical.*

Each **phospholipid molecule** of the lipid bilayer is **amphipathic** because it is composed of a **polar head**, located at the surface of the membrane, and two long **nonpolar** fatty acyl (fatty acid) tails, usually consisting of chains of 16 to 18 carbon atoms, projecting into the center of the plasmalemma (see Fig. 2.8). The nonpolar fatty acyl tails of the two layers face each other within the membrane and form weak noncovalent bonds with each other, holding the bilayer together.

The polar heads are composed of **glycerol**, to which a positively charged nitrogenous group is attached by a negatively charged **phosphate group**. The two fatty acyl tails, only one of which is usually saturated, are covalently bound to glycerol. Other amphipathic molecules—such as **glycolipids, glycosphingolipids,** and **cholesterol**—are also present in the cell membrane. The unsaturated fatty acyl molecules increase membrane fluidity, whereas cholesterol decreases it (although

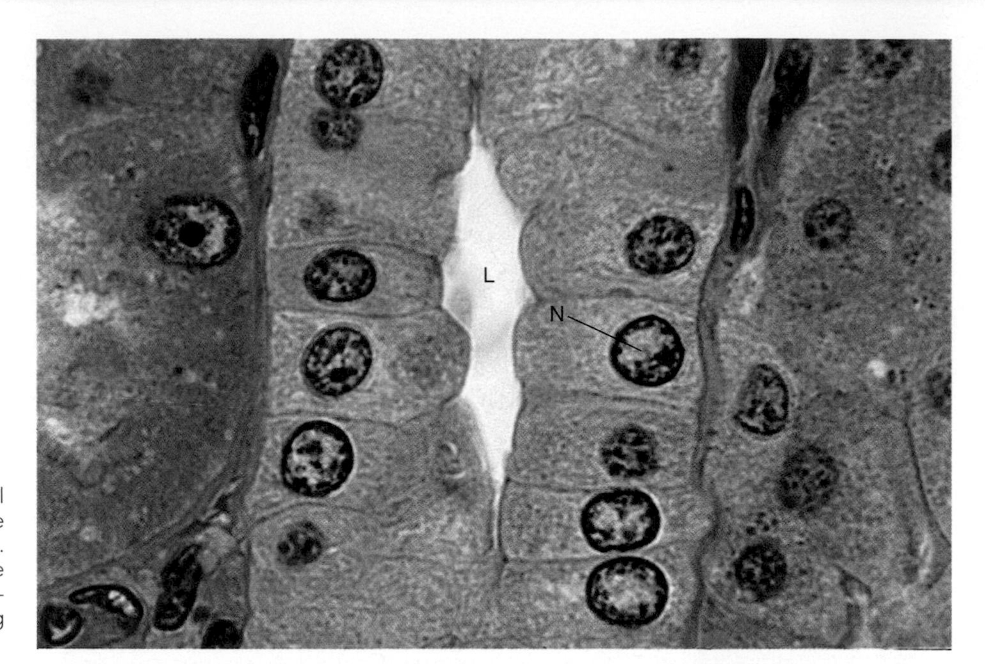

Fig. 2.1 Light photomicrograph of typical cells from the renal cortex of a monkey. Note the blue nucleus (N) and the pink cytoplasm. The boundaries (CM) of individual cells may be easily distinguished. The white area in the middle of the field is the lumen (L) of a collecting tubule. (×975)

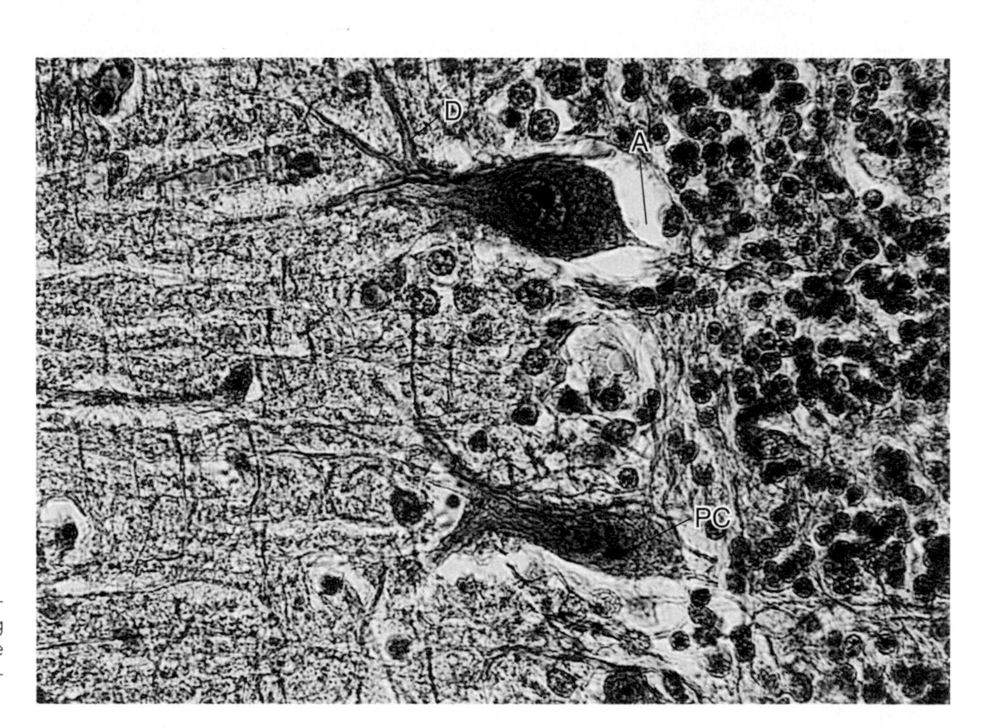

Fig. 2.2 Purkinje cells (PC) from the cerebellum of a monkey. Observe the long, branching processes, dendrites (D) and axon (A) of these cells. The nucleus is located in the widest portion of the cell. (×540)

cholesterol concentrations much lower than normal increases membrane fluidity). In fact, certain regions of the plasmalemma are so well endowed with glycosphingolipids and cholesterol that they create a bulge in the cell membrane. These thickened microdomains are known as **lipid rafts**, which form a slight bulge into the extracellular space. Frequently, lipid rafts possess protein components that participate in diverse signaling events. Therefore, lipid rafts appear to facilitate and enhance the possibilities of communications between a variety of cells.

The protein components of the plasmalemma either span the entire lipid bilayer as **integral proteins** or are attached to the cytoplasmic aspect (and, at times, the extracellular aspect) of the lipid bilayer as **peripheral proteins**. Because most integral proteins pass through the thickness of the membrane, they are also referred to as **transmembrane proteins**. Those regions of transmembrane proteins that project into the cytoplasm or the extracellular space are composed of hydrophilic amino acids, whereas the intramembrane region consists of hydrophobic amino acids. Transmembrane proteins frequently form ion channels and carrier proteins that facilitate the passage of specific ions and molecules across the cell membrane.

Many of these transmembrane proteins are quite long and are folded so that they make several passes through the membrane. Thus, they are known as **multipass proteins** and are frequently attached to the inner leaflet (and infrequently to the outer leaflet) by prenyl groups or fatty acyl groups. The cytoplasmic and extracytoplasmic aspects of these proteins commonly possess receptor sites that are specific for particular **signaling**

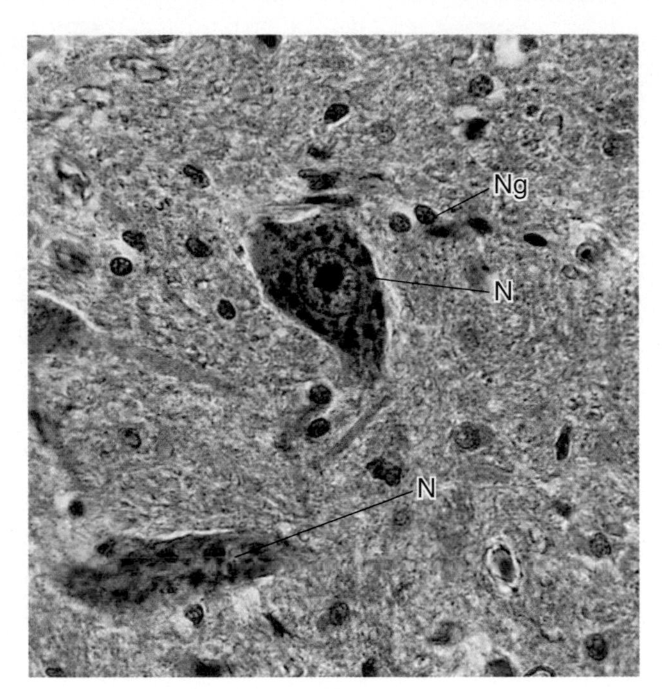

Fig. 2.3 Motor neurons from the human spinal cord. These nerve cells have numerous processes (axons and dendrites). The centrally placed nucleus and the single large nucleolus are clearly visible. The Nissl bodies (N) (rough endoplasmic reticulum) are the most conspicuous features of the cytoplasm. Observe also the small nuclei of the neuroglia cells (Ng). (×540).

molecules. Once these molecules are recognized at these receptor sites, the integral proteins can alter their conformation and can perform a specific function.

Because integral membrane proteins have the ability to float like icebergs in the sea of phospholipids, this model is referred to as the **fluid mosaic model** of membrane structure. However, the integral proteins frequently possess only limited mobility, especially in polarized cells, in which particular regions of the cell serve specialized functions.

Peripheral proteins do not usually form covalent bonds with either the integral proteins or the phospholipid components of the cell membrane. Although they are usually located on the cytoplasmic aspect of the cell membrane, they may also be on the extracellular surface. These proteins may form bonds, either with the phospholipid molecules or with the transmembrane proteins. Frequently, they are associated with the secondary messenger system of the cell (discussed below) or with the cytoskeletal apparatus.

Using freeze-fracture techniques, one can cleave the plasma membrane into its two leaflets in order to view the hydrophobic surfaces (Figs. 2.9 and 2.10). The outer surface of the inner leaflet is referred to as the **P-face** (closer to the ***protoplasm***); the inner surface of the outer leaflet is known as the **E-face** (closer to the *extracellular* space). Electron micrographs of freeze-fractured plasma membranes show that the integral proteins, visualized by shadowing replica, are more numerous on the P-face than on the E-face (see Fig. 2.10).

Glycocalyx

Glycocalyx, composed usually of carbohydrate chains, coats the cell surface.

A fuzzy coat, referred to as the **cell coat** or **glycocalyx**, is often evident in electron micrographs of the cell membrane. This coat is usually composed of carbohydrate chains that are covalently attached to transmembrane proteins and/or phospholipid molecules of the outer leaflet (see Fig. 2.8). Its intensity and thickness vary, but it may be as thick as 50 nm on some epithelial sheaths, such as those lining regions of the digestive system.

The most important function of the glycocalyx is protection of the cell from interaction with inappropriate proteins, chemical injury, and physical injury. Other cell coat functions include cell–cell recognition and adhesion, as occurs between endothelial cells and neutrophils, as well as T cells and antigen-presenting cells; facilitating blood clotting and inflammatory responses; and assisting in reducing friction between blood and the endothelial cells lining blood vessels.

Membrane Transport Proteins

Membrane transport proteins are of two types, channel proteins and carrier proteins; they facilitate the movement of aqueous molecules and ions across the plasmalemma.

Although the hydrophobic components of the plasma membrane limit the movement of polar molecules across it, the presence and activities of specialized transmembrane proteins facilitate the transfer of these hydrophilic molecules across this barrier. These transmembrane proteins and protein complexes form **channel proteins** and **carrier proteins**, which are specifically concerned with the transfer of ions and small molecules across the plasma membrane.

A number of small nonpolar molecules (e.g., benzene, oxygen, nitrogen) and uncharged polar molecules (e.g., water, glycerol) can move across the cell membrane by **simple diffusion** down their concentration gradients. Enhanced movement of most ions and small molecules across a membrane requires the aid of either channel proteins or carrier proteins. This process is known as **facilitated diffusion**. Because both types of diffusion occur without any input of energy other than that inherent in the concentration gradient, they represent **passive transport** (Fig. 2.11). By expending energy, cells can transport ions and small molecules against their concentration gradients. Only carrier proteins can mediate such energy-requiring **active transport**. The several channel proteins involved in facilitated diffusion are discussed first, followed by consideration of the more versatile carrier proteins.

Channel Proteins

Channel proteins may be gated or ungated; they are incapable of transporting substances against a concentration gradient.

Channel proteins participate in the formation of hydrophilic pores, called **ion channels**, across the plasmalemma. There are the more than 100 different types of ion channels. Some of these are specific for one particular ion; others permit the passage of several different ions and small water-soluble molecules. Although these ions and small molecules follow chemical or electrochemical concentration gradients for the direction of their passage, cells have the capability of preventing these substances from entering these hydrophilic tunnels by means of controllable **gates** that block their opening. Most channels

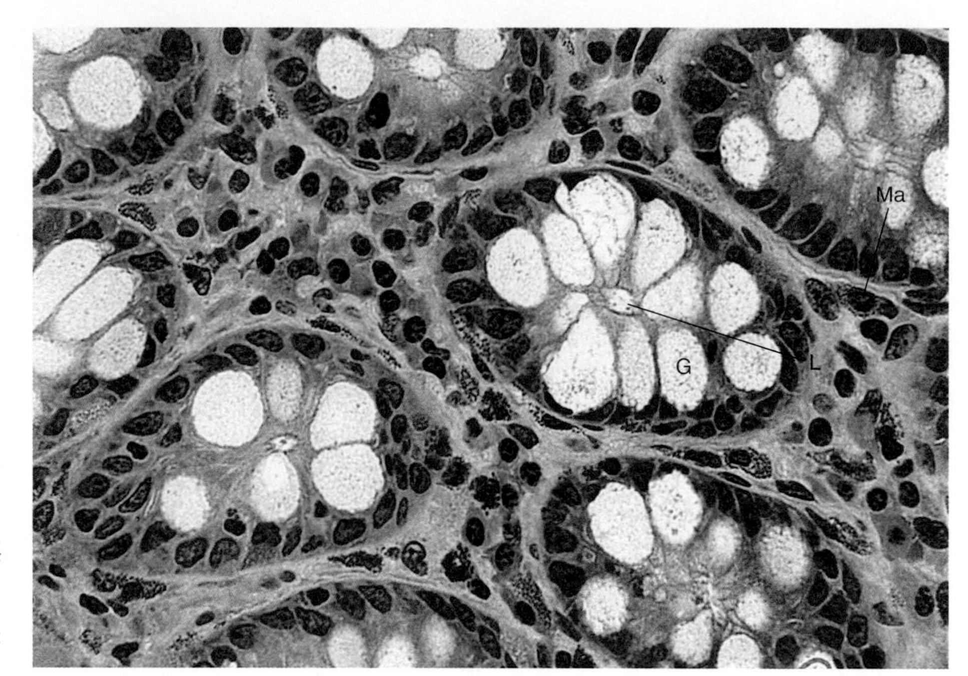

Fig. 2.4 Goblet cells (G) from a monkey colon. Some cells, such as goblet cells, specialize in secreting materials. These cells accumulate mucinogen, which occupies much of the cell's volume, and then release it into the lumen (L) of the intestine. During the processing of the tissue, the mucinogen is extracted, leaving behind empty spaces. Observe the presence of a mast cell (Ma). (×540)

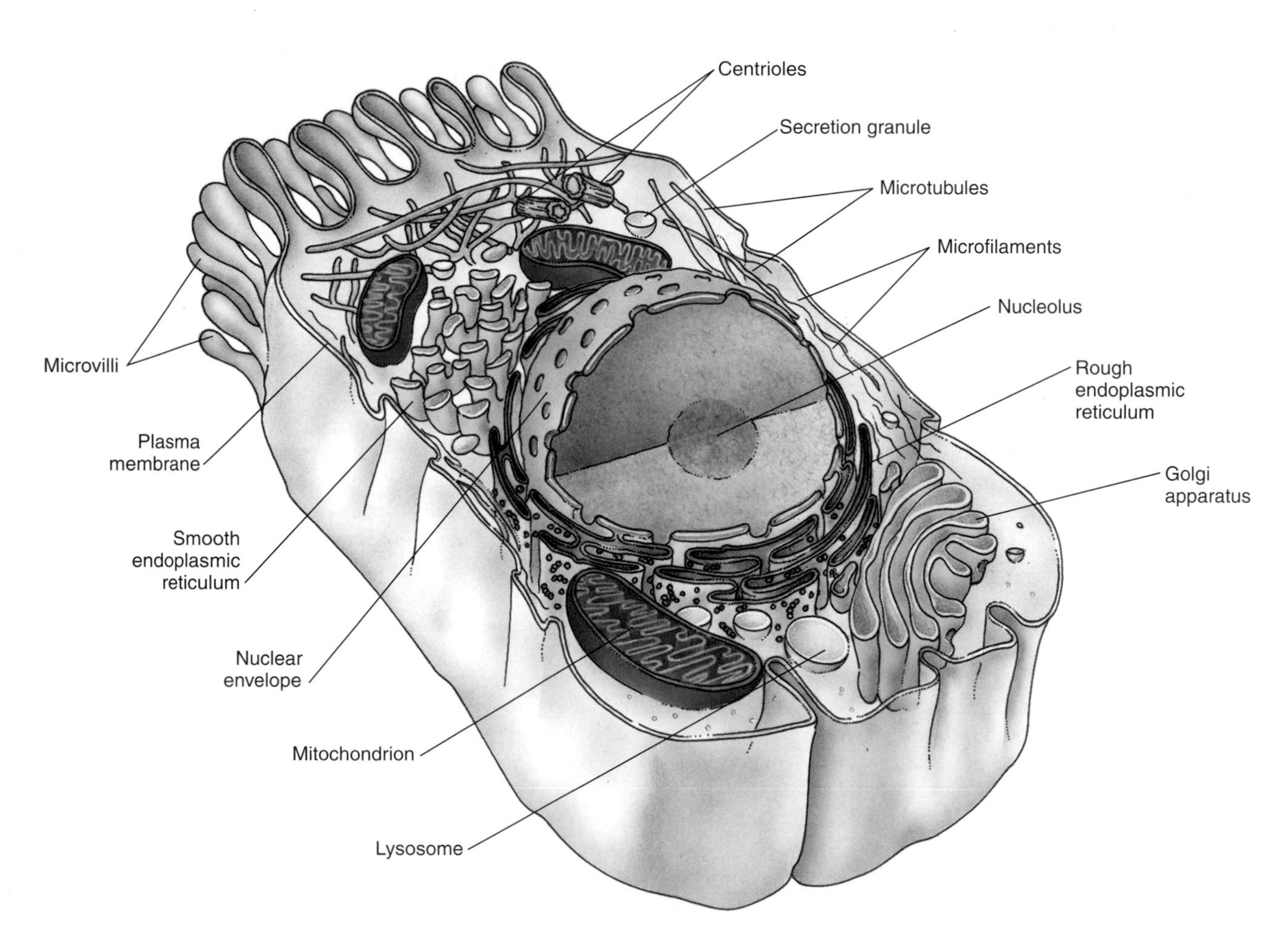

Fig. 2.5 Three-dimensional schematic diagram of an idealized cell, as visualized by transmission electron microscopy. Various organelles and cytoskeletal elements are displayed.

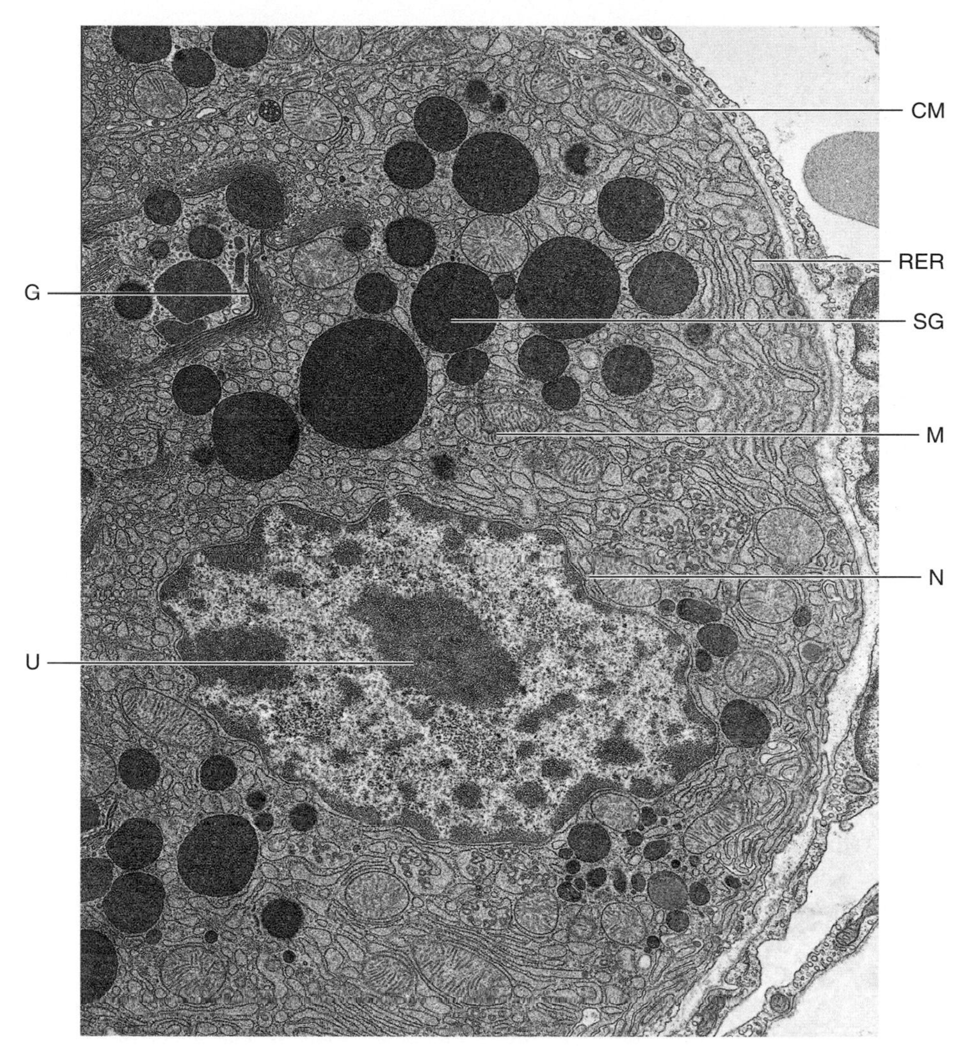

Fig. 2.6 Electron micrograph of an acinar cell from the urethral gland of a mouse, illustrating the appearance of some organelles (×11,327). M, mitochondria; G, Golgi apparatus; N, nucleus; U, nucleolus; SG, secretory granules; RER, rough endoplasmic reticulum; CM, cell membrane. (From Parr MB, Ren HP, Kepple L, et al. Ultrastructure and morphometry of the urethral glands in normal, castrated, and testosterone-treated castrated mice. *Anat Rec.* 1993;236:449–458. Copyright © 1993. Reprinted by permission of Wiley-Liss, Inc, a subsidiary of John Wiley & Sons, Inc.)

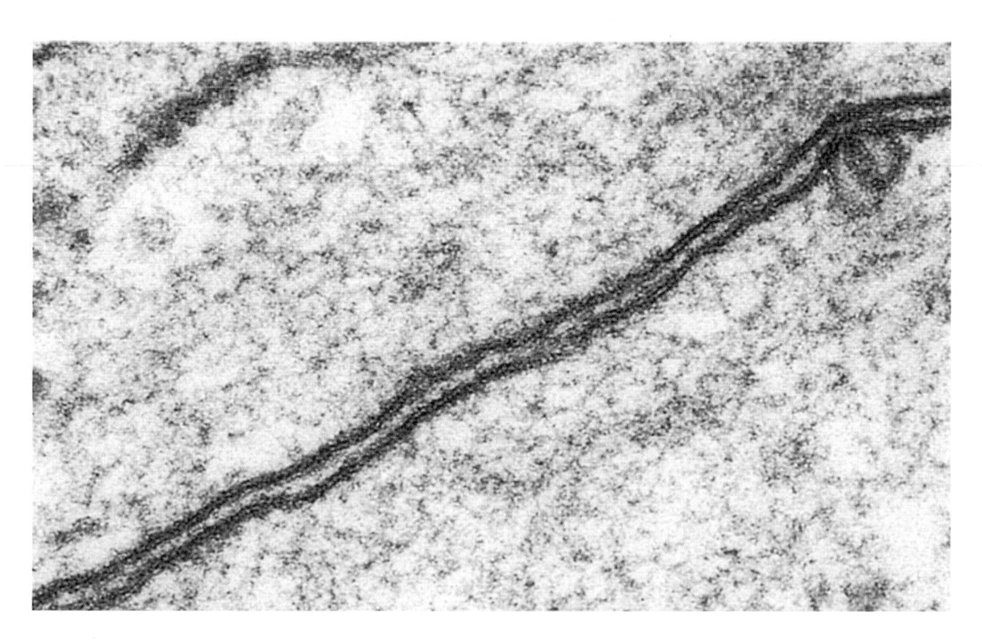

Fig. 2.7 A junction between two cells demonstrates the trilaminar structures of the two cell membranes (×240,000). (From Leeson TS, Leeson CR, Papparo AA. *Text/Atlas of Histology*. Philadelphia: WB Saunders; 1988.)

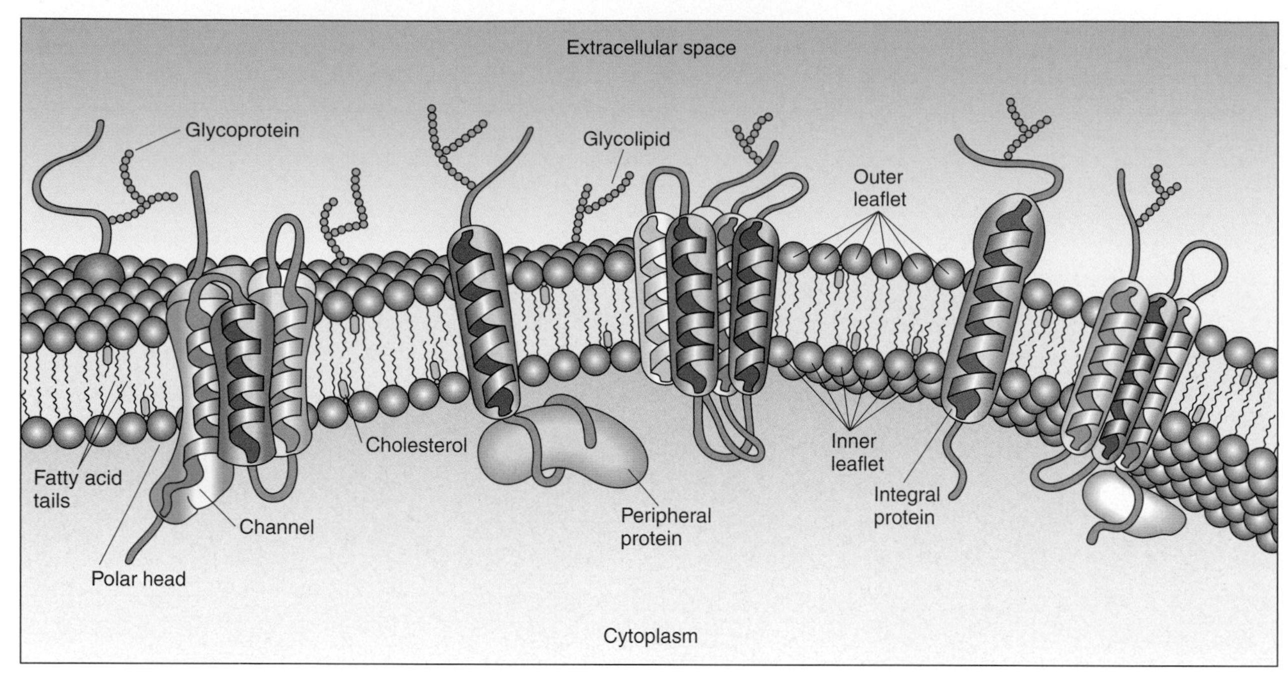

Fig. 2.8 Three-dimensional diagrammatic representation of the fluid mosaic model of the cell membrane.

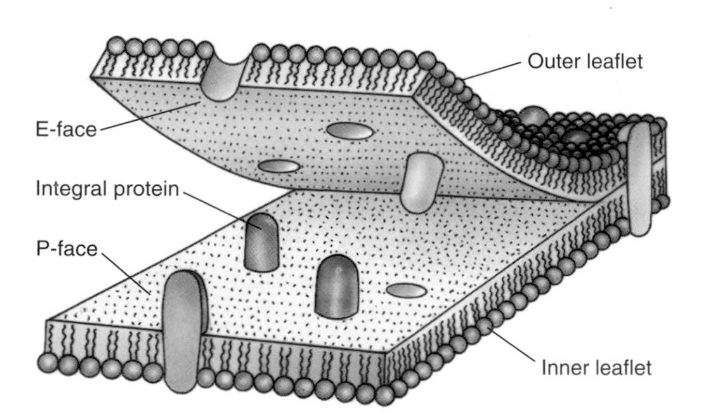

Fig. 2.9 Schematic diagram of the E-face and P-face of the cell membrane.

are **gated channels**; only a few are **ungated**. Gated channels are classified according to the control mechanism required to open the gate.

Voltage-Gated Channels. **Voltage-gated channels** go from the closed to the position, permitting the passage of ions from one side of the membrane to the other. The most common example is depolarization in the transmission of nerve impulses. In some channels, such as Na^+ channels, the open position is unstable and the channel goes from an open to **inactive position**, in which the passage of the ion is blocked and for a short time (a few milliseconds) the gate cannot be opened again. This is the **refractory period** (see Chapter 9 on the nervous system). The velocity of response to depolarization may also vary; some of those channels are referred to as **velocity-dependent**.

Ligand-Gated Channels. Channels that require the binding of a **ligand** (signaling molecule) to the channel protein to open their gate are known as **ligand-gated channels**. Unlike voltage-gated channels, these channels remain open until the ligand dissociates from the channel protein; they are referred to as **ion channel–linked receptors**. Some of the ligands controlling these gates are neurotransmitters, whereas others are nucleotides. These ligands can be neurotransmitters (neurotransmitter-gated channels), such as acetylcholine; and nucleotides (nucleotide-gated channels), such as cyclic AMP and cyclic GMP.

Mechanically Gated Channels. In **mechanically gated channels,** an actual physical manipulation is required to open the gate. An example of this mechanism is found in the hair cells of the inner ear. These cells, located on the basilar membrane, possess **stereocilia** that are embedded in a matrix known as the **tectorial membrane**. Movement of the basilar membrane causes a shift in the positions of the hair cells, resulting in the bending of the stereocilia. This physical distortion opens the mechanically gated channels of the stereocilia.

G-Protein–Gated Ion Channels. Certain gated ion channels (e.g., muscarinic acetylcholine receptors of cardiac muscle cells) require the interaction between a receptor molecule and a G-protein complex (discussed later in this chapter) with the resultant activation of the G protein. The activated G protein then interacts with the channel protein, modulating the ability of the channel to open or close.

Ungated Channels. One of the most common forms of an ungated channel is the **potassium (K^+) leak channel**, which permits the movement of K^+ ions across it and is instrumental in the creation of an **electrical potential (voltage) difference** between the two sides of the cell membrane. Because this channel is ungated, the transit of K^+ ions is not under the cell's control; rather, the direction of ion movement reflects its concentration on the two sides of the membrane.

Aquaporins. Currently, there are at least 13 different types of **aquaporins**, a family of multipass proteins that form channels designed for the passage of water from one side of the cell membrane to the other. Some of these channels are pure water transporters (e.g., AqpZ), whereas others transport glycerol (GlpF). These aquaporins discriminate in the transport of the two molecules by restricting the pore sizes in such a fashion that glycerol is too large to pass through the pore of the AqpZ channel. An interesting property of aquaporins is that they are

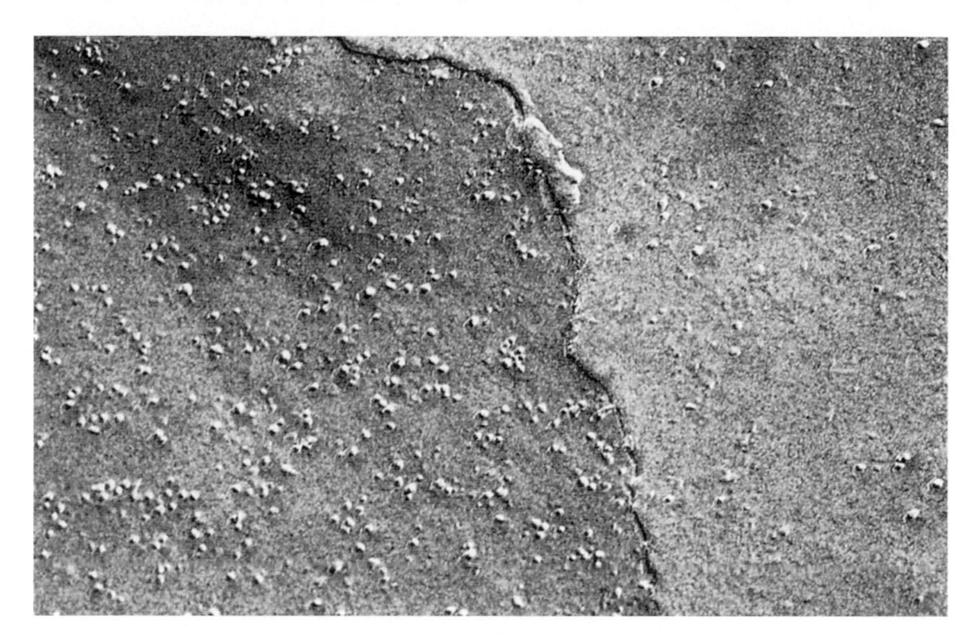

Fig. 2.10 Freeze-fracture replica of a cell membrane. The E-face (closer to the *extracellular* space) is on the right, and the P-face (closer to the *protoplasm*) is on the left. Note that the integral proteins are more numerous on the P-face (left-hand side) than on the E-face (right-hand side). (×168,000) (From Leeson TS, Leeson CR, Papparo AA. *Text/Atlas of Histology*. Philadelphia: WB Saunders; 1988.)

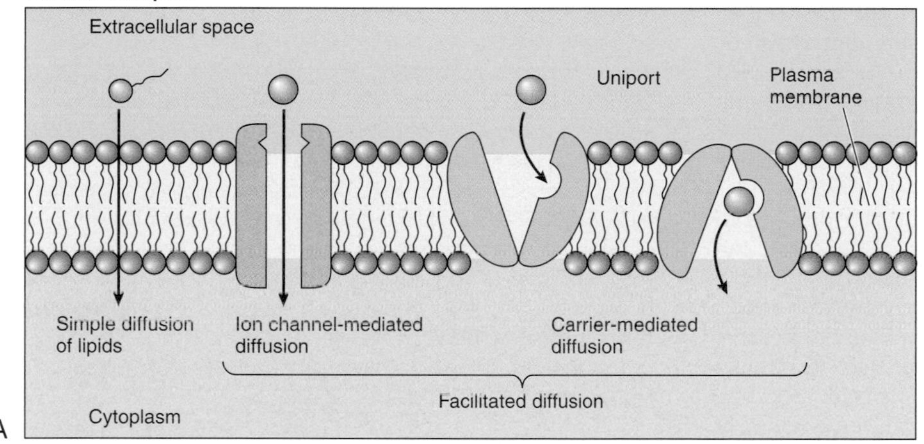

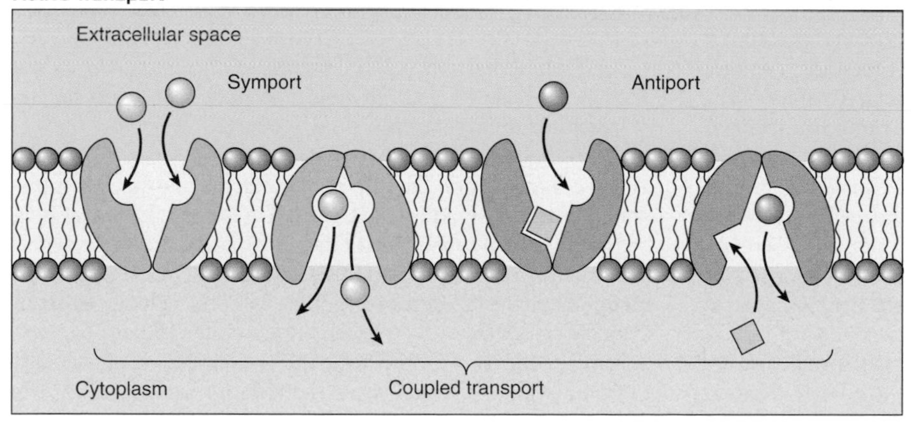

Fig. 2.11 Types of transport. (A) Passive transport: diffusion, ion channel–mediated diffusion, and carrier-mediated diffusion. (B) Active transport: coupled transport. Symport and antiport.

completely impermeable to protons, so that streams of protons cannot traverse the channel even though they readily pass through water molecules via the process of donor-acceptor configurations. Aquaporins interfere with this donor-acceptor model by forcing the water molecules to flip-flop halfway along the channel, so that water molecules enter the channel face up (hydrogen side up and oxygen side down—that is, the oxygen enters first, followed by the two hydrogens), flip over, and leave the channel face down (so that the two hydrogen molecules leave first, followed by the oxygen). Properly functioning aquaporins in the kidney may transport as much as 20 L of water per hour, whereas improperly functioning aquaporins may result in diseases such as diabetes insipidus and congenital cataracts of the eye.

Carrier Proteins

Carrier proteins can use ATP-driven transport mechanisms to ferry specific substances across the plasmalemma against a concentration gradient.

Carrier proteins are **multipass** membrane transport proteins that possess binding sites for specific ions or molecules on both sides of the phospholipid bilayer. When an ion or molecule specific to the particular carrier protein binds to the binding site, the carrier protein undergoes *reversible* conformational changes; as the ion or molecule is released on the other side of the membrane, the carrier protein returns to its previous conformation.

As stated earlier, transport by carrier proteins may be **passive**, along an electrochemical concentration gradient, or **active**, against a gradient, thereby requiring energy expenditure by the cell. Transport may be **uniport**, a single molecule moving in one direction, or **coupled**, two different molecules moving in the same (**symport**) or opposite (**antiport**) directions (see Fig. 2.11). Coupled transporters convey the solutes either simultaneously or sequentially.

Primary Active Transport by Na^+-K^+ Pump. Normally, the concentration of Na^+ is much greater outside the cell than inside, and the concentration of K^+ is much greater inside the cell than outside. The cell maintains this concentration differential by expending **adenosine triphosphate** (**ATP**) to drive a coupled antiport carrier protein known as the **Na^+-K^+** pump. This pump transports K^+ ions into and Na^+ ions out of the cell, each against a steep concentration gradient. **Na^+-K^+ ATPase** has been shown to be associated with the Na^+-K^+ pump. When three Na^+ ions bind on the cytosolic aspect of the pump, ATP is hydrolyzed to **adenosine diphosphate** (**ADP**) and the released phosphate ion is used to *phosphorylate* the ATPase, resulting in alteration of the conformation of the pump, with the consequent transfer of Na^+ ions out of the cell. Binding of two K^+ ions on the external aspect of the pump causes *dephosphorylation* of the ATPase with an ensuing return of the carrier protein to its previous conformation, resulting in the transfer of the K^+ ions into the cell. Thus, the expenditure of a single ATP molecule provides the energy for the transfer of three Na^+ ions and two K^+ ions across the cell membrane.

The constant operation of this pump reduces the intracellular ion concentration, resulting in decreased intracellular osmotic pressure. Because the binding sites on the external aspect of the pump bind not only K^+ but also the glycoside **ouabain**, this glycoside inhibits the Na^+-K^+ pump.

Secondary Active Transport by Coupled Carrier Proteins. The ATP-driven transport of Na^+ out of the cell establishes a low intracellular concentration of that ion. The energy reservoir inherent in the sodium ion gradient can be used by carrier proteins to transport ions or other molecules against a concentration gradient. Frequently, this mode of active transport is referred to as **secondary active transport**, distinct from **primary active transport**, which uses the energy released from the hydrolysis of ATP. The carrier proteins that participate in secondary active transport are either symports or antiports.

ATP-Binding Cassette Transporters (ABC-Transporters). These highly conserved transporters occur in the largest numbers of all carrier proteins. They are present in both prokaryotic organisms, such as bacteria, and in all eukaryotic organisms. The major difference is that in prokaryotic organisms, the ABC-transporters move substances in both directions (into and out of the cell) whereas in eukaryotic cells, the transport is in a single direction only, namely, out of the cell; only the eukaryotic transporters are discussed here.

ABC-transporters are transmembrane proteins, thus, protruding through both sides of the cell membrane. The intracellular portion of the transporters possesses binding sites (known as **ATP-binding cassettes**) for two ATP molecules. When ATP is not present, the intracellular binding sites for specific molecules are exposed and the particular ion or molecule adheres to the binding site. When the ATP molecules bind to the ATP-binding cassettes, the transporter's conformation becomes altered and the ion or molecule is permitted to leave at the transporter's extracellular surface. It should be stated that not all ABC-transporters are located on the plasmalemma; many are present on the membranes of intracellular membranous organelles, such as the trans-Golgi network, rough endoplasmic reticulum, and mitochondrion.

Clinical Correlations

A member of the ABC-transporters, the ***cystic fibrosis transmembrane conductance regulator protein*** ***(CFTR protein,*** *coded for by a mutated form of the CFTR gene) is responsible for the formation of abnormal chloride channel proteins, especially in the respiratory system. The channels formed by these proteins do not permit Cl^- ions to pass through them to leave the cell; thereby, the increased negative charge due to the increased concentration of chloride ions in the cytoplasm attracts Na^+ ions into the cells. The elevated NaCl content of the cell attracts water from the extracellular milieu into the cell, increasing the viscosity of the mucus lining the respiratory tract. The thickened mucus blocks the smaller bronchioles, leading to infection, debilitated lung function, and, eventually, death.*

Many ABC-transporters transport various hydrophobic toxic substances and drugs out of the cell. Various cancer cells possess specific ABC-transporters, known as ***multidrug resistance proteins*** *(****MDR proteins****), that drive anticancer drugs out of the cell, providing the malignant cells with increased resistance to chemotherapeutic agents.*

Cell Signaling

Cell signaling is the communication that occurs when signaling cells release signaling molecules that bind to cell surface receptors of target cells.

When cells communicate with each other, the one that sends the signal is called the **signaling cell**; the cell receiving the signal is called the **target cell**. Transmission of the information may occur either by the secretion or presentation of **signaling molecules**, which contact **receptors** on the target cell membrane (or intracellularly either in the cytosol or nucleus) or by the formation of intercellular pores known as **gap junctions**, which permit the movement of ions and small molecules (e.g., cyclic adenosine monophosphate [cAMP]) between the two cells. Gap junctions are discussed in Chapter 5.

The signaling molecule, or **ligand**, may be either secreted and released by the signaling cell or may remain bound to its surface and presented by the signaling cell to the target cell. A cell-surface receptor usually is a transmembrane protein; an intracellular receptor is a protein that resides in the cytosol or in the nucleus of the target cell. Ligands that bind to cell-surface receptors usually are **polar** molecules; those that bind to intracellular receptors are **hydrophobic** and, thus, can diffuse through the cell membrane (Table 2.1).

TABLE 2.1 Types of Signaling

Signaling Type	Description
Synaptic signaling	The signaling molecule, a neurotransmitter, is released so close to the target cell that only a single cell is affected by the ligand.
Paracrine signaling	The signaling molecule is released into the intercellular environment and affects cells in its immediate vicinity.
Autocrine signaling	The signaling cell is also the target cell.
Endocrine signaling	The signaling molecule enters the bloodstream to be ferried to target cells situated at a distance from the signaling cell.

Signaling Molecules

Signaling molecules bind to extracellular or intracellular receptors to elicit a specific cellular response.

Most signaling molecules are hydrophilic (e.g., **acetylcholine**) and cannot penetrate the cell membrane. Therefore, they require receptors on the cell surface. Other signaling molecules are either hydrophobic, such as **steroid hormones**, or are small nonpolar molecules, such as **nitric oxide** (**NO**), both of which have the ability to diffuse through the phospholipid bilayer. These ligands require the presence of an intracellular receptor. Hydrophilic ligands have a very short life span (a few milliseconds to minutes at most), whereas steroid hormones last for extended time periods (several hours to days).

Binding of signaling molecules to their receptors activates an intracellular **second messenger system**, initiating a cascade of reactions that result in the required response. A hormone, for example, binds to its receptors on the cell membrane of its target cell. The receptor alters its conformation, with the resultant activation of **adenylate cyclase**, a transmembrane protein whose cytoplasmic region catalyzes the transformation of **ATP** to **cAMP**, one of the most common second messengers.

The second messenger, cAMP, activates a cascade of enzymes within the cell, multiplying the effects of a very few molecules of hormones on the cell surface. The specific intracellular event depends on the enzymes located within the cell; for instance, cAMP activates one set of enzymes within an endothelial cell and another set of enzymes within a follicular cell of the thyroid gland. Therefore, the same molecule can have a different effect in different cells. The system is known as a second messenger system because the hormone is the first messenger that activates the formation of cAMP, the second messenger. Other second messengers include calcium (Ca^{2+}), cGMP, inositol triphosphate (IP_3), and diacylglycerol.

Steroid hormones (e.g., cortisol) can diffuse through the cell membrane. Once in the cytosol, they bind to **steroid hormone receptors** (members of the **intracellular receptor family**), and the ligand-receptor complex activates gene expression, or **transcription** (the formation of **messenger ribonucleic acid** [**mRNA**]). Transcription may be induced directly, resulting in a fast **primary response**, or indirectly, bringing about a slower secondary response. In the **secondary response**, the mRNA codes for the protein that is necessary to activate the expression of additional genes.

Cell-Surface Receptors

Cell-surface receptors are of three types: ion channel–linked, enzyme-linked, and G-protein–linked.

Most cell-surface receptors are integral **glycoproteins** that function in recognizing signaling molecules and in **transducing** the signal into an intracellular action. The three main classes of receptor molecules are ion channel–linked receptors, enzyme-linked receptors, and G-protein–linked receptors.

Enzyme-Linked Receptors. **Enzyme-linked receptors** are transmembrane proteins whose extracellular regions act as receptors for specific ligands. When a signaling molecule binds to the receptor site, the receptor's intracellular domain becomes activated so that it now possesses enzymatic capabilities. These enzymes then either induce the formation of second messengers, such as cGMP, or permit the assembly of intracellular signaling molecules that relay the signal intracellularly. This signal then elicits the required response by activating additional enzyme systems or by stimulating gene regulatory proteins to initiate the transcription of specific genes.

G-Protein–Linked Receptors. G-protein–linked receptors are multipass proteins whose extracellular domains act as receptor sites for ligands. Their intracellular regions have two separate sites: one that binds to G proteins and another that becomes phosphorylated during the process of receptor desensitization.

Most cells possess two types of GTPases (monomeric and trimeric), each of which has the capability of binding **guanosine triphosphate** (**GTP**) and **guanosine diphosphate** (**GDP**). Trimeric GTPases, **G proteins**, are composed of a large **α subunit** and two **small subunits**, **β** and **γ**, and can associate with G-protein–linked receptors. There are several types of G proteins, including:

- Stimulatory (G_s)
- Inhibitory (G_i)
- Pertussis toxin-sensitive (G_o)
- G_{olf}
- Pertussis toxin-insensitive (G_{Bq})
- Transducin (G_t)
- $G_{12/13}$

G proteins act by linking receptors with enzymes that modulate the levels of the intracellular signaling molecules (second messengers) cAMP or Ca^{2+}.

Signaling via G_s and G_i Proteins. G_s proteins (Fig. 2.12) are usually present in the **inactive** state, in which a **GDP** molecule is bound to the α subunit. When a ligand binds to the G-protein–linked receptor, it alters the receptor's conformation, permitting it to bind to the α subunit of the **G_s protein**, which, in turn, exchanges its GDP for a **GTP**. The binding of GTP causes the α subunit to dissociate not only from the receptor but also from the other two subunits and to bind with **adenylate cyclase**, a transmembrane protein. This binding activates adenylate cyclase to form many molecules of cAMP from ATP molecules. As the activation of adenylate cyclase is occurring, the ligand uncouples from the G-protein–linked receptor, returning the receptor to its original conformation without affecting the activity of the α subunit. Within a few seconds, the α subunit

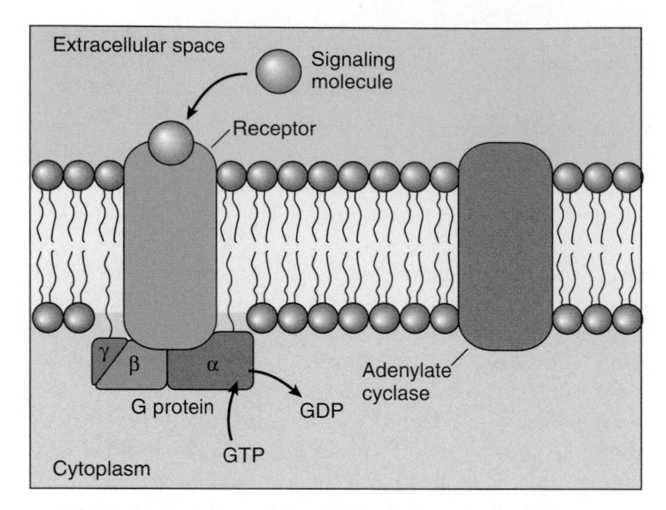

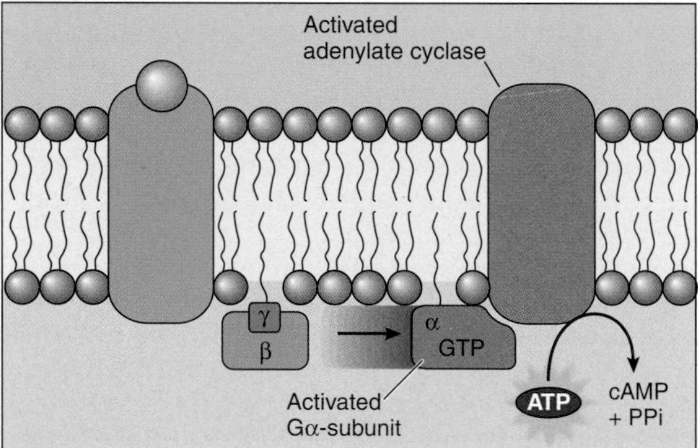

Fig. 2.12 G-protein–linked receptor. When the signaling molecule contacts its receptor, the α subunit dissociates from the G protein and contacts and activates adenylate cyclase, which converts adenosine triphosphate (ATP) to cyclic adenosine monophosphate (cAMP). GDP, guanosine diphosphate; GTP, guanosine triphosphate; PPi, pyrophosphate.

hydrolyzes its GTP to GDP, detaches from adenylate cyclase (thus, deactivating it), and reassociates the β and γ subunits.

G_i **protein** behaves similarly to G_s, but instead of activating adenylate cyclase, it inhibits it so that cAMP is not being produced. The lack of cAMP prevents the phosphorylation—thus, activation—of enzymes that would elicit a particular response. Hence, a particular ligand binding to a particular receptor may activate or inactivate the cell depending on the type of G protein that couples it to adenylate cyclase.

Cyclic AMP and Its Role as a Second Messenger. cAMP is an intracellular signaling molecule that activates cAMP-dependent protein kinase (**A-kinase**) by binding to it. The activated A-kinase dissociates into its **regulatory component** and two **active catalytic subunits**. The active catalytic subunits phosphorylate other enzymes in the cytosol, initiating a cascade of phosphorylations and resulting in a specific response. Elevated levels of cAMP in some cells result in the transcription of those genes whose regulatory regions possess **cAMP response elements** (**CREs**). A-kinase phosphorylates—and, thus, activates—a gene-regulatory protein known as **CRE-binding protein (CREB)** whose binding to the CRE stimulates the transcription of those genes.

As long as cAMP is present at a high enough concentration, a particular response is elicited from the target cell. In order to prevent responses of unduly long duration, cAMP is quickly degraded by **cAMP phosphodiesterases** to 5′-AMP, which is unable to activate A-kinase. Moreover, the enzymes phosphorylated during the cascade of phosphorylations become deactivated by becoming dephosphorylated by another series of enzymes (**serine/threonine phosphoprotein phosphatases**).

Signaling via G_o *Protein.* When a ligand becomes bound to G_o**-protein–linked receptor**, the receptor alters its conformation and binds with G_o. This trimeric protein dissociates, and its subunit activates **phospholipase C**, the enzyme responsible for cleaving the membrane phospholipid **phosphatidylinositol bisphosphate** (**PIP_2**) into **IP_3** and **diacylglycerol.** IP_3 leaves the membrane and diffuses to the endoplasmic reticulum, where it causes the release of Ca^{2+}—another second messenger—into the cytosol. Diacylglycerol remains attached to the inner leaflet of the plasma membrane and, with the assistance of Ca^{2+}, activates the enzyme protein kinase C (**C-kinase**). C-kinase, in turn, initiates a phosphorylation cascade, whose end result is the activation of gene-regulatory proteins that initiate transcription of specific genes.

IP_3 is rapidly inactivated by being dephosphorylated, and diacylglycerol is catabolized within a few seconds after its formation. These actions ensure that responses to a ligand are of limited duration.

Ca^{2+} and Calmodulin. Because cytosolic Ca^{2+} acts as an important second messenger, its cytosolic concentration must be carefully controlled by the cell. These control mechanisms include the sequestering of Ca^{2+} by the endoplasmic reticulum, specific Ca^{2+}-binding molecules in the cytosol and mitochondria, and the active transport of this ion out of the cell.

When IP_3 causes elevated cytosolic Ca^{2+} levels, the excess ions bind to **calmodulin**, a protein found in high concentration in most animal cells. The Ca^{2+}-calmodulin complex activates a group of enzymes known as **Ca^{2+}-calmodulin-dependent protein kinases** (**CaM-kinases**). CaM-kinases have numerous regulatory functions in the cell, such as initiation of glycogenolysis, synthesis of catecholamines, and contraction of smooth muscle.

Signaling via Other G Proteins. **G_{olf}** is an olfactory-specific protein that reacts to recognize specific odorants; **$G_{12/13}$** prompts actin formation in the cytosol, thus remodeling the cytoskeleton and, in that manner, facilitates cell motility. Pertussis toxin-insensitive (**G_{Bq}**) **G protein** activates substance P, which, in the brain, regulates the opening of potassium channels.

PROTEIN SYNTHETIC AND PACKAGING MACHINERY OF THE CELL

The primary components of the protein synthetic machinery of the cell are ribosomes (and polyribosomes), rough endoplasmic reticulum, and the Golgi apparatus.

Ribosomes

Ribosomes are small particles, approximately 12 nm wide and 25 nm long, composed of proteins and **ribosomal RNA** (**rRNA**). They function as a surface for the synthesis of proteins. Each ribosome is composed of a **large subunit** and a **small subunit**, both of which are manufactured or assembled in the nucleolus and released as separate entities into the cytosol. The small subunit has a sedimentation value of 40S and is composed of 33 proteins and an 18S rRNA. The sedimentation value of the large subunit is 60S, and it consists of 49 proteins and 3 rRNAs. The sedimentation values of the RNAs are 5S, 5.8S, and 28S.

The small subunit has a site for binding mRNA, a **P-site** for binding peptidyl **transfer ribonucleic acid (tRNA)**, an **A-site** for binding aminoacyl tRNAs, and an **E-site** where the tRNA that gave up its amino acid exits the ribosome. Some of the rRNAs of the large subunit are referred to as **ribozymes** since they have enzymatic activity and catalyze peptide bond formation. The small and large subunits are present in the cytosol individually and do not form a ribosome until protein synthesis begins.

Recent studies suggest that not all ribosomes are alike; instead, certain proteins have to be synthesized on specific ribosomes. In fact, an examination of the various ribosomal proteins indicated that certain ribosomal proteins are required for the ribosome to be able to translate mRNAs that code for particular proteins, but the same ribosomes cannot translate certain other mRNAs that code for other proteins.

Clinical Correlations

Mutations in ribosomal proteins are responsible for a growing constellation of genetic disorders known as ***ribosomopathies****. One of the first ones to be recognized that belong to the group of ribosomopathies is* ***Diamond-Blackfan anemia (DBA)****, characterized by the inability of the bone marrow to produce the normal amount of erythrocytes. The bone marrows of affected individuals show normal white cell and platelet production, but erythroblast numbers are greatly depressed or even completely absent. Proerythroblasts are present but in greatly repressed numbers. A large percent of the erythrocytes that are present possess fetal hemoglobin instead of the adult form. Individuals suffering with DBA also display certain skeletal anomalies and shorter statures.*

Endoplasmic Reticulum

The **endoplasmic reticulum (ER)** is the largest membranous system of the cell, comprising approximately half of the total membrane volume. It is a system of interconnected tubules and vesicles whose lumen is referred to as the **cistern**. The ER has two components: the **smooth endoplasmic reticulum (SER)** and **rough endoplasmic reticulum (RER)**.

Smooth Endoplasmic Reticulum

A system of anastomosing tubules and occasional flattened membrane-bound vesicles constitute the SER (Fig. 2.13). The lumen of the SER is assumed to be continuous with that of the RER. Except for cells active in synthesis of steroids, cholesterol, and triglycerides, and cells that function in detoxification of toxic materials (e.g., alcohol and barbiturates), most cells do not possess an abundance of SER. The SER has become specialized in some cells (e.g., skeletal muscle cells), where it is known as the **sarcoplasmic reticulum** (see Chapter 8, "Muscle"), where it functions in sequestering calcium ions from the cytosol, assisting in the control of muscle contraction. The SER has no ribosomes associated with it.

Rough Endoplasmic Reticulum

Cells that function in the synthesis of proteins that are to be exported are richly endowed with RER (see Fig. 2.6). The membranes of this organelle are somewhat different from those of its smooth counterpart: their cytoplasmic surfaces are studded with ribosomes; the membranes possess integral proteins that function in recognizing and binding these ribosomes to its cytosolic surface and maintaining, in the interior of the cell, a flattened morphology of the RER. The integral proteins of interest are (1) the **signal recognition particle receptor (docking protein)**, (2) **ribosome receptor protein** (ribophorin I and ribophorin II), and (3) **pore protein**. Their functions are discussed below.

The flattened, sheet-like appearance of the RER at the periphery of the cell is really composed of ribosomal-studded tubular membranous structures that are in constant motion; as they overlap each other, they merely *present* the appearance of flattened sheets. In order to preserve their morphological characteristics, they possess **ER-shaping proteins** that support their distinguishing configurations. There are at least three families of these proteins: (1) **reticulons**, which support the curvatures of the RER; (2) **kinectins**, which support the flat, sheet-like RER and keep the proper dimensions of the cisterna; and (3) **atlastins**, which stabilize the junctions between and among profiles of RERs.

Clinical Correlations

Mutations in genes coding for the ER-shaping proteins of the reticulon and atlastin families are responsible for ***hereditary spastic paraplegia (HSP)****, a genetic neurodegenerative condition. HSP is distinguished by disturbance of gait due to weakness and spastic condition of the lower limbs. The abnormal proteins interfere with the formation of junctions in the RER, preventing normal myelin formation involving especially axons in the pyramidal and dorsal column tracts.*

The RER participates in the synthesis of all proteins that are to be packaged or delivered to the plasma membrane, as well as proteins that are destined to remain in the RER. It also performs posttranslational modifications of these proteins within the RER cisterna (lumen), including sulfation, folding, glycosylation, and, when necessary, their degradation. Additionally, lipids and integral proteins of all membranes of the cell are manufactured by the RER. The cisterna of the RER is also continuous with the perinuclear cistern, the space between the inner and outer nuclear membranes.

Polyribosomes

Proteins to be packaged are synthesized on the RER surface, whereas proteins destined for the cytosol are manufactured within the cytosol. The information coding for the sequence of amino acids that constitute the primary structure of a protein is housed in the **deoxyribonucleic acid (DNA)** of the nucleus. This information is **transcribed** into a strand of mRNA, which leaves the nucleus and enters the cytoplasm. The sequence of **codons** of the mRNA thus represents the chain of amino acids, in which *each* codon is composed of three consecutive nucleotides. Because any three consecutive nucleotides constitute a codon, it is essential that the protein synthetic machinery recognize the beginning and end of the message; otherwise, an incorrect protein will be manufactured.

The three types of RNA play distinctive roles in protein synthesis:

- **mRNA** carries the coded instructions specifying the sequence of amino acids.

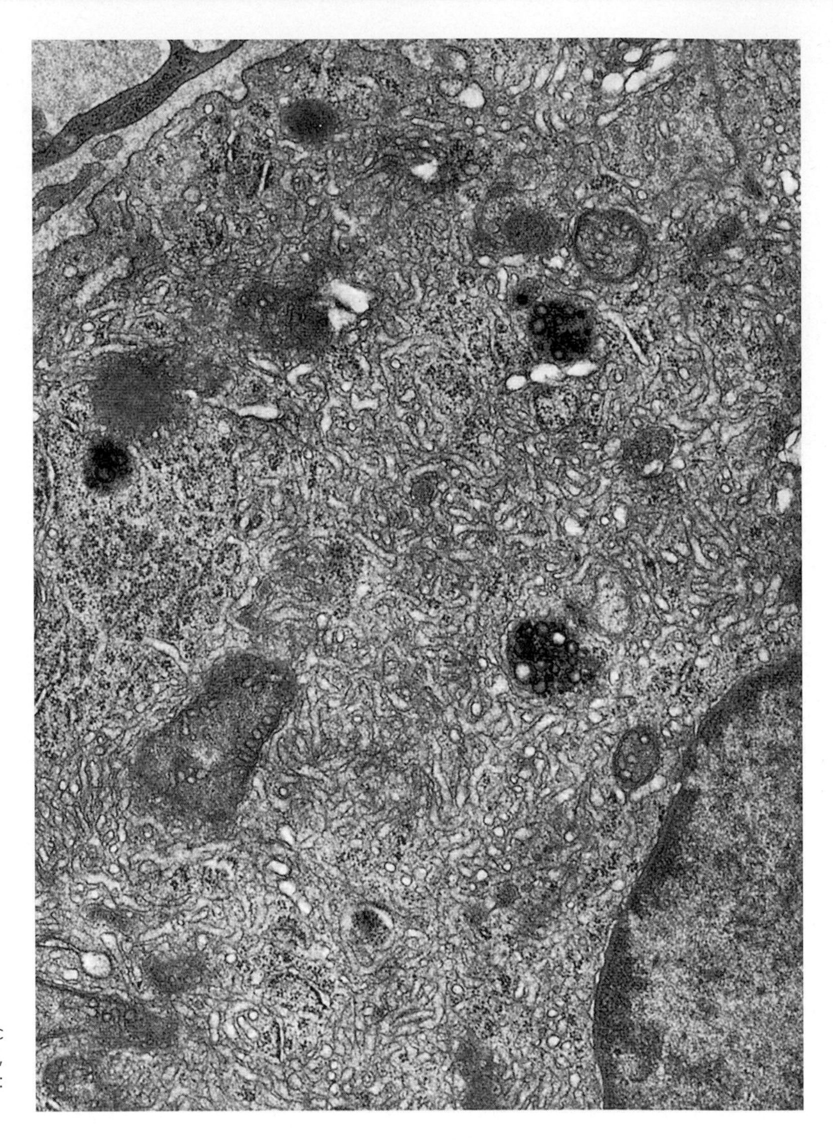

Fig. 2.13 Electron micrograph of the smooth endoplasmic reticulum of the human suprarenal cortex. (From Leeson TS, Leeson CR, Papparo AA. *Text/Atlas of Histology.* Philadelphia: WB Saunders; 1988.)

- **tRNAs** form covalent bonds with amino acids, forming **aminoacyl tRNAs.** Each tRNA also contains the **anticodon** that recognizes the codon in mRNA corresponding to the amino acid that it carries.
- Several **rRNAs** associate with a large number of proteins to form the small and large ribosomal subunits.

Protein Synthesis (Translation)

Protein synthesis (translation) occurs on ribosomes in the cytosol or on the surface of the rough endoplasmic reticulum.

The requirements for protein synthesis are:

- **mRNA** strand
- **tRNAs**, each of which carries an amino acid and possesses the anticodon that recognizes the codon of the mRNA coding for that particular amino acid
- Small and large **ribosomal subunits**

It is interesting that the approximate time of synthesis of a protein composed of 400 amino acids is about 20 seconds. Because a single strand of mRNA may have as many as 15 ribosomes translating it simultaneously, a large number of protein molecules may be synthesized in a short period of time. This conglomeration of mRNA-ribosome complex—which usually has a spiral or long, hairpin form—is referred to as a **polyribosome**, or **polysome** (Fig. 2.14).

Synthesis of Cytosolic Proteins

The general process of protein synthesis in the cytosol is outlined in Fig. 2.15.

Step 1

- The process begins when the P-site of the small ribosomal subunit is occupied by an **initiator tRNA**, whose anticodon recognizes the triplet **codon AUG**, coding for the amino acid **methionine.**
- An **mRNA** binds to the small subunit.
- The small subunit assists the anticodon of the tRNA molecule to recognize the **start codon AUG** on the mRNA molecule. This step acts as a registration step so that the next three nucleotides of the mRNA molecule may be recognized as the next codon.

Step 2

- The large ribosomal subunit binds to the small subunit and the ribosome moves along the mRNA chain, in a 5′ to 3′ direction, until the next codon lines up with the A-site of the small subunit.

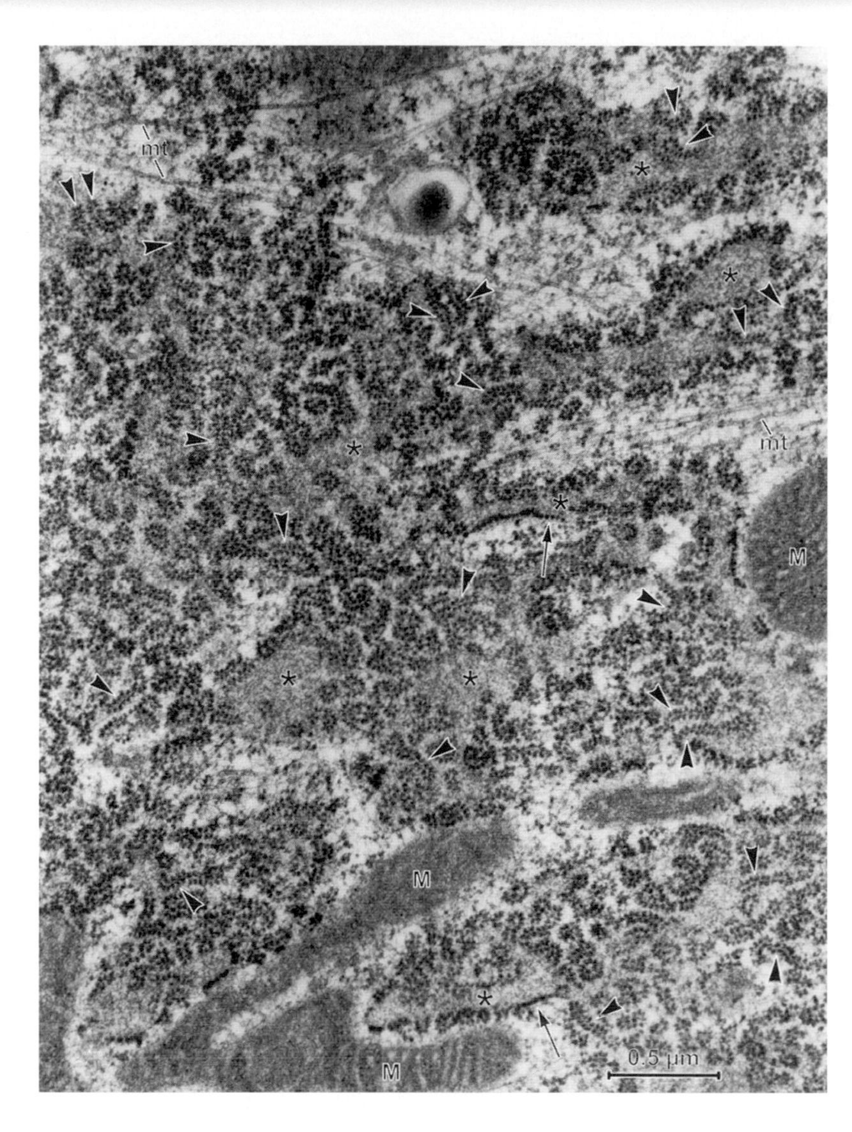

Fig. 2.14 Electron micrograph of bound polysome. (From Christensen AK, Bourne CM: Shape of large bound polysomes in cultured fibroblasts and thyroid epithelial cells. *Anat Rec.* 1999;255:116–129. Copyright © 1999. Reprinted by permission of Wiley-Liss, Inc., a subsidiary of John Wiley & Sons, Inc.)

Step 3
- An acylated tRNA (a tRNA bearing an amino acid) compares its anticodon with the codon of the mRNA; if they match, the tRNA binds to the A-site.

Step 4
- The amino acids at the A-site and P-site form a peptide bond.
- The tRNA on the P-site yields its amino acid to the tRNA at the A-site, which now has two amino acids attached to it. These reactions are catalyzed by peptidyl transferase, the rRNA-based enzyme of the large ribosomal subunit.

Step 5
- The deaminated tRNA leaves the P-site and binds to the E-site; the tRNA, with its two amino acids attached, moves from the A-site to the P-site. Concurrently, the ribosome moves along the mRNA chain until the next codon lines up with the A-site of the small ribosomal subunit and the tRNA from the E-site is ejected. The energy required by this step is derived from the hydrolysis of GTP.

Step 6
- Steps 3 through 5 are repeated, elongating the polypeptide chain until the stop codon is reached.
- There are three stop codons (**UAG**, **UAA**, and **UGA**), each of which may halt translation.

Step 7
- When the A-site of the small ribosomal subunit reaches a stop codon, the **release factors eRF1** and **eRF3** bind to the A site. eRF1 binds to the three stop codons UAG, UAA, and UGA.

Step 8
- The tRNA moves from the P-site to the E-site. eRF3, a GTPase, assists eRF1 in releasing the polypeptide from the ribosome; the ribosome leaves the mRNA and dissociates into a small and a large subunit.

Synthesis of Proteins on the Rough Endoplasmic Reticulum
Proteins that need to be packaged either for delivery to the outside of the cell, inserted into the cell membrane, sent to an cytoplasmic organelle, retained in the RER, or merely isolated from the cytosol must be identified and delivered **cotranslationally** (during the process of synthesis) into the RER cistern. The mode of identification resides in a small segment of the mRNA, located immediately following the start codon, which codes for a sequence of amino acids known as the **signal peptide.**

Employing the sequence just outlined for the synthesis of protein in the cytosol, the mRNA begins to be translated, forming the signal peptide (Fig. 2.16). This peptide is recognized by the **signal-recognition particle** (**SRP**), a ribonucleated-protein (protein-RNA complex) located in the cytosol. The SRP

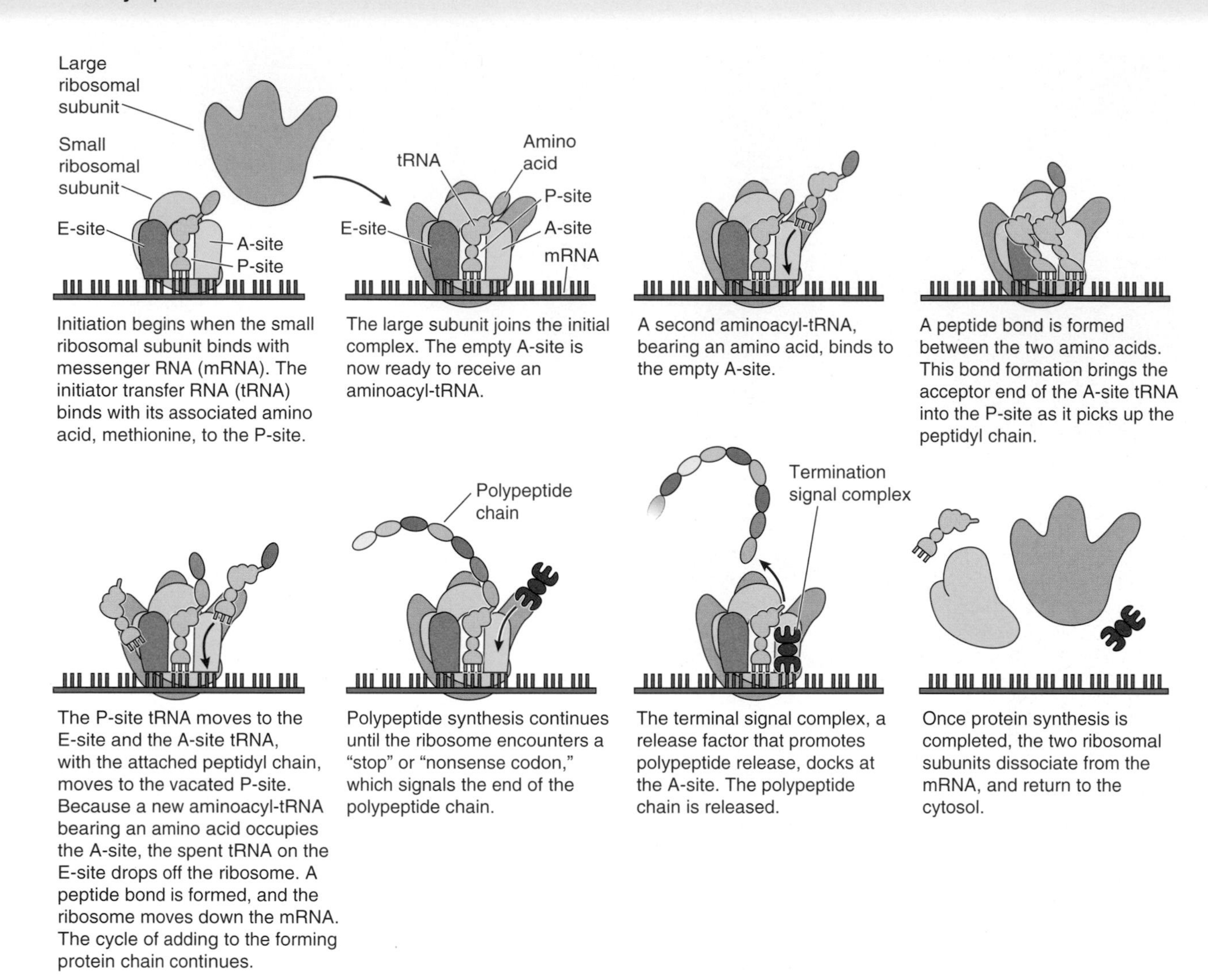

Fig. 2.15 Schematic diagram of protein synthesis in the cytosol.

becomes attached to the signal peptide and by occupying the P-site on the small subunit of the ribosome halts translation. It then directs the polysome to migrate to the RER.

The **SRP receptor protein** (**docking protein**) in the RER membrane contacts the SRP, and the ribosome receptor protein contacts the large subunit of the ribosome, attaching the polysome to the cytosolic surface of the RER. The following events then occur almost simultaneously:

1. A group of proteins, the **protein translocators**, assemble, forming a **pore** through the lipid bilayer of the RER.
2. The signal peptide contacts the pore protein and begins to be translocated (amino terminus first) into the cistern of the RER.
3. The SRP is dislodged, reenters the cytosol, and frees the P-site on the small ribosomal subunit. The ribosome remains on the RER surface.
4. As translation resumes, the nascent protein continues to be channeled into the cistern of the RER.
5. An enzyme attached to the cisternal aspect of the RER membrane, known as **signal peptidase**, cleaves the signal peptide from the forming protein. The signal peptide becomes degraded into its amino acid components.
6. As detailed earlier in STEPS 6 through 8 under the synthesis of cytosolic proteins, when the stop codon is reached, protein synthesis is completed; the small and large ribosomal subunits then dissociate and reenter the cytosol to join the pool of ribosomal subunits.
7. The newly formed proteins are sulfated, folded so that the proteins are no longer linear in shape, glycosylated, and undergo additional posttranslational modifications within the RER cisternae.
8. The modified proteins leave the cistern via small **COP II** coated (**co**at **p**rotein complex II, coatomer II) **transfer vesicles** at regions of the RER known as the **transitional endoplasmic reticulum** (**TER**). These are elements of the RER devoid of ribosomes (see later discussion).

Golgi Apparatus

The Golgi apparatus functions in the synthesis of carbohydrates and in the modification and sorting of proteins manufactured on the RER.

Proteins manufactured, modified, and packaged in the RER follow a **default pathway** to the Golgi apparatus for posttranslational modification and packaging. Proteins destined to remain in the RER or to go to a compartment other than the Golgi

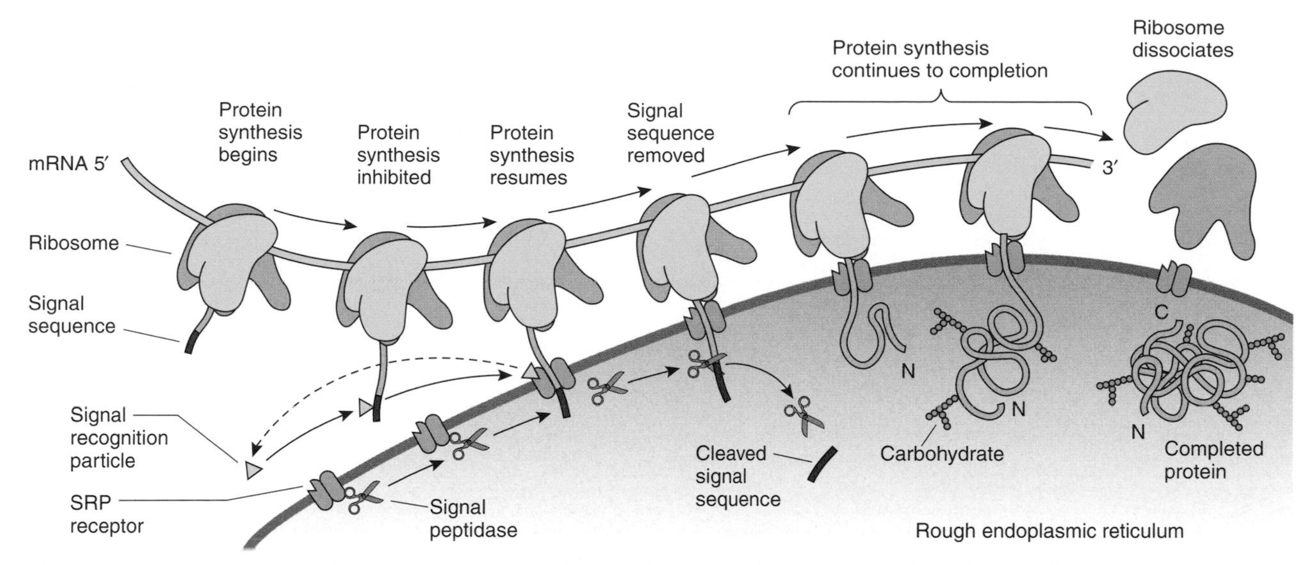

Fig. 2.16 Schematic diagram of protein synthesis on the rough endoplasmic reticulum. C, carboxyl terminus; mRNA, messenger ribonucleic acid; N, amino terminus; SRP, signal recognition particle.

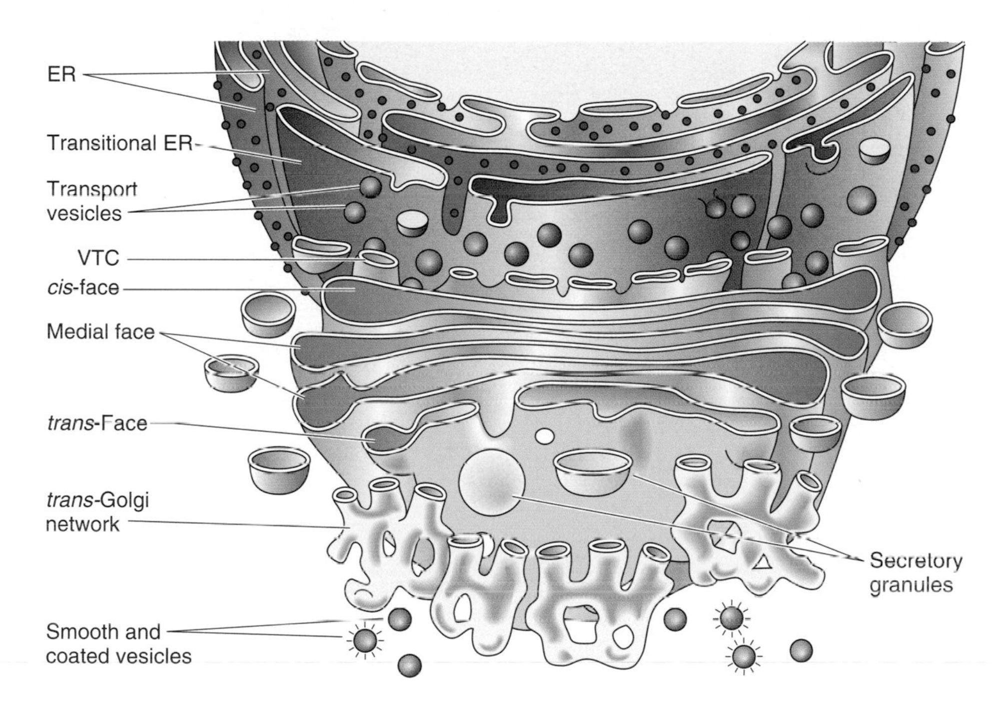

Fig. 2.17 Schematic diagram illustrating the rough endoplasmic reticulum and the Golgi apparatus. Transfer vesicles contain newly synthesized protein and are ferried to the ERGIC and from there to the Golgi apparatus. The protein is modified in the various faces of the Golgi complex and enters the *trans* Golgi network for packaging. ER, endoplasmic reticulum; VTC, endoplasmic reticulum/Golgi intermediate compartment.

apparatus possess a signal that will divert them from the default pathway.

The Golgi apparatus is composed of one or more series of flattened, slightly curved, membrane-bounded **cisternae** (known as faces), the **Golgi stack**, which resemble a stack of pita breads that do not quite contact each other (Figs. 2.17 to 2.19). The periphery of each cisterna is dilated and is rimmed with vesicles that are in the process of either fusing with or budding off that particular compartment.

Each Golgi stack has three levels of cisternae:

- The *cis*-face (or *cis* Golgi network)
- The medial face (intermediate face)
- The *trans*-face

The *cis*-face is closest to the RER. It is convex and is considered to be the entry face, because newly formed proteins from the RER enter the *cis*-face before they are permitted to enter the other cisternae of the Golgi apparatus. The *trans*-face is concave and is considered to be the exit face, because the modified protein is ready to be packaged and sent to its destination from here.

There are two additional compartments of interest: one associated with the *cis*-face and the other with the *trans*-face. Located between the RER and the *cis*-face of the Golgi apparatus is an intermediate compartment of vesicles, known as the **vesicular-tubular clusters** (**VTCs**). The second compartment, known as the ***trans* Golgi network** (**TGN**), is located at the distal side of the Golgi apparatus. The VTC is a collection of vesicles and tubules formed from the fusion of **transfer vesicles** derived from the **transitional endoplasmic reticulum** (**TER**). These transfer vesicles bud off the TER and contain nascent proteins synthesized on the surface and modified within the cisternae of the RER.

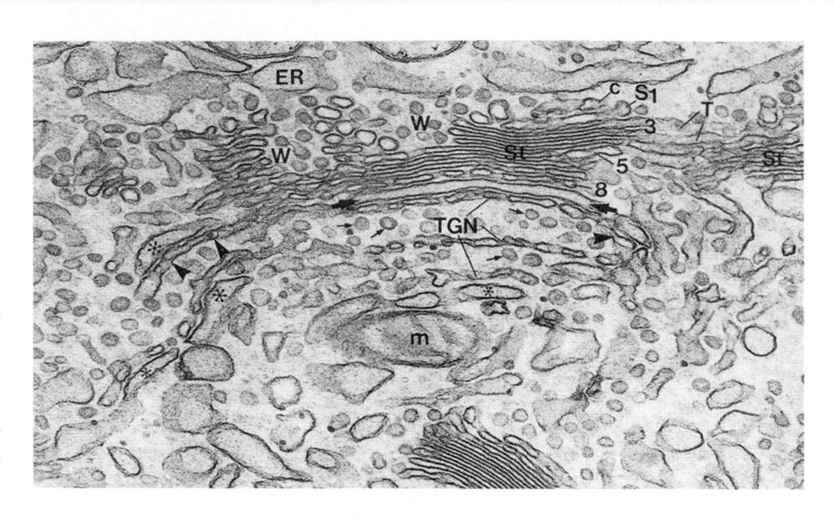

Fig. 2.18 Electron micrograph of the Golgi apparatus of the rat epididymis. ER, endoplasmic reticulum; TGN, *trans* Golgi network; m, mitochondrion; numbers represent the saccules of the Golgi apparatus. (From Hermo L, Green H, Clermont Y. Golgi apparatus of epithelial principal cells of the ependymal initial segment of the rat: Structure, relationship with endoplasmic reticulum, and role in the formation of secretory vesicles. *Anat Rec.* 1991;229:159–176. Copyright © 1991. Reprinted by permission of Wiley-Liss, Inc., a subsidiary of John Wiley & Sons, Inc.)

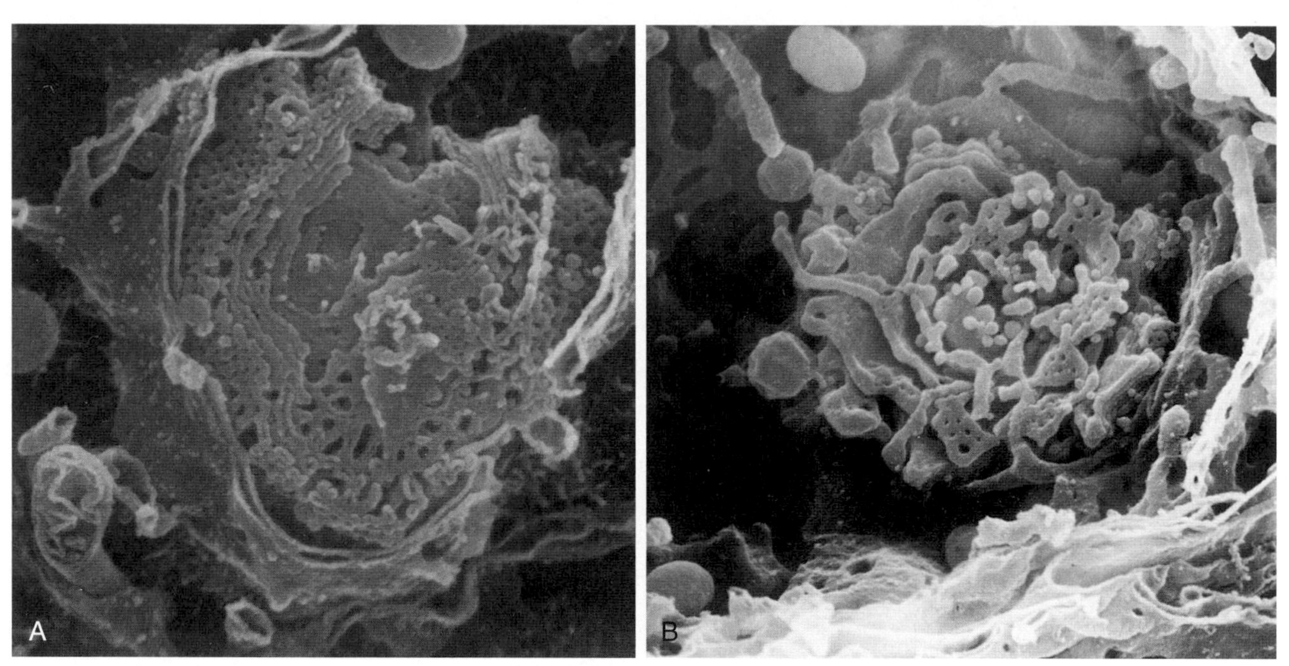

Fig. 2.19 (A) Face view of the *cis* Golgi network in a step 6 spermatid. The *cis*-most saccule is a regular network of anastomotic membranous tubules, capped by the endoplasmic reticulum. Some of the medial saccules, with fewer but larger and more irregular pores, are visible under the *cis* Golgi saccule. (B) Face view of another *cis* Golgi network in a step 6 spermatid. Note the fenestration at the edges of the irregular *trans* Golgi saccules. (From Ho HC, Tang CY, Suarez SS. Three-dimensional structure of the Golgi apparatus in mouse spermatids: A scanning electron microscopic study. *Anat Rec.* 1999;256:189–194. Copyright © 1999. Reprinted with permission of Wiley-Liss, Inc., a subsidiary of John Wiley & Sons, Inc.)

Vesicles derived from the VTC make their way to and fuse with the periphery of the *cis*-face of the Golgi apparatus, delivering the protein to this compartment for further modification. The modified proteins are transferred from the *cis* to the medial and finally to the *trans* cisternae (see later discussion) via vesicles that bud off and fuse with the rims of the particular compartment (Fig. 2.20). As the proteins pass through the Golgi apparatus, they are modified within the Golgi stacks. Proteins that form the cores of glycoprotein molecules become heavily glycosylated, whereas other proteins acquire or lose sugar moieties.

Mannose phosphorylation occurs within the *cis*-face cisterna, whereas the removal of mannose from certain proteins takes place within the *cis* and medial compartments of the Golgi stack. *N*-acetylglucosamine is added to the protein within the medial cisternae. Addition of sialic acid (*N*-acetylneuraminic acid) and galactose—as well as phosphorylation and sulfation of amino acids—occurs in the *trans*-face.

Coated Vesicles

Most vesicles possess a protein coat that assists them in reaching their destination; different protein coats are employed for different destinations in the cell.

Vesicles that transport proteins (**cargo**) between organelles and regions of organelles must have a way of budding off the organelle and must be labeled as to their destination. The process of budding is facilitated by the assembly of a proteinaceous coat on the cytosolic aspect of the organelle. Five types of proteins are known to elicit the formation of cargo-bearing vesicles: **coatomer I (COP I)**, **coatomer II (COP II)**, **clathrin**, **retromer**,

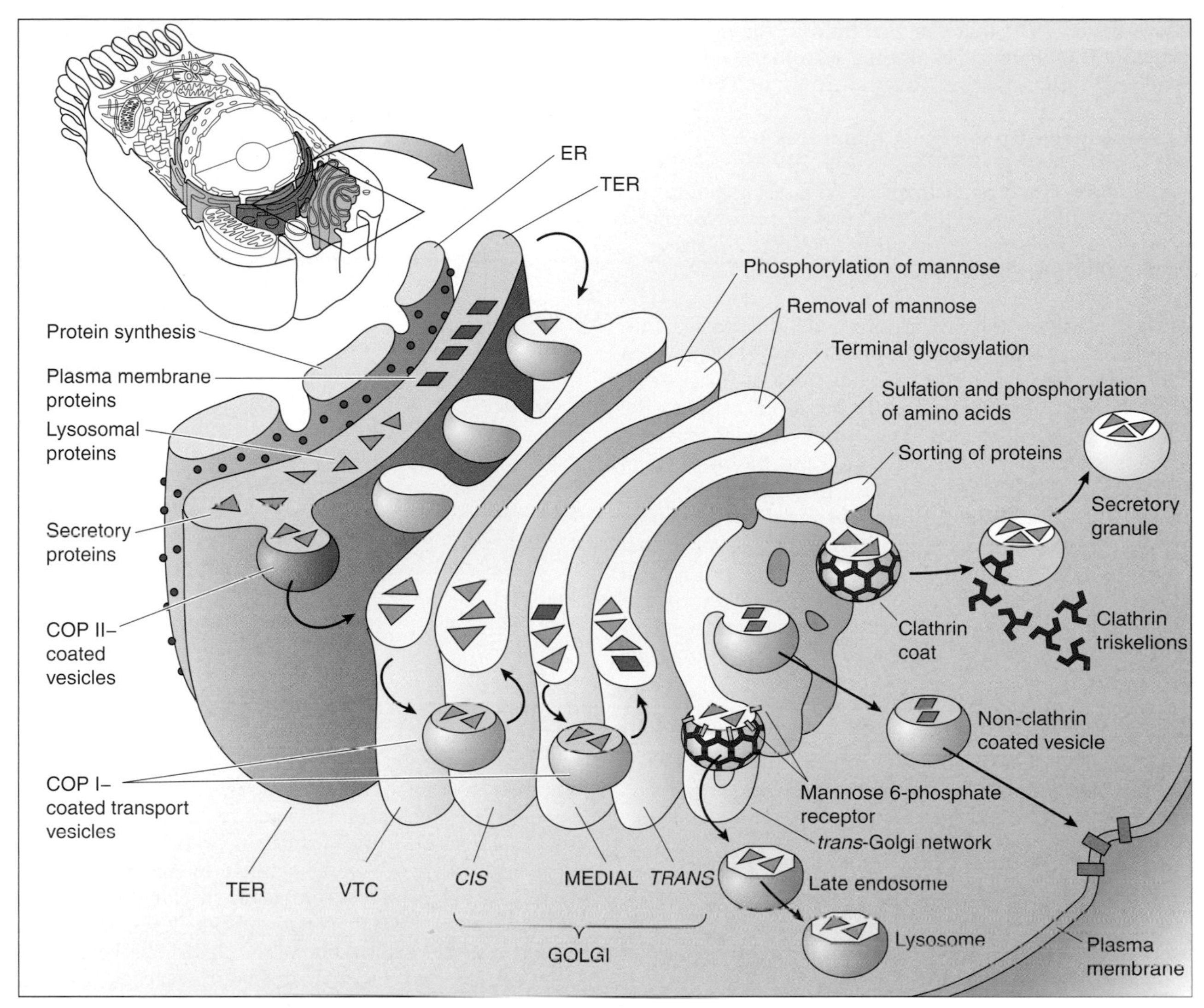

Fig. 2.20 Schematic diagram of the Golgi apparatus and packaging in the *trans* Golgi network. COP, Coatomer; ER, endoplasmic reticulum; TER, transitional endoplasmic reticulum; VTC, vesiculotubular clusters.

and **caveolin**. Thus, there are COP I–coated, COP II–coated, clathrin-coated, retromer-coated, and caveolin-coated vesicles. At the site of future vesicle formation, these proteins coalesce, attach to the membrane, draw out the vesicle, and coat its cytosolic surface.

Vesicles that arise from endosomes to be returned to the *trans* Golgi network are coated by retromer. Caveolin-coated vesicles are present in smooth muscle cells and endothelial cells. In the former, they are associated with calcium transfer (see Chapter 8, "Muscle"); in the latter, their functions appear to be those of endocytosis, transcytosis (see Chapter 11, "Circulatory System"), and cell signaling.

Vesicle and Target Recognition

The movement of vesicles from the donor site to the target site requires the presence of protein molecules embedded in the vesicle membrane, as well as in the target membrane. For the vesicles to be able to dock to the target, these molecules must recognize each other. The proteins on the vesicle membrane are known as **vesicle soluble NSF attachment protein (SNAP) receptors (v-SNAREs)**. Those that are on the target membranes are known as **t-SNAREs**. Because there are various v-SNARES and t-SNARES, they recognize each other only if they are complementary. If they recognize each other, then the vesicle is permitted to dock on the target membrane. In order to deliver the cargo carried by the vesicle—that is, fusion of the vesicle and target membranes—two additional molecules, recruited from the cytosol, are necessary. These are **N-ethylmaleimide-sensitive-fusion** (**SNF**) and **SNAP**. However, before the v-SNARES and t-SNARES can recognize each other, they must be brought into close proximity. This process of bringing the vesicle to the target membrane is performed by a large group of monomeric GTPases, known as **Rab proteins** (**Rab-GTPs**). Rab proteins of the vesicle, recognized by **tethering proteins** (**Rab effector proteins**) located in the target membrane, assist in bringing the vesicle to the target membrane so that the v-SNAREs and t-SNARES can recognize each other. In the case in which the tethering protein does not recognize the vesicle's Rab protein, docking is not permitted.

A special case of vesicle and target recognition occurs only if cargo that was delivered to the endosome has to be returned to the TGN. Such vesicles, as stated earlier, are coated with the protein **retromer** and are referred to as **retromer-coated vesicles**. In order for the retromer to assemble on the vesicle membrane, two components must be present: an appropriate **cargo receptor protein** that can bind to the retromer and the phospholipid

phosphoinositide (**PIP**) that can also bind to the retromer. If these two conditions are satisfied, then retromer can coat the vesicle and the vesicle is permitted to return to the TGN.

Vesicles Associated with the Golgi Apparatus

Nascent protein-bearing vesicles reach the Golgi apparatus from the TER and deposit the newly formed protein into the Golgi complex for modification within the Golgi cisternae, packaging, and distribution throughout the cell.

Transfer vesicles leaving the TER are always COP II coated until they reach the VTC, where they shed their COP II coat, which is recycled. It is believed by most investigators that vesicles that arise from the VTC, carrying recently delivered cargo to the *cis*-face are coated by COP I, as are all other vesicles that proceed through the medial to the *trans*-face and the *trans* Golgi network. Most of the vesicles that arise from the *trans* Golgi network, however, are coated by **clathrin** for their formation. The transport mechanism has a quality control aspect in that if RER (or TER) resident proteins are packaged in vesicles and these "stowaway" molecules reach the VTC, they are returned to the RER in **COP I–coated** vesicles. This is referred to as **retrograde transport** in contrast to **anterograde transport** of cargo, described earlier.

Sorting in the *Trans* Golgi Network

The TGN is responsible for the sorting of proteins to their respective pathways, so that they reach the plasma membrane, secretory granules, or lysosomes.

Cargo that leaves the TGN is enclosed in vesicles that may do one of the following (see Fig. 2.20):

- Insert into the cell membrane as membrane proteins and lipids
- Fuse with the cell membrane such that the protein they carry is *immediately* released into the extracellular space
- Congregate in the cytoplasm near the apical cell membrane as **secretory granules** (**vesicles**) and, upon a given signal, fuse with the cell membrane for *eventual* release of the protein outside the cell
- Fuse with **late endosomes** (see later discussion), releasing their content into that organelle, which then becomes a lysosome

The first three processes are known as **exocytosis**, because material leaves the cytoplasm proper. Neither immediate release into the extracellular space nor insertion into the cell membrane requires a particular regulatory process; thus, both processes are said to follow the **constitutive secretory pathway** (**default pathway**). In contrast, the pathways to lysosomes and to secretory vesicles are known as the **regulated secretory pathway**.

Transport of Lysosomal Proteins. The sorting process begins with the phosphorylation of mannose residues of the lysosomal proteins (lysosomal hydrolases) in the *cis* cisterna of the Golgi stack. When these proteins reach the *trans* Golgi network, their **mannose-6-phosphate** (**M6P**) is recognized as a signal, and they become bound to **mannose-6-phosphate receptors**, transmembrane proteins of the TGN membrane.

A small pit is formed with the assistance of **clathrin triskelions**, protein complexes composed of three heavy and three light chains forming a structure with three arms that radiate from a central point (Fig. 2.21; see Fig. 2.20). The triskelions self-assemble, coating the cytoplasmic aspect of the TGN rich in M6P receptors to which M6P is bound. As the pit deepens, it pinches off the TGN and forms a **clathrin-coated vesicle**. The clathrin coat, also referred to as the **clathrin basket**, is composed of 36 triskelion molecules that completely envelop the vesicle.

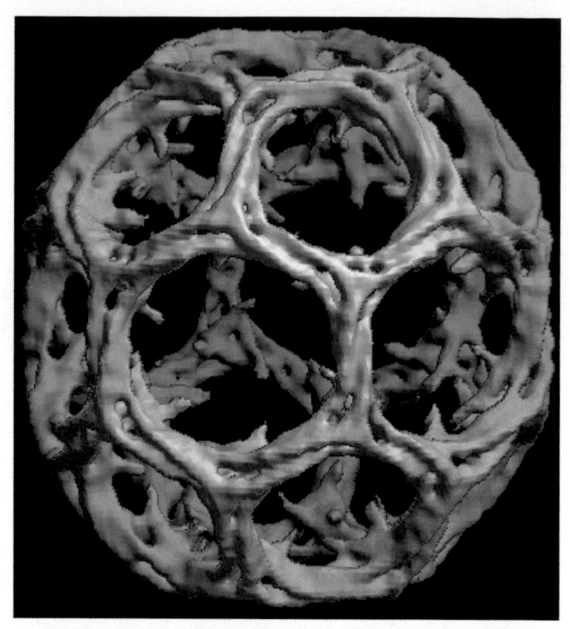

Fig. 2.21 A map of clathrin coat at 21 Å resolution. To allow a clear view of the path of the triskelion legs, the amino-terminal domain and most of the linker have been removed from this map. (From Smith CJ, Grigorieff N, Pearse BM. Clathrin coats at 21 Å resolution: A cellular assembly designed to recycle multiple membrane receptors. *Embo J.* 1998;17:4943–4953. By permission of Oxford University Press.)

The clathrin-coated vesicle quickly loses its clathrin coat, which, unlike the formation of the clathrin basket, is an energy-requiring process. The uncoated vesicle reaches, fuses with, and releases its contents into the late endosome (endosomes are discussed below).

Because clathrin coats are used for many other types of vesicles, an intermediary protein complex, known as an **adaptor** (**adaptin complex**), composed of four of the six types of the protein **adaptin**, is interposed between the cytoplasmic aspect of the receptor molecule and the clathrin. Many different types of adaptors exist; each has a binding site for a particular receptor as well as a binding site for clathrin.

Transport of Regulated Secretory Proteins. **Proteins** that are to be released into the extracellular space in a discontinuous manner also require the formation of clathrin-coated vesicles. The signal for their formation is not known; however, the mechanism is believed to be similar to that for lysosomal proteins.

Unlike vesicles that ferry lysosomal enzymes, secretory granules are quite large and carry many more proteins than there are receptors on the vesicle surface. Additionally, the contents of the secretory granules become condensed with time as a result of the loss of fluid from the secretory granules (see Figs. 2.6 and 2.20). During this process of increasing concentration, these vesicles are frequently referred to as **condensing vesicles**. Moreover, secretory granules of polarized cells remain localized in a particular region of the cell. They remain as clusters of secretory granules that, in reaction to a particular signal (e.g., neurotransmitter or hormone), fuse with the cell membrane to release their contents into the extracellular space (Fig. 2.22).

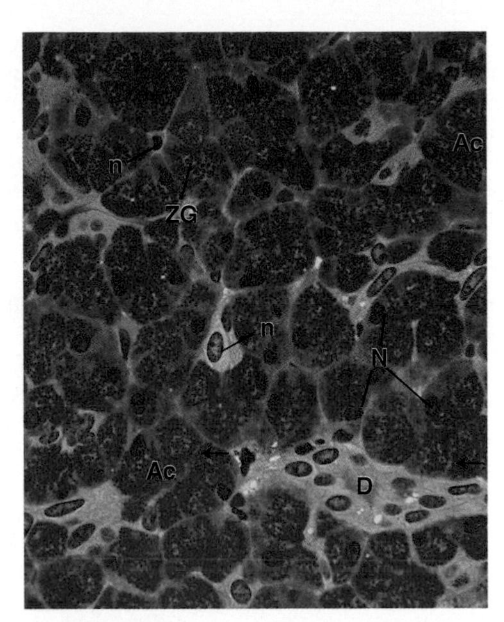

Fig. 2.22 This high-magnification photomicrograph of the exocrine pancreas displays numerous acini (Ac). The nuclei (N) of the acinar cells are basally located whereas the nucleus (n) of the centroacinar cell is located in the middle of the acinus. Centroacinar cells form the smallest part of the excretory duct system of the exocrine pancreas. Observe that the cytoplasm is filled with small pinkish-red secretory granules, known as zymogen granules (ZG). The arrow indicates the junction of two acinar cells. D, intercalated duct. (×540)

Transport Along the Constitutive Pathway. All vesicles that participate in nonselective transport, such as those passing between the RER and the *cis* Golgi network or among the cisternae of the Golgi stack or using the constitutive pathway between the TGN and the plasma membrane, also require a coated vesicle (see Fig. 2.20). However, as indicated earlier, the coating is composed of coatomer instead of clathrin.

Vesicles derived from the TGN are driven along microtubule tracts by the use of the motor protein **kinesin** and its associated protein complex. However, these vesicles also use an alternative, and perhaps their primary pathway, of actin filaments. The motor that drives these vesicles is myosin II; it is believed that myosin II is brought to the TGN subsequent to, or in conjunction with, the recruitment of the clathrin triskelions to the site of vesicle formation.

Alternative Concept of the Golgi Apparatus

An alternative concept of the Golgi apparatus suggests the occurrence of cisternal maturation instead of anterograde vesicle transport.

The two predominant theories of **anterograde vesicle transport** (already described) and **cisternal maturation** are mutually incompatible; yet, ample evidence exists to support both theories. The theory of cisternal maturation suggests that instead of the cargo being ferried through the various regions of the Golgi apparatus, it remains stationary and the various enzyme systems of the Golgi are transported in a retrograde fashion in the correct sequence and at the designated time so that a given sedentary cisterna matures into the subsequent cisternae.

At first glance, the cisternal maturation theory may appear to be dubious; however, it may be illustrated with a commonly observed phenomenon. If one is sitting in a stationary train and watches another stationary train on the neighboring railroad track when one of the trains begins to move, it is difficult initially to determine which train is moving and, without external visual aids, we cannot make a reasonable determination. The current state of research cannot determine which of the two theories is correct, but most histology and cell biology textbooks favor the anterograde vesicle transport theory.

ENDOCYTOSIS, ENDOSOMES, AND LYSOSOMES

Endocytosis, endosomes, and lysosomes are involved in the ingestion, sequestering, and degradation of substances internalized from the extracellular space.

The process whereby a cell ingests macromolecules, particulate matter, and other substances from the extracellular space is referred to as **endocytosis**. The endocytosed material is engulfed in a vesicle appropriate for its volume. If the vesicle is large (> 250 nm in diameter), the method is called **phagocytosis** (cell eating) and the vesicle is a **phagosome**. If the vesicle is small (< 150 nm in diameter), the type of endocytosis is called **pinocytosis** (cell drinking) and the vesicle is a **pinocytotic vesicle**.

Endocytotic Mechanisms

Endocytosis is divided into two categories: phagocytosis and pinocytosis.

Phagocytosis

The process of engulfing larger particulate matter, such as microorganisms, cell fragments, and cells (e.g., defunct red blood cells), is usually performed by specialized cells known as **phagocytes**. The most common phagocytes are the white blood cells, **neutrophils**, and **monocytes**. When monocytes leave the bloodstream and enter the connective tissue domain to perform their task of phagocytosis, they become known as **macrophages**.

Phagocytes can internalize particulate matter because they possess receptors that recognize certain surface features of the material to be engulfed. Two of the better understood of these surface features come from the study of immunology and are the **constant regions (Fc regions)** of antibodies and a blood-borne series of proteins known as **complement**. Because the variable region of the antibody binds to the surface of a microorganism, the Fc region projects away from its surface.

Macrophages and neutrophils possess Fc receptors that bind the Fc regions of the antibody upon contact. This relationship acts as a signal for the cell to extend pseudopods, surround the microorganism, and internalize the microorganism by forming a **phagosome**. Complement on the surface of the microorganism probably assists phagocytosis in a similar manner, because macrophages also possess complement receptors on their surface. Interaction between complement and its receptor presumably activates the cell to form pseudopods and engulf the invading microorganism.

> ***Clinical Correlations***
>
> *It is known that **macrophages**, members of the immune system of the body, have the capability of inducing inflammation, a process whereby the body combats bacterial and/or viral infections. There are instances, however, when the body initiates an inflammatory reaction in the absence of infectious agents. These occur in **autoimmune diseases**, such as inflammatory bowel syndrome and arthritis. Recently, it was discovered that macrophages can not only initiate but also retard the inflammatory process. They do that by converting glucose into itaconic acid, which blocks the factors that elicit the inflammatory process. This avenue of research may lead to the discovery of new nonsteroidal anti-inflammatory drugs.*

Pinocytosis

Because most cells export substances into the extracellular space, they continually add the membranes of vesicles that transport those substances from the TGN to the plasma membrane. These cells, in order to maintain their shape and size, must continually remove the excess membrane and return it for recycling. This cycle of membrane shuffling during exocytosis and endocytosis is known as **membrane trafficking**, the movement of membranes to and from various compartments of the cell. In most cells, pinocytosis is the most active transporting process and contributes most to the recapturing of membranes (Fig. 2.23).

Receptor-Mediated Endocytosis

Many cells specialize in the pinocytosis of several types of macromolecules. The most efficient form of capturing these substances depends on the presence of receptor proteins (**cargo receptors**) in the cell membrane. Cargo receptors are transmembrane proteins that become associated with the particular macromolecule **(ligand)** extracellularly and with a **clathrin coat** intracellularly (see Fig. 2.20).

The assembly of clathrin triskelions beneath the cargo receptors pulls on the plasma membrane, forming a clathrin-coated pit (Figs. 2.24 and 2.25), which eventually becomes a **pinocytotic vesicle**, enclosing the ligand as a droplet of fluid about to drip from a surface. To release this pinocytotic vesicle, several molecules of **dynamin**, a GTPase, surrounds the constricted neck of the vesicle, pinches its neck closed, and the pinocytotic vesicle is released from its membrane origin into the cytoplasm. This method of endocytosis, known as **receptor-mediated endocytosis**, permits the cell to increase the concentration of the ligand (e.g., low-density lipoprotein) within the pinocytotic vesicle.

A typical pinocytotic vesicle may have as many as 1000 cargo receptors of several types, for they may bind different macromolecules. Each cargo receptor is linked to its own **adaptin**, the protein with a binding site for the cytoplasmic aspect of the receptor as well as a binding site for the clathrin triskelion.

Endosomes

Endosomes are divided into two compartments: early endosomes, near the periphery of the cell, and late endosomes, situated deeper within the cytoplasm.

Shortly after their formation, pinocytotic vesicles lose their clathrin coats and fuse with **early endosomes** (Figs. 2.23 and 2.26), a system of vesicles and tubules located near the plasma membrane. If the entire content of the pinocytotic vesicle requires degradation, the material from the early endosome is

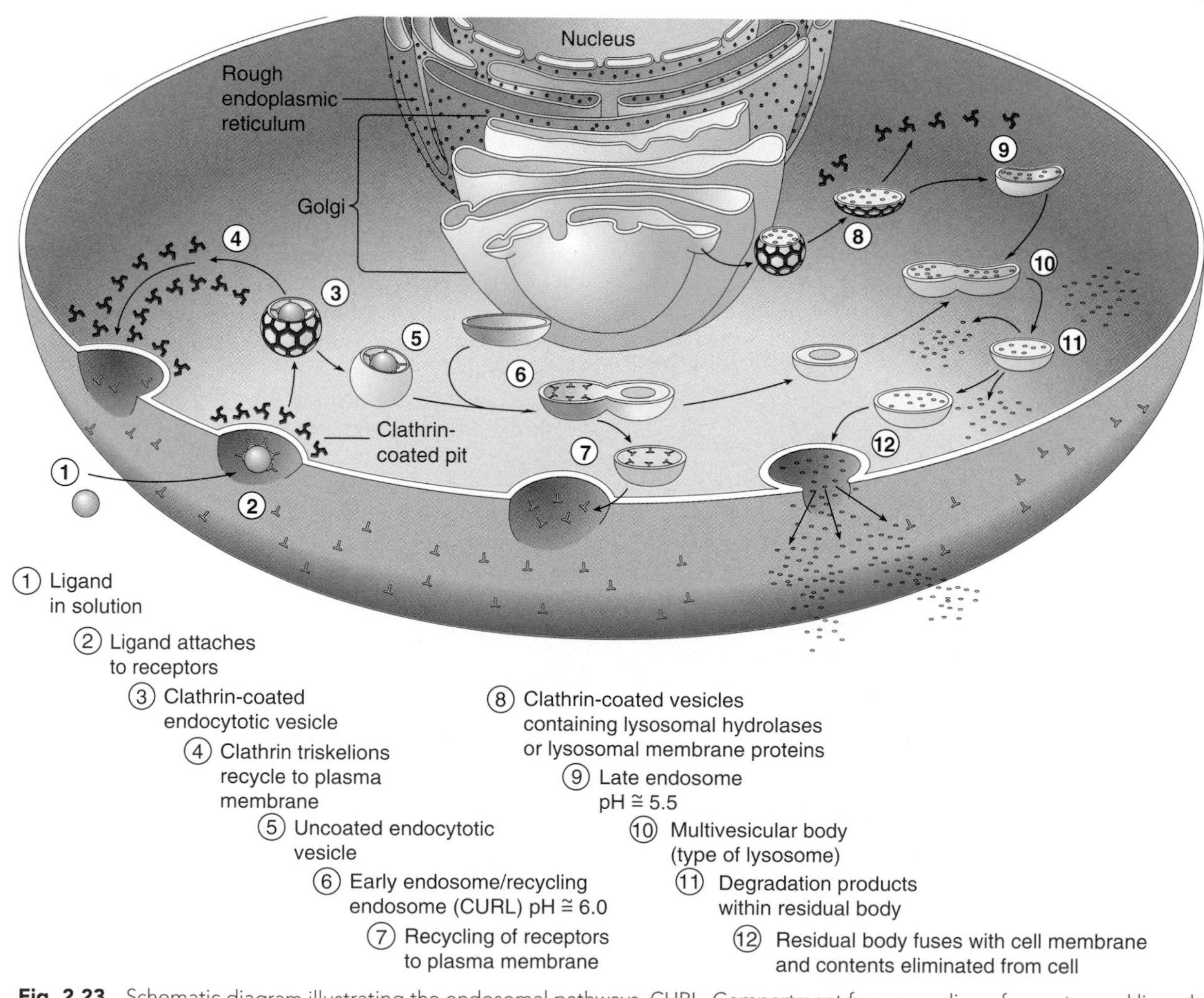

Fig. 2.23 Schematic diagram illustrating the endosomal pathways. CURL, Compartment for uncoupling of receptor and ligand.

transferred to a **late endosome**. This similar set of tubules and vesicles, located deeper in the cytoplasm near the Golgi apparatus, helps to prepare its contents for eventual destruction by lysosomes.

Early and late endosomes collectively constitute the **endosomal compartment**. The membranes of all endosomes contain ATP-linked H^+ pumps that acidify the interior of the endosomes by actively pumping H^+ ions into the interior of the endosome so that the early endosome has a pH of 6.0 and the late endosome a pH of 5.5.

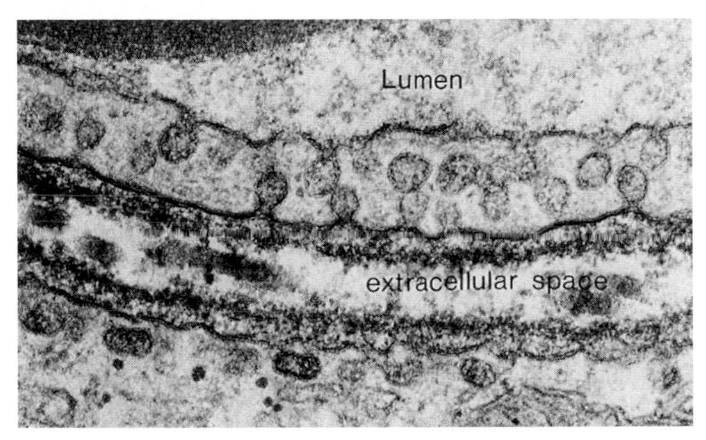

Fig. 2.24 Electron micrograph of endocytosis in a capillary. (From Hopkins CR. *Structure and Function of Cells*. Philadelphia: WB Saunders; 1978.)

Material entering the early endosome may be retrieved from that compartment and returned to its earlier location, as occurs with cargo receptors that need to be recycled. When a pinocytotic vesicle fuses with the early endosome, the acidic environment causes an uncoupling of the ligand from its receptor molecule. The ligand remains within the lumen of the early endosome, whereas the receptor molecules (e.g., low-density lipoprotein receptors) are returned to the plasma membrane where they originated or to the plasma membrane of another region of the cell, a process known as **transcytosis**. Some authors refer to this type of early endosome as a **CURL** (**c**ompartment for **u**ncoupling of **r**eceptor and **l**igand) or, more recently, as a **recycling endosome** (see Figs. 2.23 and 2.26).

Within 10 to 15 minutes of entering the early endosome, the ligand either is transferred to a late endosome (as in the case of low-density lipoprotein) or is packaged to be returned to the cell membrane, where it is released (e.g., transferrin) into the extracellular space. Occasionally, both the receptor and the ligand (e.g., epidermal growth factor and its receptor) are transferred to the late endosome, and then to a lysosome, for eventual degradation.

The transport between early and late endosomes has not been elucidated. Some authors suggest that early endosomes migrate along microtubule pathways into a deeper location within the cell and become late endosomes. Others postulate that early and late endosomes are two separate compartments and that specific **endosomal carrier vesicles** ferry material from early to late

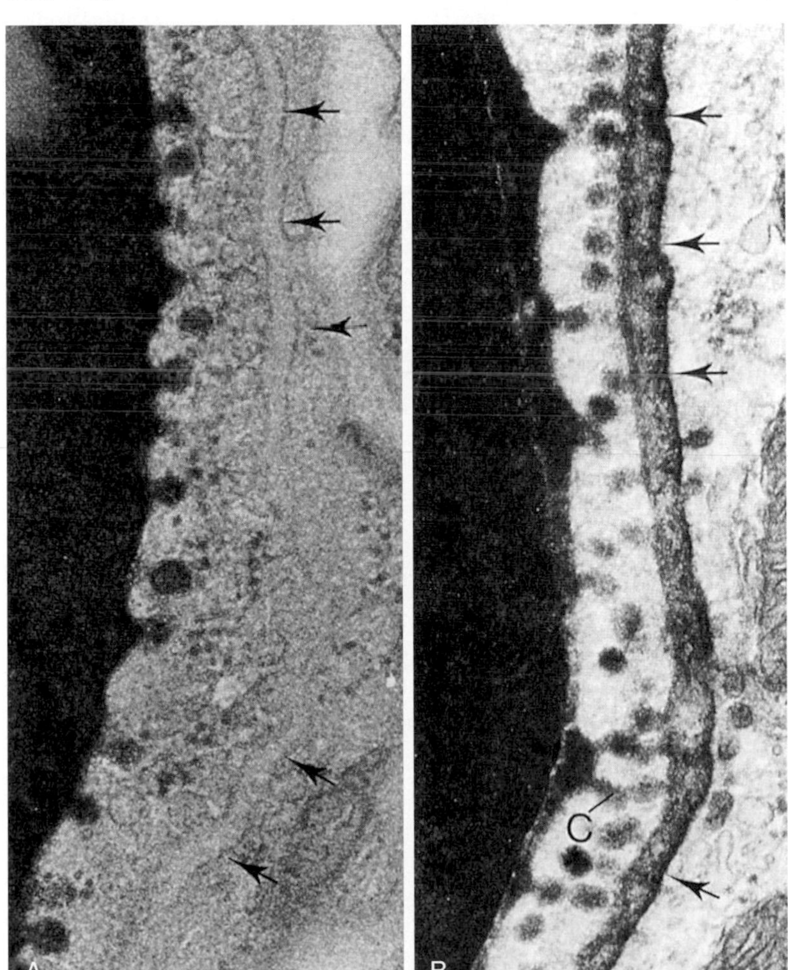

Fig. 2.25 Electron microscopy of transport of microperoxidase, a trace molecule, across the endothelial cell of a capillary (×35,840). (A) The lumen of the capillary is filled with the tracer; note its uptake of pinocytotic vesicles on the luminal aspect. (B) One minute later, the tracer has been conveyed across the endothelial cell and exocytosed on the connective tissue side into the extracellular space (demarcated by *arrows*). The letter C indicates a region of fused vesicles, forming a temporary channel between the lumen of the capillary and the extracellular space. (From Hopkins CR. *Structure and Function of Cells*. Philadelphia: WB Saunders; 1978.)

endosomes. These are believed to be large vesicles containing numerous small vesicles that have been noted as **multivesicular bodies** in electron micrographs. Both theories recognize the presence of a system of microtubules along which either the early endosome or the endosomal carrier vesicle negotiates its way to the late endosome.

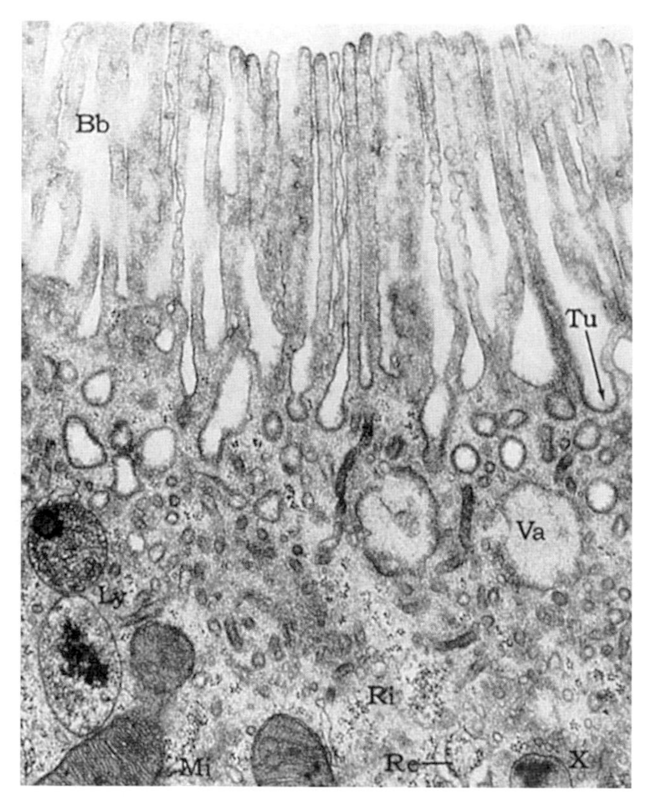

Fig. 2.26 Endocytotic vesicles (Tu) of the proximal tubule cell of the kidney cortex. Note the presence of microvilli (Bb), lysosome (Ly), mitochondria (Mi), rough endoplasmic reticulum (Re), free ribosomes (Ri), and, possibly, early endosomes (Va). (×25,000) (From Rhodin JAG. *An Atlas of Ultrastructure.* Philadelphia: WB Saunders; 1963.)

Lysosomes

Lysosomes have an acidic pH of approximately 5.0 and contain hydrolytic enzymes.

The contents of late endosomes are delivered for enzymatic digestion into the lumina of specialized organelles known as **lysosomes** (Figs. 2.26 and 2.27). Each lysosome is round to polymorphous in shape. Its average diameter is 0.3 to 0.8 μm, and it contains at least 40 different types of **acid hydrolases**, such as sulfatases, proteases, nucleases, lipases, and glycosidases, among others. Because all of these enzymes require an acid environment for optimal function, lysosomal membranes possess proton pumps that actively transport H^+ ions into the lysosome, maintaining its lumen at a pH of about 5.0.

Lysosomes aid in digesting not only macromolecules, phagocytosed microorganisms, cellular debris, and cells but also excess or senescent organelles, such as mitochondria and RER. The various enzymes digest the engulfed material into small, soluble end products that are transported by carrier proteins in the lysosomal membrane from the lysosomes into the cytosol and are either reused by the cell or exported from the cell into the extracellular space.

Formation of Lysosomes

Lysosomes receive their hydrolytic enzymes as well as their membranes from the TGN; however, they arrive in different vesicles. Although both types of vesicles possess a clathrin coat as they pinch off the TGN, the clathrin coat is lost shortly after formation. The uncoated vesicles then fuse with late endosomes.

Vesicles ferrying lysosomal enzymes possess **mannose-6-phosphate receptors**, to which these enzymes are bound. In the acidic environment of the late endosome, the lysosomal enzymes dissociate from their receptors, their mannose residue becomes dephosphorylated, and the receptors are recycled by being returned to the TGN. It should be understood that the dephosphorylated lysosomal hydrolases can no longer bind to the mannose-6-phosphate receptors and, therefore, stay in the

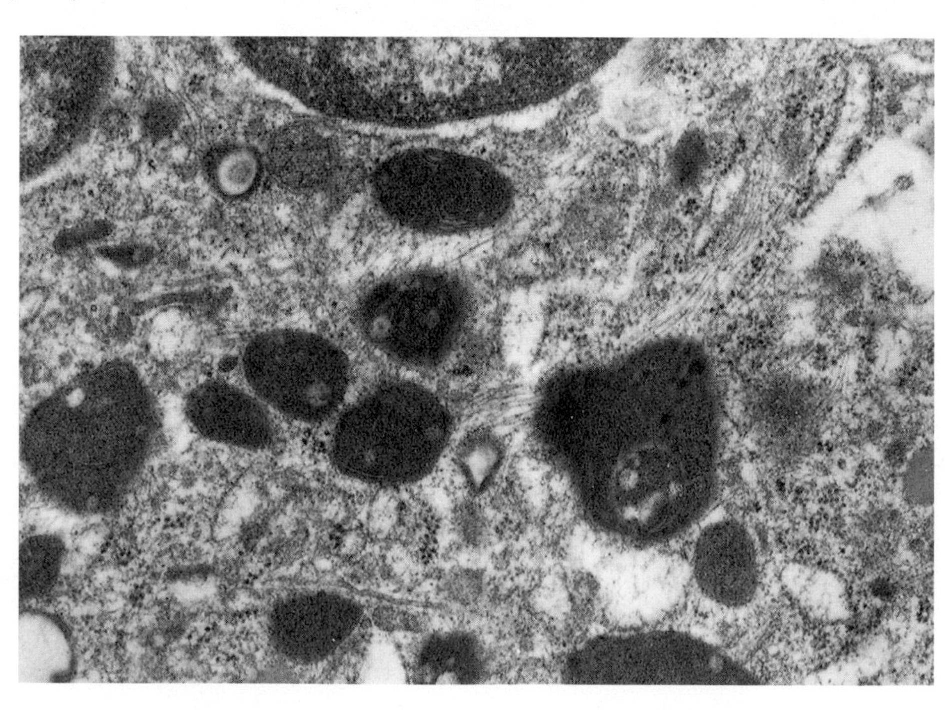

Fig. 2.27 Lysosomes of rat cultured alveolar macrophages (×45,000). (From Sakai M, Araki N, Ogawa K. Lysosomal movements during heterophagy and autophagy: With special reference to nematolysosome and wrapping lysosome. *J Electron Microsc Tech.* 1989;12:101–131. Copyright © 1989. Reprinted by permission of Wiley-Liss, Inc., a subsidiary of John Wiley & Sons, Inc.)

late endosome (see Figs. 2.20 and 2.23). Thus, proenzymes as well as lysosomal membrane proteins are present in late endosomes.

When late endosomes possess both enzymatic and membrane components, some authors hypothesize that the late endosome fuses with a lysosome. However, others suggest that it matures to become a lysosome.

Transport of Substances into Lysosomes

Substances destined for degradation within lysosomes reach these organelles in one of three ways: through phagosomes, pinocytotic vesicles, or autophagosomes (see Fig. 2.23).

Phagocytosed (or pinocytosed) material, contained within **phagosomes** (or **pinocytotic vesicles**), moves toward the interior of the cell and either joins a lysosome or a late endosome. The hydrolytic enzymes digest most of the contents of the phagosome (or pinocytotic vesicle), especially the protein and carbohydrate components. Lipids, however, are more resistant to complete digestion and remain enclosed within the spent lysosome, now referred to as a **residual body**.

Senescent organelles—such as mitochondria and organelles no longer required by the cell—need to be degraded. The organelles in question become surrounded by elements of the ER and are enclosed in vesicles called **autophagosomes**. These structures fuse either with late endosomes or with lysosomes and share the same subsequent fate as the phagosome.

Clinical Correlations

Lysosomal storage disorders

Certain individuals with hereditary enzyme deficiencies are incapable of completely degrading various macromolecules into soluble by-products. As the insoluble intermediaries of these substances become amassed within the lysosomes of their cells, the size of these lysosomes increases sufficiently to interfere with the abilities of these cells to perform their function (Table 2.2).

Probably the most commonly known of these conditions is ***Tay-Sachs disease****, occurring mostly in children of Northeast European Jewish ancestry and in certain individuals of Cajun ancestry in Louisiana. These children display a deficiency in the enzyme hexosaminidase and cannot catabolize GM_2 gangliosides. Although most cells in these children accumulate GM_2 ganglioside in the lysosomes, it is the neurons in their central and peripheral nervous systems that are the most problematic. Lysosomes of these cells become so engorged that they interfere with neuronal function, causing the children to become vegetative within the first year or two and to die by the third year of life.*

PEROXISOMES

Peroxisomes are self-replicating organelles that contain oxidative enzymes.

Peroxisomes (**microbodies**) are small (0.2–1.0 µm in diameter), spherical to ovoid membrane-bound organelles that contain more than 40 oxidative enzymes, especially **urate oxidase**, **catalase**, and **D-amino acid oxidase** (Fig. 2.28). They are present in almost all animal cells and function in the catabolism of long-chained fatty acids (**beta oxidation**), forming **acetyl coenzyme A (CoA)**, begin the manufacture of **plasmalogen** (the primary myelin phospholipid), and form **hydrogen peroxide** (**H_2O_2**) by combining hydrogen from the fatty acid with molecular oxygen. Acetyl CoA is used by the cell for its own metabolic needs or is exported into the extracellular space to be used by neighboring cells. Hydrogen peroxide detoxifies various noxious agents (e.g., ethanol) and kills microorganisms. Excess hydrogen peroxide is degraded into water and molecular oxygen by the enzyme **catalase**.

Proteins destined for peroxisomes are not manufactured on the RER but rather in the cytosol and are transported into the peroxisomes by two specific peroxisome-targeting signals that direct the protein from the cytosol to the peroxisome, where they recognize membrane-bound import receptors unique to the targeting signal. However, some peroxisomal membrane proteins may be manufactured on and targeted to the peroxisomes via the RER. Peroxisomes live for less than a week and, similar to mitochondria, they increase in size and undergo fission to form new peroxisomes. Unlike mitochondria, peroxisomes possess no genetic material of their own.

PROTEASOMES

Proteasomes are small organelles composed of protein complexes that are responsible for proteolysis of malformed and ubiquitin-tagged proteins.

The protein population of a cell is in constant flux as a result of the continuous synthesis, export, and degradation of these macromolecules. Frequently, proteins—such as those that act in metabolic regulation—have to be degraded to ensure that the metabolic response to a single stimulus is not prolonged. Additionally, proteins that have been denatured, damaged, or malformed have to be eliminated. Moreover, antigenic proteins that have been endocytosed by antigen-presenting cells (APCs) have to be cleaved into small polypeptide fragments (**epitopes**) so that they can be presented to T lymphocytes for recognition and the mounting of an immune response.

The process of cytosolic proteolysis is carefully controlled by the cell, and it requires that the protein be recognized as a potential candidate for degradation. This recognition involves **ubiquitination**, a process whereby several ubiquitin molecules (76-amino acid–long polypeptide chains) are attached to a lysine residue of the candidate protein to form a **polyubiquitinated protein**. Once a protein has been tagged in this manner, it is degraded by **proteasomes**, multisubunit protein complexes that have a molecular weight in excess of 2 million Daltons. In order to be permitted entry into the proteasome (**translocated** into the proteasome), the ubiquitin molecules must be released from the protein and the protein must be unfolded. The released ubiquitin molecules reenter the cytosolic pool. The mechanism of ubiquitination requires the following:

- The cooperation of a series of enzymes, including **ubiquitin-activating enzyme (E1)**, which activates ubiquitin
- A family of **ubiquitin-conjugating enzymes (E2)**, which attach to the candidate protein
- A number of **ubiquitin ligases (E3)**, which recognize one or more candidate proteins and attach the ubiquitin molecule to the protein

Ubiquitination, the release of ubiquitin from the candidate protein, and the mechanism of protein degradation by the proteasome are all energy-requiring processes. An average cell may

TABLE 2.2 Major Lysosomal Storage Diseases

Disease Type	Disease Name	Enzyme Deficiency	Metabolite Buildup
Glycogenosis	Pompe disease (type II)	Lysosomal glucosidase	Glycogen
Sphingolipidosis	GM_1 gangliosidoses	GM_1-ganglioside beta-galactosidase	GM_1 ganglioside; oligosaccharides containing galactose
Sphingolipidosis	GM_2 gangliosidoses (Tay-Sachs disease)	Hexosaminidase A	GM_2 ganglioside
Sphingolipidosis	GM_2 gangliosidoses (Gaucher disease)	Glucocerebrosidase	Glucocerebroside
Sphingolipidosis	GM_2 gangliosidoses (Neimann-Pick disease)	Sphingomyelinase	Sphingomyelin
Mucopolysaccharidosis	MPS I H (Hurler)	α-L-iduronidase	Heparan and dermatan sulfate
Mucopolysaccharidosis	MPS II (Hunter)	L-iduronosulfate sulfatase	Heparan and dermatan sulfate
Glycoproteinosis		Enzymes that degrade polysaccharide side chains of glycoproteins	Several, depending on enzyme

Modified from Kumar V, Cotran RS, Robbins SL. *Basic Pathology*. 5th ed. Philadelphia: WB Saunders; 1992.

have as many as 30,000 proteasomes, where each proteasome resembles a 15-nm-tall barrel, by 12 nm in diameter with a central lumen between 1.3 and 5.3 nm in diameter. Both the top and bottom of the barrel possess a **regulatory particle** that limits entrance into and exit out of the proteasome, whereas the bulk of the proteasome is known as the **core particle**. Two pairs of subunits constitute the core particle, the α units that form the top and the bottom of the core particle, each of which binds the regulatory particles, and the β units that form the bulk of the core particle. It is the β units whose internal regions digest the proteins delivered to the proteasome, into small polypeptides, 7 to 8 amino acids in length.

It should be noted that ubiquitination can be skipped under exceptional circumstances when the cell is placed into conditions of major stress; during high stress levels, proteasomes will degrade certain proteins in the absence of ubiquitination.

MITOCHONDRIA

Mitochondria possess their own DNA and perform oxidative phosphorylation and lipid synthesis.

Mitochondria are flexible, rod-shaped organelles, about 0.5 to 1 μm in girth and sometimes as much as 7 μm in length. Most animal cells possess a large number of mitochondria (as many as 2000 in each liver cell) because, via **oxidative phosphorylation**, they produce **ATP**, a stable storage form of energy that can be used by the cell for its various energy-requiring activities.

Each mitochondrion possesses a smooth **outer membrane** and a folded **inner membrane** (Fig. 2.29; see Fig. 2.6). The folds of the inner membrane, known as **cristae**, greatly increase the surface area of that membrane. The number of cristae possessed by a mitochondrion is related directly to the energy requirement of the cell; thus, a cardiac muscle cell mitochondrion has more cristae than does an osteocyte mitochondrion. The narrow space (10–20 nm in width) between the inner and outer membranes is called the **intermembrane space**, whereas the large space enclosed by the inner membrane is termed the **matrix space** (**intercristal space**). The contents of the two spaces differ somewhat and are discussed later.

Outer Mitochondrial Membrane and Intermembrane Space

The **outer mitochondrial membrane** possesses a large number of **porins**, multipass transmembrane proteins. Each porin forms a large aqueous channel through which water-soluble molecules, as large as 10 kD, may pass. Because this membrane is relatively permeable to small molecules, including proteins, the contents of the **intermembrane space** resemble that of the cytosol. Additional proteins located in the outer membrane are responsible for the formation of mitochondrial lipids.

Inner Mitochondrial Membrane

The inner mitochondrial membrane is folded into cristae to provide a larger surface area for ATP synthase and the respiratory chain.

The inner mitochondrial membrane, which encloses the matrix space, is folded to form cristae. This membrane is richly endowed with **cardiolipin**, a phospholipid that possesses four, rather than the usual two, fatty acyl chains. The presence of this phospholipid in high concentration makes the inner membrane nearly impermeable to ions, electrons, and protons.

In certain regions, the outer and inner mitochondrial membranes contact each other; these **contact sites** act as pathways for some proteins and small molecules to enter and leave the matrix space.

At additional transfer sites, the two membranes do not contact one another, but both inner and outer membranes possess receptor molecules that recognize not only the macromolecule that is being transported but also cytosolic carrier molecules (and chaperones) responsible for the delivery of that particular macromolecule. In order for most proteins destined for the mitochondrion to enter that organelle, they must have two signals: a **positively charged amino acid sequence** (amino acid presequence) at their initial terminus and an associated protein known as **heat shock**

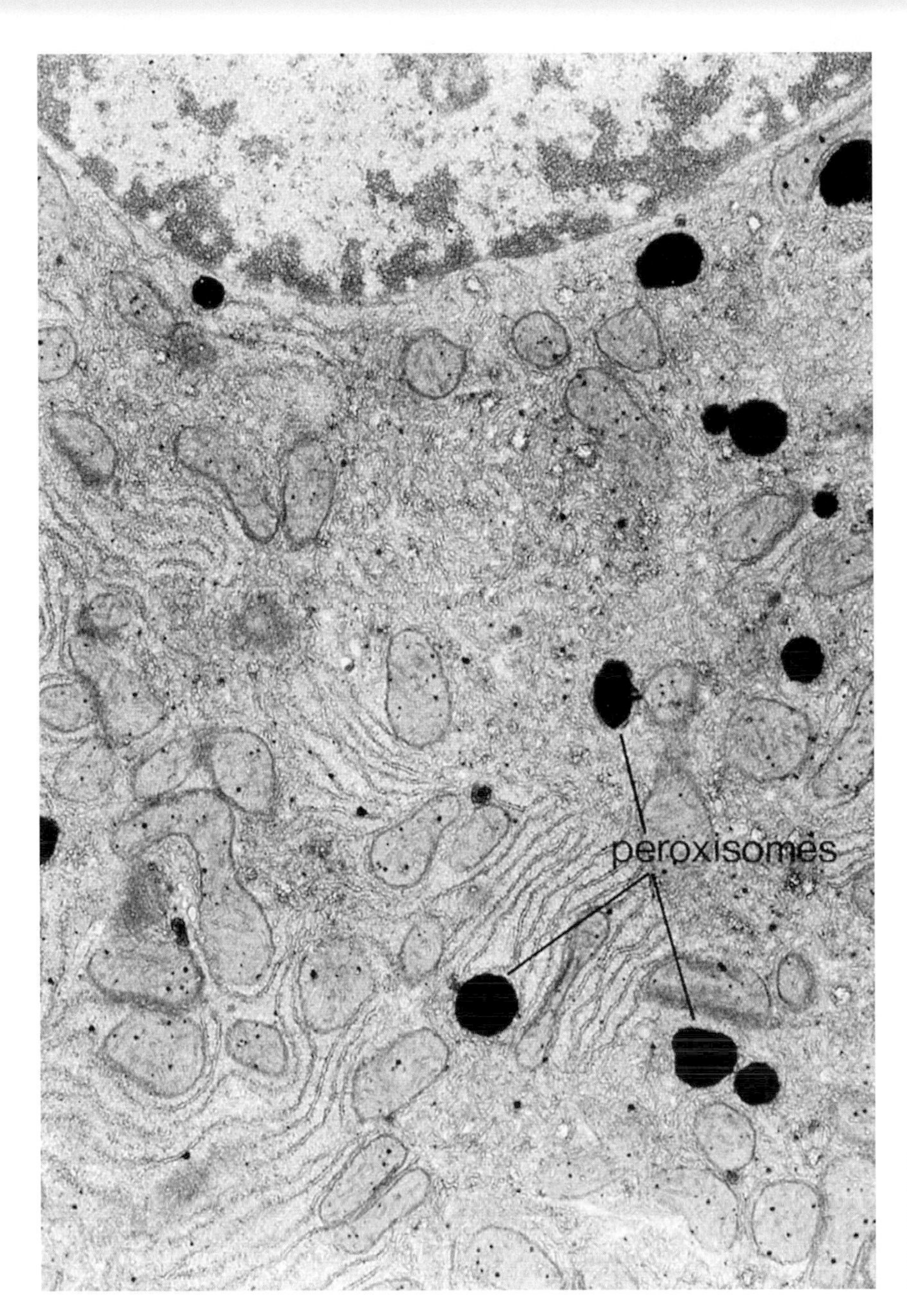

Fig. 2.28 Peroxisomes in hepatocytes (×10,700). The cells were treated with 3′,3′-diaminobenzidine and osmium tetroxide, yielding a black reaction product caused by the enzyme catalase located within peroxisomes. (From Hopkins CR. *Structure and Function of Cells*. Philadelphia: WB Saunders; 1978.)

protein 70. A carrier protein, **translocase of the outer mitochondrial membrane**, recognizes these two signals and transports the protein into the intermembrane compartment. Another carrier protein, located in the inner membrane and known as the **inner mitochondrial membrane complex**, translocates the protein from the intermembrane compartment into the matrix, where the heat shock protein 70 dissociates from the translocated protein and removes the amino acid presequence from its initial terminus.

Viewed in negatively stained preparations, the inner membrane displays the presence of a large number of lollipop-shaped inner membrane subunits, protein complexes known as **ATP synthase**, which are responsible for the generation of ATP from ADP and inorganic phosphate. The globular head of the subunit, about 10 nm in diameter, is attached to a narrow, flattened, cylinder-like stalk 4 nm wide and 5 nm long, projecting from the inner membrane into the matrix space (see Fig. 2.28).

Additionally, a large number of protein complexes, the **respiratory chains**, are present in the inner membrane. Each respiratory chain is composed of three respiratory enzyme complexes: (1) the **NADH dehydrogenase complex**, (2) **cytochrome b-**$\mathbf{c_1}$ **complex**, and (3) **cytochrome oxidase complex**. These complexes form an **electron transport chain** that is responsible for the passage of electrons along this chain and, more important, function as proton pumps that transport energy-rich H^+ from the matrix into the intermembrane space, establishing an **electrochemical gradient** that provides energy for the ATP-generating action of ATP synthase. Since ADP is required for ATP synthesis and the newly formed ATP has to leave the matrix space of the mitochondrion to enter the cytosol, both inner and outer mitochondrial membranes house the antiport carrier proteins, **ADP/ATP exchange proteins**, to import ADP into the mitochondrion and export ATP out of the mitochondrion.

Matrix

The **matrix space** is filled with a dense fluid composed of at least 50% protein, which accounts for its viscosity. Much of the protein component of the matrix is enzymes responsible for the stepwise degradation of fatty acids and pyruvate to the

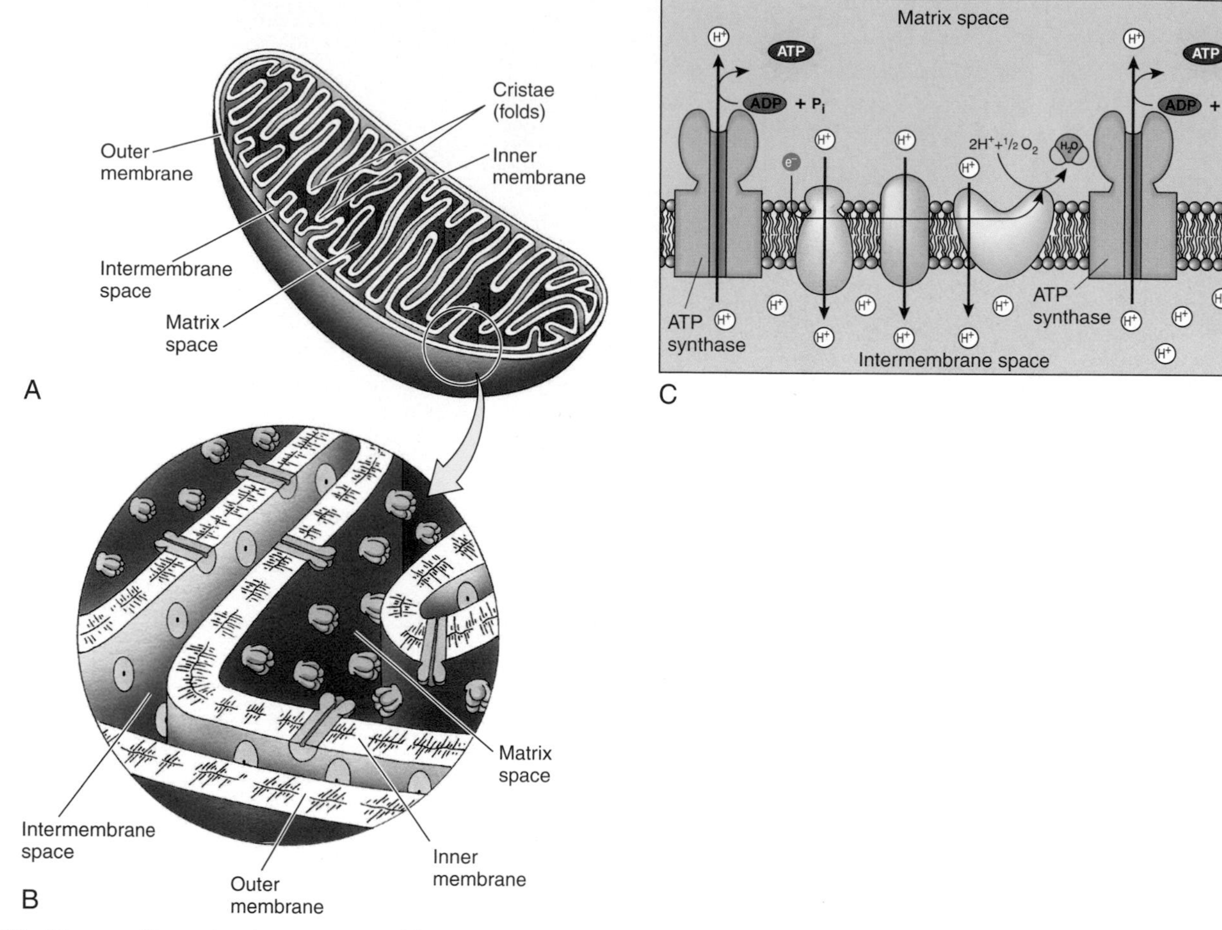

Fig. 2.29 Diagrams illustrating the structure and function of mitochondria. (A) Mitochondrion sectioned longitudinally to demonstrate its outer and folded inner membranes. (B) Diagram of a negatively stained preparation at higher magnification of the region circled in (A), displaying the inner membrane subunits, ATP synthase. (C) Diagram displaying two ATP synthase complexes and three of the five members of the electron transport chain that also function to pump hydrogen (H^+) from the matrix into the intermembrane space. ADP, Adenosine diphosphate; ATP, adenosine triphosphate.

metabolic intermediate **acetyl CoA** and the subsequent oxidation of this intermediate in the **tricarboxylic acid (Krebs) cycle**. Mitochondrial ribosomes, tRNA, mRNA, and dense spherical **matrix granules** (30–50 nm in diameter) composed of phospholipoprotein are also present in the matrix. The function of matrix granules is not understood.

The matrix also contains the double-stranded mitochondrial **circular deoxyribonucleic acid (cDNA)** and the enzymes necessary for the expression of the mitochondrial genome. cDNA contains information for the formation of only 13 mitochondrial proteins, 16S and 12S rRNA, and genes for 22 tRNAs. Therefore, most of the codes necessary for the formation and functioning of mitochondria are located in the genome of the nucleus.

Oxidative Phosphorylation

Oxidative phosphorylation is the process responsible for the formation of ATP.

Acetyl CoA, formed through the β-oxidation of fatty acids and the degradation of glucose, is oxidized in the citric acid cycle to produce, in addition to carbon dioxide (CO_2), large quantities of the reduced cofactors nicotinamide adenine dinucleotide (NADH) and flavin adenine dinucleotide ($FADH_2$). Each of these cofactors releases a hydride ion (H^-) that is stripped of its two high-energy electrons and becomes a proton (H^+). The electrons are transferred to the electron transport chain and during mitochondrial respiration reduce oxygen (O_2) to form water (H_2O).

According to the **chemiosmotic theory**, the energy released by the sequential transfer of the electrons is used to transport H^+ from the matrix into the intermembrane space, establishing a high proton concentration in that space and exerting a **proton motive force** (see Fig. 2.29). Only through ATP synthase may these protons leave the intermembrane space and reenter the matrix. As the protons pass down this electrochemical gradient, the energy differential in the proton motive force is transformed into the stable high-energy bond of ATP by the globular head of the inner membrane subunit, which catalyzes the formation of ATP from ADP + P_i, where P_i is inorganic phosphate. The newly formed ATP is either used by the mitochondrion or is transported into the cytosol through the ADP/ATP antiport system. During the entire process of glycolysis, tricarboxylic acid cycle, and electron transport, each glucose molecule yields 36 molecules of ATP.

In some cells, such as the brown fat of hibernating animals, oxidation is uncoupled from phosphorylation, resulting in the formation of heat instead of ATP. This uncoupling is dependent on the presence of proton shunts, known as **thermogenins**, that resemble ATP synthase but cannot generate ATP. As the protons pass through thermogenins to reenter the matrix, the energy of the proton motive force is transformed into heat. It is this heat that awakens the animal from its state of hibernation. Mitochondria that uncouple oxidation from phosphorylation have a somewhat different morphology and are known as **condensed mitochondria** rather than the classic mitochondria (**orthodox mitochondria**) in that they appear swollen, have a denser matrix, and present with a larger intermembrane compartment.

Origin and Replication of Mitochondria

Because of the presence of the mitochondrial genetic apparatus, it is believed that mitochondria were free-living organisms that either invaded or were phagocytosed by anaerobic eukaryotic cells, developing a **symbiotic relationship**. The mitochondrion-like organism received protection and nutrients from its host and provided its host with the capability of reducing its O_2 content and simultaneously supplying it with a stable form of chemical energy.

Mitochondria are self-replicating in that they are generated from preexisting mitochondria. These organelles enlarge in size, replicate their DNA, and undergo fission. The division usually occurs through the intracristal space of one of the centrally located cristae. The outer mitochondrial membrane of the opposing halves extends through that intracristal space; the halves meet and fuse, thus dividing the mitochondrion into two nearly equal halves. The process of fission usually takes place where mitochondria become surrounded by and contact the endoplasmic reticulum. The average life span of a mitochondrion is about 10 days.

Clinical Correlations

Pearson syndrome *is a rare mitochondrial disorder in infants due to a deletion of less than 10 kilobases in the mitochondrial DNA. The affected baby's development is poor, displays exocrine pancreatic dysfunction due to fibrosis of the gland, sideroblastic anemia due to the inability of incorporating iron into hemoglobin, type I diabetes, as well as weakened musculature and neurological problems. Unfortunately, these babies rarely survive infancy.*

ANNULATE LAMELLAE

Annulate lamellae are parallel aggregates of membranes that enclose cistern-like spaces—thus, resembling multiple copies, usually six to ten, of nuclear envelopes. They possess nuclear pore complex-like regions (**annuli**) that are in register with those of neighboring membranes. The cisternae of these organelles are relatively evenly spaced, separated by about 80 to 100 nm, and are continuous with the cisternae of the RER. They are present in oocytes, spermatocytes, and rapidly dividing cells, such as cancer cells. However, neither the function nor significance of annulate lamellae is understood.

Inclusions

Inclusions are considered to be nonliving components of the cell that do not possess metabolic activity and are not bounded by membranes. The most common inclusions are glycogen, lipid droplets, pigments, and crystals.

GLYCOGEN

Glycogen is the storage form of glucose.

Glycogen is the most common storage form of glucose in animals and is especially abundant in cells of muscle and the liver. It appears in electron micrographs as clusters, or **rosettes**, of β particles (and larger α particles in the liver) that resemble ribosomes, located in the vicinity of the SER. On demand, enzymes responsible for glycogenolysis degrade glycogen into individual molecules of glucose.

Clinical Correlations

glycogen storage disorders

Some individuals suffer from glycogen storage disorders as a result of their inability to degrade glycogen, resulting in excess accumulation of this substance in the cells. There are three classifications of this disease: (1) hepatic, (2) myopathic, and (3) miscellaneous. The lack or malfunction of one of the enzymes responsible for the degradation is responsible for these disorders (Table 2.3).

LIPIDS

Lipids are storage forms of triglycerides.

Lipids, triglycerides in storage form, not only are stored in specialized cells (**adipocytes**) but also are located as individual droplets in various cell types, especially **hepatocytes**. Most

TABLE 2.3 Major Subgroups of Glycogen Storage Disorders

Type	Deficient enzyme	Tissue changes	Clinical signs
Hepatic Hepatorenal (von Gierke disease)	Glucose-6-phosphatase	Intracellular accumulation of glycogen in hepatocytes and cortical tubules of kidneys	Enlarged liver and kidneys; hypoglycemia with subsequent convulsions; gout; bleeding; 50% mortality
Myopathic McArdle syndrome	Muscle phosphorylase	Glycogen accumulation in skeletal muscle cells	Cramps following vigorous exercise; adult onset
Miscellaneous Pompe disease	Lysosomal acid maltase	Glycogen accumulation Enlarged lysosomes in hepatocytes	Massively enlarged heart; cardiac and respiratory failure within 2 years of onset; adults have milder form involving only skeletal muscle

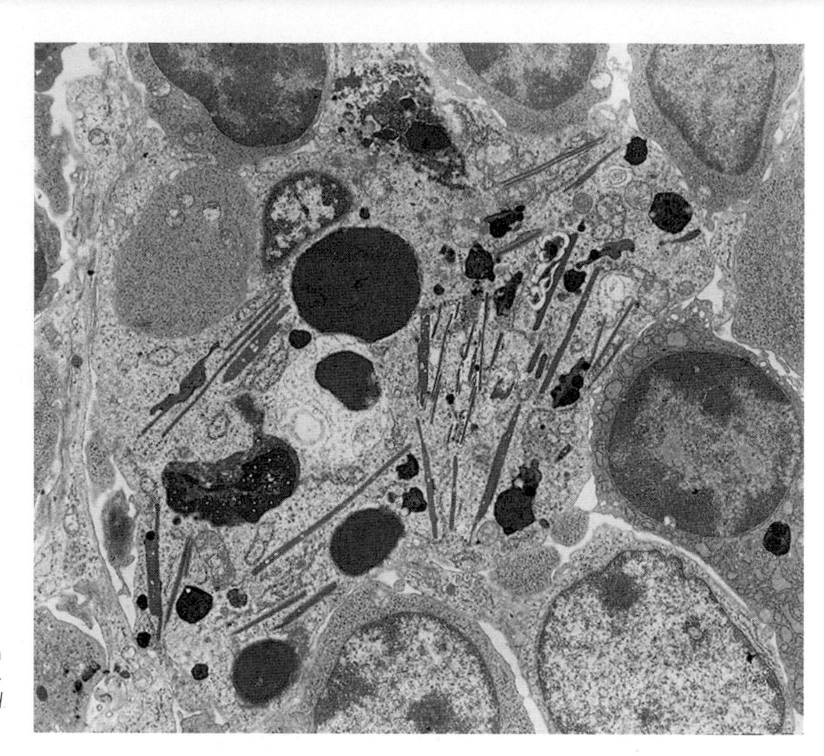

Fig. 2.30 Electron micrograph of crystalloid inclusions in a macrophage (×5100). (From Yamazaki K. Isolated cilia and crystalloid inclusions in murine bone marrow stromal cells. *Blood Cells*. 1988;13:407–416.)

solvents used in histological preparations extract triglycerides from cells, leaving empty spaces indicative of the locations of lipids. However, with the use of osmium and glutaraldehyde, the lipids (and cholesterol) may be fixed in position as gray-to-black intracellular droplets. Lipids are very efficient forms of energy reserves; twice as many ATPs are derived from 1 g of fat as from 1 g of glycogen.

PIGMENTS

The most common pigment in the body, besides **hemoglobin** of red blood cells, is **melanin**, manufactured by melanocytes of skin and hair, pigment cells of the retina, and specialized nerve cells in the substantia nigra of the brain. These pigments have protective functions in skin and aid in the sense of sight in the retina, but their role in hair and neurons is not understood. Additionally, in long-lived cells, such as neurons of the central nervous system and cardiac muscle cells, a yellow-to-brown pigment, **lipofuscin**, has been demonstrated. Unlike other inclusions, lipofuscin pigments are membrane bound and are believed to represent the undigestible remnants of lysosomal activity. They are formed from fusion of several **residual bodies**.

CRYSTALS

Crystals are not commonly found in cells, with the exception of Sertoli cells (**crystals of Charcot-Böttcher**), interstitial cells (**crystals of Reinke**) of the testes, and occasionally in macrophages (Fig. 2.30). It is believed that these structures are crystalline forms of certain proteins.

Cytoskeleton

The cytoskeleton has three major components: thin filaments, intermediate filaments, and microtubules.

The cytoplasm of animal cells contains a **cytoskeleton**, an intricate three-dimensional meshwork of protein filaments that are responsible for the maintenance of cellular morphology. Additionally, the cytoskeleton is an active participant in cellular motion, whether of organelles or vesicles within the cytoplasm, regions of the cell, or the entire cell. The cytoskeleton has three components: thin filaments (microfilaments), intermediate filaments, and microtubules.

THIN FILAMENTS

Thin filaments are actin filaments that interact with myosin to bring about intracellular or cellular movement.

Thin filaments (microfilaments) are composed of two chains of globular subunits, G-actin, coiled around each other to form a filamentous protein, F-actin", referred to as actin" (Figs. 2.31 and 2.32). Actin constitutes about 15% of the total protein content of nonmuscle cells. Only about half of their total actin is in the filamentous form, because the monomeric G-actin form is bound by small proteins, such as profilin and thymosin, which prevent their polymerization. Actin molecules, present in the cells of many different vertebrate and invertebrate species, are very similar to each other in their amino acid sequence, attesting to their highly conserved nature.

Thin filaments are 7 nm thick and possess a faster-growing **plus end** (**barbed end**) and a slower-growing **minus end** (**pointed end**). When the actin filament reaches its desired length, members of a family of small proteins, **capping proteins**, attach to the plus end, terminating the lengthening of the filament. The process of shortening of actin filaments is regulated in the presence of ATP, ADP, and Ca^{2+} by capping proteins such as gelsolin, which prevent polymerization of the filament.

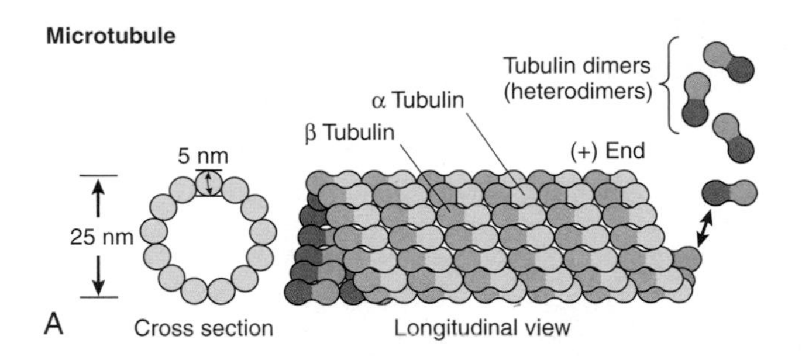

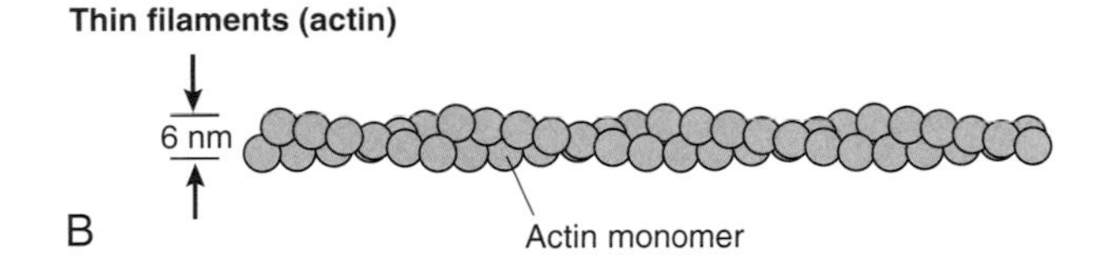

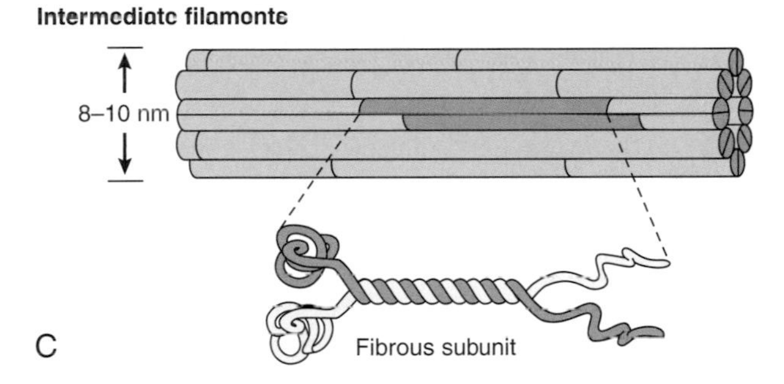

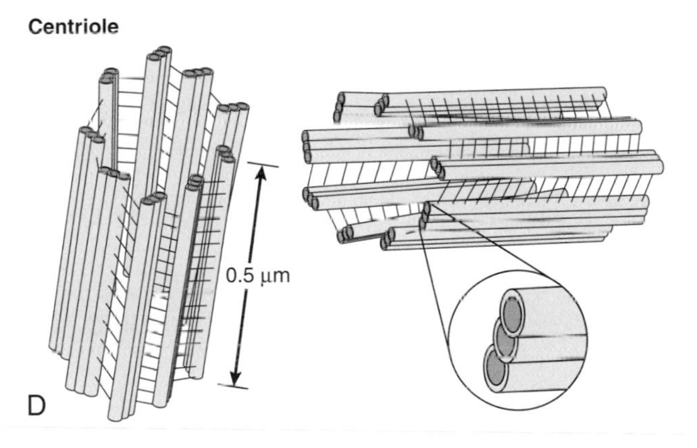

Fig. 2.31 (A–D) Diagram of the elements of the cytoskeleton and centriole.

The cell membrane phospholipid **polyphosphoinositide** has the opposite effect; it removes the gelsolin cap, permitting elongation of the actin filament.

Depending on their isoelectric point, there are three classes of actin: **α-actin** of muscle, and **β-actin** and **γ-actin** of nonmuscle cells. Although actin participates in the formation of various cellular extensions as well as in assembling structures responsible for motility, its basic composition is unaltered. It is capable of fulfilling its many roles via its association with different actin-binding proteins. The most commonly known of these proteins is **myosin**, but numerous other proteins—such as α-actinin, spectrin, fimbrin, filamin, gelsolin, and talin—also bind to actin to perform essential cellular functions (Table 2.4). Actin filaments form bundles of varied lengths, depending on the function that they perform in nonmuscle cells. These bundles form three types of associations: contractile bundles, gel-like networks, and parallel bundles.

Contractile bundles, such as those responsible for the formation of cleavage furrows (contractile rings) during mitotic division, are usually associated with myosin. Their actin filaments are arranged loosely, parallel to each other, with the plus and minus ends alternating in direction. These assemblies are responsible for movement not only of organelles and vesicles within the cell but also for cellular activities, such as exocytosis and endocytosis, as well as the extension of filopodia and cell migration.

Gel-like networks provide the structural foundation of much of the cell cortex. Their stiffness is due to the protein filamin, which assists in the establishment of a loosely organized network of actin filaments, resulting in localized high viscosity. During the formation of filopodia, the gel is liquefied by proteins such as **gelsolin**, which, in the presence of ATP and high Ca^{2+}, cleaves the actin filaments and, by forming a cap over their plus end, prevents them from lengthening.

The proteins **fimbrin** and **villin** are responsible for forming actin filaments into closely packed **parallel bundles** that form the core of microspikes and microvilli, respectively. These bundles of actin filaments are anchored in the **terminal web**, a region of the cell cortex composed of a network of intermediate filaments and the protein **spectrin**. Spectrin molecules are flexible, rod-like tetramers that assist the cell in maintaining the structural integrity of the cortex.

Actin is also important in the establishment and maintenance of **focal contacts** of the cell with extracellular matrix (Fig. 2.33). At focal contacts, the **integrin** (a transmembrane protein) of the cell membrane binds to structural glycoproteins, such as **fibronectin**, of the extracellular matrix, permitting the cell to maintain its attachment. Simultaneously, the intracellular region of the integrin contacts the cytoskeleton via intermediary proteins that attach it to actin filaments. The mode of attachment involves integrin binding to **talin**, which contacts both **vinculin** and the actin filament. Vinculin binds to α-actinin, the actin-binding protein that assembles actin into contractile bundles.

INTERMEDIATE FILAMENTS

Intermediate filaments and their associated proteins assist in the establishment and maintenance of the three-dimensional framework of the cell.

Electron micrographs display a category of filaments in the cytoskeleton, whose diameter of 8 to 10 nm places them between thick and thin filaments and are consequently named **intermediate filaments** (see Fig. 2.31). These filaments and their associated proteins accomplish the following:

- Provide structural support for the cell
- Form a deformable three-dimensional structural framework for the cell
- Anchor the nucleus in place
- Provide an adaptable connection between the cell membrane and the cytoskeleton
- Furnish a structural framework for the maintenance of the nuclear envelope, as well as its reorganization subsequent to mitosis

When microbeads bound to integrin molecules of the cell membrane are micromanipulated, as when one pulls on them,

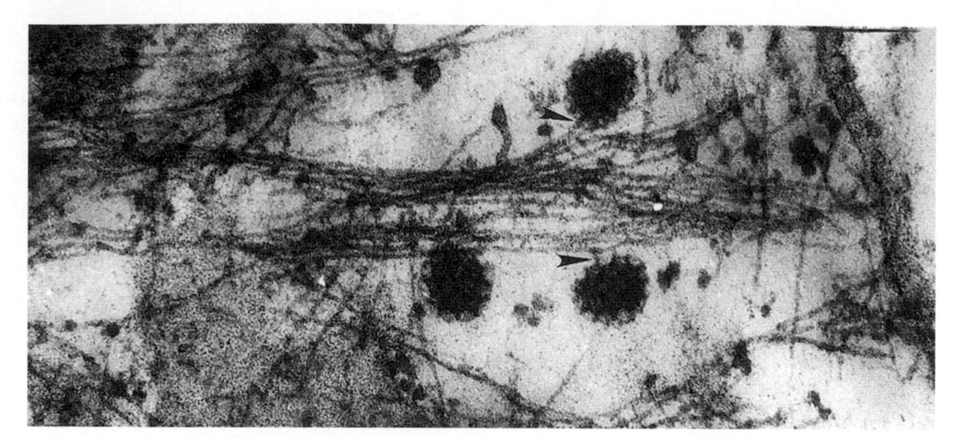

Fig. 2.32 Electron micrograph of clathrin-coated vesicles contacting filaments *(arrowheads)* in granulosa cells of the rat ovary (×35,000). (From Batten BE, Anderson E: The distribution of actin in cultured ovarian granulosa cells. *Am J Anat.* 1983;167:395–404. Copyright 1983. Reprinted by permission of John Wiley & Sons, Inc.)

TABLE 2.4 Actin-Binding Proteins

Protein	Molecular Mass of Each Subunit (D)	Function
α-Actinin	100,000	Bundling actin filaments for contractile bundles
Capping protein	74,000	Attaches to the growing (barbed) end of the actin filament, stabilizing its length
Cofilin	19,000	Active in depolymerization of the actin filament, especially during filopodia formation
Fimbrin	68,000	Bundling actin filaments for parallel bundles
Filamin	270,000	Cross-link actin filaments into gel-like network
Formin	22,000	Attaches to growing (barbed) end and promotes the filament polymerization
Myosin-II	260,000	Contraction by sliding actin filaments
Myosin-V	150,000	Movement of vesicles and organelles along actin filaments
Prolifin	15,000	Restructuring of the cytoskeleton by increasing actin polymerization
SPECTRIN		
α β	265,000 260,000	Forms supporting network for plasma membrane of red blood cell
Gelsolin	90,000	Cleaves and caps actin filaments
Thymosin	5,000	Binds to G-actin subunits, maintaining them in monomeric form

the tensile forces produce distortion of the cytoskeleton, with resultant deformation of the nucleus and rearrangement of the nucleoli. Thus, it appears that the cytoskeleton, specifically the intermediate filaments, react to forces generated in the extracellular matrix. By forcing modulations in the shape and location of cellular constituents, they protect the structural and functional integrity of the cell from external stresses and strains.

Biochemical investigations have determined that there are several categories of intermediate filaments that share the same morphological and structural characteristics. These rope-like intermediate filaments are constructed of eight tetramers of rod-like proteins that are tightly bundled into long helical arrays. The individual subunit, the **monomer**, of each tetramer differs considerably for each type of intermediate filament, but their morphology is similar in that each monomer has an N-terminus (**head**) and C-terminus (**tail**) that are both folded into globular domains whereas its central region, the **central domain**, is composed of an elongated alpha helix. The categories of intermediate filaments include keratins, desmin, vimentin, glial fibrillary acidic protein, neurofilaments, and nuclear lamins (Table 2.5).

Several intermediate filament-binding proteins have been discovered. As they bind to intermediate filaments, they link them into a three-dimensional network that facilitates the formation of the cytoskeleton. The best known of these proteins are as follows:

- **Filaggrin** binds keratin filaments into bundles.
- **Synamin** and **plectin** bind desmin and vimentin, respectively, into three-dimensional intracellular meshworks.
- **Plakins** assist the maintenance of contact between the keratin intermediate filaments and hemidesmosomes of epithelial cells, as well as actin filaments with neurofilaments of sensory neurons.

Clinical Correlations

Immunocytochemical methods, using specific immunofluorescent antibodies, are employed to distinguish intermediate filament types in tumors of unknown origin. Knowledge of the source of these tumors assists not only in their diagnosis but also in devising effective treatment plans.

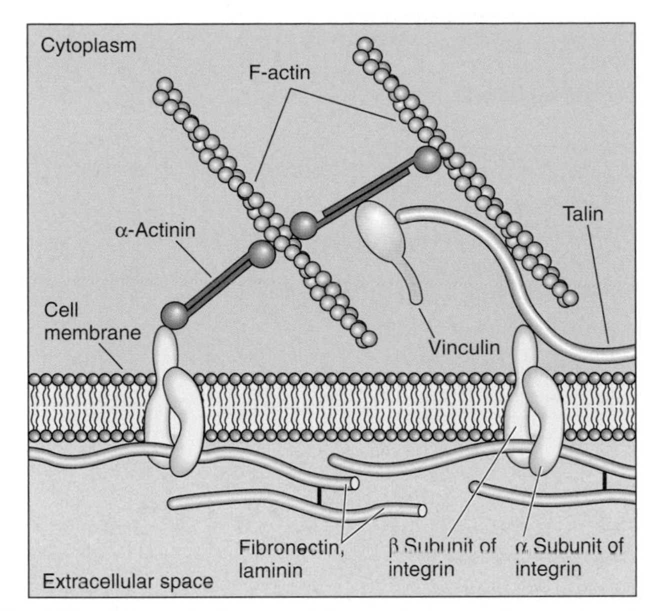

Fig. 2.33 Schematic diagram of the cytoskeleton. Fibronectin or laminin receptor regions of integrin molecules bind to fibronectin or laminin, respectively, in the extracellular space. Intracellular talin or α-actinin binding regions of integrin molecules bind to talin or α-actinin, respectively. Thus, integrin molecules bridge the cytoskeleton to an extracellular support framework.

MICROTUBULES

Microtubules are long, straight, rigid tubular-appearing structures that act as intracellular pathways.

The **centrosome** is the region of the cell in the vicinity of the nucleus that houses the centrioles as well as several hundred ring-shaped γ-**tubulin ring complex** molecules. These γ-tubulin molecules act as nucleation sites for **microtubules**, long, straight, rigid, hollow-like cylindrical structures 25 nm in outer diameter, with a luminal diameter of 15 nm (Fig. 2.34; see Fig. 2.31). Therefore, the centrosome is considered to be the **microtubule-organizing center** (**MTOC**) of the cell.

A microtubule is polarized, having a **plus end** (β-tubulin) and a **minus end** (α-tubulin), which must be stabilized or it will depolymerize, thus shortening the microtubule. The minus end is stabilized by being embedded in a γ-tubulin ring complex. A microtubule is a dynamic structure that frequently changes its length by undergoing growth spurts and then becomes shorter; both processes occur at the plus end so that the average half-life of a microtubule is only about 10 minutes. The main functions of microtubules are to:

- Provide rigidity and maintain cell shape
- Regulate intracellular movement of organelles and vesicles
- Establish intracellular compartments
- Provide the capability of ciliary (and flagellar) motion

Each microtubule consists of 13 parallel **protofilaments** composed of heterodimers of the globular polypeptide α- and

TABLE 2.5 Predominant Types of Intermediate Filaments

Type	Filament	Polypeptide Component Size (Da)	Cell Type	Function
I II	Acidic keratins Basic keratins	40,000–70,000 40,000–70,000	Epithelial cells Cells of hair and nails	Support cell assemblies and provide tensile strength to cytoskeleton
III	Desmin	53,000	All types of muscle cells	Links myofibrils in striated muscle (around Z disks); attaches to cytoplasmic densities in smooth muscle
III	Vimentin	54,000	Cells of embryo as well as cells of mesenchymal origin: fibroblasts, leukocytes, endothelial cells	Surrounds nuclear envelope; is associated with cytoplasmic aspect of nuclear pore complex
III	Glial fibrillary acidic protein (GFAP)	50,000	Astrocytes, Schwann cells, oligodendroglia	Supports glial cell structure
IV	Neurofilaments NF-L: low-molecular-weight NF-M: medium-molecular-weight NF-H: high-molecular-weight	 68,000 160,000 210,000	Neurons	Form cytoskeleton of axons and dendrites; assist in the formation of the gel state of the cytoplasm; cross-linking responsible for great tensile strength
IV	Syncoilin	64,000	Skeletal muscle cells	Forms bonds with dystrobrevin in skeletal muscle
V	Nuclear lamins A B C	65,000–75,000	Lining nuclear envelopes of all cells	Control and assembly of the nuclear envelope; organization of perinuclear chromatin
VI	Phakinin and Filensin	49,000 94,000	Lens fiber cells of the eyeball	Sustain the transparency of the lens

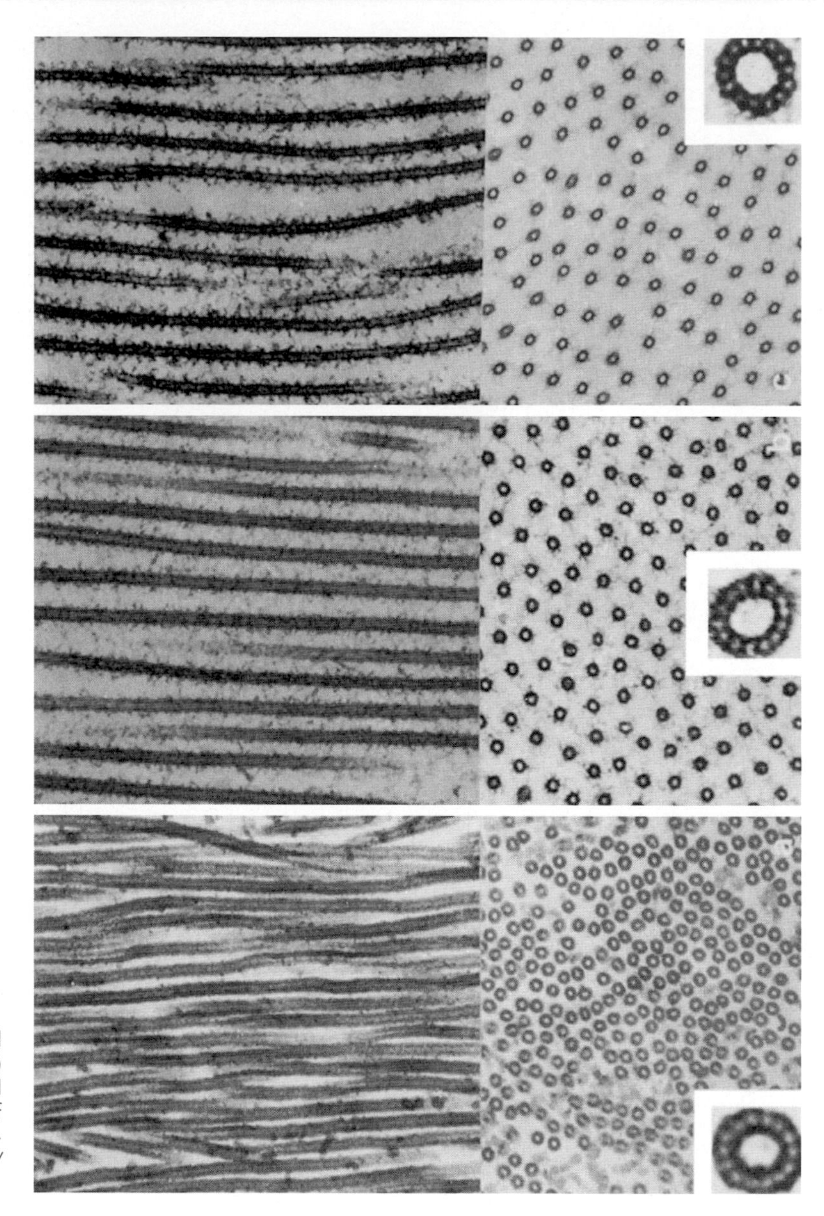

Fig. 2.34 Electron micrograph of microtubules assembled with and without microtubule-associated proteins (MAPs) (×65,790). *Top,* Microtubules assembled from unfractionated MAPs. *Center,* Microtubules assembled in the presence of MAP_2 subfraction only. *Bottom,* Microtubules assembled without MAPs. (From Leeson TS, Leeson CR, and Papparo AA. *Text/Atlas of Histology*. Philadelphia: WB Saunders; 1988.)

β-tubulin subunits, each consisting of about 450 amino acids and each having a molecular mass of about 50,000 Daltons (see Fig. 2.31). Polymerization of the heterodimers requires the presence of magnesium (Mg^{2+}) and GTP. During cell division, rapid polymerization of existing as well as new microtubules is responsible for the formation of the spindle apparatus.

Clinical Correlations

Disruption of the polymerization process of microtubules by antimitotic drugs such as colchicine blocks the mitotic event by binding to the tubulin molecules, preventing their assembly into the protofilament.

Microtubule-Associated Proteins

Microtubule-associated proteins are motor proteins that assist in the translocation of organelles and vesicles inside the cell.

In addition to tubulin heterodimers, microtubules also possess **microtubule-associated proteins (MAPs)** bound to their periphery at 32-nm intervals. There are various types of MAPs (MAP1, MAP2, MAP3, MAP4, MAP tau, and Lis 1), ranging in molecular weight from about 50,000 to more than 300,000 Daltons. Their primary functions are to prevent depolymerization of microtubules and to assist in the intracellular movement of organelles and vesicles, whereas Lis 1 functions during brain development and is responsible for the formation of sulci and gyri of the cerebral hemispheres.

Movement along a microtubule occurs in both directions, that is, toward both the **plus end** and the **minus end**. The two major families of microtubule motor proteins, the MAPs **dynein** and **kinesin**, both bind to the microtubule as well as to vesicles (and organelles). It is believed that different members of each motor protein family transport their cargo at disparate, meticulously controlled rates and that different organelles have their own particular motor protein. In the presence of ATP, dynein moves the vesicle toward the minus end of the microtubule (toward the MTOC). Kinesin effects vesicular (and organelle) transport in the opposite direction, toward the plus end. The mechanism of ATP utilization by these MAPs is not understood.

Centrioles and Centrosome

Centrioles are small, cylindrical structures composed of nine microtubule triplets; two centrioles, embedded in a matrix of pericentriolar material, constitute the core of the MTOC, or the centrosome.

Centrioles are small, cylindrical structures, 0.2 μm in diameter and 0.5 μm in length (see Fig. 2.31). Usually, centrioles are paired structures, arranged perpendicular to each other, and are embedded in a matrix of **pericentriolar material**. The entire complex is known as the **centrosome** or **microtubule organizing center** (**MTOC**) and is located in the vicinity of the Golgi apparatus. The pericentriolar material is composed of the proteins **γ-tubulin** and **pericentrin**, both of which interact with the minus ends of the microtubules and anchor them into the centrosome. The centrosome assists in the formation and organization of microtubules as well as in its self-duplication before cell division.

Centrioles are composed of a specific arrangement of nine triplets of microtubules arranged around a central axis (9 + 0 pattern). Each microtubule triplet consists of one complete and two incomplete microtubules fused to each other so that the incomplete ones share three protofilaments. The complete microtubule "A" is positioned closest to the center of the cylinder; "C" is the farthest away. Adjacent triplets are connected to each other by a fibrous substance of unknown composition, extending from microtubule A to microtubule C. Each triplet is arranged so that it forms an oblique angle with the adjacent and a straight angle with the fifth triplet. Centrioles are also associated with the calcium binding proteins called **centrins** (**caltrectins**), which function in centriole duplication.

During the S phase of the cell cycle, each centriole of the pair replicates, forming a procentriole in some unknown manner, at 90 degrees to itself. This procentriole initially possesses no microtubules, but tubulin molecules begin to polymerize closest to the parent centriole, with the plus end growing away from the parent. The actual replication of the centriole requires the presence of γ-tubulin rings, structures that do not become part of but serve to direct the elongation of the forming microtubules by occupying the forming plus and minus ends. It is believed that the γ-tubulin rings and pericentrin serve as beams that support the developing centriole. Each γ-tubulin initiates the formation of a single microtubule. Additionally, δ-tubulins, related to the α- and β-tubulin superfamily, are also required to form the triplet structure of the microtubule arrays.

Centrioles function in the formation of the centrosome, and during mitotic activity they are responsible for the formation of the spindle apparatus. Additionally, centrioles are the basal bodies that guide the formation of cilia and flagella.

Pathological Considerations

See Figs. 2.35 and 2.36.

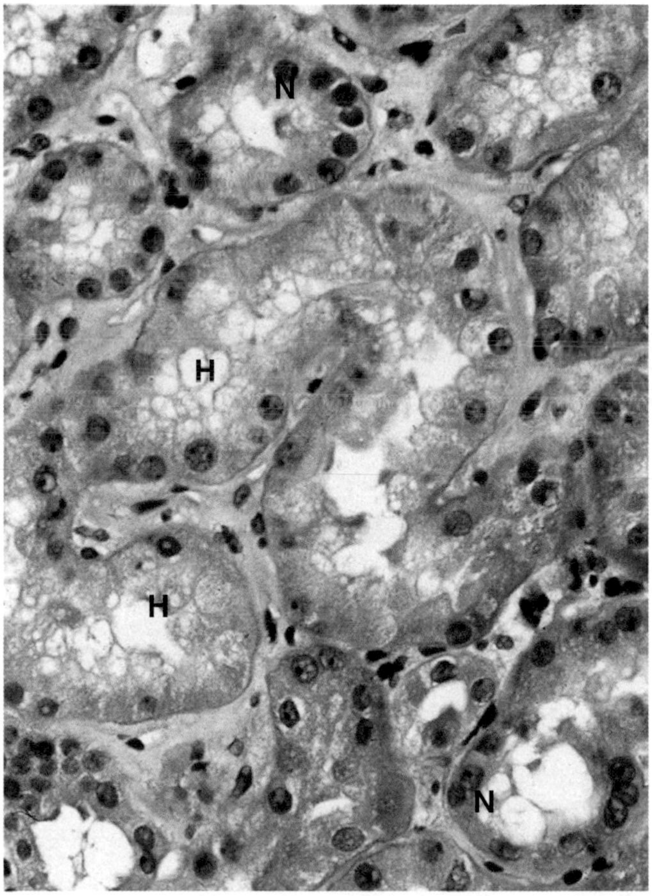

Fig. 2.35 Hydropic degeneration. Blood flow to the cortex of this kidney was diminished due to severe hypotension. Note that the cells have a pale, vacuolated appearance with enlarged nuclei. If the hypotension is not corrected, the patient could succumb to acute renal failure. H = cells undergoing hydropic degeneration; N = normal appearing cell. (From Young B, Stewart W, O'Dowd G. *Wheather's Basic Pathology: A Text, Atlas and Review of Histopathology*. 5th ed. Oxford: Churchill Livingstone/Elsevier Limited; 2011:6, Fig. 1.5B.)

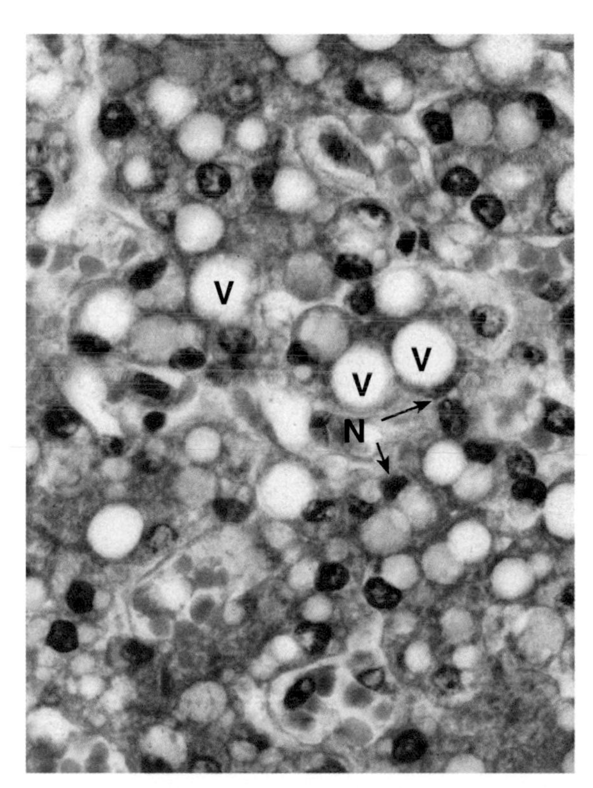

Fig. 2.36 Steatosis. Fatty alteration, steatosis, is most common in the liver, frequently due to exposure to toxins, especially alcohol abuse. Other causes are obesity, diabetes mellitus, and chronic hypoxia. This particular specimen is from an individual suffering with long-term alcohol addiction. In the living individual, the vacuoles (V) were filled with lipid and, frequently, the enlarged vacuoles displaced the nuclei (N) that, in a healthy hepatocyte, normally occupies the center of the cell. (From Young B, Stewart W, O'Dowd G. *Wheather's Basic Pathology: A Text, Atlas and Review of Histopathology*. 5th ed. Oxford: Churchill Livingstone/Elsevier Limited; 2011:7, Fig. 1.6.)

3 Nucleus

Summary

The **nucleus**, the largest organelle of the cell, houses the **nucleoplasm**, **nucleolus,** and the **chromatin**. The nucleus is separated from the cytoplasm by a double membrane, known as the ***nuclear envelope***, which is perforated by numerous openings, known as ***nuclear pores*** and their associated structures that, together with the pore, form the **nuclear pore complex** that functions in a bidirectional nucleocytoplasmic transport. Chromatin is a complex of **DNA** and associated proteins that, during cell division, are folded to form **chromosomes**. It is the DNA that comprises the genetic material of the cell and acts as a template for **RNA transcription**. The **nucleolus** is the deeply staining region within the nucleus where ribosomal RNA synthesis and **ribosome** assembly occur. The cell cycle is a series of exquisitely controlled events that prepare the somatic cell for **mitosis** and the gametes for a unique nuclear division known as ***meiosis***.

The **nucleus**, the largest organelle of the cell (Fig. 3.1), contains nearly all of the **deoxyribonucleic acid** (**DNA**) possessed by the cell, as well as the mechanisms for **ribonucleic acid** (**RNA**) synthesis. Its resident **nucleolus** is the location for rRNA synthesis and for the assembly of the ribosomal subunits. The nucleus, bounded by the **nuclear envelope**, composed of two concentric phospholipid bilayer membranes, houses three major components: **chromatin**, **nucleoplasm**, and the **nucleolus**.

The nucleus is usually spherical and is centrally located in the cell. In some cells, however, it may be spindle-shaped to oblong-shaped, twisted, lobulated, or even disk-shaped (Figs. 3.2 and 3.3). Although each cell usually has a single nucleus, some cells (such as osteoclasts) possess several nuclei, whereas mature red blood cells have extruded their nuclei and are anucleated. The size, shape, and form of the nucleus are generally constant for a particular cell type, a fact useful in clinical diagnoses of the degree of malignancy of certain cancerous cells.

Nuclear Envelope

The nuclear envelope is composed of two parallel unit membranes that fuse at certain regions to form perforations known as nuclear pores.

The nucleus is surrounded by the **nuclear envelope**, composed of two concentric parallel unit membranes: the **inner** and **outer nuclear membranes**, separated from each other by a 20- to 40-nm space called the **perinuclear cisterna** (Figs. 3.4 and 3.5).

INNER NUCLEAR MEMBRANE

The **inner nuclear membrane** is about 6 nm thick and faces the nuclear contents. It is in close contact with the **nuclear lamins**, an interwoven meshwork of **intermediate filaments**, 80 to 300 nm thick, composed of **lamins A, B_1, B_2,** and **C** and located at the periphery of the nucleoplasm. The nuclear lamins bind to integral membrane proteins, such as **lamina-associated polypeptides** and **emerin**, of the inner nuclear membrane. They function in organizing and providing support to the lipid bilayer membrane and the perinuclear chromatin, assist in the formation of nuclear pore complexes, and aid in the assembly of vesicles to reform the nuclear envelope subsequent to cell division.

OUTER NUCLEAR MEMBRANE

The **outer nuclear membrane** is also about 6 nm thick, faces the cytoplasm, is continuous with the rough endoplasmic reticulum (RER), and is considered by some authors as a specialized region of the RER, whose lumen is continuous with the perinuclear cistern (see Figs. 3.4, 3.5, and 3.6). Its cytoplasmic surface—surrounded by a thin, loose meshwork of the intermediate filaments, **vimentin**—usually possesses ribosomes actively synthesizing transmembrane proteins that are destined for the outer or inner nuclear membranes.

NUCLEAR PORE AND NUCLEAR PORE COMPLEX

The nuclear pores are circular openings in the nuclear envelope, each plugged by a complex of proteins known as the nuclear pore complex, providing controlled passage between the nucleus and the cytoplasm.

The nuclear envelope is perforated at various intervals by **nuclear pores**, where the inner and outer nuclear membranes are continuous with one another. In order to regulate the movement of larger molecules across the nuclear pore, a complex of proteins, collectively known as the **nuclear pore complex**, is inserted into each nuclear pore. Some cells may have as many as 4000 nuclear pores, with associated nuclear pore complexes.

The **nuclear pore complex** is about 100 to 125 nm in diameter, spans the two nuclear membranes, and has an average molecular weight of 125 MDa. It is composed of about 500 different proteins, collectively known as **nucleoporins**, arranged in three ring-like arrays of proteins stacked one on top of the other. Each ring displays an eightfold symmetry and is interconnected by a series of spokes arranged in a vertical fashion. In addition, the nuclear pore complex has cytoplasmic fibers, a central plug, and a nuclear basket (Figs. 3.7 through 3.9).

The **cytoplasmic ring**, composed of eight subunits, is located on the rim of the cytoplasmic aspect of the nuclear pore. Each subunit possesses a cytoplasmic filament believed to be a Ran-binding protein (a family of guanosine triphosphate [GTP]–binding proteins), that extends into the cytoplasm and may mediate access to the nucleus through the nuclear pore complex by moving substrates along their length toward the center of the pore.

The **luminal spoke ring** (**middle ring**), a set of eight transmembrane proteins, projects into the lumen of the nuclear pore, as well as into the perinuclear cistern, probably anchoring the glycoprotein components of the nuclear pore complex into the rim of the nuclear pore.

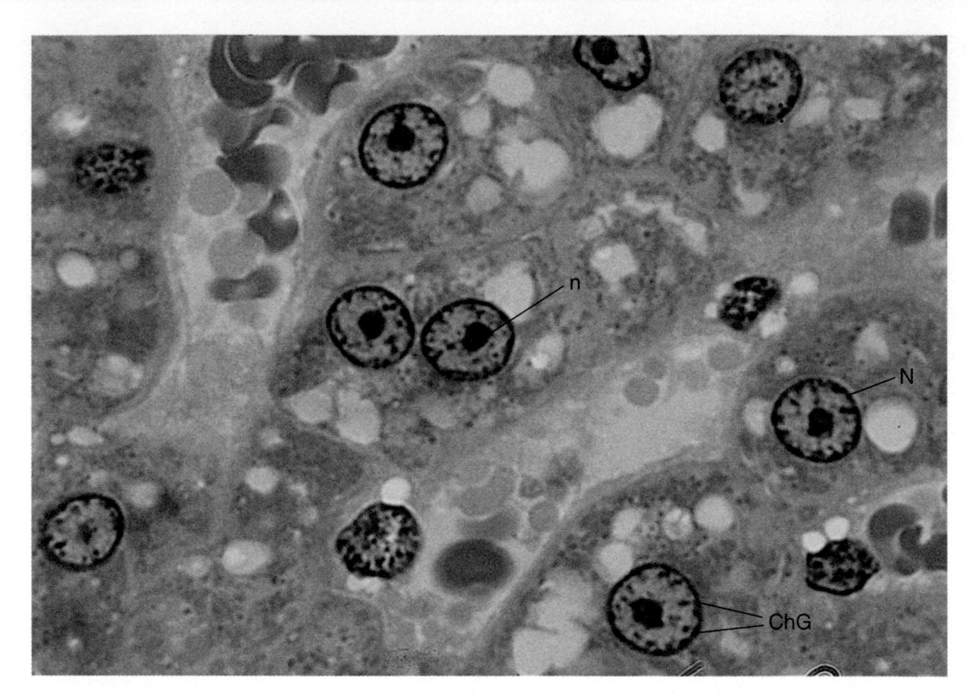

Fig. 3.1 Cell nuclei. Light micrograph (×1323). Typical cells, each containing a spherical nucleus (N). Observe the chromatin granules (ChG) and the nucleolus (n).

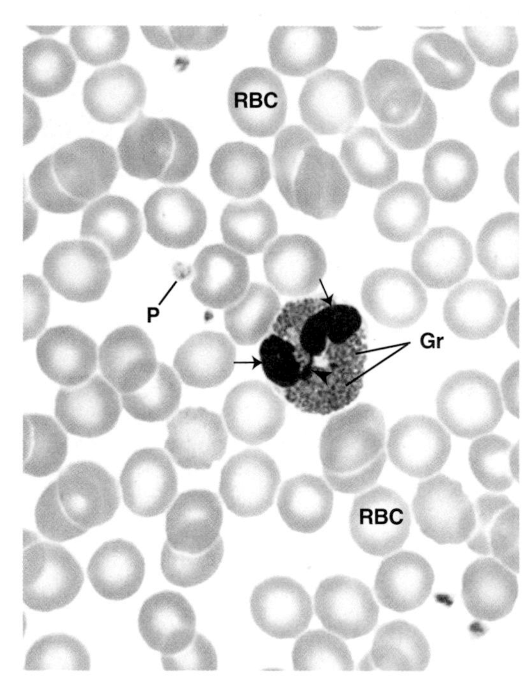

Fig. 3.2 Note that the nucleus of the eosinophil has two lobes *(arrows)* that are connected to each other by a slender filament *(arrowhead)* and that its cytoplasm is filled with specific granules (Gr). The red blood cells (RBC) extruded their nuclei during development and platelets (P) are cell fragments that have no nuclei. (×1,325)

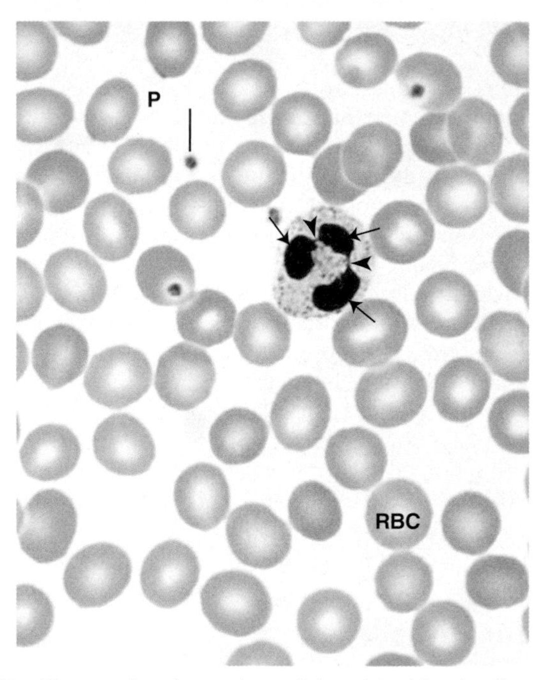

Fig. 3.3 Observe that the nucleus of the white blood cell neutrophil has several lobes *(arrows)* connected to each other by slender filaments *(arrowheads)*. The red blood cells (RBC) extruded their nuclei during development; therefore, they are anucleated. The platelets (P) are cell fragments and have no nuclei. (×1,325)

The central lumen of the middle ring is believed to be a gated channel that restricts passive diffusion between the cytoplasm and the nucleoplasm. It is associated with additional protein complexes that facilitate the regulated transport of materials across the nuclear pore complex.

A **nuclear ring** (**nucleoplasmic ring**), analogous to the cytoplasmic ring, is located on the rim of the nucleoplasmic aspect of the nuclear pore and assists in the export of several types of RNA. A filamentous, flexible, basket-like structure, the **nuclear basket**, which becomes deformed during the process of nuclear export, appears to be suspended from the nucleoplasmic ring, protruding into the nucleoplasm. Attached to the distal aspect of the nuclear basket is the **distal ring**.

Function of the Nuclear Pore Complex

The nuclear pore complex functions in bidirectional nucleocytoplasmic transport.

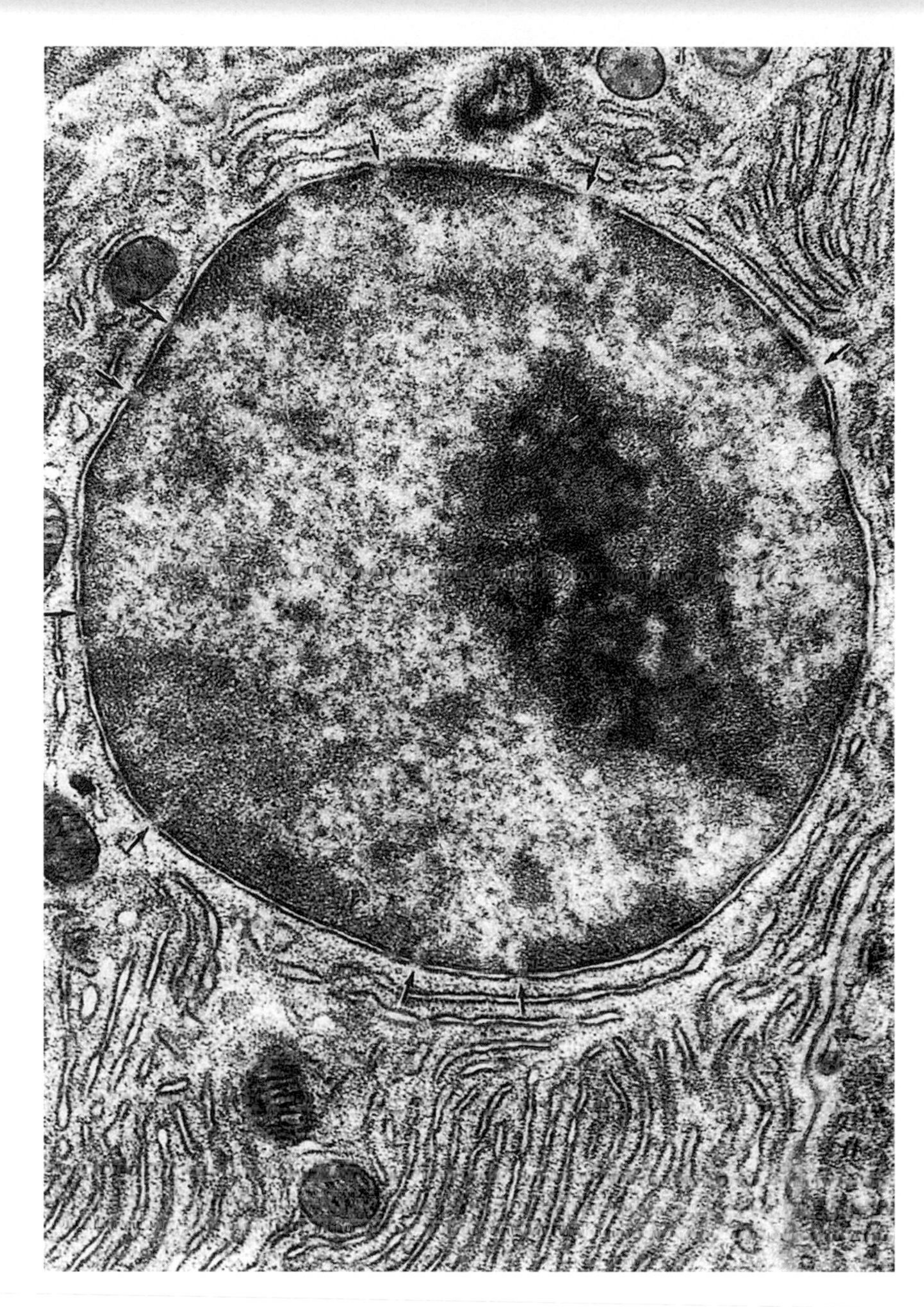

Fig. 3.4 Cell nucleus. Electron micrograph (×16,762). Observe the electron-dense nucleolus, peripherally located dense heterochromatin, and light euchromatin. The nuclear envelope surrounding the nucleus is composed of an inner nuclear membrane and an outer nuclear membrane that is interrupted by the nuclear pores *(arrows)*. (From Fawcett DW. *The Cell*. Philadelphia: WB Saunders; 1981.)

Although the nuclear pore is relatively large, it is nearly filled with the structures constituting the nuclear pore complex; as many as 1000 molecules may pass through any one of these pores every second. Because of the structural conformation of those subunits, several 9- to 11-nm-wide channels are available for simple diffusion of ions and small molecules. However, macromolecules and particles larger than 11 nm cannot reach or leave the nuclear compartment via simple diffusion. Instead, they are selectively transported via a **receptor-mediated transport** process. Signal sequences of molecules to be transported through the nuclear pores must be recognized by one of the many receptor sites of the nuclear pore complex. Transport across the nuclear pore complex is frequently an energy-requiring process.

The bidirectional traffic between the nucleus and the cytoplasm is mediated by a group of target proteins containing **nuclear localization signals** (**NLSs**) known as **importins** and **nuclear export signals** (**NESs**) known as **exportins** (also known as **karyopherins**, **PTACs**, **transportins**, and **Ran-binding proteins**). **Exportins** transport macromolecules (e.g., RNA) from the nucleus into the cytoplasm, whereas **importins** transport cargo (e.g., protein subunits of ribosomes) from the cytoplasm into the nucleus. Exportin and importin transport is regulated by a family of GTP-binding proteins known as **Ran** (see Fig. 3.9). These specialized proteins, along with other **nucleoporins** located along receptor sites in the nuclear pore complex, facilitate the signal-mediated import and export processes. Some protein trafficking is more like shuttling, because some proteins pass back and forth between the cytoplasm and the nucleus in a continuous fashion. Recently, it has been reported that certain other transport mechanisms literally shuttle in both directions. These transport signals are called **nucleocytoplasmic shuttling** (**NS**) signals. Proteins that carry this signal interact with messenger ribonucleic acid (mRNA).

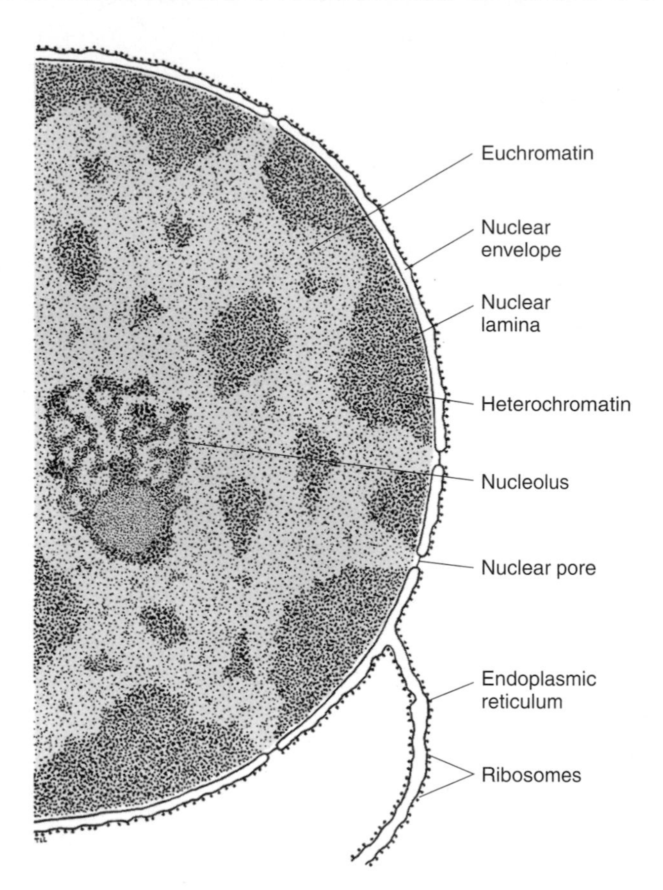

Fig. 3.5 Nucleus. The outer nuclear membrane is studded with ribosomes on its cytoplasmic surface, and it is continuous with the rough endoplasmic reticulum. The space between the inner and outer nuclear membranes is the perinuclear cistern. Observe that the two membranes are united at the nuclear pores.

Clinical Correlations

A number of diseases are associated with mutations in genes coding for various nucleoporin components of the nuclear pore complex, such as ***infantile bilateral striatal necrosis*** ***(IBSN****). There are two forms of this condition, the less common familial and the more prevalent sporadic. The familial form is a mitochondrial disorder, in which the malformation occurs in the ATP-synthase-6 molecule. In the sporadic form, the mutation is in one of the nucleoporin genes (specifically, NUP62). The sporadic form usually follows an occurrence of high fever as a result of various acute systemic conditions, such as measles or bacterial infections. As such, it has a sudden onset anytime during the first few years of life (in some instances, even during adolescence). Clinical manifestations include spasticity, rigidity, nystagmus, weakness in the arms and legs, as well as other musculoskeletal symptoms. Prospects for the familial form are poor, with quick degeneration of skeletal muscles, followed by early death. The sporadic form has a much better rate of recovery once the cause of the high fever is eradicated. The patient may recover completely; however, in some instances, the patient may suffer various neurological complications.*

Chromatin

Chromatin is a complex of DNA and proteins and represents the relaxed, uncoiled chromosomes of the interphase nucleus.

DNA, the cell's genetic material, resides in the nucleus in the form of **chromosomes**, which are clearly visible during cell division. In the interval between cell divisions, the chromosomes are unwound or partially unwound in the form of **chromatin** (see Figs. 3.4, 3.5, 3.7, and 3.10), specifically, heterochromatin or euchromatin.

Heterochromatin, a condensed and inactive form of chromatin, stains deeply with basic stains such as hematoxylin, which make it visible with the light microscope. It is located mostly at the periphery of the nucleus, comprises almost 90% of the total chromatin of the nucleus, and is not being transcribed. The remainder of the chromatin scattered throughout the nucleus and not visible with the light microscope is **euchromatin**. This represents the active form of chromatin, in which the genetic material of the DNA molecules is being transcribed into some forms of RNA.

When euchromatin is examined with electron microscopy, it is seen to be composed of a thread-like material 30 nm thick. More careful evaluation indicates that these threads may be unwound, resulting in a 10 to 11-nm-wide structure resembling "beads on a string." The beads are termed **nucleosomes**, and the string, which is the **DNA molecule**, appears as a thin filament 2 nm in diameter (see Fig. 3.10).

Each nucleosome is composed of an octomer of proteins, duplicates of each of four types of **histones** (**H_2 A, H_2 B, H_3**, and **H_4**). The nucleosome is also wrapped with two complete turns (~150 nucleotide pairs) of the DNA molecule that continues as **linker DNA** extending to the next "bead."

Electron microscopic studies of the nuclear contents following more careful manipulation have revealed chromatin fibers exhibiting diameters of 30 nm. Packaging of chromatin into 30-nm threads is believed to occur by helical coiling of consecutive nucleosomes at six nucleosomes per turn of the coil and cooperatively bound there with **histone H_1** (see Fig. 3.8). Nonhistone proteins are also associated with the chromatin, but their function is not clear.

CHROMOSOMES

Chromosomes are chromatin fibers that become so condensed and tightly coiled during mitosis and meiosis that they are visible with the light microscope.

As the cell leaves the interphase stage and prepares to undergo mitotic or meiotic activity, the chromatin fibers are extensively condensed to form **chromosomes**, visible with light microscopy. The process of packing the long, 30-nm-wide fibers into chromosomes occurs with the assistance of two large ring-shaped protein complexes known as **condensin I** and **condensin II**. Condensin II is located in the nucleus; it begins the process during the prophase of the mitotic division by forming large 300-nm-wide loops of the 30-nm fibers and, by forming a helical scaffold, causing these loops to wind around the scaffold. During prometaphase, the nuclear membrane disappears and the helically arranged loops become exposed to condensin I that is located in the cytoplasm. Condensin I partitions the 300-nm-wide loops into smaller, nested loops that can be packaged into the compact cylindrical structures, the metaphase chromosomes (Fig. 3.11). Amazingly, the majority of this packaging takes place in about 15 minutes; 45 more minutes are spent on quality control of this remarkable process.

The number of chromosomes in somatic cells is specific for the species and is called the **genome**, the total genetic makeup. In humans, the genome consists of 46 chromosomes, representing 23 homologous pairs of chromosomes. One member of each of the chromosome pairs is derived from the mother; the other

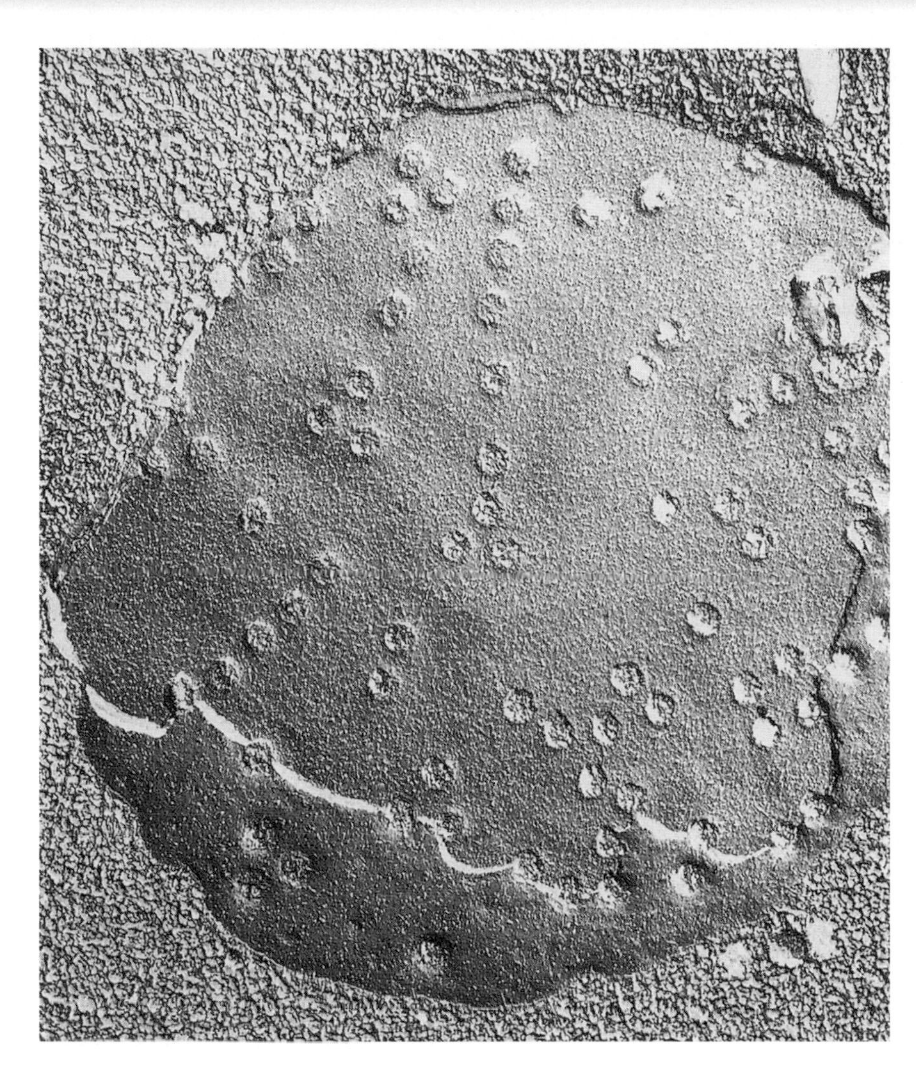

Fig. 3.6 Nuclear pores. Electron micrograph (×47,778). Many nuclear pores may be observed in this freeze-fractured preparation of a nucleus. (From Leeson TS, Leeson CR, Paparo AA. *Text/Atlas of Histology*. Philadelphia: WB Saunders; 1988.)

comes from the father. Of the 23 pairs, 22 are called **autosomes**; the remaining pair that determines gender is the **sex chromosomes**. The sex chromosomes of the female are two X chromosomes (**XX**); those of a male are the X and Y chromosomes (**XY**; see Fig. 3.11).

Telomeres are short, repeated DNA sequences at the ends of chromosomes. They appear to protect the ends of the chromosomes from degradation and, in oocytes and spermatogonia, as well as in stem cells, an enzyme-RNA complex known as **telomerase**, maintains the telomere length. Interestingly, the RNA portion of the enzyme is used as a template to synthesize the additional DNA necessary to maintain telomere length. Somatic cells do not possess telomerase. With each successive cell division, the telomeres become shorter; eventually, they become short enough that they can no longer protect the chromosome and the cell becomes unable to replicate itself. This built-in senescence is absent in cancer cells because many malignant cells are able to express the gene that codes for telomerase.

Sex Chromatin

Only one of the two X chromosomes in female somatic cells is transcriptionally active. The inactive X chromosome, randomly determined early in development, remains inactive throughout the life of that individual (see discussion in this chapter: section on RNA) as a clump of chromatin, the **sex chromatin** (**Barr body**), at the periphery of the nucleus.

Clinical Correlations

It has been reported that individuals who exercise and people with higher education appear to possess longer ***telomeres,*** *whereas people who are long-term smokers, individuals who drink alcohol excessively, and those who are under very high stress levels have shorter telomeres. It has been suggested that people with shorter telomeres tend to have a shorter life span.*

In some individuals, mostly males, the X chromosome displays a narrowed region near its terminus. About 80% of the males possessing such X chromosomes are mentally challenged, display a decreased ability to accomplish certain tasks, are hyperactive, and display anxious behavior. This condition is known as the ***fragile X syndrome*** *owing to the morphology of the X chromosome, whose tip appears to be almost broken. The altered region of the X chromosome is the locus for the* ***FMR1 gene*** *(****fragile X mental retardation 1 gene****) that codes for the* ***FMR protein****. This protein represses translation of certain mRNAs, thereby inhibiting the formation of cytoskeletal elements at synapses and, in that fashion, interfering with neuronal plasticity.*

Microscopic study of interphase nuclei of cells from females displays a very tightly coiled clump of chromatin, the **sex chromatin** (**Barr body**), the inactive counterpart of the two X chromosomes. Epithelial cells obtained from the lining of the cheek

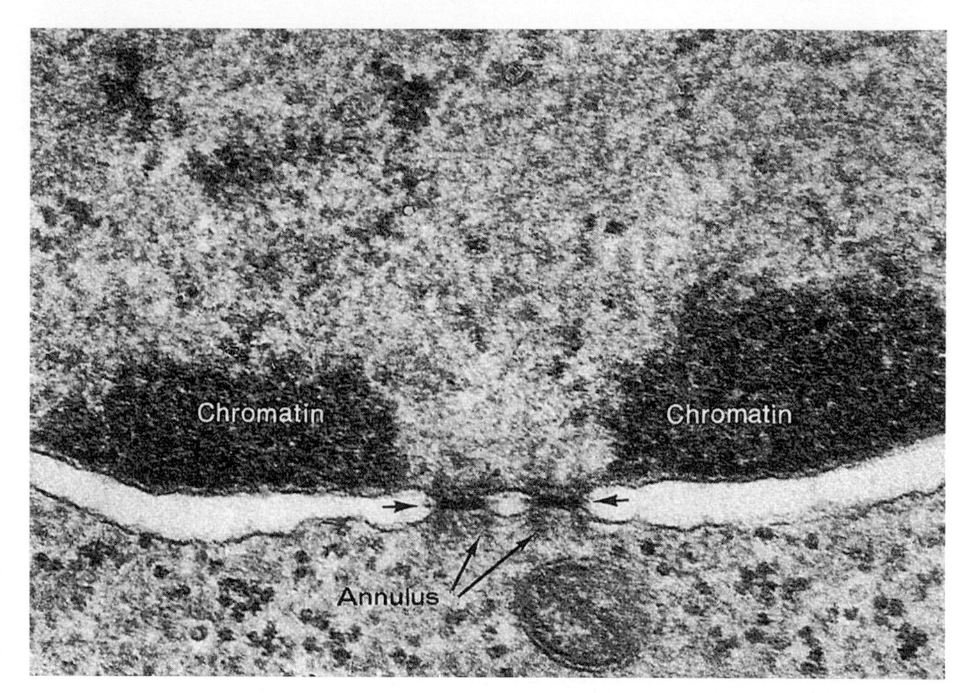

Fig. 3.7 Nuclear pore. Electron micrograph (×24,828). Note the heterochromatin adjacent to the inner nuclear membrane and that the inner and outer nuclear membranes are continuous at the nuclear pore. (From Fawcett DW. *The Cell*. Philadelphia: WB Saunders; 1981.)

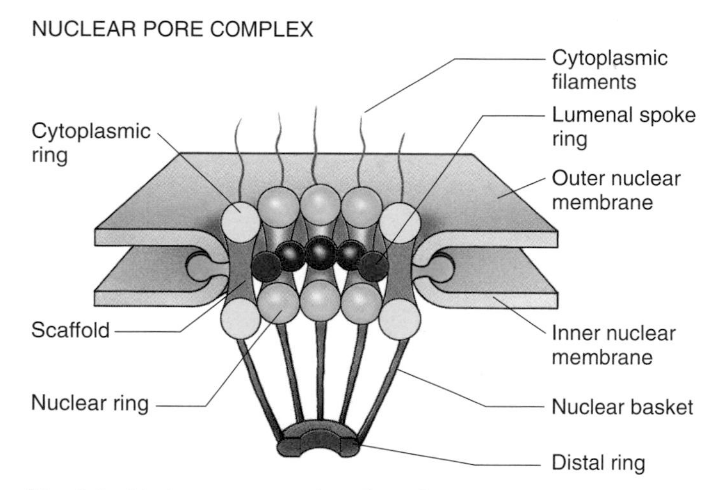

Fig. 3.8 Nuclear pore complex. This schematic representation of the current understanding of the structure of the nuclear pore complex demonstrates that it is made up of several combinations of eight units each. Note that the model does not include a transporter (see text). (Modified from Alberts B, Bray D, Lewis J, et al. *Molecular Biology of the Cell*. 3rd ed. New York: Garland Publishing; 1994.)

and neutrophils from blood smears are especially useful for studying sex chromatin. The sex chromatin is observed at the edge of the nuclear envelope in smears of the oral epithelial cells and as a small drumstick-like evagination of the nuclei of the neutrophils. A number of cells must be examined to observe sex chromatin because the X chromosome must be in the proper orientation to be displayed for observation.

Ploidy

Cells containing the full complement of chromosomes (46) are said to be **diploid (2n)**. Germ cells (mature ova or spermatozoa) are said to be **haploid (1n)**; that is, only one member of each of the homologous pairs of chromosomes is present. Upon fertilization, the chromosomal number is restored to the diploid (2n) amount as the nuclei of the two germ cells unite.

Certain alkaloids, such as colchicine, a plant derivative, arrest a dividing cell in the metaphase stage of mitosis when the chromosomes are maximally condensed, thus permitting the pairing and numbering of the chromosomes via a conventional system of **karyotyping**, an analysis of chromosome number (see Fig. 3.11).

Clinical Correlations

*One item that may be observed from the karyotype is **aneuploidy**, an abnormal chromosome number. Individuals with **Down syndrome**, for example, have an extra chromosome 21 (**trisomy 21**); they exhibit intellectual disability, stubby hands, and many congenital malformations, especially of the heart, among other manifestations.*

*Certain syndromes are associated with abnormalities in the number of sex chromosomes. **Klinefelter syndrome** results when an individual possesses three sex chromosomes (**XXY**). These persons exhibit the male phenotype, but they do not develop secondary sexual characteristics and are usually sterile. **Turner syndrome** is another example of aneuploidy, called **monosomy** of the sex chromosomes. The karyotype exhibits only one sex chromosome (**XO**). These individuals are females whose ovaries never develop and who have undeveloped breasts, a small uterus, and intellectual disability.*

Deoxyribonucleic Acid (DNA)

DNA, the genetic material of the cell, is located in the nucleus, where it acts as a template for RNA transcription.

DNA is composed of two types of bases: **purines** (adenine and guanine) and **pyrimidines** (cytosine and thymine). A double helix is established by the formation of hydrogen bonds between complementary bases on each strand of

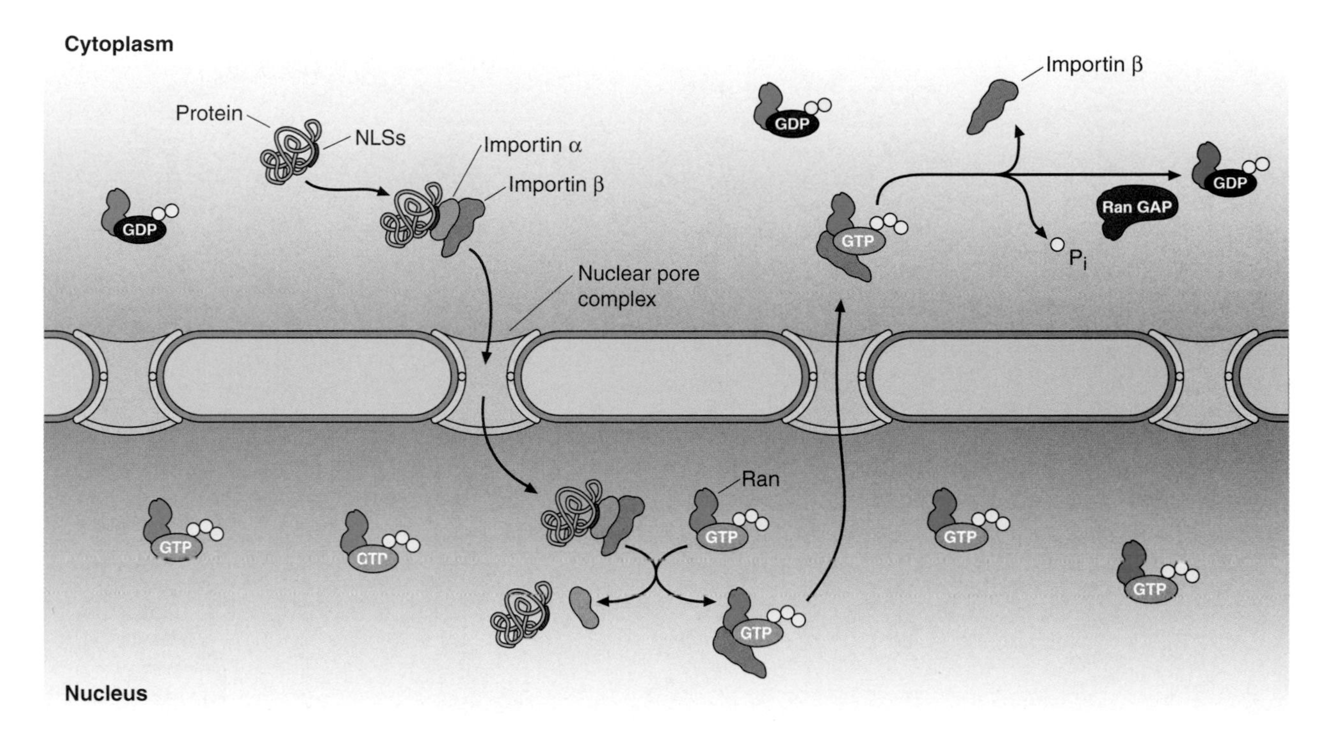

Fig. 3.9 Role of Ran in nuclear import. Ran/GDP is present in high concentration in the cytoplasm, whereas Ran/GTP is present in high concentration in the nucleus. Proteins to be imported into the nucleus form complexes with nuclear localization signals (NLS) importin α and importin β. Upon importation through the nuclear pore complex, Ran/GTP binds to importin β, thus releasing importin α and the imported protein. To complete the cycle, the Ran/GTP/importin β complex exits the nucleus to enter the cytoplasm via the nuclear pore complex. Here, the Ran/GTPase activating protein (Ran GAP) hydrolyzes the GTP, forming Ran GDP, thus releasing importin β back into the cytoplasm. *GDP,* Guanosine diphosphate; *GTP,* guanosine triphosphate.

the DNA molecule. These bonds are formed between **adenine** (A) and **thymine** (T) and between **guanine** (G) and **cytosine** (C).

Genes

The biological information that is passed from one cell generation to the next—the units of heredity—are located at specific regions on the DNA molecule called **genes**. Each gene represents a specific segment of the DNA molecule that codes for the synthesis of a particular protein, as well as for the regulatory sequences responsible for their expression. The sequential arrangement of bases constituting the gene represents the sequence of amino acids of the protein. The genetic code is designed in such a manner that a triplet of consecutive bases, a **codon**, denotes a particular amino acid. Each amino acid is represented by a different codon. The complete set of genes—that is, both the **coding** and **noncoding segments** of the DNA—are known as the **genome**. Coding segments possess the codons that determine the sequence of amino acids in a protein (or polypeptide) and noncoding segments possess regulatory or other functions.

Currently, the data indicates that the human genome contains about 25,000 genes, all of which were sequenced and mapped, which represents only 2% of the genome; 98% of the genome has regulatory or other functions.

EPIGENETICS

Epigenetics is a relatively new field of study that explores chemically induced heritable changes that occur to the genome without altering the sequence of nucleotides of the DNA molecule. These changes are caused by the addition of small molecules, such as **methyl groups** or **acetyl groups**, to the histones that compose the core of the chromatid. These small molecules act as markers that either silence the genes or cause the expression of the genes that are wrapped around the methylated or acetylated histones. The addition of these small molecules can transpire not only during embryogenesis but also in the adult individual. They may be caused by various environmental insults, such as toxic agents, or environmental stimuli, such as stress. It is important to realize that these are inheritable alterations in the same fashion that mutations in the sequence of DNA nucleotides are inheritable. Methylation tends to silence genes, whereas acetylation facilitates gene expression.

Clinical Correlations

Recent evidence has demonstrated that individuals who committed suicide had a much greater degree of ***methylation of the chromosomes*** *of their* ***hippocampus*** *(the part of the brain responsible for memory formation) than did members of the control group who died suddenly but not due to suicide.*

In a related study, it was shown that children who grew up in an orphanage exhibited a greater degree of ***chromosome methylation*** *than did the control group consisting of children who grew up in the home of their biological parents. Most of the methylated genes were related to* ***brain development*** *and* ***neural function****. Although the inheritance of these traits has not been proven in humans, mouse studies have shown that stress-related epigenetic alterations are transmitted from parents to pups.*

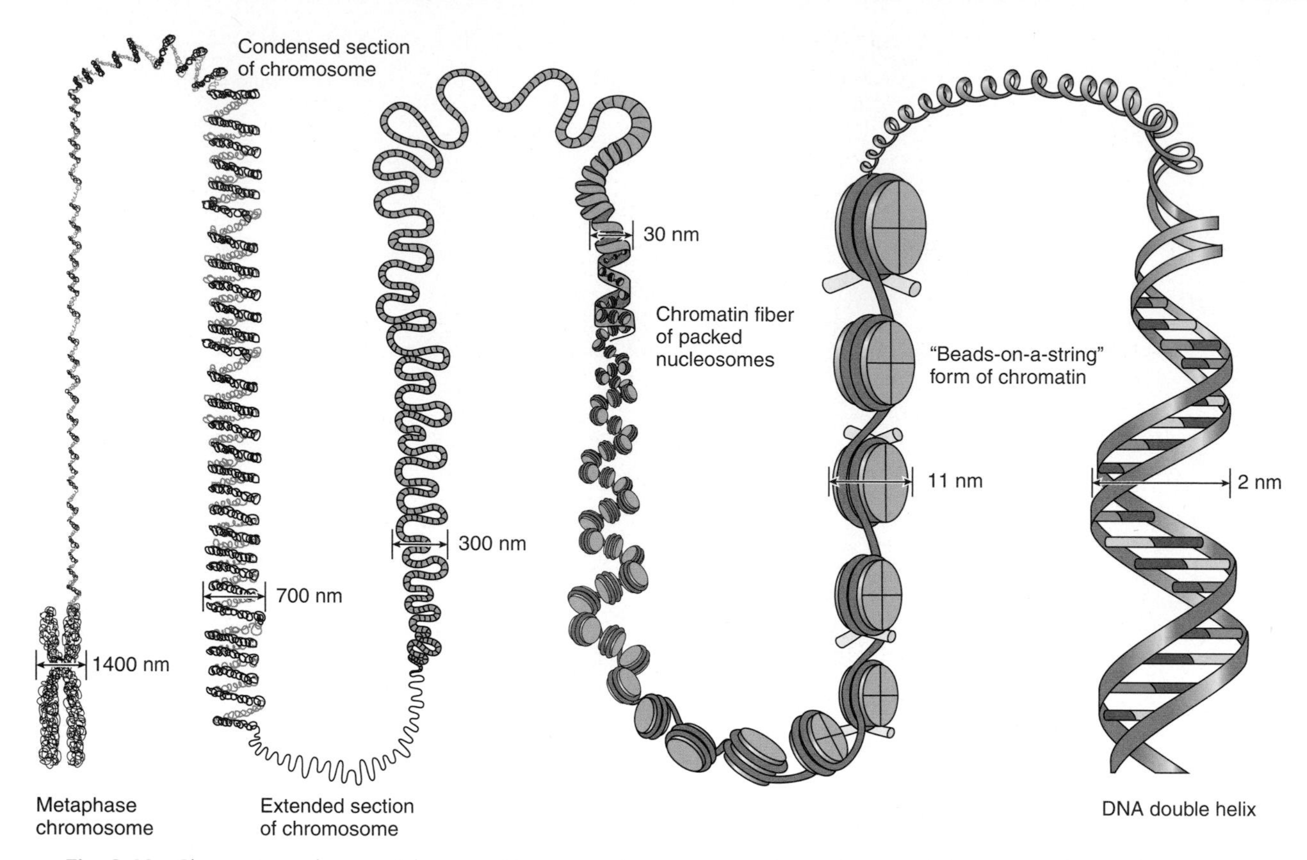

Fig. 3.10 Chromatin packaging. Schematic diagram displaying the complex packaging of chromatin to form a chromosome.

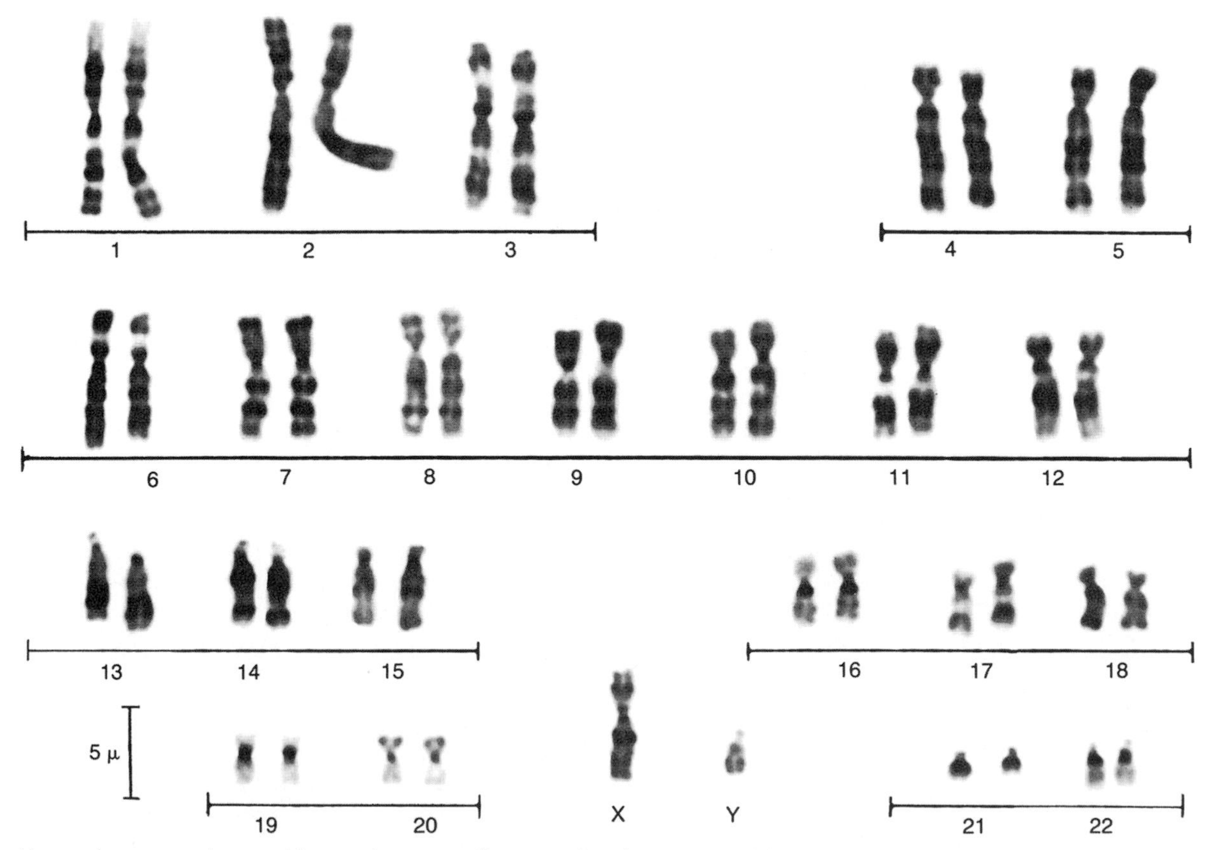

Fig. 3.11 Human karyotype. A normal human karyotype illustrating banding. (From Bibbo M. *Comprehensive Cytopathology*. Philadelphia: WB Saunders; 1991.)

TABLE 3.1 Types of RNA

Abbreviation	Name	Function
mRNA	Messenger RNA	A coding RNA that functions as the template for protein synthesis
rRNA	Ribosomal RNA	Combines with proteins to form the two ribosomal subunits to function in protein synthesis
tRNA	Transfer RNA	Binds to amino acids to carry them to the correct sites on the mRNA in protein synthesis
miRNA	Micro RNA	Short RNA segments (19–25 nucleotides) that have regulatory functions by blocking protein synthesis; they also promote cancerogenesis by blocking apoptotic pathways
siRNA	Small interfering RNA, also known as Silencing RNA	Short, double-stranded RNA segments (20–22 nucleotides) that interfere with protein synthesis. They are released by viruses or are transposons that enter the cell. There are synthetic siRNAs that are manufactured for therapeutic purposes.
lincRNA, also known as lncRNA	Long intergenic noncoding RNA Long noncoding RNA	Long-chain RNA (≥200 nucleotides) that regulate cancerogenesis and embryogenesis and also inactivate the second X chromosomes in females
piRNA	Piwi-interacting RNA	Interferes with the expression of transposons; facilitates the placement of epigenetic markers on chromosomes

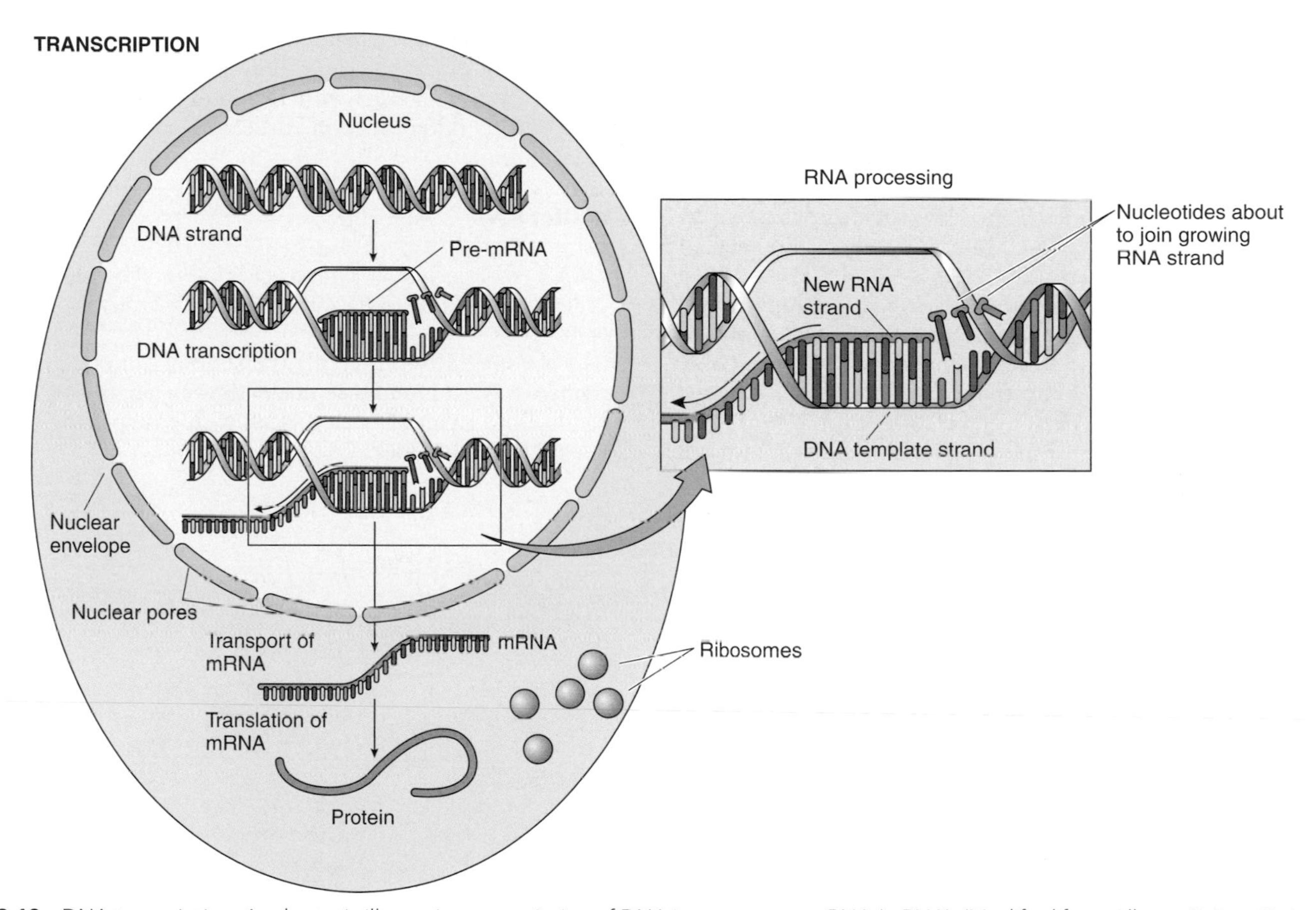

Fig. 3.12 DNA transcription. A schematic illustrating transcription of DNA into messenger RNA (mRNA). (Modified from Alberts B, Bray D, Lewis J, et al. *Molecular Biology of the Cell*. 3rd ed. New York: Garland Publishing; 1994.)

Ribonucleic Acid

RNA is similar to DNA except that it is single stranded, one of its bases is uracil instead of thymine, and its sugar is ribose instead of deoxyribose.

RNA is similar to DNA, with both composed of a linear sequence of nucleotides, but RNA is single stranded and the sugar in RNA is ribose, not deoxyribose. One of the bases, thymine, is replaced by uracil (U), which, similar to thymine, is complementary to adenine. There are two major types of RNA, **coding RNA** and **noncoding RNAs**. Coding RNA—namely, mRNA—carries the code for protein synthesis. Noncoding RNAs assist in protein synthesis (transfer RNA and ribosomal RNA) as well as in regulatory functions (Table 3.1).

The DNA in the nucleus serves as a template for synthesis of a complementary strand of RNA, a process called **transcription**. Synthesis of three of the various types of RNA is catalyzed by three different **RNA polymerases**:

- **Messenger RNA (mRNA)** by RNA polymerase II
- **Transfer RNA (tRNA)** by RNA polymerase III
- **Ribosomal RNA (rRNA)** by RNA polymerase I

The mechanism of transcription is generally the same for all three types of RNA. It should be noted that only mRNA is transcribed from the **coding segments** of the DNA. rRNA, tRNA, and regulatory RNAs are transcribed from the **noncoding segments** of the DNA.

Messenger RNA

Messenger RNA carries the genetic code from the nucleus to the cytoplasm to act as a template for protein synthesis.

mRNA serves as an intermediary for carrying the genetic information encoded in DNA that specifies the primary sequence of proteins from the nucleus to the protein-synthesizing machinery in the cytoplasm (Fig. 3.12). Each mRNA is a complementary copy of the region of the DNA molecule that codes for a single protein or a combination of proteins. An mRNA molecule thus consists of a series of codons in which each codon corresponds to particular amino acids. It also contains a **start codon** (AUG), which is necessary for initiating protein synthesis, and one or more **stop codons** (UAA, UAG, or UGA), which act to terminate protein synthesis. Once formed in the nucleus, mRNA is transported to the cytoplasm, where it is translated into protein (see Chapter 2).

Transcription. Transcription begins at a DNA triplet corresponding to the **start codon** AUG and is concluded when the enzyme RNA polymerase II recognizes a **chain-terminator** site complementary to the stop codons UAA, UAG, or UGA. When the enzyme reaches the chain terminator, it is released from the DNA molecule, permitting it to repeat the process of transcription. Simultaneously, the newly formed RNA strand (known as the **primary transcript**) is released from the DNA molecule, leaving it free in the nucleoplasm.

The primary transcript is the **precursor messenger RNA (pre-mRNA)**, which contains both **exons** (coding segments) and **introns** (noncoding segments). In order to remove the introns and splice together the exons, pre-mRNA, and nuclear processing proteins must form complexes known as **heterogenous nuclear ribonucleoprotein particles (hnRNPs)** that begin **RNA splicing,** thus reducing the length of the pre-mRNA molecule. Additional processing involves **spliceosomes**, complexes of five **small nuclear ribonucleoprotein particles (snRNPs)** and a large number of **non-snRNP splicing factors** that assist in the splicing mechanism to produce **messenger ribonucleoprotein (mRNP).** Finally, the nuclear processing proteins are removed from the complex, leaving mRNA ready to be transported out of the nucleus via the nuclear pore complexes (see Fig. 3.12).

The introns that were removed from the primary RNA transcript were thought to have no function, even though they represent about 95% or more of the RNA than the protein-coding genes. It is now known that although these intronic RNA segments do not encode protein, they perform regulatory functions that are in parallel with regulatory proteins. Their role may relate to differentiation, development, gene expression, and evolution.

Transfer RNA

tRNA ferries activated amino acids to the ribosome/mRNA complex, resulting in the formation of the protein.

tRNA is a small RNA molecule transcribed from DNA by RNA polymerase III. It is about 80 nucleotides in length and is folded upon itself to resemble a cloverleaf, with base pairing between some of the nucleotides.

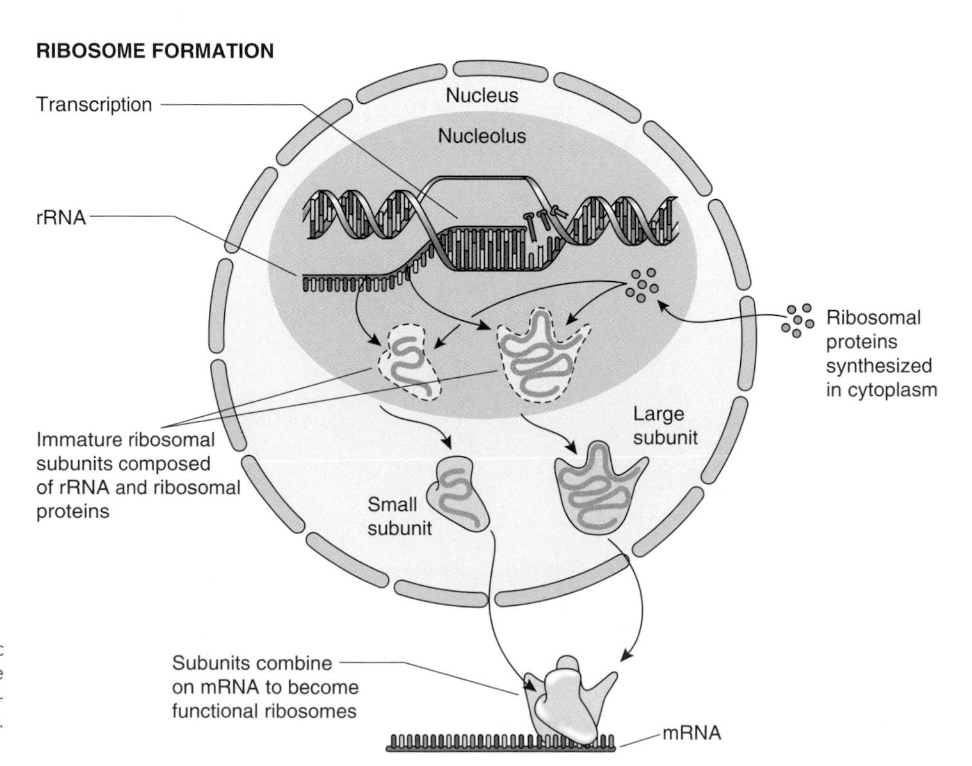

Fig. 3.13 Ribosome formation. A schematic presentation of the nuclear events in ribosome formation. (Modified from Alberts B, Bray D, Lewis J, et al. *Molecular Biology of the Cell*. 3rd ed. New York: Garland Publishing; 1994.)

Two regions of the tRNA are of special significance. One of these, the **anticodon**, recognizes the codon of the mRNA; the other is the amino acid–bearing region, which resides at the 3′ end of the molecule. tRNA is aminoacylated not only in the cytoplasm but also in the nucleus. This is believed to be a "proofreading" step that facilitates functional readiness in the cytoplasm. tRNA then transfers activated amino acids to the ribosome-mRNA complex, where they are incorporated into the polypeptide chain forming the protein (see Chapter 2).

Ribosomal RNA

rRNA forms associations with proteins and enzymes in the nucleus to form ribosomes.

rRNA is synthesized in the nucleolus by RNA polymerase I (Fig. 3.13). The primary transcript is called **45S rRNA (pre-rRNA)**, a huge molecule composed of about 13,000 nucleotides. Ribosomal proteins, synthesized in the cytoplasm, are transported through the nuclear pore complexes into the nucleus and from there into the nucleolus to join a 5S rRNA molecule. Once there, they associate with the 45S rRNA molecules, forming a very large **ribonucleoprotein particle** (**RNP**). This RNP is processed by several resident molecules into precursors of the large and small ribosomal subunits in the nucleolus. Thereafter, assembled small ribosomal subunits, made up of 18S rRNAs and ribosomal proteins, make their way from the nucleolus to the cytoplasm by transport via the nuclear pore complexes. The remaining 28S, 5.8S, and 5S rRNAs "as well as ribosomal proteins", are assembled into large ribosomal subunits and are transported out of the nucleus to the cytoplasm by way of the nuclear pore complexes.

Regulatory RNAs

There are several types of regulatory RNAs, such as micro RNA (miRNA), small interfering (also known as silencing) RNA (siRNA), large intergenic noncoding RNA (lincRNA, also known as long noncoding RNA [lncRNA]), and piwi interacting RNA (piRNA). All of these are noncoding, meaning that none of these RNAs are translated into proteins (see Table 3.1).

miRNAs, as their name implies, are usually very short RNA segments, composed of only 19 to 25 nucleotides. They comprise a very large group of regulatory RNAs, consisting of over 1000 members each with a specific function. miRNAs are either transcribed from DNA or are formed from the introns that are spliced from the pre-RNA as long nucleotide sequences, known as **primary miRNA** (**pri-miRNA**). The pri-miRNAs are processed in the nucleus to form **pre-miRNAs** that are about 70 nucleotides long and are exported through the nuclear pore complex, an energy-requiring process using the shuttle protein **exportin-5**. Once in the cytoplasm, the pre-miRNA is modified by the **RNAse III enzyme** known as **dicer**, forming two strands of nucleotides, each with two free ends. The two strands become separated and one of the strands is destroyed, whereas dicer facilitates the other strand, now known as **miRNA**, to form an miRNA-protein complex, known as **RNA-induced silencing complex-miRNA** (**RISC-miRNA**). It is the RISC-miRNA that accomplishes the attachment of the miRNA to the mRNA by way of the formation of complementary nucleotide bonds. The nucleotides of the miRNA do not have to match perfectly with the nucleotide sequence of the mRNA; in fact, in mammals, the match is usually imperfect. The presence of the RISC-miRNA complex on the mRNA not only blocks protein synthesis but it also facilitates the rapid degradation of the mRNA and, in that fashion, inhibits gene expression. In addition to blocking protein synthesis, miRNAs interfere with the ability of cells to enter the apoptotic pathway, making those cells "immortal" and, thereby, promoting cancerogenesis. Other miRNAs have been shown to suppress metastasis in some human breast cancers. miRNAs also function in facilitating some and interfering with other cellular signaling activities.

Clinical Correlations

Not all miRNAs are synthesized by cells of the individual organism; in fact, some enter the body as part of the digestive process. It has been demonstrated that certain plant miRNAs that were ingested by patients were present in their native state in the blood of these individuals. An example of an miRNA, known as ***MIR168a****, present in rice has been noted to be abundant in human blood of individuals whose diet contains rice. This miRNA binds with* **low-density lipoprotein (LDL) receptor adapter protein 1 mRNA** *in the liver, whose protein product is responsible for LDL clearing from the bloodstream.*

Recently, investigators have created ***siRNAs*** *that act as naturally introduced siRNAs in that they form* ***RNA-induced silencing complex-siRNA (RISC-siRNA)*** *that complement regions of the mRNA that the investigators want silenced. It is believed that these synthetic siRNAs will have therapeutic benefits in fighting certain diseases.*

A form of genetic engineering that involves the synthesis of an RNA molecule whose nucleotides complement the region of interest of the human genome is performed by proteins known as ***Cas proteins (CRSPR-associated proteins—*** *the acronym stands for* ***clustered regularly interspaced short palindromic repeats****). The Cas proteins associated with the synthetic RNA molecule seek out the complementary regions of the DNA molecule, and the complex excises the targeted DNA nucleotide sequence. Future therapeutic modalities include replacing the excised DNA region with the corrected patch of DNA sequence, thus not only eliminating the disease-causing sequence but also supplying the corrective action to repair the mutated gene.*

Small interfering RNAs (**siRNAs**), also known as **silencing RNAs** (**siRNAs**), are similar to miRNAs in that they are initially double stranded and are about 20 to 22 nucleotides in length. They are usually released by viruses or are transposons that enter the cell and are attached to the RISC, forming an RISC-siRNA complex. These complexes bind, in a complementary fashion, to mRNAs and interfere with protein synthesis. Additionally, just as RISC-miRNA complexes, they expedite the degradation of the mRNAs to which they are attached and inhibit gene expression.

Large intergenic noncoding RNA (**lincRNA**, also known as **long noncoding RNA** [**lncRNA**]) are long chains composed of 200 or more nucleotides. Although some investigators believe these lincRNAs to have no function and are destined to be degraded, others have demonstrated that there are at least 35,000 known lincRNAs, some present in the nucleus and others located in the cytoplasm. This suggests that many of them must have metabolic roles; otherwise, they would not have been conserved during evolution. It is known that at least two lincRNAs—H19 and Xist (X-inactive specific transcript)—have important functions, the former in carcinogenesis and embryogenesis and the latter in inactivating the second X chromosomes of females.

Clinical Correlations

***H19**, although present on both maternally and paternally derived chromosomes, is expressed only on the maternally derived chromosome. It is believed to act as a regulator of gene expression at the chromosomal level by specifically enlisting groups of regulatory proteins to those sites of the genes that control transcription, thereby enhancing or inhibiting mRNA formation. The RNA gene product of H19 is especially present in high concentration in malignant cells derived from cancers of the esophagus, colon, bladder, liver, ovary, lung, testis, breast, and uterus.*

*The lincRNA, **Xist**, is especially active in females as a product of one of the two X chromosomes, specifically the one that will become silenced. Although the process of inactivating the second X chromosome in females is not understood completely, it is known that Xist binds with a protein complex known as **polycomb repressive complex 2 (PRC2)**, which inactivates the chromosome in question by forming a microscopically visible "enclosure" around the entire chromosome that is attached to specific sites on the chromosome. Interestingly, some of the genes are permitted to be expressed; these chromosomal segments are noted to be protruding outside the physical "enclosure."*

Piwi-interacting RNAs (piRNA) are about 25 to 30 nucleotides in length and comprise a very large group of RNA in mammals, consisting of more than 50,000 members. In mammals, they are located primarily in the testes and in the ovaries, housed both in the cytosol and nucleus. The precise functions of piRNAs are not known but they are believed to repress gene expression and are believed to function in the formation of spermatozoa.

piRNA has been shown to recruit and bind to **piwi protein**. The piRNA-piwi protein complex migrates to specific sites on the DNA and recruits a host of proteins that place **epigenetic marks** on the histones at that position. These epigenetic marks become permanent marks on the chromosomes that cause that particular gene to be silenced or expressed.

Clinical Correlations

*In 2015, a molecular genome editing instrument named **CRSPR/Cas9** (**c**lustered **r**egularly **i**nterspaced **s**hort **pal**indromic **r**epeats/**CR**ISPR **as**sociated protein 9) was developed and adapted from microorganisms. CRSPR/Cas9 is a molecular DNA slicing tool in which the enzyme Cas9 has the ability to excise any specific region of the DNA molecule and replace it by other nucleotides. Although genome editing tools have been available for a number of years, CRSPR/Cas9 is a much faster, cheaper, and more reliable tool. In fact, recent modifications of this system have allowed researchers to replace single nucleotides; it is hoped that, eventually, the repair of point mutations such as the one responsible for sickle cell anemia becomes feasible, thus, curing patients with that anomaly. Or "single-gene anomalies," such as hemophilia and cystic fibrosis, as well as more multigene anomalies, such as cancer, cardiovascular disease, are beginning to and autoimmune diseases, benefit from the use of this genome editor.*

NUCLEOPLASM

The nucleoplasm consists of interchromatin and perichromatin granules, water, snRNPs, Cajal bodies, and the nuclear matrix.

Nucleoplasm, separated from the cytoplasm by the nuclear envelope, is a somewhat viscous substance that surrounds the chromosomes and nucleoli and is composed of interchromatin and perichromatin granules, water, snRNPs, Cajal bodies, ribonucleoproteins (RNPs), and the nuclear matrix.

Interchromatin granules (**IGs**), located in clusters scattered throughout the nucleus among the chromatin material, appear to be connected to each other by thin fibrils which are 20 to 25 nm in diameter. They are composed of ribonuclear proteins and a number of enzymes, including ATPase, GTPase, β-glycerophosphatase, and NAD-pyrophosphatase. Their function is unclear.

Perichromatin granules (**PCGs**) are electron-dense particles 30 to 50 nm in diameter located at the margins of the heterochromatin. These are surrounded by a 25-nm-wide halo of a less dense region. They are composed of densely packed fibrils of 4.7S low-molecular-weight RNA complexed to two peptides, resembling **heterogeneous nuclear ribonucleoproteins** (**hnRNPs**).

Small nuclear ribonucleoprotein particles (**snRNPs**) participate in splicing, cleaving, and transporting hnRNPs. Although most snRNPs are located in the nucleus, some are limited to nucleoli. **Ribonucleoproteins** are RNA with its associated protein, such as mRNA and its protective proteins.

Cajal (**coiled**) **bodies** are small structures in the close vicinity of the nucleolus. They are associated with the formation of the enzyme telomerase, which they probably direct to the tips of chromosomes. They may also organize components of the nucleus in preparation for transcription.

Nuclear Matrix

The structural components of the **nuclear matrix** include the nuclear pore–nuclear lamina complex, residual nucleoli, residual RNP networks, and fibrillar elements. The nucleus possesses a nucleoplasmic reticulum that is continuous with the ER of the cytoplasm and the nuclear envelope. This reticulum houses calcium ions that are localized to and function within the nucleus. Further, this reticulum possesses receptors for inositol 1,4,5-triphosphate which ultimately regulate calcium signaling within certain compartments of the nucleus, specifically regions dedicated to protein transport, transcription of certain genes, and possibly others.

Functionally, the nuclear matrix is associated with DNA replication sites, rRNA and mRNA transcription and processing, steroid receptor binding, heat shock proteins, carcinogen binding, DNA viruses, and viral proteins. This list is not inclusive and does not address the functional natures of each of these associations because they are still unclear. It has been suggested, however, that the nucleus may contain many interactive subcompartments that function spatially and temporally in a tightly coordinated fashion to facilitate gene expression.

NUCLEOLUS

The nucleolus is the deeply staining non–membrane-bounded structure within the nucleus that is involved in rRNA synthesis and in the assembly of small and large ribosomal subunits.

The **nucleolus**, a dense nonmembranous structure located in the nucleus, is observed only during interphase because it dissipates during cell division. It stains basophilic with hematoxylin and eosin, being rich in rRNA and protein. The nucleolus contains only small amounts of DNA, which is also inactive and thus does not stain with Feulgen stains. Usually, there are no more than two or three nucleoli per cell; however, their number, size, and shape are generally species specific and relate to the synthetic activity of the cell. In cells that are actively synthesizing protein, the nucleolus may occupy up to 25% of the nuclear volume. Densely staining regions are the **nucleolus-associated chromatin**, which is being transcribed into rRNA (see Figs. 3.4 and 3.5). Also located in the pale-staining regions are the tips of chromosomes 13, 14, 15, 21, and 22 (in humans), containing the **nucleolar-organizing regions (NORs)**, where gene loci that encode rRNA are located.

The cell's ribosomal subunits are organized and assembled within the nucleolus, except those located in the mitochondria. Additionally, the nucleolus is the site of the synthesis of some of the regulatory RNAs; regulation of some of the events in the cell cycle such as cytokinesis; the inactivation of mitotic cyclin-dependent kinases by sequestering cell cycle regulatory proteins, thus inactivating them; modification of small RNAs, that moderate and alter pre-rRNA; assembly of RNP; engagement in nuclear export; and participation in the control of the aging process.

Clinical Correlation

Some suggest that the region of the DNA that codes for ribosomal RNA in the nucleolus may become unstable, thereby accelerating the aging process. In malignant cells, the nucleolus may become hypertrophic. Further, it is known that in tumor cells the nucleolar-organizing regions become larger and more numerous, indicating a poorer clinical prognosis.

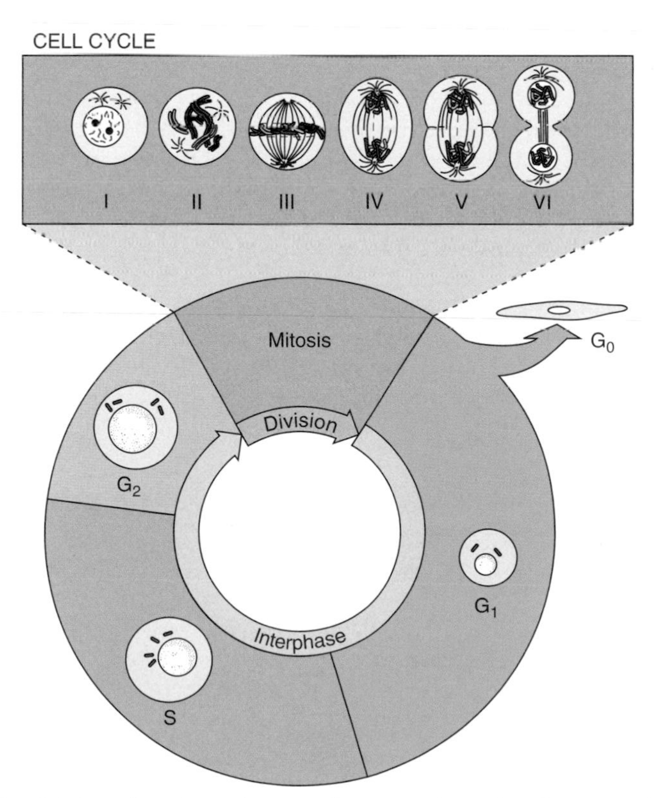

Fig. 3.14 Cell cycle. A diagram illustrating the cell cycle in actively dividing cells. Nondividing cells, such as neurons, leave the cycle to enter the G_0 phase (resting stage). Other cells, such as lymphocytes, may return to the cell cycle.

The Cell Cycle

The cell cycle is a series of events within the cell that prepare it for dividing into two daughter cells.

The **cell cycle** is divided into two major events: **mitosis**, the short period of time during which the cell divides its nucleus and cytoplasm, giving rise to two **daughter cells**; and **interphase,** a longer period of time during which the cell increases its size and content and replicates its genetic material (Fig. 3.14). In order for a cell to enter the cell cycle, it must be prompted by a signaling molecule known as a **mitogen**. There are at least 50 different molecules that serve as mitogens. Some are very specific in that they can promote only a single population of cells, such as **erythropoietin**, which promotes cell division in erythroid progenitor cells that are responsible for the formation of red blood cells. Others are less specific and can induce mitosis in a variety of cells, such as **epidermal growth factor**, which can induce epithelial as well as other cells to enter the cell cycle. Most mitogens bind to cell surface receptors that transduce the signal intracellularly, causing a second messenger system to respond by activating the synthesis of **transcription regulatory proteins**, such as **Myc**, which is responsible for prompting the cell to produce factors that initiate entry into the cell cycle.

The cell cycle may be thought of as beginning at the conclusion of the telophase stage in **mitosis (M)**, after which the cell enters interphase. Interphase is subdivided into three phases:

- **G_1 (gap) phase**, when the synthesis of macromolecules essential for DNA duplication begins
- **S (synthetic) phase**, when the DNA is duplicated
- **G_2 phase**, when the cell undergoes preparations for mitosis

Cells that have left the cell cycle are said to be in a resting stage, the **G_0 (outside) phase**, or the **stable phase**. Those cells that become highly differentiated after the last mitotic event may cease to undergo mitosis either for a very long time (e.g., neurons and skeletal muscle cells are said to be in a **terminally differentiated** G_0 state) or for a short period of time (e.g., certain hematopoietic stem cells) and return to the cell cycle at a later time.

INTERPHASE

Interphase, the time between mitotic events, is subdivided into three phases: gap 1, synthesis, and gap 2.

Gap 1

G_1 phase (gap 1) is a period of cell growth, RNA synthesis, and other events in preparation for the next mitosis.

Daughter cells formed during mitosis enter the **G_1 phase**. During this phase, the cells synthesize RNA, regulatory proteins essential to DNA replication, and enzymes necessary to carry out these synthetic activities. Thus, the cell volume, reduced by dividing the cell in half during mitosis, is restored to normal. Additionally, the nucleoli are reestablished during the G_1 phase. It is during this time that the centrioles begin to duplicate themselves, a process that is completed by the **G_2 phase.**

The triggers inducing the cell to enter the cell cycle may be (1) a mechanical force (e.g., stretching of smooth muscle), (2) injury to the tissue (e.g., ischemia), and (3) cell death. All of these incidents

TABLE 3.2 Cyclins, Cyclin-Dependent Kinases (CDKs), and the Cell Cycle

Phase	Cyclin binds to CDKs	Effect
Early G_1 phase	Cyclin D to CDK4 and CDK6	The cell may enter and progress through the S phase.
Late G_1 phase	Cyclin E to CDK2	
S phase	Cyclin A to CDK2 and CDK1	The cell may leave the S phase and induce formation of cyclin B.
G_2 phase	Cyclin B to CDK1	The cell is allowed to leave the G_2 phase and enter the M phase.

TABLE 3.3 Cell Cycle Checkpoints and Their Functions

Checkpoint and Its Phase	Function
G_1 DNA damage checkpoint in G_1 phase	DNA replication is monitored; if an error has occurred, the cell may not enter the S phase.
S DNA damage checkpoint in S phase	DNA replication is monitored; if an error has occurred, the cell may not leave the S phase.
Unreplicated DNA checkpoint in G_2 phase	If not all of the DNA was replicated, the cell may not leave the G_2 phase.
G2 damage checkpoint in G_2 phase	If there are errors in the duplicated DNA, the cell may not leave the G_2 phase.
Spindle assembly checkpoint	If the spindle apparatus is not assembled correctly, the cell may not leave the M phase.
Chromosome segregation checkpoint	If the chromosome has not separated correctly (chromosome stickiness), the cell may not leave the M phase.

cause the release of ligands by signaling cells in the involved tissue. Frequently, these ligands are growth factors that indirectly induce the expression of **proto-oncogenes**, genes that are responsible for controlling the proliferative pathways of the cell. Mutations in the proto-oncogenes that enable the cell to escape control and divide in an unrestrained fashion are responsible for many cancers. Such mutated proto-oncogenes are known as **oncogenes**.

Signaling molecules that stimulate proliferation bind to cell surface receptor proteins of the target cell and activate one of the **signal transduction pathways** described in Chapter 2. Hence, extracellular signals that are perceived at the cell surface are transduced into intracellular events, most of which involve the sequential activation of a cascade of cytoplasmic **protein kinases**. These kinases activate a series of intranuclear **transcription factors** that regulate the expression of proto-oncogenes, resulting in cell division.

The capability of the cell to begin and advance through the cell cycle is governed by the presence and interactions of a group of related proteins known as **cyclins**, with specific **cyclin-dependent kinases (CDKs)** as listed in Table 3.2.

Once the cyclins have performed their specific functions, they enter the ubiquitin-proteasome pathway, where they are degraded into their component molecules. The cell also employs quality control mechanisms, known as **checkpoints**, to safeguard against early transition between the phases (Table 3.3). These checkpoints ensure that the essential events are completed properly before the cell is permitted to progress from one phase to the next. If the quality control mechanism discovers an

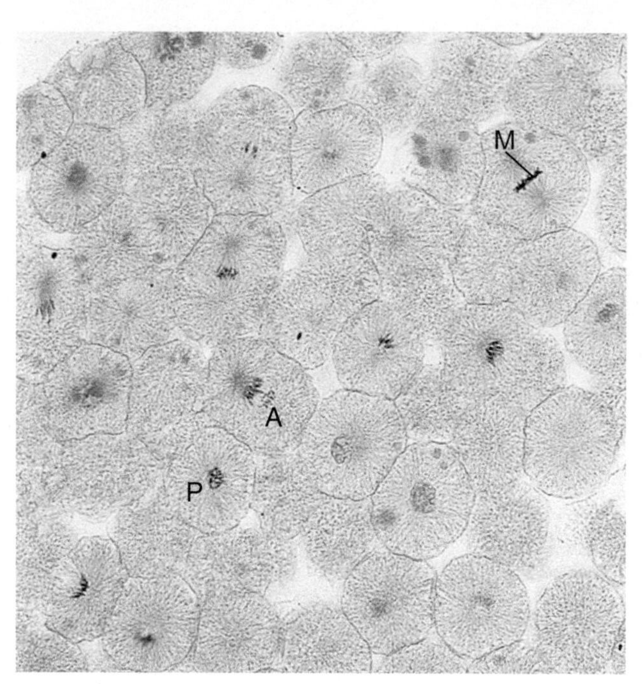

Fig. 3.15 Stages of mitosis. Light micrograph (×270). Note the various stages: A, anaphase; M, metaphase; and P, prophase.

error, the cell may not leave its current phase unless the problem is corrected. If the problem cannot be corrected, the cell is ushered back into the G_0 phase.

The actual control mechanisms are considerably involved and complicated; for more details, see relevant textbooks of cell biology, as well as the current literature of the cell cycle.

S Phase

DNA synthesis occurs during the S phase.

During the **S phase**, the synthetic phase of the cell cycle, the **centrosomes** and **genome** are duplicated. All of the requisite nucleoproteins, including the histones, are imported and incorporated into the DNA molecule, forming the chromatin material. The cell now contains twice the normal complement of its DNA. The amount of DNA present in autosomal and germ cells also varies. Autosomal cells contain the diploid (2n) amount of DNA before the synthetic (S) phase of the cell cycle when the (2n) amount of DNA is doubled (4n) in preparation for cell division. In contrast, germ cells produced by meiosis possess the haploid (1n) number of chromosomes and also the (1n) amount of DNA.

G_2 Phase

The gap 2 phase (G_2 phase) is the period between the end of DNA synthesis and the beginning of mitosis.

During the **G_2 phase**, the RNA and proteins essential to cell division are synthesized, the energy for mitosis is stored, tubulin is synthesized for assembly into microtubules required for mitosis, DNA replication is analyzed for possible errors, and these errors are corrected.

MITOSIS

Mitosis is the process of cell division that results in the formation of two identical daughter cells.

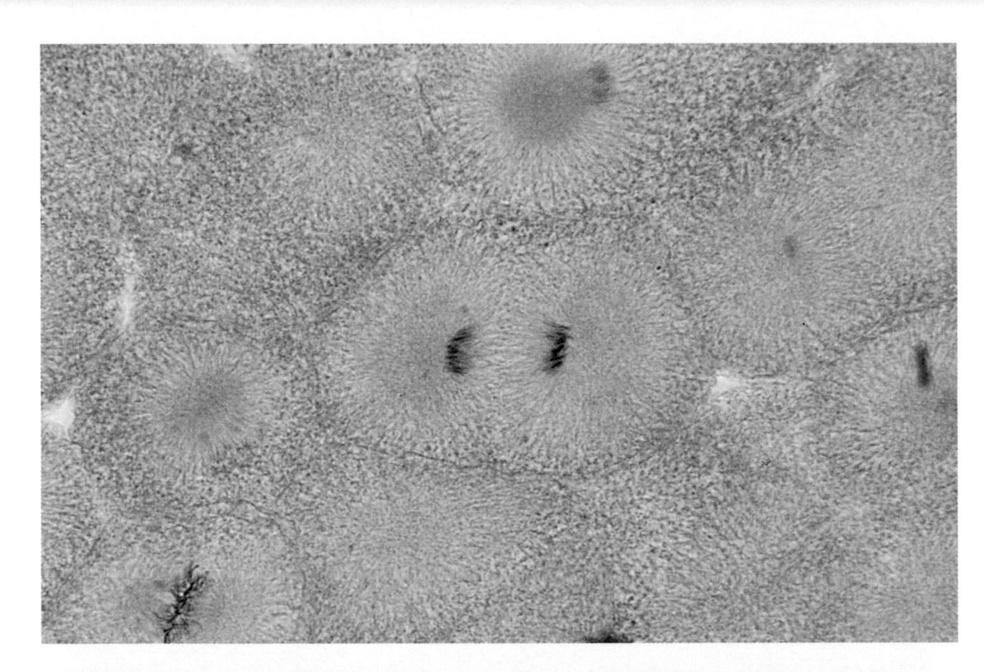

Fig. 3.16 Anaphase stage of mitosis (×540). Sister chromatids have separated from the metaphase plate and are now migrating away from each other to opposite poles.

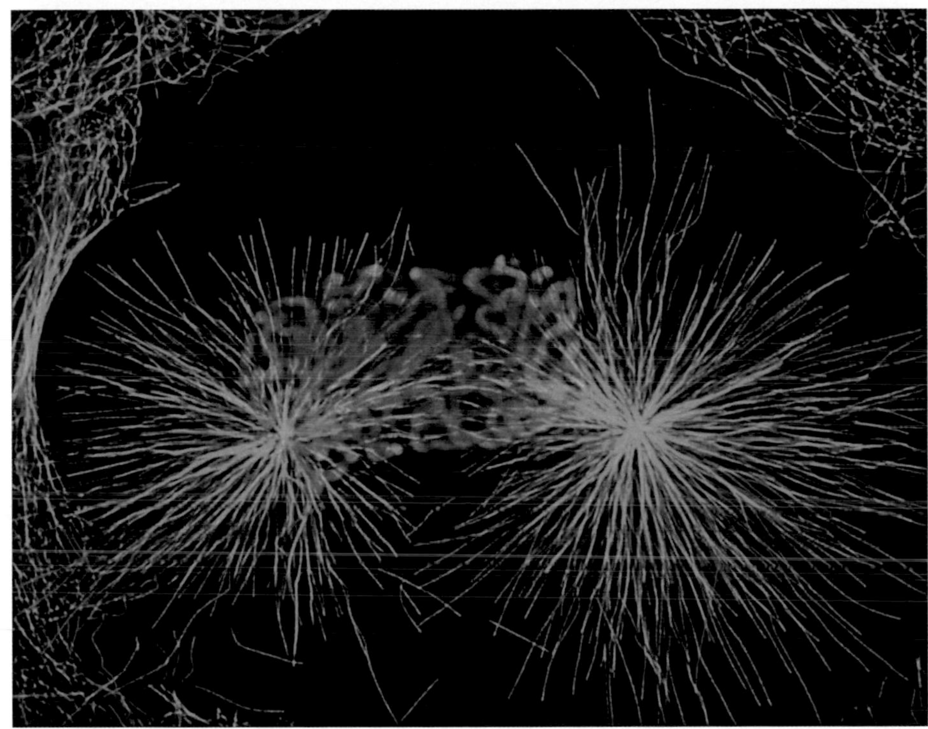

Fig. 3.17 Immunofluorescence image of a cell in the prometaphase stage of mitosis. Note the spindle microtubules *(green)* and the chromosomes *(blue)*. (© 1999, Alexey Khodjakov, MD)

Mitosis (**M**) occurs at the conclusion of the **G_2 phase** and, thus, completes the cell cycle. Mitosis is the process whereby the cytoplasm and the nucleus of the cell are divided equally into two identical daughter cells (Figs. 3.15 to 3.17). First, the nuclear material is divided in a process called **karyokinesis**, followed by division of the cytoplasm, called **cytokinesis**. The process of mitosis is divided into five distinct stages: **prophase**, **prometaphase**, **metaphase**, **anaphase**, and **telophase** (Fig. 3.18).

Prophase

During prophase, the chromosomes condense and the nucleolus disappears.

At the beginning of prophase, the chromosomes are condensing to become visible microscopically. Each chromosome consists of two parallel **sister chromatids**, joined together at one point along their length at the **centromere**. As chromosomes condense, the nucleolus disappears. The **centrosome** also divides into two regions, each half containing a pair of **centrioles** in a sea of **γ-tubulin rings**. It is the **microtubule-organizing center** (**MTOC**) of the cell (see Chapter 2). The centrosomes migrate away from each other to opposite poles of the cell, where they each form a new MTOC.

From each MTOC, astral microtubules, kinetochore microtubules, and polar microtubules develop, giving rise to the mitotic spindle apparatus.

- It is thought that the **astral microtubules** that radiate out from the pole of the spindle may assist in retaining each

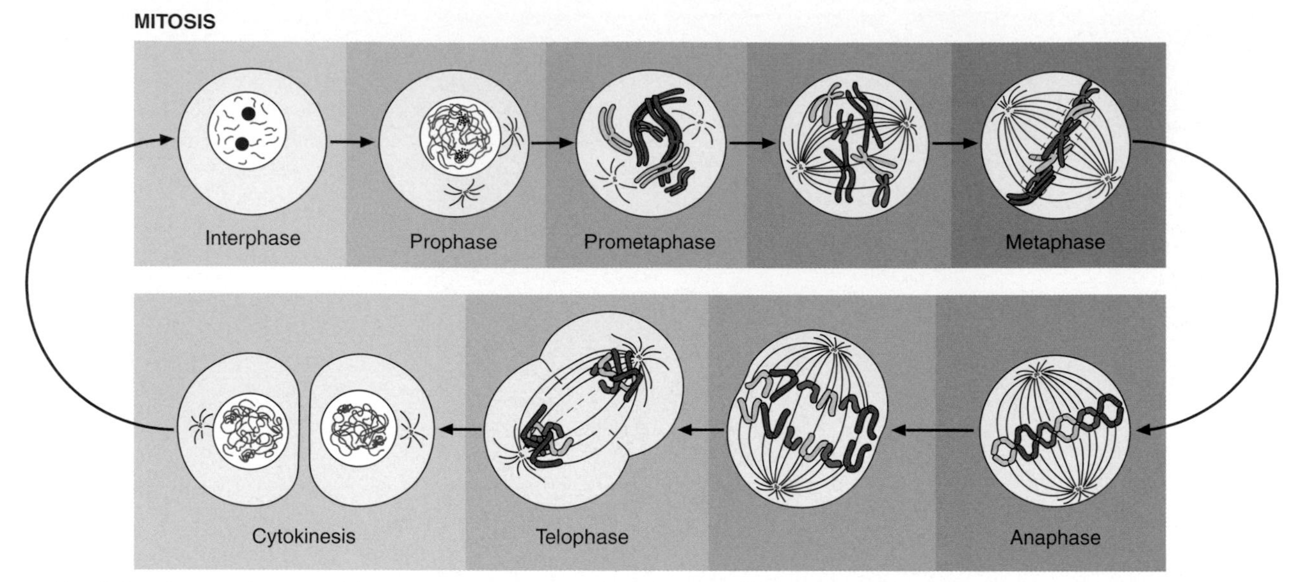

Fig. 3.18 Stages of mitosis. Schematic representation of mitosis in a cell containing a diploid (2n) number of 6 chromosomes.

MTOC at its pole of the cell and ensure that the spindle apparatus is oriented in the correct fashion.

- Those microtubules that attach to the kinetochores assembled on the centromere of each sister chromatid are **kinetochore microtubules.** They assist in separating the sister chromatids from each other during anaphase and pulling them to opposite poles of the cell. In the absence of centrioles, the microtubule-nucleating material is dispersed within the cytoplasm, astral microtubules and kinetochore microtubules do not form properly, and mitosis does not proceed in the appropriate manner.
- **Polar microtubules** originate from the two MTOCs located at opposite poles of the cell; as these polar microtubules elongate, they meet at the center of the cell. In this manner, they ensure that the two MTOCs maintain their respective locations at opposite poles of the cell and do not migrate toward each other.

Prometaphase

Prometaphase begins when the nuclear envelope disappears.

Prometaphase begins as the nuclear lamins are phosphorylated, resulting in the breakdown and disappearance of the nuclear envelope. During this phase, the chromosomes are arranged randomly throughout the cytoplasm; each chromosome is composed of two sister chromatids held to each other by a complex of proteins, known as **cohesins** and **condensins**. Microtubules that become attached to the kinetochores are known as **kinetochore microtubules**, whereas microtubules that do not become incorporated into the spindle apparatus are called **polar microtubules**.

Metaphase

Metaphase begins as the newly duplicated chromosomes align themselves on the equator of the mitotic spindle.

During **metaphase**, the chromosomes become maximally condensed and are lined up at the equator of the mitotic spindle (**metaphase plate** configuration). Each chromatid parallels the equator, and kinetochore microtubules are attached to their kinetochore, radiating to the spindle pole. Sister chromatids must be maintained in close proximity as the chromosome condenses and aligns on the metaphase mitotic spindle.

Anaphase

During anaphase, the sister chromatids separate and begin to migrate to opposite poles of the cell, and a cleavage furrow begins to develop.

Anaphase begins when the cohesion proteins located between the sister chromatids disappear; the sister chromatids, located at the equator of the metaphase plate, separate and begin their migration toward the opposite poles of the mitotic spindle. The spindle/kinetochore attachment site leads the way, with the arms of the chromatids simply trailing, contributing nothing to the migration or its pathway.

It has been postulated that the observed movement of the chromatids toward the pole in anaphase may be the result of shortening of the microtubules via depolymerization at the kinetochore end. This, coupled with the discovery of dynein associated with the kinetochore, may be analogous to vesicle transport along microtubules. In **late anaphase**, a cleavage furrow begins to form at the plasmalemma, indicating the region where the cell will be divided during cytokinesis.

Telophase

Telophase, the terminal phase of mitosis, is characterized by cytokinesis, reconstitution of the nucleus and nuclear envelope, disappearance of the mitotic spindle apparatus, and unwinding of the chromosomes into chromatin.

At **telophase**, each set of chromosomes has reached its respective pole, the nuclear lamins are dephosphorylated, and the nuclear envelope is reconstituted. The chromosomes uncoil and become organized into heterochromatin and euchromatin of the interphase cell. The nucleolus is developed from the **nucleolar organizing regions** on each of five pairs of chromosomes.

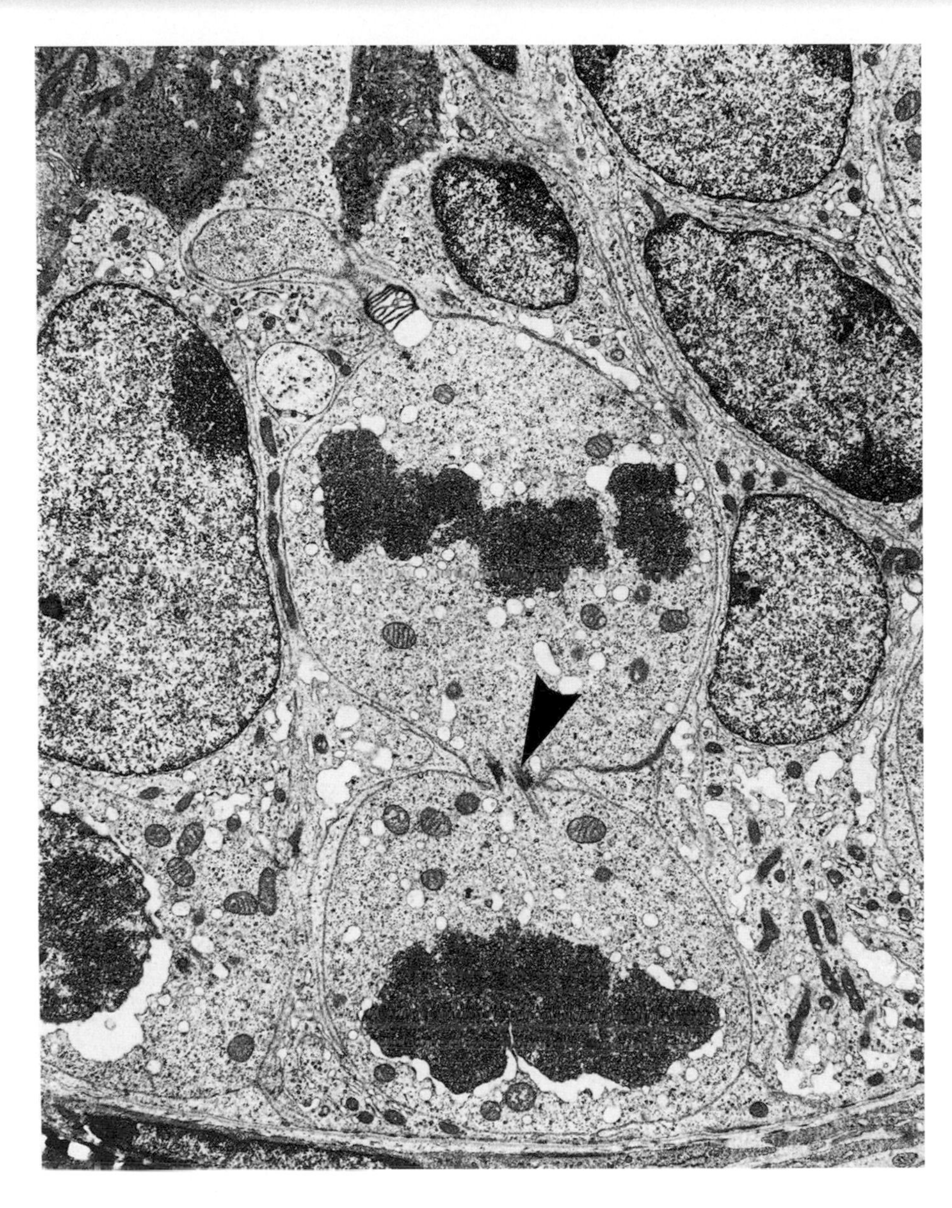

Fig. 3.19 Cytokinesis. Electron micrograph (×8092). A spermatogonium in late telophase demonstrating the forming midbody *(arrowhead)*. The chromosomes in the daughter nuclei are beginning to uncoil. From Miething A. Intercellular bridges between germ cells in the immature golden hamster testis: Evidence for clonal and nonclonal mode of proliferation. *Cell Tissue Res.* 1990;262:559–567.

CYTOKINESIS

Cytokinesis is the division of the cytoplasm into two equal parts during mitosis.

The cleavage furrow continues to deepen until only the **midbody**, a small bridge of cytoplasm, and remaining polar microtubules connect the two daughter cells (Fig. 3.19). The polar microtubules are surrounded by a **contractile ring**, which lies just inside the plasma membrane. The contractile ring is composed of **actin** and **myosin filaments** attached to the plasma membrane. Constriction of the ring is followed by depolymerization of the remaining polar microtubules separating the two daughter cells. During separation of the daughter cells and shortly thereafter, the elements of the contractile ring and the remaining microtubules of the mitotic apparatus are disassembled, concluding cytokinesis.

Each daughter cell resulting from mitosis is identical in every respect, including the entire genome, and each daughter cell possesses a diploid (2n) number of chromosomes.

Clinical Correlations

A more complete understanding of mitosis and the cell cycle has greatly aided cancer chemotherapy, making it possible to use drugs at a time when the cells are in a particular stage of the cell cycle. For example, ***vincristine*** *and similar drugs disrupt the mitotic spindle, arresting the cell in mitosis.* ***Colchicine****, another plant alkaloid that produces the same effect, has been used extensively in studies of individual chromosomes and karyotyping.* ***Methotrexate****, which inhibits purine synthesis, and* ***5-fluorouracil****, which inhibits pyrimidine synthesis, both halt the cell cycle in the S phase, preventing cell division; both are common chemotherapy agents.*

Oncogenes *are mutated forms of normal genes called proto-oncogenes, which code for proteins that control cell division. Oncogenes may result from a viral infection or random genetic accidents. When present in a cell, oncogenes dominate genes over the normal proto-oncogene alleles, causing unregulated cell division and proliferation. Examples of cancer cells arising from oncogenes include* ***bladder cancer*** *and* ***acute myelogenous leukemia****.*

MEIOSIS

Meiosis is a special type of cell division resulting in the formation of gametes, cells whose chromosome number is reduced from the diploid (2n) to the haploid (1n) number.

Meiosis is a specialized type of cell division that results in the formation of germ cells—the **gametes** ova and spermatozoa. This process has two crucial results:

1. The number of chromosomes is reduced from the **diploid** (**2n**) to the **haploid** (**1n**) number, ensuring that each gamete carries the haploid amount of DNA and the haploid number of chromosomes.
2. **Recombination** of genes promotes genetic variability and diversity of the gene pool.

Meiosis is divided into two separate events:

Meiosis I, the **reductional division** (first event). Homologous pairs of chromosomes line up, members of each pair separate and go to opposite poles and the cell divides; thus, each daughter cell receives half the number of chromosomes (haploid number).

Meiosis II, the **equatorial division** (second event). The two **sister chromatids** of each chromosome are separated, as in mitosis, followed by migration of the chromatids to opposite poles and the formation of two daughter cells. These two events produce four cells, each with the haploid number of chromosomes and haploid DNA content.

Meiosis I

Meiosis I (reductional division) separates the homologous pairs of chromosomes, thus reducing the number from diploid (2n) to haploid (1n).

Meiosis begins at the conclusion of interphase in the cell cycle. In gametogenesis, when the germ cells are in the **S phase** of the cell cycle preceding meiosis, the amount of DNA is doubled to **4n**, whereas the chromosome number remains at **2n** (46 chromosomes). Meiosis I proceeds as outlined in Fig. 3.20.

Prophase I

Prophase I, the commencement of meiosis, begins after the DNA has been doubled to 4n in the S phase.

Prophase of meiosis I takes a long time and is subdivided into the following five phases:

1. *Leptotene.* Individual chromosomes, composed of two chromatids joined at the centromere, begin to condense, forming long strands in the nucleus.
2. *Zygotene.* Homologous pairs of chromosomes approximate each other, lining up in register (gene locus to gene locus), and make synapses via the **synaptonemal complex**, forming a tetrad.
3. *Pachytene.* Chromosomes continue to condense, becoming thicker and shorter; **chiasmata** (crossing over sites) are formed as random exchange of genetic material occurs between homologous chromosomes.
4. *Diplotene.* Chromosomes continue to condense; as they separate, chiasmata are revealed.
5. *Diakinesis.* Chromosomes condense maximally and the nucleolus disappears, as does the nuclear envelope, freeing the chromosomes into the cytoplasm.

Metaphase I

Metaphase I is characterized by homologous pairs of chromosomes, each composed of two chromatids, lining up on the equatorial plate of the meiotic spindle.

During **metaphase I**, homologous chromosomes align as pairs on the equatorial plate of the spindle apparatus in random order, ensuring a subsequent reshuffling of the maternal and paternal chromosomes. Kinetochore microtubules become attached to the kinetochores of the chromosomes, but the four sister chromatids are attached to each other.

Anaphase I

Anaphase I is evident when the homologous pairs of chromosomes begin to pull apart, commencing their migrations to opposite poles of the cell.

In **anaphase I**, homologous chromosomes migrate away from each other, going to opposite poles. Unlike in mitotic anaphase,

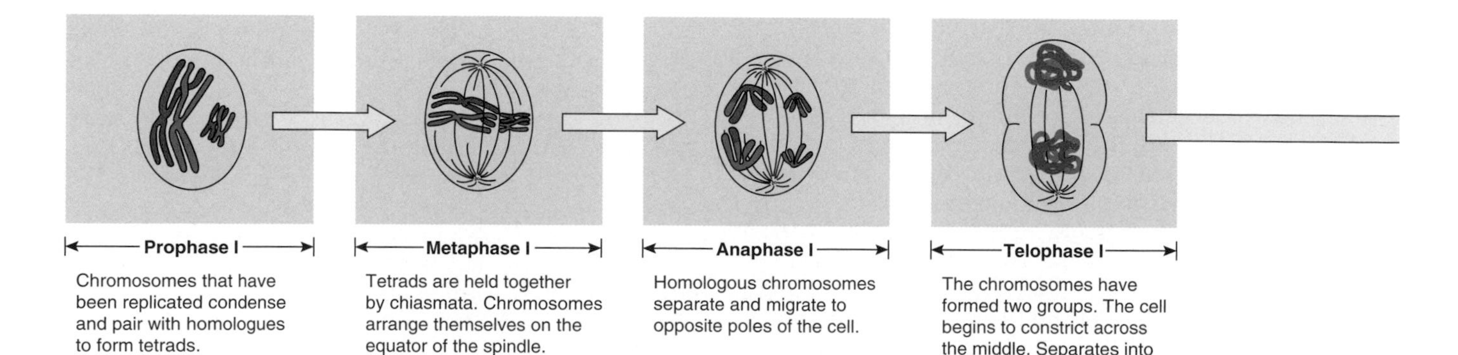

Fig. 3.20 Stages of meiosis. Schematic presentation of the events in meiosis in an idealized cell containing a diploid (2n) number of 4 chromosomes.

in which the sister chromatids are separated from each other, in meiosis the four sister chromatids are separated to form two pairs of sister chromatids. Each pair of sister chromatids is pulled to opposing poles of the cell.

Telophase I

During telophase I, the migrating chromosomes, each consisting of two chromatids, reach opposite poles.

Telophase I is similar to telophase of mitosis. The chromosomes reach the opposing poles, nuclei are re-formed, and cytokinesis occurs, giving rise to two daughter cells. Each cell possesses 23 chromosomes, the haploid (**1n**) number. However, because each chromosome is composed of two sister chromatids, the DNA content is still diploid. Each of the two newly formed daughter cells enters meiosis II.

Meiosis II

Meiosis II (equatorial division) occurs without DNA synthesis and proceeds rapidly through four phases and cytokinesis to form the four daughter cells from the original diploid germ cell, each with the haploid chromosome number.

The **equatorial division** is not preceded by an **S** phase. It is very similar to mitosis and is subdivided into **prophase II, metaphase II**, **anaphase II**, **telophase II,** and **cytokinesis** (see Fig. 3.20). The chromosomes line up at the equator; the kinetochores attach to kinetochore microtubules, followed by the now separated sister chromatids migrating to opposite poles, and cytokinesis divides each of the *two* cells, giving a total of four daughter cells from the original diploid germ cell. Each of the four cells contains a haploid amount of DNA content and a haploid chromosome number.

Unlike the daughter cells resulting from mitosis, each of which contains the diploid number of chromosomes and is an identical copy of the other, the four cells resulting from meiosis contain the haploid number of chromosomes and are genetically distinct because of reshuffling of the chromosomes and crossing over. Thus, every gamete contains its own unique genetic complement.

Clinical Correlations

Abnormalities in chromosome numbers may occur during meiosis. During meiosis I, when homologous pairs normally separate, **nondisjunction** may occur. Thus, one daughter cell will have both rather than just the one chromosome of the homologous pair, resulting in 24 chromosomes, whereas the other daughter cell will have only 22 chromosomes. At fertilization with a normal gamete (containing 23 chromosomes), the resultant zygote will have either 47 chromosomes (**trisomy**) or 45 chromosomes (**monosomy**). Nondisjunction occurs more frequently with certain chromosomes (i.e., trisomy of chromosomes 8, 9, 13, 18, 21) that produce unique characteristics (e.g., the characteristics of Down syndrome [trisomy 21]).

TABLE 3.4 Histological Signs of Apoptosis Versus Necrosis

Apoptosis	Necrosis
Caspase-induced destruction of cytoskeletal elements results in rounded cells.	Cells become swollen and bleb formation ensues.
Pyknotic nuclei due to chromatin condensation is followed by nuclear fragmentation as a result of DNA degradation (karyorrhexis).	Cellular contents are freely present in the extracellular space.
Blebs form at the cell periphery.	Nuclei become pyknotic and become lysed, a process known as karyolysis.
Cytoplasm becomes condensed and consequently stains darker.	Necrotic cells and their remnants are not phagocytosed.
Cell becomes fragmented into apoptotic bodies that are phagocytosed by macrophages.	The immune system does not react to necrotic tissues.

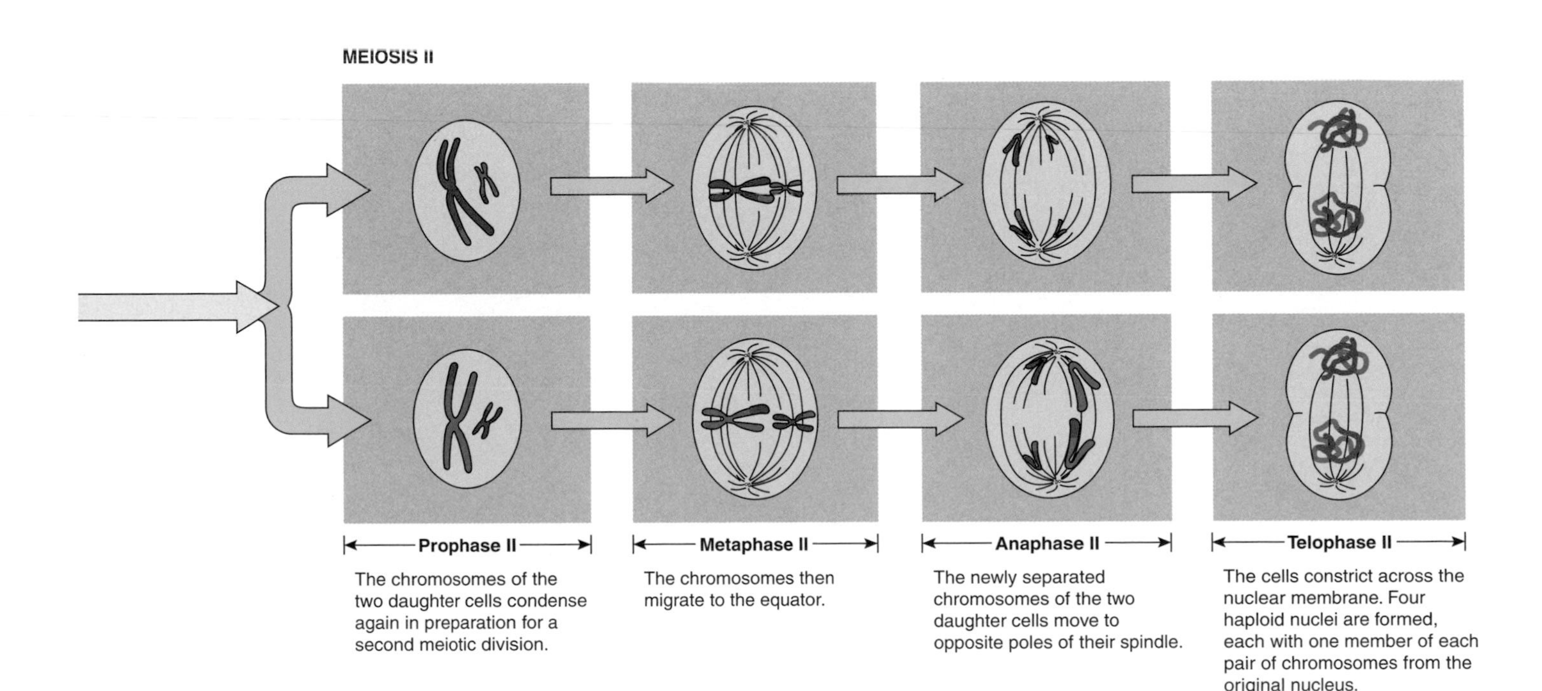

Apoptosis and Necrosis

Cells die as a result of various factors, including (1) acute injury, (2) accidents, (3) lack of a vascular supply, (4) destruction by pathogens or by the immune system, and (5) genetic programming. During embryogenesis, many cells, such as those that would give rise to a tail in the human embryo, are driven into the genetically determined process of dying. This process continues on throughout adult life to establish a balance between cell proliferation and cell death. For example, in the adult human, billions of cells die each hour within the bone marrow and digestive tract to balance cell proliferation in these tissues. Cell death by this means is called **apoptosis (programmed cell death)**. In contrast to apoptosis, during **necrosis** the cell dies in an unregulated fashion because of attack or traumatic injury, causing the cell to rupture. This process exposes its contents to neighboring cells, thus, initiating an inflammatory response. Unlike apoptosis, which has beneficial effects for the organism, necrosis almost always harms the organism and may even cause death (Table 3.4). Because apoptosis has formidable consequences for the cell involved as well as for the organism, it must be carefully regulated, controlled, and monitored.

The process of apoptosis is regulated by a number of highly conserved genes that code for a family of enzymes known as **caspases (cysteine-aspartic acid proteases)**, which degrade regulatory and structural proteins in the nucleus and in the cytoplasm, whereas **necrosis is caspase independent**.

Activation of caspases is induced in at least two ways, the **extrinsic** and **intrinsic pathways**.

- The **extrinsic pathway** is activated when extracellular conditions cause the release of certain cytokines, such as **tumor necrosis factor** (**TNF**), by signaling cells, which then binds to the TNF receptor of the target cell. These TNF receptors are transmembrane proteins whose cytoplasmic aspect binds to adapter molecules to which caspases are bound. Once TNF binds to the extracellular moiety of its receptor, the signal is transduced and caspase becomes activated. The activated caspase is released and, in turn, triggers a cascade of caspases that results in the degradation of chromosomes, nuclear lamins, and cytoskeletal proteins. Finally, the entire cell becomes fragmented. The cell fragments, known as **apoptotic bodies**, are then phagocytosed by macrophages. However, these macrophages do not release cytokines that would initiate an inflammatory response.
- The **intrinsic pathway** can be activated when injury occurs intracellularly; it is essential that the immune system does not become involved and that the inflammatory reaction does not occur. The best understood type of the intrinsic pathway is **mitochondrial apoptosis**, which occurs as a result of damage to the DNA, damage to the endoplasmic reticulum, or other intracellular stresses. Numerous intracellular proteins interact with each other to form a complex, known as the **death-inducing signaling complex** (**DISC**). This activates a pathway that results in the formation of factors that are transported into mitochondria, where they cause the leakage of cytochrome C into the cytosol. Once in the cytosol, cytochrome C activates the apoptotic pathway and the cell enters apoptosis.

Pathological Considerations

See Figs. 3.21 and 3.22.

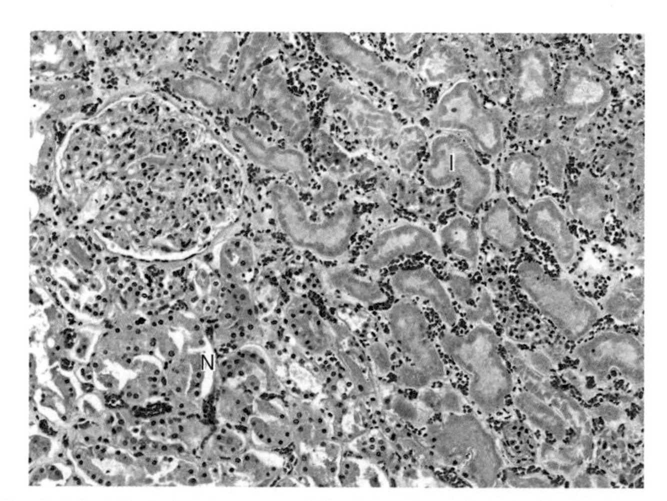

Fig. 3.21 Microscopic image of the boundary of normal kidney cortex (N) on the left side and kidney infarct (I) on the right side. Observe that the necrotic side displays cellular blebs and the absence of nuclei in the cells of the tubules. Note the presence of inflammatory infiltrate in the connective tissue between the tubules. (From Kumar V, Abbas AK, Aster JC. *Robbins and Cotran Pathologic Basis of Disease*. 9th ed. Philadelphia: Elsevier; 2015:43, Fig. 2.11B.)

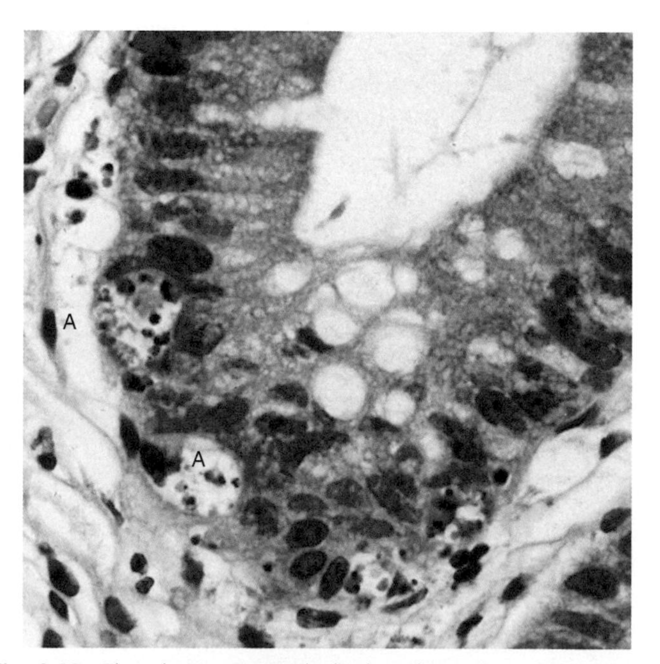

Fig. 3.22 This photomicrograph displays the presence of apoptotic bodies (A) in the colon of a patient who is suffering from graft-versus-host disease. (From Young B, Stewart W, O'Dowd G. *Wheater's Basic Pathology: A Text, Atlas and Review of Histopathology*. 5th ed. Oxford: Churchill Livingstone/Elsevier Limited; 2011:10, Fig. 1.9C.)

4 Extracellular Matrix

Cells of similar structure and function assemble to form structural and functional associations, known as **tissues**, in all multicellular organisms. Groups of these tissues are assembled in various organizational and functional arrangements into **organs**, which carry out functions of the body. The four basic tissue types are **epithelium**, **connective tissue**, **muscle**, and **nervous tissue**. Each of these tissues and their component cells possess specific, defined characteristics and traits, which are detailed in subsequent chapters. These traits include the **cells** themselves and the **extracellular matrix** (**ECM**), a complex of nonliving macromolecules that they manufacture and export into the **extracellular space**, which is the space between cells.

The extent of ECM located in the extracellular space varies with the particular tissue type. Epithelia, for instance, form sheets of cells with only a scant amount of ECM, whereas connective tissue is composed mostly of ECM, with a limited number of cells scattered throughout the matrix. Cells maintain their associations with the ECM by forming specialized junctions that hold them to the surrounding macromolecules. This chapter explores the nature of the ECM and its functions, not only as it relates to the tissues that house it but also its relationship with the cells contained within it. Although it was initially believed that the ECM forms merely the skeletal elements of the tissue in which it resides, it is now known that it has additional functions, such as:

- Modifying the morphology and functions of cells
- Modulating the survival of cells
- Influencing the development of cells
- Regulating the migration of cells
- Directing mitotic activity of the cells
- Forming junctional associations with cells
- Providing a milieu for the immune defense of the body
- Resisting forces of compression and tensile forces acting on tissues

The ECM of connective tissue proper, the most common connective tissue of the body, is composed of a hydrated gel-like **ground substance** with **fibers** embedded in it. Ground substance resists forces of compression, whereas fibers withstand tensile forces. The water of hydration permits the rapid exchange of nutrients and waste products carried by the extracellular fluid as it percolates through the ground substance (Fig. 4.1).

Ground Substance

Ground substance is an amorphous, gel-like material composed of glycosaminoglycans, proteoglycans, and glycoproteins.

Extracellular fluid (derived from the fluid components of blood) percolates through **ground substance**, which is composed of **glycosaminoglycans (GAGs)**, **proteoglycans**, and **cell adhesive glycoproteins**. These three families of macromolecules form various interactions with each other, with fibers, and with the cells of connective tissue and epithelium (Fig. 4.2).

GLYCOSAMINOGLYCANS

GAGs are negatively charged, long, rod-like chains of repeating disaccharides that have the capability of binding large quantities of water.

GAGs are long, inflexible, unbranched polysaccharides composed of chains of repeating disaccharide units. One of the two repeating disaccharides is always an **amino sugar** (*N*-acetylglucosamine or *N*-acetylgalactosamine); the other one is typically a **uronic acid** (iduronic or glucuronic). GAGs are classified into 4 groups, depending on their core disaccharide constituents (Table 4.1).

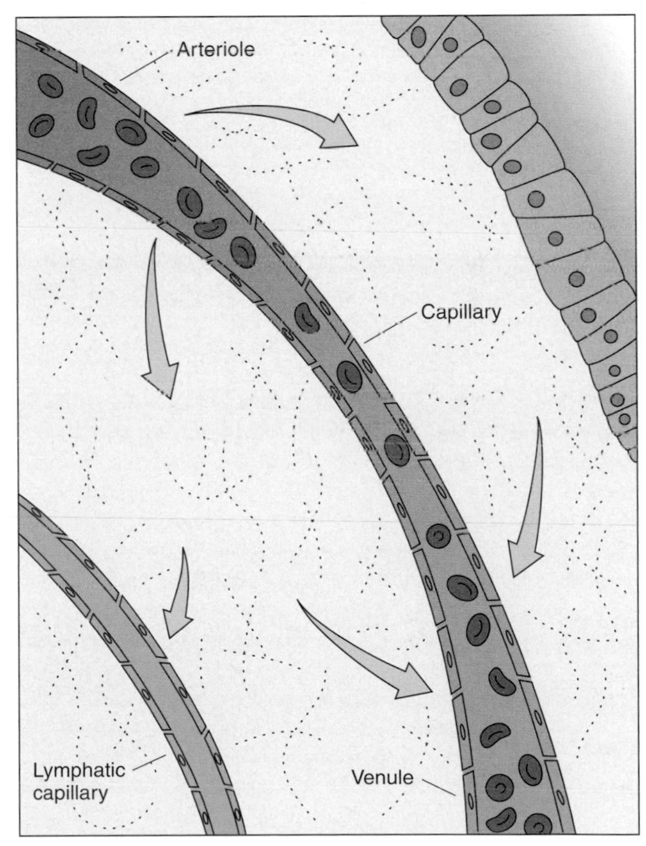

Fig. 4.1 Schematic diagram of extracellular fluid flow. Fluid from the higher-pressure arterial ends of the capillary bed enters the connective tissue spaces and becomes what is known as *extracellular fluid*, which percolates through the ground substance. Some, but not all, of the extracellular fluid then reenters the blood circulatory system at the lower pressure venous end of the capillary bed and venules. The extracellular fluid that did not reenter the blood vascular system will enter the even lower-pressure lymphatic system, which will eventually deliver it to the blood vascular system.

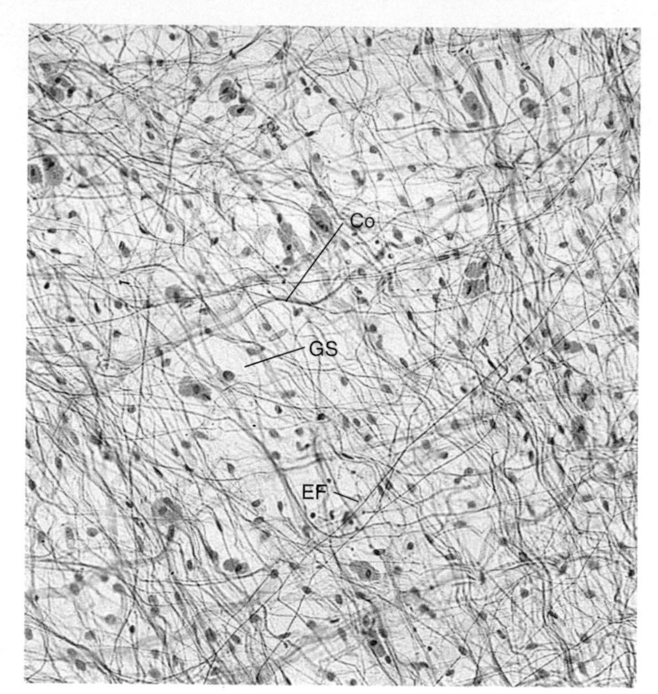

Fig. 4.2 Light micrograph of areolar connective tissue, displaying cells, collagen fibers (Co), elastic fibers (EF), and ground substance (GS). Observe that, in this very loose type of connective tissue, the fibers, although interwoven, present a relatively haphazard arrangement. This permits the stretching of the tissue in any direction. The cells of areolar connective tissue are principally of three types: fibroblast, macrophages, and mast cells. The extensive extracellular spaces are occupied by ground substance composed mainly of glycosaminoglycans and proteoglycans, a large component of which is aggrecan aggregate, a highly hydrated macromolecule. (×132)

Because the amino sugar is usually sulfated and these sugars also have carboxyl groups projecting from them, they are negatively charged and, thus, attract cations, such as sodium (Na^+).

A high-sodium concentration in the ground substance attracts extracellular fluid, which (by hydrating the intercellular matrix) assists in the resistance to forces of compression. As these molecules come into close proximity to each other, their negative charges repel one another, which gives them a slippery texture, as evidenced by the slickness of mucus (such as the mucus of the nasal cavity), vitreous humor of the eye, and synovial fluid.

With the exception of hyaluronic acid, the major GAGs of ECM are sulfated, each consisting of fewer than 300 repeating disaccharide units (see Table 4.1). The sulfated GAGs include **keratan sulfate**, **heparan sulfate**, **heparin**, **chondroitin 4-sulfate**, **chondroitin 6-sulfate**, and **dermatan sulfate**. These GAGs are usually linked covalently to protein molecules to form proteoglycans. The only nonsulfated GAG, **hyaluronic acid** (**hyaluronan**), may have as many as 10,000 repeating disaccharide units. It is a very large macromolecule (up to 10,000 kDa) that does *not* form covalent links to protein molecules (although proteoglycans do become attached to it via link proteins). All GAGs are synthesized within the Golgi apparatus by resident enzymes except for hyaluronic acid, which is synthesized as a free linear polymer at the cytoplasmic face of the plasma membrane by **hyaluronan synthases**. These enzymes are integral membrane proteins that not only catalyze the polymerization but also facilitate the transfer of the newly formed macromolecule into the ECM. It has been suggested that hyaluronic acid also has intracellular functions. Some of the newly released hyaluronic acid is endocytosed by some cells,

TABLE 4.1 Types of Glycosaminoglycans (GAGs)

GAG	Molecular Mass (Da)	Repeating Disaccharides	Covalent Linkage to Protein	Location in Body
GROUP I				
Hyaluronic acid	10^7–10^8	D-glucuronic acid-β-1,3-*N*-acetyl-D-glucosamine	No	Most connective tissue, synovial fluid, cartilage, dermis
GROUP II				
Chondroitin 4-sulfate	10,000–30,000	D-Glucuronic acid-β-1,3-*N*-acetylgalactosamine-4-SO_4	Yes	Cartilage, bone, cornea, blood vessels
Chondroitin 6-sulfate	10,000–30,000	D-Glucuronic acid-β-1,3-*N*-acetylgalactosamine-6-SO_4	Yes	Cartilage, Wharton jelly, blood vessels
Dermatan sulfate	10,000–30,000	L-Iduronic acid-α-1,3- and *N*-acetylglucosamine-4-SO_4	Yes	Heart valves, skin, blood vessels
GROUP III				
Heparan sulfate	15,000–20,000	D-Glucuronic acid-β-1,3-*N*-acetyl-galactosamine L-Iduronic acid-2-SO_4-β-1,3-N-acetyl-D-galactosamine	Yes	Blood vessels, lung, basal lamina
Heparin (90%)	15,000–20,000	L-Iduronic acid-beta-1,4-sulfo-D-Glucosamine-6-SO_4	No	Mast cell granule, liver, lung, skin
(10%)		*D-Glucuronic acid-β-1,4-N*-acetylglucosamine-6-SO_4		
GROUP IV				
Keratan sulfate I and II	10,000–30,000	Galactose-β-1,4-*N*-acetyl-D-glucosamine-6-SO_4	Yes	Cornea (keratan sulfate I), cartilage (keratan sulfate II)

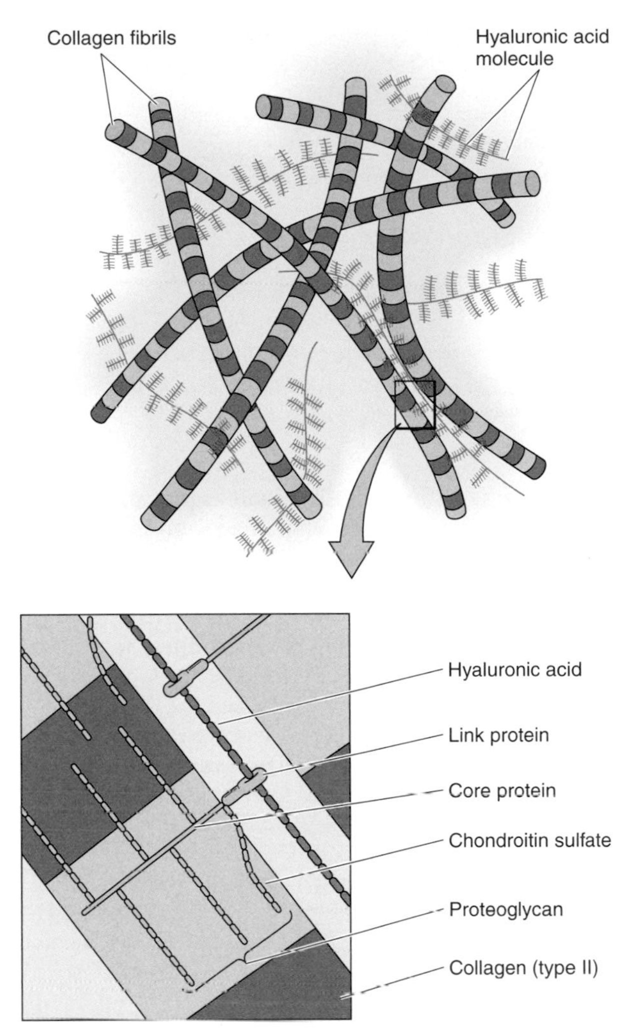

Fig. 4.3 Schematic diagram of the association of aggrecan molecules with collagen fibers. The *inset* displays a higher magnification of the aggrecan molecule, indicating the core protein of the proteoglycan molecule to which glycosaminoglycans are attached. The core protein is attached to the hyaluronic acid by link proteins. (Modified from Fawcett DW. *Bloom and Fawcett A Textbook of Histology.* 11th ed. Philadelphia: WB Saunders; 1986.)

especially during the cell cycle, where it appears to have a role in maintaining space and modulating microtubular activities during metaphase and anaphase stages of mitosis, thus, facilitating chromosomal movements. Additional intracellular roles may involve the directing of intracellular trafficking and influencing intracytoplasmic- and intranuclear-specific kinases.

PROTEOGLYCANS

Proteoglycans constitute a family of macromolecules; each is composed of a protein core to which GAGs are covalently bonded.

When sulfated GAGs form covalent bonds with a protein core, they form a family of macromolecules known as **proteoglycans**, many of which occupy huge domains. These large structures look like a bottle brush, with the protein core resembling the wire stem and the various sulfated GAGs projecting from its surface in three-dimensional space, as do the bristles of the brush (Fig. 4.3).

Proteoglycans range from about 50,000 Da (**decorin** and **betaglycan**) to as large as 3 million Da (**aggrecan**). When the protein cores of proteoglycans, manufactured on the rough endoplasmic reticulum (RER), reach the Golgi apparatus, resident enzymes there covalently bind **bridge tetrasaccharides** (a series of four saccharides) to its serine side chains. Then, the GAG is assembled by the addition of sugars one at a time. Sulfation, catalyzed by sulfotransferases and epimerization (rearrangement of various groups around the carbon atoms of the sugar units), also occurs in the Golgi apparatus.

Many proteoglycans, especially **aggrecan**, a macromolecule present in cartilage and connective tissue proper, attach to hyaluronic acid (see Fig. 4.3). The mode of attachment involves a noncovalent ionic interaction between the sugar groups of the hyaluronic acid and the core protein of the proteoglycan molecule. The connection is reinforced by small **link proteins** that form bonds with both the core protein of aggrecan and the sugar groups of hyaluronic acid. Because hyaluronic acid may be as much as 20 μm in length, the result of this association is an aggrecan composite that occupies a very large volume and may have a molecular mass as large as several hundred million daltons. This immense molecule is responsible for the gel state of the ECM and acts as a barrier to fast diffusion of aqueous deposits, as when one observes the slow disappearance of an aqueous bubble after its subdermal injection.

Clinical Correlations

Many pathogenic bacteria, such as Staphylococcus aureus, secrete ***hyaluronidase****, an enzyme that cleaves hyaluronic acid into numerous small fragments, thus converting the gel state of the ECM to a sol (liquid) state. The consequence of this reaction is to permit the rapid spread of the bacteria through the connective tissue spaces. This is the case in the condition known as* ***necrotizing fasciitis****, when methicillin-resistant Staphylococcus aureus, frequently in combination with other microorganisms, such as Streptococcus pyogenes and/or one of the Clostridium species, enters the connective tissue spaces through a wound and destroys the gel-like state of the connective tissue, permitting rapid spread of the infection. Most of the patients afflicted by necrotizing fasciitis are older, immunosuppressed, or diabetic. Others afflicted have chronic diseases or are abusers of alcohol, tobacco, or drugs. However, about 25% to 30% of patients are healthy and have no predisposing factors in their medical history. If the condition is discovered and diagnosed early enough in the infection process and extensive debridement is performed along with the administration of appropriate antibiotic therapy, the patient's prognosis is very good. Contrary to popular belief, necrotizing fasciitis is not a new disease; its symptoms have been described over 2500 years ago in the fifth century BCE by Hippocrates.*

Functions of Proteoglycans

By occupying a large volume, proteoglycans resist compression and retard the rapid movement of microorganisms and metastatic cells. However, in the same fashion, they facilitate normal cellular locomotion by permitting migrating cells to move into the space that these hydrated macromolecules occupied. Proteoglycans, in association with the basal lamina, form molecular filters of varying pore sizes and charge distributions that selectively screen and retard macromolecules as they pass through them.

TABLE 4.2 The Major Types of Cell Adhesive Glycoproteins

Glycoprotein	Size (Da)	Location	Function
Fibronectin	440,000	Connective tissue	Assists cells in binding to the extracellular matrix
Laminin	950,000	Basal laminae and external laminae	Binds cells to basal lamina and external lamina
Entactin	150,000	Basal laminae and external laminae	Binds laminin to type IV collagen
Tenascin	250,000–300,000	Embryonic connective tissue	Assists cells in binding to the extracellular matrix during their migration
Chondronectin	40,000	Cartilage	Facilitates the binding of cartilage cells to their matrix
Osteonectin	40,000	Bone	Facilitates the binding of bone cells to their matrix; assists in bone matrix mineralization

Proteoglycans also possess binding sites for certain signaling molecules, whereby they can either prevent them from reaching their destinations or they can enhance the function of signaling molecules by concentrating them in a specific location near their targets. Proteoglycans, such as decorins, assist in the formation of collagen fibers; skins of mice that cannot produce decorins or those that produce defective decorins have reduced tensile strength.

Some proteoglycans, such as **syndecans**, instead of being released into the ECM remain attached to the cell membrane. The core proteins of syndecans act as transmembrane proteins and are attached to the actin filaments of the cytoskeleton. Their extracellular moieties bind to components of the ECM, thus permitting the cell to become attached to macromolecular components of the matrix. In addition, syndecans of fibroblasts function as coreceptors because they bind **fibroblast growth factor** and present it to **cell membrane fibroblast growth factor receptors** in their vicinity.

CELL ADHESIVE GLYCOPROTEINS (GLYCOPROTEINS)

Cell adhesive glycoproteins have binding sites for several components of the ECM, as well as for integrin molecules of the cell membrane that facilitate the attachment of cells to the ECM.

Cell adhesive glycoproteins are large macromolecules that have several domains, at least one of which usually binds to cell surface proteins called ***integrins***, one to collagen fibers, and one to proteoglycans. In this manner, adhesive glycoproteins not only assist cells to adhere to the extracellular matrix but also aid in fastening the various components of tissues to each other. The major types of adhesive glycoproteins are fibronectin, laminin, entactin, tenascin, chondronectin, and osteonectin (Table 4.2).

Fibronectin is a large, V-shaped dimer about 440,000 Da in molecular weight composed of two similar polypeptide subunits that are attached to each other at their carboxyl ends by disulfide bonds. Each subunit has binding sites for various extracellular components (e.g., collagen, heparin, heparan sulfate, and hyaluronic acid) and for specific **fibronectin receptors** (**integrins**), of the cell membrane. Fibronectin is produced mainly by connective tissue cells known as **fibroblasts**. The actin components of the cytoskeleton of these cells and their associated myosin counterparts interact, placing tension on their plasmalemma. The integrin molecules relay the tensile forces to the newly exocytosed fibronectin molecules, stretching them just enough to expose hidden binding sites that permit fibronectins to bind to each other, thus forming the fibronectin matrix.

Fibronectin is also present in blood as **plasma fibronectin**, where it facilitates wound healing, phagocytosis, and coagulation. Fibronectin may be temporarily attached to the plasma membrane as **cell-surface fibronectin**. In the embryo, fibronectin marks migratory pathways for cells so that the migrating cells of the developing organism can reach their destination.

Laminin is a very large glycoprotein (950,000 Da) composed of three large polypeptide chains: A, B_1, and B_2. The B chains wrap around the A chain, forming a cross-like pattern, held in position by disulfide bonds at the point where the three chains diverge from each other, thereby forming the two arms and head of the cross-like pattern. There are at least 15 different types of laminins, depending on the amino acid composition of the three chains. The location of laminin is almost strictly limited to basal laminae (and external laminae); therefore, this glycoprotein has binding sites for heparan sulfate, type IV collagen, entactin, and the cell membrane.

Clinical Correlations

*In **nephritic syndrome**, the presence of an **abnormal laminin** results in the inability of the proximal tubules of nephrons from preventing proteins from entering urine. The symptoms of this condition include swollen ankles, feet, and the region of the eyes; reduced appetite; foamy urine; fatigue; and weight gain. Diagnosing of the condition is done by urine and blood tests to look for proteinurea, as well as hypoalbuminemia.*

Entactin, a sulfated glycoprotein (also known as **nidogen**) is about 150,000 Da in weight. It binds to the laminin molecule where the three short arms of that molecule meet each other. Entactin also binds to type IV collagen, thus facilitating the binding of laminin to the collagen meshwork.

Tenascin is a large glycoprotein (250,000–300,000 Da) composed of six polypeptide chains held together by disulfide bonds. It resembles an insect whose six legs project radially from a central body and has binding sites for the transmembrane proteoglycan syndecan and for fibronectin. Tenascin's distribution is usually limited to embryonic tissue, where it marks migratory pathways for specific cells.

Chondronectin and **osteonectin** (about 40,000 Da) are similar to fibronectin. The former has binding sites for type II collagen, chondroitin sulfates, hyaluronic acid, and integrins of chondroblasts and chondrocytes. Osteonectin possesses domains for type I collagen, proteoglycans, and integrins of osteoblasts and osteocytes. In addition, it may facilitate the binding of calcium hydroxyapatite crystals to type I collagen in bone.

Fibers

Collagen and elastic fibers, the two major fibrous proteins of connective tissue, have distinctive biochemical and mechanical properties as a consequence of their structural characteristics.

The fibers of the ECM provide tensile strength and elasticity to this substance. Classical histologists have described three types of fibers on the basis of their morphology and reactivity with histological stains: **collagen**, **reticular**, and **elastic** (see Fig. 4.2). Although it is now known that reticular fibers are type III collagen fibers, many histologists retain the term *reticular fibers* not only for historical reasons but also for convenience when describing organs that possess large quantities of this particular collagen type.

COLLAGEN FIBERS: STRUCTURE AND FUNCTION

Collagen fibers are composed of tropocollagen subunits whose α-chain amino acid sequences permit the classification of collagen into at least 30 different fiber types.

The capability of the ECM to withstand compressive forces is due to the presence of the hydrated matrix formed by GAGs and proteoglycans. Tensile forces are resisted by fibers of the tough, firm, inelastic protein **collagen**. This family of proteins is very abundant, constituting about 25% to 30% of all the proteins in the body. The subunit of the collagen fiber is a protein known as **tropocollagen**, composed of three **α-chains** intertwined about each other. Although at least 30 different types of collagen are known, depending on the amino acid sequence of their α-chains, only 12 are of interest in this textbook. Each α-chain is coded by a separate mRNA. These different collagen types are located in specific regions of the body, where they serve various functions (Table 4.3).

When describing the collagen that forms about 80% of all collagen types—namely, type I collagen (Fig. 4.4)—it forms flexible fibers whose tensile strength is greater than that of stainless steel of comparable diameter. Large collections of type I collagen fibers appear glistening white in the living individual; therefore, collagen fiber bundles are occasionally referred to as *white fibers*. Collagen fibers of connective tissue are usually less than 10 μm in diameter and are colorless when unstained. Stained with hematoxylin and eosin, they appear as long, wavy, pink fiber bundles.

Electron micrographs of type I collagen fibers, stained with heavy metals, display cross-banding at regular intervals of 67 nm, a characteristic property of these fibers. They are formed from parallel aggregates of thinner fibrils 10 to 300 nm in diameter and many micrometers in length (Figs. 4.5 and 4.6). As indicated earlier, collagen fibers are fashioned from a highly regular assembly of **tropocollagen (collagen) molecules**, each about 280 nm long and 1.5 nm in diameter, where each tropocollagen molecule is composed of three polypeptide chains, called ***α-chains***, wrapped around each other in a triple helical configuration.

Each α-chain is composed of approximately 1000 amino acid residues, in which every third amino acid is **glycine** and most of the remaining amino acids are composed of **proline**, **hydroxyproline**, and **hydroxylysine**. Because of its small size, glycine permits the close association of the three α-chains; the hydrogen bonds of hydroxyproline hold the three α-chains together; and hydroxylysine permits the formation of fibrils by binding the tropocollagen molecules to each other. Before discussing further the four different categories of collagen, their properties, and their functions, the synthesis of type I collagen will be detailed.

General Aspects of Collagen Synthesis

The synthesis of all collagen occurs on the RER as individual preprocollagen chains (α-chains).

The synthesis of collagen occurs on the RER where individual **preprocollagen** molecules (Fig. 4.7), α-chains possessing additional amino acid sequences known as ***propeptides***, at both the amino and carboxyl ends, are manufactured. As the mRNA coding for preprocollagen molecule is being translated, the nascent protein enters the cisterna of the RER where it becomes modified. First, the signal sequence directing the molecule to the RER is removed. Then, some of the proline and lysine residues are hydroxylated (by the enzymes peptidyl proline hydroxylase and peptidyl lysine hydroxylase) in a process known as *posttranslational modification* to form hydroxyproline and hydroxylysine, respectively. Subsequently, selected hydroxylysines are glycosylated by the addition of glucose and galactose.

Three preprocollagen molecules align with each other within the RER cisterna and assemble to form a tight helical configuration known as a ***procollagen molecule***. It is believed that the precision of their alignment is directed by the propeptides that do not wrap around each other; the procollagen molecule resembles a tightly wound rope whose two ends are frayed. The propeptides not only function in the precise alignment of the three α-chains but also keep the procollagen molecules soluble, thus preventing their spontaneous aggregation into collagen fibers within the cell.

The procollagen molecules leave the RER via transfer vesicles that transport them to the Golgi apparatus, where they are further modified by the addition of oligosaccharides. The modified procollagen molecules are packaged in the *trans* Golgi network into clathrin-coated vesicles and are immediately ferried out of the cell.

As procollagen enters the extracellular environment, proteolytic enzymes, **procollagen peptidases**, endopeptidases located on the extracellular side of the plasmalemma, cleave the propeptides (removing a portion of the frayed ends) from both amino and carboxyl ends (see Fig. 4.7). The newly formed molecule is shorter (280 nm in length) and is known as a ***tropocollagen* (collagen) *molecule***. Tropocollagen molecules spontaneously self-assemble (see Fig. 4.7) in specific head-to-tail direction into a regularly staggered array, fashioning fibrils that display a 67-nm banding representative of collagen types I, II, III, V, and XI (see Fig. 4.5). The formation and maintenance of the fibrillar structure are augmented by covalent bonds formed between lysine and hydroxylysine residues of neighboring tropocollagen molecules.

As the tropocollagen molecules self-assemble in a three-dimensional array, the spaces between the heads and tails of successive molecules in a single row line up as repeating **gap regions** (every 67 nm), not in adjoining but in neighboring rows (see Figs. 4.5 and 4.7). Similarly, the overlaps of heads and tails in neighboring rows are in register with one another as the **overlap regions**. Heavy-metal stains used in electron microscopy preferentially deposit in the gap regions. Consequently,

TABLE 4.3 Major Types and Characteristics of Collagen

Molecular Type	Molecular Formula	Synthesizing Cells	Function	Location in Body
I (Fibril-forming). Most common of all collagens.	$[\alpha 1(I)]_2\alpha 2(I)$	Fibroblast, osteoblast, odontoblast, cementoblast	Resists tension	Dermis, tendon, ligaments, capsules of organs, bone, dentin, cementum
II (Fibril-forming)	$[\alpha 1(II)]_3$	Chondroblasts	Resists pressure	Hyaline cartilage, elastic cartilage
III (Fibril-forming) Also known as reticular fibers; they are highly glycosylated.	$[\alpha 1(III)]_3$	Fibroblast, reticular cell, smooth muscle cell, hepatocyte	Forms structural framework of spleen, liver, lymph nodes, smooth muscle, adipose tissue	Lymphatic system, spleen, liver, cardiovascular system, lung, skin
IV (Network-forming) They do not display 67-nm periodicity and the α-chains retain their propeptides.	$[\alpha 1(IV)]_2\alpha 2(IV)$	Epithelial cells, muscle cells, Schwann cells	Forms meshwork of the lamina densa of the basal lamina to provide support and filtration	Basal lamina
V (Fibril-forming)	$[\alpha 1(V)]_2\alpha 2(V)$	Fibroblasts, mesenchymal cells	Associated with type I collagen, also with placental ground substance	Dermis, tendon, ligaments, capsules of organs, bone, cementum, placenta
VII (Network-forming) They form dimers that assemble into anchoring fibrils.	$[\alpha 1(VII)]_3$	Epidermal cells	Forms anchoring fibrils that fasten lamina densa to underlying lamina reticularis	Junction of epidermis and dermis
VIII (Network-forming)	$[\alpha 1(VIII)]_2\alpha 2(VIII)$	Endothelial cells, epidermal cells, mast cells	Promotes migration of smooth muscle cells Limits stretching of elastic fibers, thereby protecting them from becoming overstretched	Corneal epithelium basal lamina Associated with elastic fibers
IX (Fibril-associated) They decorate the surface of type II collagen fibers.	$[\alpha 1(IX)\alpha 2(IX)\alpha 3(IX)]$	Epithelial cells	Associated with type II collagen fibers	Cartilage
XI (Fibril-forming) They occupy the center of type I cartilage and stabilize cartilage matrix.	$[\alpha 1(XI)]_2\alpha 2(II)$	Chondrocytes	Associated with type I collagen as well as type II collagen fibers	Collagenous connective tissue; cartilage
XII (Fibril-associated) They decorate the surface of type I collagen fibers.	$[\alpha 1(XII)]_3$	Fibroblasts	Associated with type I collagen fibers	Tendons, ligaments, and aponeuroses
XVII (Collagen-like protein) A transmembrane protein, formerly known as bullous pemphigoid antigen.	$[\alpha 1(XVII)]_3$	Epithelial cells	?	Hemidesmosomes
XVIII (Collagen-like protein) Cleavage of its C-terminal forms endostatin and angiogenesis inhibitor.	$[\alpha 1(XVIII)]_3$	Endothelial cells	?	Basal lamina of endothelial cells

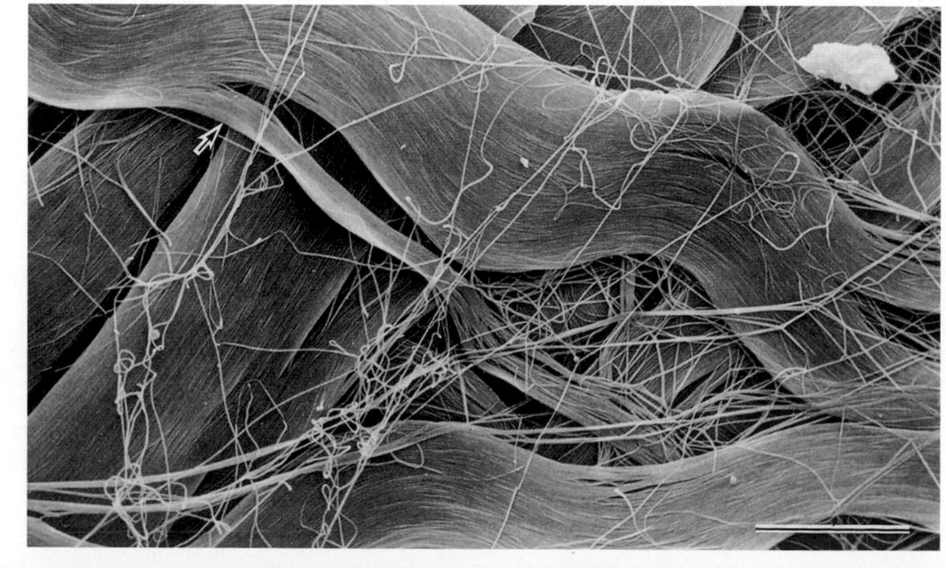

Fig. 4.4 Scanning electron micrograph of collagen fiber bundles from the epineurium of the rat sciatic nerve. Note that the thick fiber bundles are interwoven and arranged in an almost haphazard manner. Also, fiber bundles split into thinner bundles (or thinner bundles coalesce to form larger bundles). Moreover, each of the thick fiber bundles is composed of numerous fine fibrils that run a parallel course in each bundle. (×2034) (From Ushiki T, Ide C. Three-dimensional organization of the collagen fibrils in the rat sciatic nerve as revealed by transmission and scanning electron microscopy. *Cell Tissue Res.* 1990;260:175–184.)

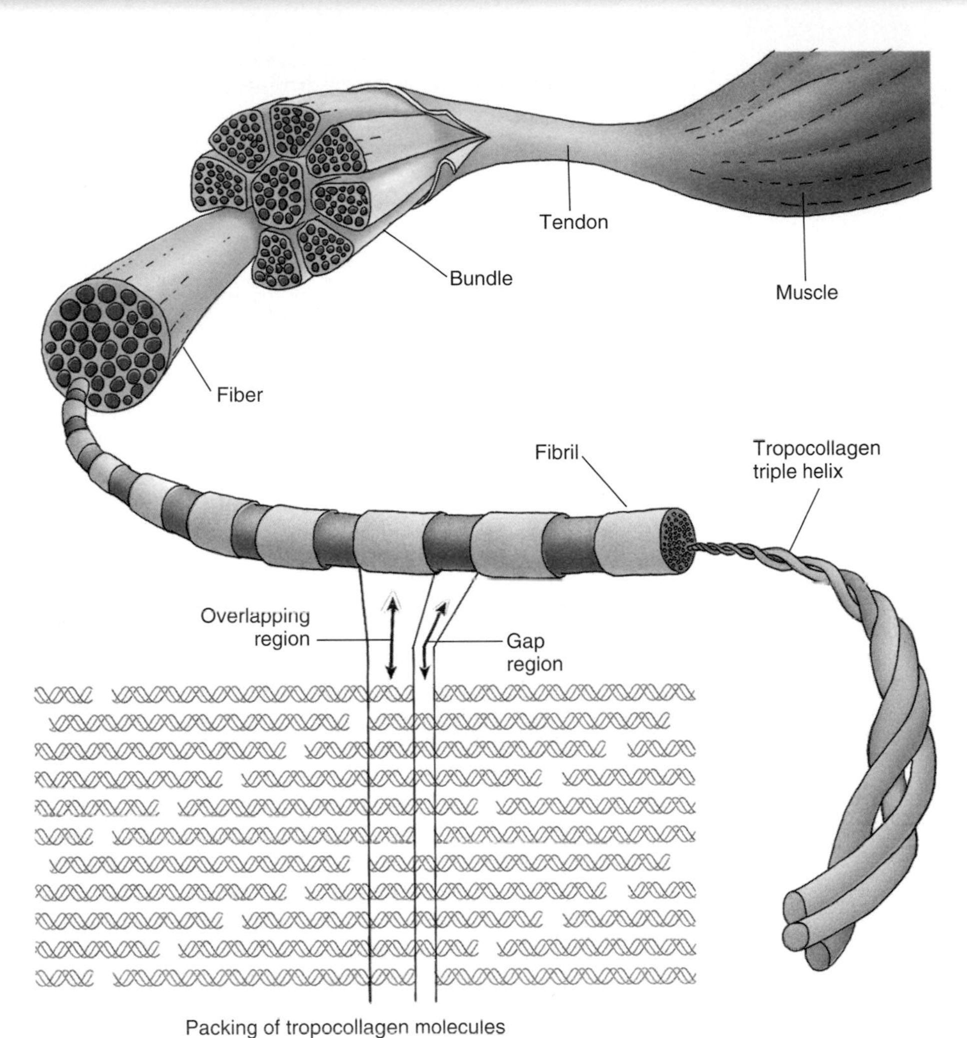

Fig. 4.5 Schematic representation of the components of a collagen fiber. The ordered arrangement of the tropocollagen molecules gives rise to the gap and overlap regions, responsible for the 67-nm cross-banding of type I collagen. The gap region is the area between the head of one and the tail of the next tropocollagen molecule. The overlap region is where the tail of one tropocollagen molecule overlaps the tail of a tropocollagen molecule in the row above or below that tropocollagen. In three dimensions, the overlap region coincides with numerous other overlap regions, and the gap regions coincide with numerous other gap regions. The heavy metals that are used in electron microscopy precipitate into the gap regions; therefore, the large number of these coinciding gaps are filled with heavy-metal precipitates and are visible as the 67-nm cross-banding. Type I collagen is composed of two identical α1(I) chains *(blue)* and one α2(I) chain *(pink)*.

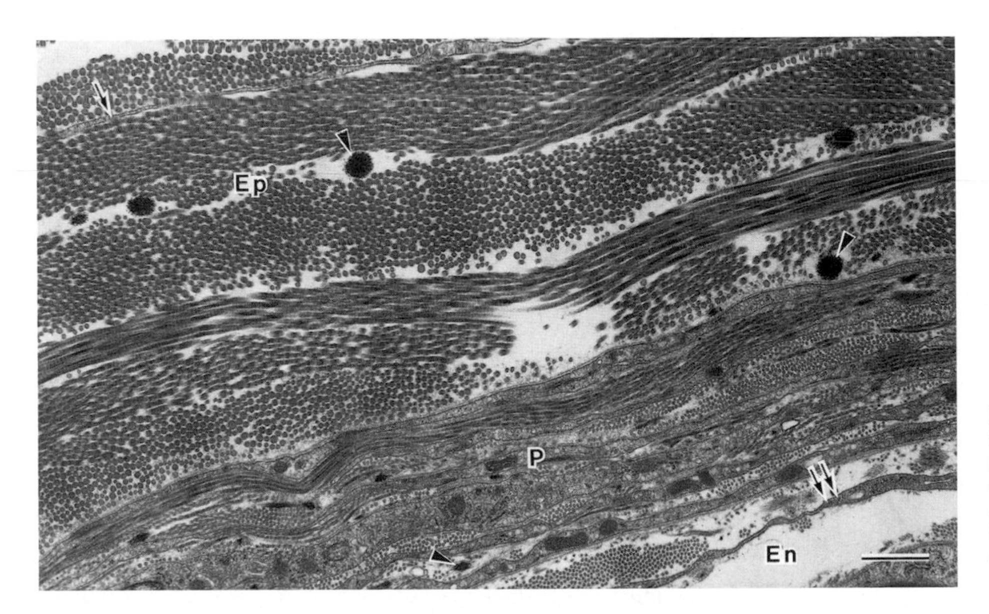

Fig. 4.6 Electron micrograph of collagen fibers from the perineurium of the rat sciatic nerve (×22463). En, Endoneurium; Ep, epineurium; P, perineurium. (From Ushiki T, Ide C. Three-dimensional organization of the collagen fibrils in the rat sciatic nerve, as revealed by transmission and scanning electron microscopy. *Cell Tissue Res.* 1990;260:175–184.)

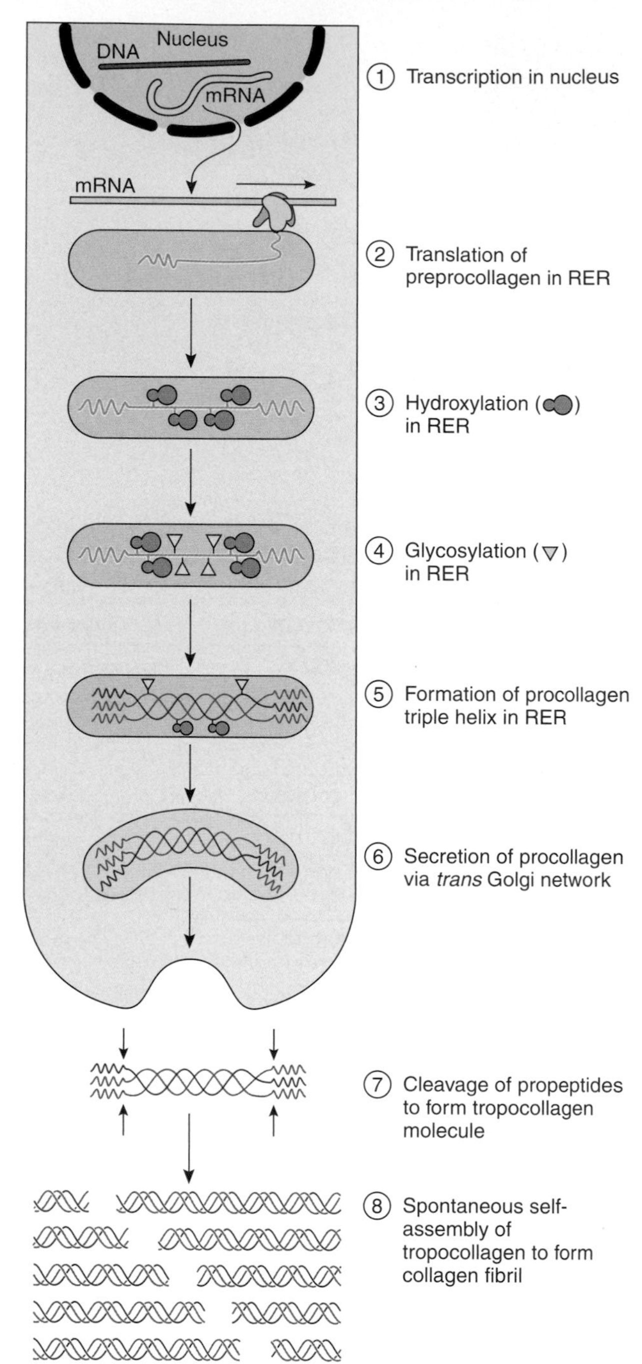

Fig. 4.7 Schematic diagram of the sequence of events in the synthesis of type I collagen. Messenger RNA leaves the nucleus and attracts small and large subunits of ribosomes. As translation begins, the polysome complex translocates to the rough endoplasmic reticulum (RER), and the nascent α-chains enter the lumen of the RER. Within the lumen, some proline and lysine residues of the α-chains are hydroxylated, and the preprocollagen molecule is also glycosylated. Three α-chains form a helical configuration, and the procollagen triple helix is formed. The procollagen is packaged and transferred to the Golgi complex, where further modification occurs. At the *trans* Golgi network, the procollagen is packaged in clathrin-coated vesicles, and the procollagen is exocytosed. As the procollagen leaves the cell, the membrane-bound enzyme, procollagen peptidase, cleaves the propeptides from both the carboxyl- and the amino-end of procollagen, transforming it into tropocollagen. These newly formed macromolecules self-assemble into collagen fibrils.

viewed in the electron microscope, collagen displays alternating dark and light bands. The dark bands represent the gap regions filled with heavy metal and the light bands represent overlap regions, where the heavy metal cannot be deposited (see Fig. 4.6). The formation of some of the collagen types requires the presence of other collagens, such as type XI, which forms the core of type I collagen.

The alignment of the collagen fibrils and fiber bundles is determined by the cells that synthesize them. The procollagen is released into folds and furrows of the plasmalemma, which act as molds that arrange the forming fibrils in the proper direction. The fibril orientation is further enhanced as the cells tug on the fibrils and physically drag them to fit the required pattern.

Fibrillar structure is absent in **types IV** and **VII collagen** because the propeptides are not removed from the procollagen molecule. Its procollagen molecules assemble into dimers, which then form a felt-like meshwork.

Clinical Correlations

Hydroxylation of proline residues requires the presence of vitamin C. In individuals with a deficiency of this vitamin, the α-chains of the tropocollagen molecules are unable to form stable helices, and the tropocollagen molecules are incapable of aggregating into fibrils. This condition, known as ***scurvy****, first affects connective tissues with high turnover of collagen, such as the periodontal ligament and gingiva (Fig. 4.8). Because these two structures are responsible for maintaining teeth in their sockets, the symptoms of scurvy include bleeding gums and loose teeth. If the vitamin C deficiency is prolonged, other sites are also affected. These symptoms may be alleviated by eating foods rich in vitamin C.*

Types of Collagen

The 30 types of collagen may be placed into at least four categories: fibril-forming, fibril-associated, network-forming, and transmembrane collagens.

The 30 types of collagen fibers are classified into four categories: fibril-forming, fibril-associated, network-forming, and transmembrane collagens. The last category is also known as *collagen-like proteins*.

1. **Fibril-forming collagens**, whose synthesis was just described, are types I, II, III, V, and XI.

Type I collagen is the most common, constituting approximately 80% of all collagens in the body. It is located in the dermis of the skin, capsules of organs, matrix of bone, ligaments, tendons, and fibrocartilage. It functions to resist tensile forces and connects muscle to bone via tendons, and bone to bone via ligaments. Type I collagen has a core of type XI collagen and types V and XII collagens are incorporated into its fibrillar structure during its synthesis. **Type II collagen** is located in the ECM of hyaline and elastic cartilage and also functions in resisting tension. During the formation of type II collagen, type IX collagen fibers augmented with chondroitin sulfate are incorporated into its fibrillar structure. **Type III collagen** was known as reticular fiber but is a fibril-forming collagen type that forms the structural framework of organs such as the liver, lymph nodes, spleen, lung, and scaffolding of tissues, such as muscle and adipose tissue. **Type V collagen** is prevalent in the embryo and also assists in the development of types I and III collagens by coassembling with both.

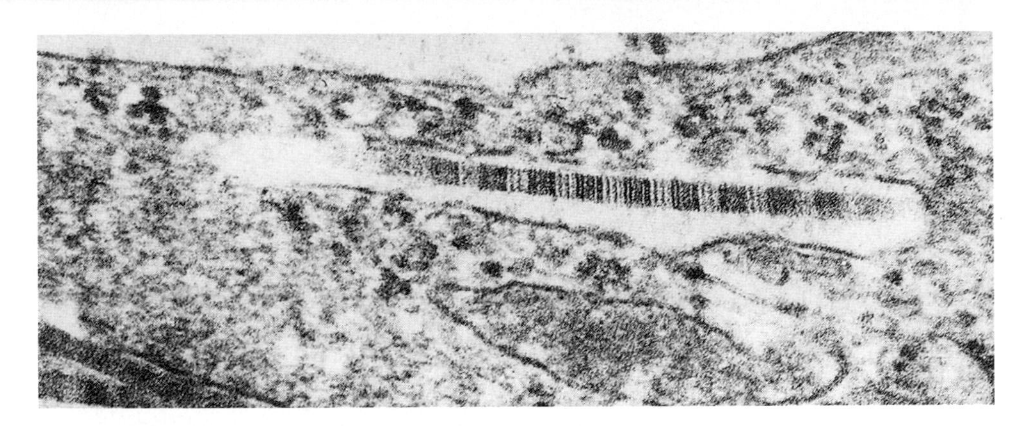

Fig. 4.8 Degradation of type I collagen by fibroblasts. Collagen turnover is relatively slow in some regions of the body (e.g., bone, where it may be stable for as long as 10 years). In other regions, such as the gingiva and the periodontal ligament, the half-life of collagen may be a matter of weeks or months. Fibroblasts of the gingiva and periodontal ligament are responsible not only for the synthesis but also for the resorption of collagen. (From Ten Cate AR. *Oral Histology: Development, Structure, and Function.* 4th ed. St. Louis: Mosby-Year Book; 1994.)

Clinical Correlations

Deficiency of the enzyme ***lysyl hydroxylase****, as well as in Type V collagen with correlated mutations in the α1(V) and /or α2(V) chains, results in abnormal cross-links among tropocollagen molecules, with the consequent genetic disorder known as* ***Ehlers-Danlos syndrome****. Individuals afflicted with this anomalous condition possess abnormal collagen fibers that result in hypermobile joints and hyperextensive skin. In many instances, the skin of affected patients is readily traumatized, and the patient is subject to dislocation of the affected joints.*

Type XI collagen forms the center core on which type I collagen is assembled and also stabilizes type II collagens of hyaline and elastic cartilages.

2. **Fibril-associated collagens** have been recognized as stabilizing collagens because they form molecular bridges between fibril-forming collagens and components of the ground substance. There are two types of fibril-associated collagens:

Type XII collagen binds to type I collagen of the dermis of the skin and connective tissues of the placenta.

Type IX collagen binds to type II collagens of cartilage.

3. **Network-forming collagens** are formed by epithelial cells and, unlike fibrous collagen types, are not exposed to **procollagen peptidase**, the enzyme that cleaves the telopeptides off the ends of the **procollagen molecules.** Therefore, instead of **tropocollagen molecules** that form the basic units of fibrous collagens, **procollagen** molecules form the basic unit of network-forming collagens. Procollagen units cannot associate to form fibers; instead, they form **dimers** that assemble with other dimers to form an interlocking **network of thin three-dimensional sheets.** There are two types of network-forming collagens:

Type IV collagen forms the sheet-like lamina densa of the basal lamina (and external lamina).

Type VII collagen aggregates in sheaves to form **anchoring fibers** whose function is to attach the basal lamina to the lamina reticularis of the basement membrane.

4. **Transmembrane collagens** (also known as ***collagen-like proteins***) are integral proteins, one of which, **type XVII**, functions in the adherence of the epidermis to the dermis. As such, these transmembrane collagens are components of the hemidesmosomes. There are three other types of transmembrane collagens, types XIII, XXIII, and XXV, whose functions are not as yet understood.

Clinical Correlations

1. *At the end of surgery, the cut surfaces of skin are carefully sutured; usually, a week or so later, the sutures are removed. The tensile strength of the dermis at that point is only about 10% that of normal skin. Within the next 4 weeks, the tensile strength increases to about 80% of normal, but in many cases, it never reaches 100%. The initial weakness is attributed to the formation of type III collagen during early wound healing. The later improvement in tensile strength is due to scar maturation, when type III collagen is replaced by type I collagen.*
2. *Some individuals, especially blacks, are predisposed to an excessive accumulation of collagen during wound healing. In these patients, the scar forms an elevated growth known as a* ***keloid****.*
3. *Malformation of* ***type XVII*** *collagens, previously known as bullous pemphigoid antigen, results in blistering of the skin and mucous membranes due to incomplete adherence of the epithelium to the underlying connective tissue, a condition known as* ***epidermolysis bullosa****.*
4. *Malformation of* ***types II*** *and* ***XI collagens*** *results in* ***Stickler syndrome****, a genetic condition that causes defects in the formation of bone and connective tissue proper. Depending on the degree of the mutation in the genes coding for types II and XI collagens, as well as additional attributing mutations, the severity of Stickler syndrome may vary from no symptoms at all to serious malformations. These severe symptoms may include oral defects, such as cleft palate, decrease in mandibular size, and enlarged tongue; ocular defects, such as retinal detachment, myopia, glaucoma, and malformed vitreous humor; defects in the auditory apparatus, resulting in partial or complete hearing loss; and early onset arthritis.*

ELASTIC FIBERS

Elastic fibers, unlike collagen, are highly accommodating and may be stretched one and a half times their resting length without breaking. When the force is released, elastic fibers return to their resting length.

The presence of **elastic fibers** in the ECM provides for much of the elasticity of connective tissue (Figs. 4.9 and 4.10; also see Fig. 4.2). In loose connective tissue, the elastic fibers are usually slender, long, and branching, whereas in ligaments and fenestrated sheets, they congregate to form coarse bundles. Thick collections of elastic fibers are found in the ligamentum flava of the vertebral column and in the walls of larger blood vessels; in fact, elastic fibers constitute about 50% of the aorta by dry weight.

Fibroblasts of connective tissue and smooth muscle cells of blood vessels can both manufacture elastic fibers. These fibers are composed of **elastin**, **fibrillin-1**, and **fibulin-5**, as well as **type VIII collagen**.

- **Elastin** is a protein that is rich in glycine, lysine, alanine, valine, and proline residues but has no hydroxylysine. Elastin is derived from a soluble protein precursor, **tropoelastin**, which becomes insoluble owing to the cross-linking of its lysine residues by the enzyme lysyl oxidase. In this manner, the elastin chains that are formed are held together because four lysine molecules, each belonging to a different elastin chain, form covalent bonds with each other to form what are known as ***desmosine cross-links.*** Because desmosine bonds are highly deformable, they impart a high degree of elasticity to elastic fibers; in fact, these fibers may be stretched to about 150% of their resting lengths before breaking. After being stretched, elastic fibers return to their resting length.
- The elastin core of elastic fibers is surrounded by a sheath of **microfibrils**; each microfibril is about 10 nm in diameter and is composed of the glycoprotein **fibrillin-1** (Fig. 4.11). During the synthesis of elastic fibers, the fibrillin-1 molecules are elaborated first and are arranged head to tail in rod-shaped configuration to form a microfibril. A number of microfibrils gather to form a hollow cylinder, and the tropoelastin is deposited in the space surrounded by the microfibrils (Fig. 4.12). The soluble tropoelastin, which forms chemical bonds to fibrillin-1, is converted into **elastin** by the action of lysine oxidase.
- Integrin molecules of cells that synthesize elastic fibers bind to **fibulin-5**, a protein that facilitates the formation of elastic fibers and has an affinity to itself as well as to tropoelastin and fibrillin-1.

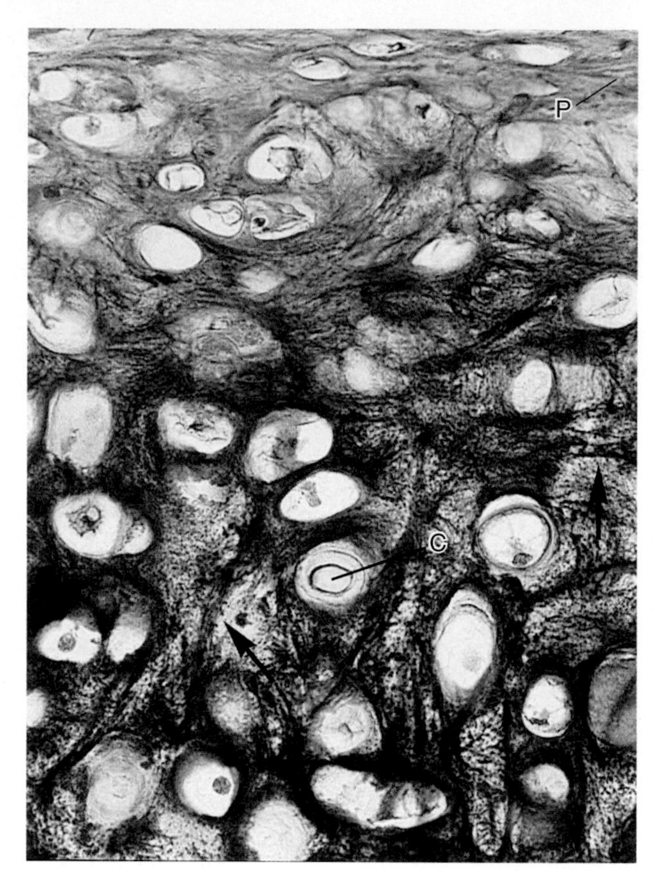

Fig. 4.9 Note the presence of elastic fibers *(arrows)* in the matrix in this photomicrograph of elastic cartilage. The large chondrocytes of elastic cartilage occupy spaces, known as *lacunae*, in the proteoglycan-rich matrix. The large bundles of elastic fibers are clearly evident and appear to be arranged in a haphazard fashion. Observe that the thicker elastic fibers are composed of fine fibrils. C, Chondrocyte; P, perichondrium. (×270)

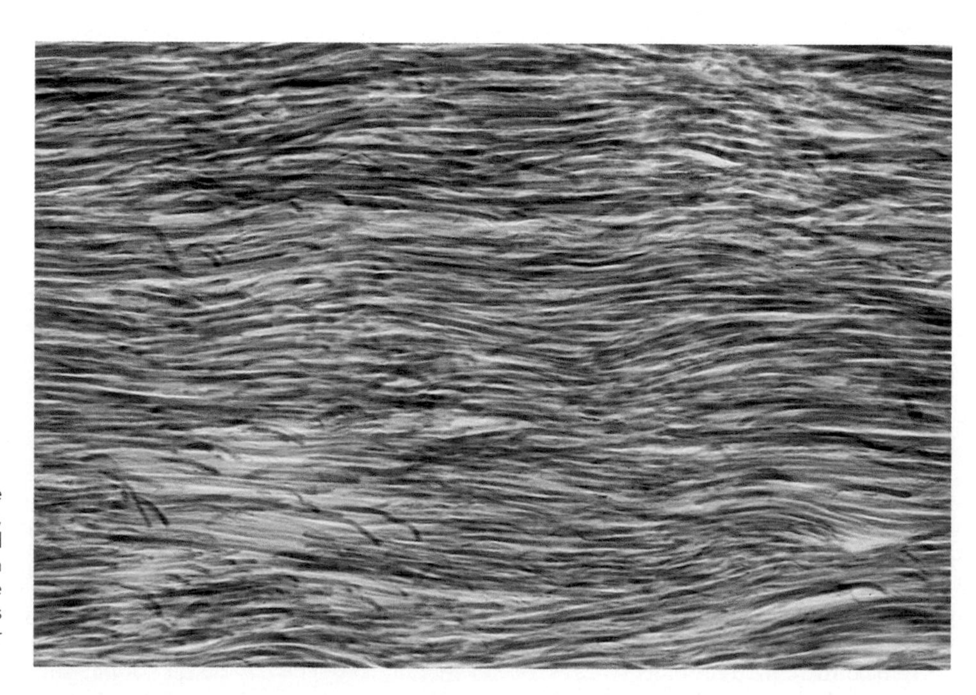

Fig. 4.10 Dense, regular elastic connective tissue. Note that the elastic fibers are short, arranged almost parallel with each other, and their ends are somewhat curled. Unlike collagen fibers of dense regular collagenous connective tissue, where the collagen fibrils and fibers closely parallel each other, elastic fibers appear somewhat misaligned. (×270)

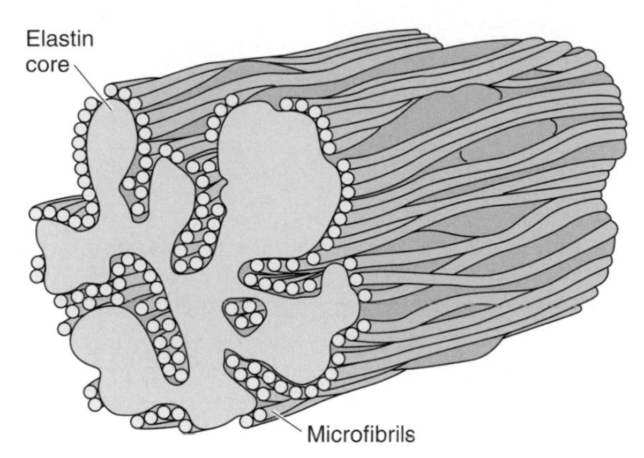

Fig. 4.11 Schematic diagram of elastic fiber. Microfibrils surround the amorphous elastin.

- **Type VIII collagen** has also been demonstrated to form a part of elastic fibers. Because collagen is inelastic, it is believed that type VIII collagen acts to limit the amount of stretching that elastic fibers are permitted to undergo.

Clinical Correlations

The integrity of elastic fibers depends on the presence of microfibrils. Patients with ***Marfan syndrome*** *have a defect in the gene on chromosome 15 that codes for fibrillin; therefore, their elastic fibers do not develop normally. People who are severely affected with this condition are predisposed to fatal rupture of the aorta.*

Basement Membrane

The basement membrane of light microscopy is shown by electron microscopy to be composed of the basal lamina and lamina reticularis.

The **basement membrane**, which is well stained by the periodic acid Schiff reaction and by other histological stains that detect GAGs, forms the interface between epithelium and connective tissue as a narrow, acellular region. A structure similar to the basement membrane, the **external lamina**, surrounds smooth and skeletal muscle cells, adipocytes, and Schwann cells.

Viewed by electron microscopy, the basement membrane displays two constituents: the **basal lamina**, a product of epithelial cells, and the **lamina reticularis**, produced by connective tissue cells (Fig. 4.13).

BASAL LAMINA

The basal lamina, a product of the epithelium, has two components: the lamina lucida and the lamina densa.

Electron micrographs of the **basal lamina** display its two regions: the **lamina lucida**, a 50-nm-thick electron-lucent region just beneath the epithelium, and the **lamina densa**, a 50-nm-thick electron-dense region (see Figs 4.13, 4.14, and 4.15).

The **lamina lucida** consists mainly of the extracellular glycoproteins **laminin** and **entactin**, as well as those moieties of **integrins** and **dystroglycans** (i.e., transmembrane laminin

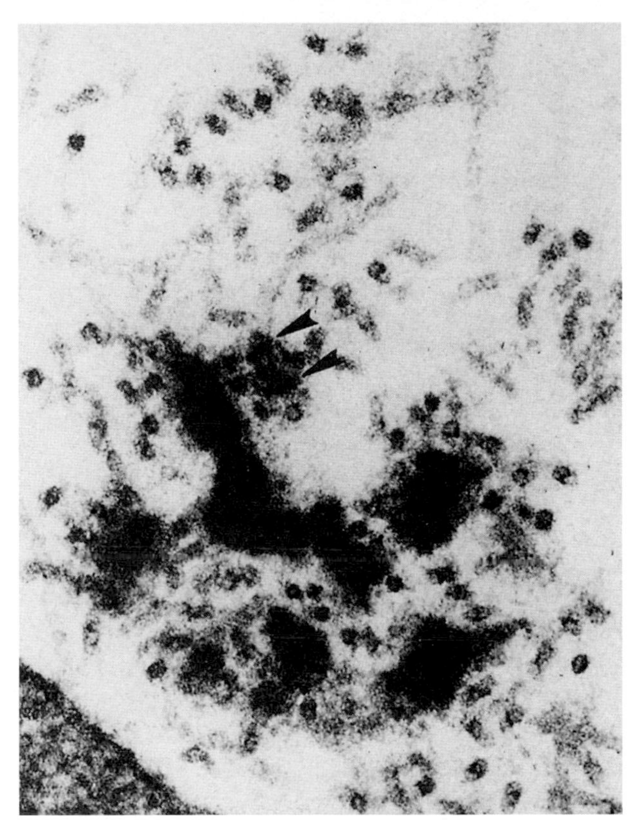

Fig. 4.12 Electron micrograph of elastic fiber development. Note the presence of microfibrils surrounding the amorphous matrix of elastin as if a small space were to be delineated by slats of a picket fence *(arrowheads)*. These fibrillin-containing microfibrils are elaborated and released first. Then, the manufacturing cell, be it a fibroblast of connective tissue proper or smooth muscle cell of a blood vessel, releases elastin into the space enclosed by the microfibrils. (From Fukuda Y, Ferrans VJ, Crystal RG. Development of elastic fibers of nuchal ligament, aorta, and lung of fetal and postnatal sheep: an ultrastructural and electron microscopic immunohistochemical study. *Am J Anat.* 1984;170:597–629. Reprinted with permission of Wiley-Liss, Inc., a subsidiary of John Wiley & Sons, Inc.)

receptors, both discussed later in this chapter) that project from the epithelial cell membrane into the basal lamina. In rapidly frozen tissues, the lamina lucida is frequently absent. This suggests that it may be an artifact of fixation, and the lamina densa may be closer to the integrins and dystroglycans of the basal cell membrane than previously believed.

The **lamina densa** is composed of a type IV collagen, and is coated on both the lamina lucida and lamina reticularis surfaces by the proteoglycan **perlacan**. The **heparan sulfate** side chains projecting from the protein core of perlacan form a polyanion. The lamina reticularis aspect of the lamina densa also possesses **fibronectin**.

Laminin has domains that bind to type IV collagen, heparan sulfate, and the integrins and dystroglycans of the epithelial basal cell membrane, thus anchoring the epithelial cell to the basal lamina. The basal lamina appears to be well anchored to the reticular lamina by several substances, including fibronectin, anchoring fibrils (type VII collagen) and microfibrils (fibrillin-1), all elaborated by fibroblasts of connective tissue (Fig. 4.16).

The basal lamina functions both as a molecular filter and as a flexible, firm support for the overlying epithelium. The filtering aspect is due not only to the type IV collagen, whose

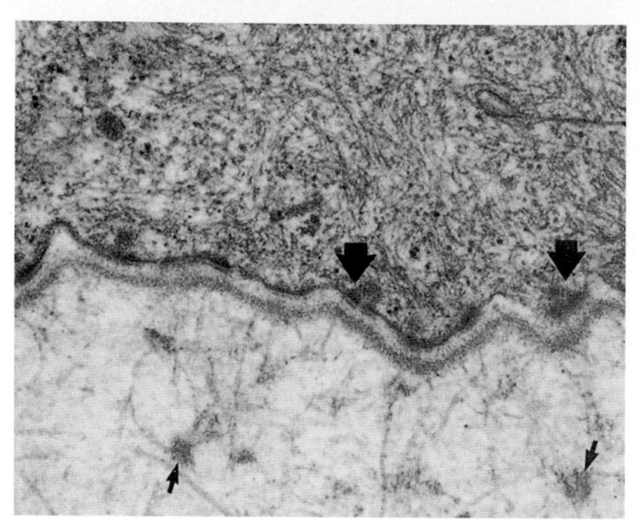

Fig. 4.13 Electron micrograph of the basal lamina of the human cornea. Note the hemidesmosomes *(large arrows)* and the anchoring plaques among the anchoring fibrils *(small arrows)*. Observe that the basal cell membrane is clearly visible and that the plaques of the hemidesmosomes are attached to the cytoplasmic surface of the basal plasmalemma. The dense, amorphous-appearing line that follows the contour of the basal plasma membrane is the lamina densa; the clear area between it and the basal cell membrane is the lamina lucida. These two laminae constitute the epithelially derived basal lamina. The region that is located beneath the lamina densa is the connective tissue–derived lamina reticularis. (×50,000) (From Albert D, Jakobiec FA. *Principles and Practice of Ophthalmology: Basic Sciences*. Philadelphia: WB Saunders; 1994.)

interwoven meshwork forms a physical filter of specific pore sizes, but also to the negative charges of its heparan sulfate constituent, which preferentially restricts the passage of negatively charged molecules. Additional functions of the basal lamina include facilitation of mitotic activity and cell differentiation, modulating cellular metabolism, assisting in the establishment of cell polarity, playing a role in the modification of the arrangement of the integral proteins localized in the basal cell membrane, and acting as a path for cellular migration, as in reepithelialization during wound repair or in the reestablishment of myoneural junctions during regeneration of motor nerves.

Clinical Correlations

*The basement membrane that forms a capsule around the lens of the eye, known as the **lens basement membrane (LBM)**, aids in supporting the lens in its position in the eyeball. During cataract surgery, the cloudy natural lens is replaced by an artificial lens in such a fashion that the lens capsule is undisturbed so that it can now form a supporting element for the artificial lens. In about 30% of the patients, the posterior aspect of the LBM becomes somewhat opaque within a few years after surgery. This posterior capsule opacification (PCO), known also as **secondary cataract formation**, is the result of mitotic activity of the lens epithelial cells that remained after the removal of the opaque, natural lens. Fortunately, a simple office procedure of burning a hole in the postsurgically formed lens epithelial cells using a laser beam alleviates the problem.*

LAMINA RETICULARIS

The lamina reticularis is derived from the connective tissue component and is responsible for affixing the lamina densa to the underlying connective tissue.

The **lamina reticularis** (see Figs. 4.13, 4.14, and 4.16) is manufactured by fibroblasts and is composed of **types III, VII (anchoring fibrils)**, and **XVIII** and a slight amount of **type I collagens**; additionally, a slight amount of **microfibrils** is also present. The lamina reticularis forms the interface between the basal lamina and the underlying connective tissue, and its thickness varies with the amount of frictional force on the overlying epithelium. Thus, it is quite thick in skin and very thin beneath the epithelial lining of the alveolus of the lung; however, in most cases it is about 200 nm in thickness.

Type I and type III collagen fibers of the connective tissue loop into the lamina reticularis, where they interact with and are bound to the microfibrils and anchoring fibrils and type XVIII collagen of the lamina reticularis. Moreover, the basic groups of the collagen fibers form bonds with the acidic groups

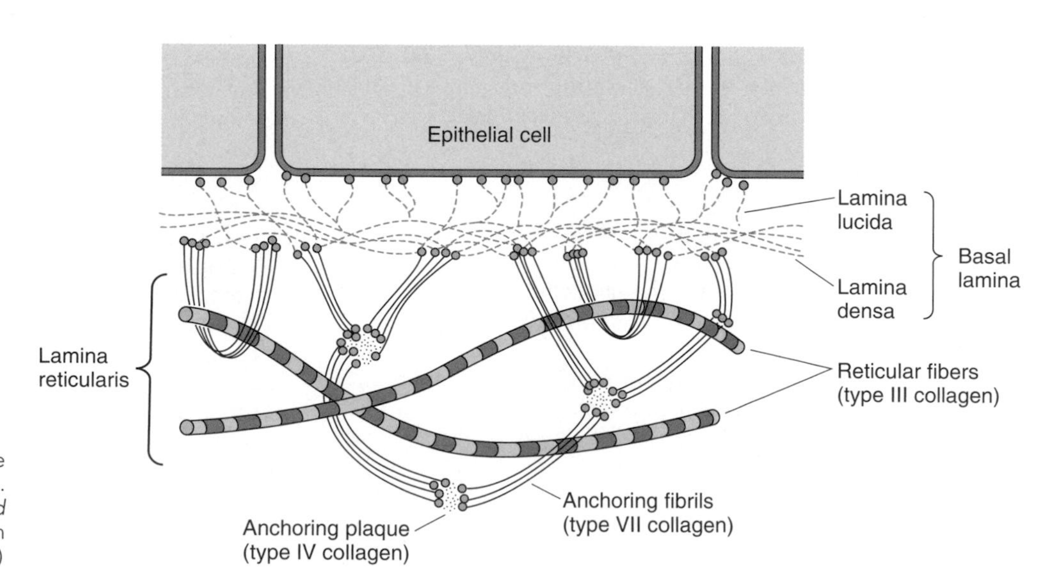

Fig. 4.14 Schematic diagram of the basal lamina and the lamina reticularis. (Modified from Fawcett DW. *Bloom and Fawcett A Textbook of Histology*. 12th ed. New York: Chapman and Hall; 1994.)

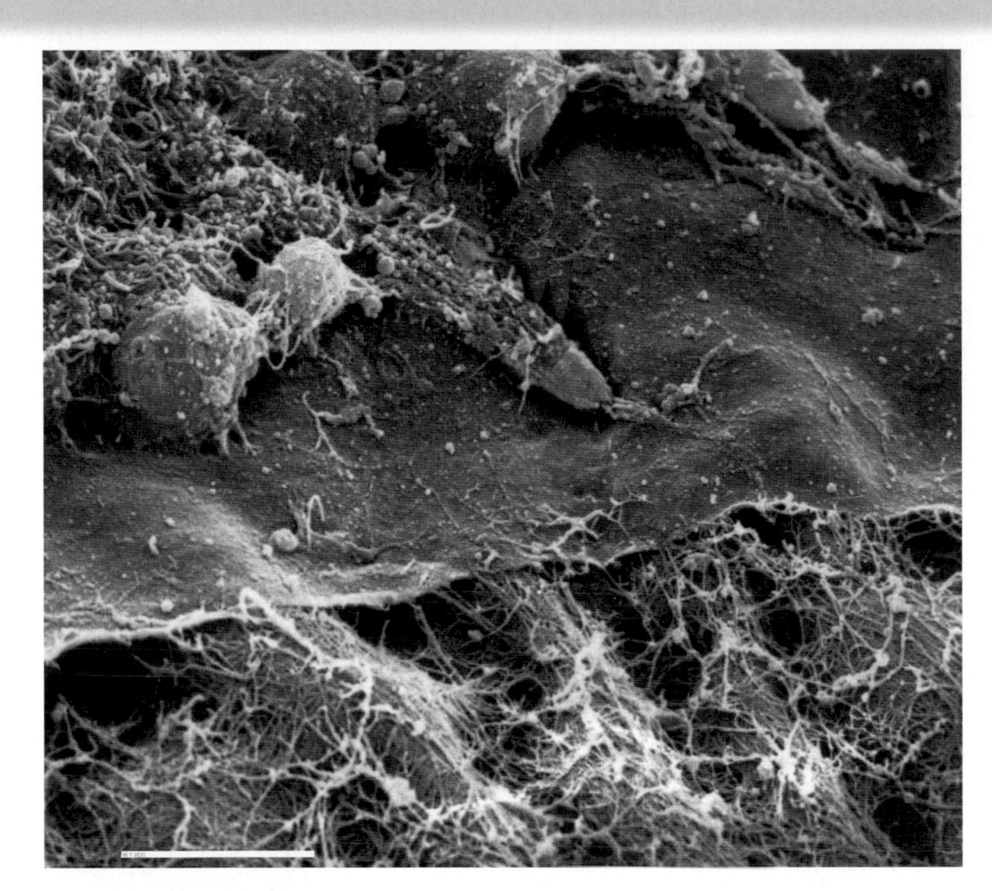

Fig. 4.15 Image from a 6-day chick embryo cornea from which a portion of the epithelium has been removed, exposing epithelial cells on the underlying basement membrane. The membrane itself has been partially removed, revealing the underlying primary corneal stroma composed of orthogonally arrayed collagen fibrils. The *white bar* at the lower left is the 10-μm mark. (Courtesy Robert L. Trelstad.)

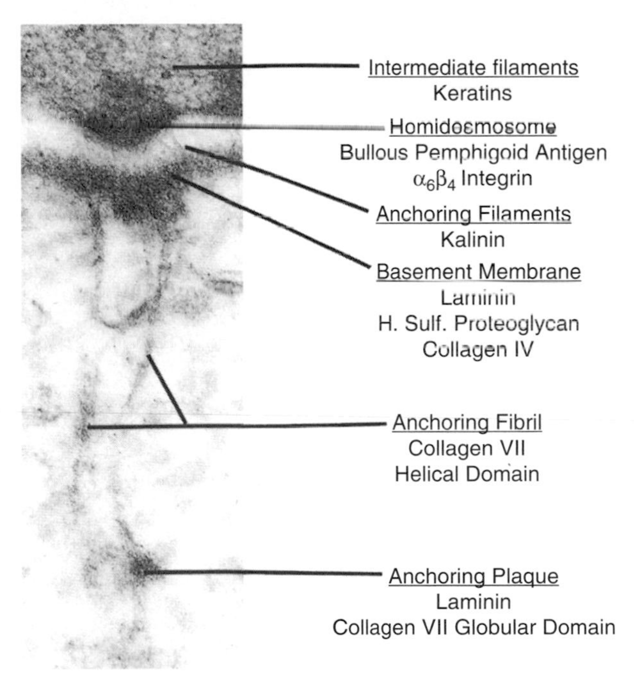

Fig. 4.16 Electron micrograph of the basal lamina of the corneal epithelium. (×165,000) (From Albert D, Jakobiec FA. *Principles and Practice of Ophthalmology: Basic Sciences*. Philadelphia: WB Saunders; 1994.)

of the GAGs of the lamina densa. In addition, collagen-binding domains and GAG domains of fibronectin further assist in anchoring the basal lamina to the lamina reticularis. Thus, the epithelial sheath is bound to the underlying connective tissue by these resilient, flexible, acellular interfaces, the basal lamina and lamina reticularis.

Integrins and Dystroglycans

Integrins and dystroglycans are transmembrane glycoproteins that act as laminin receptors, as well as organizers of basal lamina assembly.

Integrins are transmembrane proteins that are similar to cell membrane receptors in that they form bonds with ligands. However, unlike those of receptors, their cytoplasmic regions are linked to the cytoskeleton and their *ligands* are not signaling molecules but are rather structural members of the ECM, such as collagen, laminin, and fibronectin. Moreover, the association between an integrin and its ligand is much weaker than that between a receptor and its ligand. Integrins are much more numerous than receptors, thus compensating for the bond weakness; simultaneously, they facilitate the migration of cells along the ECM surface.

Integrins are heterodimers (~250,000 Da) composed of **α and β glycoprotein** chains whose carboxyl ends are linked to **talin**, **paxillin**, **vinculin**, and **α-actinin** of the cytoskeleton, which, in turn, form bonds with **actin filaments**. Their amino ends possess binding sites for macromolecules of the ECM (see Chapter 2, Fig. 2.33). Because integrins link the cytoskeleton to the ECM, they are also called ***transmembrane linkers***. The α-chain of the integrin molecule binds Ca^{2+} or Mg^{2+}, divalent cations necessary for the maintenance of proper binding with the ligand. In this fashion, the integrin molecules form a large number of **focal adhesions** (**anchoring junctions**) that help secure the epithelium to the basal lamina.

Many integrins differ in their ligand specificity, cellular distribution, and function. Some are commonly referred to as *receptors* for their ligand (e.g., laminin receptor, fibronectin receptor). Cells can modulate the affinity of their receptor for its ligand by regulating the availability of divalent cations, modifying the conformation of the integrin, or otherwise altering the integrin's affinity for the ligand. In this manner, cells are not locked into a particular position once their integrins bind to the macromolecules of the ECM but can release their integrin–ligand bonds and move away from that particular location.

In addition to their roles in adhesion, integrins function in transducing biochemical signals into intracellular events by activating second messenger system cascades. The versatility of integrins in biochemical transduction is evidenced by their ability to stimulate diverse signaling pathways, including mitogen-activated protein kinase, protein kinase C, and phosphoinositide pathways that lead to activation of the cell cycle, cell differentiation, cytoskeletal reorganization, regulation of gene expression, and even programmed cell death via apoptosis. Frequently, integrins have to be activated by **focal adhesion kinase**, a protein tyrosine kinase; otherwise, they cannot initiate their signaling functions.

Dystroglycans are glycoproteins that are also composed of two subunits, a **transmembrane β-dystroglycan** and an **extracellular α-dystroglycan**. The α-dystroglycan binds to the laminin of the basal lamina, but at different sites than does the integrin molecule. The intracellular moiety of the β-dystroglycan binds to the actin-binding protein **dystrophin**, which, in turn, binds to α-actinin of the cytoskeleton.

Dystroglycans and integrins have significant roles in the assembly of basal laminae because embryos lacking in either or both of these glycoproteins are unable to form normal basal laminae.

Pathological Considerations

See Figs. 4.17 and 4.18.

Clinical Correlations

Individuals with the autosomal recessive disorder ***leukocyte adhesion deficiency*** *are incapable of synthesizing the β-chain of the white blood cell integrins. Their leukocytes are incapable of adhering to the endothelial cells of blood vessels and, thus, cannot migrate to sites of inflammation. Patients with this disease have difficulty in fighting bacterial infections.*

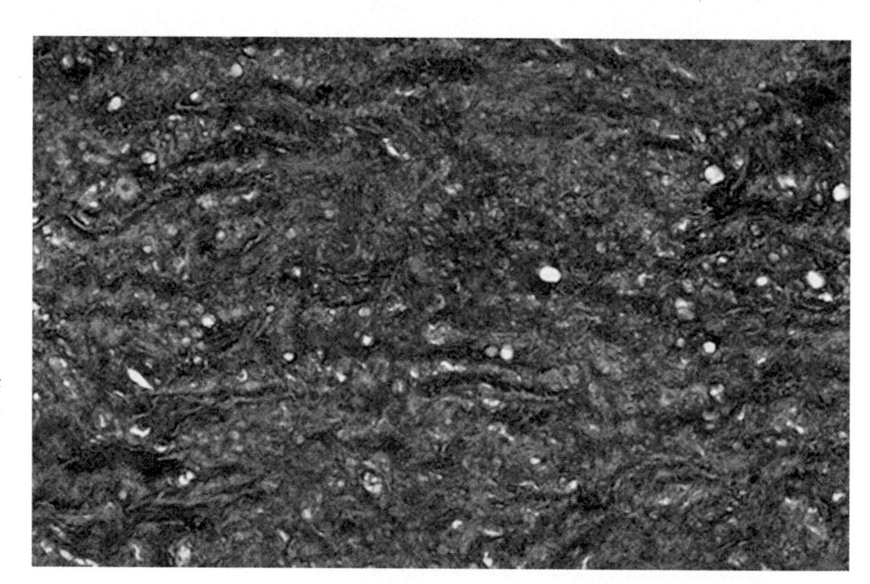

Fig. 4.17 This mucin stain of the aortic media shows cystic medial degeneration. Pink elastic fibers, instead of running in parallel arrays, are seen here to be disrupted by pools of blue ground substance. This is typical for Marfan syndrome affecting connective tissues containing elastin. This causes the connective tissue weakness that explains the propensity for aortic dissection. (From Klatt EC. *Robbins and Cotran: Atlas of Pathology*. 2nd ed. Philadelphia: Elsevier; 2010.)

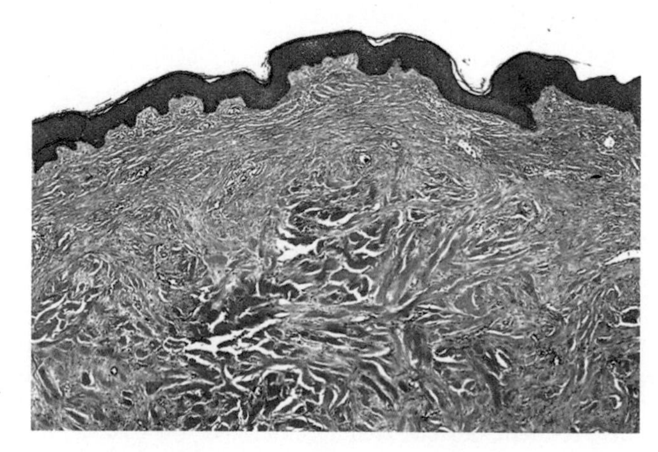

Fig. 4.18 Microscopic image of a keloid. Note the thick collagen deposition in the dermis. (From Kumar V, et al. *Robbins and Cotran Pathologic Basis of Disease*. 9th ed. Philadelphia: Elsevier; 2015:110.)

5 Epithelium and Glands

Epithelium

Epithelial tissue forms two distinct structural and functional forms: sheets of contiguous cells (**epithelia**), which cover the external and internal surfaces of the body, and clusters of cells (**glands**), which originate from invaginated epithelial cells.

All three germ layers give rise to epithelia. The oral and nasal mucosae, cornea, epidermis of skin, and glands of the skin and mammary glands are derived from **ectoderm**; liver, pancreas, and lining of the respiratory and gastrointestinal tract are derived from the **endoderm**; and the uriniferous tubules of the kidney, lining of the male and female reproductive systems, endothelial lining of the circulatory system, and mesothelium of the body cavities develop from the **mesoderm**.

Epithelial tissues have numerous functions:

- **Protection** of underlying tissues of the body from abrasion and injury
- **Transcellular transport** of molecules across epithelial sheets
- **Secretion** of mucinogen (the precursor of mucus), hormones, enzymes, and other molecules from various glands
- **Absorption** of material from a lumen (i.e., intestinal tract or certain kidney tubules)
- **Selective permeability**, that is, the control of movement of materials between body compartments
- **Detection of sensations** via taste buds, retina of the eye, and specialized hair cells in the ear

EPITHELIUM

Tightly bound contiguous cells forming sheets covering or lining the body are known as an epithelium.

The sheets of contiguous cells in the epithelium are tightly bound together by junctional complexes. Epithelia possess little extracellular space and little extracellular matrix. Epithelium is separated from the underlying connective tissue by an extracellular matrix, the **basement membrane**, composed of the **basal lamina** and the **lamina reticularis** (discussed in Chapter 4), synthesized by the epithelial cells and cells of the connective tissue. Because epithelium is avascular, the adjacent supporting connective tissue through its capillary beds supplies nourishment and oxygen via diffusion through the basement membrane.

Classification of Epithelial Membranes

Cell arrangement and morphology are the bases of classification of epithelium.

Epithelial membranes are classified according to the number of cell layers between the basal lamina and the free surface and by the morphology of the surface-most epithelial cells (Table 5.1). If the membrane is composed of a **single layer of cells**, it is called ***simple epithelium***; if it is composed of **more than one cell layer**, it is called ***stratified epithelium*** (Fig. 5.1). The morphology of the cells may be squamous (flat), cuboidal, or columnar when viewed in sections taken perpendicular to the basement membrane. Stratified epithelia are classified by the morphology of the cells in their *superficial layer only*. In addition to these two major classes of epithelia, which are further identified by cellular morphology, there are two other distinct types: pseudostratified and transitional (see Fig. 5.1).

- **Simple squamous epithelium** is composed of a single layer of tightly packed, thin, or low-profile polygonal cells. When viewed from the surface, the epithelial sheet looks much like a tile floor with a centrally placed bulging nucleus in each cell (Figs. 5.2A, 5.3). Viewed in section, however, only some cells display nuclei because the plane of section frequently does not encounter the nucleus. Simple squamous epithelia line pulmonary alveoli, compose the loop of Henle and the parietal layer of Bowman capsule in the kidney, and form the endothelial lining of blood and lymph vessels as well as the mesothelium of the pleural, pericardial, and peritoneal cavities.
- A single layer of polygon-shaped cells constitutes **simple cuboidal epithelium** (see Figs. 5.2A and 5.3). When viewed in a section cut perpendicular to the surface, the cells present a square profile with a centrally placed round nucleus. Simple cuboidal epithelia form the ducts of many glands of the body, the covering of the ovary, and many kidney tubules.
- The cells of **simple columnar epithelium**, when viewed in longitudinal section, are tall, rectangular cells whose ovoid nuclei are usually located essentially at the same level in the basal half of the cell (see Fig. 5.2B). Simple columnar epithelium may exhibit a striated border composed of **microvilli**, narrow, finger-like cytoplasmic processes that project from the apical surface of the cells into the lumen. Simple columnar epithelium lines much of the digestive tract, gallbladder, and large ducts of glands; those that line the uterus, oviducts, ductuli efferentes, and small bronchi are ciliated. In these organs, **cilia** (hair-like structures) project from the apical surface of the columnar cells into the lumen.
- **Stratified squamous (nonkeratinized) epithelium** is thick; because it is composed of several layers of cells, only the deepest layer is in contact with the basal lamina (Fig. 5.4A). The most basal (deepest) cells of this epithelium are cuboidal in shape, those located in the middle of the epithelium are polymorphous, and the cells composing the free surface of the epithelium are flattened (squamous)—hence, the name *stratified squamous.* Because the surface cells are nucleated, this epithelium is called *nonkeratinized.* It is wet and lines the mouth, oral pharynx, esophagus, true vocal folds, and vagina.

TABLE 5.1 Classification of Epithelia

Type	Shape of Surface Cells	Sample Locations	Functions
SIMPLE			
Simple squamous	Flattened	*Lining:* Pulmonary alveoli, loop of Henle, parietal layer of Bowman capsule, inner and middle ear, blood and lymphatic vessels, pleural and peritoneal cavities	Limiting membrane, fluid transport, gaseous exchange, lubrication, reducing friction (thus aiding movement of viscera), lining membrane
Simple cuboidal	Cuboidal	Ducts of many glands, covering of ovary, form kidney tubules	Secretion, absorption, protection
Simple columnar	Columnar	*Lining:* Oviducts, ductuli efferentes of testis, uterus, small bronchi, much of digestive tract, gallbladder, and large ducts of some glands	Transportation, absorption, secretion, protection
Pseudostratified	All cells rest on basal lamina but not all reach epithelial surface; surface cells are columnar.	*Lining:* Most of trachea, primary bronchi, epididymis and ductus deferens, auditory tube, part of tympanic cavity, nasal cavity, lacrimal sac, male urethra, large excretory ducts	Secretion, absorption lubrication, protection, transportation
STRATIFIED			
Stratified squamous (nonkeratinized)	Flattened (with nuclei)	*Lining:* Mouth, epiglottis, esophagus, vocal folds, vagina	Protection, secretion
Stratified squamous (keratinized)	Flattened (without nuclei)	Epidermis of skin	Protection
Stratified cuboidal	Cuboidal	*Lining:* Ducts of sweat glands	Absorption, secretion
Stratified columnar	Columnar	Conjunctiva of eye, some large excretory ducts, portions of male urethra	Secretion, absorption, protection
Transitional	Dome shaped (relaxed), flattened (distended)	*Lining:* Urinary tract from renal calyces to urethra	Protection, distensible

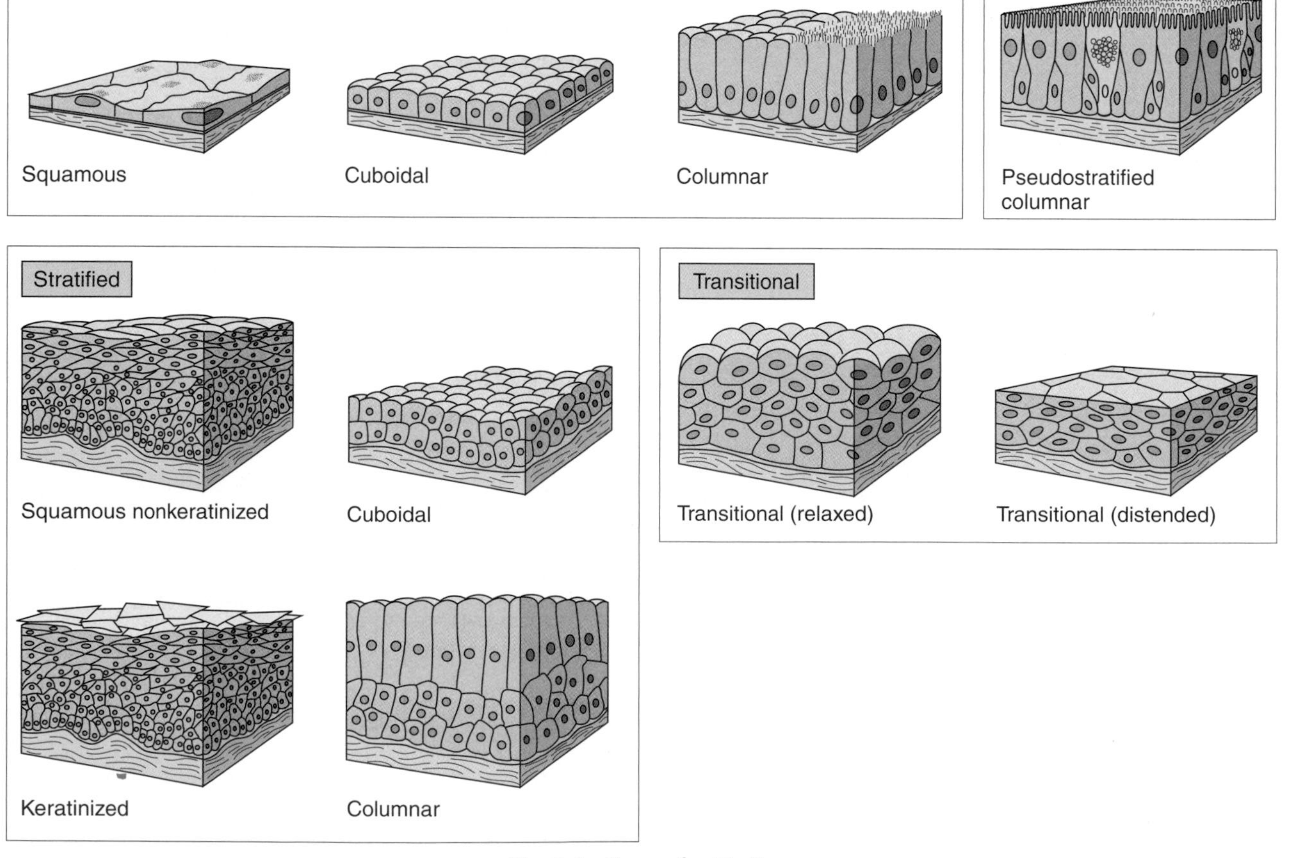

Fig. 5.1 Types of epithelia.

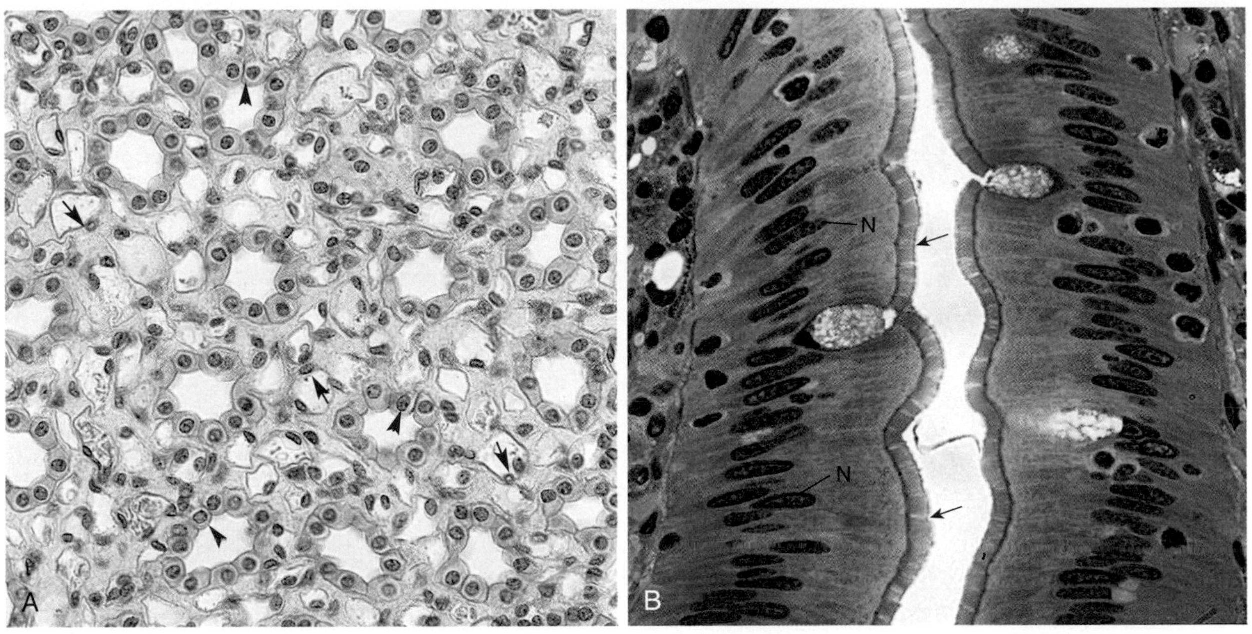

Fig. 5.2 Light micrographs of simple epithelia. (A) Simple squamous epithelium *(arrows)*. Note the morphology of the cells and their nuclei. Simple cuboidal epithelium *(arrowheads)*. Note the round, centrally placed nuclei (×270). (B) Simple columnar epithelium. Observe the oblong nuclei (N) and the striated border *(arrows)* (×540).

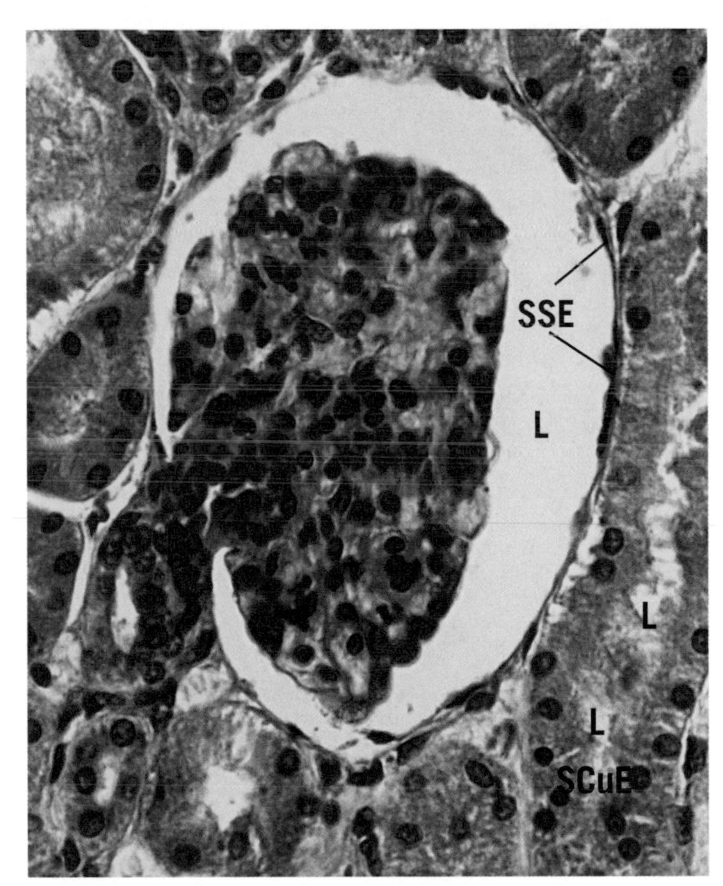

Fig. 5.3 Light micrograph of the kidney cortex displaying simple squamous epithelium (SSE) and simple cuboidal epithelium (SCuE). L, lumen. Note that the nuclei of the simple squamous epithelial cells—when in the plane of the section—bulge into the lumen and that the cytoplasm of the cell is highly attenuated. In three dimensions, it would resemble a fried egg (over medium). The nuclei of cuboidal epithelial cells are round and mostly basally located (away from the lumen). In three dimensions, it would resemble a square glass with a round ice cube at the bottom. (×540)

- **Stratified squamous (keratinized) epithelium** is similar to stratified squamous (nonkeratinized) epithelium except that the superficial layers of the epithelium are composed of dead cells whose nuclei and cytoplasm have been replaced with keratin (see Fig. 5.4B). This epithelium constitutes the epidermis of skin, a tough layer that resists friction and is impermeable to water. There is another category of stratified squamous epithelium—namely, stratified squamous parakeratinized epithelium—which is discussed in Chapter 16.
- **Stratified cuboidal epithelium**, which contains only two layers of cuboidal cells, lines the ducts of sweat glands (see Fig. 5.4C).
- **Stratified columnar epithelium** is composed of a low polyhedral to cuboidal deeper layer in contact with the basal lamina and a superficial layer of columnar cells. This epithelium is found in only a few places in the body: the conjunctiva of the eye, some large excretory ducts, and regions of the male urethra.
- **Transitional epithelium** is composed of many layers of cells; those located basally are either low columnar or cuboidal cells. Polyhedral cells compose several layers above the basal cells. This epithelium is located exclusively in the urinary system, where it lines the urinary tract from the renal calyces to the urethra. The most superficial cells of the empty bladder are large, occasionally binucleated, and exhibit rounded dome tops that bulge into the lumen (see Figs. 5.4D and 5.5). These dome-shaped cells become flattened, and the epithelium becomes thinner when the bladder is distended with urine.
- **Pseudostratified columnar epithelium** appears to be stratified, but it is actually composed of a single layer of cells. All of the cells in pseudostratified columnar epithelium are in contact with the basal lamina, but only some cells reach the surface of the epithelium (Fig. 5.6). Cells not extending to the surface usually have a broad base

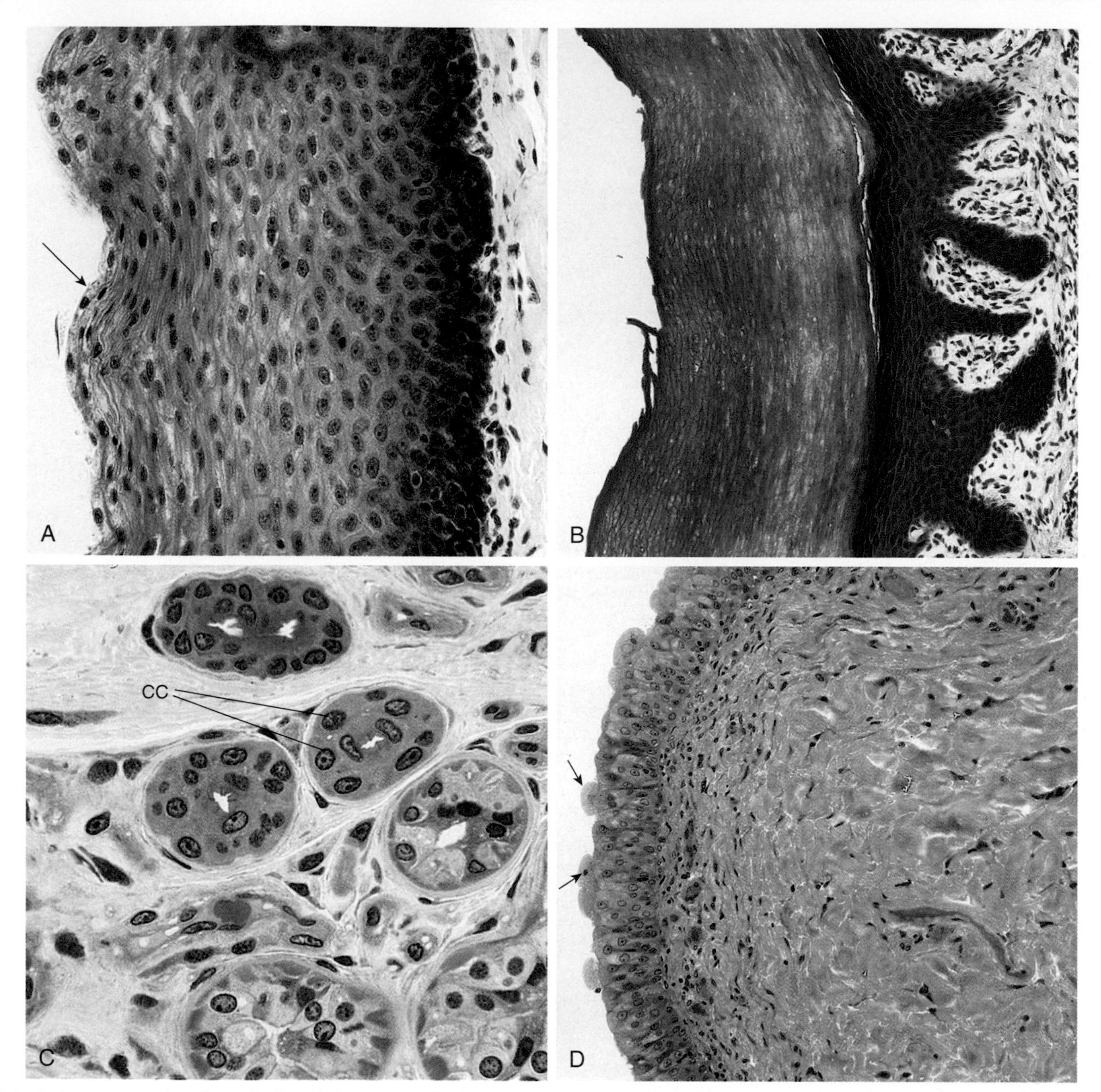

Fig. 5.4 Light micrographs of stratified epithelia. (A) Stratified squamous nonkeratinized epithelium. Observe the many layers of cells and flattened (squamous), nucleated cells in the top layer *(arrow)* (×509). (B) Stratified squamous keratinized epithelium (×125). (C) Stratified cuboidal epithelium of the duct of a sweat gland (CC) (×509). (D) Transitional epithelium. Observe that the surface cells facing the lumen of the bladder are dome shaped *(arrows)*, which characterize transitional epithelium (×125).

and become narrow at their apical end. Taller cells reach the surface and possess a narrow base in contact with the basal lamina and a broadened apical surface. Because the cells of this epithelium are of different heights, their nuclei are located at different levels, giving the impression of a stratified epithelium, even though it is composed of a single layer of cells. Pseudostratified columnar epithelium is found in the male urethra, epididymis, and larger excretory ducts of glands. The most widespread type of pseudostratified columnar epithelium is **ciliated**, having cilia on the apical surface of the cells that reach the epithelial surface. Pseudostratified ciliated columnar epithelium is found lining most of the trachea and primary bronchi, the auditory tube, part of the tympanic cavity, the nasal cavity, and the lacrimal sac.

Polarity and Cell-Surface Specializations

Epithelial cell polarity and cell-surface specializations are related to cellular morphology and function.

Epithelial cells have distinct morphological, biochemical, and functional domains and, thus, commonly display a polarity support these various regions. Consequently, many epithelial cells possess an **apical domain** that faces a lumen and a **basolateral domain** whose basal component is in contact with the basal lamina. The functional distinctions of these regions are responsible

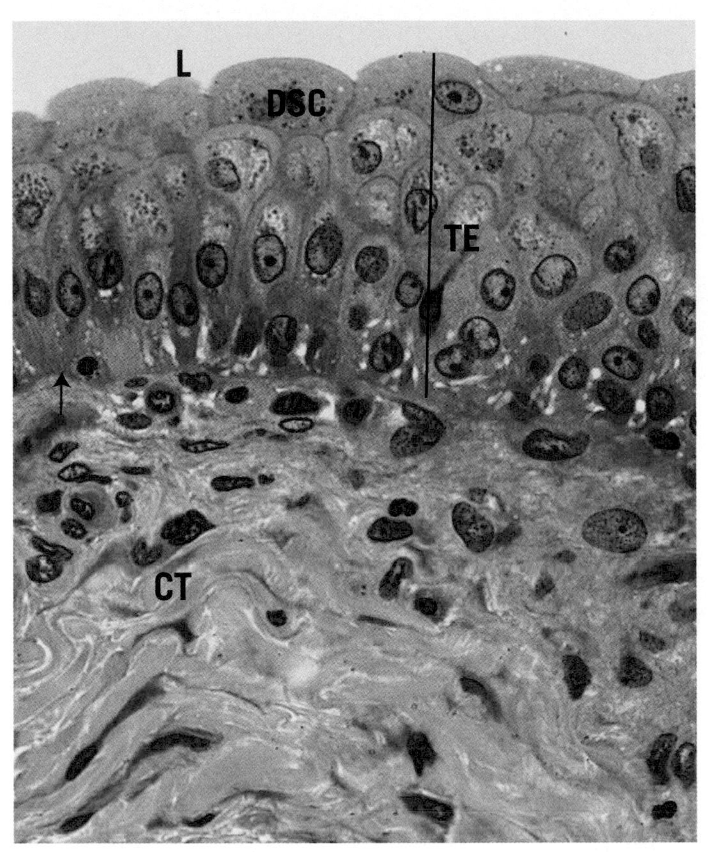

Fig. 5.5 This is a photomicrograph of the lining of an empty human urinary bladder. Note that the transitional epithelium (TE) that lines the lumen (L) is composed of several cell layers and that the superficial layer of cells are plump and dome shaped (DSC). The basement membrane *(arrow)* separates the epithelium from the urinary bladder connective tissue (CT). The epithelial cells between the basement membrane and the dome-shaped cells vary from cuboidal to low columnar in shape. (×540)

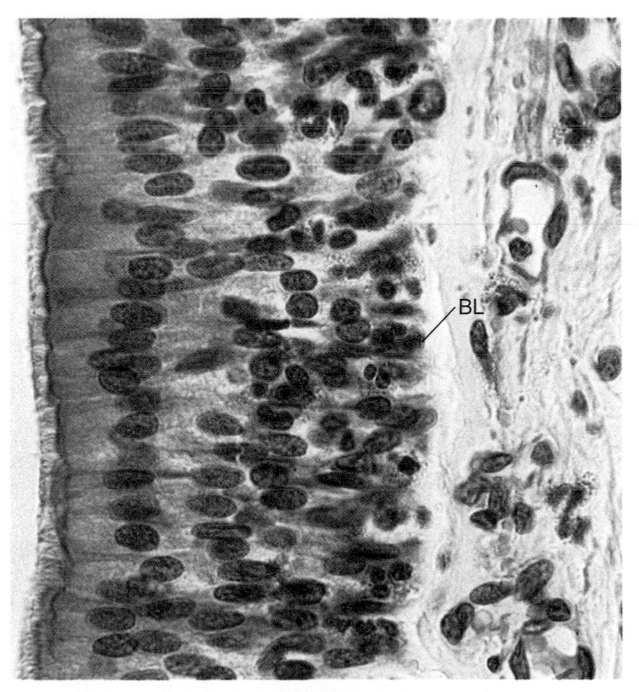

Fig. 5.6 Light micrograph of pseudostratified epithelia. This type of epithelium appears to be stratified; however, all of the epithelial cells in this figure stand on the basal lamina (BL) (×540).

for the presence of surface modifications and specializations of these domains in that the apical surfaces of many epithelial cells may possess microvilli or cilia, whereas their basolateral regions may exhibit various junctional specializations and intercellular interdigitations. The apical and basolateral domains are isolated from each other by tight junctions that encircle the apical aspect of the cell.

Apical Domain

The apical domain represents the free surface of the epithelial cells.

The **apical domain** is that region of the epithelial cell that abuts the lumen; it is rich in ion channels, carrier proteins, ATPase (adenosine triphosphatase, transmembrane ATPase), glycoproteins, and hydrolytic enzymes as well as **aquaporins**, proteins that form channels that regulate the water balance of the cell. Regulated secretory products are released from the epithelial cells at the apical domains. Modifications of the apical surface that facilitate many of the functions of epithelial cells include microvilli (and associated glycocalyx) as well as stereocilia, cilia, and flagella.

Microvilli.

Microvilli are small, finger-like cytoplasmic projections emanating from the free surface of the cell into the lumen.

Microvilli represent the **striated border** of the intestinal absorptive cells and the **brush border** of the kidney proximal tubule cells observed by light microscopy. Electron microscopy demonstrated these closely packed **microvilli** to be 1 to 2 μm long cylindrical, membrane-bound projections that greatly increase the surface areas of these cells (Fig. 5.7). In other, less active cells, microvilli may be sparse and short. Each microvillus contains a core bundle of 25 to 30 **actin filaments**, whose members are cross-linked to each other by a number of actin-binding proteins, such as **espin**, **fascin**, **villin**, and **fimbrin**. The plus ends of the actin filaments are embedded in an amorphous region composed mostly of villin, at the tip of the microvillus. The minus ends of the actin filaments are embedded in and attached to the **terminal web**, which is a complex of **actin** and **spectrin** molecules, as well as **intermediate filaments** located at the cortex of the epithelial cells (Figs. 5.8, 5.9, and 5.10). **Myosin-I** and **calmodulin** provide structural support by connecting the actin filaments at the periphery of the bundle to the plasma membrane of the microvillus. **Tropomyosin** and **myosin II**, located in the terminal web, act on the **actin filaments**, causing contraction of the apical aspect of the cell, thereby spreading the microvilli apart, increasing the space available for molecular transport at the cell apex. Epithelia not functioning in absorption or transport may exhibit microvilli without cores of actin filaments.

An amorphous, fuzzy coating over the tips of the microvilli, the **glycocalyx** is composed of carbohydrate residues attached to the transmembrane proteins of the plasmalemma. These glycoproteins function in the realms of protection and cell recognition (see Chapter 2).

Stereocilia (not to be confused with cilia) are long, rigid, nonmotile microvilli present only in the epididymis and on the sensory hair cells of the cochlea (inner ear). The core actin filaments of stereocilia are held together by **fimbrin**. The peripheral-most members of the actin filament bundle are bound to the stereocilia's membrane by **ezrin** and **villin-2**; there is no villin at the tip of the stereocilia where the plus ends of the

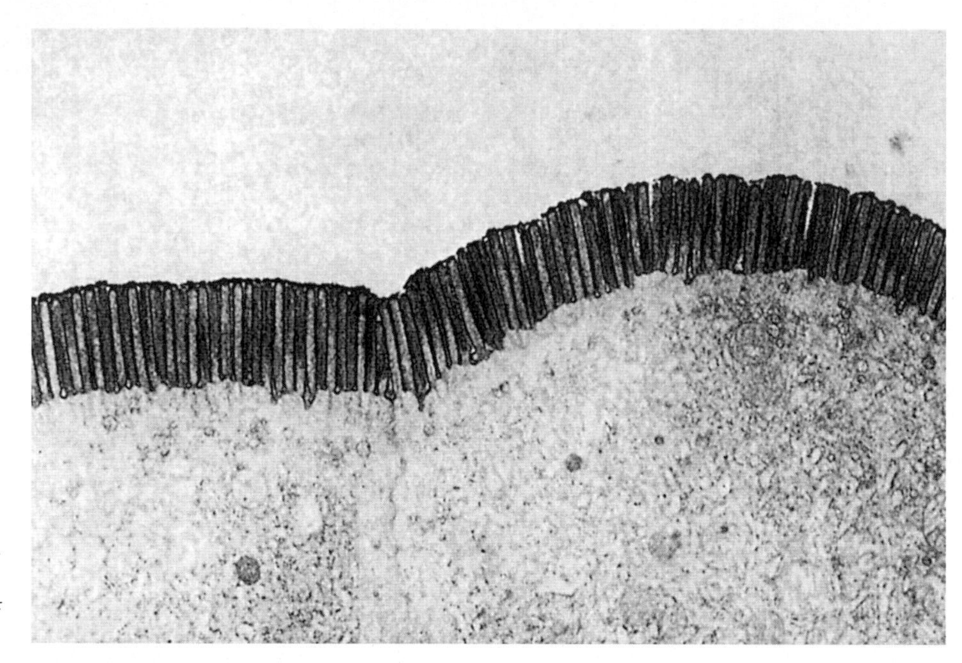

Fig. 5.7 Electron micrograph of microvilli of epithelial cells from the small intestine (×2800). (From Hopkins CR. *Structure and Function of Cells*. Philadelphia: WB Saunders; 1978.)

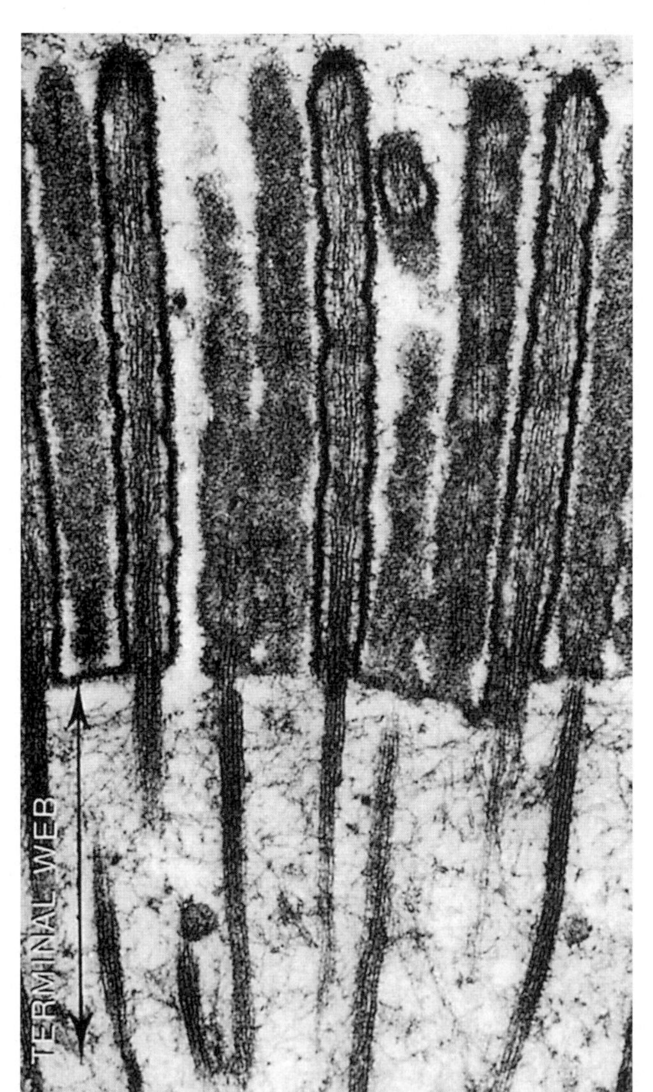

Fig. 5.8 High-magnification electron micrograph of microvilli (×60800). From Hopkins CR. *Structure and Function of Cells*. Philadelphia: WB Saunders; 1978.

actin filaments terminate. The minus ends of the actin filaments terminate in the terminal web. In the epididymis, stereocilia probably function in increasing the surface area; in the hair cells of the ear, they function in signal generation.

> ***Cilia.***
> *Cilia are of two types: long, motile, hair-like structures emanating from the apical cell surface (whose core is composed of a complex arrangement of microtubules known as the axoneme) and primary cilia, which are similar but are nonmotile.*

Motile cilia (called ***cilia*** in this textbook) are hair-like projections that emanate from the surface of certain epithelial cells. Usually, they are 7 to 10 µm long and 0.2 µm in diameter. Cilia of the respiratory tree, for example, move mucus and debris toward the oropharynx via rapid, rhythmic oscillations, where they may be swallowed or expectorated. Cilia of the oviduct move the fertilized ovum toward the uterus.

The internal structure of cilia, as demonstrated by electron microscopy, reveals that the core of the cilium contains complex microtubules called the ***axoneme***, which is composed of a constant number of longitudinal microtubules arranged in a specific 9 + 2 organization (Figs. 5.11 and 5.12). Two centrally placed microtubules (**singlets**) are surrounded by nine **doublets** of microtubules. The singlets are separated from one another, both display a circular profile in cross-section, and each is composed of 13 protofilaments. The nine doublets are each composed of two subunits. In cross-section, **subunit A** is a microtubule composed of 13 protofilaments, exhibiting a circular profile. **Subunit B** possesses 10 protofilaments, exhibits an incomplete circular profile in cross-section, and shares three protofilaments of subunit A.

Several elastic protein complexes are associated with the axoneme. **Radial spokes** project from subunit A of each doublet inward toward the **central sheath** surrounding the two singlets. Neighboring doublets are connected by **nexin**, another elastic protein, extending from subunit A of one doublet to subunit B of the adjacent doublet (see Fig. 5.11).

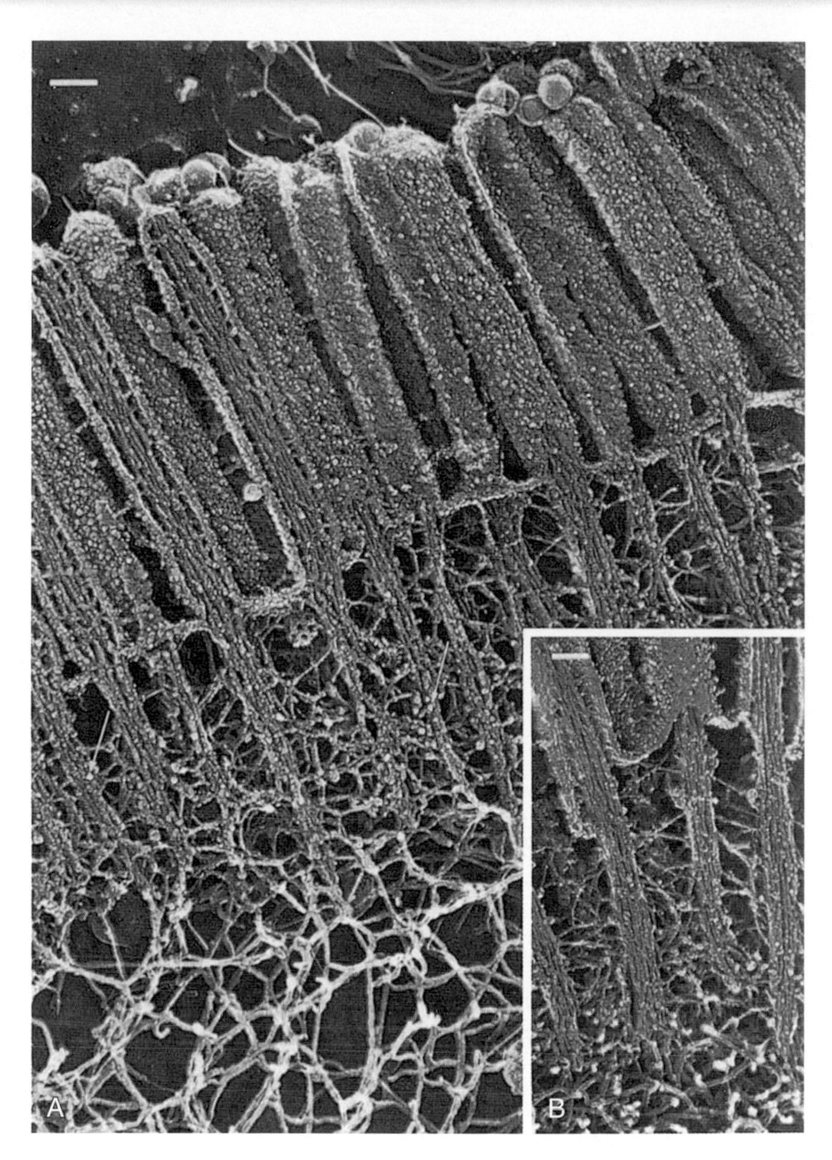

Fig. 5.9 Electron micrograph of the terminal web and microvillus. Observe that the actin filaments of the microvilli are attached to the terminal web (A, ×83060; B, *inset*, ×66,400). (From Hirokana N, Tilney LG, Fujiwara K, Heuser JE. Organization of actin, myosin, and intermediate filaments in the brush border of intestinal epithelial cells. *J Cell Biol*. 1982;94:425-443. Reprinted with the permission of The Rockefeller University Press.)

The microtubule-associated protein **dynein** has ATPase activity and is known as the ***ciliary dynein arm***. Two dynein arms, an **inner** and an **outer**, radiate from subunit A of one doublet toward subunit B of the neighboring doublet. These dynein arms are arranged at 24-nm intervals along the length of subunit A so that subunit A resembles a millipede and its numerous bilaterally symmetrical legs. Dynein ATPase, by hydrolyzing ATP, provides the energy for the ciliary bending. Movement of the cilia is initiated by the dynein arms transiently attaching to specific sites on the protofilaments of the adjacent doublets, sliding them toward the tip of the cilium. However, **nexin**, an elastic protein extending between adjacent doublets, restrains this action to some degree, thus translating the sliding movement into a bending motion. As the cilium bends, *an energy-requiring process*, the elastic protein complex is stretched. When the dynein arms release their hold on the B subunit, the stretched elastic protein complex returns to its original length, thereby snapping the cilium back to its straight position (*requiring no energy*). This snapping movement of the cilium back to its original position causes the movement of the material at the tip of the cilium. An additional protein, **tektin**, which resembles a rod and is approximately 2 to 3 nm in diameter, assembles head to tail to form a "rod" along the entire doublet microtubule. This **tektin rod** is located at the junction of microtubules A and B, close to the outer dynein arm, acting as a support for the doublet and preventing the cilium from bending too far.

Clinical Correlations

Kartagener syndrome results from hereditary defects in the ciliary dynein that would normally provide the energy for ciliary bending. Thus, ciliated cells without functional dynein are prohibited from functioning. Persons having this syndrome are susceptible to lung infections because their ciliated respiratory cells fail to clear the tact of debris and bacteria. Additionally, males with this syndrome are sterile because their sperm are immotile.

The 9 + 2 microtubule arrangement within the axoneme continues throughout most of the length of the cilium except at its base, where it is attached to the basal body (see Fig. 5.11). The morphology of the **basal body** is similar to that of a centriole in that, instead of nine doublets and a pair of singlets, it is composed only of nine **triplets** and no singlets. The basal body and its associated components are responsible for the adherence of the cilium to the cell and for the ability of all of the cilia of the cell to beat in a uniform fashion and in the identical direction.

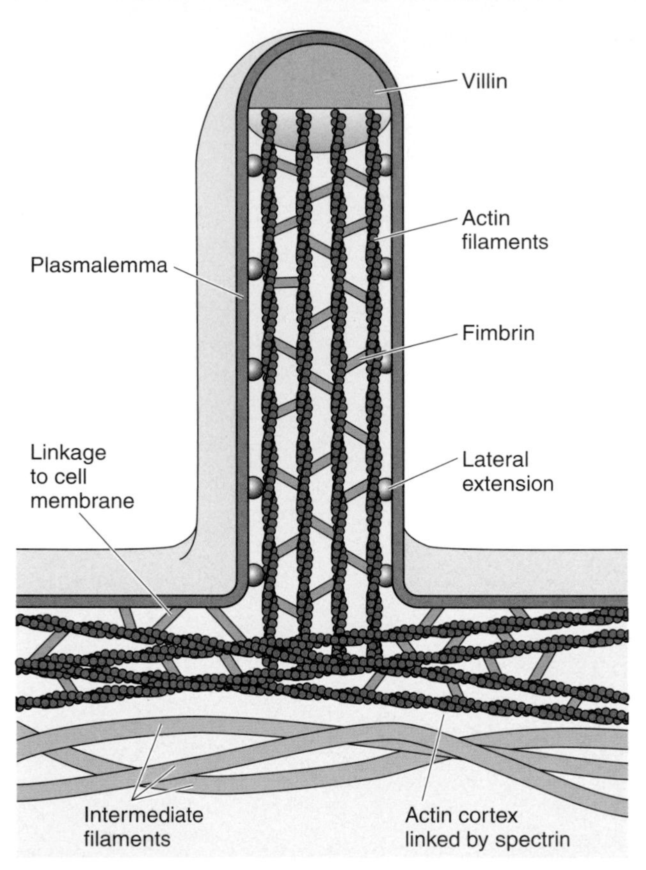

Fig. 5.10 Schematic diagram of the structure of a microvillus.

Basal bodies develop from **procentriole organizers**. As the procentriole lengthens, a third microtubule, **microtubule C**, is added to microtubule B. The new microtubule is also composed of 10 protofilaments and shares 3 of microtubule B's protofilaments. Once formed, the basal body migrates to the apical plasmalemma and gives rise to a cilium. At this junction of the basal body and the axoneme, known as the **transition zone**, nine doublet microtubules develop from the nine triplets of the basal body, and a pair of central microtubules, the two **singlets**, forms to give the cilium's axoneme its characteristic 9 + 2 microtubule arrangement. Arising from this transition zone and attached to microtubule C is the **alar sheath**, a fibrous *semipermeable membrane* that forms an upside-down, tent-like cover whose tip encloses microtubule C and whose base attaches to the cell membrane around the region where the cilium emerges from the cell, effectively separating the cytoplasm of the cilium from that of the cell. Two additional structures are associated with the basal body: the **basal foot**, which is responsible for orienting the cilia so that all cilia face and beat in the same direction, and the **striated rootlet**, which is believed to anchor the basal body into the apical cytoplasm.

Cilia (as well as flagella) require the constant transport of various substances in and out of their cytoplasm. Generally, this movement is known as ***axonemal transport***; however, within cilia, it is referred to as ***intraciliary transport*** (***intraflagellar transport*** in flagella). If it occurs from the basal body toward the tip of the cilium, it is known as ***anterograde intraciliary transport***; in the opposite direction, it is known as ***retrograde***

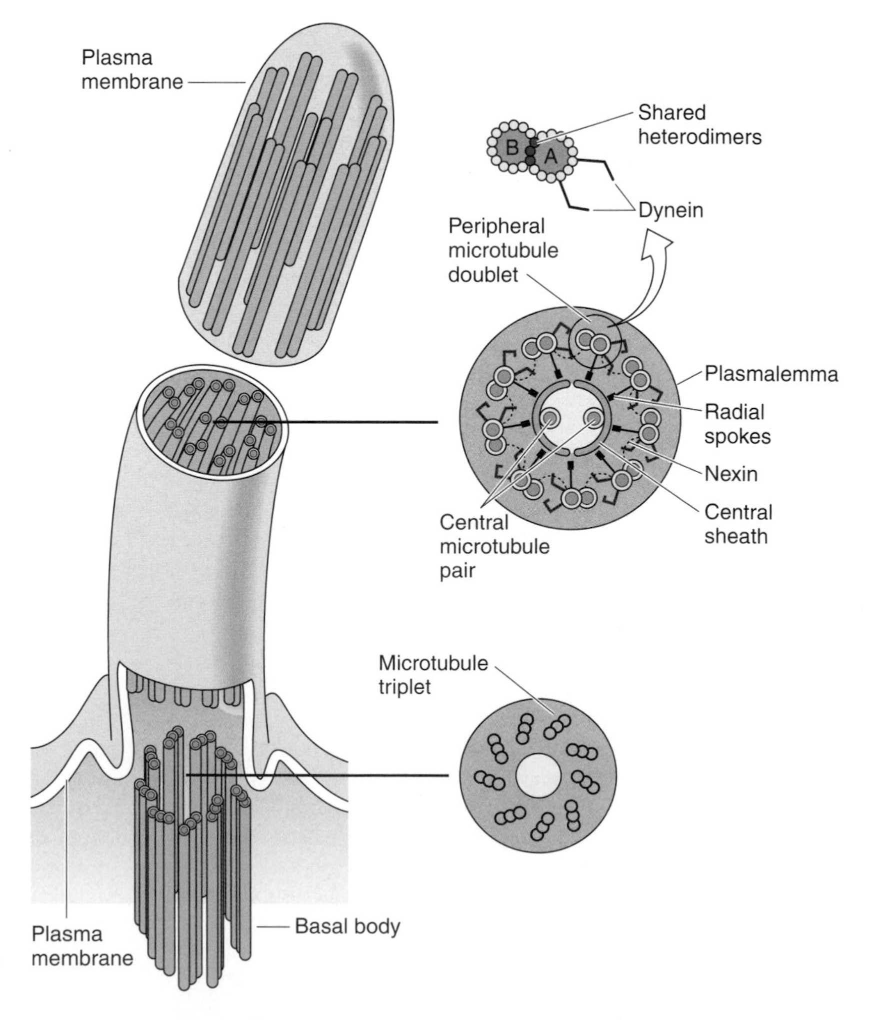

Fig. 5.11 Schematic diagram of the microtubular arrangement of the axoneme in the cilium.

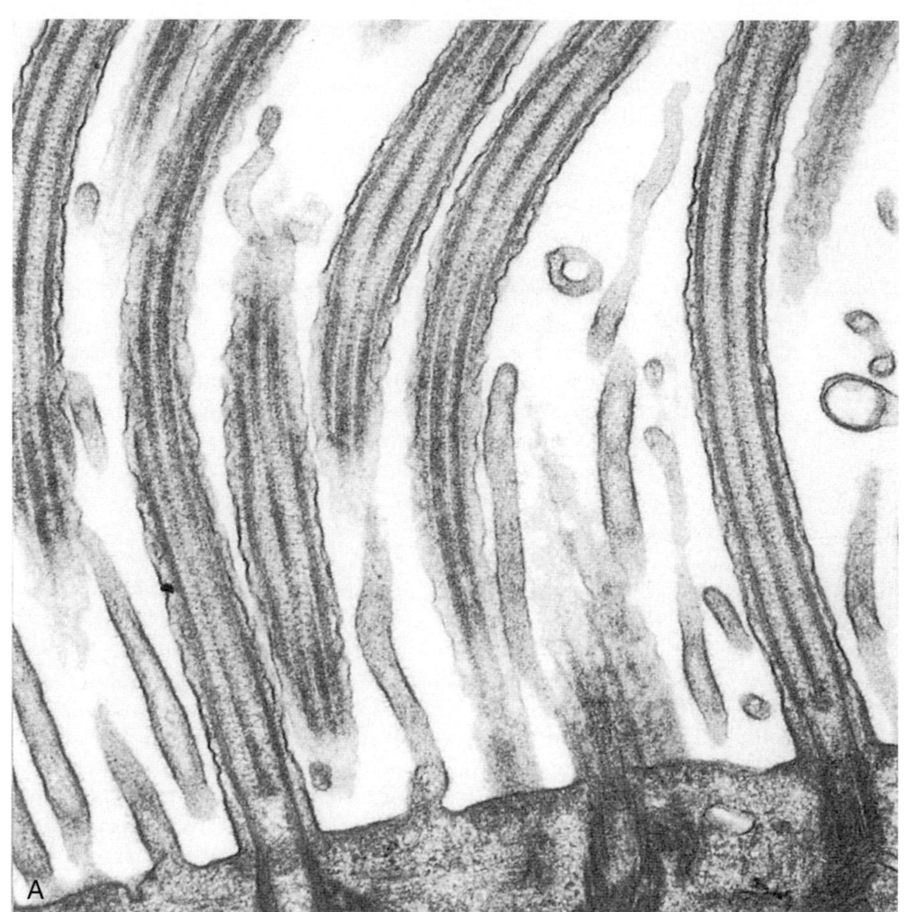

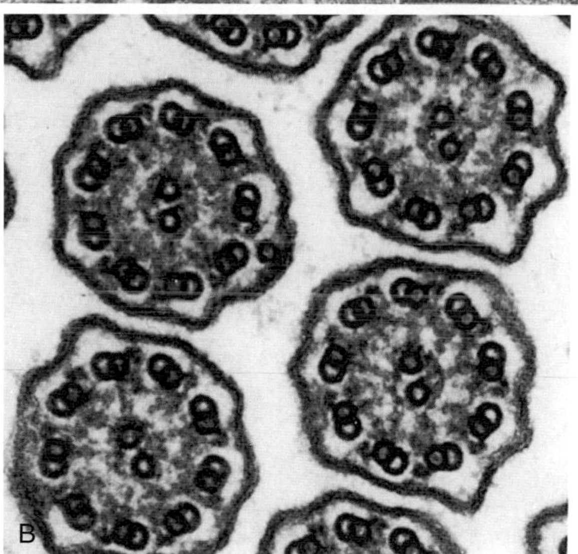

Fig. 5.12 Electron micrographs of cilia. (A) Longitudinal section of cilia (×36000). (B) Cross-sectional view demonstrating microtubular arrangement in cilia (×88000). (From Leeson TS, Leeson CR, Paparo AA. *Text/Atlas of Histology*. Philadelphia: WB Saunders; 1988.)

intraciliary transport. The material to be transported (e.g., tubulin molecules) is referred to as ***cargo***. The transport of cargo is performed by carrier proteins known as ***raft proteins***, which are ferried in the anterograde direction by **kinesin-2** and in the retrograde direction by **dynein-2** along the outer aspect (facing the plasmalemma of the cilia) of the axoneme microtubules. The change of direction from anterograde to retrograde intraciliary transport occurs at the distal tip of the cilia and depends on the presence of the enzyme **intestinal cell kinase (ICK)**, which phosphorylates a subunit of kinesin-2, a motor-protein that functions not only in intraciliary transport but also in ciliogenesis, the formation of cilia. In the absence of ICK, intraciliary transport ceases, and ciliogenesis does not occur in the proper fashion.

Clinical Correlations

*Individuals with **Majewski polydactyly** syndrome, a recessive autosomal defect, have been shown to have abnormally developed chondrocyte cilia. These individuals display abnormal chondrogenesis, as well as abnormal osteogenesis, resulting in shortened limbs, narrowed thoracic cage, fused fingers and toes, genital malformations, cardiovascular problems, and respiratory insufficiency, among numerous other congenital defects. It appears that the chondrocyte cilia of these individuals are foreshortened and display a bulbous expansion, and their **intraciliary retrograde transport** was disrupted.*

Primary Cilia. **Primary cilia** are nonmotile and are noted to be present on most mammalian cells that are not participating in the cell cycle, that is, they are in the G_0 state. Each cell possesses a single primary cilium that functions in surveying its immediate environment and in eliciting the cell to respond to changes in that milieu. The axoneme of primary cilia has no central singlets, dynein arms, central sheath, or radial spokes. Their nine doublets resemble those of the motile cilia's axoneme. Primary cilia display the presence of a protein complex, known as the ***BBSome complex*** **(Bardet-Biedl syndrome protein complex)** at the junction of the basal body with the basal foot. The BBSome complex, in a fashion similar to COP I, COP II, and clathrin, forms a membrane coat that sorts, binds to, and ferries membrane proteins (e.g., membrane-bound receptors), into the cytoplasm of primary cilia to be inserted into their plasmalemma.

The **basal foot** serves a similar role in primary cilia as it does in motile cilia; it ensures that primary cilia of all cells in the region are aligned in the same direction, thus, they are exposed to the same conditions.

Clinical Correlations

*A number of genetic disorders that involve primary and motile cilia are known as **ciliopathies**. These involve various mutations that result in disturbances in the intraciliary transport and may be lethal during fetal life or early in postnatal development. Some of these mutations involve the **MKS1 gene (Meckel syndrome, type 1)** that codes for **MKS1 protein**. This protein, in conjunction with another protein known as **meckelin**, is associated with the basal body and is essential for ciliogenesis, and its mutant form is responsible for the lethal genetic ciliopathy known as **Meckel syndrome**. The symptoms of this condition include aberrant formation of the central nervous system, defects in hepatogenesis, polydactyly, and the formation of renal cysts that cause an enormous enlargement of the kidneys.*

*Other mutations involve genes coding for **melanocortin-4 receptor** (**MC4R**), a protein that associates with the enzyme **adenylate cyclase 3** (**ADCY3**) on the primary cilia of certain neurons of the paraventricular nucleus of the hypothalamus. These neurons regulate body weight by monitoring the energy storage of the body and adjusting energy outflow and ingestion of food. Mutated MC4R cannot join with ADCY3; as a consequence, adenylyl-cyclase signaling is inhibited, resulting in severe obesity in the affected individuals.*

Flagella. The only cells in the human body that possess **flagella** are the spermatozoa. The structure of flagella is discussed in Chapter 21, which covers the male reproductive system.

Basolateral Domain

The basolateral domain includes the basal and lateral aspects of the cell membrane.

The **basolateral domain** may be subdivided into two regions: the lateral plasma membrane and the basal plasma membrane. Each region possesses its own junctional specializations and receptors for hormones and neurotransmitters. In addition, these regions are rich in Na^+-K^+ ATPase and ion channels and are sites for constitutive secretion.

Lateral Membrane Specializations.

Lateral membrane specializations reveal the presence of junctional complexes.

Light microscopy reveals zones, called ***terminal bars***, where epithelial cells are in contact and, presumably, attach to each other. These terminal bars are quite evident in the apical region of the simple columnar epithelium lining the gut. Horizontal sections through the terminal bars demonstrated that they are continuous around the entire circumference of each cell, indicating that each cell is attached to every cell adjacent to it. Electron microscopy has revealed that terminal bars are, in fact, composed of intricate **junctional complexes** that possess **cell adhesion molecules** that assist in holding contiguous epithelial cells to each other. Junctional complexes may be classified into three types, schematically depicted in Fig. 5.13:

- **Occluding junctions** function in joining cells to form an impermeable barrier, preventing material from taking an intercellular route (**paracellular route**) in passing across the epithelial sheath.
- **Anchoring junctions** function in maintaining cell-to-cell or cell-to-basal lamina adherence.
- **Communicating junctions** function in coupling adjacent cells both electrically and metabolically by facilitating the movement of ions or small signaling molecules between cells.

Zonulae Occludentes (tight junctions).

Zonulae occludentes, the only type of occluding junction, prevent movement of membrane proteins and function to prevent intercellular movement of water-soluble molecules.

Zonulae occludentes (**zonula occludens** is the singular form) are located between adjacent plasma membranes and are the most apically located junction between the cells of the epithelia (see Fig. 5.13 and Table 5.2). They form a belt-like junction that encircles the entire circumference of the cell. It should be appreciated that the formation of a zonula adherens requires the interaction of *several adjoining cells*.

In electron micrographs, the adjoining cell membranes approximate each other; their outer leaflets fuse, then diverge, and then fuse again several times within a distance of 0.1 to 0.3 μm (Fig. 5.14). At the fusion sites, the extracellular moieties of the four types of transmembrane proteins (**claudins**, **occludins**, **nectins**, and **junctional adhesive molecules [JAMs]**) of the two membranes bind to each other, forming a seal occluding the extracellular space between adjoining cells participating in the

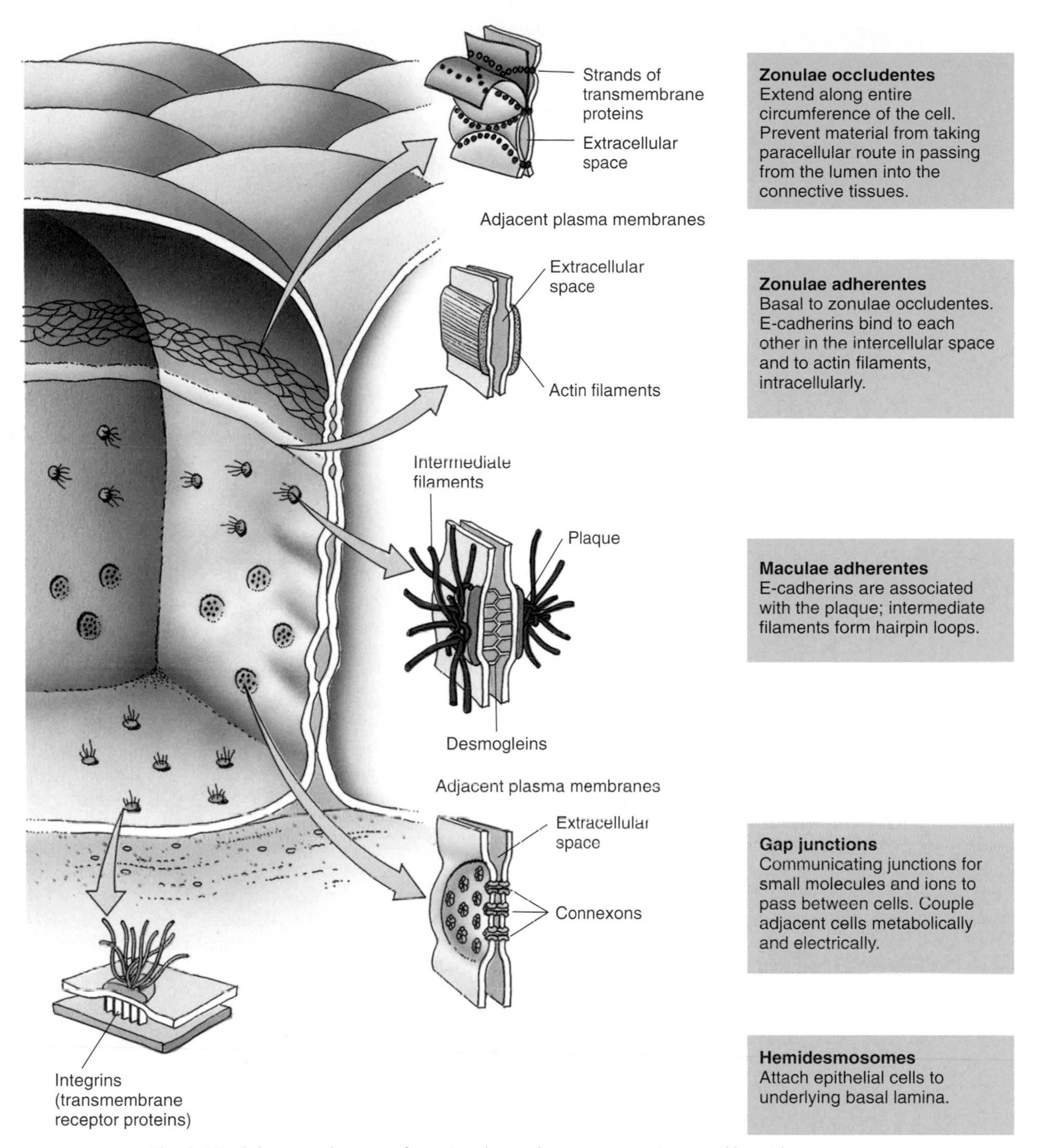

Fig. 5.13 Schematic diagram of junctional complexes, gap junctions, and hemidesmosomes.

TABLE 5.2 Junctions that Cells Make with Each Other

Protein	Type	Distance Between Adjoining Cells	Function
ZONULA OCCLUDENS			
Claudins	Transmembrane	0 nm	Occludes paracellular routes
Occludins	Transmembrane	0 nm	Occludes paracellular routes (?)
Nectins	Transmembrane	0 nm	Occludes paracellular routes
JAMs	Transmembrane	0 nm	Occludes paracellular routes (?)
Actin	Intracellular	NP	Supports transmembrane proteins
Afadin	Intracellular	NP	Supports transmembrane proteins
ZO-1, ZO-2, ZO-3	Intracellular	NP	Supports transmembrane proteins

TABLE 5.2 Junctions that Cells Make with Each Other—cont'd

Protein	Type	Distance Between Adjoining Cells	Function
ZONULA ADHERENS			
E-cadherins	Transmembrane	10-20 nm	Adheres to its counterpart
Actin	Intracellular	NP	Supports E-cadherins
α-Actinin	Intracellular	NP	Binds to actin
Catenin	Intracellular	NP	Binds to vinculin and E-cadherin
Vinculin	Intracellular	NP	Binds to catenin and actin
MACULA ADHERENS (DESMOSOME)			
Desmogleins	Transmembrane	30 nm	Binds to its counterpart
Desmocollins	Transmembrane	30 nm	Binds to its counterpart
Plakoglobins	Intracellular	NP	Binds to desmogleins and desmocollins
Plakophilins	Intracellular	NP	Binds to desmogleins and desmocollins
Desmoplakins	Intracellular	NP	Binds to plakoglobins and plakophilins
Keratin	Intracellular	NP	Binds to desmoplakins
GAP JUNCTIONS			
Connexon[a]	Transmembrane	2-4 nm	Bind to connexon counterpart to form an aqueous channel through which ions and small molecules can move between cells

JAMs, Junctional adhesive molecules; NP, not pertinent.
[a]Each connexon is formed by 6 connexin subunits (cell membranes are 2 nm apart).

formation of the occluding junction. Freeze-fracture analysis of cell membranes at the zonulae occludentes displays a "quilted" appearance of anastomosing strands, known as ***tight junction strands***, on the P-face and a corresponding network of **grooves** on the E-face (Fig. 5.15). These tight junction strands are the extracellular components of the transmembrane proteins of the two adjacent membranes that contact each other to obliterate the extracellular space between the two cells.

The roles of nectins, occludins, and JAMs are as yet not known; however, **claudins**, by forming the greatest portion of the tight junction strands, are known to bear the brunt of the responsibility in blocking movement of material through the intercellular space. However, because claudins are calcium independent, they do not form strong cell adhesions; therefore, their contact must be reinforced by **cadherins**, as well as by the four cytoplasmic zonula occludens proteins, **ZO-1**, **ZO-2**, **ZO-3**, and **afadin**. These four proteins bind to the cytoplasmic moieties of the transmembrane proteins participating in the formation of the zonula occludens and bind to the actin filaments of the cell's cytoskeleton, providing stability to the tight junction.

Tight junctions have two major functions: (1) preventing the movement of membrane proteins from the apical domain to the basolateral domain (and vice versa); and (2) fusing plasma membranes of adjacent cells to each other, thereby prohibiting molecules from passing between cells. Depending on the numbers and patterns of these *sealing strands* in the zonula, some tight junctions are said to be "tight," whereas others are "leaky." These terms reflect the efficiency of the epithelial cells in maintaining the integrity of the epithelial barrier between two adjacent body compartments.

Zonulae Adherentes.

Zonulae adherentes, one of the four types of anchoring junctions, are belt-like junctions that assist adjoining cells to adhere to one another.

Zonulae adherentes (singular: **zonula adherens**), one of the four types of **anchoring junctions** of epithelial cells, are located just basal to the zonulae occludentes. As their name implies, they also encircle the cell (see Fig. 5.13 and Table 5.2). The intercellular space of 15 to 20 nm between the outer leaflets of the two adjacent cell membranes is occupied by the extracellular moieties of **E-cadherins** (whose name comes from *epithelial-calcium-dependent adhesion*), also known as **transmembrane linker proteins** (see Fig. 5.14), Ca^{2+}-dependent integral proteins of the cell membrane. Their intracytoplasmic aspect binds to bundles of actin filaments that run parallel to and along the cytoplasmic aspect of the cell membrane. The actin filaments are attached to each other by **α-actinin** and to the intracytoplasmic moieties of the E-cadherins by the anchor proteins **vinculin** and **catenins** (see Chapter 2). In the presence of calcium ions, the extracellular region of the cadherins of one cell forms bonds with those of the adjoining cell participating in the formation of the zonula adherens. Thus, this junction not only links the cell membranes to each other but also links the cytoskeletons of the two cells via the transmembrane linker proteins. It should be appreciated that the formation of a zonula adherens requires the interaction of *several adjoining cells.*

Fascia adherens is similar to zonula adherens but does not go around the entire circumference of the cell. Instead of being belt-like, it is ribbon-like. Cardiac muscle cells, for example, are attached to each other at their longitudinal terminals via the fascia adherens.

Desmosomes (Maculae Adherentes [singular: macula adherens]).

Desmosomes, one of the four types of anchoring junctions, are weld-like junctions along the lateral cell membranes that help resist shearing forces.

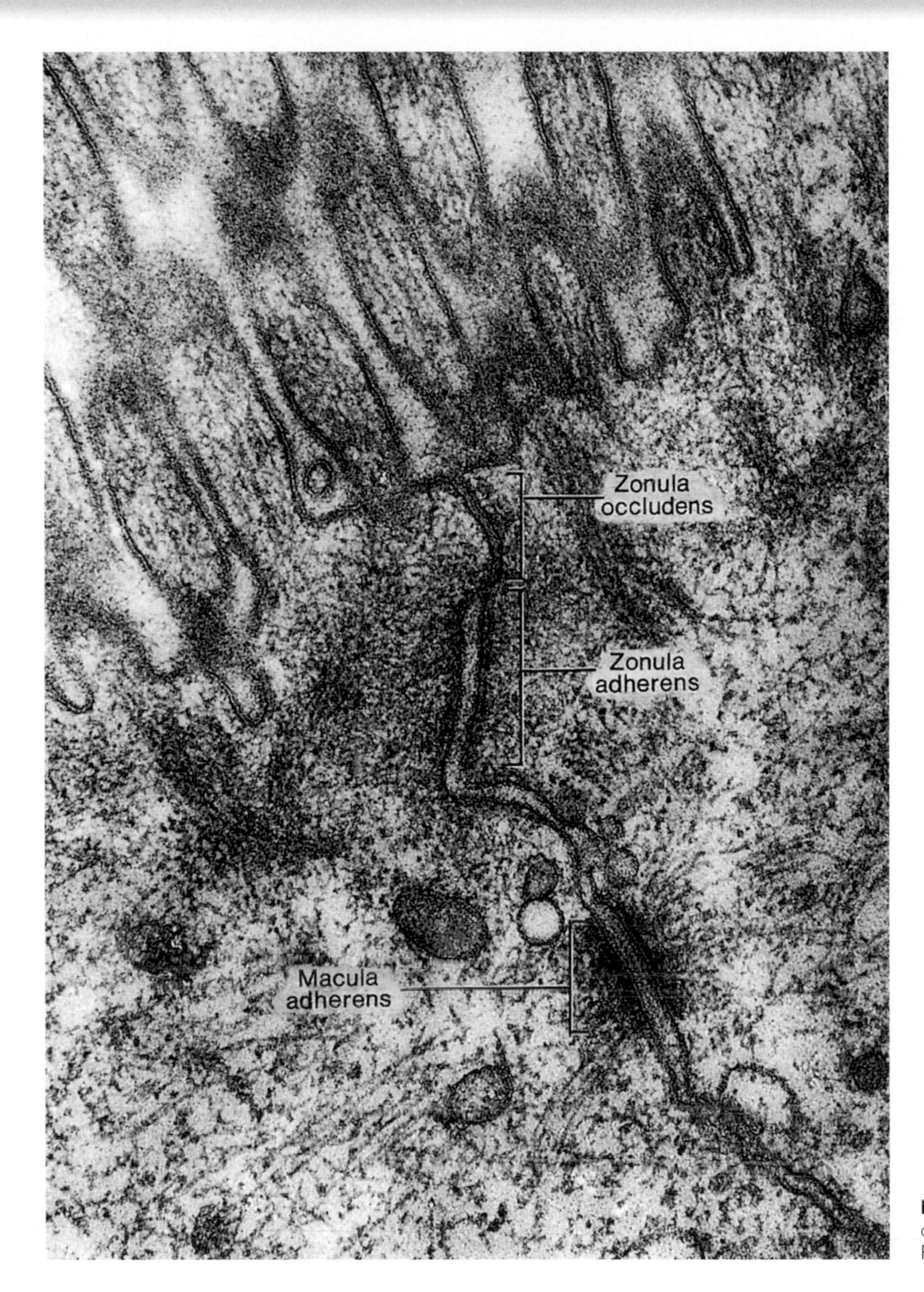

Fig. 5.14 Electron micrograph of the junctional complex. (From Fawcett DW. *The Cell*. 2nd ed. Philadelphia: WB Saunders; 1981.)

Desmosomes (see Table 5.2) are the last of the three components of the junctional complex. These spot-weld–like junctions also appear to be randomly distributed along the lateral cell membranes of simple epithelia and throughout the cell membranes of stratified squamous epithelia, especially in the epidermis.

A pair of disk-shaped **attachment plaques**, the **inner** and **outer dense plaques** (combined dimensions of ~ 400 × 250 × 10 nm) are located opposite each other on the cytoplasmic aspects of the plasma membranes of each of the adjacent epithelial cells (see Figs. 5.13, 5.14, and Fig. 5.16). The extracellular space between the two cells is approximately 30 nm in width and is occupied by the extracellular regions of **desmocollins**, **desmogleins**, and **cadherins** (**transmembrane proteins**) that project from both participating cell membranes into this space. In the presence of calcium ions, the extracellular portions of these cadherins contact each other and form bonds that attach these adjacent cells to one another. This extracellular contact is evident with electron microscopy as an electron-dense line and is known as the ***extracellular core***.

The **outer dense plaque** closely adheres to the cytoplasmic aspect of the plasmalemma. This plaque is composed of the glycoproteins **plakoglobins** and **plakophilins**, held together by proteins known as ***desmoplakins***. The intracellular components of the desmocollins and desmogleins contact and are stabilized by the plakoglobins and plakophilins. Additionally, the desmoplakins contact the **keratin intermediate filaments** located somewhat deeper in the cytoplasm. This region of contact, visible with the electron microscope, forms the **inner dense plaque**

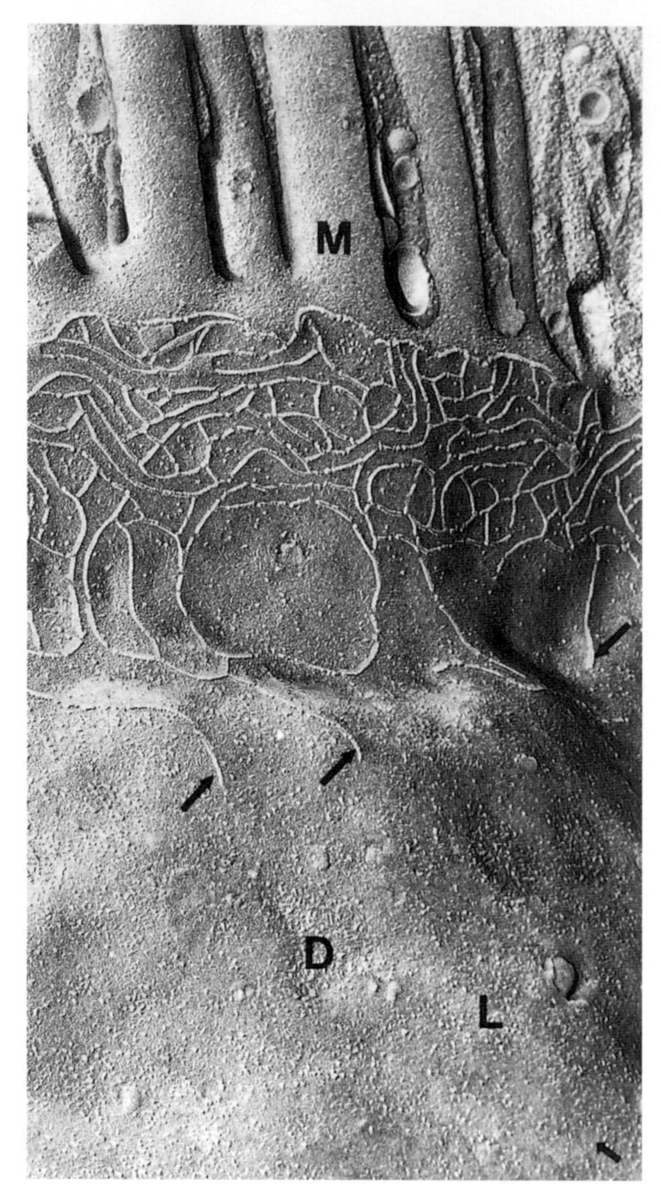

Fig. 5.15 Freeze-fracture replica displaying the tight junction (zonula occludens) in a guinea pig's small intestine. The P-face of the microvillar membrane (M) possesses fewer intramembrane particles than the P-face of the lateral cell membrane (L). *Arrows* point to free terminal ridge–shaped protrusions. A desmosome (D) is shown (×60,000). (From Trier JS, Allan CH, Marcial MA, Madara JL. Structural features of the apical and tubulovesicular membranes of rodent small intestinal tuft cells. *Anat Rec.* 1987;219:69-77. Reprinted by permission of Wiley-Liss, Inc., a subsidiary of John Wiley & Sons, Inc.)

that stabilizes the outer plaque, which, in turn, stabilizes the extracellular core. It is in this fashion that the desmosome is able to maintain the adherence of the two cells to each other, as if they were spot welded to each other. It should be appreciated that the formation of a desmosome requires the interaction of *two adjoining cells.*

Clinical Correlations

1. *Some people produce autoantibodies against desmosomal proteins, especially those in the skin, resulting in a skin disease called* ***pemphigus vulgaris****. Binding of the autoantibodies to desmosomal proteins disrupts cell adhesion, leading to widespread blistering and consequent loss of extracellular fluids. If untreated, this condition leads to death. Treatment with systemic steroids and immunosuppressive agents usually controls the condition.*

Clinical Correlations—cont'd

2. ***Naxos syndrome****, a genetic anomaly prevalent in the Greek islands in the vicinity of Naxos as well as in regions of the Middle East, is due to malformed* ***plakoglobins*** *and* ***desmoplakins****. It causes keratoderma of the palms of the hands and soles of the feet, wooly hair, and cardiomyopathy involving right ventricular arrhythmia. A similar condition that affects the left ventricles and is prevalent in parts of the Indian subcontinent and Ecuador is known as* ***Carvajal syndrome****. Both conditions have a high degree of mortality, but patients' lives may be prolonged by the administration of antiarrhythmic medications and, at the end stages of the disease, a heart transplant.*

Gap Junctions.

Gap junctions, also called nexus, communicating junctions, or gap junction channel, are regions of intercellular communication.

Gap junctions (see Table 5.2) are widespread in epithelial tissues throughout the body, as well as in cardiac muscle cells, smooth muscle cells, and neurons but not in skeletal muscle cells. They differ from the occluding and anchoring junctions in that they mediate intercellular communication by permitting the passage of various small molecules between adjacent cells. The intercellular cleft at the gap junction is narrow and constant at about 2 to 4 nm. Note that the formation of gap junctions requires the cooperation of *two adjoining cells.* When a connexon of one plasma membrane is in register with its counterpart of the adjacent plasma membrane, the two connexons fuse, forming a functional intercellular hydrophilic communication channel (Fig. 5.17). With a diameter of 1.5 to 2.0 nm, the hydrophilic channel permits the passage of ions, amino acids, vitamins, small second messenger molecules (e.g., cyclic adenosine monophosphate), certain hormones, and molecules smaller than 490 Da. At the same time, the channel created by the fused connexons thwarts the escape of the transiting material from the channel, preventing it from entering the space between the cells.

Gap junctions are regulated and may be opened or closed rapidly. Although the opening and closing mechanism is not fully understood, it has been shown experimentally that a decrease in cytosolic pH or an increase in cytosolic Ca^{2+} concentrations closes gap junctions. Conversely, high pH or low Ca^{2+} concentration opens the channels.

Gap junctions are built by six closely packed transmembrane channel-forming proteins (**connexins**) that assemble to form a channel-like structure called a **connexon** (**hemichannel**), which extends through the plasma membrane by about 1.5 nm into the extracellular space (see Fig. 5.13). Two connexons, one in each adjacent cell, align precisely and fuse with one another, to form a **gap junction**. Presently, it is believed that there may be more than 20 different connexins that can assemble into many different arrays of connexons. There are **homotypic** gap junctions, where both connexons of the gap junction are composed of identical connexins, or **heteromeric**, where the two connexons of

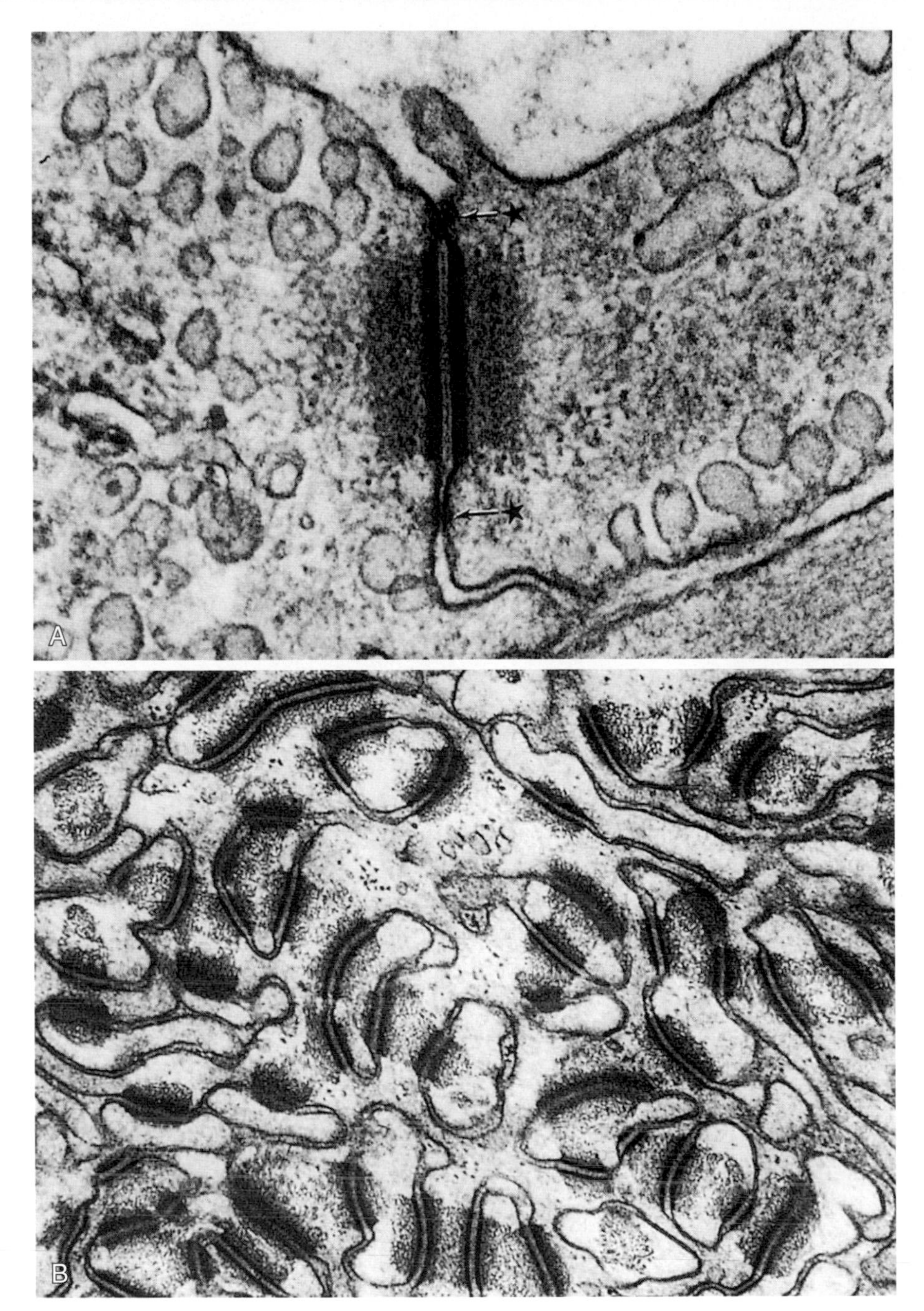

Fig. 5.16 Electron micrograph of a desmosome. Observe the dense accumulation of intracellular intermediate filaments inserting into the plaque of each cell. (From Fawcett DW. *The Cell*. 2nd ed. Philadelphia: WB Saunders; 1981.)

the gap junction are not composed of identical connexins. Clusters of gap junctions may be composed of a few to many thousands of connexons; these are referred to as **gap junction plaques**.

Gap junctions exhibit many diverse functions within the body, including cellular sharing of molecules for coordinating physiological continuity within a particular tissue. For example, when glucose is needed in the bloodstream, the nervous system stimulates liver cells (hepatocytes) to initiate glycogen breakdown. Because not all hepatocytes are individually stimulated, the signal is dispersed to other hepatocytes via gap junctions, thus, coupling the hepatocytes. Gap junctions also function in electrical coupling of cells (i.e., in heart muscle and in smooth muscle cells of the gut during peristalsis), coordinating the activities of these cells. Also, gap junctions are important during embryogenesis in coupling the cells of the developing embryo electrically and in distributing informational molecules throughout the migrating cell masses, keeping them coordinated in the proper development pathway. Mutations in the genes coding for connexins may cause an X-linked form of Charcot-Marie-Tooth syndrome.

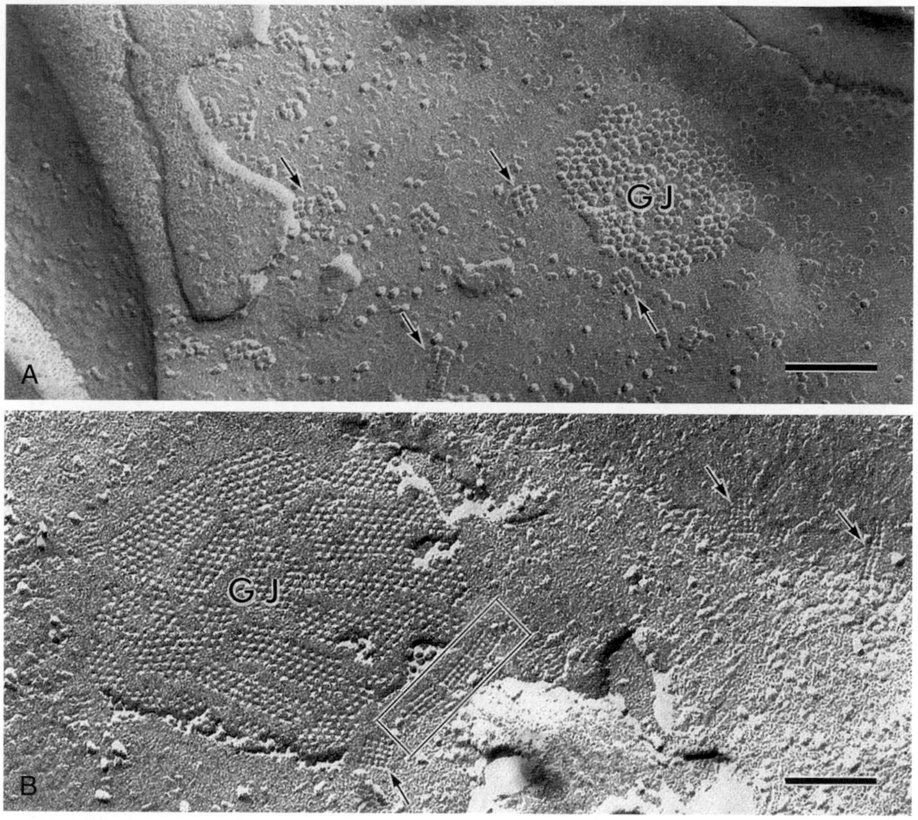

Fig. 5.17 Electron micrographs of freeze-fracture replica showing the intramembrane particles of the astrocyte. (A) Protoplasmic fracture face. Orthogonal arrays of particles (OAPs) *(arrows)* are observed near the gap junction (GJ). Note the differences between OAPs and GJ particles in shape *(square* and *circle)*, size (30 nm^2 and 45 nm^2 on average), and arrangement *(orthogonal* and *hexagonal)*. (B) Ectoplasmic fracture face. Corresponding pits of OAP are oriented into columns *(arrows)* near the GJ pits. Three OAPs show gathering *(squared)*. Scale bar = 0.1 µm. (From Yakushigawa H, Tokunaga Y, Inanobe A, et al. A novel junction-like membrane complex in the optic nerve astrocyte of the Japanese macaque with a possible relation to a potassium channel. *Anat Rec*. 1998;250:465-474. Reprinted by permission of Wiley-Liss, Inc., a subsidiary of John Wiley & Sons, Inc.)

Clinical Correlations

1. *Mutations in connexin genes have been linked to genetically based* **nonsyndromic deafness** *and to* **erythrokeratodermia variabilis**, *a skin disorder. In addition, dysfunctional migration of neural crest cells during development have been linked to mutations in the connexin genes, resulting in defects in the formation of the pulmonary vessels of the heart.*
2. *A number of* **cardiac arrhythmias** *have been attributed to gap junction anomalies. In certain diseased ventricular cardiac myocardial cells, the number of* **gap junction plaques** *and the cellular locations of these plaques were different from those of healthy ventricular myocardial cells. Specifically, the gap junction plaques, instead of being in the ends of the cells, were located in the lateral plasma membranes.*

Basal Surface Specializations.
Basal surface specializations include the basement membrane, plasma membrane infoldings, and hemidesmosomes.

Three important features mark the basal surface of epithelia: the basement membrane, plasma membrane infoldings, and hemidesmosomes, which anchor the basal plasma membrane to the basement membrane. The basement membrane is an extracellular supporting structure secreted by the epithelium and cells of the connective tissue and is located at the boundary between the tissues. The structure and appearance of the basement membrane are discussed in Chapter 4.

Plasma Membrane Infoldings.
Infoldings of the basal plasma membrane increase the surface area available for transport.

Epithelial cells that function in ion transport along their basal surface create numerous infoldings of their basal membranes. These infoldings increase the surface area of the basal membrane and the segmented cytoplasm house numerous mitochondria, which provide the energy required for active transport of ions in establishing osmotic gradients to ensure the movement of water across the epithelium, such as those of the kidney tubules. The compactness of the infolded plasma membranes coupled with the arrangement of the mitochondria within the infoldings gives a striated appearance when viewed with the light microscope; this is the origin of the term ***striated ducts*** for certain ducts of the pancreas and salivary glands.

Hemidesmosomes.
Hemidesmosomes attach the basal cell membrane to the underlying basal lamina; they have strong adhesive properties.

There are two types of **hemidesmosomes**: type I hemidesmosome (classical type) and type II hemidesmosome. They both resemble half of a desmosome and serve to attach firmly and for an extended period of time the basal cell membrane to the basement membrane (Fig. 5.18; see Fig. 5.13).

Type I hemidesmosome is more complex than type II and is present in the basal layers of cells of the stratified squamous and pseudostratified epithelia; they have a number of component molecules.

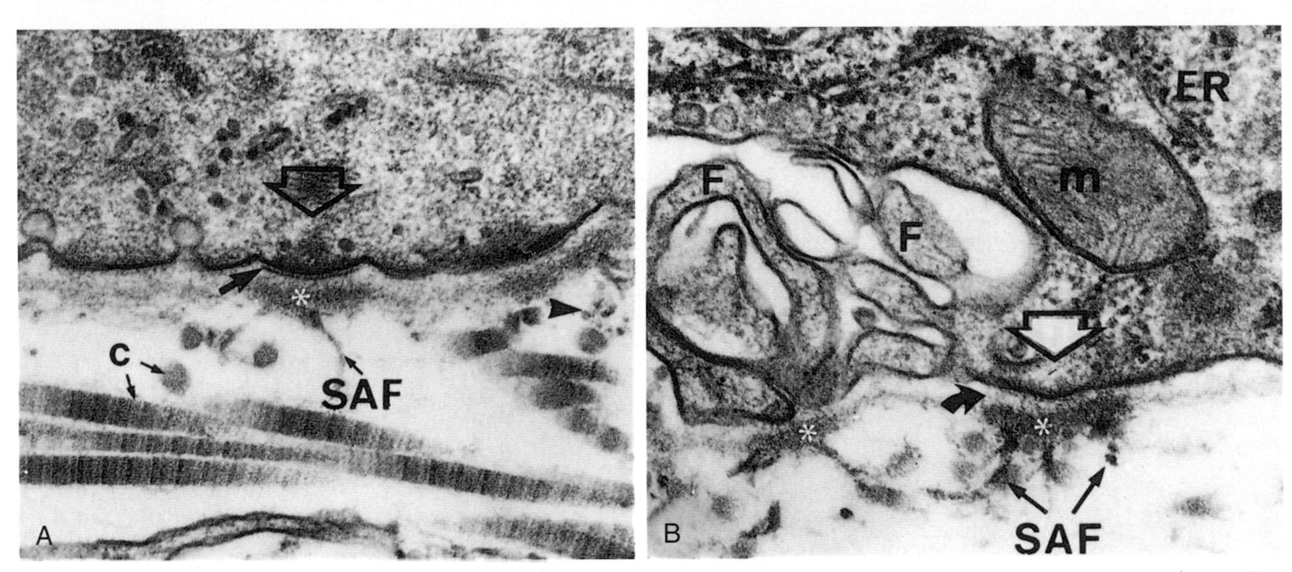

Fig. 5.18 Electron micrograph of hemidesmosomes illustrating the relationship of striated anchoring fibers (SAF), composed of type VII collagen, with the lamina densa and type III collagen of the lamina reticularis. c, Collagen fibers; ER, rough endoplasmic reticulum; F, cell extensions; m, mitochondria. *Open arrowheads* indicate the cytoplasmic aspect of hemidesmosomes; *asterisk* (*) indicates SAF plaque. (From Clermont Y, Xia L, Turner JD, Hermo L. Striated anchoring fibrils–anchoring plaque complexes and their relation to hemidesmosomes of myoepithelial and secretory cells in mammary glands of lactating rats. *Anat Rec.* 1993;237:318-325. Reprinted by permission of Wiley-Liss, Inc., subsidiary of John Wiley & Sons, Inc.)

The ***intracellular components of a type I desmosome***, starting at the plasmalemma, include:

- Numerous $\alpha_6\beta_4$ **integrin molecules** (transmembrane proteins) aligned close to each other
- **Tonofilaments** (**keratin-5** and **keratin-14 intermediate filaments**)
- **Plakin proteins** (**bullous pemphigoid antigen 230 [BP230]** and **plectin**); these form bonds not only with the tonofilaments but also with the intracytoplasmic aspects of $\alpha_6\beta_4$ integrin molecules
- **Erbin** molecules, which cross-bind $\alpha_6\beta_4$ integrin molecules to BP230
- **CD 151** (**tetraspanin protein CD 151**), which not only forms bonds with the α_6 component of $\alpha_6\beta_4$ integrin molecules but also recruits other $\alpha_6\beta_4$ integrin molecules to the region, providing a proper concentration of these integrins for hemidesmosome formation.

All of these structures together form the dense **intracytoplasmic plaque** observed with the electron microscope.

The ***extracellular components***, starting at the plasmalemma, include:

- The extracellular moieties of the $\alpha_6\beta_4$ **integrin molecules**
- **Bullous pemphigoid antigen 180 (BP180)**, a transmembrane protein (also referred to as *type XVII collagen*), whose intracellular moiety binds to the *intracellular portion* of the α_6 component of the integrin molecules, as well as to **plectin.** Extracellularly, it binds to the extracellular component of the α_6 portion of the integrin molecules and to the **laminin** and **type IV collagen** of the **basal lamina.**

Type II hemidesmosomes are less complex than type I, and they are present in the basal plasma membranes of the simple columnar epithelial lining of the small and large intestines. Just as in type I hemidesmosomes, the most numerous components of type II hemidesmosomes are a large concentration of $\alpha_6\beta_4$ **integrin molecules**. The intracellular moieties of these integrin molecules attach to **plectin**, which then form bonds with **keratin-8** and **keratin-18** intermediate filaments, forming a dense **intracellular plaque** similar to that of the type I hemidesmosome.

Both type I and type II hemidesmosomes require the presence of calcium ions to maintain an attachment to the basal lamina. Because most of these cells will move at one time or another, the cells have access to complex and well-regulated molecular pathways, whereby they are able to modulate the extracellular calcium ion concentration in the vicinity of the hemidesmosome and, in that fashion, affix the cell to or release it from the basal lamina.

Focal Adhesions.

Focal adhesions are anchoring junctions that attach the basal cell membranes of epithelial cells to the basal lamina; however, these are relatively transient and weak attachments.

Focal adhesions are present in clusters on the basal cell membranes of epithelial cells. They form weak anchoring junctions with the basal lamina and participate in the cell signaling pathways by acting as receptors for signaling molecules. Each focal adhesion is formed by clusters of **α and β integrins** whose *extracellular moieties* form weak interactions with **laminin, type IV collagen,** and **fibronectin molecules** of the basal lamina. The *intracytoplasmic moieties* of the α and β integrins bind to the actin-binding proteins **vinculin, α-actinin, paxillin,** and **talin,** which, by binding to **actin filaments**, anchor the integrins into the cytoplasm. These focal adhesions can be modified by intracellular and extracellular molecular signals severing the attachment of the α and β integrins to the basal lamina as well as to the actin filaments, thus freeing the cell from its attachment and permitting it to migrate from its previous location.

Renewal of Epithelial Cells

Cells constituting the epithelial tissues generally exhibit a high turnover rate, which is related to their location and function. The time frame for cell renewal remains constant for a particular epithelium.

Cells of the **epidermis**, for example, are constantly being renewed at the basal layer by cell division. From here, the cells begin their migration from the germinal layer to the surface, being keratinized on their route until they reach the surface, die, and are sloughed, the total event taking approximately 28 days. Other epithelial cells are renewed in a shorter period of time.

Cells lining the **small intestine** are replaced every 4 to 6 days by regenerative cells in the base of the crypts. The new cells then migrate to the tips of the villi, die, and are sloughed. Still other epithelia, for example, are renewed periodically until adulthood is reached; subsequently, the cell population remains for life. Even then, however, when a large number of cells are lost because of injury or acute toxic destruction, cell proliferation is triggered, and the cell population is restored.

Clinical Correlations

Each epithelium within the body has its own unique characteristics, location, and cell morphology, all of which are related to function. In certain pathological conditions, the cell population of an epithelium may undergo ***metaplasia****, transforming it into another epithelial type.*

Pseudostratified ciliated columnar epithelium of the bronchi of heavy smokers may undergo ***squamous metaplasia****, transforming it into stratified squamous epithelium. This change impairs function, but the process may be reversed when the pathological insult (smoking) is removed.*

Tumors that arise from epithelial cells may be benign (nonmalignant) or malignant. Malignant tumors arising from epithelia are called ***carcinomas****; those arising from glandular epithelial cells are called* ***adenocarcinomas****. It is interesting to note that cancers in adults are most often adenocarcinomas and, after age 45 years, about 90% are of epithelial cell origin. However, in children younger than 10 years of age, epithelial-derived cancers are the least prevalent type of cancer.*

Glands

Glands are derived from epithelial cells that, as they penetrate into the underlying connective tissue, manufacture a basal lamina that envelops them. The secretory units, along with their ducts, are the **parenchyma** of the gland, whereas the elements of connective tissue that invade and support the parenchyma are known as the **stroma**.

Cells of the secretory units manufacture their product intracellularly, usually packaging and storing these products in vesicles called ***secretory granules***. The secretory product may be a polypeptide hormone (e.g., from the pituitary gland); a waxy substance (e.g., from the ceruminous glands of the ear canal); a mucinogen (e.g., from the goblet cells); or milk, a combination of protein, lipid, and carbohydrates from the mammary glands. Other glands (e.g., sweat glands) secrete little besides the modified exudate that they receive from the bloodstream. In addition, cells of striated ducts (e.g., those of the major salivary glands) act as ion pumps that modify the substances produced by their secretory units.

Glands are classified into two major categories on the basis of the method of distribution of their secretory products:

1. **Exocrine glands** secrete their products via ducts onto the external or internal epithelial surface from which they originated.
2. **Endocrine glands** are **ductless**, having lost their connections to the originating epithelium, and thus secrete their products into the surrounding connective tissue, from where they enter blood or lymphatic vessels for distribution.

Many cell types secrete signaling molecules called ***cytokines***, which perform the function of cell-to-cell communication. Cytokines are released by **signaling cells** and act on **target cells**, which possess receptors for the specific signaling molecule. (Hormone signaling is discussed in detail in Chapter 2.)

Depending on the distance the cytokine must travel to reach its target cell, its effect may be one of the following:

- **Autocrine.** The signaling cell is its own target; thus, the cell stimulates itself.
- **Paracrine.** The target cell is located in the vicinity of the signaling cell; thus, the cytokine does not have to enter the vascular system for distribution to its target.
- **Endocrine.** The target cell and signaling cell are far from each other; thus, the cytokine has to be transported either by the blood or by the lymph vascular system.

Glands that secrete their products via a **constitutive secretory pathway** do so continuously, releasing their secretory products immediately without storage and without requiring a prompt by signaling molecules. Glands that exhibit a **regulated secretory pathway** concentrate and store their secretory products until the proper signaling molecule for its release is received (see Chapter 2, Figs. 2.20 and 2.23).

EXOCRINE GLANDS

Exocrine glands secrete their products via a duct to the surface of their epithelial origin.

Exocrine glands are classified according to the nature of their secretion, their mode of secretion, and the number of cells (unicellular or multicellular). Many exocrine glands in the digestive, respiratory, and urogenital systems secrete substances that are described as mucous, serous, or mixed (both) types.

Mucous glands secrete **mucinogens**, large glycosylated proteins that, upon hydration, swell to become a thick, viscous, gel-like protective lubricant known as **mucin**, a major component of **mucus**. Examples of mucous glands include goblet cells and the minor salivary glands of the hard and soft palates.

Serous glands (Fig. 5.19), such as the exocrine pancreas, secrete an enzyme-rich watery fluid.

Mixed glands contain acini (secretory units) that produce mucous secretions, as well as acini that produce serous secretions. In addition, some of their mucous acini possess **serous demilunes**, a group of cells that secrete a serous fluid (it is now believed that serous demilunes are artifacts of fixation; see Chapter 18). The sublingual and submandibular glands are examples of mixed glands (Fig. 5.20).

Cells of exocrine glands exhibit three different mechanisms for releasing their secretory products: (1) merocrine, (2) apocrine, and (3) holocrine (Fig. 5.21). The release of the secretory product of **merocrine glands** (e.g., parotid gland) occurs via exocytosis; as a result, neither cell membrane nor cytoplasm becomes a part of the secretion. Although many investigators question the existence of the apocrine mode of secretion, historically, it was believed that in **apocrine glands** (e.g., lactating mammary gland), a small portion of the apical cytoplasm is

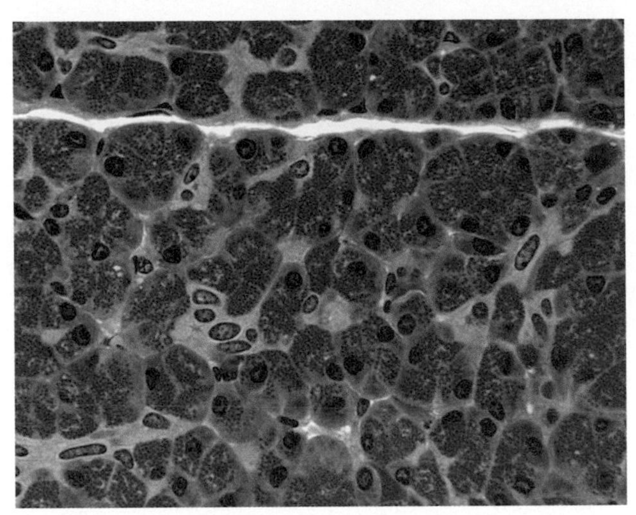

Fig. 5.19 Serous gland. Light micrograph of a plastic-embedded monkey pancreas. (×540)

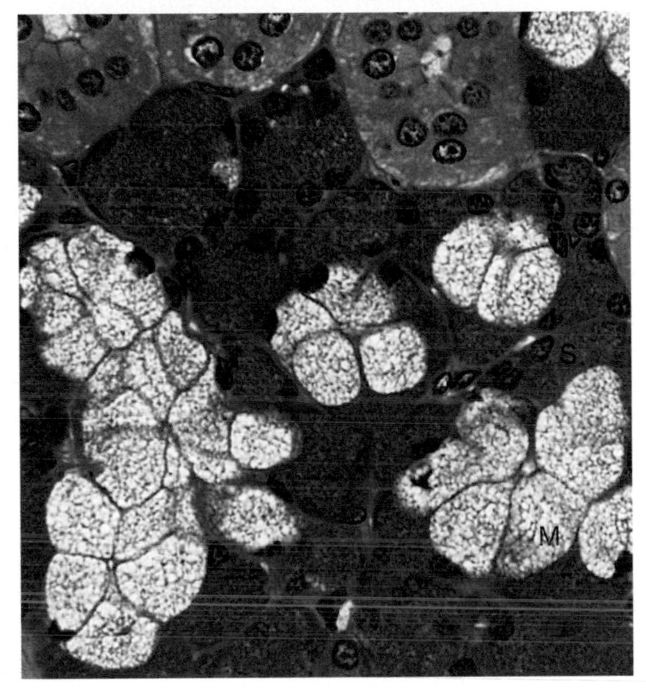

Fig. 5.20 Light micrograph of the monkey submandibular gland. (×540)

released along with the secretory product. In **holocrine glands** (e.g., sebaceous gland), as a secretory cell matures, it dies and becomes the secretory product.

Unicellular Exocrine Glands

Unicellular exocrine glands represent the simplest form of exocrine gland.

Unicellular exocrine glands are individual secretory cells that are interspersed among the epithelial cells. The classical example is the **goblet cell**, present throughout the epithelial lining of regions of the digestive and segments of the respiratory tracts (Figs. 5.22 and 5.23).

Goblet cells are named according to their shape, which resembles a goblet (see Figs. 5.2 and 5.24). The thin **basal region** sits on the basal lamina, whereas their expanded apical portion, the **theca**, faces the lumen of the digestive tube or respiratory tract. The theca is filled with membrane-bound secretory droplets containing **mucinogen**, which displace the cytoplasm to the cell's periphery and the nucleus toward its base. The process of mucinogen release is regulated and stimulated by chemical irritation and parasympathetic innervation, resulting in exocytosis of the entire secretory contents of the cell, lubricating and protecting the epithelial sheet.

Multicellular Exocrine Glands

Multicellular exocrine glands exist as organized clusters of secretory units.

Multicellular exocrine glands consist of clusters of secretory cells arranged in varying degrees of organization. These secretory cells do not act independently but instead function as secretory organs. Multicellular glands may have a simple structure, exemplified by the glandular epithelium of the uterus and gastric mucosa, or a complex structure composed of various types of secretory units and organized in a compound branching fashion.

Because of their structural arrangement, multicellular glands are subclassified according to the organization of their secretory and duct components, as well as according to the shape of their secretory units (Fig. 5.25).

Multicellular glands are classified as **simple** if their ducts do not branch and **compound** if their ducts do branch. They are

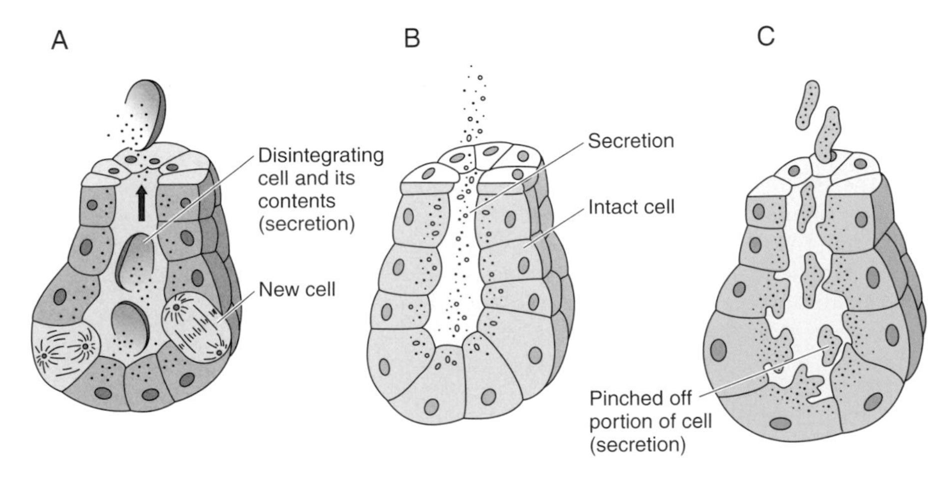

Fig. 5.21 Schematic diagram of modes of secretion. (A) Holocrine, (B) merocrine, (C) apocrine.

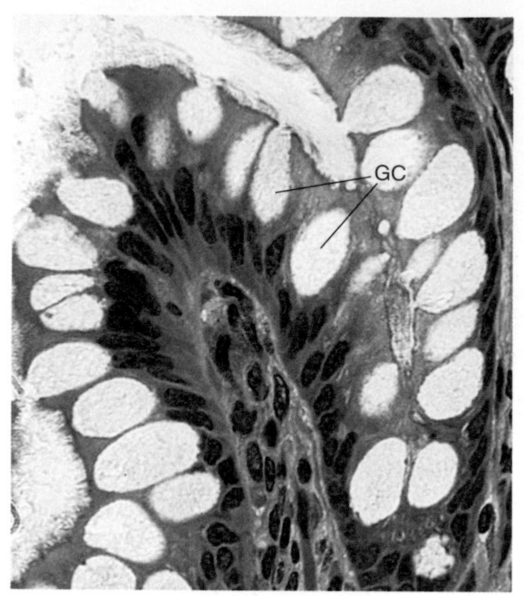

Fig. 5.22 Light micrograph of goblet cells (GC) in the epithelial lining of the monkey ileum. (×540)

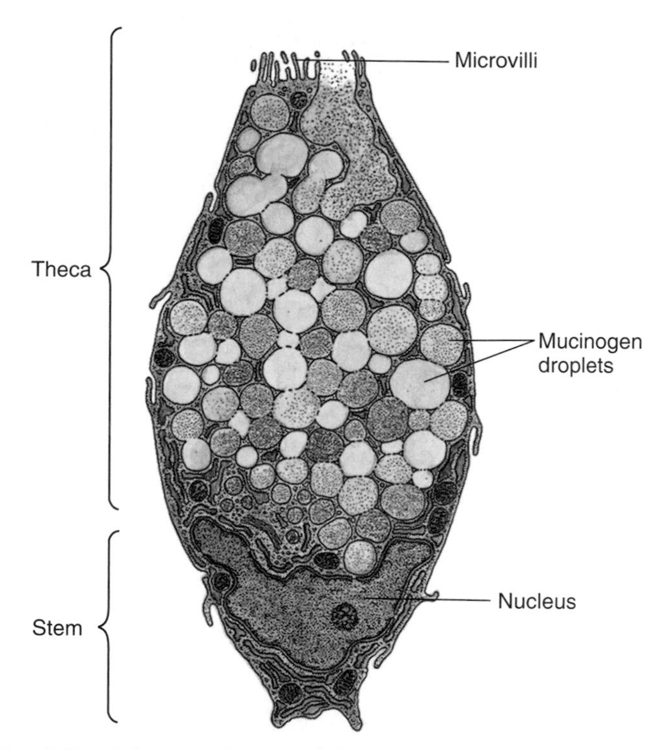

Fig. 5.23 Schematic diagram of the ultrastructure of a goblet cell illustrating the tightly packed secretory granules of the theca. From Lentz TL. *Cell Fine Structure: An Atlas of Drawings of Whole-Cell Structure.* Philadelphia: WB Saunders; 1971.

further categorized according to the morphology of their secretory units as ***tubular***, ***acinar*** (resembling a grape), or ***tubuloacinar*** (Fig. 5.26).

Larger multicellular glands are surrounded by a collagenous connective tissue **capsule**, which sends strands of connective tissue, known as **septa**, into the gland. The connective tissue elements provide support for the gland and subdivide the gland into smaller segments known as ***lobes*** and ***lobules***. Vascular elements, nerves, and ducts use the connective tissue septa to enter and exit the gland.

Acini of many multicellular exocrine glands, such as sweat glands and major salivary glands, possess **myoepithelial cells** that share the basal lamina of the acinar cells. Myoepithelial cells are of epithelial origin; they have small nuclei and sparse fibrillar cytoplasm radiating out from the cell body, wrapping around the acini and some of the small ducts (Fig. 5.27; see Fig. 5.26). They resemble smooth muscle cells because of their contractile abilities, which aid in expressing secretions from the acini and from some small ducts into the larger excretory ducts of the gland.

ENDOCRINE GLANDS

Endocrine glands are without ducts; their secretory products are thus released into the connective tissue and from there into the bloodstream or the lymphatic system.

Endocrine glands release their secretions, **hormones**, into richly vascularized connective tissue whose blood or lymphatic vessels distribute them to the target organs. The major endocrine glands of the body include the pituitary, suprarenal (adrenal), thyroid, parathyroid, and pineal glands, as well as the ovaries, placenta, and testes.

The islets of Langerhans and the interstitial cells of Leydig are unusual because they are composed of clusters of cells ensconced within the connective tissue stroma of other organs (the pancreas and testes, respectively). Hormones secreted by endocrine glands include peptides, proteins, modified amino acids, steroids, and glycoproteins. Because of their complexity and important role in regulating bodily processes, the endocrine glands are discussed in detail in Chapter 13.

Some glands of the body are mixed; for example, the parenchyma contains both exocrine and endocrine secretory units. In these mixed glands (e.g., pancreas, ovary, and testes), the exocrine portion of the gland secretes its product into a duct, whereas the endocrine portion of the gland secretes its product into the bloodstream.

Diffuse Neuroendocrine System

The diffuse neuroendocrine system functions to produce paracrine and endocrine hormones.

Widespread throughout the digestive tract and in the respiratory system are endocrine cells interspersed among the epithelial cells; these are members of the **diffuse neuroendocrine system (DNES)** which manufactures various paracrine and endocrine hormones (Fig. 5.28). DNES cells are described in greater detail in Chapter 17.

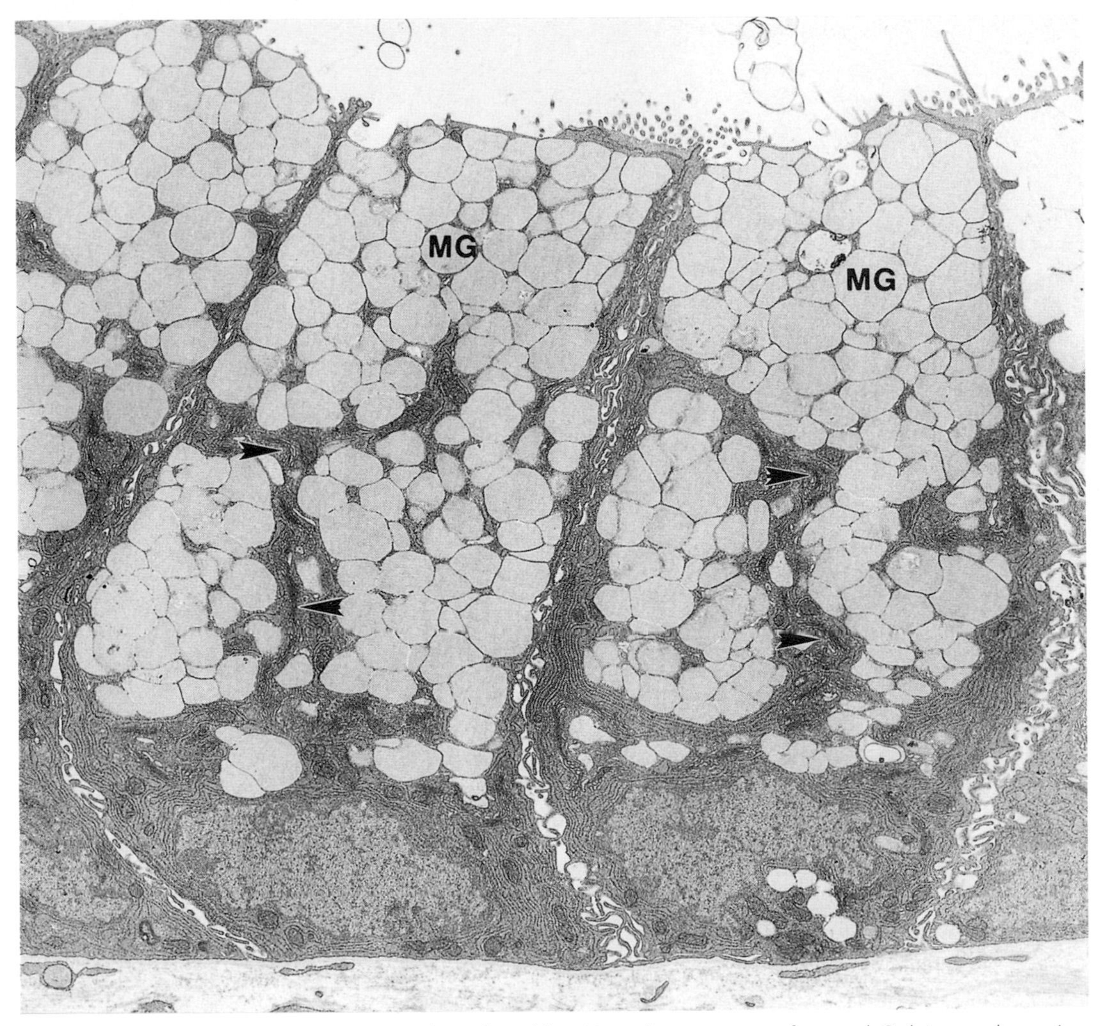

Fig. 5.24 Electron micrograph of goblet cells from the colon of a rabbit. Note the presence of several Golgi complexes *(arrowheads)* and the numerous compactly packed mucinogen granules (MGs) that occupy much of the apical portion of the cells (×9114). (From Radwan KA, Oliver MG, Specian RD. Cytoarchitectural reorganization of rabbit colonic goblet cells during baseline secretion. *Am J Anat.* 1990;198:365-376. Reprinted by permission of Wiley-Liss, Inc., a subsidiary of John Wiley & Sons, Inc.)

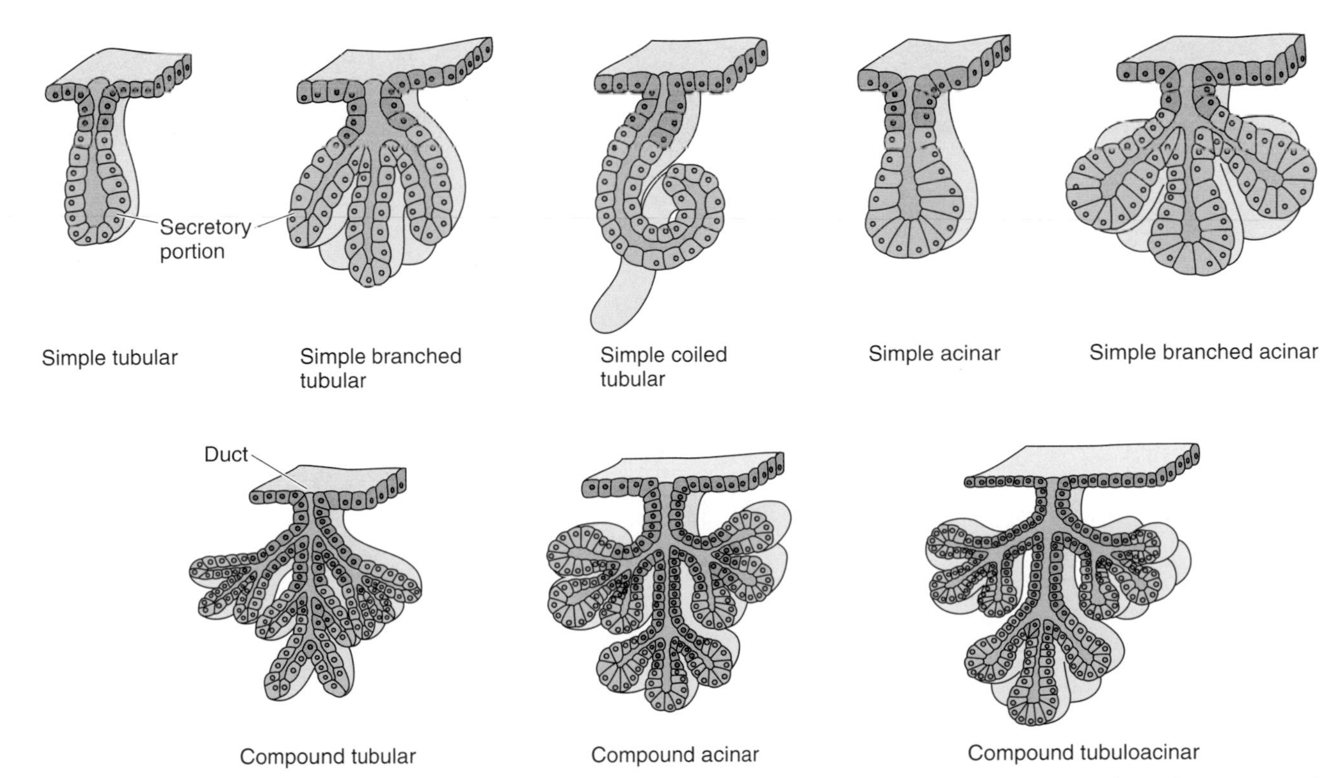

Fig. 5.25 Schematic diagram of the classification of multicellular exocrine glands. *Green* represents secretory portion; *lavender* represents the duct portion of the gland.

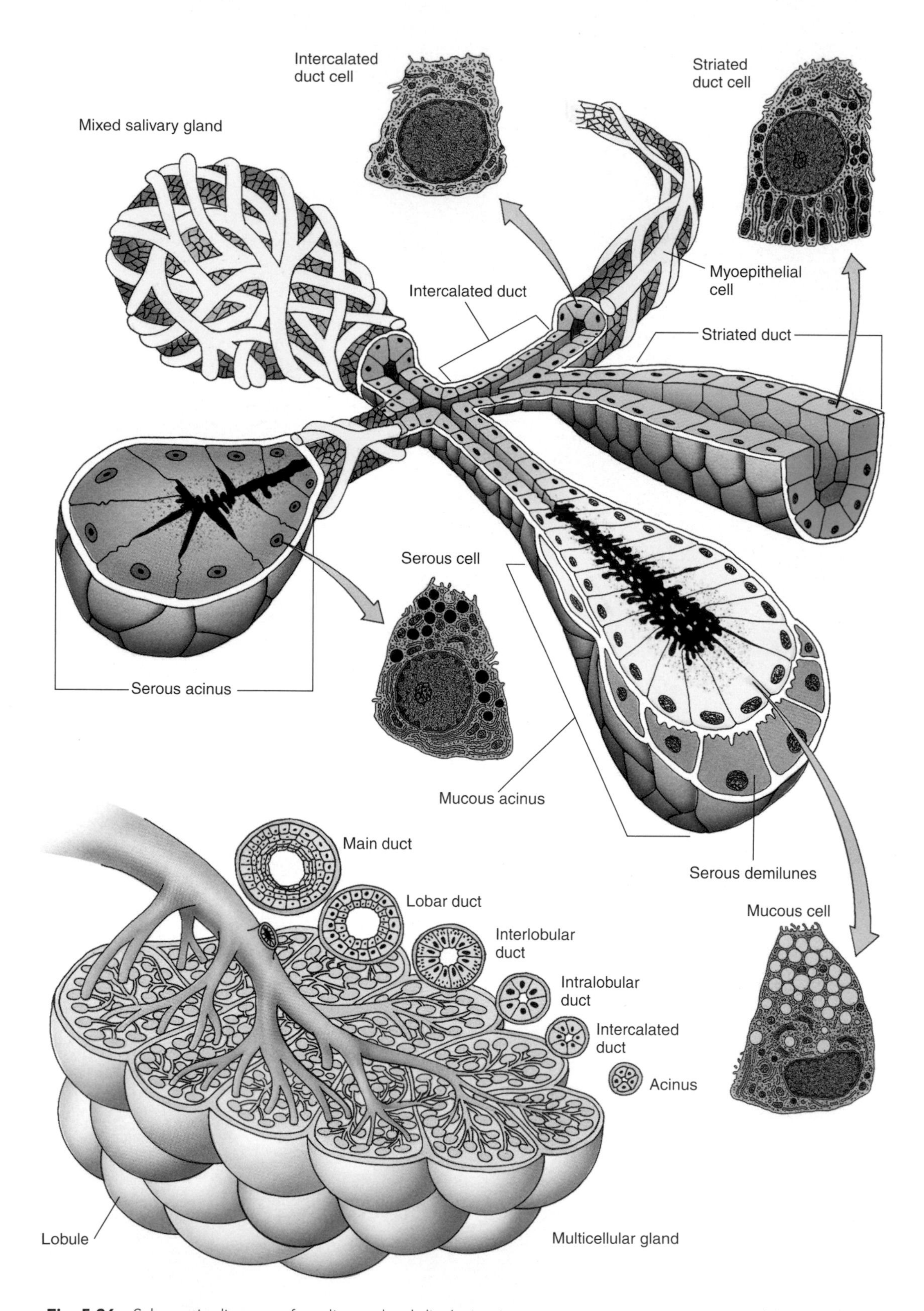

Fig. 5.26 Schematic diagram of a salivary gland displaying its organization, secretory units, and system of ducts.

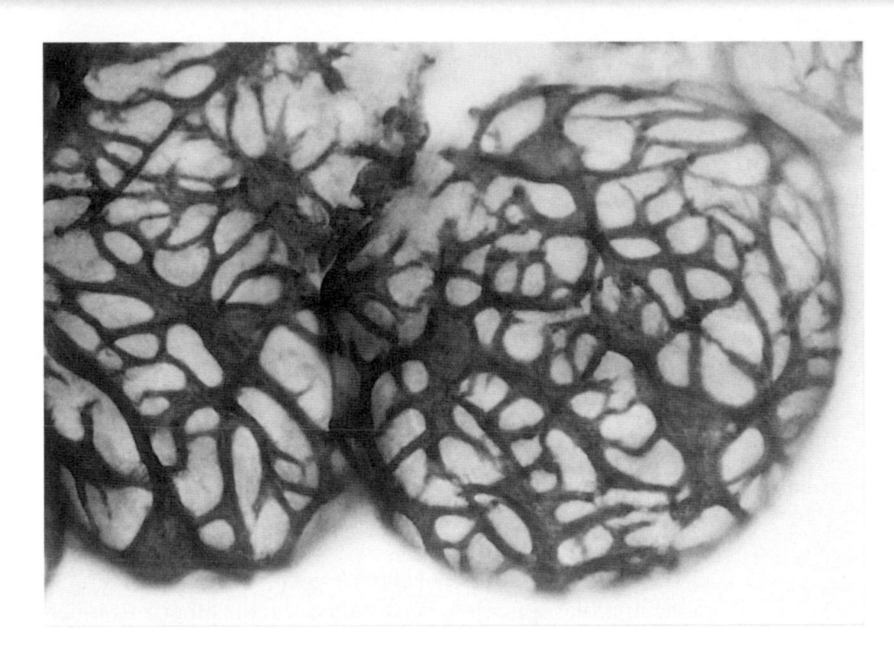

Fig. 5.27 Light micrograph of myoepithelial cells immunostained for actin. Myoepithelial cells surround the acini (×640). (From Satoh Y, Habara Y, Kanno T, Ono K. Carbamylcholine-induced morphological changes and spatial dynamics of $[Ca^{2+}]c$ in Harderian glands of guinea pigs: calcium-dependent lipid secretion and contraction of myoepithelial cells. *Cell Tissue Res.* 1993;274:1-14.)

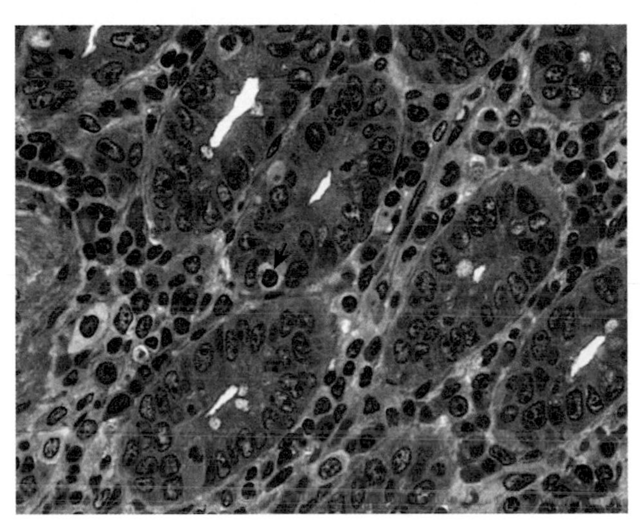

Fig. 5.28 Diffuse neuroendocrine system (DNES) cell. Note the pale-staining DNES cell *(arrow)* located in the mucosa of the ileum. (×540)

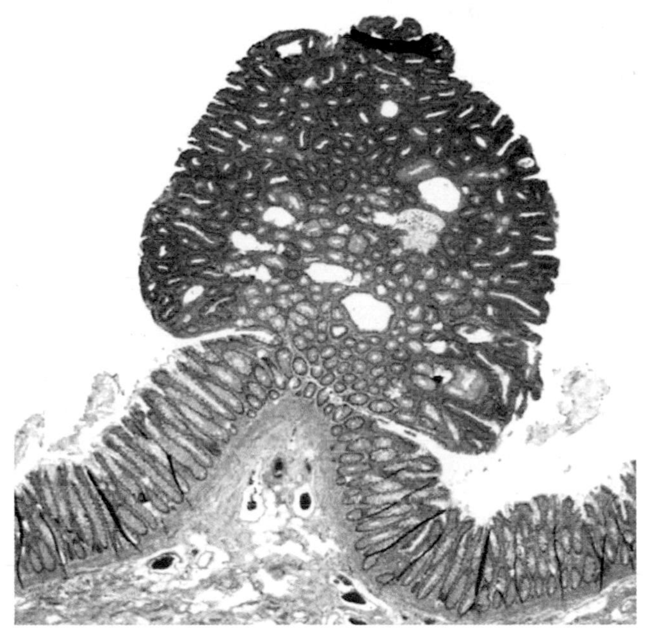

Fig. 5.29 A colonic polyp that is jutting into the lumen of the colon. Note that it is connected to the mucosa by a slender stalk. (From Kumar V, Abbas AK, Aster JC. *Robbins and Cotran Pathologic Basis of Disease.* 9th ed. Philadelphia: Elsevier; 2015: 267.)

Pathological Considerations

See Figs. 5.29 through 5.31.

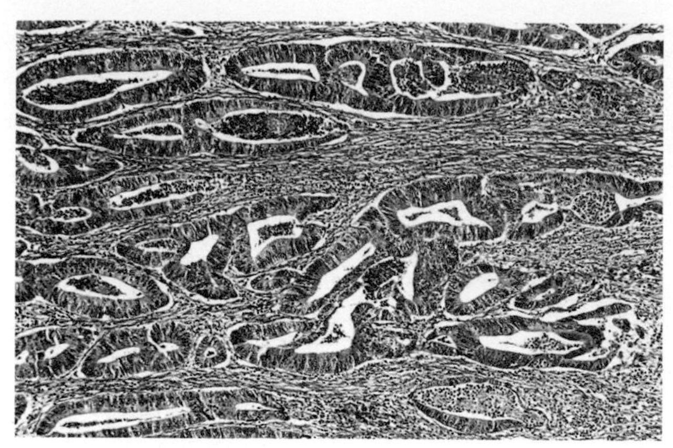

Fig. 5.30 Adenocarcinoma (glandular carcinoma) of the colon. Observe that the malignant glands that appear in this photomicrograph are irregular in morphology and appear completely different from the normal glands of a healthy colon. (From Kumar V, Abbas AK, Aster JC. *Robbins and Cotran Pathologic Basis of Disease*. 9th ed. Philadelphia: Elsevier; 2015:269.)

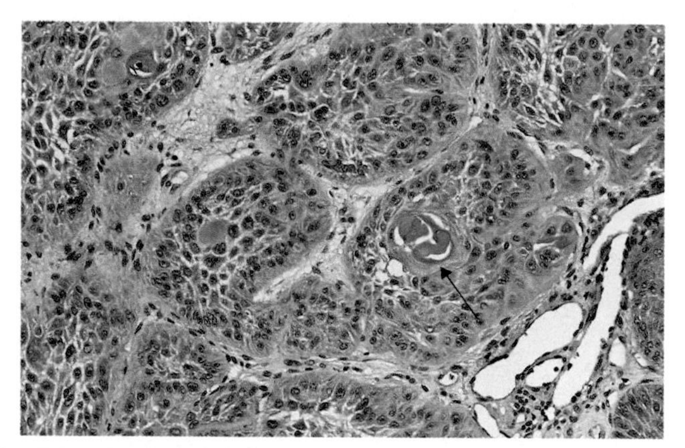

Fig. 5.31 Note that this photomicrograph of a squamous cell carcinoma of the skin displays a keratin pearl *(arrow)*. (From Kumar V, Abbas AK, Aster JC. *Robbins and Cotran Pathologic Basis of Disease*. 9th ed. Philadelphia: Elsevier; 2015:269.)

Histology Laboratory Instructions

EPITHELIUM AND GLANDS

Epithelium

When viewing microscope slides—whether real or virtual—you should look for empty spaces that are lined or covered by epithelia. Remember that these descriptions refer to two-dimensional images. See the drawing in Fig. 5.1 for their two- and three-dimensional appearances.

To find *simple squamous epithelia,* select the kidney medulla, where you will see circular profiles (Fig. 5.2A, *arrows*) of a single layer of thin cells with somewhat flattened nuclei. Another good place to observe simple squamous epithelium is in the kidney cortex. Look for rounded circular structures, known as renal *corpuscles*, and find the parietal layer of Bowman capsule (Fig. 5.3, SSE). *Simple cuboidal epithelium* is also present in both kidney cortex and kidney medulla (Figs. 5.3, SCuE; and 5.2, *arrowheads*). Note that the cells of this epithelium appear to be a single layer of little squares, each with a round, centrally placed nucleus. Simple columnar epithelial cells are best seen in the lining of the intestines; these cells form a single layer and resemble rectangular structures with oval nuclei (Fig. 5.2B).

Stratified squamous nonkeratinized epithelium is best located in the esophagus (Fig. 5.4A). It has numerous layers, and the cells on the free surface are flat and possess healthy nuclei *(arrow)*. *Stratified squamous keratinized epithelium* is best seen in skin (Fig. 5.4B), where the cells of the free surface are dead and no longer possess nuclei. Cells of the deeper layer display the presence of nuclei. *Stratified cuboidal epithelia* are best seen in the dermis of the skin, where they form the ducts of sweat glands (Fig. 5.4C, CC). Note that the two cell layers are evident because of the clearly observable nuclei of the cells. *Stratified columnar epithelia* are infrequent in humans and are not displayed in this textbook.

There are two additional types of epithelia: one is a simple epithelium that appears to be stratified and the other a stratified epithelium that resembles, superficially, stratified squamous nonkeratinized epithelium.

Pseudostratified columnar epithelium (Fig. 5.6) is best represented in the trachea. It is a simple epithelium because all of the cells form a single layer but the nuclei of the cells appear to be placed haphazardly so that the shortest cells have their nuclei basally and the nuclei of medium tall cells appear to be in the middle of the epithelium, whereas the nuclei of the tallest cells are positioned apically. Looking at just the nuclei, the epithelium appears to be stratified; therefore, this epithelium is named *pseudostratified*. *Transitional epithelium* is stratified and has a superficial resemblance to stratified squamous nonkeratinized epithelium. The best place to see this epithelium is the lining of the urinary bladder. When the bladder is empty, the epithelium is thicker and the cells at the free surface appear dome shaped (Figs. 5.4D, *arrows*; and 5.5, DSC).

Glands (Exocrine only)

The most common example of unicellular glands is the *goblet cell.* It is interspersed among the epithelial cells lining the small and large intestines and the larger pathways of the conducting portion of the respiratory tract. The theca of the goblet cell appears empty because the mucinogen is extracted during slide preparation (Figs. 5.22, GC; 5.23; and 5.24). Multicellular glands are of various conformations (Fig. 5.25); the mode and type of their secretions can be determined due to histological appearance of their cells (Figs. 5.21 and 5.25). The acini of purely *serous glands*, such as the exocrine pancreas (Fig. 5.19), form round clusters with round, basally displaced nuclei (resembling a pepperoni pizza with a single pepperoni per slice). *Mucous acini* of mixed glands, such as those of the submandibular gland (Fig. 5.20, M) also form round clusters but the cells appear foamy and their nuclei, also basally oriented, are flattened (resembling an anchovy pizza with a single anchovy per slice). Mucous acini of mixed glands also sport serous demilunes (Fig. 5.26 and unlabeled in Fig. 5.20).

6 Connective Tissue

Connective tissue is derived from **mesoderm**, the middle germ layer of the embryonic tissue, except in certain areas of the head and neck, where mesenchyme develops from neural crest cells of the developing embryo and is known as *ectomesenchyme*. Mesenchyme and ectomesenchyme give rise to multipotential cells of the embryo, known as **mesenchymal cells**, which migrate throughout the body, giving rise to the connective tissues and their cells, including those of bone, cartilage, tendons, capsules, blood and hemopoietic cells, and lymphoid cells (Fig. 6.1).

Mature connective tissue is classified as **connective tissue proper**, the major subject of this chapter, or **specialized connective tissue** (i.e., cartilage and bone, detailed in Chapter 7; and blood, detailed in Chapter 10).

Connective tissue is composed of cells and extracellular matrix (ECM), consisting of ground substance and fibers (Figs. 6.2, 6.3, and 6.4).

Some types of connective tissue are recognized because of the preponderance of their fibers, whereas other connective tissues are distinguished by the predominance of their cells. From a functional perspective, fibroblasts are the most important component of loose connective tissue because they manufacture and maintain the fibers and ground substance composing the ECM. In contrast, fibers are the most important component of tendons and ligaments because they function in attaching muscle to bone and bone to bone, respectively. In still other connective tissues, the ground substance is the most important component because it is where certain specialized connective tissue cells, such as extravasated white blood cells, carry out their functions.

Functions of Connective Tissue

The primary functions of connective tissue include structural **support**; serving as a **medium for exchange** of nutrients and waste products, as well as signaling molecules; aiding in the **defense**, **protection**, and **repair** of the body; and acting as a site for **storage of fat.** Connective tissues also help protect the body by forming a physical barrier to invasion and dissemination of microorganisms. **Repair** is performed mostly by fibroblasts that manufacture fibrous connective tissue and by **cells of bone** that mend broken or fractured bones.

Extracellular Matrix

The **ECM**, a nonliving material, is composed of ground substance and fibers designed to resist compressive and stretching forces. The components of the ECM are **ground substance** and **fibers**, as described in Chapter 4; the reader is directed to that chapter to review their features.

Cellular Components

The cells in connective tissues are grouped into two categories: **fixed cells** and **transient cells** (see Fig. 6.1). Fixed cells remain mostly stationary within the connective tissue, where they were formed; it is there that they perform their functions. **Transient cells** (free or wandering cells) originate mainly in the bone marrow and circulate in the bloodstream, which they leave to enter the connective tissue spaces to perform their specific functions.

FIXED CONNECTIVE TISSUE CELLS

The connective tissue cell types that are clearly fixed (fibroblasts, adipose cells, pericytes, mast cells, and macrophages, which exhibit both fixed and transient properties) are described in this section.

Fibroblasts

Fibroblasts, the most abundant cell type in the connective tissue, are responsible for the synthesis of almost the entire ECM.

Fibroblasts form the largest and most profusely distributed cell types of connective tissue proper. They are the least specialized cellular components of connective tissue. They may be active, fibroblasts that manufacture ECM (Figs. 6.1, 6.3, 6.4, and 6.5), or inactive, fibroblasts that do not manufacture ECM.

Active fibroblasts (see Fig. 6.5) often reside in close association with type I collagen bundles, where they lie parallel to the long axis of the fibers (Fig. 6.6). Such fibroblasts are elongated, fusiform cells possessing pale-staining cytoplasm, which is often difficult to distinguish from collagen when stained with hematoxylin and eosin. The most obvious portion of the cell is the darker-stained, large, granular, ovoid nucleus containing a well-defined nucleolus. Electron microscopy reveals a prominent Golgi apparatus and abundant rough endoplasmic reticulum (RER) in the fibroblast, especially when the cell is actively manufacturing matrix, as in wound healing.

Inactive fibroblasts (sometimes called fibrocytes) are smaller and more ovoid and possess an acidophilic cytoplasm. Their nuclei are smaller, elongated, and more deeply stained. Electron microscopy reveals sparse amounts of RER but an abundance of free ribosomes.

Clinical Correlations

Although considered to be fixed cells in the connective tissues, fibroblasts are capable of some movement. These cells seldom undergo cell division but may do so during wound healing and may differentiate into adipose cells, chondrocytes (during formation of fibrocartilage), and osteoblasts (under pathological conditions).

Myofibroblasts

Myofibroblasts are modified fibroblasts that demonstrate characteristics similar to those of both fibroblasts and smooth muscle cells.

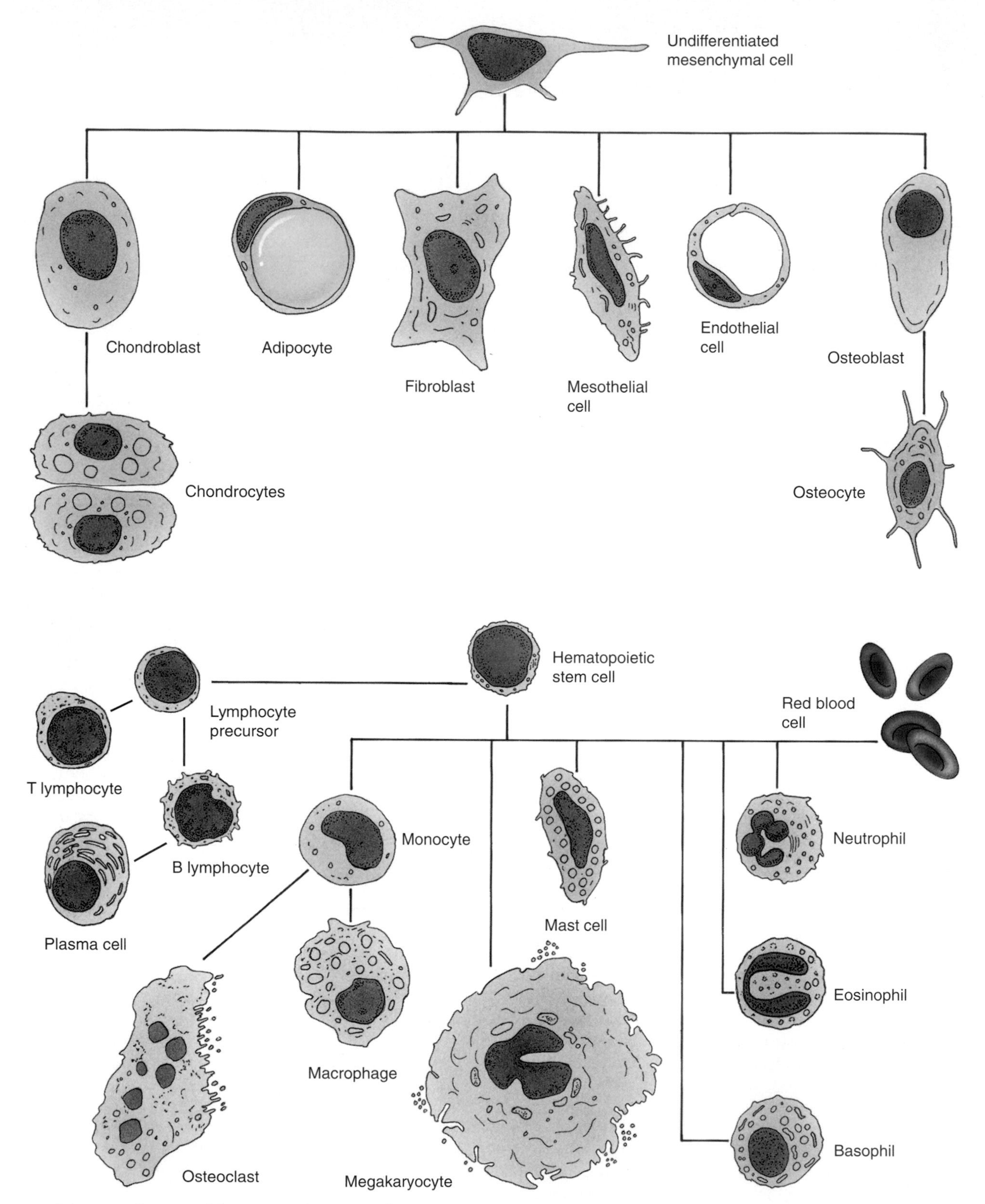

Fig. 6.1 Schematic diagram of the origins of the cells of connective tissue. Top: Fixed cells; bottom: transient cells. Cells are not drawn to scale.

Histologically, fibroblasts and **myofibroblasts** are not easily distinguished by routine light microscopy. Electron microscopy, however, reveals that myofibroblasts have bundles of actin filaments and myosin and dense bodies similar to those of smooth muscle cells. Additionally, the surface profile of the nucleus resembles that of a smooth muscle cell; however, myofibroblasts are not surrounded by an external lamina (basal lamina). Myofibroblasts, transitional modifications of fibroblasts, are abundant in areas undergoing wound healing, where they function in wound contraction.

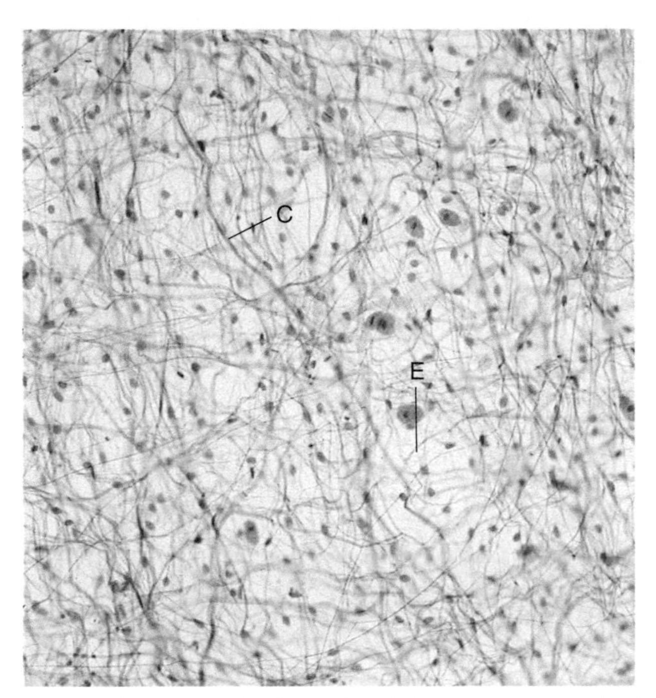

Fig. 6.2 Light micrograph of loose (areolar) connective tissue displaying collagen (C) and elastic (E) fibers and some of the cell types common to loose connective tissue (×132).

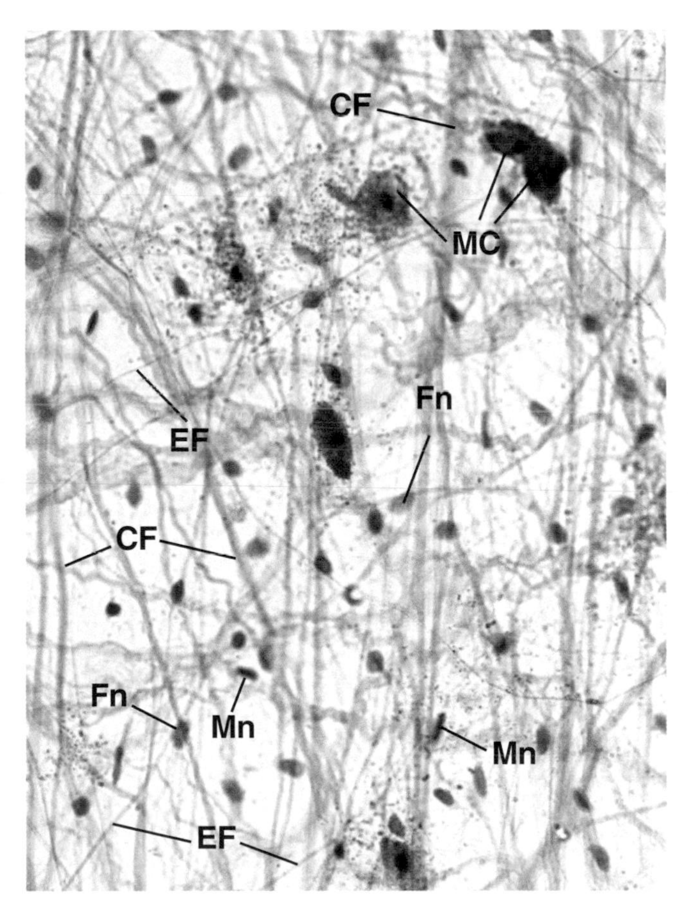

Fig. 6.3 This is a higher magnification of an area of Fig. 6.2. Note that the fibroblast nuclei (Fn) are oval and that they are larger and paler than the macrophage nuclei (Mn). Mast cells (MC) are the largest cells; they are red because of their numerous, closely packed granules. The thin elastic fibers (EF) and the thicker collagen fibers (CF) are easily distinguishable from each other. (×270).

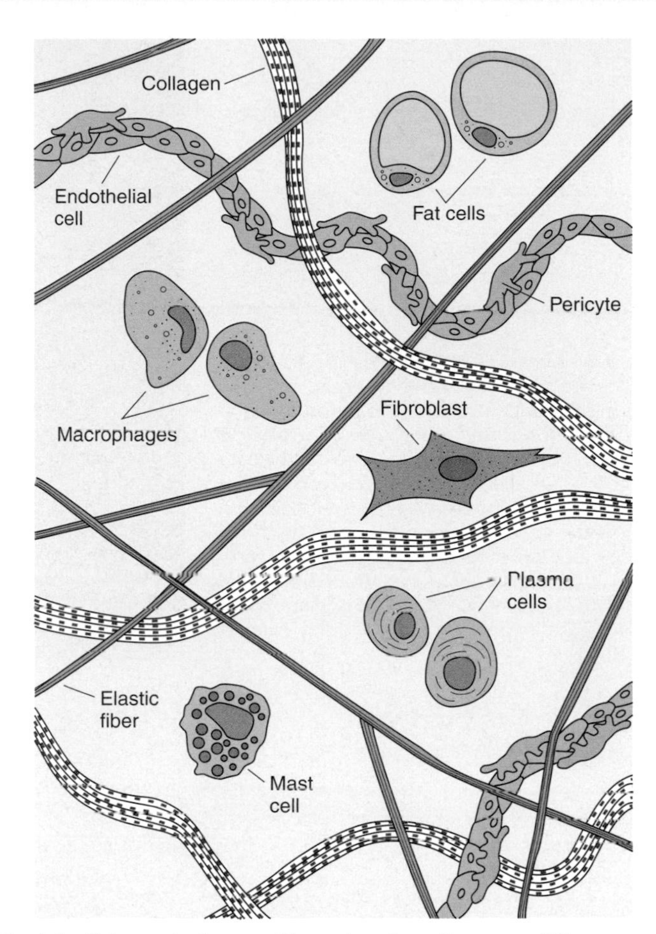

Fig. 6.4 Schematic diagram illustrating the cell types and fiber types in loose connective tissue. Cells are not drawn to scale.

Pericytes

Pericytes surround endothelial cells of capillaries and small venules and technically reside outside of the connective tissue compartment because they possess their own basal lamina.

Pericytes (also known as *perivascular cells* and *adventitial cells*), derived from undifferentiated mesenchymal cells, partly surround the endothelial cells of capillaries and small venules (see Fig. 6.4). These cells are outside of the connective tissue compartment because they are surrounded by their own basal lamina, which is usually fused with that of the endothelial cells. Pericytes possess some characteristics of smooth muscle cells in that they contain actin, myosin, and tropomyosin, suggesting that they may function in contraction. They are multipotential cells that, under certain conditions, are able to differentiate into other cells, including vascular smooth muscle cells, endothelial cells, and fibroblasts. Pericytes are discussed more fully in Chapter 11.

Adipose Cells

Adipose cells are fully differentiated cells that function in the synthesis, storage, and release of fat.

Fat cells, or **adipocytes**, are derived from undifferentiated fibroblast-like mesenchymal cells (Fig. 6.7), although, under certain conditions, they may arise from fibroblasts.

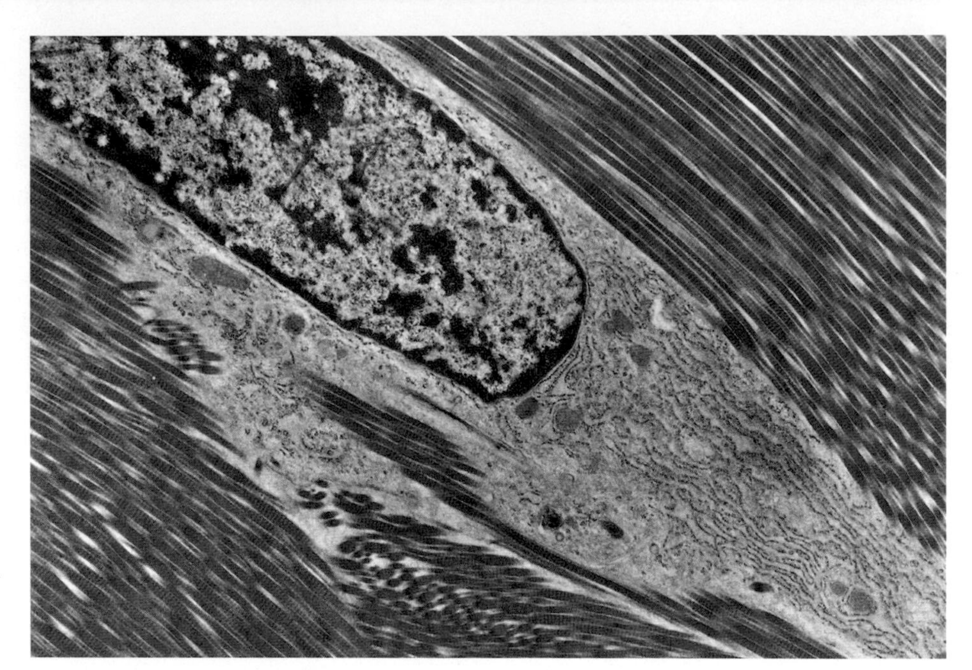

Fig. 6.5 Electron micrograph displaying a portion of a fibroblast and the packed collagen fibers in rat tendon. Observe the heterochromatin in the nucleus and the rough endoplasmic reticulum in the cytoplasm. Banding in the collagen fibers may also be observed. (From Ralphs JR, Benjamin M, Thornett A. Cell and matrix biology of the suprapatellar in the rat: a structural and immunocytochemical study of fibrocartilage in a tendon subject to compression. *Anat Rec.* 1991;231:167-177. Reprinted by permission of Wiley-Liss, Inc., a subsidiary of John Wiley & Sons, Inc.)

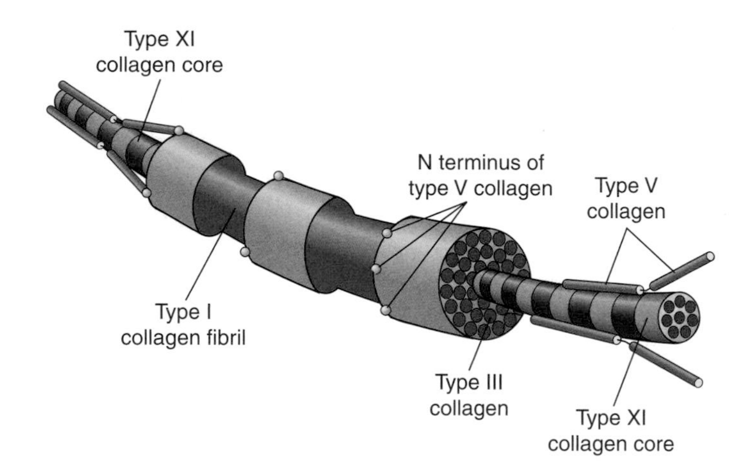

Fig. 6.6 Schematic diagram of type I collagen, demonstrating that it has a core of type XI and type V collagen. The bulk of type I collagen is interspersed with type II and type III collagen fibers.

Fat cells rarely undergo cell division. They manufacture, store, and release triglycerides, as well as synthesize and release hormones called ***adipokines*** (see white adipose tissue section in this chapter). There are two types of fat cells: (1) those with a single, large lipid droplet, called ***unilocular fat cells***, which congregate to form **white adipose tissue**; and (2) cells with multiple, small lipid droplets, called ***multilocular fat cells***, which congregate to form **brown adipose tissue**. White fat is much more abundant than brown fat, is distributed differently, and its physiology is different. Here, we describe the histological characteristics of the adipocytes themselves.

Unilocular adipocytes are large spherical cells, up to 120 µm in diameter, which become polyhedral when crowded into adipose tissue (Fig. 6.8). They store fat as a single droplet, which continues to increase in size so that the cytoplasm and nucleus are displaced peripherally against the plasma membrane; the cell resembles a "signet ring" when viewed by light microscopy. Electron micrographs reveal a small Golgi complex situated adjacent to the nucleus, only a few mitochondria, and sparse RER, but an abundance of free ribosomes. Additionally, adipocytes have their own basal lamina. That the fat droplet is not bound by a membrane is clear in electron micrographs but unclear in light micrographs. Their plasma membranes possess receptors for glucocorticoids, growth hormone, insulin, and norepinephrine, which regulate free fatty acid, glycerol, and triglyceride transport into and out of the cell. Minute pinocytotic vesicles of unknown function have been noted on the surface of the plasma membrane. During fasting, the cell surface becomes irregular, displaying pseudopod-like projections. Individual unilocular fat cells are located throughout the body in loose connective tissue and are concentrated along blood vessels. They may also accumulate into masses, forming white adipose tissue.

Multilocular adipocytes are smaller and more polygonal than white fat cells. They store lipids in several small droplets; therefore, their spherical nucleus is not squeezed up against the plasma membrane. Moreover, they house more mitochondria and smooth ER but fewer free ribosomes than unilocular fat

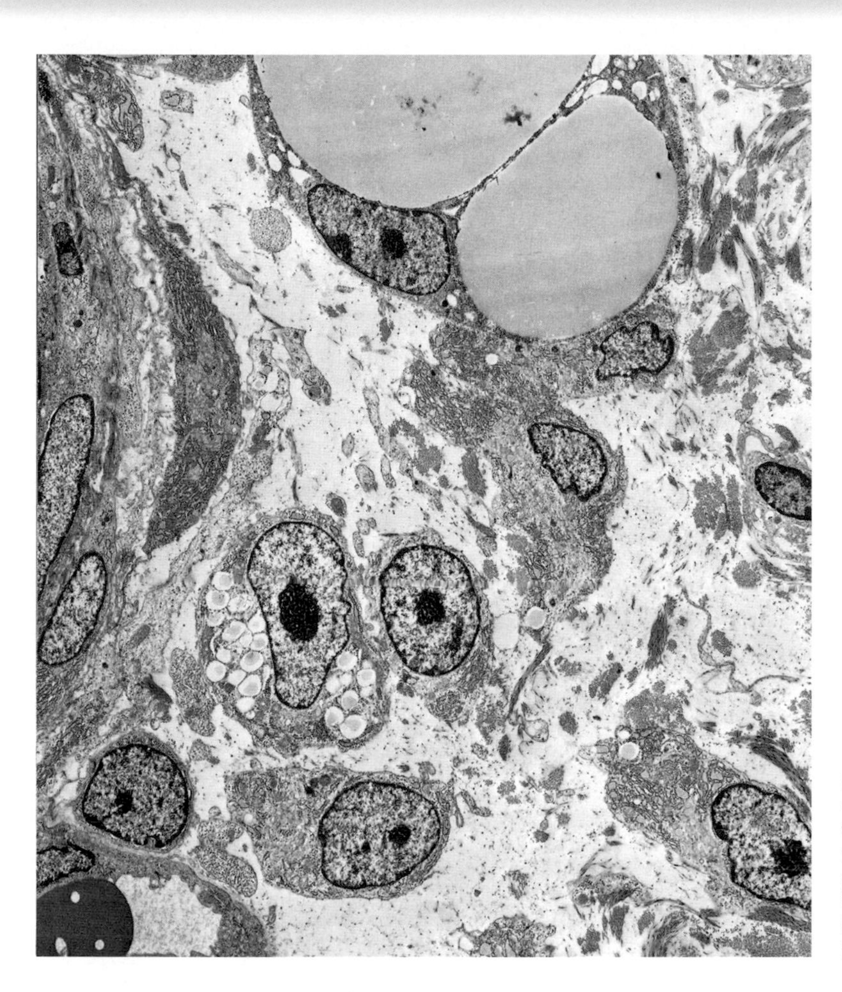

Fig. 6.7 Electron micrograph of adipocytes in various stages of maturation in rat hypodermis. Observe the adipocyte at the top of the micrograph, with its nucleus and cytoplasm crowded to the periphery by the fat droplet. From Hausman GJ, Campion DR, Richardson RL, Martin RJ. Adipocyte development in the rat hypodermis. *Am J Anat.* 1981;161:85-100. Reprinted by permission of Wiley-Liss, Inc., a subsidiary of John Wiley & Sons, Inc.

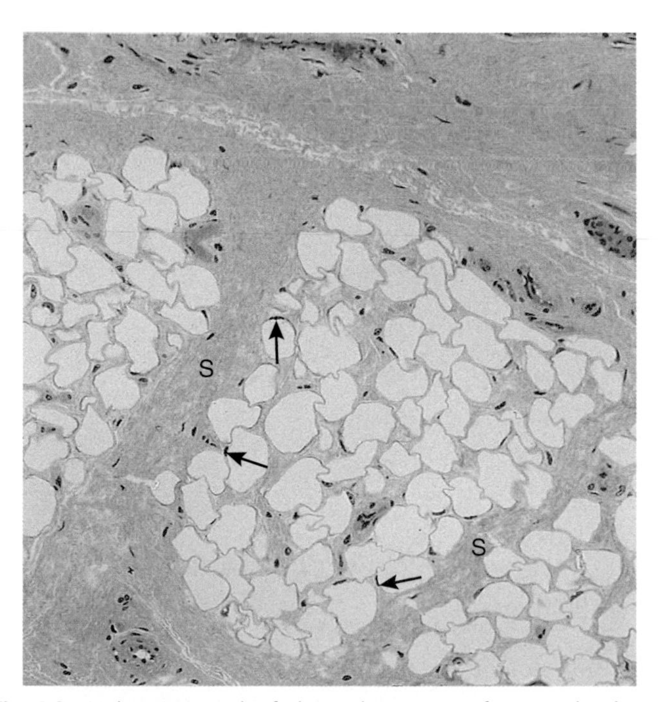

Fig. 6.8 Light micrograph of white adipose tissue from monkey hypodermis (×132). The lipid was extracted during tissue processing. Note how the cytoplasm and nuclei *(arrows)* are crowded to the periphery. Septa (S) divide the fat into lobules.

cells (Fig. 6.9). By uncoupling oxidation from phosphorylation, these cells generate heat.

Beige adipose cells (**brite adipose cells**), a form of multilocular fat cells, are present among unilocular adipocytes of the inguinal region; they function in heat generation and lipid storage.

Mast Cells

Mast cells arise from bone marrow stem cells and function in mediating the inflammatory process and immediate hypersensitivity reactions.

Mast cells, among the largest of the fixed cells of the connective tissue, are 20 to 30 μm in diameter. They are ovoid and possess a centrally placed, spherical nucleus (Figs. 6.10 and 6.11). Unlike the three types of fixed cells discussed earlier, mast cells probably derive from precursors in the bone marrow (see Fig. 6.1).

Electron microscopic studies of mast cells demonstrate that they possess numerous granules of various sizes (0.3-0.8 μm in diameter) in their cytoplasm (Fig. 6.12), as well as a few mitochondria, a sparse number of RER profiles, and a relatively small Golgi complex.

Mast cell granules contain various pharmacological agents, including **heparin**, **histamine** (or **chondroitin sulfates**),

neutral proteases (tryptase, chymase, and carboxypeptidases), **aryl sulfatase** (as well as other enzymes, such as β-glucuronidase, kininogenase, peroxidase, and superoxide dismutase), **eosinophil chemotactic factor** (ECF), and **neutrophil chemotactic factor** (NCF). Because they are present within the granules, they are referred to as the ***primary mediators*** (***preformed mediators***). Mast cells also synthesize a number of pharmacological agents *as needed* and these are known as ***secondary mediators*** (or ***newly synthesized mediators***). Some are manufactured from membrane arachidonic acid precursors and include **leukotrienes** (C_4, D_4, and E_4), **thromboxanes** (**TXA_2** and **TXB_2**), and **prostaglandins** (PGD_2). Others are *not derived* from arachidonic acid precursors, such as **platelet-activating factor** (**PAF**), **bradykinins**, **interleukins** (**IL-4**, **IL-5**, **IL-6**), and **tumor necrosis factor-alpha** (TNF-α). These pharmacological agents, whether primary or secondary, function in the immune system by the initiation of an **inflammatory response** (discussed later).

Mast Cell Development and Distribution

Basophils and mast cells share some characteristics, but they are different cells and have different precursors (see Fig. 6.1). Mast cells have a life span of less than a few months and, occasionally, undergo cell division. There are two types of mast cells: those concentrated along small blood vessels, which are known as ***connective tissue mast cells***; and those that are present in the subepithelial connective tissue of the respiratory and digestive systems, which are called ***mucosal mast cells***. Mast cells in connective tissue contain the sulfated glycosaminoglycan (GAG) heparin in their granules, whereas those located in the alimentary tract mucosa house the GAG chondroitin sulfate. GAGs stain metachromatically with toluidine blue (i.e., toluidine blue stains the granules purple), a characteristic feature of mast cells.

Clinical Correlations

The central nervous system is devoid of mast cells, most probably to prevent swelling of the brain and spinal cord.

Mucosal mast cells release histamine to facilitate the activation of parietal cells of the stomach to produce hydrochloric acid.

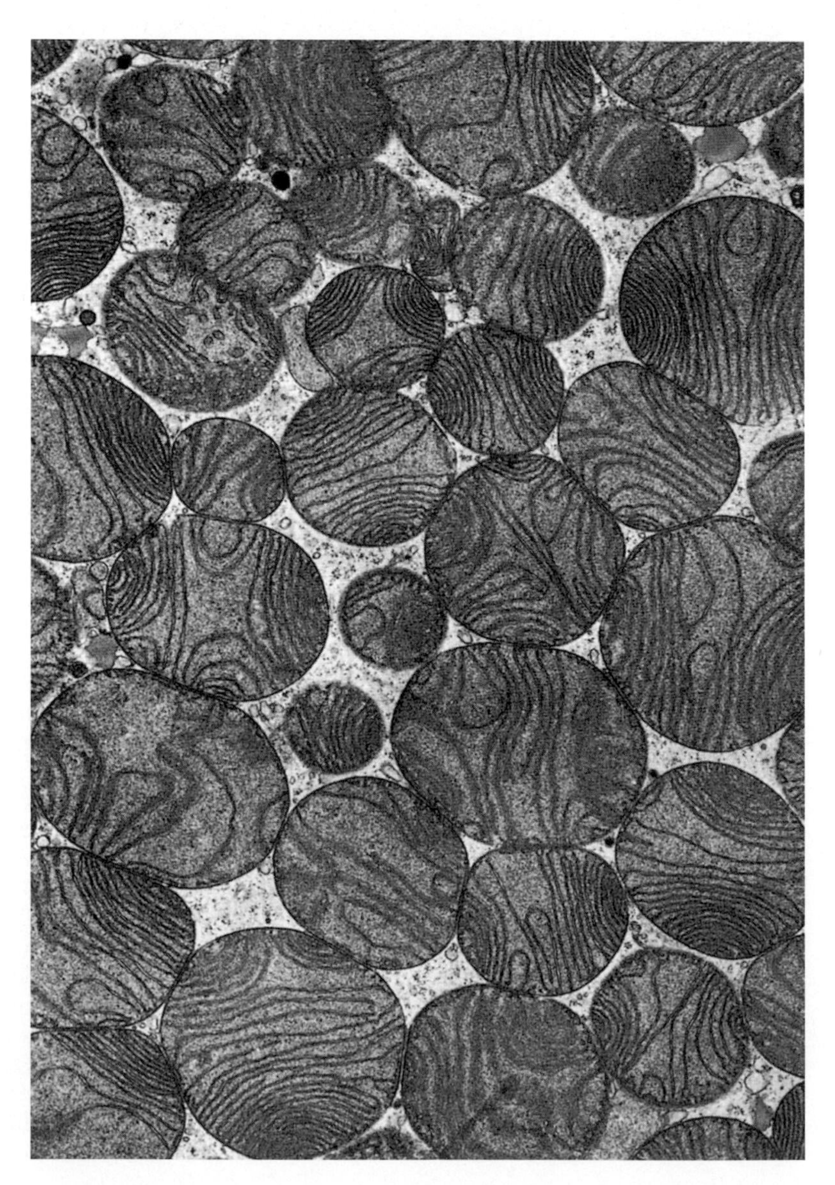

Fig. 6.9 Multilocular fat cells (brown fat) in the bat (×11,000). Note the numerous mitochondria dispersed throughout the cell. From Fawcett DW. *An Atlas of Fine Structure. The Cell.* Philadelphia: WB Saunders; 1966.

Mast Cell Activation and Degranulation

Mast cells possess high-affinity cell-surface Fc receptors (**FcεRI**) for immunoglobulin E (IgE). These cells function in the immune system by initiating an inflammatory response known as the ***immediate hypersensitivity reaction*** (whose systemic form, known as an ***anaphylactic reaction***, may have lethal consequences). This response commonly is induced by foreign molecules (antigens) such as bee venom, pollen, and certain drugs, as follows:

1. The first exposure to any of these antigens elicits formation of IgE antibodies by plasma cells. The IgE binds to the FcεRI receptors of the plasmalemma of mast cells, thereby **sensitizing** these cells.
2. On subsequent exposure to the *same* antigen, the antigen binds to the IgE on the mast cell surface, causing cross-linking of the bound IgE antibodies and clustering of the receptors (Fig. 6.13).
3. Cross-linking and clustering activate membrane-bound **receptor coupling factors**, which, in turn, initiate at least two independent processes, the release of **primary mediators** from the granules and synthesis and release of the **secondary mediators** (Table 6.1).
4. The primary and secondary mediators released by mast cells during immediate hypersensitivity reactions initiate the inflammatory response, activate the body's defense system by attracting leukocytes to the site of inflammation, and modulate the degree of inflammation (see Fig. 6.13).

Sequence of Events in the Inflammatory Response.

1. **Histamine** dilates and increases the permeability of nearby blood vessels. It also causes bronchospasms and increases mucus production in the respiratory tract.
2. Complement components that escaped blood vessels are cleaved by **neutral proteases** to form additional inflammatory agents.

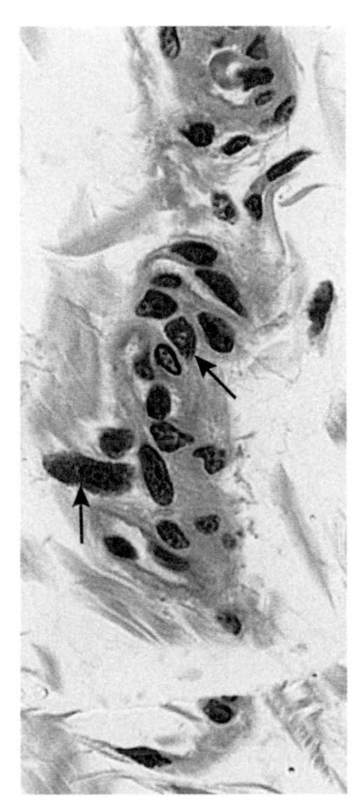

Fig. 6.10 Light micrograph of mast cells *(arrows)* in monkey connective tissue (540). The granules within the mast cells contain histamine and other preformed pharmacological agents.

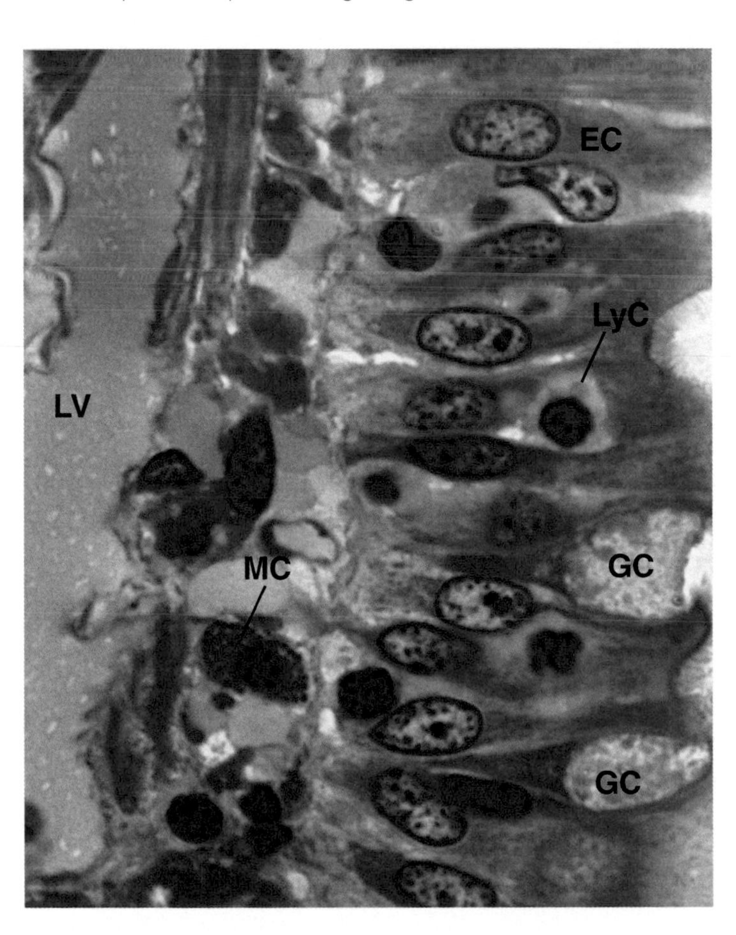

Fig. 6.11 A high-magnification light micrograph of the monkey duodenum displaying a mast cell (MC) whose central nucleus and large number of granules are housing the primary mediators. The simple columnar epithelium (EC) has lymphocytes (LyC) migrating through it. Observe the expanded theca of the goblet cells (GC) as well as the lymph vessel (LV) deep to the epithelium. (×1,325)

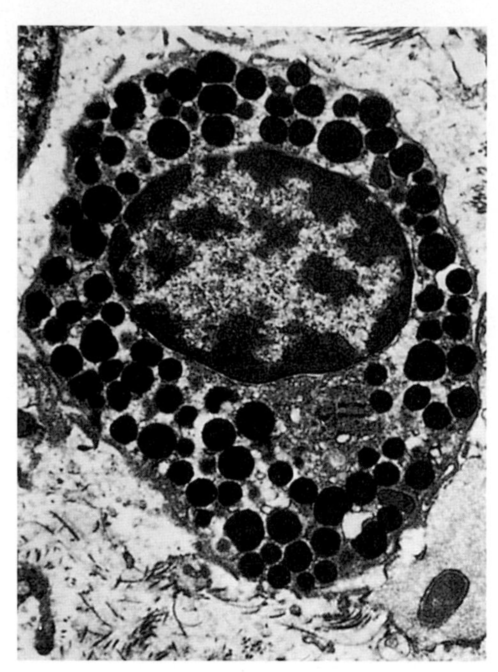

Fig. 6.12 Electron micrograph of a mast cell in the rat (×5500). Observe the dense granules filling the cytoplasm. From Leeson TS, Leeson CR, Paparo AA. *Text/Atlas of Histology*. Philadelphia: WB Saunders; 1988.

3. **ECF** attracts eosinophils to the site of inflammation. These cells phagocytose antigen–antibody complexes, destroy any parasites present, and limit the inflammatory response.
4. **NCF** attracts neutrophils to the site of inflammation. These cells phagocytose and kill microorganisms, if present.
5. **Leukotrienes C_4, D_4,** and **E_4** increase vascular permeability and cause bronchospasms. They are several thousand times more potent than histamine in their vasoactive effects.
6. **Prostaglandin D_2** causes bronchospasms and increases secretion of mucus by the bronchial mucosa.
7. **PAF** causes greater vascular permeability.
8. **Thromboxane A_2** is a vigorous platelet-aggregating mediator that also causes vasoconstriction. It is quickly transformed into **thromboxane B_2**, its inactive form.
9. **Bradykinin** is a powerful vascular dilator that causes vascular permeability. It is also responsible for pain.

Macrophages

Macrophages belong to the mononuclear phagocytic system and are subdivided into two groups of cells: phagocytes and antigen-presenting cells.

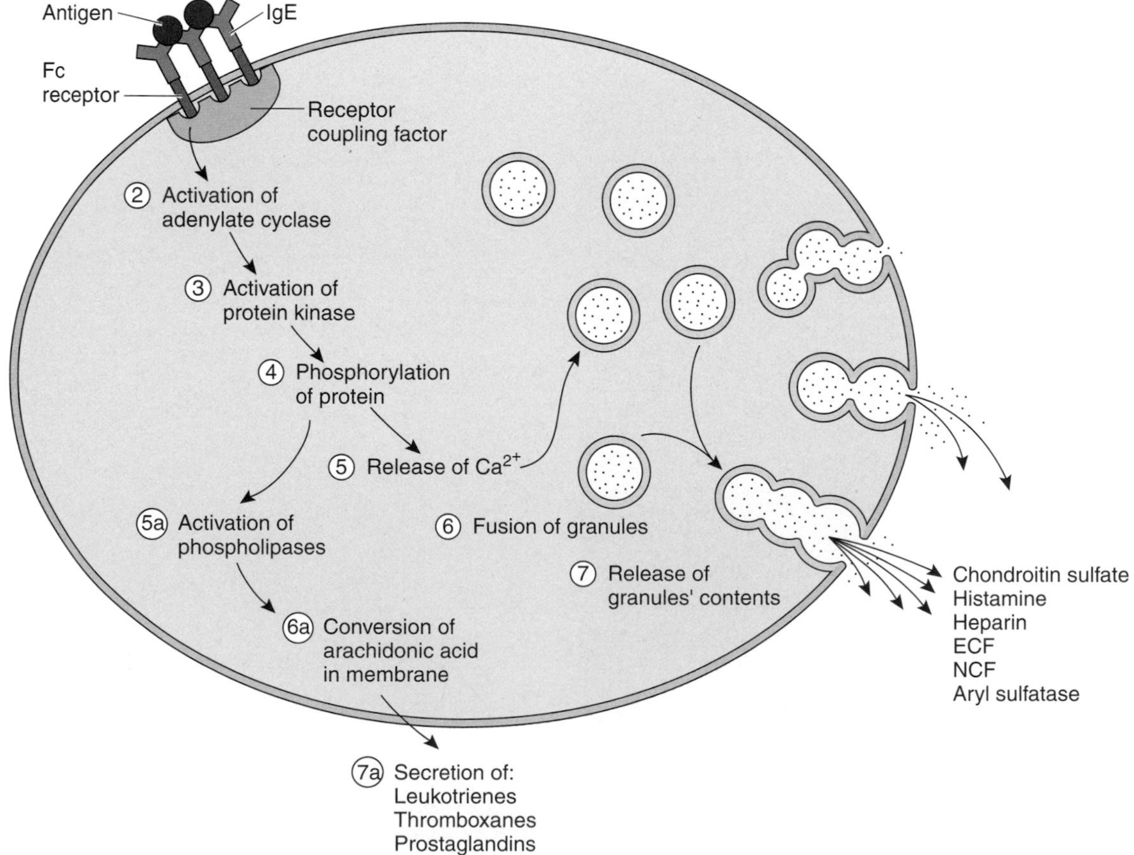

Fig. 6.13 Schematic diagram illustrating the binding of antigens and cross-linking of immunoglobulin E (IgE)–receptor complexes on the mast cell plasma membrane. This event triggers a cascade that ultimately results in the synthesis and release of leukotrienes and prostaglandins, as well as in degranulation, thus releasing histamine, heparin, eosinophil chemotactic factor (ECF), and neutrophil chemotactic factor (NCF).

Clinical Correlations

1. *People suffering from **hay fever** attacks experience the effects of **histamine** being released by the mast cells of the nasal mucosa, which causes localized edema from increased permeability of the small blood vessels. The swelling of the mucosa results in feeling "stuffed up" and hinders breathing.*
2. *People experiencing **asthma** attacks have difficulty breathing as a result of bronchospasms caused by **leukotrienes** released in the lungs.*
3. *Because degranulation of mast cells usually is a localized phenomenon, the typical inflammatory response is mild and site specific. However, a risk also exists for **hyperallergic persons** who may experience a systemic and severe immediate hypersensitivity reaction (**systemic anaphylaxis**) following a secondary exposure to an allergen (i.e., insect stings, antibiotics, or other antigens). This reaction (**anaphylactic shock**) may occur within seconds to a few minutes, including shortness of breath, decreasing blood pressure, and the symptoms of shock, which may result in the person's death (in a matter of a few hours) if left untreated. Persons susceptible to this condition often wear a medical emergency bracelet informing the first responder giving assistance to get them immediate medical attention and carry an epinephrine auto-injection device to self-inject a predetermined amount of epinephrine to stop the anaphylactic reaction.*
4. ***Mastocytosis** is a rare condition in which the patient possesses too many mast cells. The most common form of this disease is a skin disorder known as urticaria pigmentosa, a condition limited to the skin in neonates that exhibits itself, upon irritation, as hives or splotchy reddish-brown discoloration of the skin. This condition is caused by an autosomal point mutation that alters a transmembrane protein on mast cell precursors, which become hypersensitive to the chemokine, known as mast cell growth factor. This hypersensitivity to mast cell growth factor greatly enhances the proliferative ability of these cells, resulting in an increased number of mast cells in the dermis.*

As noted earlier, some macrophages behave both as fixed cells and as transient cells. Because macrophages are active phagocytes, they function in removing cellular debris and in protecting the body against foreign invaders.

Macrophages are irregularly shaped cells with a diameter of about 10 to 30 μm (Fig. 6.14). They present in various ways, from short and blunt to finger-like projections from their surface, whereas macrophages that are motile or are actively phagocytosing particular matter display pleats and folds of their plasma membranes. Macrophage cytoplasm is basophilic, with many small vacuoles and small, dense granules. Their eccentric nuclei are small, kidney-shaped, and are usually void of nucleoli. Viewed with the electron microscope, a well-developed Golgi apparatus, prominent RER, and abundance of lysosomes are evident. As macrophages mature, they increase not only in size but also in their organelle population.

Macrophage Development and Distribution

Macrophages have an average life span of about 2 months and are derived from **monocytes** of the **mononuclear phagocyte system** (Table 6.2) whose members arise from a common stem cell in the bone marrow, possess lysosomes, are capable of phagocytosis, and display complement and FcεRI receptors.

Macrophages localized in certain regions of the body were given specific names before their origin was completely understood. Thus, **Kupffer cells** of the liver (Fig. 6.15); **dust cells** of the lung; **Langerhans cells** of the skin; **monocytes** of the blood; **macrophages** of the connective tissue, spleen, lymph nodes, thymus, and bone marrow; **osteoclasts** of bone; and **microglia** of the brain are all members of the mononuclear phagocyte system and possess similar morphology and functions. Under chronic inflammatory conditions, macrophages congregate, greatly enlarge, and become polygonal **epithelioid cells.** When the particulate matter to be disposed of is excessively large, a number of macrophages may fuse to form a very large multinucleated macrophage, known as **foreign-body giant cells.**

Macrophages residing in the connective tissues were previously called ***fixed macrophages***, and those that developed as a result of an exogenous stimulus and migrated to the particular

TABLE 6.1 Principal Primary and Secondary Mediators Released by Mast Cells

Substance	Type of Mediator	Source	Action
Histamine	Primary	Granule	Increases vascular permeability; vasodilation; smooth muscle contraction of bronchi; increases mucus production
Heparin	Primary	Granule (of CT mast cells)	Anticoagulant; binds to and inactivates histamine
Chondroitin sulfate	Primary	Granule (of mucosal mast cells)	Binds to and inactivates histamine
Aryl sulfatase	Primary	Granule	Inactivates leukotriene C_4, thus limiting the inflammatory response
Neutral proteases	Primary	Granule	Protein cleavage to activate complement (especially C3a); increases inflammatory response
Eosinophil chemotactic factor	Primary	Granule	Attracts eosinophils to site of inflammation
Neutrophil chemotactic factor	Primary	Granule	Attracts neutrophils to site of inflammation
Leukotrienes C_4, D_4, and E_4	Secondary	Membrane lipid	Vasodilator; increases vascular permeability; bronchial smooth muscle contractant
Prostaglandin D_2	Secondary	Membrane lipid	Causes contraction of bronchial smooth muscle; increases mucus secretion; vasoconstriction
Thromboxane A_2	Secondary	Membrane lipid	Causes platelet aggregation; vasoconstriction
Bradykinins	Secondary	Formed by activity of enzymes located in granules	Causes vascular permeability and is responsible for pain sensation
Platelet-activating factor	Secondary	Activated by phospholipase A_2	Attracts neutrophils and eosinophils; causes vascular permeability and contraction of bronchial smooth muscle

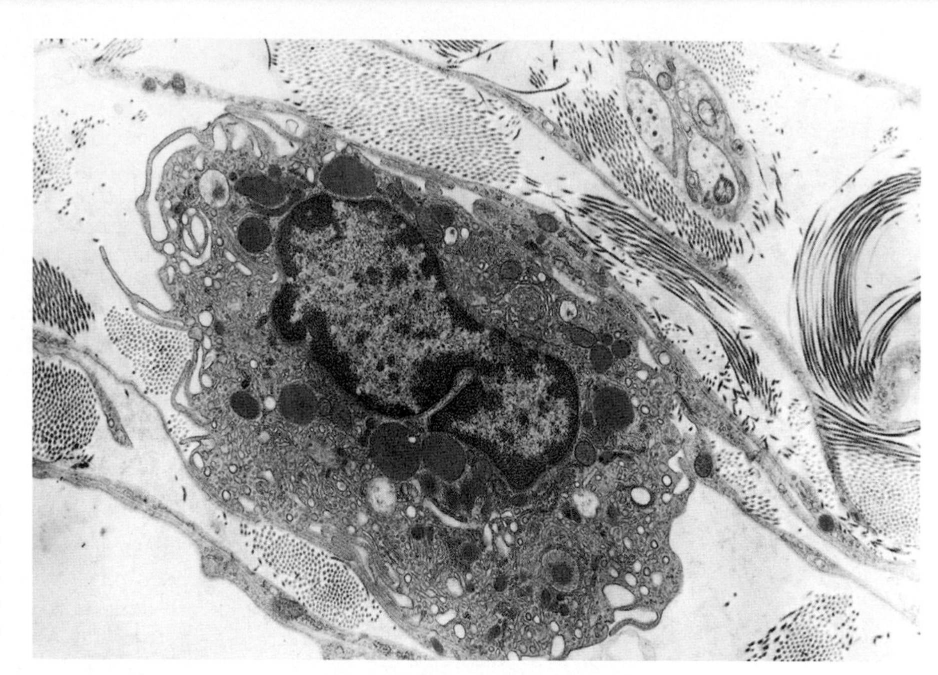

Fig. 6.14 Electron micrograph of a macrophage in the rat epididymis. From Flickinger CJ, Herr CJ, Sisak JR, Howards SS. Ultrastructure of epididymal interstitial reactions following vasectomy and vasovasostomy. *Anat Rec.* 1993;235:61-73. Reprinted by permission of Wiley-Liss, Inc., a subsidiary of John Wiley & Sons, Inc.

TABLE 6.2 Cells of the Mononuclear Phagocyte System

Cells	Classification	Location	Function
Macrophages	Transient and fixed	Connective tissue proper, lymph nodes, spleen	Phagocytosis, antigen presenting, manufacture and release of cytokines and inflammatory agents, participation in immune reactions
Foreign-body giant cells	Transient	Connective tissue proper	Macrophages can fuse with each other to form giant cells to phagocytose large particulate matter
Dust cells	Transient	Alveoli of lung	Phagocytosis of inhaled particulate matter; surfactant uptake; act as anti-inflammatory agents
Langerhans cells	Fixed	Stratum spinosum of skin	Phagocytose and process antigens that enter the epidermis and present the epitopes to T lymphocytes in lymph nodes
Kupffer cells	Fixed	Sinusoids of liver	Phagocytose particulate matter, especially defunct red blood cells
Monocytes	Wandering	Bloodstream	Leave the vascular system to differentiate into macrophages
Osteoclasts	Fixed	Bone	Resorb bone by decalcifying it and phagocytosing bone matrix
Microglia	Fixed	Central nervous system (CNS)	Phagocytose debris and damaged structures in the CNS; present epitopes to T cells; also destroy unnecessary synapses

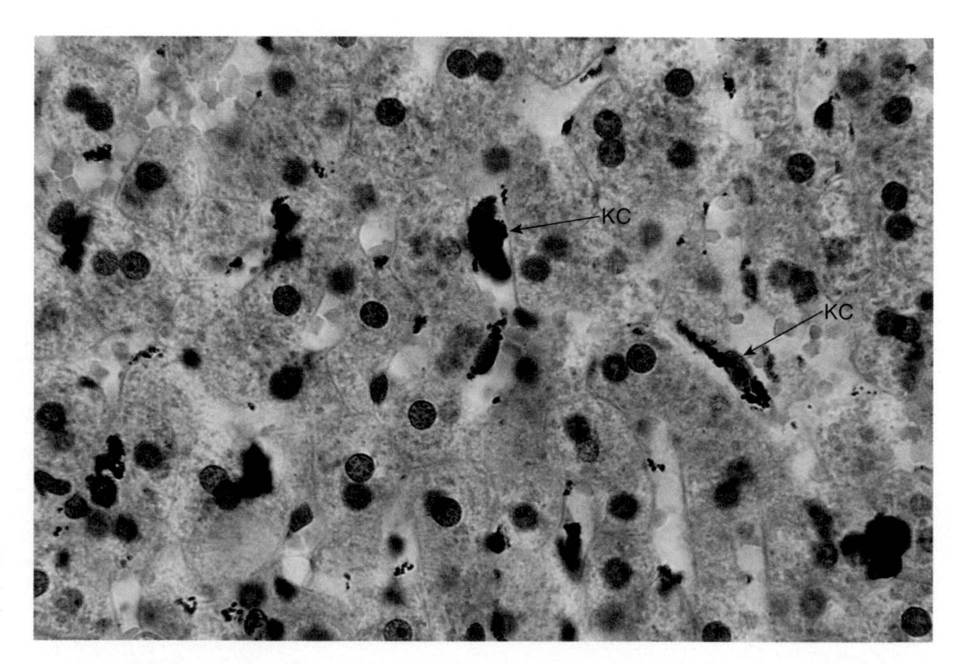

Fig. 6.15 Light micrograph of liver of an animal injected with India ink demonstrating the presence of cells known as Kupffer cells (KC) that preferentially phagocytose the ink (×540).

site were called ***free macrophages***. These names have been replaced by the more descriptive terms ***resident macrophages*** and ***elicited macrophages***, respectively.

Macrophage Function

Macrophages phagocytose foreign substances and damaged and senescent cells, as well as cellular debris; they also assist in the initiation of the immune response.

Macrophages phagocytose senescent, damaged, and dead cells, cellular debris, and foreign substance (including microorganisms) and digest the phagocytosed material via their endolysosomal system (see Chapter 2). During an immune response, cytokines released by lymphocytes activate macrophages, thereby increasing their phagocytic activity. **Activated macrophages** vary considerably in shape, possess microvilli and lamellipodia, and exhibit more locomotion compared with inactivated macrophages. Macrophages also phagocytose foreign proteins and cleave them into short peptide sequences known as *epitopes*, complexing these epitopes with their major histocompatibility complex molecules (major histocompatibility complex [MHC] I or MHC II), placing them on their cell membranes, and presenting the epitope-MHC complex to T cells. Thus, they are also known as antigen-presenting cells (see Chapter 12 for a more complete description of this process).

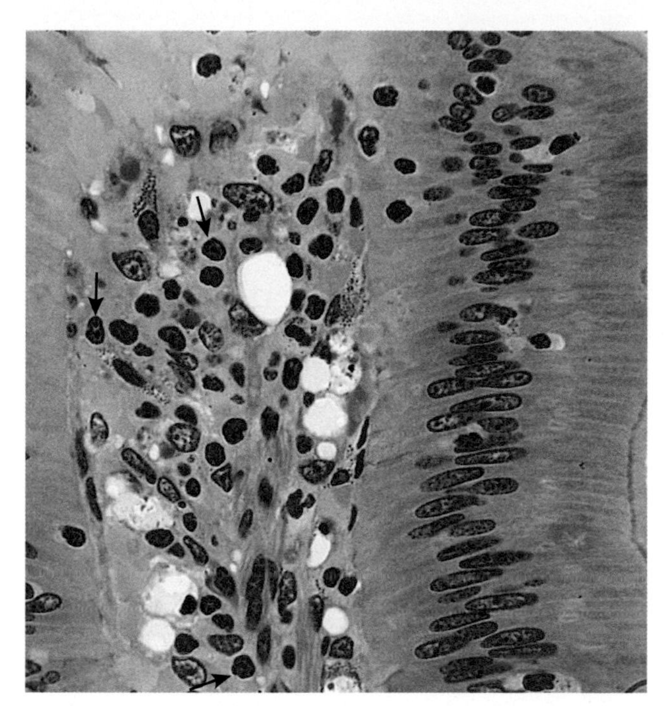

Fig. 6.16 Light micrograph of plasma cells in the lamina propria of the monkey jejunum (×540). Observe the "clock face" nucleus *(arrows)* and clear perinuclear zone.

TRANSIENT CONNECTIVE TISSUE CELLS

Transient connective tissue cells are derived from precursors in the bone marrow (see Fig. 6.1) and are discussed in more detail in other chapters.

Plasma Cells

Plasma cells are derived from B lymphocytes and manufacture antibodies.

Plasma cells, derived from B lymphocytes that have interacted with antigen, produce and secrete antibodies and are responsible for **humorally mediated immunity**. These processes are discussed in later chapters (see Chapters 10 and 12). These large ovoid cells have a relatively short life span of less than 3 weeks. They are about 20 μm in diameter and have an eccentrically placed spherical nucleus that displays heterochromatin radiating out from the center, giving it a characteristic "clock face" or "spoke wheel" appearance under the light microscope. Adjacent to the nucleus is a clear area occupied by the Golgi complex (Figs. 6.16 and 6.17).

Electron microscopy displays a well-developed RER with closely spaced cisternae, only a few mitochondria, a large juxtanuclear Golgi complex, and a pair of centrioles located in the same vicinity (Figs. 6.18 and 6.19).

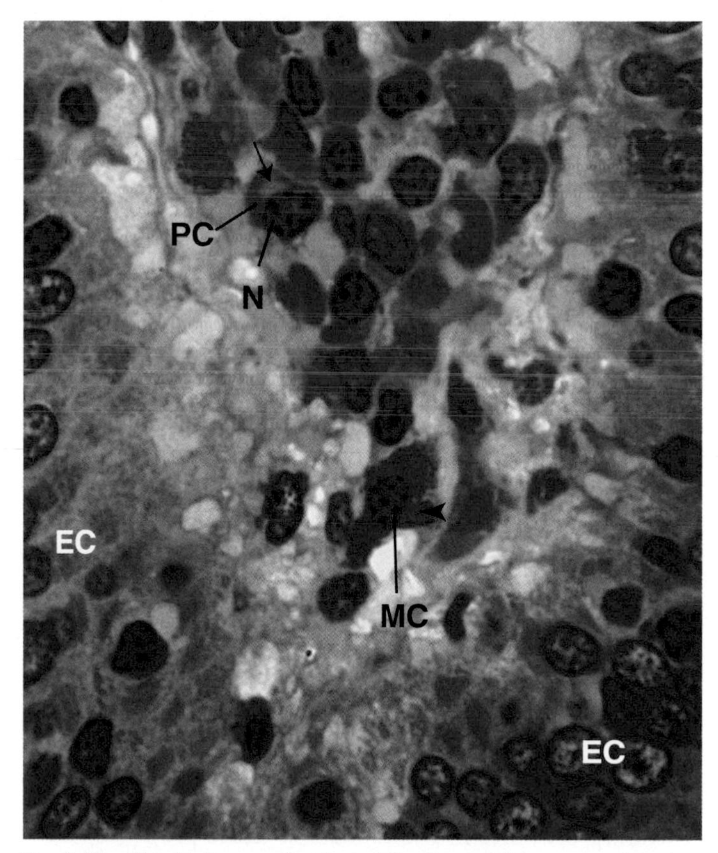

Fig. 6.17 This high magnification of the mucosa from a monkey duodenum displays the simple columnar epithelial cells (EC) lining the organ. The lamina propria, a loose connective tissue, demonstrates the presence of plasma cells (PC) recognizable by the "clock-face" nucleus (N) and the clear Golgi zone *(arrow)* near the nucleus. A mast cell (MC) is also evident, displaying its numerous granules *(arrowhead)*. (×1325)

Leukocytes

Leukocytes exit the bloodstream during inflammation, invasion by foreign elements, and immune responses to perform various functions.

Leukocytes are white blood cells (monocytes, neutrophils, eosinophils, basophils, and lymphocytes) that circulate in the

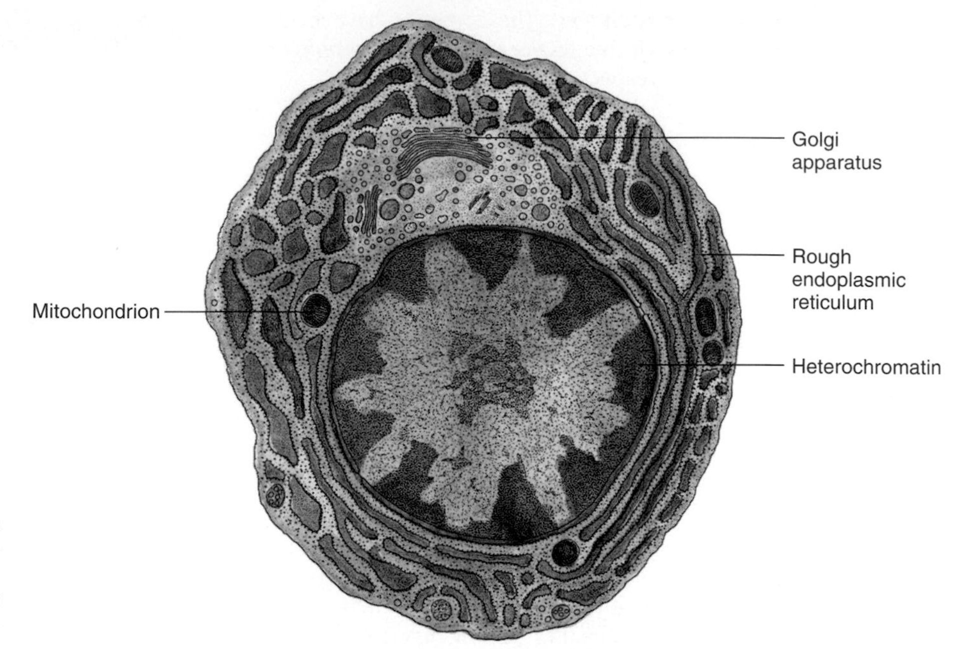

Fig. 6.18 Drawing of a plasma cell from an electron micrograph. The arrangement of heterochromatin gives the nucleus the "clock face" appearance. From Lentz TL. *Cell Fine Structure: An Atlas of Drawings of Whole-Cell Structure.* Philadelphia: WB Saunders; 1971.

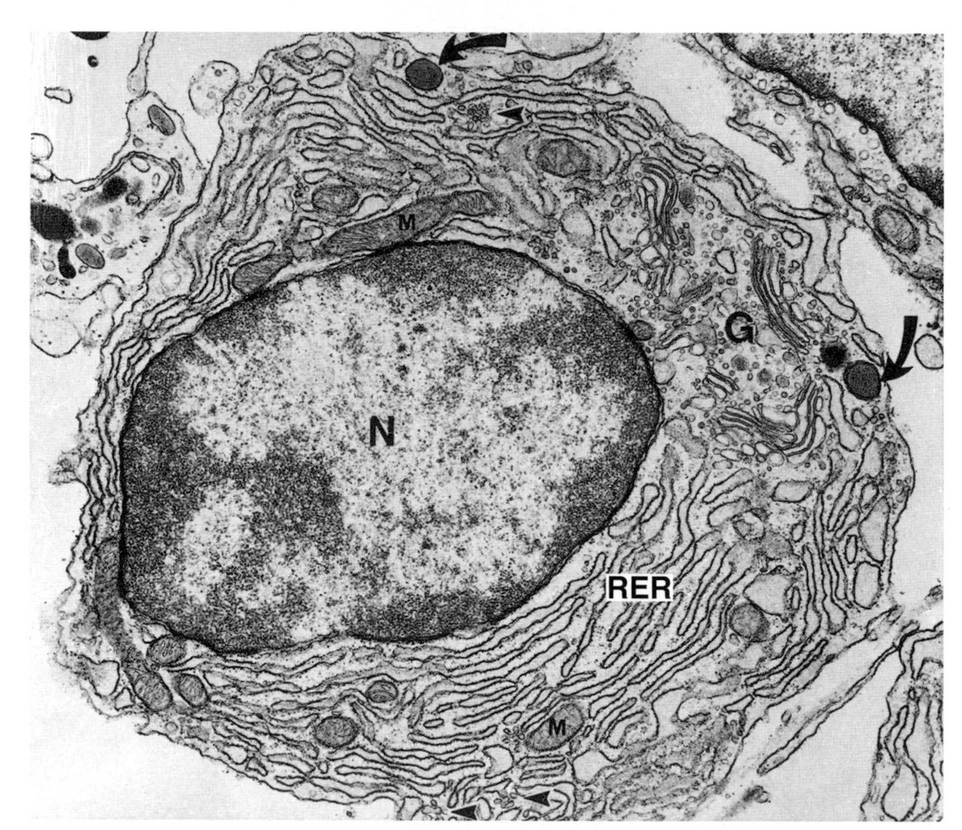

Fig. 6.19 Electron micrograph of a plasma cell from the lamina propria of the rat duodenum displaying abundant rough endoplasmic reticulum (RER) and prominent Golgi complex (×10,300). *Arrowheads* represent small vesicles; *arrows* represent dense granules. G, Golgi apparatus; M, mitochondria; N, nucleus. From Rambourg A, Clermont Y, Hermo L, Chretien M. Formation of secretion granules in the Golgi apparatus of plasma cells in the rat. *Am J Anat.* 1988;184:52-61. Reprinted by permission of Wiley-Liss, Inc., a subsidiary of John Wiley & Sons, Inc.

bloodstream. However, they frequently migrate through small venule and capillary walls to enter the connective tissues, especially during inflammation, where they carry out their various functions.

Monocytes, once in the connective tissue proper, differentiate into macrophages. **Neutrophils** phagocytose and digest bacteria in areas of acute inflammation, forming **pus**, an accumulation of dead neutrophils, extracellular fluid, and debris. **Eosinophils** combat parasites by releasing cytotoxins. They also are attracted to sites of allergic inflammation, where they moderate the allergic reaction and phagocytose antibody–antigen complexes. **Basophils** are similar to mast cells in that they release preformed and newly synthesized pharmacological agents that initiate, maintain, and control the inflammatory process. **Lymphocytes** (T lymphocytes, B lymphocytes, natural killer cells) assemble at sites of chronic inflammation; they also congregate in lymph nodules, lymph nodes, and the spleen. Chapter 10 describes leukocytes in more detail, and Chapter 12 discusses macrophages and lymphocytes in their roles as immune responders.

BOX 6.1 Classification of Connective Tissues

A. Embryonic connective tissues
    1. Mesenchymal connective tissue
    2. Mucous connective tissue
B. Connective tissue proper
    1. Loose (areolar) connective tissue
    2. Dense connective tissue
        a. Dense irregular connective tissue
        b. Dense regular connective tissue
            • Collagenous
            • Elastic
    3. Reticular tissue
    4. Adipose tissue
C. Specialized connective tissue
    1. Cartilage
    2. Bone
    3. Blood

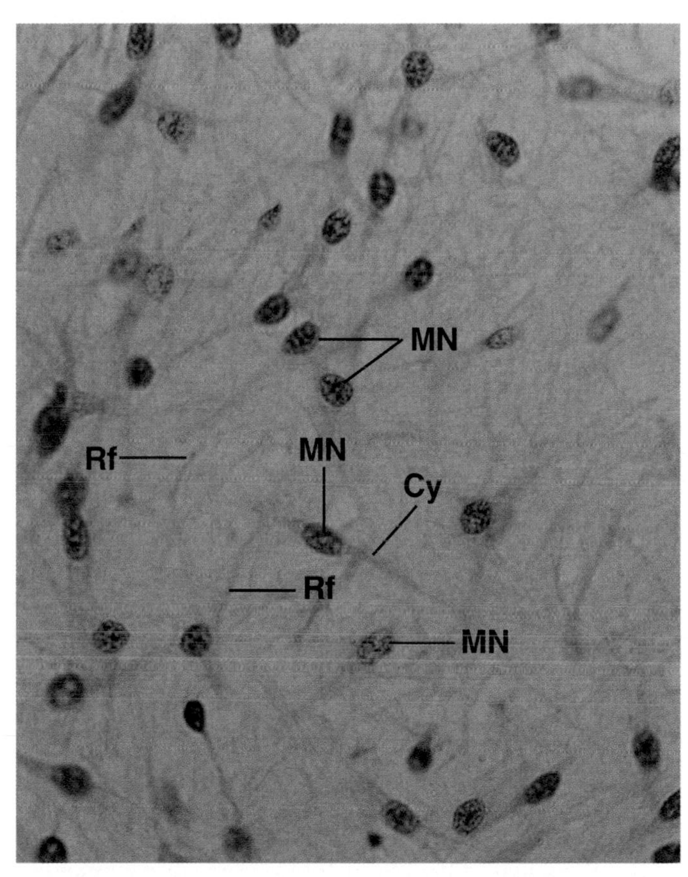

Fig. 6.20 Light micrograph of mesenchymal connective tissue displaying the oval, centrally placed nuclei (MN), and the clear spindle-shaped cytoplasm (Cy) of mesenchymal cells. The matrix is composed of gelatinous ground substance enriched with slender reticular fibers (Rf). (×270)

Classification of Connective Tissue

Connective tissue is classified into connective tissue proper—the major subject of this chapter—and the specialized connective tissues: cartilage, bone, and blood. The third recognized category of connective tissue is **embryonic connective tissue**. Box 6.1 summarizes the major classes of connective tissue and their subclasses.

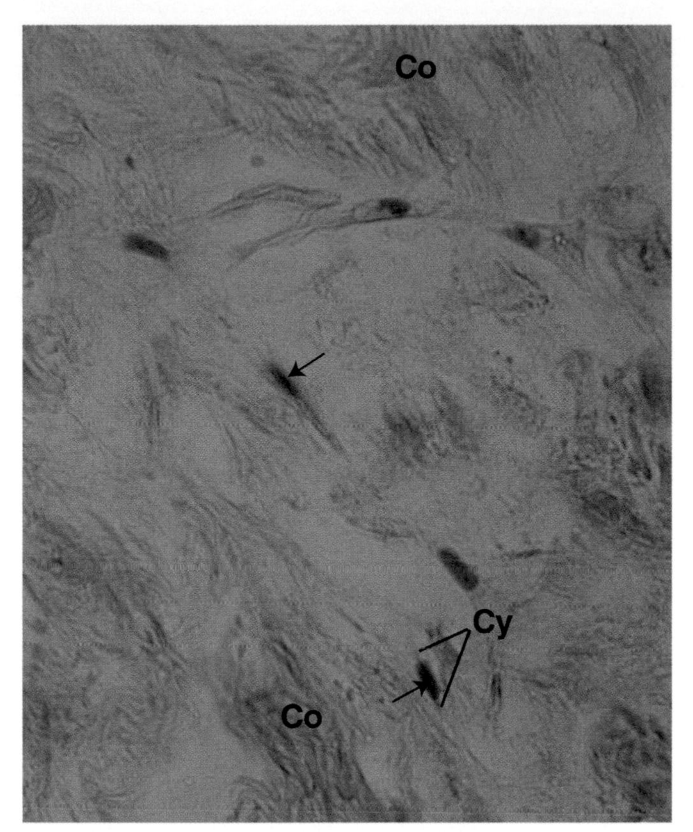

Fig. 6.21 Light micrograph of mucous connective tissue displaying the nuclei *(arrows)* of fibroblasts. Although the cytoplasm (Cy) of these cells blends in with the surrounding matrix, occasionally they can be observed. Bundles of types II and III collagen fibers (Co) are clearly evident. The empty-appearing spaces that occupy much of the photomicrograph were occupied by the ground substance that was dissolved during slide preparation. (×270).

EMBRYONIC CONNECTIVE TISSUE

Embryonic connective tissue includes both mesenchymal tissue and mucous tissue.

Mesenchymal connective tissue (Fig. 6.20) is present only in the embryo and consists of mesenchymal cells in a gel-like, amorphous ground substance containing scattered reticular fibers. **Mesenchymal cells** possess an oval nucleus exhibiting a fine chromatin network and prominent nucleoli. The sparse, pale-staining cytoplasm extends small processes in several directions. Mitotic figures are frequently observed in mesenchymal cells because they give rise to most of the cells of loose connective tissue. It is generally believed that most, if not all, of the mesenchymal cells, once scattered throughout the embryo, are eventually depleted and do not exist as such in the adult except in the pulp of teeth. In adults, however, pluripotential pericytes, which reside along capillaries, can differentiate into certain other cells of connective tissue.

Mucous tissue (Fig. 6.21) is a loose, amorphous connective tissue exhibiting a jelly-like matrix primarily composed of hyaluronic acid and sparsely populated with type I and type III collagen fibers and fibroblasts. This tissue, also known as *Wharton jelly*, is found only in the umbilical cord and subdermal connective tissue of embryos.

CONNECTIVE TISSUE PROPER

The four recognized types of connective tissue proper (**loose, dense, reticular connective tissues**, and **adipose tissue**) differ in their histology, location, and functions.

Loose (Areolar) Connective Tissue

Loose (areolar) connective tissue is composed of a loose arrangement of fibers and dispersed cells embedded in a gel-like ground substance.

Loose connective tissue, also known as ***areolar connective tissue*** (see Figs. 6.2 and 6.3), is widely distributed throughout the body, specifically just deep to the skin and the mesothelial lining of the internal body cavities. It is associated with the adventitia of blood vessels and surrounds the parenchyma of glands; the loose connective tissue of mucous membranes (as in the alimentary canal) is called the ***lamina propria***.

This tissue has abundant **ground substance** housing loosely woven **collagen**, **reticular**, and **elastic fibers** surrounding the fixed connective tissue cells: **fibroblasts**, **adipose cells**, **macrophages**, and **mast cells**, as well as some **undifferentiated cells**. Small nerve fibers and blood vessels course through loose connective tissue.

Because this tissue lies immediately beneath the thin epithelia of the digestive and respiratory tracts, it is here that the body first attacks antigens, bacteria, and other foreign invaders. Therefore, loose connective tissue has many transient cells that are responsible for inflammation, allergic reactions, and the immune response. These cells, which originally circulate in the bloodstream, are released from blood vessels in response to an inflammatory stimulus. Pharmacological agents released by mast cells increase the permeability of small vessels so that excess plasma enters the loose connective tissue spaces, causing it to become swollen.

Clinical Correlations

1. *Under normal circumstances, extracellular fluid returns to the blood capillaries or enters lymph vessels to be returned to the blood. A potent and prolonged inflammatory response, however, causes accumulation of excess tissue fluid within loose connective tissue beyond what can be returned via the capillaries and lymph vessels. This results in gross swelling, or edema, in the affected area. Edema can result from excessive release of histamine and leukotrienes C_4 and D_4, which all increase capillary permeability, as well as from the obstruction of venous or lymphatic vessels.*
2. ***Sarcomas**, unlike carcinomas that have epithelial origins, are cancers that arise from mesenchymal cell derivatives. Therefore, sarcomas include cancers of bone, or osteosarcomas; cancers of muscle, such as leiomyosarcomas and rhabdomyosarcomas; cancers of cartilage, or chondrosarcomas; cancers of adipose cells, or liposarcomas; cancers of fibrous connective tissues, or fibrosarcomas; and cancers of the endothelial cells of blood vessels, or angiosarcomas.*

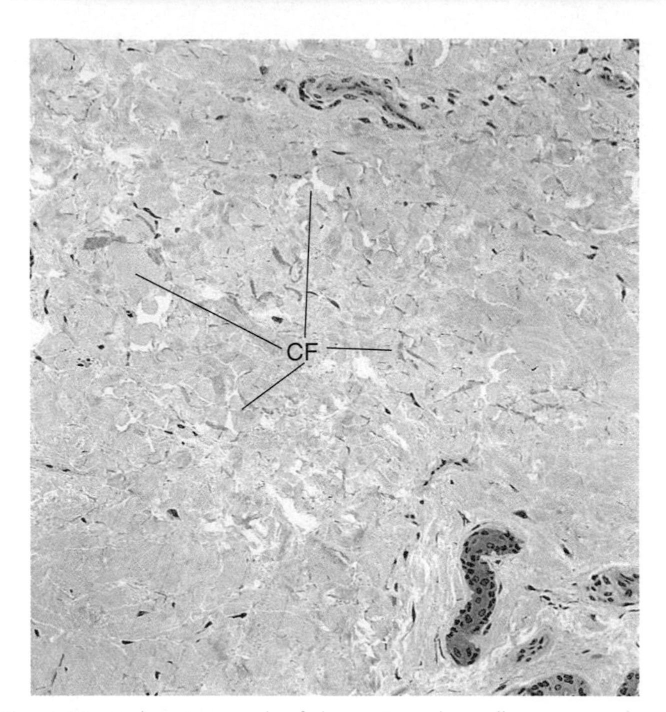

Fig. 6.22 Light micrograph of dense, irregular, collagenous connective tissue from monkey skin (×132). Observe the many bundles of collagen (CF) in random orientation.

Dense Connective Tissue

Dense connective tissue contains a greater abundance of fibers and fewer cells than loose connective tissue.

Dense connective tissue contains most of the same components found in loose connective tissue, except that it has many more fibers and fewer cells. The orientation and arrangements of the bundles of collagen fibers in this tissue make it resistant to stress. When the collagen fiber bundles are arranged randomly, the tissue is called ***dense irregular connective tissue***. When fiber bundles of the tissue are arranged in parallel or organized fashion, the tissue is called ***dense regular connective tissue***, which is divided into **collagenous** and **elastic** types.

Dense irregular connective tissue contains mostly coarse collagen fibers interwoven into a meshwork that resists stress from all directions (Fig. 6.22). The collagen bundles are packed so tightly that space is limited for ground substance and cells. Fine networks of elastic fibers are often scattered about the collagen bundles. Fibroblasts, the most abundant cells of this tissue, are located in the interstices between collagen bundles. Dense irregular connective tissue constitutes the dermis of skin; the sheaths of nerves; and the capsules of spleen, testes, ovary, kidney, and lymph nodes.

Using probe-based confocal laser endomicroscopy (pCLE), previously unrecognized microscopic tissue spaces were discovered in dense irregular collagenous connective tissue (Fig. 6.23). These fluid-filled **interstitial spaces**, bolstered by bundles of collagen fibers, appear to be lined by highly attenuated cells bearing CD34 molecules on their cell membranes. The fluid contained in these spaces is believed to be prelymphatic fluid that probably makes its way to lymph vessels. It is postulated that this tissue compartment has not been observed because the fluid is drained from the tissues during excision and the tissue collapses onto itself during routine histological

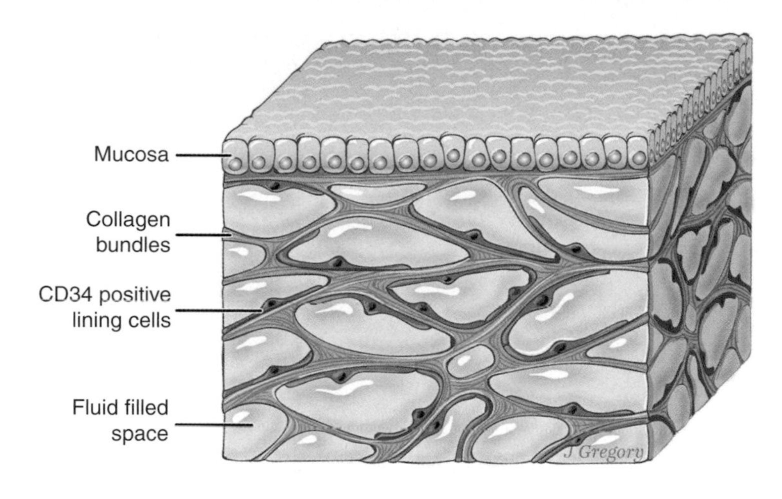

Fig. 6.23 Artist's rendition of fluid-filled spaces in the bile duct connective tissue as visualized by probe-based confocal laser endomicroscopy. Using regular histological preparation of connective tissue proper, the collagen fiber bundles are pressed against each other, obscuring the fluid-filled spaces revealed by probe-based confocal laser endomicroscopy. These spaces are lined by CD34 positive lining cells. Illustration by Jill K. Gregory, CMI. Printed with permission from Mount Sinai Health System, licensed under CC-BY-ND.

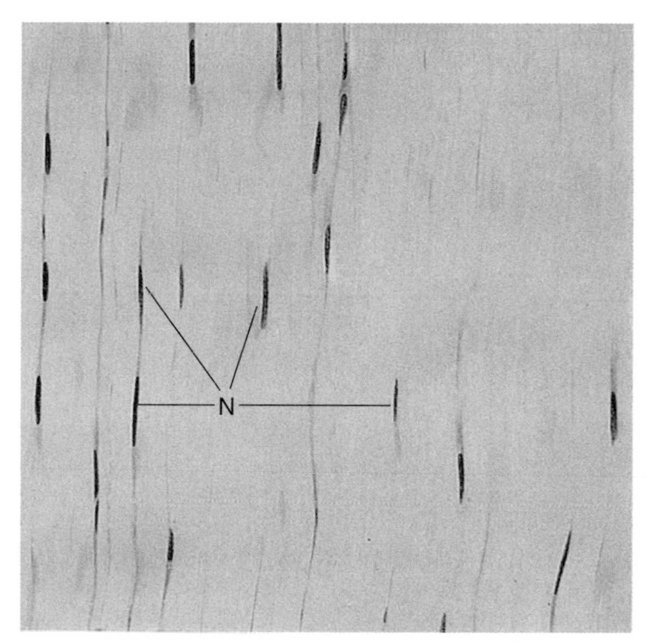

Fig. 6.24 Light micrograph of dense regular collagenous connective tissue from monkey tendon (×270). Note the ordered, parallel array of collagen bundles and the elongated nuclei (N) of the fibroblasts lying between collagen bundles.

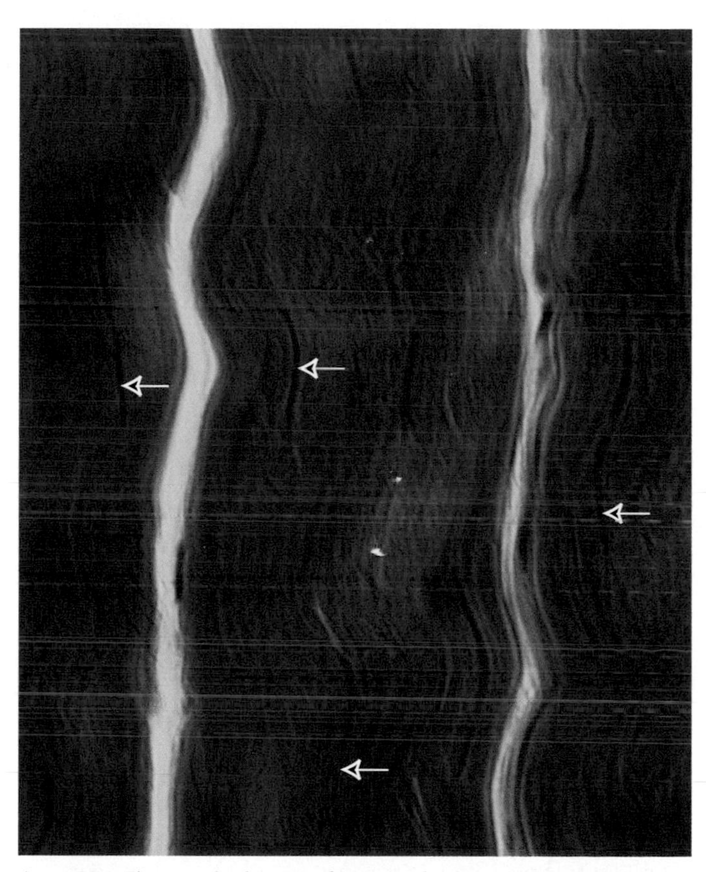

Fig. 6.25 This is a high magnification of a longitudinal section of a tendon similar to that in Fig. 6.24. Note that the fibroblast nuclei *(arrows)* are compressed among the closely packed type I collagen fibers. The cytoplasms of these cells are flattened and are essentially invisible because they stain the same color as the collagen fibers. (×540)

preparation. In the living organism, these prelymphatic fluid-filled interstitial spaces act as "shock absorbers" that counter forces of compression.

Dense regular collagenous connective tissue is composed of coarse collagen bundles densely packed and oriented into parallel cylinders or sheets that resist tensile forces (Figs. 6.24 to 6.27). Because of the tight packing of the collagen fibers, little space can be occupied by ground substance and cells. Thin, sheet-like fibroblasts are located between bundles of collagen, with their long axes parallel to the bundles. Tendons, ligaments, and aponeuroses are examples of dense regular collagenous connective tissue.

Dense regular elastic connective tissue possesses coarse branching elastic fibers, with only a few collagen fibers forming networks (Fig. 6.28). Scattered throughout the interstitial spaces are fibroblasts. The elastic fibers are arranged parallel to one another and form either thin sheets or fenestrated membranes. The latter are present in large blood vessels, ligamenta flava of the vertebral column, and the suspensory ligament of the penis.

Reticular Tissue

Type III collagen is the major fiber component of reticular tissue (Figs. 6.29 and 6.30). The collagen fibers form mesh-like networks interspersed with fibroblasts and macrophages. It is the fibroblasts that synthesize the type III collagen. Reticular tissue forms the architectural framework of liver sinusoids, adipose tissue, bone marrow, lymph nodes, spleen, smooth muscle, and the islets of Langerhans.

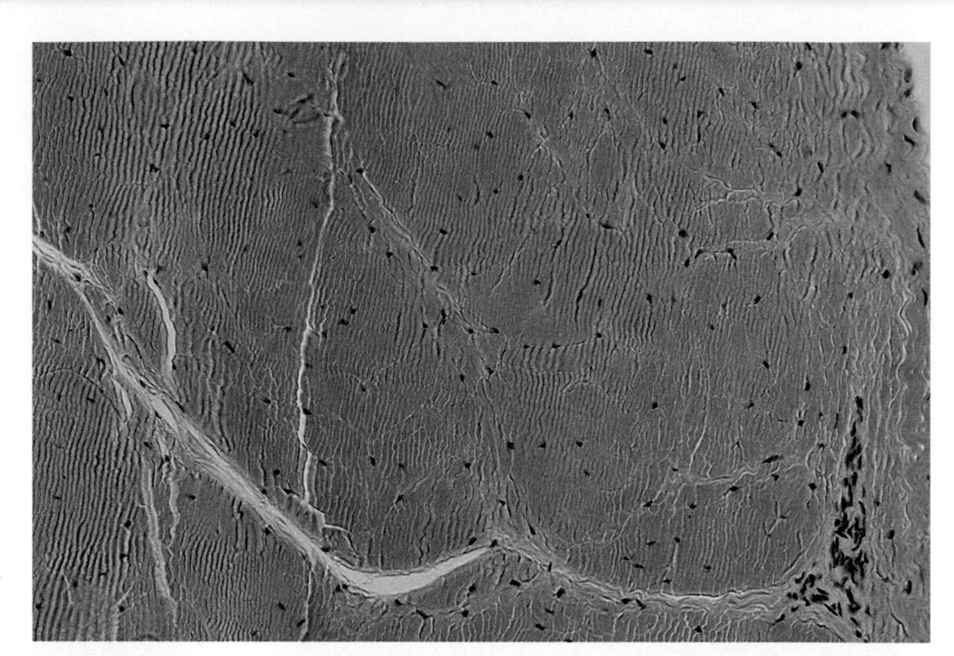

Fig. 6.26 Light micrograph of a cross-section of monkey tendon. The scattered small black structures represent nuclei of fibroblasts. (×270)

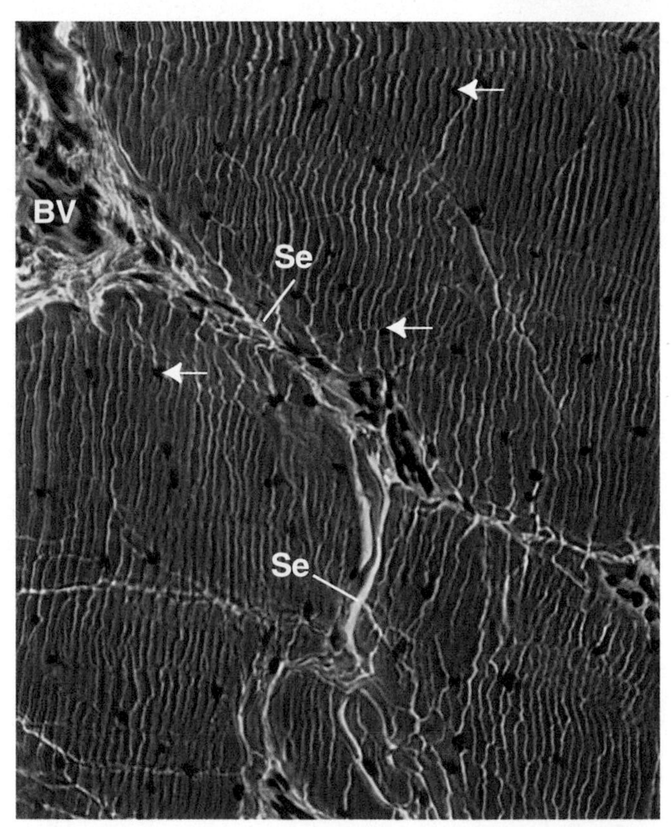

Fig. 6.27 This is a high magnification of a cross-section of a tendon similar to that in Fig. 6.26. Note that the fibroblast nuclei *(arrows)* appear as dark dots among the closely packed type I collagen fibers. The cytoplasms of these cells are flattened and are essentially invisible because they stain the same color as the collagen fibers. Observe the connective tissue septa (Se) that subdivide the tendon and in areas in which the septa expand and are occupied by blood vessels (BV) and nerves. (×540)

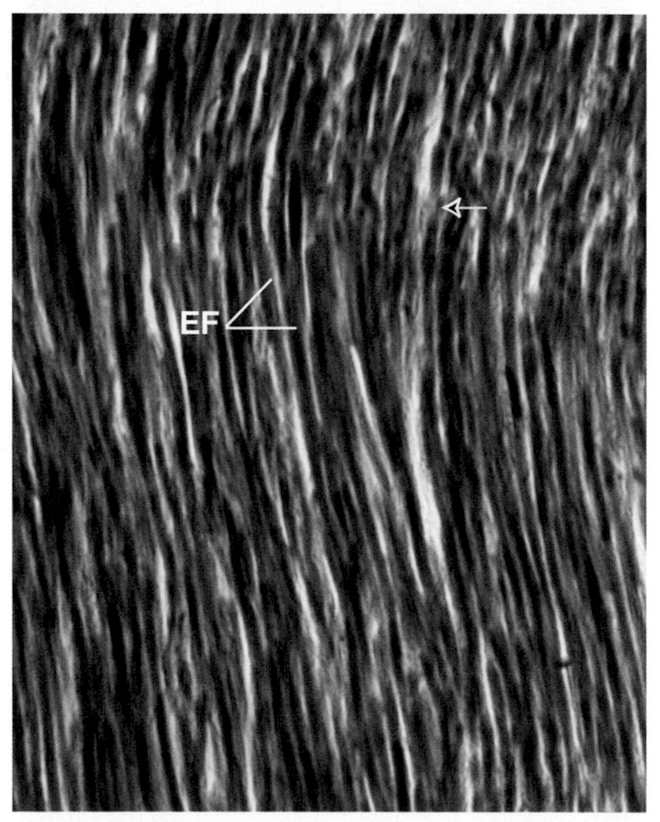

Fig. 6.28 This is a high magnification of a longitudinal section of dense regular elastic tissue. Note that the fibroblasts, although present, cannot be seen because they stain the same color as the elastic fibers (EF). The ends of the fibers form curls *(arrow)*. (×540)

Adipose Tissue

There are two categories of **adipose tissue**, depending on whether it is composed of **unilocular** or **multilocular** adipocytes. Other differences between the two types of adipose tissue are color, degree of vascularity, and type of metabolic activity.

White (Unilocular) Adipose Tissue

Each **unilocular** fat cell contains a large, single lipid droplet, giving the adipose tissue composed of such cells a white color, although a diet rich in carotenes may alter it to be orange. **White adipose tissue** has an exceptionally rich vascular and nerve supply. The blood vessels and nerve fibers gain access via connective tissue **septa** that partition the fat into **lobules** resembling clusters of grapes closely

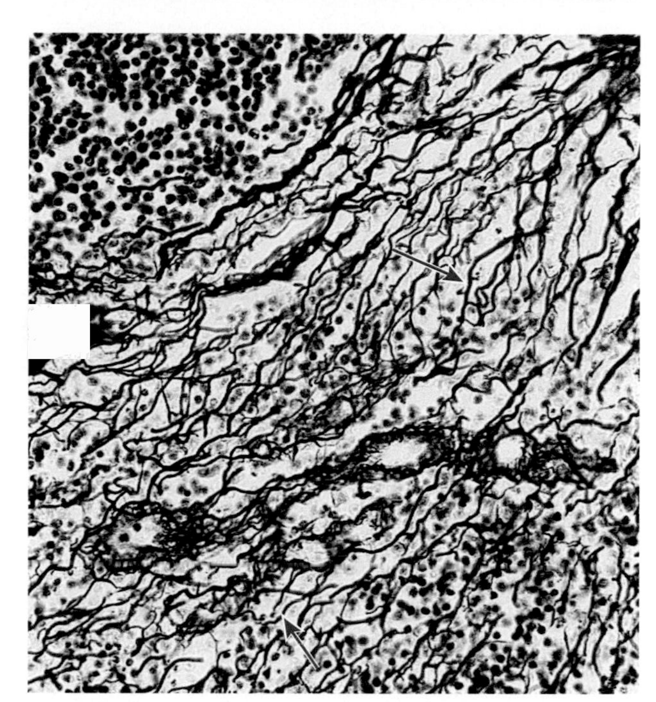

Fig. 6.29 Light micrograph of reticular tissue (stained with silver) displaying the networks of reticular fibers (×270). Many lymphoid cells are interspersed between the reticular fibers *(arrows)*.

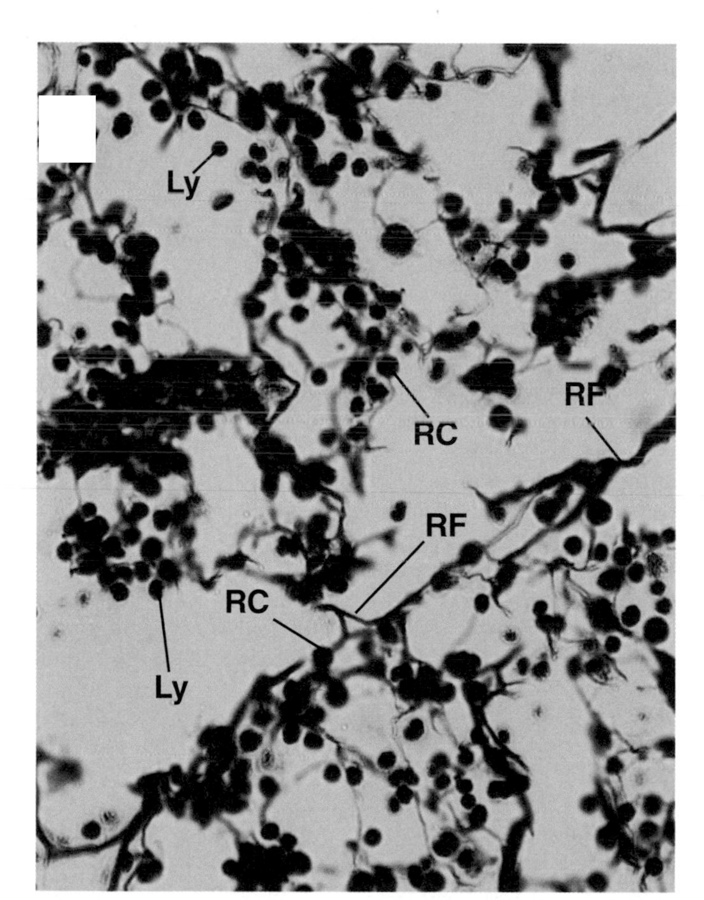

Fig. 6.30 This is a high magnification of reticular tissue stained with silver stain. Note that the reticular fibers (RC) are narrow, straight fibers that branch elaborately, forming a meshwork of fibers. Two types of cells are evident, the smaller and more numerous lymphoid cells (Ly) and the larger reticular cells (RC) that are usually in the close vicinity of reticular fibers. (×540)

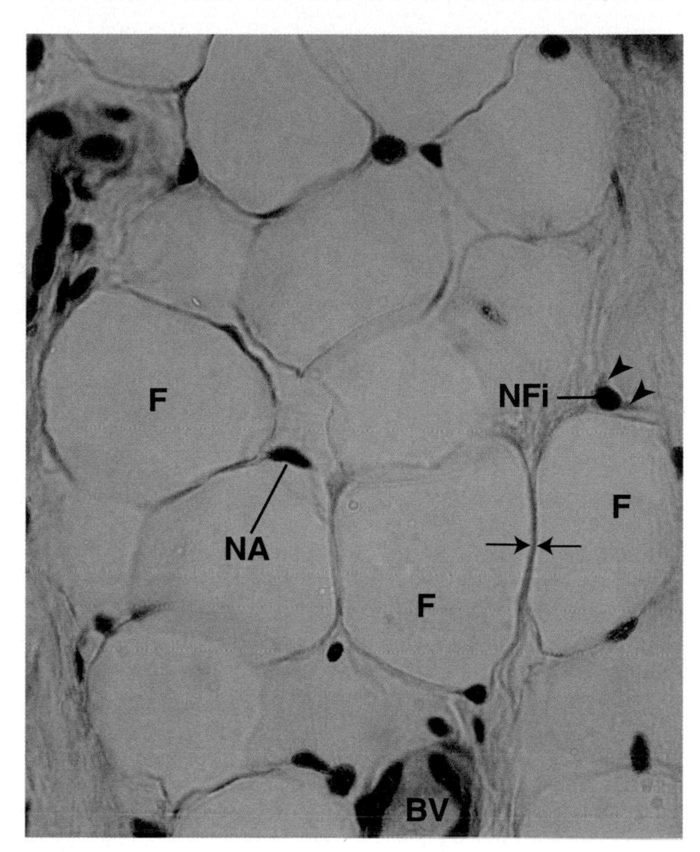

Fig. 6.31 This is a high magnification of white adipose tissue. Note that the cells are closely packed and that each cell has a large fat droplet (F) that presses the adipocyte nucleus (NA) to the periphery of the cell. The cytoplasm and cell membrane form a thin rim that can be differentiated where two fat cells contact each other *(arrows)*. The thin reticular fibers expand in areas to house blood vessels (BV) and nerve fibers, and even nuclei (NFi) and cytoplasm *(arrowheads)* of fibroblasts may be observed. (×540)

packed together (see Figs. 6.8 and 6.31). Each fat cell is enveloped by slender connective tissue elements that convey capillary networks and nerve fibers into its immediate vicinity. Unilocular adipose cells contain **insulin**, **growth hormone**, **norepinephrine**, and **glucocorticoid** receptors on their cell membranes, which modulate their uptake and release of free fatty acids and glycerol, thereby regulating the metabolic state of the body's fatty acid levels. White adipose tissue also produces endocrine hormones. Adipocytes constitute only about half of the cells in adipose tissue; the remainder of the cells are composed of macrophages, mast cells, fibroblasts, lymphoid elements, and stem cells that reside in the connective tissue (**stroma**).

Clinical Correlations

*It appears that white adipose tissue has a richer supply of stem cells than bone marrow. These **adipose-derived stem cells** are reprogrammed relatively easily to give rise not only to adipocytes but also to osteoblasts, myoblasts, and chondrocytes. In fact, animal studies have demonstrated that three-dimensional printing technology can use chondroblasts, reprogrammed from adipose-derived stem cells, to manufacture artificial cartilage that can be implanted into osteoarthritic joints. Osteoarthritic goats treated in this manner regained the ability to move their joints without experiencing pain; researchers hope eventually to apply these techniques to humans suffering from osteoarthritis.*

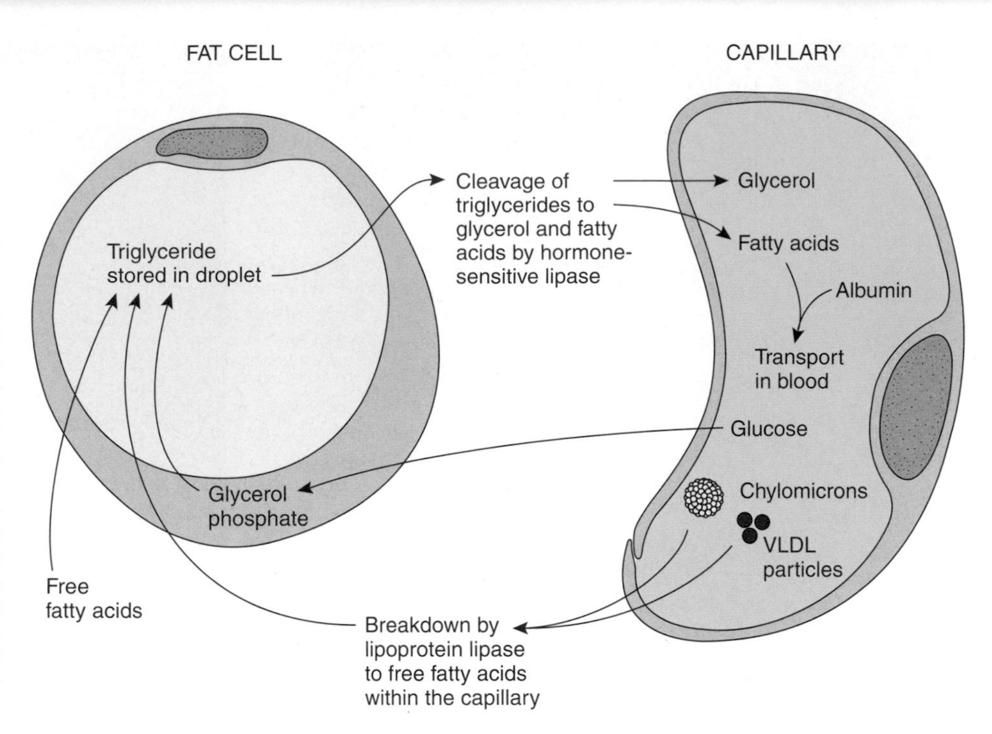

Fig. 6.32 Schematic diagram of the transport of lipid between a capillary and an adipocyte. Lipids are transported in the bloodstream in the form of chylomicrons and very-low-density lipoproteins (VLDLs). The enzyme lipoprotein lipase, manufactured by the fat cell and transported to the capillary lumen, hydrolyzes the lipids to fatty acids and glycerol. Fatty acids diffuse into the connective tissue of the adipose tissue and into the lipocytes, where they are reesterified into triglycerides for storage. When required, triglycerides stored within the adipocyte are hydrolyzed by *hormone-sensitive lipase* into fatty acids and glycerol. These then enter the connective tissue spaces of adipose tissue and from there enter into a capillary, where they are bound to albumin and transported in the blood. Glucose from the capillary can be transported to adipocytes, which can manufacture lipids from carbohydrate sources.

Unilocular fat is present in the subcutaneous layers throughout the body. It also occurs in masses in characteristic sites influenced by sex and age. In men, fat is stored in the neck, in the shoulders, about the hips, and in the buttocks. As men age, the abdominal wall becomes an additional storage area. In women, fat is stored in the breasts, buttocks, hips, and lateral aspects of the thighs. Additionally, fat is stored in both sexes in the abdominal cavity about the omental apron and the mesenteries.

Storage and Release of Fat by Adipose Cells

In the capillaries of adipose tissue, very-low-density lipoprotein synthesized by the liver, fatty acids, and chylomicrons are exposed to the enzyme **lipoprotein lipase** (manufactured and released by fat cells and delivered to blood vessels), which breaks it down into free fatty acids and glycerol (Fig. 6.32). The fatty acids leave the blood vessels, enter the connective tissue, and diffuse through the cell membranes of adipocytes. These cells then combine their own glycerol phosphate with the imported fatty acids to form triglycerides, which are added to the forming lipid droplets within the adipocytes. Under the influence of insulin, adipocytes can convert glucose and amino acids into fatty acids, thereby increasing their lipid storage.

Norepinephrine is released from nerve endings of postganglionic sympathetic neurons in the vicinity of fat cells. Also, during strenuous exercise, **epinephrine** and **norepinephrine** are released from the suprarenal medulla. These two hormones bind to their respective receptors of fat cell membranes, activating **adenylate cyclase** to form **cyclic adenosine monophosphate** (**cAMP**), a second messenger, resulting in activation of two enzymes, **adipose triglyceride lipase (ATL)**, which converts triglycerides to diglycerides, and **hormone-sensitive lipase (HSL)**, which completes the hydrolysis, forming glycerol and fatty acids. It appears that in primates, including humans, **natriuretic peptides**, formed by cardiac muscle cells, can also induce ATL and HSL activities. The fatty acids and glycerol leave the adipocyte, entering the connective tissue from which they gain entry into the bloodstream.

Adipokines Produced by White Adipose Tissue

As indicated previously, adipose tissue plays a major role in controlling the body's fatty acid equilibrium. When food is readily available, the body stores the bulk of its free fatty acids as triglycerides in fat cells of adipose tissue. When food is not available, the triglyceride depot is degraded into fatty acids and glycerol and is released for the body's use. This control mechanism is performed by macromolecules known as ***adipokines***. Some of these molecules influence the immune system but others *do not*; therefore, they are probably better designated as **hormones**. However, whether they act as hormones or not, the term ***adipokines*** will be used in this textbook. Adipocytes manufacture and release **leptin**, **adiponectin**, **retinol-binding protein-4 (RBP-4)**, **vaspin**, and **apelin**. **Resistin**, **TNF-α**, **adipocyte-fatty acid binding protein**, and **interleukin-6** are derived from macrophages resident in adipose tissue (Table 6.3).

Adipokines Manufactured by Fat Cells

Leptin serum levels are lowest in the afternoon and highest in mid-morning. Leptin binds to **neuropeptide Y**, inhibiting it from triggering the appetite control center of the hypothalamus to induce the feeling of hunger. Instead, leptin binds to leptin receptors of the hypothalamus to induce ATL and HSL to break down triglycerides and release fatty acids from the adipocytes. Leptin also induces an increased level of **α-melanocyte-stimulating hormone**, which also acts on the appetite control center to suppress appetite.

Adiponectin forms various combinations as multimers, as many as 18 individual molecules (octadecamers) bound to each other. Obese individuals have low plasma levels of adiponectin, whereas lean individuals have high plasma adiponectin levels. Adiponectin trimers act on the appetite control center of the hypothalamus to repress hunger and octadecamers of adiponectin increase the **insulin sensitivity** of

TABLE 6.3 Adipokines of Human White Adipose Tissue

ADIPOKINE	Molecular Weight (kDa)[a]	Cells of Origin	Function in Fatty Acid Metabolism
Leptin	16	Adipocytes	Reduces appetite
Adiponectin	30	Adipocytes	Increases insulin sensitivity of skeletal muscle cells; decreases glucose release by the liver
Retinol-binding protein-4	21	Adipocytes	Increases insulin resistance; amplifies glucose production and release by the liver
Vaspin	45.1	Adipocytes	Enhances insulin sensitivity in rodents but its effect on insulin in humans is not known
Apelin	1.5	Adipocytes	Apelin synthesis by fat cells is enhanced by insulin
Resistin	12.5	Macrophages	Increases insulin resistance; amplifies glucose production and release by the liver
Tumor necrosis factor-α	17	Macrophages	Primary cause of insulin resistance; interferes with fatty acid oxidation by hepatocytes
Interleukin-6	21	Macrophages	Increases insulin resistance; induces glucose uptake and fatty acid oxidation by skeletal muscle cells

[a]Monomeric form.

Clinical Correlations

1. *Obese individuals usually have a condition known as* ***metabolic syndrome****, a constellation of diseases that include type II diabetes, insulin resistance, cardiovascular problems, fatty liver disease, and chronic inflammation in the adipose tissue. It was noted that in some mice and rats, obesity can be induced by their intestinal bacterial flora, because these microorganisms synthesize and release the short chained fatty acid, acetate, that enters the rodent bloodstream and is conveyed to the brain. Acetate prompts certain nuclei of the brain to signal the pancreas to release insulin, which then signals fat cells to store more lipid, resulting in obesity. Additionally, acetate also induces DNES cells of the stomach to release ghrelin, a hormone that acts on the brain to induce hunger, thereby increasing food intake and resulting in an even greater degree of obesity. As of this writing, it is not known whether acetate is manufactured by human bacterial flora and whether the human metabolism reacts in the same fashion.*
2. *In some cases, there appears to be a genetic basis of obesity. Mutations in the gene responsible for the coding for* ***leptin*** *produce an inactive form of that hormone. Because leptin regulates the appetite center of the hypothalamus, people who either do not produce leptin or who produce a biologically inactive form of this hormone have a voracious appetite, leading to an almost uncontrollable weight gain. Additionally, even though obese individuals have a much higher leptin serum concentration than lean individuals that should decrease their appetite, there appears to be a* ***leptin resistance*** *in obese people, thus, they do not respond to the higher leptin levels.*

skeletal muscle cells, thereby causing these cells to internalize glucose and oxidize fatty acids. Octadecamers also activate hepatic **adenosine monophosphate (AMP)-activated protein kinase**, repressing glucose release and increasing gluconeogenesis by the liver.

RBP-4 interferes with the ability of insulin to cause glucose uptake by skeletal muscle cells and to amplify glucose production and release by hepatocytes. Obese individuals possess increased insulin resistance believed to be effected by RBP-4, and this adipokine may be partly responsible for the presence of chronic inflammation and fatty liver disease in these individuals.

Vaspin (visceral adipose tissue-derived serine protease inhibitor) is known to enhance insulin sensitivity in mice and rats, but its effects on insulin sensitivity in humans is not understood.

Apelin synthesis by fat cells is enhanced by insulin; this adipokine appears to protect cardiac function by its antihypertensive actions and also induces nitric oxide–dependent vasodilation. Obese individuals have an elevated serum apelin level, probably due to their higher serum insulin levels.

Adipokines Manufactured By Macrophages Resident In Adipose Tissue

Resistin, similar to RBP-4, is partly responsible for the establishment of **insulin resistance** in obese individuals. This peptide is similar in structure to adiponectin and also circulates in the multimeric form, where six monomers join each other to form hexamers. Resistin represses hepatic **AMP-activated protein kinase**, elevating glucose release by the liver. This results in hyperglycemia and contributes to obesity, chronic inflammation, and type II diabetes mellitus.

TNF-α has two major functions in the body's fatty acid homeostasis. It is the primary cause of insulin resistance and interferes with fatty acid oxidation by hepatocytes.

Interleukin-6, another product of macrophages in the stroma of adipose tissue of obese individuals, contributes to insulin resistance and induces glucose uptake and fatty acid oxidation by skeletal muscle cells.

Brown (Multilocular) Adipose Tissue

Brown adipose tissue (brown fat) has an extensive neural and vascular supply and is composed of **multilocular adipocytes** that display numerous small droplets of fat, as well as an abundance of mitochondria rich in cytochromes (see Fig. 6.7). Its vascularity and cytochrome-rich mitochondria impart a reddish-brown color to this tissue.

The lobular organization of multilocular adipose tissue displays a rich trabecular network of connective tissue proper that permits its unmyelinated nerve fibers to synapse with blood vessels, as well as with fat cells. In white fat tissue, the neurons end on the blood vessels only.

Multilocular fat is present in many mammalian species, especially those that hibernate, and in the infants of most mammals, including newborn humans, where brown fat is located in the neck and interscapular regions. As humans mature, the fat droplets in brown fat cells coalesce and form into one droplet (similar to the droplets in white fat cells), and the cells become more similar to those in unilocular fat tissue. Thus, although adults appear to contain unilocular fat only, there is evidence that they also possess brown fat. This feature can be demonstrated in some of the wasting diseases of older people, in which multilocular fat tissue forms again and in the same areas as in a newborn.

Clinical Correlations

1. *Obesity increases the risks for many health problems, including non–insulin-dependent diabetes mellitus and problems involving the cardiovascular system. In adults, obesity develops in two ways.* ***Hypertrophic obesity*** *results from the accumulation and storage of fat in unilocular fat cells, which may increase their size by as much as four times.* ***Hypercellular obesity****, a severe form of obesity, results from an overabundance of adipocytes. Although mature adipocytes do not divide, their precursors proliferate in early postnatal life. There is substantial evidence that overfeeding newborn infants even for a few weeks may actually increase the number of adipocyte precursors, leading to an increase in the number of adipocytes and setting the stage for hypercellular obesity in the adult. Overweight infants are at least three times more likely to exhibit obesity as adults than infants of average weight. Presently, it is understood that persons exhibiting severe obesity also exhibit an increase in the adipocyte population, although it is not understood how this recruitment is driven.*
2. ***Cachexia*** *is one of the wasting disorders that accompanies cancers of the digestive tract and displays severe loss of muscle and fat tissues, resulting in unmanageable weight loss and a high degree of mortality. The loss of fat tissue is due not to the death of white adipocytes but to the reduction of the fat droplet within each adipocyte. It is believed that this loss of lipids is due to increased lipase activity that depletes the triglyceride deposits. Apparently, the malignant cells release certain factors that result in cardiac insufficiency. This may cause an increase in the release of natriuretic peptides that enhance the production of both adipose-triglyceride lipase and hormone sensitive lipase, resulting in the depletion of the triglyceride content of unilocular fat cells.*

Brown adipose tissue is associated with production of body heat because of the large number of mitochondria in the multilocular adipocytes composing this tissue. These cells can oxidize fatty acids at up to 20 times the rate of white fat, increasing body heat production threefold in cold environments. Sensory receptors in the skin send signals to the temperature-regulating center of the brain, resulting in the relaying of sympathetic nerve impulses directly to the brown fat cells. The neurotransmitter norepinephrine activates the enzyme that cleaves triglycerides into fatty acids and glycerol, initiating heat production by oxidation of fatty acids in the mitochondria. **Uncoupling protein-1 (UCP-1; thermogenin)**, a transmembrane protein located on the inner membrane of mitochondria, is usually inhibited by the presence of ADP and GDP. However, an ample supply of free fatty acids overrides the inhibitory activity of these purine nucleotides, resulting in the backflow of protons, and UCP-1 uncouples oxidation from phosphorylation. The proton flow generates energy that is dispersed as heat. When heat generation is no longer required the cell stops the production of free fatty acids, UCP-1 becomes inhibited, and the mitochondria produce ATP.

Beige (Brite) Adipose Cells

Ensconced among white adipose cells of white adipose tissue is a small population of cells, known as **beige (brite) adipocytes** that appear to be unilocular adipocytes; but, unlike white fat cells, they display low levels of UCP-1. When beige fat cells receive the proper stimulus, they can increase their UCP-1 content, accumulate free fatty acids, and begin to generate heat.

Clinical Correlations

1. *Tumors of the adipose tissues may be benign or malignant.* ***Lipomas*** *are common benign tumors of adipocytes, whereas* ***liposarcomas*** *are malignant tumors of adipocytes. The latter form most commonly in the leg and in retroperitoneal tissues, although they may form anywhere in the body. The tumor cells may resemble either unilocular adipocytes or multilocular adipocytes, another indication that adult humans do indeed possess the two kinds of adipose tissue.*
2. *Brown fat has been demonstrated to be present in small quantities in adults in the neck, as well as in the region of the clavicle. Interestingly, the amount of brown fat detected was inversely proportional to the degree to which an individual is overweight. That is, thin young men had more brown fat than did overweight young men.*

Pathological Considerations

See Figs. 6.33 and 6.34.

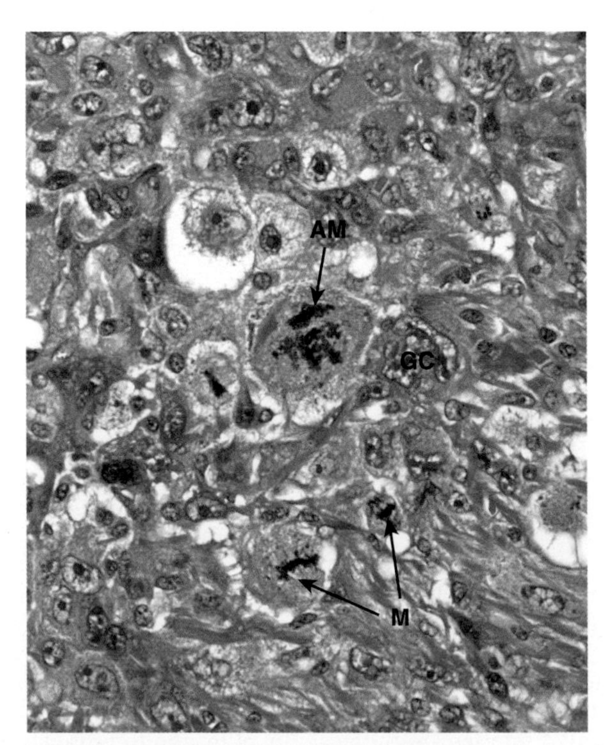

Fig. 6.33 Photomicrograph of a highly pleomorphic sarcoma. Note the presence of some very large cells (GC) as well as numerous mitotic figures (M), some of which are atypical (AM). start here From Young B, et al.*Wheater's Basic Pathology*. 5th ed. Philadelphia: Elsevier; 2010:295, with permission.

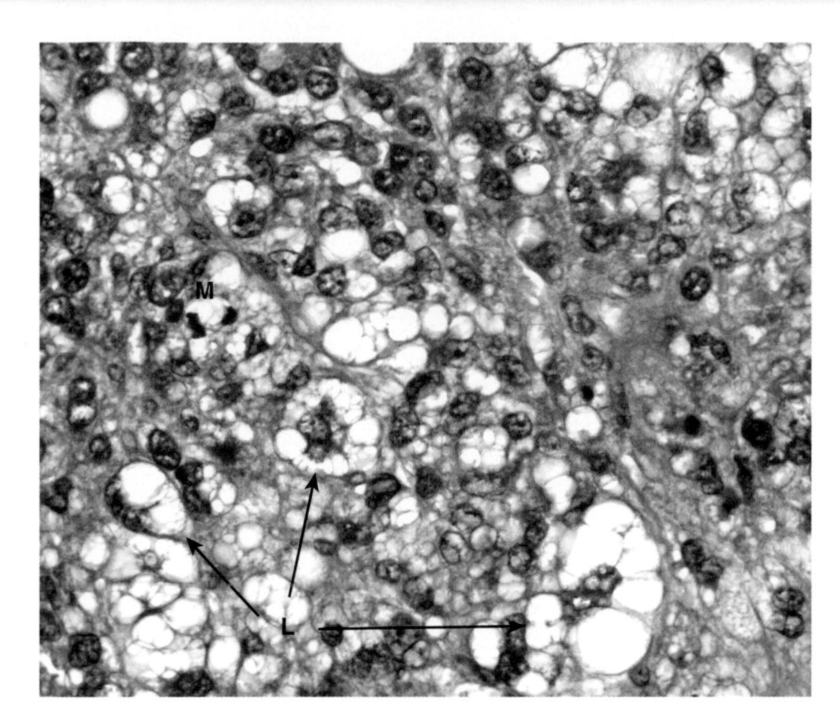

Fig. 6.34 Liposarcomas are characterized by vacuolated tumor cells, known as lipoblasts (Ls). Note the presence of a cell undergoing mitosis (M). From From Young B, Stewart W, O'Dowd G. *Wheater's Basic Pathology: A Text, Atlas and Review of Histopathology*. 5th ed. Oxford: Churchill Livingstone/Elsevier Limited; 2011:294, with permission.

Histology Laboratory Instructions

Embryonic Connective Tissue and Connective Tissue Proper

Embryonic Connective Tissue

Mesenchymal connective tissue (Fig. 6.20) is best seen in a slide of the head of a fetal mouse or fetal pig. The ECM appears empty because the ground substance was dissolved during slide preparation. Slender reticular fibers (Rf) are present and most of the cell population is composed of mesenchymal cells (MN) whose processes contact each other. *Mucous connective tissue* (Fig. 6.21) is present deep to the embryonic dermis and in the umbilical cord. Its ECM also appears empty because of the dissolved ground substance, but there are thick bundles of types II and III collagen fibers (Co) distributed throughout the extracellular space. Usually, the only cells that are present are fibroblasts *(arrows)*.

Connective Tissue Proper

Loose (areolar) connective tissue lies deep to the skin, lamina propria of the alimentary canal, and other places. Select the slide called "Loose Connective tissue" (Figs. 6.2 and 6.3) and observe the thin elastic fibers (E) and the thicker collagen fibers (C). There are three cell types that are usually present: the large, reddish mast cells (MC); fibroblasts, whose nuclei (Fn) are paler and larger than the nuclei (Mn) of macrophages. In the lamina propria of the digestive tract, look for more mast cells (Figs. 6.11 and 6.17, MC) and plasma cells (Fig. 6.17, PC).

Dense irregular connective tissue constitutes the dermis of the skin and capsules of many organs. If you look at a slide of skin, observe the dermis (Fig. 6.22), where the haphazard arrangement of the thick type I collagen fibers (CF) is clearly evident. Nuclei mostly of fibroblasts and macrophages appear as small dark dots at low magnification. Other cells are also present but are usually difficult to distinguish because the collagen fibers hide their cytoplasm.

Dense regular collagenous connective tissue is best observed in slides of tendons and ligaments. Type I collagen fibers are so densely packed that fibroblasts—the predominant cell type—appear flattened and only their nuclei (Fig. 6.24, N; and Fig. 6.25, *arrows*) are evident. In cross-section (Figs 6.26 and 6.27), the fibroblast nuclei appear as small circular profiles (Fig. 6.27, *arrows*) and slender elements of connective tissue septa (Fig. 6.27, Se) are seen to subdivide the tendon into fascicles.

Dense regular elastic connective tissue is best observed in the ligamentum flava of the spinal cord (Fig. 6.28). These elastic fibers (EF) form curls at their ends *(arrow)*. Because they are stained with elastic stain, their fibroblasts are hidden from sight.

Reticular connective tissue is composed mostly of highly branched type III collagen fibers that form the framework of lymphoid structures such as lymph nodes and the spleen as well as of the liver, adipose tissue, and smooth muscle, among others. They are best observed when stained with silver stain that precipitates on the fibers, displaying their meshwork configuration. These fibers are clearly evident in lymph nodes (Fig. 6.29, *arrows*; and Fig. 6.30, RF). The cells in lymph nodes are mostly lymphoid cells (Fig. 6.30, Ly) and reticular cells (Fig. 6.30, RC).

White adipose tissue is one of the most vascular tissues in the body and is composed of closely packed unilocular fat cells that are subdivided into lobes and lobules by connective tissue septa (Fig. 6.8, S). Each adipocyte houses a single globule of lipid that displaces the nucleus (Fig. 6.8, *arrows*) and cytoplasm to the periphery of the cell. At high magnifications, it is evident that the cytoplasm of the cells is exceptionally thin (Fig. 6.31, *arrows*) and its nucleus, pressed against the cell membrane, conforms to the shape of the lipid droplet (Fig. 6.31, NA).

7 Cartilage and Bone

Cartilage and bone are both specialized connective tissues that function in supporting parts of the body. The former has a firm pliable matrix that resists mechanical stresses; the latter is one of the hardest tissues of the body, and protects vital organs such as the brain, spinal cord, bone marrow, and heart. Both cartilage and bone have cells that are specialized to secrete the matrix in which the very same cells become trapped. Most cartilage and all bones are surrounded by a connective tissue capsule, the **perichondrium** and the **periosteum**, respectively.

Cartilage

Cells of cartilage, known as **chondrocytes**, occupy small cavities called **lacunae** within the cartilage **extracellular matrix (ECM)**. Cartilage is avascular, has no nerve supply, and does not have lymphatic vessels. Chondrocytes receive oxygen and nourishment from blood vessels of the perichondrium by diffusion through the ECM, which is composed of **glycosaminoglycans** (GAGs) and **proteoglycans** that are intimately associated with the collagen and elastic fibers embedded within the matrix. The flexibility and resistance of cartilage to compression permit it to function as a shock absorber, and its smooth surface permits almost friction-free movement of the joints of the body as it covers the articulating surfaces of the bones.

There are three types of cartilage, based on the types of fibers present in the matrix (Fig. 7.1 and Table 7.1). **Hyaline cartilage** contains **type II** collagen fibers in its matrix; it is the most abundant cartilage in the body. **Elastic cartilage** contains, in addition to the **type II** collagen fibers, an abundance of **elastic fibers** scattered throughout its matrix, giving it more pliability. **Fibrocartilage** possesses dense, coarse **type I** collagen fibers in its matrix, which aids it in withstanding tensile forces.

HYALINE CARTILAGE

Hyaline cartilage, the most abundant cartilage in the body, forms the template for endochondral bone formation.

Hyaline cartilage, a semitranslucent, bluish-gray, pliable substance, is the most abundant cartilage of the body. It is located in the nose and larynx, on the ventral ends of the ribs where they articulate with the sternum, in the tracheal rings and bronchi, and on the articulating surfaces of the movable joints of the body. It is hyaline cartilage that forms the cartilaginous template of long bones during embryonic development and constitutes the epiphyseal plates of growing long bones (see Table 7.1).

Histogenesis and Growth of Hyaline Cartilage

Cells responsible for hyaline cartilage formation differentiate from mesenchymal cells.

In the region where cartilage is to form, individual mesenchymal cells retract their processes and congregate in cell clusters to form ***chondrification centers***. Under the influence of a small molecule called ***kartogenin***, cells in the chondrification centers differentiate into **chondroblasts** and secrete cartilage matrix, entrapping themselves within small individual compartments called ***lacunae***. Once surrounded by this matrix, these cells are known as ***chondrocytes*** (Figs. 7.2 to 7.4). These cells are still capable of cell division, forming a cluster of two to four or more cells in a lacuna. These groups are known as **isogenous groups** and represent one, two, or more cell divisions from an original chondrocyte (see Fig. 7.1). As the cells of an isogenous group manufacture matrix, they are pushed away from each other, forming separate lacunae and, thus, enlarging the cartilage from within. This type of growth is called **interstitial growth**.

Mesenchymal cells at the periphery of developing cartilage differentiate to form fibroblasts that manufacture a dense irregular collagenous connective tissue, the **perichondrium**, responsible for the maintenance and growth of cartilage. The perichondrium has two layers: an **outer fibrous layer** composed of type I collagen, fibroblasts, and blood vessels; and an **inner cellular layer** composed mostly of **chondrogenic cells** that divide, then differentiate into **chondroblasts**. (Note that under increased oxygen tension, these cells become transformed into osteoprogenitor cells that give rise to bone-forming cells, known as **osteoblasts**.) These newly formed cells elaborate matrix; in this way, cartilage also grows by adding to its periphery a process called **appositional growth**.

Interstitial growth occurs only in the early phase of hyaline cartilage formation. Articular cartilage lacks a perichondrium and increases in size by interstitial growth only. This type of growth also occurs in the **epiphyseal plates** of long bones, where the lacunae are arranged in a longitudinal orientation parallel to the long axis of the bone; in this case, interstitial growth serves to lengthen the bone. The cartilage in the remainder of the body grows mostly by apposition, a controlled process that may continue during the life of the cartilage.

Clinical Correlations

1. *Mesenchymal cells located within the chondrification centers are induced to become secreting chondroblasts by their attachments and the chemistry of the surrounding extracellular matrix. Also, if chondroblasts are removed from their secreted cartilage matrix and are grown in a monolayer in a low-density substrate, they will cease to secrete cartilage matrix containing type II collagen. Instead, they will become fibroblast-like and start secreting type I collagen.*
2. *It has been demonstrated in animal experiments that mice with arthritic-like knee joints when treated with kartogenin developed more cartilage and were able to move their joints freely and without pain.*

Continued

Clinical Correlations—cont'd

3. *Because osteoarthritis does not damage bone until after the cartilage is completely worn down and bone articulates directly against bone, an artificial cartilage could be constructed to replace the damaged cartilage and assuage joint pain. Recently, a hydrogel composed of 70% to 90% water and nanofibers of aramid—the material used in bulletproof vests—has been tested to replace the damaged cartilage in animals. The hydrogel satisfied many of the requirements for artificial cartilage but clinical studies have to be conducted to see how well the material adheres to bone and how it interacts with the surrounding tissues.*

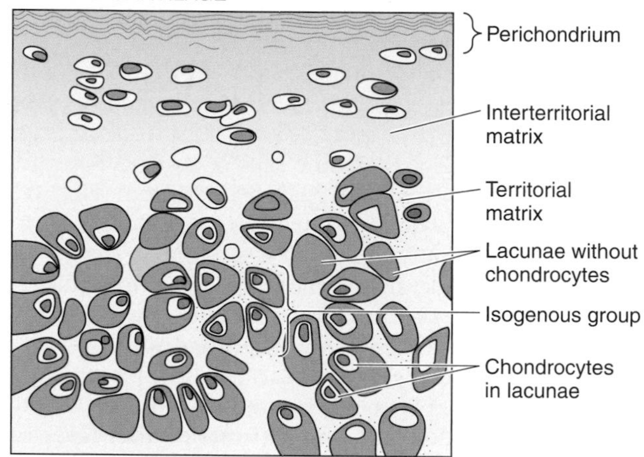

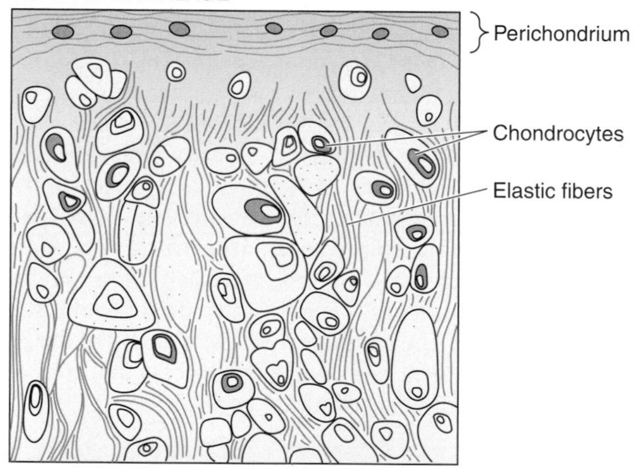

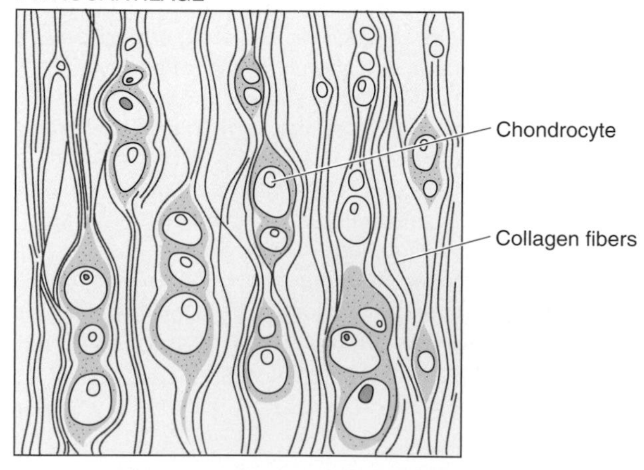

Fig. 7.1 Diagram of the types of cartilage.

Matrix of Hyaline Cartilage

The matrix of hyaline cartilage is composed of type II collagen, proteoglycans, glycoproteins, and extracellular fluid.

The semitranslucent blue-gray matrix of hyaline cartilage contains up to 40% of its dry weight in collagen. In addition, it contains proteoglycan aggregates (mostly in the form of aggrecans), glycoproteins (mostly chondronectin), and extracellular fluid. Because the refractive index of the collagen fibrils and that of the ground substance are nearly the same, the matrix appears to be an amorphous, homogeneous mass, as seen with the light microscope.

The matrix of hyaline cartilage contains primarily **type II collagen**, but types IX, X, and XI and other minor collagens are also present in small quantities. Type II collagen does not form large bundles, although the bundle thickness increases with distance from the lacunae. The matrix is subdivided into two regions: the **territorial matrix**, around each lacuna, and the **interterritorial matrix** (see Fig. 7.4). The territorial matrix, a 50-μm-wide band, is poor in collagen and rich in chondroitin sulfate, which contributes to its basophilic and intense staining. The bulk of the matrix is **interterritorial matrix**, which is richer in type II collagen and poorer in proteoglycans than the territorial matrix.

A small region of the matrix—1 to 3 μm thick, immediately surrounding the lacuna—is known as the ***pericellular capsule***. It displays a fine meshwork of collagen fibers embedded in a basal lamina–like substance. These fibers may represent some of the other minor collagens present in hyaline cartilage; it has been suggested that the pericellular capsule may protect chondrocytes from mechanical stresses.

Cartilage matrix is rich in **aggrecans**, large proteoglycan molecules composed of protein cores to which chondroitin 4-sulfate, chondroitin 6-sulfate, and heparan sulfate are covalently linked. The abundant negative charges associated with these exceedingly large proteoglycan molecules attract cations, predominantly Na^+ ions, which, in turn, attract water molecules. In this way, the cartilage matrix becomes hydrated to such an extent that up to 80% of the wet weight of cartilage is water, accounting for the ability of cartilage to resist forces of compression.

Not only do hydrated proteoglycans fill the interstices among the collagen fiber bundles but also their GAG side chains form electrostatic bonds with the collagen. Thus, the ground substance and fibers of the matrix form a cross-linked molecular framework that resists tensile forces.

Cartilage matrix also contains the adhesive glycoprotein **chondronectin**. This large molecule, similar to fibronectin, has binding sites for type II collagen, chondroitin 4-sulfate, chondroitin 6-sulfate, hyaluronic acid, and integrins (transmembrane proteins) of chondroblasts and chondrocytes. Chondronectin thus assists these cells in maintaining their contact with the fibrous and amorphous components of the matrix.

Histophysiology of Hyaline Cartilage

The smoothness of hyaline cartilage and its ability to resist forces of both compression and tension are essential to its function at the articular surfaces of joints. Because cartilage is avascular, nutrients and oxygen must diffuse through the water of hydration present in the matrix. The inefficiency of such a system necessitates a limit on the width of cartilage. There is a constant turnover in the proteoglycans of cartilage that changes

TABLE 7.1 Types, Characteristics, and Locations

Type of Cartilage	Identifying Characteristics	Perichondrium	Location
Hyaline	Type II collagen, basophilic matrix, chondrocytes usually arranged in groups	Perichondrium present in most places. Exceptions: articular cartilages and epiphyses	Articular ends of long bones, nose, larynx, trachea, bronchi, ventral ends of ribs
Elastic	Type II collagen, elastic fibers	Perichondrium present	Pinna of ear, walls of auditory canal, auditory tube, epiglottis, cuneiform cartilage of larynx
Fibrocartilage	Type I collagen, acidophilic matrix, chondrocytes arranged in parallel rows between bundles of collagen, always associated with dense, regular collagenous connective tissue or hyaline cartilage	Perichondrium absent	Intervertebral disks, articular disks, pubic symphysis, insertion of some tendons

with age. Hormones and vitamins also exert influence over the growth, development, and function of cartilage. Many of these substances also affect skeletal formation and growth (Table 7.2).

Clinical Correlations

Hyaline cartilage degenerates when the chondrocytes hypertrophy and die and the matrix begins to calcify. This process is a normal and integral part of endochondral bone formation. However, it is also a natural process of aging, often resulting in less mobility and pain in the joints.

Cartilage regeneration is usually poor, except in children. Chondrogenic cells from the perichondrium enter the defect and form new cartilage. If the defect is large, the cells form dense connective tissue to repair the scar.

ELASTIC CARTILAGE

Elastic cartilage greatly resembles hyaline cartilage except that its matrix and perichondrium possess elastic fibers.

Elastic cartilage is located in the pinna of the ear, external and internal auditory tubes, epiglottis, and larynx (cuneiform cartilage). In the fresh state, owing to the presence of elastic fibers, elastic cartilage is somewhat yellow in appearance and is more opaque than hyaline cartilage (see Table 7.1).

The outer fibrous layer of the perichondrium is rich in elastic fibers. The matrix of elastic cartilage possesses abundant fine-to-coarse branching elastic fibers interspersed with type II collagen fiber bundles, giving it much more flexibility than the matrix of hyaline cartilage (Figs. 7.5 and 7.6). Chondrocytes of elastic cartilage are more abundant and larger than those of hyaline cartilage. The matrix is not as ample as in hyaline cartilage, and the elastic fiber bundles of the territorial matrix are larger and coarser than those of the interterritorial matrix.

FIBROCARTILAGE

Fibrocartilage, unlike hyaline and elastic cartilage, does not possess a perichondrium and its matrix possesses type I collagen.

Fibrocartilage, present in intervertebral disks, in the pubic symphysis, and in articular disks, does not possess a perichondrium. It displays a scant amount of matrix (rich in chondroitin sulfate and dermatan sulfate) and exhibits bundles of type I

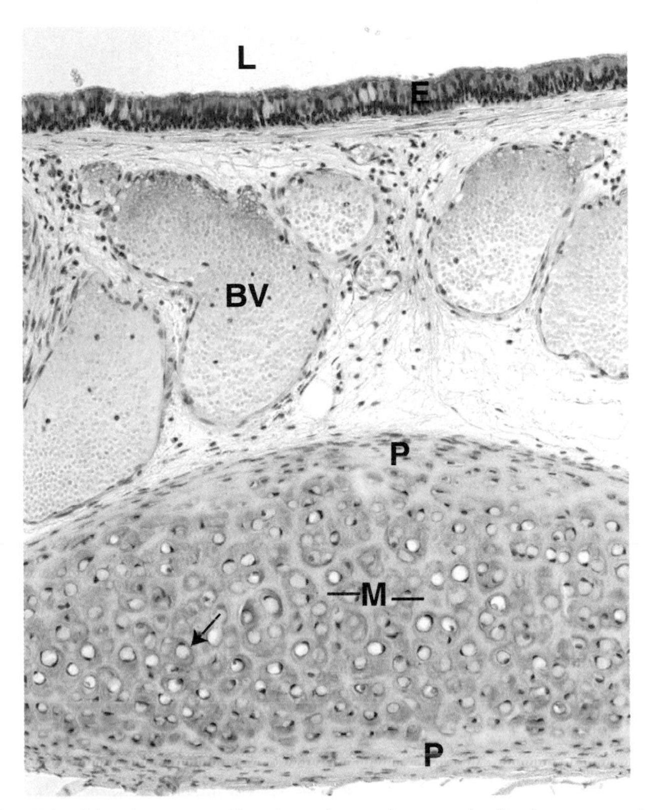

Fig. 7.2 This low-magnification photomicrograph displays a monkey trachea with its pseudostratified ciliated columnar epithelium (E) lining its lumen (L). Observe the perichondrium (P) surrounding the hyaline cartilage and chondrocytes *(arrow)* housed within the lacunae surrounded by the cartilage matrix (M). Large blood vessels (BV) are located deep to the epithelium. (×125)

collagen, which stain acidophilic (Fig. 7.7). Chondrocytes are often aligned in alternating parallel rows with the thick, coarse bundles of collagen, which parallel the tensile forces attendant on this tissue (see Table 7.1).

Chondrocytes of fibrocartilage usually arise from fibroblasts that experience increasing tensile forces and, therefore, begin to manufacture proteoglycans. As the ground substance surrounds the fibroblast, the cell becomes incarcerated in its own matrix and differentiates into a chondrocyte.

Intervertebral disks represent an example of the organization of fibrocartilage. They are interposed between the hyaline cartilage coverings of the articular surface of successive vertebrae. Each disk contains a gelatinous center, called the ***nucleus pulposus***, which is composed of notochord-derived cells lying within

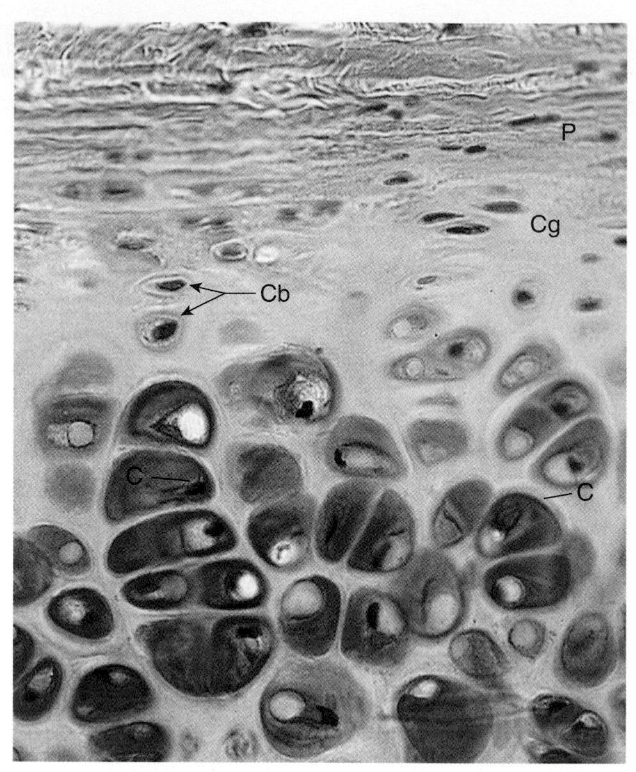

Fig. 7.3 Light micrograph of hyaline cartilage (×270). Observe the large ovoid chondrocytes (C) trapped in their lacunae. Directly above them are the elongated chondroblasts (Cb). At the very top is the perichondrium (P) and the underlying chondrogenic (Cg) cell layer.

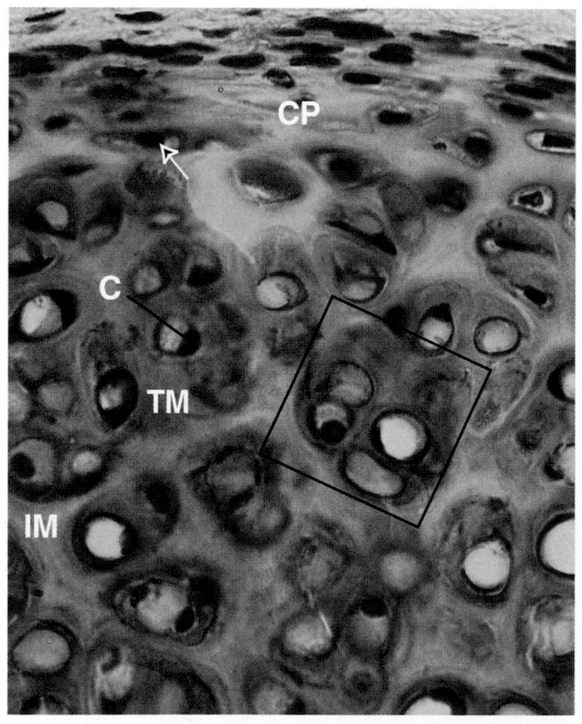

Fig. 7.4 High-magnification light micrograph of hyaline cartilage. Observe the cellular perichondrium (CP) housing chondrogenic cells and chondroblasts *(arrow)*. Note the nuclei of chondrocytes (C) in their lacunae. This cartilage is growing larger, as is evident by the presence of cell nests *(boxed area)*. The darker territorial matrix (TM) is clearly distinguishable from the lighter interterritorial matrix (IM). The intense red line at the circumference of each lacuna is the pericellular capsule. (×540)

TABLE 7.2 Effects of Hormones and Vitamins on Hyaline Cartilage

Hormone	Effects
Thyroxine, testosterone, and somatotropin (via insulin-like growth factors)	Stimulate cartilage growth and matrix formation
Cortisone, hydrocortisone, and estradiol	Inhibit cartilage growth and matrix formation
Vitamin	
Hypovitaminosis A	Reduces width of epiphyseal plates
Hypervitaminosis A	Accelerates ossification of epiphyseal plates
Hypovitaminosis C	Inhibits matrix synthesis and deforms architecture of epiphyseal plate; leads to scurvy
Absence of vitamin D, resulting in deficiency in absorption of calcium and phosphorus	Proliferation of chondrocytes is normal but matrix does not become calcified properly; results in rickets

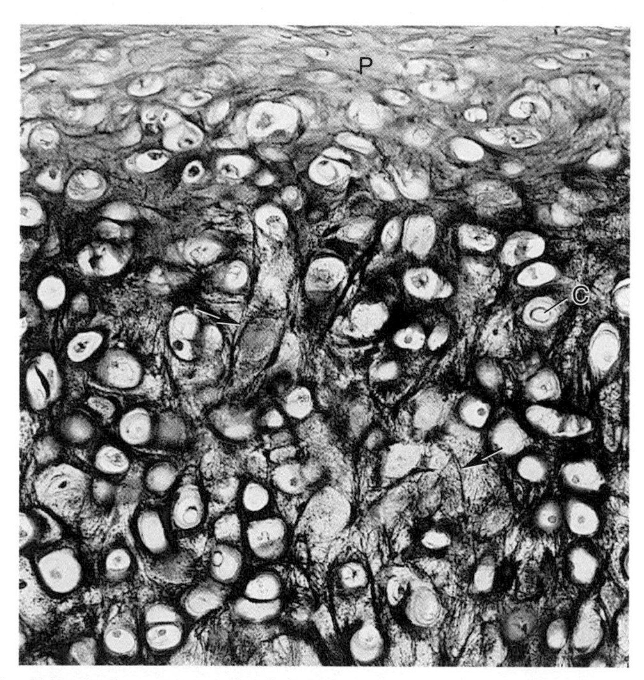

Fig. 7.5 Light micrograph of elastic cartilage (×132). Observe the perichondrium (P) and the chondrocytes (C) in their lacunae (shrunken from the walls because of processing), some of which contain more than one cell, evidence of interstitial growth. Elastic fibers *(arrows)* are scattered throughout.

a hyaluronic acid–rich matrix. These cells disappear by the 20th year of life. Much of the nucleus pulposus is surrounded by the **annulus fibrosus**, layers of fibrocartilage whose type I collagen fibers run vertically between the hyaline cartilages of the two vertebrae. The fibers of adjacent lamellae are oriented obliquely to each other, providing support to the gelatinous **nucleus pulposus**. The annulus fibrosus provides resistance against tensile forces, whereas the nucleus pulposus resists forces of compression.

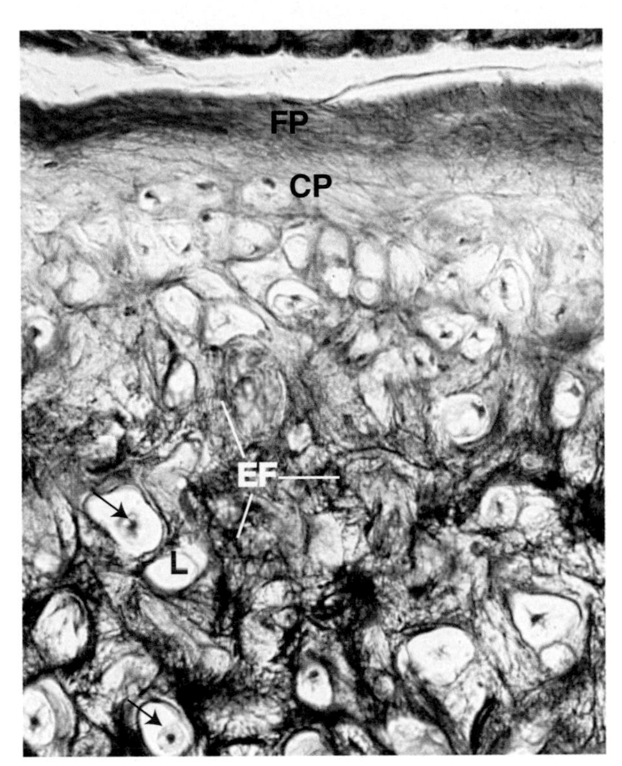

Fig. 7.6 Medium magnification of a light micrograph of elastic cartilage. Note the fibrous (FP) and the cellular (CP) perichondrium and the differences in their cell population. The lacunae (L) of the cartilage have chondrocytes (arrows) that shrunk during preparation so they do not occupy the entire lacuna as they would in living cartilage. Numerous elastic fibers (EF) are embedded in the gelatinous matrix. (x270)

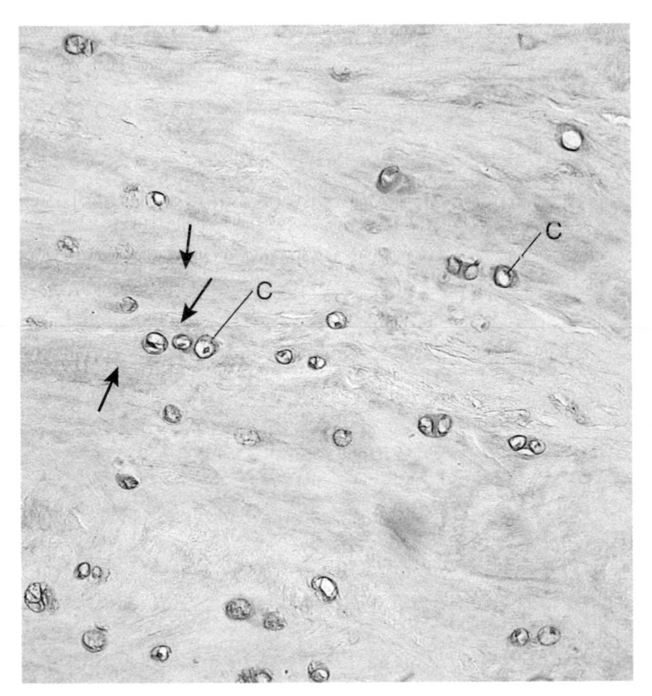

Fig. 7.7 Light micrograph of fibrocartilage (×132). Note alignment of the chondrocytes (C) in rows interspersed with thick bundles of collagen fibers *(arrows)*.

Clinical Correlations

A ruptured disk refers to a tear or break in the laminae of the annulus fibrosus through which the gel-like nucleus pulposus extrudes. This condition occurs more often on the posterior portions of the intervertebral disks, particularly in the lumbar portion of the back, where the disk may dislocate, or slip. A "slipped disk" leads to severe, intense pain in the lower back and extremities because the displaced disk compresses the lower spinal nerves.

Bone

Bone is a specialized connective tissue whose extracellular matrix is calcified, incarcerating the cells that secreted it.

Bone is the primary structural framework for support and protection of the organs of the body, including the brain and spinal cord and the structures within the thoracic cavity—the lungs and heart. It also contains a central cavity, the **marrow cavity**, which houses the **bone marrow**, a hemopoietic organ. Bones also serve as levers for the muscles attached to them, thereby multiplying the force of the muscles to attain movement. Additionally, bone is a reservoir for several minerals of the body; for example, it stores about 99% of the body's calcium.

Although **bone** is one of the hardest substances of the body, it is a dynamic tissue that constantly changes shape in relation to the stresses placed on it. Thus, pressures applied to bone lead to its resorption, and tension applied to it results in development of new bone.

Bone is covered on its external surface, except at synovial articulations, with a **periosteum**, which consists of an outer layer of dense fibrous connective tissue and an inner cellular layer containing **osteoprogenitor (osteogenic) cells** as well as occasional **osteoblasts**. Bundles of collagen fibers from the periosteum, known as **Sharpey fibers**, are embedded into the outer surface of bone, thereby securing the periosteum to the bone surface. The central cavity of a bone is lined with **endosteum**, a specialized thin connective tissue composed of a monolayer of **osteoprogenitor cells** and **osteoblasts**.

The cells of bone include **osteoprogenitor cells**, which differentiate into **osteoblasts**. Osteoblasts are responsible for secreting and eventually calcifying bone matrix. When these cells are surrounded by that matrix, they become quiescent and are known as **osteocytes**, housed in spaces known as **lacunae**. Additional cells of bone, known as **osteoclasts**, are multinucleated giant cells derived from fused bone marrow precursors. Osteoclasts are responsible for bone resorption and remodeling.

Because bone is such a hard tissue, two methods are employed to prepare it for study. **Decalcified sections** can be prepared by decalcifying the bone in an acid solution to remove the calcium salts. The tissue can then be embedded, sectioned, and routinely stained for study. **Ground sections** are prepared by sawing the undecalcified bone into thin slices, followed by grinding the sections with abrasives between glass plates. When the section is sufficiently thin, it is mounted for study with light microscopy. Each system has disadvantages. In decalcified sections, osteocytes are distorted by the decalcifying acid bath; in ground sections, the cells are destroyed, and the lacunae and canaliculi are filled in with bone debris.

BONE MATRIX

Bone matrix has inorganic and organic constituents.

Inorganic Component

The inorganic constituents of bone are crystals of calcium hydroxyapatite, composed mostly of calcium and phosphorus.

The inorganic portion of bone, which constitutes about 65% of its dry weight, is composed mainly of calcium and phosphorus along with other components, including bicarbonate, citrate, magnesium, sodium, and potassium. Calcium and phosphorus exist primarily in the form of **hydroxyapatite crystals** [$Ca_{10}(PO_4)_6(OH)_2$], but calcium phosphate is also present in an amorphous form. Hydroxyapatite crystals (40 nm in length by 25 nm in width and 1.5–3 nm in thickness) are arranged in an ordered fashion along the type I collagen fibers. They are deposited into the gap regions of the collagen but also are present along the overlap region. The free surface of the crystals is surrounded by amorphous ground substance. The surface ions of the crystals attract H_2O molecules, forming a **hydration shell** around the crystals that permits ion exchange with the extracellular fluid.

When bone is decalcified (i.e., all mineral is removed from the bone), it still retains its original shape but becomes so flexible that it can be bent like a piece of tough rubber. If the organic component is extracted from bone, the mineralized skeleton still retains its original shape but becomes extremely brittle and can be fractured with ease.

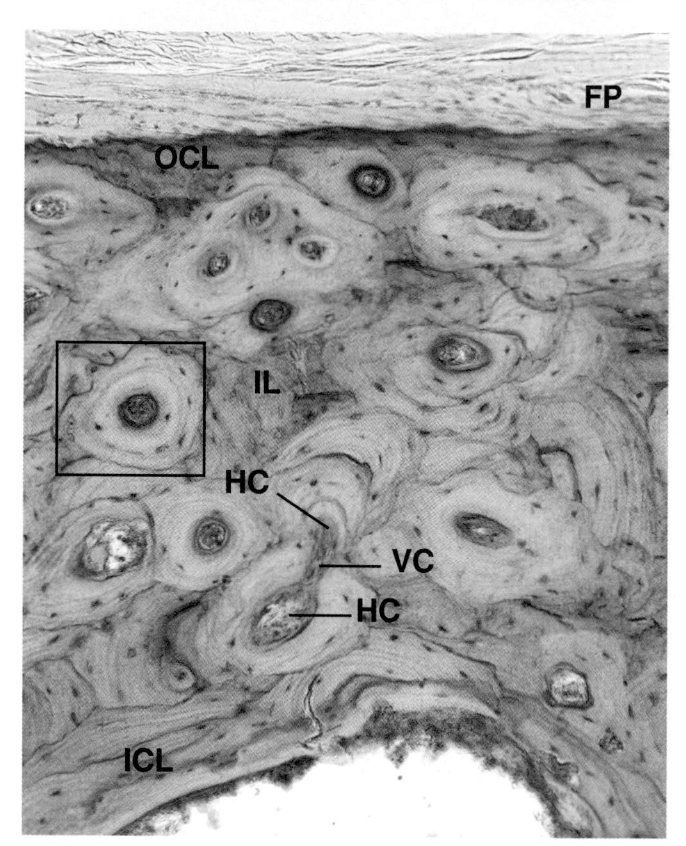

Fig. 7.8 This is a low-magnification cross-section of a decalcified human rib. Observe that the four lamellar systems are clearly evident: the outer circumferential lamellae (OCL) just deep to the periosteum (FP); the inner circumferential lamellae (ICL), encircling the marrow cavity; the numerous osteons, one of which is enclosed by the box; and the interstitial lamellae (IL) interposed among the osteons. Each osteon has its own haversian canal (HC) and haversian canals are interconnected by occasional Volkmann canals (VC).

Organic Component

The predominant organic component of bone is type I collagen.

The **organic component** of bone matrix constitutes approximately 35% of the dry weight of bone; it includes fibers that are almost exclusively type I collagen (with a small amount of type V, VII, XI, and XII collagen).

Collagen comprises about 80% to 90% of the organic component of bone. It is formed in large (50–70 nm in diameter) bundles displaying the typical 67-nm periodicity. Type I collagen in bone is highly cross-linked, which prevents it from being easily extracted.

The fact that bone matrix stains with periodic acid–Schiff (PAS) reagent and displays slight metachromasia indicates the presence of sulfated GAGs, predominantly chondroitin sulfate and keratan sulfate. These form small proteoglycan molecules with short protein cores to which the GAGs are covalently bound. The proteoglycans are noncovalently bound via link proteins to **hyaluronic acid**, forming very large **aggrecan composites**. The abundance of collagen, however, causes the matrix to be acidophilic.

Several glycoproteins are also present in the bone matrix. These appear to be restricted to bone and include **osteocalcin** (which binds to hydroxyapatite) and **osteopontin**, which also binds to hydroxyapatite but has additional binding sites for other components as well as for integrins present on osteoblasts and osteoclasts. Vitamin D stimulates the synthesis of these glycoproteins. **Bone sialoprotein**, another matrix protein, has binding sites for matrix components and integrins of osteoblasts and osteocytes, suggesting its involvement in the adherence of these cells to bone matrix.

Cells of Bone

The cells of bone are osteoprogenitor cells, osteoblasts, osteocytes, and osteoclasts (Figs. 7.8 and 7.9).

Osteoprogenitor Cells

Osteoprogenitor cells are derived from embryonic mesenchymal cells and retain their ability to undergo mitosis.

Osteoprogenitor cells are located in the inner cellular layer of the periosteum, lining haversian canals, and in the endosteum (see Fig. 7.9). These cells, derived from embryonic mesenchyme, remain in place throughout postnatal life and can undergo mitotic division and have the potential to differentiate into osteoblasts. Moreover, under certain conditions of low oxygen tension, these cells may differentiate into chondrogenic cells. Osteoprogenitor cells are spindle shaped and have a pale-staining oval nucleus. Their scant pale-staining cytoplasm displays sparse rough endoplasmic reticulum (RER) and a poorly developed Golgi apparatus but has an abundance of free ribosomes. These cells are most active during the period of intense bone growth.

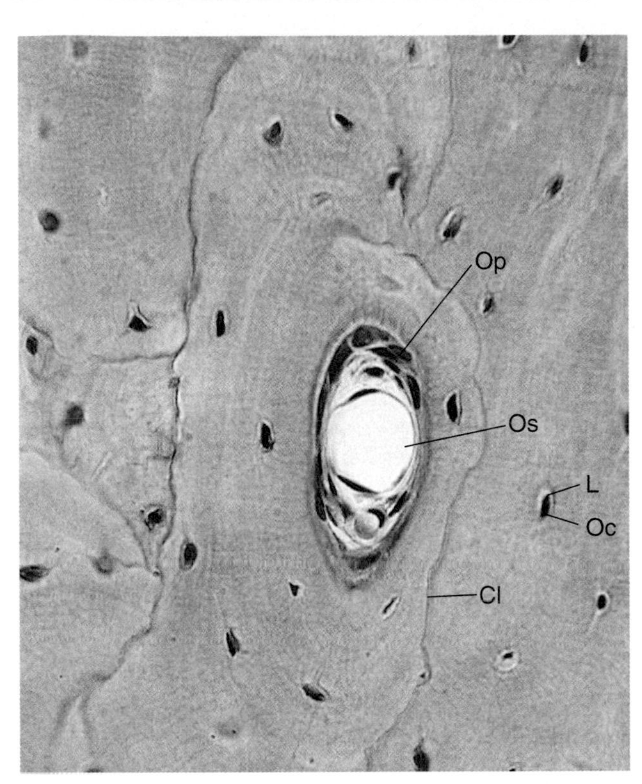

Fig. 7.9 Light micrograph of decalcified compact bone (×540). Osteocytes (Oc) may be observed in lacunae (L). Also note the blood vessel (Os) and osteoprogenitor cells (Op) in the haversian canal of the osteon, and observe the cementing lines (Cl) that completely surround osteons.

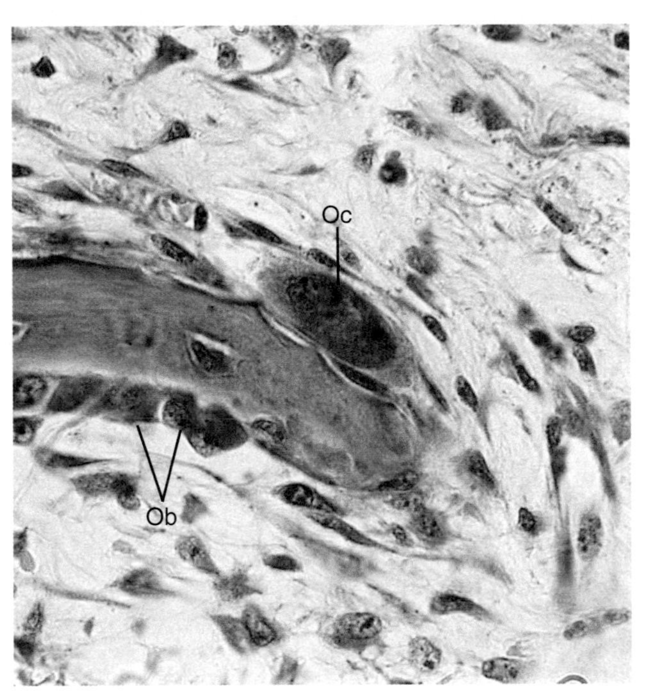

Fig. 7.10 Light micrograph of intramembranous ossification (×540). Osteoblasts (Ob) line the bony spicule, where they are secreting osteoid onto the bone. Osteoclasts (Oc) may be observed housed in a Howship lacuna.

Osteoblasts

Osteoblasts not only synthesize the organic matrix of bone but also possess receptors for parathyroid hormone.

Bone morphogenic protein-6 (BMP-6)—as well as, to some extent, BMP-2 and BMP-4—and **transforming growth factor-β (TGF-β)** induce osteoprogenitor cells to differentiate into **osteoblasts**, cells that manufacture and secrete the organic components of **bone matrix (osteoid)**: type I collagen and some type V collagen, glycoproteins, and proteoglycans. Osteoblasts also synthesize the **receptor for the activation of nuclear factor kappa B ligand (RANKL)**, **macrophage colony-stimulating factor (M-CSF)**, **alkaline phosphatase**, **insulin-like growth factor-1 (IGF-1) receptors**, and **parathyroid hormone (PTH) receptors**, all of which they place on their cell membranes. These cells also manufacture and release a number of additional macromolecules, such as

- **Osteocalcin**, a signaling molecule responsible for mineralization of bone
- **Osteonectin**, a glycoprotein that assists in the binding of calcium hydroxyl apatite crystals to collagen
- **Osteopontin**, which aids in the formation of the sealing zone of osteoclasts (see section on the morphology of osteoclasts)
- **Bone sialoprotein**, which assists osteoblasts in adhering to the bone matrix, and
- **Osteoprotegerin (OPG)**, a glycoprotein that can bind to RANKL and, thus, interfere with osteoclast formation.

Osteoblasts are located on the surface of the bone in a sheet-like arrangement of cuboidal to columnar cells (Fig. 7.10). When actively secreting matrix, they exhibit a basophilic cytoplasm.

The organelles of osteoblasts are polarized so that the nucleus is located away from the region of secretory activity, which houses secretory granules believed to contain matrix precursors. Electron micrographs exhibit abundant RER, a well-developed Golgi complex (Fig. 7.11A), and numerous secretory vesicles containing flocculent material. Osteoblasts extend short processes that contact those of neighboring osteoblasts and long processes that form contacts with processes of osteocytes. Although these processes form **gap junctions** with one another, the number of gap junctions between osteoblasts is much fewer than those between osteocytes. As osteoblasts exocytose their secretory products, each cell surrounds itself with the bone matrix that it has just produced. When this occurs, the incarcerated cell is referred to as an **osteocyte**, and the space it occupies is known as a **lacuna**. Most of the bone matrix becomes calcified; however, osteoblasts as well as osteocytes are always separated from the calcified substance by a thin, noncalcified layer known as the **osteoid** (uncalcified bone matrix).

Surface osteoblasts that cease to form matrix revert to a more flattened-shaped quiescent state and are called **bone-lining cells**. Although these cells appear to be similar to osteoprogenitor cells, they are most likely incapable of dividing but can be reactivated to the secreting form with the proper stimulus (Table 7.3).

Clinical Correlations

1. *Osteoblast cell membranes are rich in the enzyme* ***alkaline phosphatase.*** *During active bone formation, these cells secrete high levels of alkaline phosphatase, elevating the levels of this enzyme in the blood. Thus, the clinician can monitor bone formation by measuring the blood alkaline phosphatase level.*

Continued

Clinical Correlations—cont'd

2. *Individuals who have the type of mutations in the genes that code for TGF-β, in which the factor is always active, have the rare autosomal-dominant inherited disorder known as* **Camurati-Engelmann disease**. *This ailment usually manifests itself in late adolescence or early adulthood, characterized by an excess of highly active osteoblasts, resulting in very thick bones of the extremities. In some patients, the bones of the skull and hip may also be involved. The individual experiences intense pain in the bones and muscles of the leg. Additionally, the muscles of the extremities may be weakened; that, with the additional factor of pain, causes many affected individuals to "waddle" as they walk.*

Osteoblasts have several factors on their cell membranes, the most significant of which are integrins and ***PTH receptors***. When PTH binds to these receptors, it stimulates osteoblasts to secrete ***RANKL***, a factor that induces the differentiation of preosteoclasts into osteoclasts. Also, osteoblasts secrete an ***osteoclast-stimulating factor***, which activates osteoclasts to resorb bone. Osteoblasts also secrete enzymes responsible for removing osteoid so that osteoclasts can make contact with the mineralized bone surface.

Osteocytes

Osteocytes are mature bone cells derived from osteoblasts that became trapped in their lacunae.

Osteocytes are mature bone cells, transformed from osteoblasts under the influence of two transcription factors, **Cbfa1/Runx2** and **osterix**, both of which appear to be dependent on the presence of BMP-2. As osteoblasts transform into osteocytes, they no longer express alkaline phosphatase on their cell membranes. They become flat, lenticular-shaped cells trapped in their **lacunae** within the calcified bony matrix (see Figs. 7.9 and 7.11B). Their nucleus is flattened and their cytoplasm is poor in organelles, displaying scant RER and a greatly reduced Golgi apparatus.

Radiating out in all directions from the lacuna are narrow, tunnel-like spaces (**canaliculi**) that house cytoplasmic processes of the osteocyte. These processes make contact with similar processes of neighboring osteocytes, forming **gap junctions**. The canaliculi also contain extracellular fluid carrying nutrients and metabolites, which nourish the osteocytes.

The space between the osteocyte plasmalemma and the walls of the lacuna and canaliculi, known as the ***periosteocytic space***, is occupied by extracellular fluid. Considering the extensive network of the canaliculi and the sheer number of osteocytes present in the skeleton of an average person (as many as 20,000–30,000 osteocytes per mm^3 of bone), the volume of the periosteocytic space and the surface area of the walls have been calculated to be a staggering 1.3 L and as much as 5000 m^2, respectively. It has been suggested that the 1.3 L of extracellular fluid occupying the periosteocytic space is exposed to as much as 20 g of exchangeable calcium that can be resorbed from the walls of these spaces. If the calcium level in the extracellular fluid in their lacunae is low (which reflects the level of calcium in blood), osteocytes secrete **sclerostin**, a paracrine hormone that inhibits bone formation and encourages bone resorption, thereby elevating blood-calcium levels. The resorbed calcium gains access to the bloodstream and ensures the maintenance of adequate blood calcium levels.

Although osteocytes appear to be inactive cells, they secrete substances necessary for bone maintenance. These cells have also been implicated in **mechanotransduction** in that they respond to stimuli that place tension on bone by releasing **cyclic adenosine monophosphate (cAMP)**, **osteocalcin**, and **IGF**. The release of these and other factors facilitates the recruitment of **osteoprogenitor cells** to assist in the remodeling of the skeleton (adding more bone) not only during growth and development but also during the long-term redistribution of forces acting on the skeleton. An example of such remodeling is evident in the comparison of male and female skeletons, in which the muscle attachments of the male skeleton are usually better defined than those of the female skeleton.

Clinical Correlations

Although bone is constantly remodeled during an individual's life and osteocytes have a very long life span of approximately 25 years, these cells undergo apoptosis as an individual ages. By the time a person is about 80 years old, 75% of the bone's osteocyte population is dead. As osteocytes undergo apoptosis and disintegrate into apoptotic bodies, they release RANKL, a cytokine that stimulates the formation and activation of osteoclasts. Young osteocytes release TGF-β, which suppresses bone resorption. However, as these cells age, they release increasingly reduced quantities of TGF-β, permitting an increase in osteoclastic activity that results in increased bone resorption. Thus, the aging individual loses bone mass as a result of age-related osteocytic alterations.

Osteoclasts

Osteoclasts are multinucleated cells originating from granulocyte-macrophage progenitors and play a role in bone resorption.

The precursor of the osteoclast originates in the bone marrow. Osteoclasts have receptors for osteoclast-stimulating factor, colony-stimulating factor-1, OPG, receptor for activation of nuclear factor kappa B (RANK), and calcitonin, among others. Osteoclasts are responsible for resorbing bone; after they finish doing so, these cells probably undergo apoptosis.

Morphology of Osteoclasts. Osteoclasts are large, motile, multinucleated cells 150 µm in diameter, with as many as 50 nuclei and an acidophilic cytoplasm (see Fig. 7.10). These cells arise from a bone marrow precursor, the **preosteoclast**, a member of the ***cells of the mononuclear-phagocyte system***, from which monocytes arise. The fate of **preosteoclasts** is under the influence of osteoblasts, which secrete four signaling molecules that regulate their differentiation into osteoclasts.

- The first of these signals, **M-CSF**, binds to a receptor on the osteoclast precursor, inducing it to proliferate and to express the **RANK** on the osteoclast precursor cell membrane. Another signaling molecule, **RANKL**, bound to the osteoblast cell membrane, binds to the **RANK** receptor on the osteoclast precursor cell membrane, inducing the precursor cell to differentiate into the multinucleated osteoclast and, along

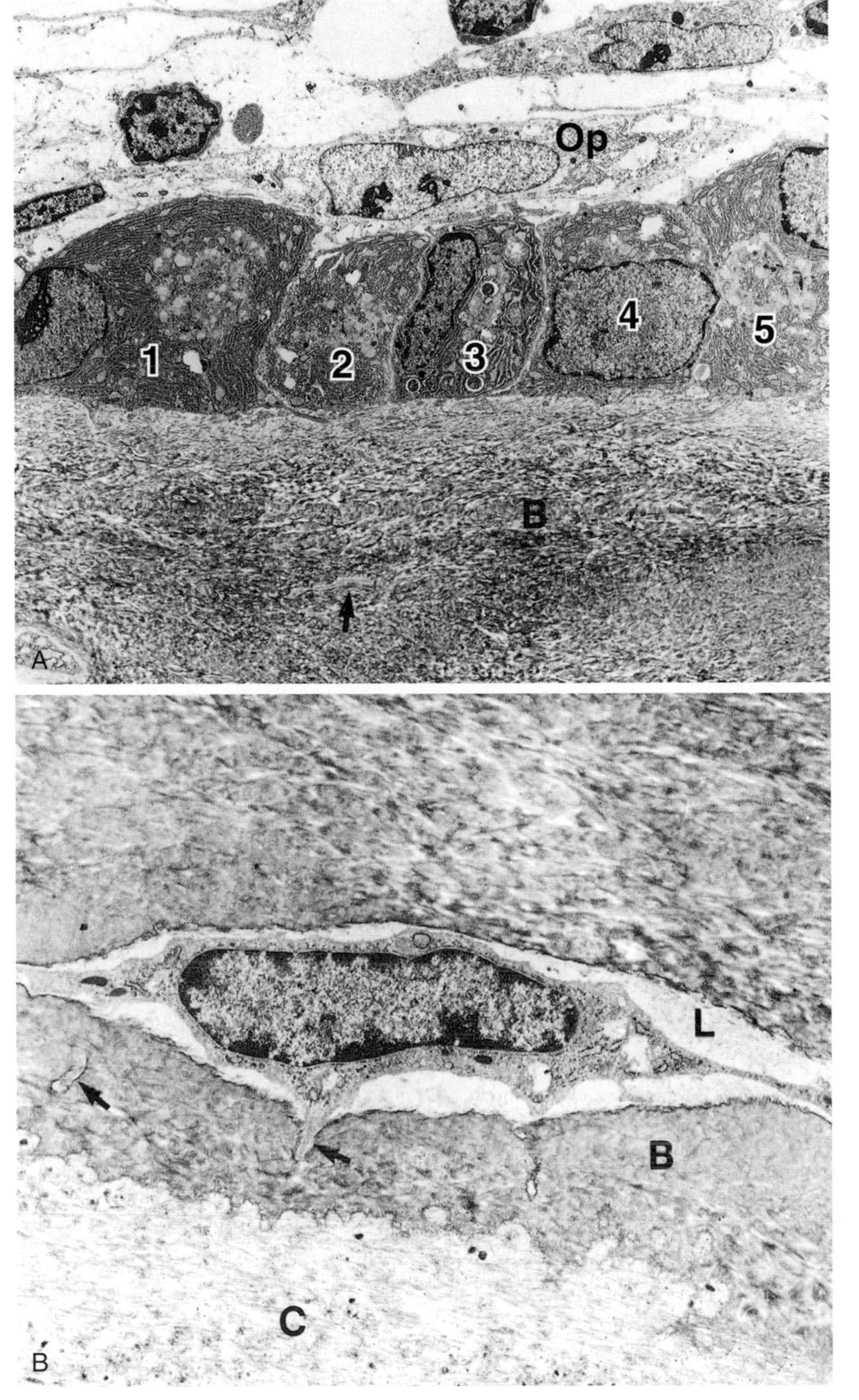

Fig. 7.11 Electron micrograph of bone-forming cells. (A) Observe the five osteoblasts (numbered 1 to 5) lined up on the surface of bone (B) displaying abundant rough endoplasmic reticulum. The *arrow* indicates the process of an osteocyte in a canaliculus. The cell with the elongated nucleus lying above the osteoblasts is an osteoprogenitor cell (op) (×2500). (B) Note the osteocyte in its lacuna (L) with its processes extending into canaliculi (×1000). B, bone; C, cartilage. (From Marks SC Jr, Popoff SN. Bone cell biology: the regulation of development, structure, and function in the skeleton. *Am J Anat.* 1988;183:1-44. Reprinted by permission of Wiley-Liss, Inc., a subsidiary of John Wiley & Sons, Inc.)

with osteoclast-stimulating factor, activating it and enhancing bone resorption.

- The second osteoblast-derived signaling molecule, the growth factor **interleukin-6 (IL-6)**, facilitates the recruitment and differentiation of osteoclasts.
- The third signaling molecule released by the osteoblast is **interleukin-1 (IL-1)**, which induces osteoclast precursors to proliferate.
- The fourth signaling molecule, **osteoprotegerin**, a member of the **tumor necrosis factor receptor (TNFR)** family, can serve as a decoy by interacting with RANKL, thus prohibiting it from binding to the macrophage and inhibiting osteoclast formation.

Therefore, RANKL, RANK, and OPG regulate bone metabolism and osteoclastic activity. **OPG** is produced not only by osteoblasts but also by cells of many other tissues, including the cardiovascular system, lung, kidney, intestines, hematopoietic cells, and in immune cells. Therefore, it is not surprising that its expression is modulated by various cytokines, peptides, hormones, and drugs. In bone, OPG not only inhibits the differentiation of osteoclasts but also suppresses the osteoclast's bone-resorbing capabilities.

TABLE 7.3 Osteoblast-Derived Cytokines

Cytokine	Function
Alkaline phosphatase	Encourages bone matrix mineralization
Bone morphogenic protein	Stimulates osteoprogenitor cells to become osteoblasts
Bone sialoprotein	Assists the adherence of osteoblasts to bone matrix
Insulin-like growth factor-1	Encourages bone formation
Interleukin-1	Stimulates osteoclast precursors to undergo mitosis
Interleukin-6	Recruits and induces osteoclast precursors to become osteoclasts
Macrophage colony-stimulating factor	Stimulates osteoclast precursor formation and induces them to express RANK on their cell membrane
Osteocalcin	Stimulates mineralization of bone matrix
Osteoclast-stimulating factor	Stimulates osteoclast to become active and resorb bone
Osteonectin	Encourages calcium hydroxyapatite binding to type I collagen
Osteopontin	Aids osteoclasts in their formation of sealing zone
Osteoprotegerin	Inhibits osteoclast formation by forming bonds with RANKL
PTH receptor	Parathyroid hormone binding induces osteoblasts to secrete RANKL
RANKL	Encourages preosteoclast differentiation into osteoclast
TGF-β	Stimulates osteoprogenitor cells to become osteoblasts

RANK, Receptor for the activation of nuclear factor κ; *RANKL*, receptor for the activation of nuclear factor κ-β ligand; *TGF-β*, transforming growth factor-alpha.

Osteoclasts occupy shallow depressions on the bone surface, called ***Howship lacunae*** (**resorption bays**), that identify regions of bone resorption. An osteoclast active in bone resorption may be subdivided into four morphologically recognizable regions:

1. **The basal zone**, located farthest from the Howship lacuna, houses most of the organelles, including nuclei, Golgi complexes, and centrioles. Mitochondria, RER, and polysomes are distributed throughout the cell but are more numerous near the ruffled border.
2. **The ruffled border** is the portion of the cell that is directly involved in resorption of bone. Its finger-like processes are active and dynamic, changing their configuration continually as they project into the resorption compartment, known as the ***subosteoclastic compartment***. The cytoplasmic aspect of the ruffled border plasmalemma displays a regularly spaced, bristle-like coat that increases the thickness of the plasma membrane of this region. As resorption progresses and the subosteoclastic compartment increases in size, it becomes known as the **Howship lacuna.**
3. **The clear zone** is the region of the cell that immediately surrounds the periphery of the ruffled border. It is organelle free but contains many actin filaments that form an **actin ring** and appear to function in helping integrins of the clear zone plasmalemma maintain contact with the bony periphery of the Howship lacuna. In fact, the plasma membrane of this region is so closely applied to the bone that its integrin molecules, in concert with **osteopontin,** form the **sealing zone** of the subosteoclastic compartment. Thus, the clear zone isolates the subosteoclastic compartment from the surrounding region, establishing a microenvironment whose contents may be modulated by cellular activities. For the osteoclast to be able to resorb bone, the actin ring must first be formed; its formation may be facilitated by **RANKL.** Then, the ruffled border is formed, whose finger-like processes increase the surface area of the plasmalemma in the region of bone resorption, facilitating the resorptive process.
4. **The vesicular zone** of the osteoclast is between the basal zone and the ruffled border. It consists of numerous endocytotic and exocytotic vesicles that ferry lysosomal enzymes and metalloproteinases into the subosteoclastic compartment and the products of bone degradation into the cell (Figs. 7.12 and 7.13).

Mechanism of Bone Resorption. Osteoclasts must be activated by osteoclast-stimulating factor before they are able to resorb bone. Additionally, the osteoblasts must resorb the osteoid that separates them from the calcified bony surface; then, the osteoblasts have to migrate from that surface. Activated osteoclasts can then occupy the newly freed bone surface and alter their morphology to display the four zones described earlier. The sealing zone has to be established, isolating the subosteoclastic compartment from the external milieu; then, the ruffled border can be formed. The finger-like processes express aquaporins, proton pumps, and Cl^- channels on their plasmalemmae.

Within the cytosol of the osteoclasts, the enzyme carbonic anhydrase catalyzes the intracellular formation of carbonic acid (H_2CO_3) from carbon dioxide and water. Carbonic acid dissociates within the cells into H^+ ions and bicarbonate ions, HCO_3^-. The bicarbonate ions, accompanied by Na^+ ions, cross the plasmalemma of the basal zone, where they act to buffer any hydrochloric acid that may escape from the subosteoclastic compartment; excess bicarbonate will enter nearby capillaries. Proton pumps in the plasmalemma of the ruffled border of the osteoclasts actively transport H^+ ions into the subosteoclastic compartment. Cl^- ions follow passively and the two then form HCl, thus reducing the pH of the microenvironment of the subosteoclastic compartment. Water from the cell enters the subosteoclastic compartment through aquaporins of the ruffled border plasmalemma. The inorganic component of the bone matrix is dissolved as the environment becomes acidic; the liberated minerals enter the osteoclast cytoplasm to be delivered to nearby capillaries.

Lysosomal hydrolases, **cathepsin K**, and **matrix metalloproteinases**, such as **collagenase** and **gelatinase**, are secreted by osteoclasts into the subosteoclastic compartment to degrade the organic components of the decalcified bone matrix. The degradation products are endocytosed by the osteoclasts and digested in the osteoclasts' cytoplasm, forming amino acids, monosaccharides, and disaccharides, which then are released into nearby capillaries (see Fig. 7.13).

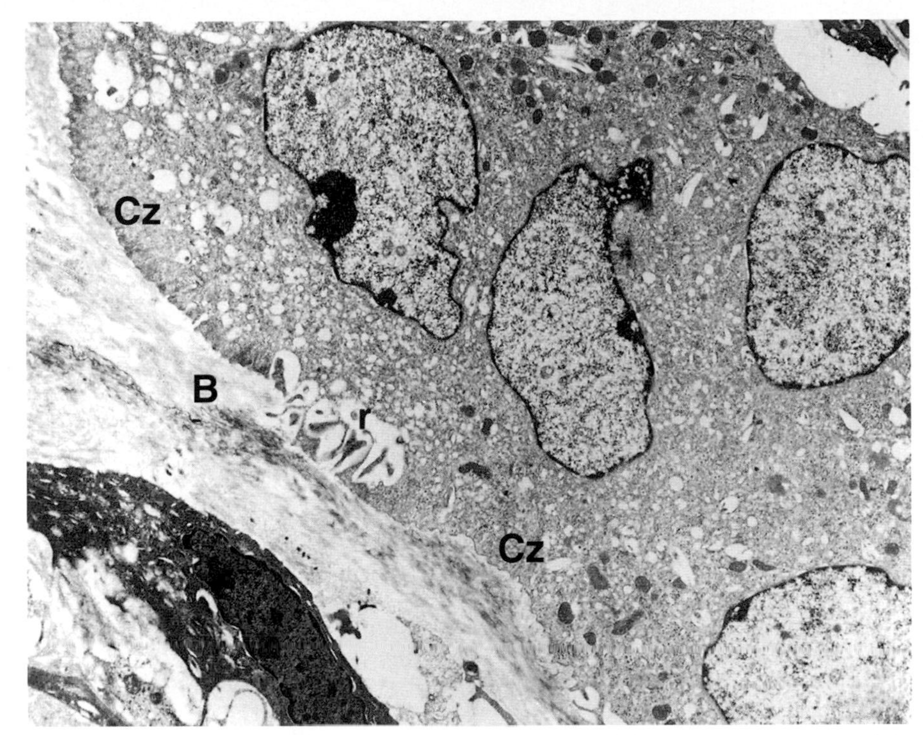

Fig. 7.12 Electron micrograph of an osteoclast. Note the clear zone (Cz) on either side of the ruffled border (B) of this multinucleated cell. (From Marks SC Jr, Walker DG. The hematogenous origin of osteoclasts. Experimental evidence from osteopetrotic [microphthalmic] mice treated with spleen cells from beige mouse donors. *Am J Anat.* 1981;161:1-10. Reprinted by permission of Wiley-Liss, Inc., a subsidiary of John Wiley & Sons, Inc.)

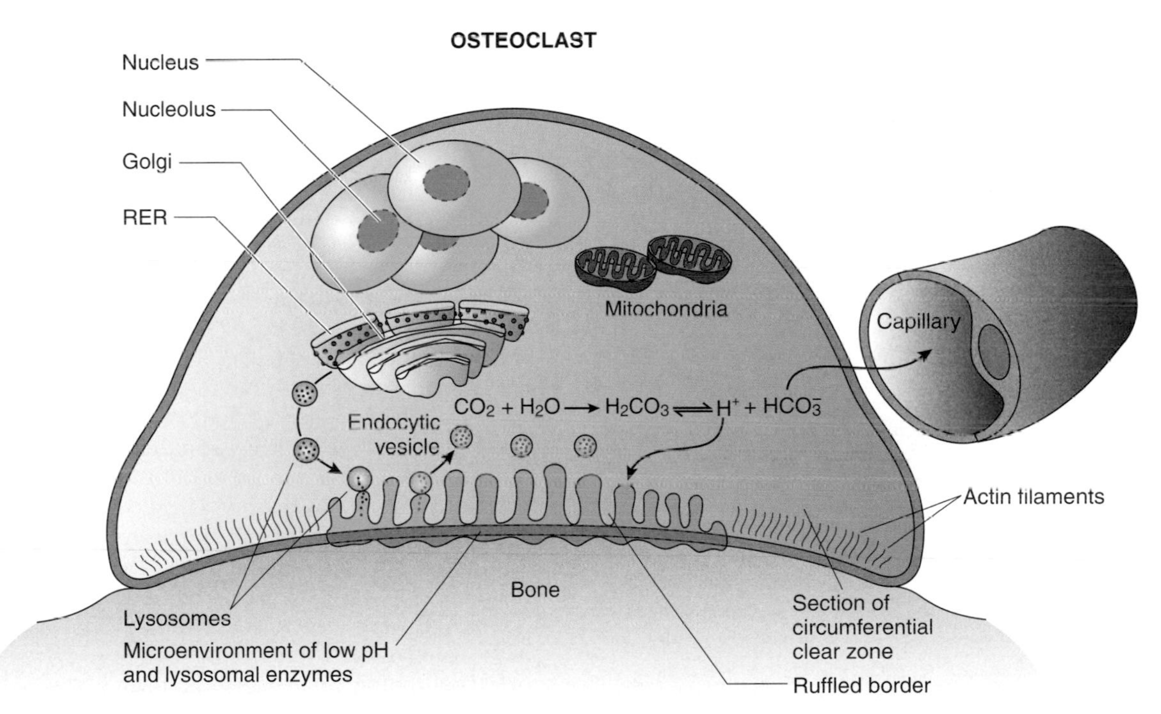

Fig. 7.13 Schematic diagram illustrating osteoclastic function. RER, Rough endoplasmic reticulum. (From Gartner LP, Hiatt JL, Strum JM. *Cell Biology and Histology [Board Review Series].* Philadelphia: Lippincott Williams & Wilkins; 1998:100.)

Clinical Correlations

Osteoporosis *is a disorder of the skeletal system in which the mineral density of the bone is reduced to such an extent that the possibility of fracture has increased. Individuals who are possible candidates for this disorder are postmenopausal women and aged men. There are approximately 200 million or so individuals who have been diagnosed with osteoporosis, of whom almost 9 million have suffered fractures, usually of the vertebrae, hip, or arm. Because of the aging population, these numbers are certain to increase in the future. There are two categories of osteoporosis:* ***primary osteoporosis****, which includes type I (postmenopausal) and type II (senile); and* ***secondary osteoporosis****, which is due to medical conditions such as malabsorption, vitamin D deficiency, or calcium deficiency; prescription drug use, such as glucocorticoids, aromatase inhibitors, or chemotherapeutic medications; or endocrine disorders, such as hyperparathyroidism, hypogonadism, or early ovarian failure. Individuals who are at risk, including*

Clinical Correlations—cont'd

all women 65 and men 70 years or older, should have **bone mineral density (BMD)** *measurements performed to prevent risk of fractures. The frequency of BMD measurements depends on the results of the first measurement and the physician's evaluation of test results. Treatment of osteoporosis is severalfold: preventive measures to alleviate hazards at home; corrective measures to improve eyesight and balance of the elderly patient; monitoring and possibly eliminating medications that can interfere with alertness and balance; and altering lifestyles, such as initiating smoking cessation, reducing alcohol consumption, and ensuring a properly balanced diet. Additionally, the patient should be placed on one of two types of osteoporosis medications:* **anabolic agents** *(increase bone formation) or* **antiresorptive agents** *(decrease bone resorption). Unfortunately, all of these agents have side effects that include risks such as cancer, cardiovascular problems, atypical femoral fractures, stroke, thromboembolism, and other conditions.*

Hormones of the Endocrine System That Control Bone Resorption. The bone-resorbing activity of osteoclasts is regulated by two hormones, **PTH** and **calcitonin**. PTH is released from the **parathyroid gland** when calcium blood levels fall below approximately 8.8 mg/dL (in adults). It acts in an indirect fashion by binding to PTH receptors on osteoblasts. Those cells respond by releasing factors noted earlier to recruit and activate osteoclasts to resorb bone, thereby increasing blood calcium levels. Calcitonin, released by **C cells (parafollicular cells)** of the **thyroid gland**, has an opposite effect. When calcium blood levels are above approximately 10.5 mg/dL (in adults), calcitonin is released and binds directly to calcitonin receptors on osteoclasts, causing them to undergo apoptosis, thereby increasing blood calcium levels.

Clinical Correlations

Osteopetrosis, *not to be confused with osteoporosis, is a genetic disorder in which osteoclasts do not possess ruffled borders, possibly because of the presence of mutations in the gene that codes for IL-6. Consequently, these osteoclasts cannot resorb bone and persons with osteopetrosis display increased bone density. Individuals with this disease may exhibit anemia resulting from decreased marrow space, as well as blindness, deafness, and cranial nerve involvement because of impingement of the nerves caused by narrowing of the foramina housing these nerves.*

Osteonecrosis (avascular necrosis) *is a disease of bone due to vascular problems in which blood supply to a region of the bone is obstructed, resulting in the death and eventual collapse of that portion of the bone. Osteonecrosis occurs most commonly in individuals who are between 30 and 50 years of age and affects the humerus, shoulder, femur, knees, and ankles. Unfortunately, osteonecrosis is often asymptomatic until the situation becomes more severe. Then, the region of the bone may develop pain that progresses in a gradual fashion, indicative of worsening conditions. The cause of this condition is diminished or complete interruption of blood flow that can result from various medical conditions, including the lysosomal storage disease known as Gaucher disease, sickle cell anemia, diabetes, and pancreatitis; fracture or dislocation of joints, which can harm the regional vascular supply; and diseases such as arteriosclerosis and atherosclerosis. There are certain risk factors that may contribute to the development of osteonecrosis, which include the long-term use of high doses of corticosteroids, alcoholism, smoking, radiation therapy, and kidney transplantation.*

BONE STRUCTURE

Bones are classified according to their anatomical shape: long, short, flat, irregular, and sesamoid.

Bones are classified according to their shape. **Long bones** display a shaft located between two heads (e.g., tibia). **Short bones** have more or less the same width and length (e.g., carpal bones of the wrist). **Flat bones** are flat, thin, and plate-like (e.g., bones forming the brain case of the skull). **Irregular bones** have an irregular shape that does not fit into the other classes (e.g., sphenoid and ethmoid bones within the skull). **Sesamoid bones**, shaped like sesame seeds, develop within tendons, where they increase the mechanical advantage for the muscle (e.g., patella) across a joint.

Gross Observation of Bone

Gross observations of a long bone, such as the femur, cut in longitudinal section reveal two different types of bone structure. The very dense bone on the outside surface is **compact bone**; the porous portion lining the marrow cavity is **cancellous bone**, also known as **spongy bone** (Fig. 7.14).

Trabeculae and **spicules**, composed of lamellae of bone arranged in an apparently random order, protrude from the internal surface of the compact bone into the marrow cavity to form cancellous bone. These lamellae of bone contain lacunae housing osteocytes that are nourished by diffusion from the marrow cavity.

The shaft of a long bone is called the ***diaphysis***, and the articular ends are called the ***epiphyses*** (singular, **epiphysis**). In a growing individual, both ends of the diaphysis are separated from the epiphysis by the cartilaginous **epiphyseal plate**, which is resorbed when the growth is finished. The articulating surface of the epiphysis is covered with only a thin layer of compact bone overlying spongy bone, which, in turn, is covered by the highly polished **articular hyaline cartilage**. This smoothly polished cartilage reduces friction as it moves against the articular cartilage of the bony counterpart of the joint. The area of transition between the epiphyseal plate and diaphysis is called the **metaphysis**, where columns of spongy bone are located. It is from the epiphyseal plate and metaphysis that bone grows in length.

The flat bones of the skull develop by a different method from most of the long bones of the body. The inner and outer surfaces of the calvaria (**skull cap**) possess two relatively thick layers of compact bone called the ***inner*** and ***outer tables***, which surround the spongy bone (**diploë**) sandwiched between them. The outer table possesses a periosteum, identified as the **pericranium**. Internally, the inner table is lined with **dura mater**, whose outer leaflet serves as a periosteum for the inner table, as well as a protective covering for the brain.

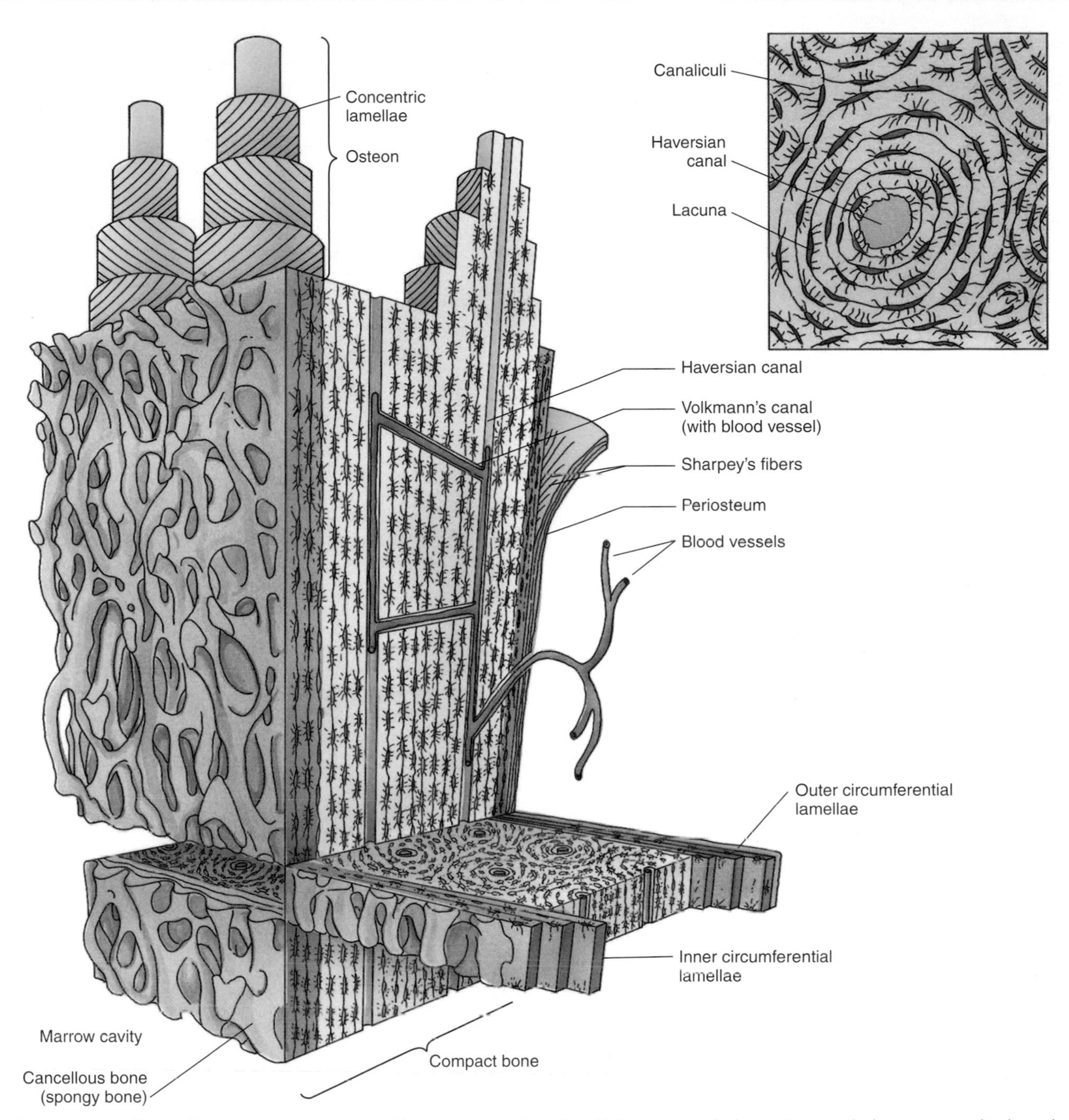

Fig. 7.14 Diagram of bone illustrating compact cortical bone, osteons, lamellae, Volkmann canals, haversian canals, lacunae, canaliculi, and spongy bone.

Bone Types Based on Microscopic Observations

Microscopically, bone is classified as either primary (immature) or secondary (mature) bone.

Microscopic observations reveal two types of bone: primary bone (immature or woven bone) and secondary bone (mature or lamellar bone).

Primary bone is immature in that it is the first bone to form during fetal development and during bone repair. It has abundant osteocytes and irregular bundles of collagen, which are later replaced and organized as secondary bone, except in certain areas (e.g., at sutures of the calvaria, insertion sites of tendons, and bony alveoli surrounding the teeth). The mineral content of primary bone is also much less than that of secondary bone.

Secondary bone is mature bone composed of parallel or concentric bony lamellae, where each lamella is 3 to 7 μm thick. Osteocytes in their lacunae are arranged at regular intervals between, or occasionally within, lamellae. **Canaliculi**, housing osteocytic processes, connect neighboring lacunae with one another, forming a network of intercommunicating channels that facilitate the flow of nutrients, hormones, ions, and waste products to and from osteocytes. In addition, osteocytic processes within these canaliculi make contact with similar processes of neighboring osteocytes and form gap junctions, permitting these cells to communicate with each other.

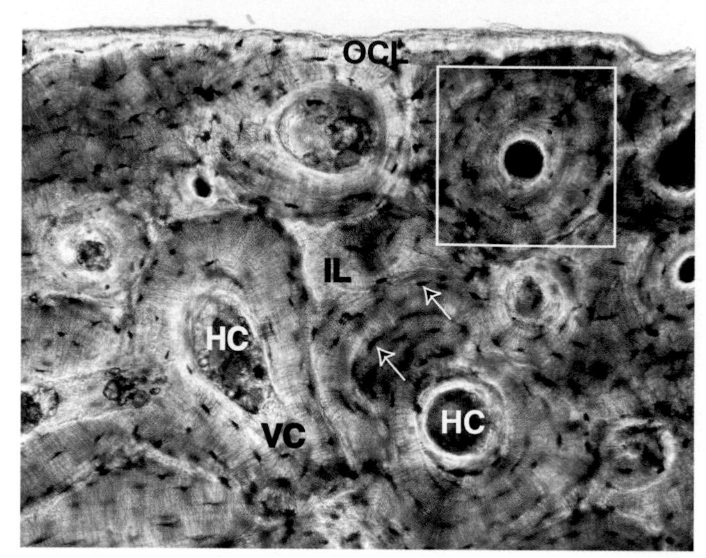

Fig. 7.15 This low-magnification light micrograph of a ground section of bone displays three of the four lamellar systems: the outer circumferential lamellar system (OCL), haversian canal system *(boxed area)*, and the interstitial lamellar system (IL). Arrows indicate the dust-filled lacunae. HC, haversian canal; VC, Volkmann canal. An image similar to the boxed area is shown at a higher magnification in Fig. 7.16.

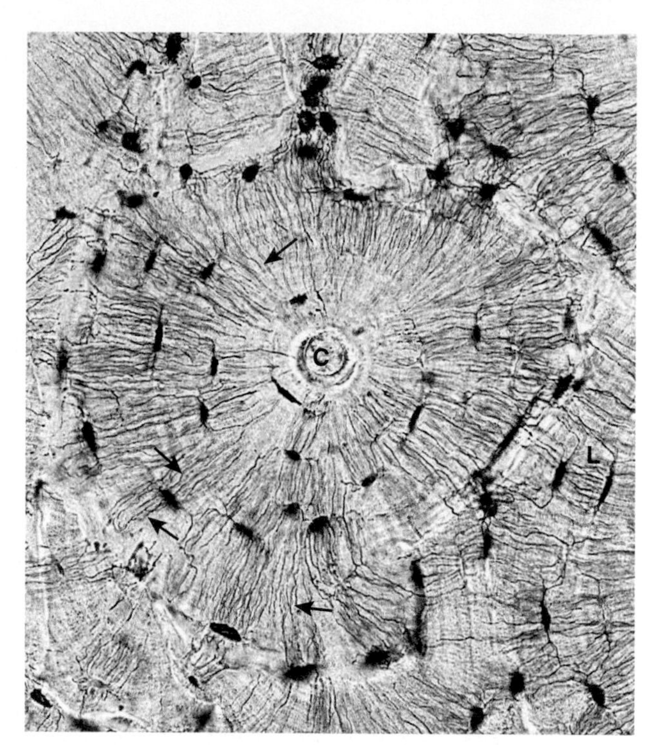

Fig. 7.16 Light micrograph of nondecalcified ground bone (×270). Observe the haversian system containing the haversian canal (C) and concentric lamellae with lacunae with their canaliculi *(arrows)*.

Because secondary bone is more calcified, it is stronger than primary bone. In addition, the collagen fibers of secondary bone are arranged so that they parallel each other within a given lamella, conferring still greater strength on secondary bone.

Lamellar Systems of Compact Bone

There are four lamellar systems in compact bone: outer circumferential lamellae, inner circumferential lamellae, osteons, and interstitial lamellae.

Compact bone is composed of wafer-like thin layers of bone, **lamellae**, that are arranged in lamellar systems and are especially evident in the diaphyses of long bones. These lamellar systems are the outer circumferential lamellae, inner circumferential lamellae, osteons (haversian canal systems), and interstitial lamellae.

Outer and Inner Circumferential Lamellae. The outer circumferential lamellae (see Figs. 7.8, 7.14, and 7.15) are just deep to the periosteum, forming the outermost region of the diaphysis, and contain Sharpey fibers anchoring the periosteum to the bone.

The **inner circumferential lamellae**—analogous to, but not as extensive as, outer circumferential lamellae—completely encircle the marrow cavity. Trabeculae of spongy bone extend from the inner circumferential lamellae into the marrow cavity, interrupting the endosteal lining of the inner circumferential lamellae.

Haversian Canal System (Osteon) and Interstitial Lamellae. The bulk of compact bone is composed of an abundance of **haversian canal systems** (**osteons**). Each system is composed of cylinders of **lamellae**, concentrically arranged around a vascular space known as the ***haversian canal*** (see Figs. 7.8, 7.16, and 7.17). Frequently, osteons bifurcate along their considerable length. Each osteon is bounded by a thin **cementing line**, composed mostly of calcified ground substance with a scant amount of collagen fibers (see Fig. 7.9).

Collagen fiber bundles line up parallel to each other within any one lamella but are oriented almost perpendicular to those of adjacent lamellae. This arrangement is possible because the collagen fibers follow a helical arrangement around the haversian canal within each lamella but are pitched differently in adjacent lamellae.

Each haversian canal, lined by a layer of osteoblasts and osteoprogenitor cells, houses a neurovascular bundle with its associated connective tissue. Haversian canals of adjacent osteons are connected to each other by **Volkmann canals** (see Figs. 7.8, 7.14, and 7.17), vascular spaces that are oriented oblique or perpendicular to haversian canals.

The diameter of haversian canals varies from approximately 20 µm to about 100 µm. During the formation of osteons, the lamella closest to the cementing line is the first one to be formed. As additional lamellae are added to the system, the diameter of the haversian canal is reduced and the thickness of the osteon wall increases. Because nutrients from blood vessels of the haversian canal must traverse canaliculi to reach osteocytes, a rather inefficient process, most osteons possess no more than 4 to 20 lamellae.

As bone is being remodeled, osteoclasts resorb portions of osteons, and osteoblasts form new haversian canal systems. Remnants of osteons remain as irregular arcs of lamellar fragments, known as ***interstitial lamellae***, surrounded by osteons. Similar to osteons, interstitial lamellae are also surrounded by cementing lines.

Histogenesis of Bone

Although during embryogenesis bone may be formed in two different ways, **intramembranous** and **endochondral**, the two bones types are identical histologically. In both instances, the first bone formed is **primary bone**, which is later resorbed and replaced by **secondary bone**. Secondary bone continues to be resorbed throughout life, although at a slower rate.

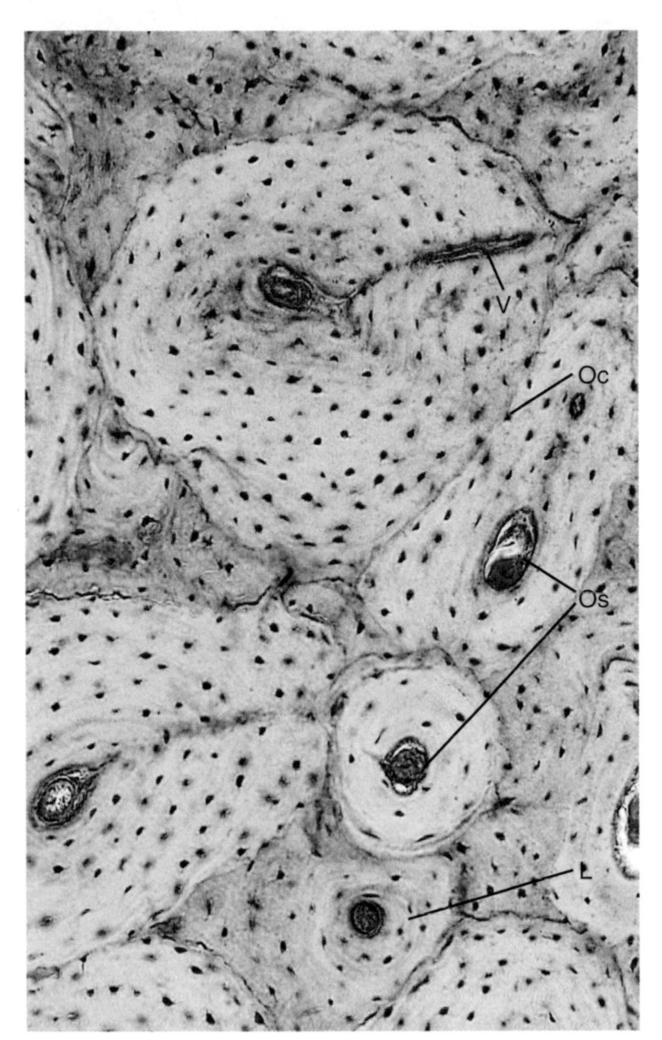

Fig. 7.17 Light micrograph of decalcified compact bone (×162). The haversian canals (Os) of several osteons are displayed with their concentric lamellae (L). A Volkmann canal (V) is also denoted. The dark-staining structures scattered throughout represent nuclei of osteocytes (Oc).

Intramembranous Bone Formation

Intramembranous bone formation occurs within mesenchymal tissue.

Most flat bones develop by **intramembranous bone formation**. This process occurs in a richly vascularized mesenchymal tissue whose cells make contact with each other via long processes.

Mesenchymal cells, under the influence of **Cbfa1/Runx2** and **osterix**, differentiate into **osteoblasts** that secrete **bone matrix**, forming a network of **spicules** and **trabeculae** whose surfaces are populated by these cells (Figs. 7.18 to 7.20). This region of initial osteogenesis is known as the **ossification center**. As expected in primary bone, the type I collagen fibers of these developing spicules and trabeculae are oriented in a random fashion. Calcification quickly follows osteoid formation, and osteoblasts trapped in their matrices become osteocytes. The processes of these osteocytes contact one another and are also surrounded by forming bone, establishing a system of canaliculi. Continuous mitotic activity of mesenchymal cells provides a constant supply of undifferentiated **osteoprogenitor cells**, which differentiate into osteoblasts that will continue bone formation.

As the sponge-like network of trabeculae is established, the vascular connective tissue in their interstices is transformed into bone marrow. The addition of trabeculae to the periphery increases the size of the forming bone. Larger bones, such as the occipital bone of the base of the skull, have several ossification centers, which enlarge and fuse with one another to form a single bone. The **fontanelles** ("soft spots") on the frontal and parietal bones of a newborn infant represent ossification centers that did not fuse prior to birth.

Regions of the mesenchymal tissues that remain uncalcified differentiate into the periosteum and endosteum of developing bone. The spongy bone deep to the periosteum and the periosteal layer of the dura mater of flat bones are transformed into compact bone, forming the **inner** and **outer tables** with the intervening **diploë**.

Endochondral Bone Formation

Endochondral bone formation requires the presence of a cartilage template.

Most of the long and short bones of the body develop by **endochondral bone formation**, which occurs in two steps: (1) a miniature hyaline cartilage model is formed and (2) the cartilage model continues to grow, serving as a structural scaffold for bone development, and is eventually resorbed and replaced by bone (Table 7.4 and Fig. 7.21)

Clinical Correlations

It has been shown that mesenchymal cells of mouse embryos that are ***osterix null****—that is, they do not express osterix—cannot differentiate into osteoblasts and, as a consequence, cannot form bone.*

Events in Endochondral Bone Formation (Primary Center of Ossification).

1. A **hyaline cartilage template** develops in the region of future bone formation. As the cartilage model grows, the chondrocytes in its center hypertrophy, accumulate glycogen in their cytoplasm, and become vacuolated (Fig. 7.22). Hypertrophy of the chondrocytes forces enlargement of their lacunae, and the cartilage matrix septa, which became decreased in thickness, becomes calcified.
2. Concurrently, the perichondrium at the **midriff of the diaphysis of cartilage becomes vascularized** (Fig. 7.23) and, due to the increased oxygen tension, chondrogenic cells become osteoprogenitor cells. Therefore, this small region of the perichondrium becomes a periosteum.
3. Osteoprogenitor cells differentiate into **osteoblasts** that secrete bone matrix, forming the **subperiosteal bone collar** on the surface of the cartilage template by *intramembranous bone formation* (see Fig. 7.23).
4. The subperiosteal bone collar prevents the diffusion of nutrients to the hypertrophied chondrocytes within the core of the cartilage model, causing them to die. The empty, confluent lacunae become the future marrow cavity in the center of the cartilage model.
5. Holes etched in the bone collar by osteoclasts permit **periosteal buds** (osteogenic buds)—composed of osteoprogenitor cells, hemopoietic cells, and blood vessels—to enter the concavities within the cartilage model (see Fig. 7.21).

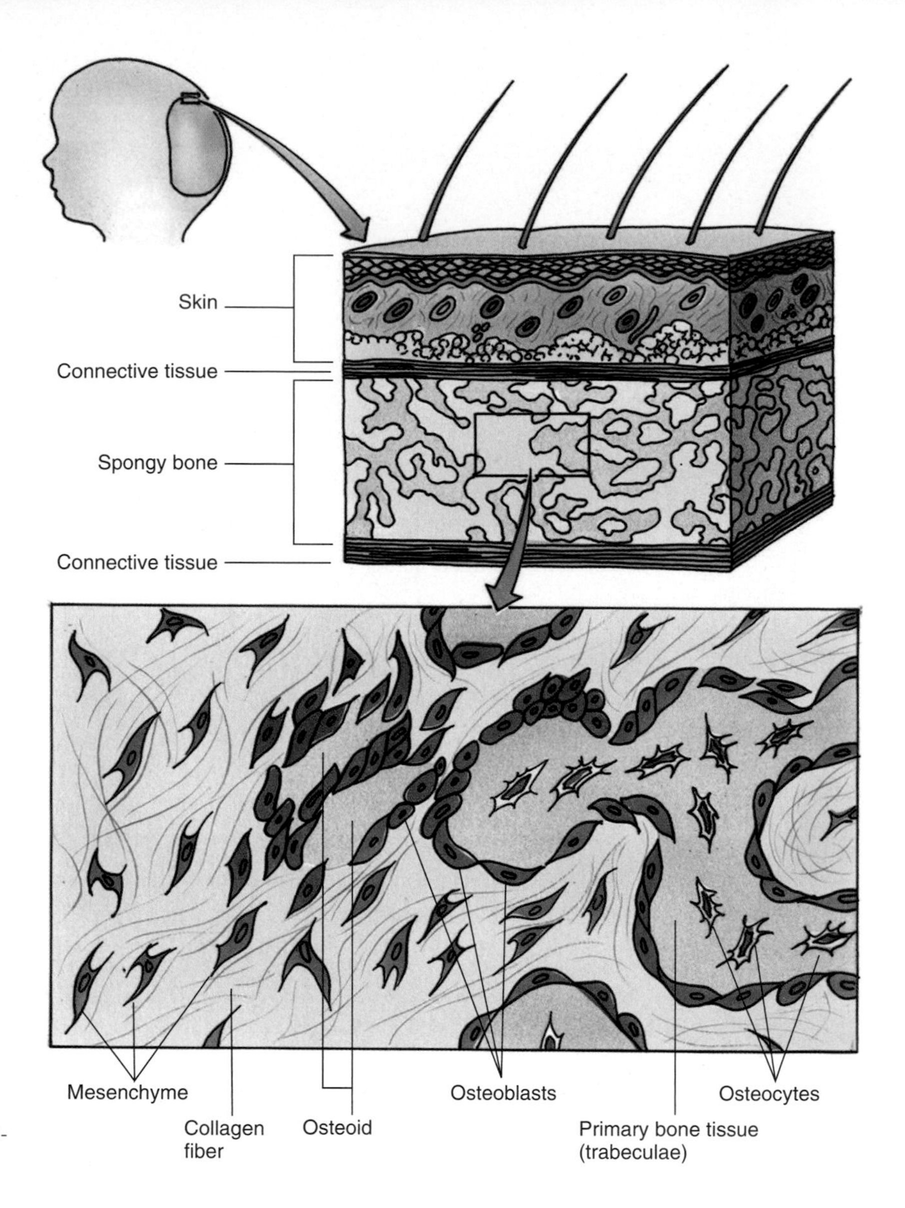

Fig. 7.18 Diagram of intramembranous bone formation.

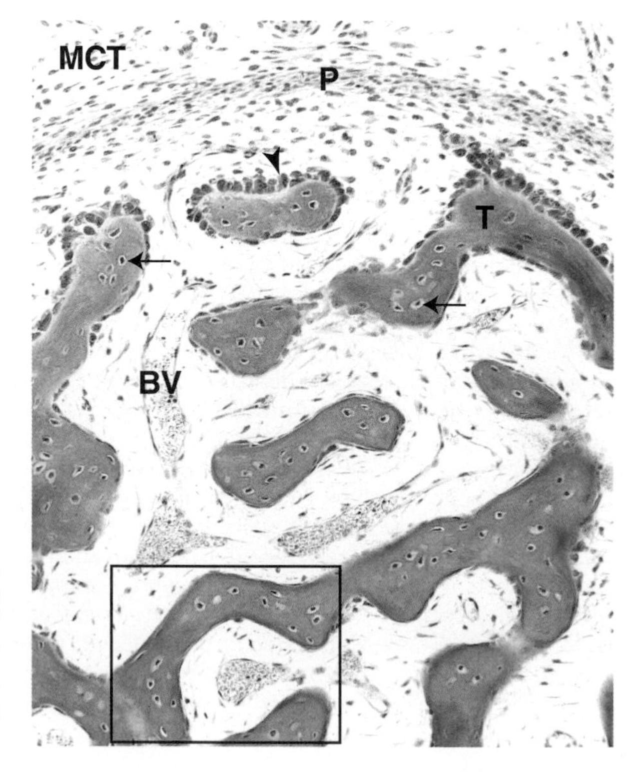

Fig. 7.19 This low-magnification light micrograph of the head of a pig embryo displays the mesenchymal connective tissue (MCT), which is a site of bone formation. Note the mesenchymal condensation of the future periosteum (P) as well as the formation of the bony trabeculae (T) that are being transformed into future osteons *(boxed area)*. Within the trabeculae, note the presence of numerous osteocytes *(arrows)* in their lacunae. On the trabecular surfaces, note the presence of a single layer of closely packed osteoblasts *(arrowheads)*. The entire ossification center is richly endowed with blood vessels (BV). (×135).

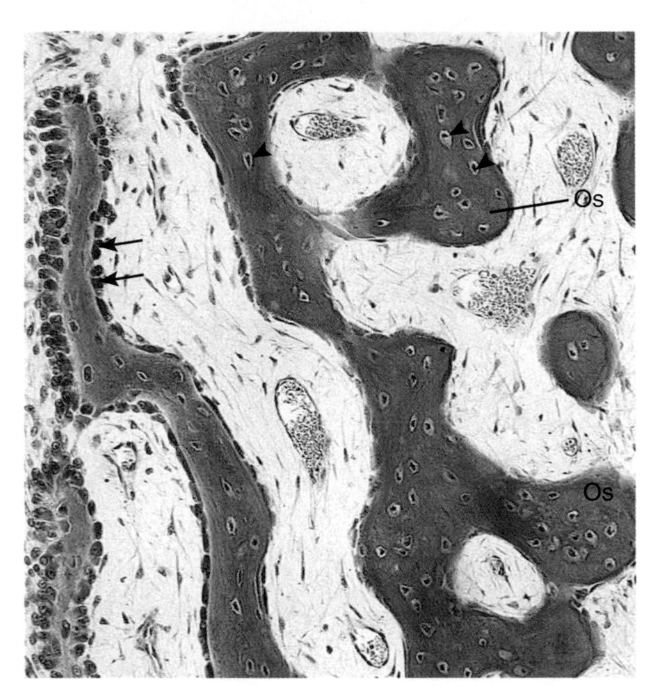

Fig. 7.20 Light micrograph of intramembranous ossification (×270). Trabeculae of bone are being formed by osteoblasts lining their surface *(arrows)*. Observe osteocytes trapped in lacunae *(arrowheads)*. Primitive osteons (Os) are beginning to form.

6. More osteoprogenitor cells differentiate into osteoblasts, which elaborate bone matrix on the surface of the calcified cartilage. The bone matrix becomes calcified to form a **calcified cartilage–calcified bone complex** (calcified bone is acidophilic, whereas calcified cartilage is basophilic). This complex can be appreciated in routinely stained histological sections because calcified cartilage stains blue, whereas calcified bone stains pink with hematoxylin and eosin (see Figs. 7.23-7.25)
7. As the subperiosteal bone collar increases in thickness and grows in each direction from the midriff of the diaphysis toward the two epiphyses, osteoclasts continue resorbing the calcified cartilage–calcified bone complex, enlarging the marrow cavity. Eventually, all of the cartilage of the diaphysis is replaced by bone, except for the **epiphyseal plates**, which are responsible for the continued lengthening of the bone for the next 18 to 20 years.

Events Occurring at Secondary Centers of Ossification. **Secondary centers of ossification** begin to form at the epiphysis at each end of the forming bone by a process similar to that in the diaphysis, except that a bone collar is not formed. Rather, osteoprogenitor cells invade the cartilage of the epiphysis, differentiate into osteoblasts, and begin secreting matrix on the cartilage scaffold (see Fig. 7.21). These events take place and progress much as they do in the diaphysis. Eventually, the cartilage of the epiphysis is replaced with bone, except at the articular surface

TABLE 7.4 Events in Endochondral Bone Formation

Event	Description
Hyaline cartilage model formed	Miniature hyaline cartilage model formed in region of developing embryo where bone is to develop. Some chondrocytes mature, hypertrophy, and die. Cartilage matrix becomes calcified.
PRIMARY CENTER OF OSSIFICATION	
Perichondrium at the midriff of diaphysis becomes vascularized.	Vascularization of perichondrium changes it to periosteum. Chondrogenic cells become osteoprogenitor cells.
Osteoblasts secrete matrix, forming subperiosteal bone collar.	The subperiosteal bone collar is formed of primary bone (intramembranous bone formation).
Chondrocytes within the diaphysis core hypertrophy, die, and degenerate.	Presence of periosteum and bone prevents diffusion of nutrients to chondrocytes. Their degeneration leaves lacunae, opening large spaces in cartilage.
Osteoclasts etch holes in subperiosteal bone collar, permitting entrance of osteogenic bud.	Holes permit osteoprogenitor cells and capillaries to invade cartilage model, now calcified, and begin elaborating bone matrix.
Formation of calcified cartilage–calcified bone complex	Bone matrix laid down on septa of calcified cartilage forms this complex. Histologically, calcified cartilage stains blue and calcified bone stains red.
Osteoclasts begin resorbing the calcified cartilage–calcified bone complex.	Destruction of the calcified cartilage–calcified bone complex enlarges the marrow cavity.
Subperiosteal bone collar thickens, begins growing toward epiphyses.	This event, over a period of time, completely replaces diaphyseal cartilage with bone.
SECONDARY CENTER OF OSSIFICATION	
Ossification begins at epiphysis.	Begins in same way as primary center except that there is no bone collar. Osteoblasts lay down bone matrix on calcified cartilage scaffold.
Growth of bone at epiphyseal plate.	Cartilaginous articular surface of bone remains. Epiphyseal plate persists—growth added at epiphyseal end of plate. Bone added at diaphyseal end of plate.
Epiphysis and diaphysis become continuous.	At end of bone growth, cartilage of epiphyseal plate ceases proliferation. Bone development continues to unite the diaphysis and epiphysis.

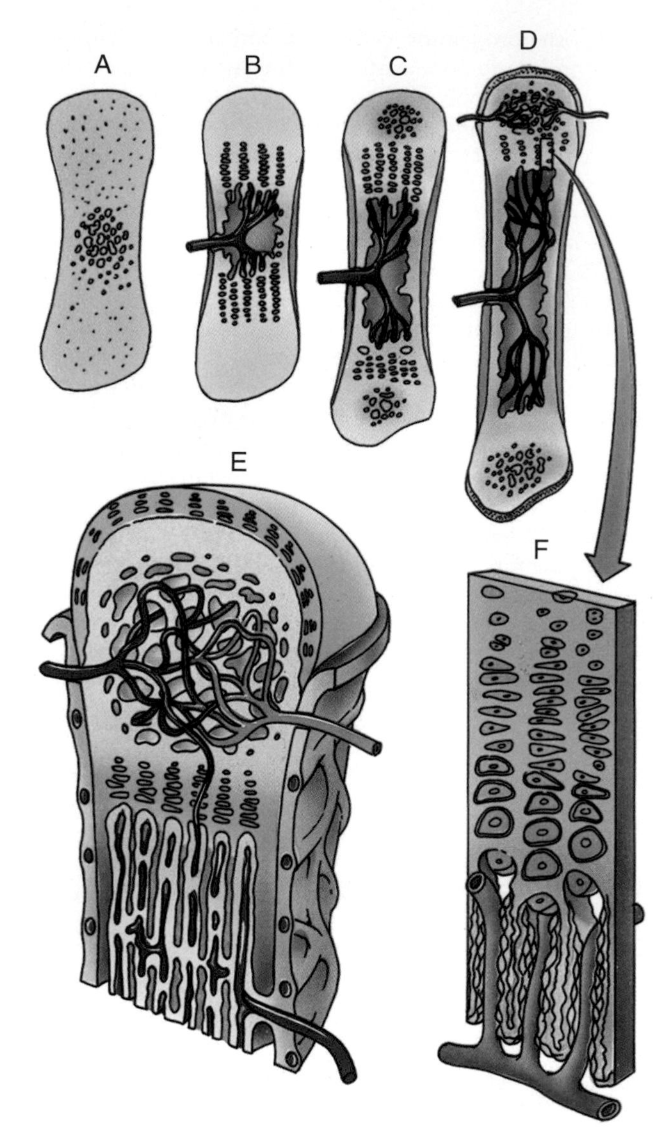

Fig. 7.21 Diagram of endochondral bone formation. *Blue* represents the cartilage model upon which bone is formed, replacing the cartilage.

and at the epiphyseal plate. The articular surface of the bone remains cartilaginous throughout life. The process at the epiphyseal plate, which controls bone length, is described in the next section.

These events form a dynamic continuum that is completed over a number of years as bone growth and development progress toward the growing epiphyses at each end of the bone (see Table 7.4). At the same time, the bone is constantly being remodeled to meet the changing forces placed on it.

Bone Growth in Length.

The continued lengthening of bone depends on the epiphyseal plate.

The chondrocytes of the epiphyseal plate proliferate and participate in the process of endochondral bone formation. Proliferation occurs at the epiphyseal aspect, and replacement by bone takes place at the diaphyseal side of the plate. Histologically, the epiphyseal plate is divided into five recognizable zones. These zones, beginning at the epiphyseal side, are as follows:

- **Zone of reserve cartilage.** Chondrocytes randomly distributed throughout the matrix are mitotically active (interstitial cartilage growth).
- **Zone of proliferation.** Chondrocytes, rapidly proliferating, form rows of isogenous cells that parallel the direction of bone growth. This proliferation rate is under the control of a signaling molecule, a paracrine hormone known as ***Indian hedgehog***, manufactured and released by the chondrocytes of this zone to act on all of the chondrocytes in their immediate vicinity. This factor not only induces proliferation of the chondrocytes but also delays chondrocytic hypertrophy, thus maintaining the requisite thickness of the epiphyseal plate. The chondrocytes of this zone are also sensitive to **IGF-1** and, to a very limited extent, to IGF-2. IGF-1 is a hormone manufactured by hepatocytes in response to **growth hormone** secreted by the pituitary gland. Chondrocytes of this zone proliferate in response to being exposed to IGF-1. Although osteocytes also manufacture and release IFG-1, in the case of the epiphyseal plate, it is the hepatocyte-produced IGF-1 that acts on the chondrocytes.
- **Zone of maturation and hypertrophy.** Chondrocytes mature, hypertrophy, and accumulate glycogen in their cytoplasm (see Fig. 7.21). The interterritorial matrix between their lacunae narrows, with a corresponding enlargement of the chondrocytes within the lacunae. The chondrocytes of this zone eventually undergo apoptosis and die. However, while enlarging, they secrete **vascular endothelial growth factor**, a cytokine that encourages the invasion of blood vessels, which bring calcium ions and specialized macrophage precursors into the area.
- **Zone of calcification.** Lacunae become confluent, hypertrophied chondrocytes die, and cartilage matrix becomes calcified using the calcium ions brought in by the blood vessels.
- **Zone of ossification.** Osteoprogenitor cells invade the area and differentiate into osteoblasts, which elaborate matrix on the surface of calcified cartilage. This is followed by calcification of the bone matrix and the resorption of the calcified cartilage–calcified bone complex by the specialized macrophages recruited by the hypertrophied chondrocytes.

As long as the rate of mitotic activity in the zone of proliferation equals the rate of resorption in the zone of ossification, the epiphyseal plate remains the same thickness and the bone continues to grow longer. At about 20 years old, the rate of mitosis decreases in the zone of proliferation, and the zone of ossification overtakes the zones of proliferation and the zone of reserve cartilage. The cartilage of the epiphyseal plate is replaced by a plate of calcified cartilage–calcified bone complex, which becomes resorbed by osteoclastic activity, and the marrow cavity of the diaphysis becomes confluent with the bone marrow cavity of the epiphysis. After the epiphyseal plate is resorbed, growth in length is no longer possible.

Bone Growth in Width. Growth of the diaphysis in girth occurs via **appositional growth**. **Osteoprogenitor cells** of the periosteum proliferate and differentiate into osteoblasts that begin elaborating bone matrix on the subperiosteal bone surface. This process occurs continuously throughout the total period of bone growth and development so that, in a mature vlong bone, the diaphysis becomes wider via subperiosteal intramembranous bone formation.

During bone growth and development, bone resorption is as important as bone deposition. Formation of bone on the outside of the shaft must be accompanied by osteoclastic activity internally so that the marrow space can be enlarged (Fig. 7.24).

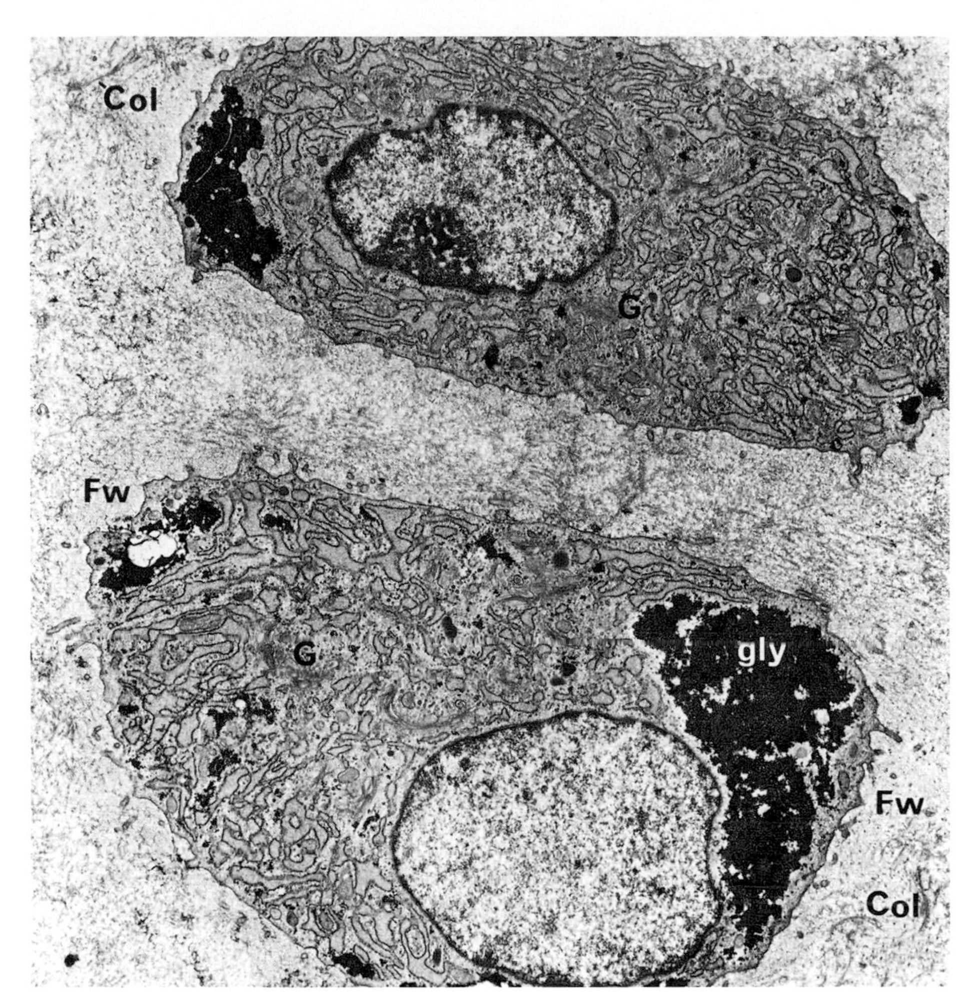

Fig. 7.22 Electron micrograph of hypertrophic chondrocytes in the growing mandibular condyle (×83,000). Observe the abundant rough endoplasmic reticulum and developing Golgi apparatus (G). Note also glycogen (gly) deposits in one end of the cells, a characteristic of these cells shortly before death. Col, Collagen fibers; Fw, territorial matrix. (From Marchi F, Luder HU, Leblond CP. Changes in cells' secretory organelles and extracellular matrix during endochondral ossification in the mandibular condyle of the growing rat. *Am J Anat*. 1991;190:41-73. Reprinted by permission of Wiley-Liss, Inc., a subsidiary of John Wiley & Sons, Inc.)

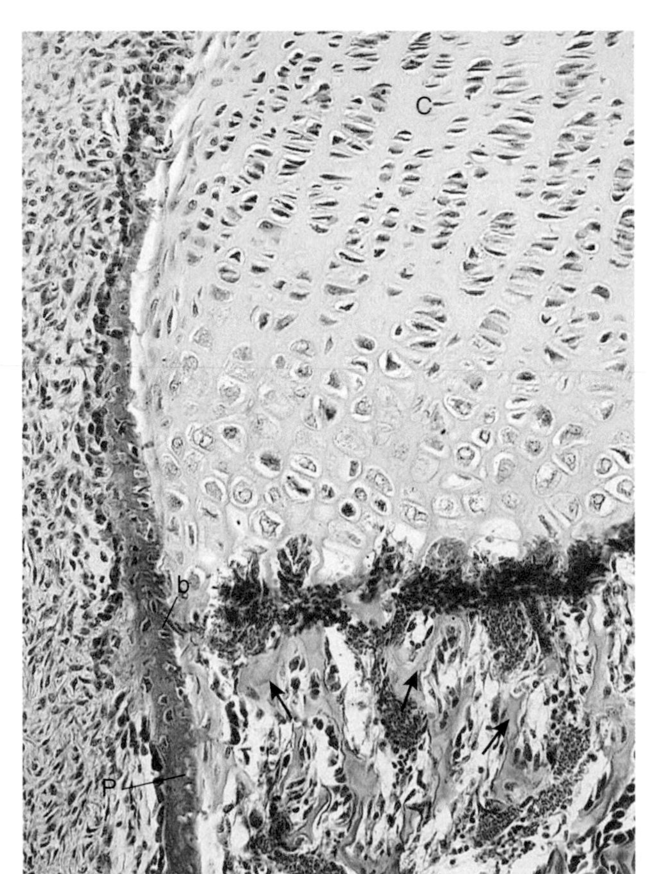

Fig. 7.23 Light micrograph of endochondral bone formation (×14). The *upper half* of the photograph demonstrates cartilage (C) containing chondrocytes that mature, hypertrophy, and calcify at the interface; the *lower half* shows where calcified cartilage–bone complex *(arrows)* is being resorbed and bone (b) is being formed. P, Subperiosteal bone collar.

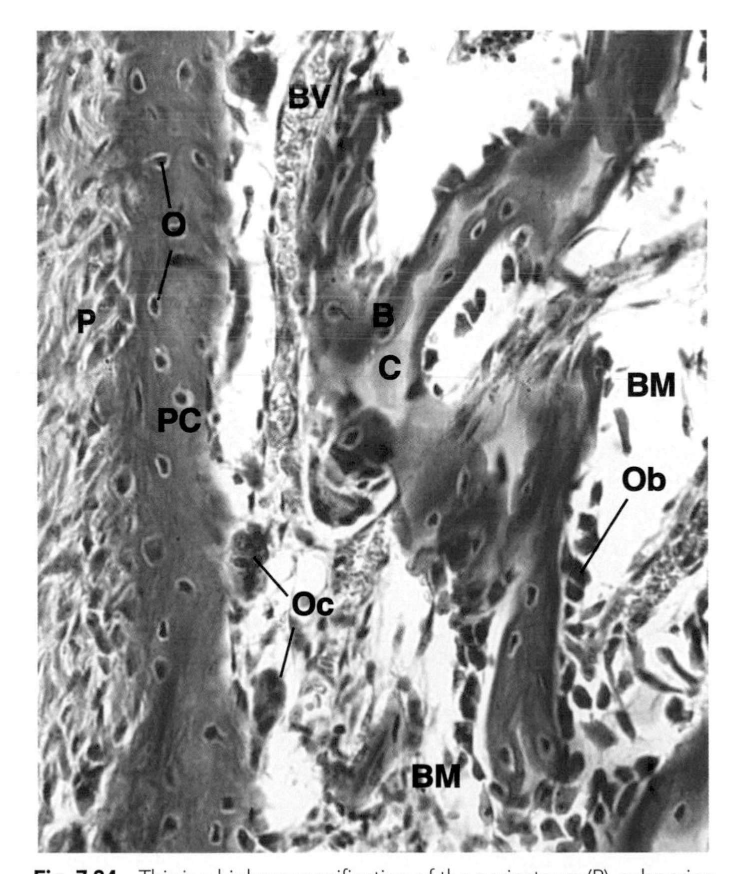

Fig. 7.24 This is a higher magnification of the periosteum (P), subperiosteal bone collar (PC), and the trabecular region of a slide similar to Fig. 7.23. Observe the osteocytes (O) within their lacunae as well as the osteoblasts (Ob) and osteoclasts (Oc) as they are making the diaphysis wider and at the same time enlarging the marrow cavity. The developing bone marrow (BM) surrounds the calcified bone (B)–calcified cartilage (C) complex. (×270)

Calcification of Bone.

Calcification begins when there are deposits of calcium phosphate on the collagen fibril.

Calcification of bone is stimulated by certain proteoglycans and the Ca^2-binding glycoprotein **osteonectin**, as well as **bone sialoprotein**. One possibility, called ***heterogeneous nucleation***, states that once metastable calcium and phosphate are deposited into the gap region of the collagen, calcification proceeds.

The most commonly accepted theory of calcification is based on the presence of membrane-bound **matrix vesicles** released by osteoblasts into the osteoid. These small vesicles, 100 to 200 nm in diameter, contain a high concentration of Ca^{2+} and PO_4^{3-} ions, cAMP, adenosine triphosphate (ATP), adenosine triphosphatase (ATPase), alkaline phosphatase, pyrophosphatase, calcium-binding proteins, and phosphoserine. Additionally, the matrix vesicle membrane possesses numerous calcium pumps, which transport Ca^{2+} ions from the bone matrix into the vesicle. The increasing Ca^{2+} ion concentration within the vesicle results in the formation and growth of calcium hydroxyapatite crystals that pierce the matrix vesicle membrane, bursting it and releasing its contents. Simultaneously, **alkaline phosphatase** cleaves **pyrophosphate groups** from the macromolecules of the matrix. The liberated pyrophosphate molecules are inhibitors of calcification, but they are cleaved by the enzyme pyrophosphatase into individual PO_4^{3-} ions, increasing the concentration of this ion in the microenvironment.

The calcium hydroxyapatite crystals released from the matrix vesicles act as **nidi of crystallization**. The high concentration of ions in their vicinity, along with the presence of calcification factors and calcium-binding proteins, fosters calcification of the bone matrix; concurrently, water is resorbed from the matrix. As mineralization spreads along the various closely spaced nidi of crystallization, these nidi fuse and increasingly larger regions of bone matrix are dehydrated and calcified.

Bone Remodeling

In adults, bone development is balanced with bone resorption as bone is remodeled to meet stresses placed on it.

In a young person who has not finished growing, bone development exceeds the rate of bone resorption because more haversian systems are being added than resorbed. In normal physiological conditions after the requisite bone growth has been attained, the rate of bone formation equals the rate of bone resorption.

Growing bones largely retain their general architectural shape from the beginning of bone development in a fetus to the end of bone growth in an adult. This is accomplished by **surface remodeling**, a process involving bone deposition under certain regions of the periosteum, with concomitant bone resorption under other regions of the periosteum. Similarly, bone is being deposited in certain regions of the endosteal surface while being resorbed in other regions. The bones of the calvaria are being reshaped in a similar way to accommodate the growing brain; how this process is regulated is unclear.

Because bone-forming/resorbing cells of cancellous bone are located within the bone marrow cavity, they respond to **local factors** such as IL-6, tumor necrosis factor-α (TNF-α), M-CSF, OPG, RANKL, and transforming growth factor- β (TGF-β) that are released by nearby bone marrow cells. Most of the bone-forming/resorbing cells of compact bone are located in the cellular layer of the periosteum and in the lining of haversian canals. Thus, they are too far from the bone marrow cells to be under their direct influence. Therefore, unlike bone-forming/resorbing cells of cancellous bone, those cells of compact bone respond to **systemic factors**, such as calcitonin and parathyroid hormone.

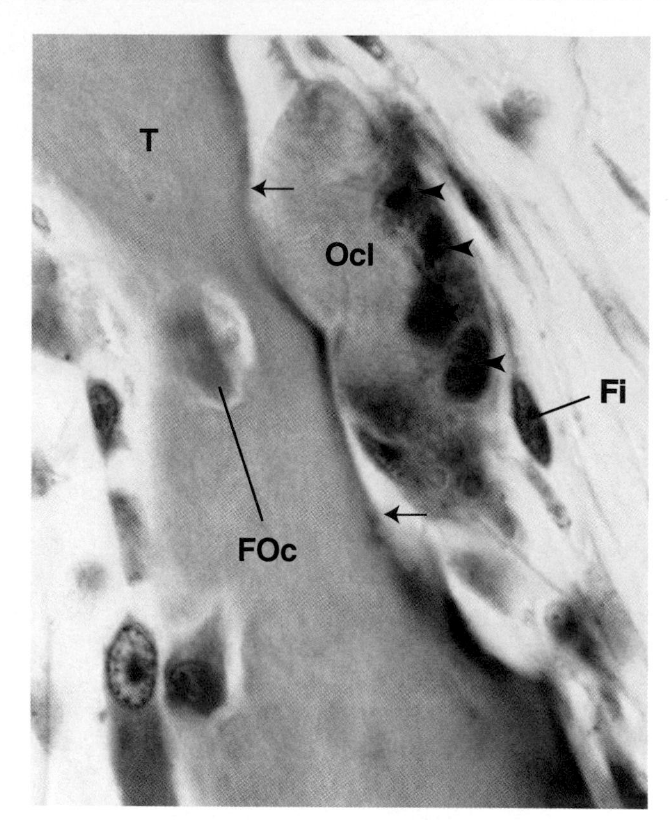

Fig. 7.25 This is a high magnification of an osteoclast (Ocl) in endochondral bone formation as it is remodeling a forming trabecula (T). The *arrows* point to a Howship lacuna being formed by the osteoclast, whose nuclei are indicated by *arrowheads*. Observe that an osteoblast is being trapped in its matrix and is now a future osteocyte (FOc). A mesenchymal cell (Fi) is evident in the forming bone marrow. (×540)

The internal structure of adult bone is continually being altered because bone must be resorbed from one area and added to another to meet changing stresses that are placed on it, such as weight changes, postural alterations, or microfractures of bone involving individual osteons. This process is known as ***internal remodeling*** and is performed by the **bone remodeling unit** (Fig. 7.26) whose two elements are the **cutting cone** (**resorption cavity**) and the **closing cone** (**lamellar formation**).

In regions where compact bone is to be remodeled, osteoclasts are recruited to the area to resorb the bone, forming cone-shaped tunnels in compact bone, known as ***cutting cones*** (**resorption cavities**). Continual osteoclastic activity increases the diameter and length of these cutting cones, which may reach as much as 1.5 mm in length and 100 μm in radius. After these tunnels reach their maximum size, they are invaded by blood vessels, osteoblasts, and osteoprogenitor cells. At this point, bone resorption ceases and osteoblasts deposit new concentric lamellae around the blood vessels, forming new haversian systems (**closing cone**). Not only is primary bone remodeled in this fashion, which strengthens the bone by establishing ordered collagen alignment about the haversian system, but also remodeling continues throughout life as resorption is replaced by deposition and the formation of new haversian systems. This process of bone resorption, followed by bone replacement, is known as a ***coupled system of activation***, ***resorption***, and ***formation*** (**coupling**). The interstitial lamellae that are observed in adult bone are remnants of remodeled haversian systems.

Bone Repair

Bone repair involves both intramembranous and endochondral bone formation.

A bone fracture causes damage and destruction to the bone matrix, death to cells, tears in the periosteum and endosteum, and possible displacement of the ends of the broken bone (fragments). Blood vessels are severed near the break and localized hemorrhaging fills in the zone of the break, resulting in blood clot formation at the site of injury. Soon, the blood supply is shut down in a retrograde fashion from the injury site back to regions of anastomosing vessels, which can establish a new circulation route. As a consequence of the cessation of circulation, there is a widening zone of injury on either side of the original break owing to the lack of blood supply to many haversian systems, thus causing the zone of dead and dying osteocytes to increase appreciably. Because bone marrow and the periosteum are highly vascularized, the initial injury site in either of these two areas does not grow significantly, and there is no notable increase in dead and dying cells much beyond the original injury site. Wherever the bone's haversian systems are without a blood supply, osteocytes become pyknotic, undergo lysis, and leave empty lacunae behind.

The blood clot filling the site of the fracture is invaded by small capillaries and fibroblasts from the surrounding connective tissue, forming **granulation tissue**. Approximately 48 hours after injury, osteoprogenitor cells build up because of increased mitotic activity of the osteogenic layer of the periosteum. The deepest layer of proliferating osteoprogenitor cells of the periosteum (those closest to the bone), which are in the vicinity of capillaries, differentiate into osteoblasts and begin elaborating a collar of bone, cementing it to the dead bone about the injury site. Although the capillaries are growing, their rate of proliferation is much slower than that of the osteoprogenitor cells. Thus, the osteoprogenitor cells in the middle of the proliferating mass are now without a profuse capillary bed, resulting in lowered oxygen tension, causing these osteoprogenitor cells to become chondrogenic cells. The chondroblasts that are derived from chondrogenic cells form cartilage in the outer parts of the bony collar.

Osteoprogenitor cells adjacent to the fibrous layer of the periosteum have intact blood vessels in their vicinity; therefore, they continue to proliferate as osteoprogenitor cells. Thus, the collar under the periosteum exhibits three zones that blend together: (1) the deepest stratum consists of a layer of new bone cemented to the bone of the fragment, (2) an intermediate layer of cartilage, and (3) a proliferating osteogenic layer on the surface. In the meantime, the collars formed on the ends of each fragment fuse into a single, combined collar, known as the ***external callus***, leading to an external union of the fragments. Continued growth of the external collar is derived mainly from proliferation of osteoprogenitor cells and, to some degree, from interstitial growth of the cartilage in its intermediate zone.

The cartilage matrix adjacent to the new bone formed in the deepest region of the external collar becomes calcified and is eventually replaced with cancellous bone. Ultimately, all of the cartilage is replaced with primary bone via endochondral bone formation.

A similar event occurs in the marrow cavities as a clot forms; the clot is soon invaded by osteoprogenitor cells of the endosteum and multipotential cells of the bone marrow, forming an ***internal callus*** of bony trabeculae within 1 week or so subsequent to the break (Fig. 7.27).

After the fragments of bone are united by bridging with cancellous bone both on the external and the marrow surfaces, it is necessary to remodel the injury site by replacing the primary bone with secondary bone and resolving the callus.

The first bone elaborated against injured bone develops by intramembranous bone formation, and the new trabeculae become firmly cemented to the injured or dead bone. Matrices of dead bone, located in the empty spaces between newly developing bony trabeculae, are resorbed and the spaces are filled in by new bone. Eventually, all of the dead bone is resorbed and replaced. These events are concurrent, resulting in repair of the fracture with cancellous bone surrounded by a bony callus.

Through the events of remodeling, the primary bone of intramembranous bone formation is replaced with secondary bone, further reinforcing the mended fracture zone. At the same time, the callus is resorbed. It appears that the healing and remodeling processes at the fracture site are in direct response to the stresses placed on it; eventually, the repaired zone is restored to its original shape and strength.

Clinical Correlations

1. *If segments of bone are lost or damaged so severely that they have to be removed, a "**bony union**" is not possible; that is, the process of bone repair cannot occur because a bony callus does not form. In cases of this sort, a bone graft is required. Since the 1970s, bone banks have become available to supply viable bone for grafting purposes. The bone fragments are harvested and frozen to preserve their osteogenic potential and are then used as transplants by orthopedic surgeons. **Autografts** are the most successful because the transplant recipient is also the donor. **Homografts** are from different individuals of the same species and may be rejected because of an immunological response. **Heterografts**, grafts from different species, are least successful, although it has been shown that calf bone loses some of its antigenicity after being refrigerated, making it a worthy bone graft when necessary.*
2. *Skeletal maturation is also influenced by hormones produced in the male and female gonads. Closure of the epiphyseal plates is normally rather stable and constant and is related to sexual maturation. For example, precocious sexual maturation stunts skeletal development because the epiphyseal plates are stimulated to close too early. In other people whose sexual maturation is retarded, skeletal growth continues beyond normal because the epiphyseal plates do not close.*
3. ***Acromegaly** occurs in adults who produce an excess of somatotropin, causing an abnormal increase in bone deposition without normal bone resorption. This condition creates thickening of the bones, especially those of the face, in addition to disfiguring soft tissue.*

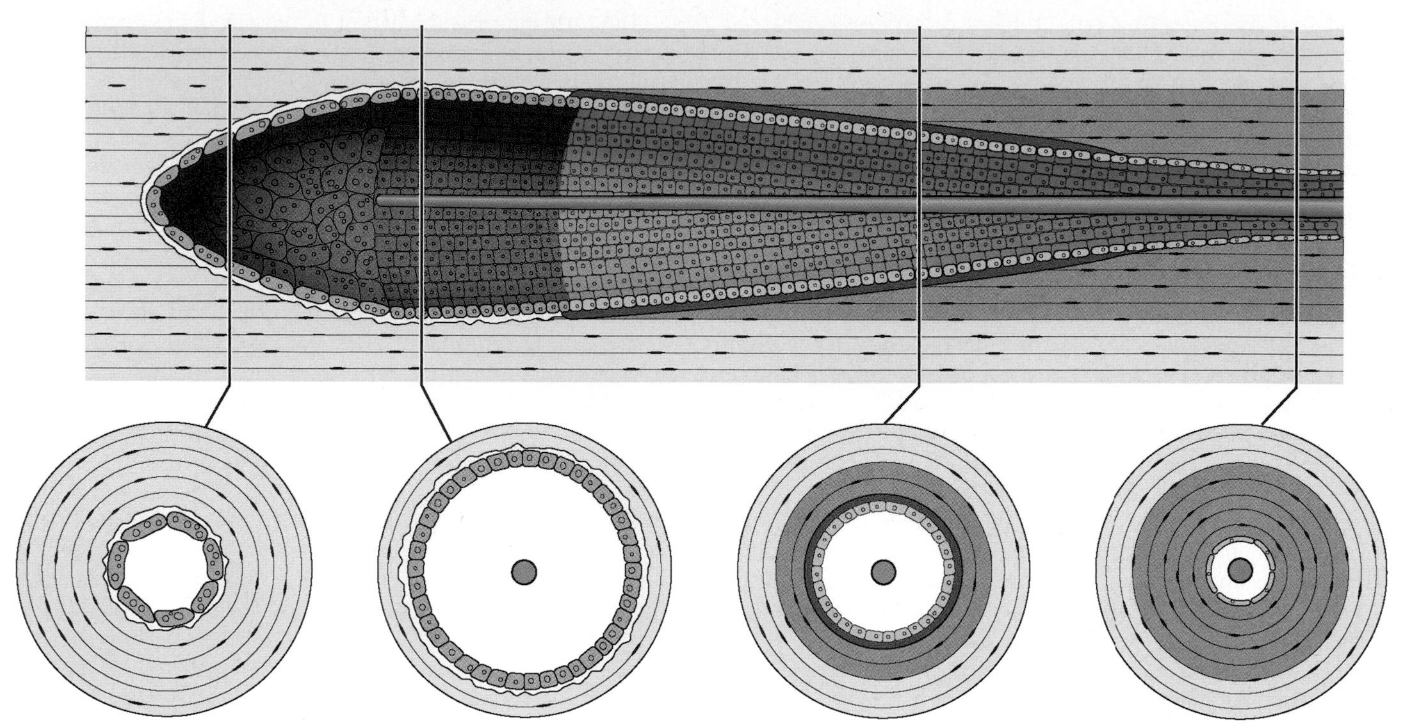

Fig. 7.26 An artist's diagram of the process known as internal remodeling. Observe that in the purple region of the haversian canal system *(far left)* osteoclasts are resorbing bone, forming a cutting cone (resorption cavity). Once all of the lamellae that are to be resorbed are gone (red zone), osteoblasts begin to elaborate new lamellae (green zone), remodeling the original haversian system. Note that the cutting cone progresses to the left and the closing cone is catching up with it. When the cutting zones reach their maximum size, they become invaded by blood vessels (blue dot in the center), osteoblasts, and osteoprogenitor cells. At this point, bone resorption ceases, and osteoblasts deposit new concentric lamellae around the blood vessels, forming new haversian systems.

Recapitulation of the Principal Hormones and Factors Affecting Bone

The following systemic hormones affect bone:

- PTH is released from the chief cells of the parathyroid gland when calcium blood levels fall below approximately 8.8 mg/dL (in adults). It acts in an indirect fashion by binding to PTH receptors on osteoblasts; those cells respond by releasing factors noted previously to recruit and activate osteoclasts to resorb bone, thereby increasing blood calcium levels.
- Calcitonin, released by C cells (parafollicular cells) of the thyroid gland, has an opposite effect. When calcium blood levels are above approximately 10.5 mg/dL (in adults), calcitonin is released and binds directly to calcitonin receptors on osteoclasts and causes them to undergo apoptosis, thereby decreasing blood calcium levels.

The following local factors and cytokines affect bone:

- BMP-6 (also, to a limited extent, BMP-2 and BMP-4) and TGF-β induce osteoprogenitor cells to differentiate into osteoblasts.
- Osteoblasts synthesize RANKL, M-CSF, alkaline phosphatase, IGF-1, and PTH receptors, all of which they place on their cell membranes.
- Osteoblasts synthesize and release: osteocalcin, a signaling molecule responsible for mineralization of bone; osteonectin, a glycoprotein that assists in the binding of calcium hydroxyl apatite crystals to collagen; osteopontin, which assists in the formation of the sealing zone of osteoclasts; bone sialoprotein, which assists osteoblasts to adhere to the bone matrix; and OPG, a glycoprotein that can bind to RANKL and, thus, interfere with osteoclast formation.
- Osteoblasts are transformed into osteocytes under the influence of two transcription factors, Cbfa1/Runx2 and osterix, both of which appear to be dependent on BMP-2 to be expressed. This is especially evident during intramembranous bone formation.
- Osteocytes release cAMP, osteocalcin, and IGF-1 in response to tension placed on bone to facilitate the recruitment of osteoprogenitor cells.
- In response to low calcium levels in the extracellular fluid in their lacunae, osteocytes secrete sclerostin, a paracrine hormone that inhibits bone formation and encourages bone resorption, thereby elevating blood calcium levels.
- Osteoblasts secrete four signaling molecules: (1) M-CSF, which binds to a receptor on the osteoclast precursor, inducing it to proliferate and to express RANK on the osteoclast precursor cell membrane; when the signaling molecule RANKL on the osteoblast cell membrane binds to the RANK receptor on the osteoclast precursor cell membrane, the osteoclast precursor is induced to differentiate into the multinucleated osteoclast, activating it and enhancing bone resorption. (2) IL-6 facilitates the recruitment and differentiation of osteoclasts. (3) IL-1 activates osteoclast precursors to proliferate; it also has an indirect role in osteoclast stimulation. (4) Signaling molecule, OPG, a member of the TNFR family, can serve as a decoy by interacting with RANKL, prohibiting it from binding to the macrophage and thereby inhibiting osteoclast formation.

TABLE 7.5 Vitamins and Their Effects on Skeletal Development

Vitamin	Effects on Skeletal Development
Vitamin A deficiency	Inhibits proper bone formation as coordination of osteoblast and osteoclast activities fails. Failure of resorption and remodeling of cranial vault to accommodate the brain, with serious damage to the central nervous system.
Hypervitaminosis A	Erosion of cartilage columns without increases of cells in proliferation zone. Epiphyseal plates may become obliterated, ceasing growth prematurely.
Vitamin C deficiency	Mesenchymal tissue affected as connective tissue is unable to produce and maintain extracellular matrix. Deficient production of collagen and bone matrix results in retarded growth and delayed healing. Scurvy.
Vitamin D deficiency	Ossification of epiphyseal cartilages disturbed. Cells become disordered at metaphysis, leading to poorly calcified bones, which become deformed by weight bearing. In children—rickets. In adults—osteomalacia.

- Osteoclasts have receptors for osteoclast-stimulating factor, colony-stimulating factor, OPG, RANK, and calcitonin, among others.
- TNF-α, released by activated macrophages, acts in a fashion similar to IL-1.
- Interferon-γ, released by T lymphocytes, inhibits differentiation of osteoclast precursors into osteoclasts.
- TGF-β, liberated from bone matrix during bone resorption by osteoclasts, induces osteoblasts to manufacture bone matrix and enhances the process of matrix mineralization. Also, it inhibits proliferation of osteoclast precursors and their differentiation into mature osteoclasts.

The following factors and cytokines affect the epiphyseal plate:

- Chondrocytes of the zone of proliferation of the epiphyseal plate release a paracrine hormone known as **Indian hedgehog** to act on all of the chondrocytes in the immediate vicinity, inducing not only the proliferation of the chondrocytes but also delaying chondrocytic hypertrophy. This maintains the requisite breadth of the epiphyseal plate.
- The chondrocytes of the zone of proliferation are also sensitive to **IGF-1** and, to a very limited extent, to IGF-2. IGF-1 is a hormone manufactured by hepatocytes in response to **growth hormone** secreted by the pituitary gland, and chondrocytes of this zone proliferate in response to being exposed to IGF-1. Although osteocytes also manufacture and release IFG-1, in the case of the epiphyseal plate, it is the hepatocyte-produced IFG-1 that acts on the chondrocytes.
- The chondrocytes of the zone of maturation and hypertrophy eventually undergo apoptosis and die. Before they die, they secrete vascular endothelial growth factor, a signaling molecule that encourages the invasion of blood vessels, which bring calcium ions and specialized macrophage precursors into the area.

NUTRITIONAL EFFECTS

Normal bone growth is dependent on several nutritional factors. Unless a person's intake of protein, minerals, and vitamins is sufficient, the amino acids essential for collagen synthesis by osteoblasts are lacking, and collagen formation is reduced. Insufficient intake of calcium or phosphorus leads to poorly calcified bone, which is subject to fracture. A deficiency of vitamin D prevents calcium absorption from the intestines, causing **osteomalacia** in adults and **rickets** in children. Vitamins A and C are also necessary for proper skeletal development (Table 7.5). The consequence of excess or insufficient vitamin A availability results in a decreased height of the affected individual. Vitamin C is required for collagen production; therefore, a deficiency of vitamin C results in the condition known as *scurvy*.

Clinical Correlations

Rickets *is a disease in children who are deficient in vitamin D. Without vitamin D, the intestinal mucosa cannot absorb calcium even though there may be adequate dietary intake. This results in disturbances in ossification of the epiphyseal cartilages and disorientation of the cells at the metaphysis, giving rise to poorly calcified bone matrix. Children with rickets display deformed bones, particularly in the legs, simply because the bones cannot bear their weight.*

Osteomalacia*, or adult rickets, results from prolonged deficiency of vitamin D. When this occurs, the newly formed bone in the process of remodeling does not calcify properly. This condition may become severe during pregnancy because the fetus requires calcium, which must be supplied by the mother.*

Scurvy *is a condition resulting from a deficiency of vitamin C. One effect is deficient collagen production, causing a reduction in formation of bone matrix and bone development. Healing is also delayed.*

Joints

Bones articulate or come into close proximity with one another at joints, which are classified according to the degree of movement available between the bones of the joint. Those that are closely bound together with only a minimum of movement between them are called ***synarthroses***; joints in which the bones are free to articulate over a fairly wide range of motion are classified as ***diarthroses***.

There are three types of **synarthrosis joints** according to the tissue making up the union:

1. **Synostosis.** There is little if any movement, and joint-uniting tissue is bone (e.g., skull bones in adults).
2. **Synchondrosis.** There is little movement, and joint-uniting tissue is hyaline cartilage (e.g., joint of the first rib and sternum).

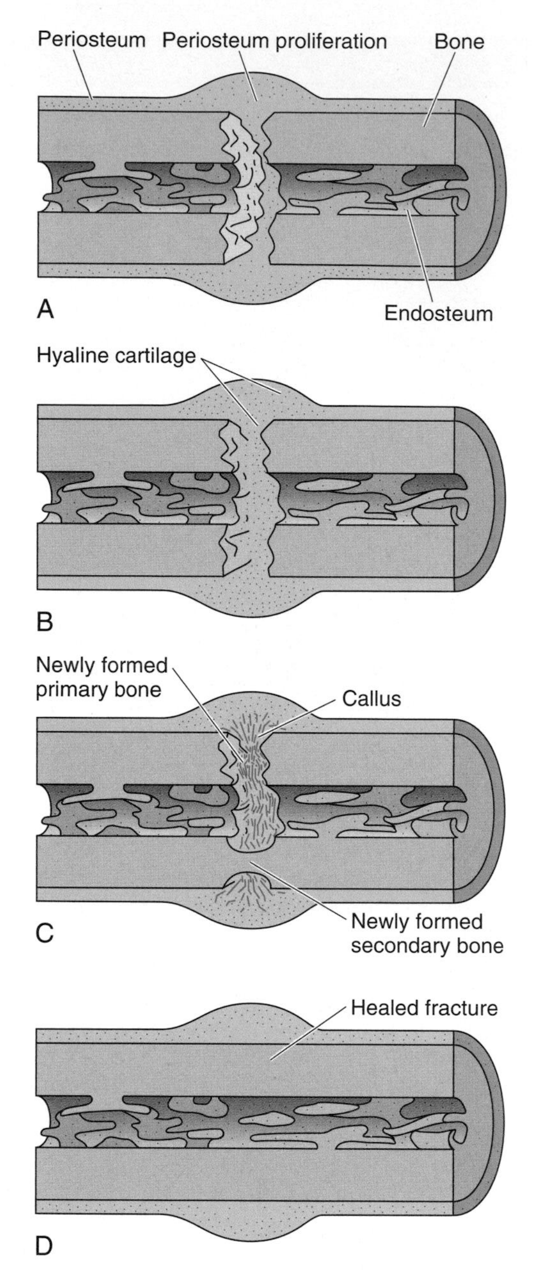

Fig. 7.27 Diagram of the events in bone fracture repair. (A) Osteoprogenitor cells of the inner (cellular) layer of the periosteum proliferate. (B) Because the osteoprogenitor cells do not have adequate blood supply, they differentiate into chondrogenic cells and form a callus composed mostly of hyaline cartilage. (C) As the blood supply is reestablished, the cartilaginous callus is transformed into an osseous callus via chondrogenic bone formation. (D) As the osseous callus is remodeled, the fracture is repaired. Refer to the text for complete information about bone repair.

3. **Syndesmosis.** There is little movement, and bones are joined by dense connective tissue (e.g., pubic symphysis).

Most of the joints of the extremities are diarthroses (Fig. 7.28). The bones making up these joints are covered by persistent hyaline cartilage or articular cartilage. Usually, ligaments maintain the contact between the bones of the joint, which is sealed by the joint capsule. The capsule is composed of an outer fibrous layer of dense connective tissue, which is continuous with the periosteum of the bones, and an inner cellular synovial layer, which covers all nonarticular surfaces. Some prefer to call this a *synovial membrane.*

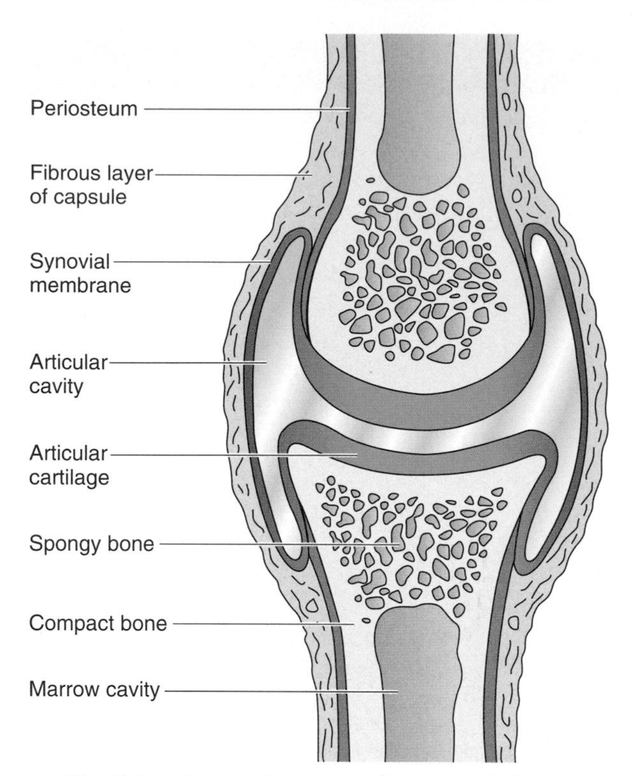

Fig. 7.28 Illustrated anatomy of a diarthrodial joint.

Two kinds of cells are located in the synovial layer: **Type A cells** are macrophages displaying a well-developed Golgi apparatus and many lysosomes but only a small amount of RER. These phagocytic cells are responsible for removing debris from the joint space. **Type B cells** resemble fibroblasts, exhibiting a well-developed RER; these cells are thought to secrete the **synovial fluid**.

Synovial fluid contains a high concentration of **hyaluronic acid** and the glycoprotein **lubricin** combined with filtrate of plasma. In addition to supplying nutrients and oxygen to the chondrocytes of the articular cartilage, this fluid has a high content of hyaluronic acid and lubricin that permits it to function as a lubricant for the joint. Moreover, macrophages in the synovial fluid act to phagocytose debris in the joint space.

Pathological Considerations

See Figs. 7.29 through 7.32.

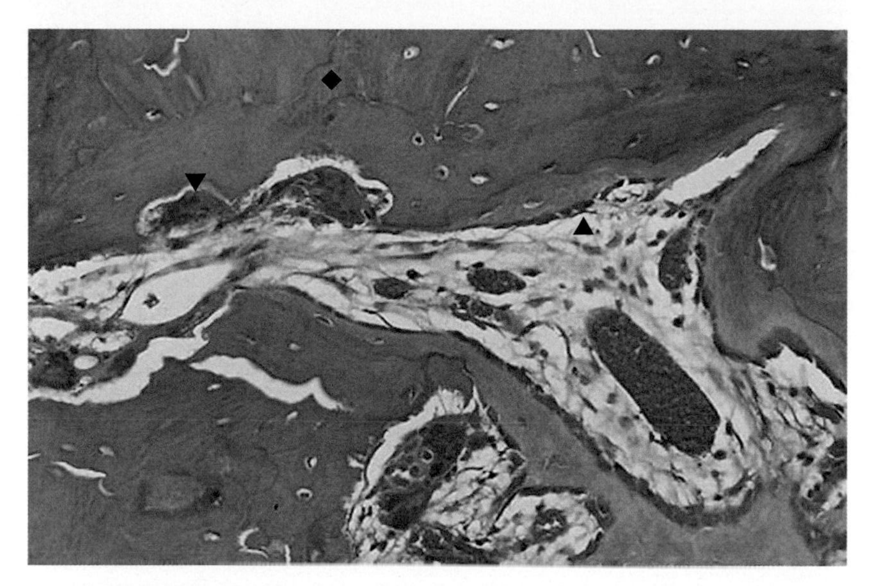

Fig. 7.29 Photomicrograph of Paget disease of bone. Note that there is an active osteoclastic *(down arrowhead)* and osteoblastic *(up arrowhead)* activity, leading to a disorganized microscopic appearance of the lamellar pattern of the bone. Note also the irregularly arranged cement line *(diamond)*. (From Klatt EC. *Robbins and Cotran Atlas of Pathology*. 2nd ed. Philadelphia: Elsevier; 2010:446, with permission.)

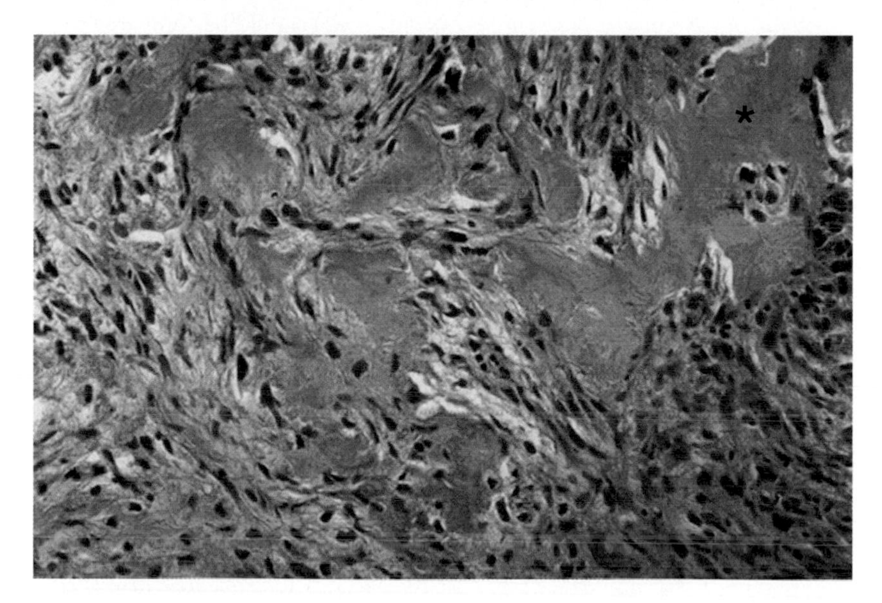

Fig. 7.30 Photomicrograph of osteosarcoma. Note that the neoplastic spindle-shaped cells are manufacturing a pinkish osteoid (*asterisk*), a characteristic feature of osteosarcoma. (From Klatt EC. *Robbins and Cotran Atlas of Pathology*. 2nd ed. Philadelphia: Elsevier; 2010:453, with permission.)

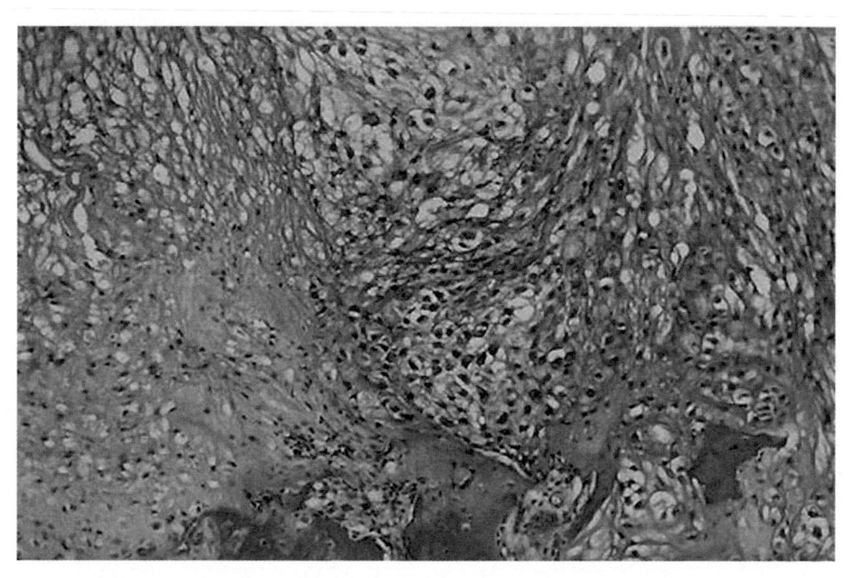

Fig. 7.31 Photomicrograph of chondrosarcoma. Note that the chondrocytes of the cartilage are haphazardly arranged and that the bone at the bottom of the photomicrograph is being invaded and destroyed by the malignant cells. (From Klatt EC. *Robbins and Cotran Atlas of Pathology*. 2nd ed. Philadelphia: Elsevier; 2010:456, with permission.)

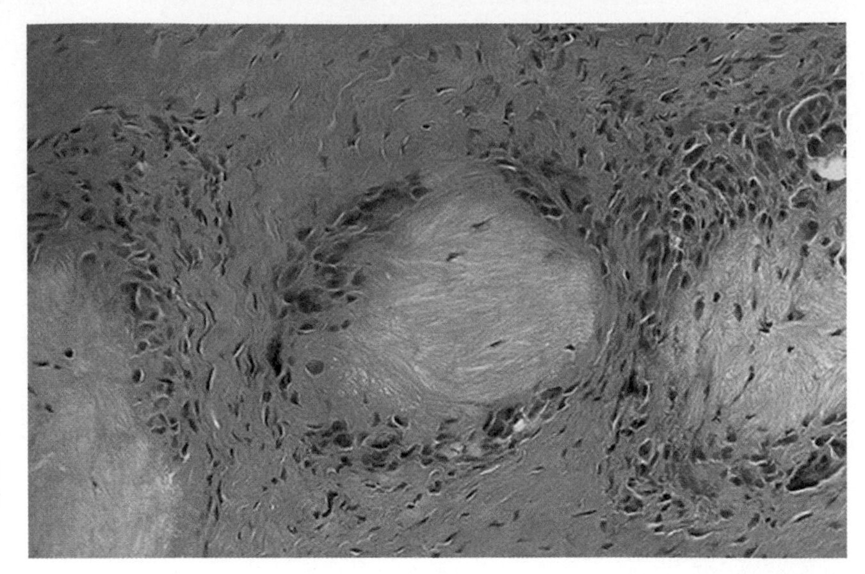

Fig. 7.32 Photomicrograph of gouty arthritis of a joint. Note that the pale areas in the center of the photomicrograph are regions of urate crystal deposition. The urate crystals elicit an inflammatory response, as evidenced by the chronic inflammatory cells surrounding the crystal deposits. (From Klatt EC. *Robbins and Cotran Atlas of Pathology*. 2nd ed. Philadelphia: Elsevier; 2010:464, with permission.)

 Histology Laboratory Instructions: Cartilage and Bone

Cartilage

Hyaline cartilage is best seen in the C-ring of the trachea. At low magnification, the perichondrium the entire width of the cartilage may be observed and the perichondrium may easily be differentiated from the substance of the cartilage with its lacunae, distributed throughout the smooth-appearing matrix, housing chondrocytes (see Fig. 7.2, P, M, *arrow*). At medium magnification, chondrogenic cells and chondroblasts are evident in the cellular layer of the perichondrium and chondrocytes are clearly evident in their lacunae (see Fig. 7.3, Cg, Cb, P, C). At high magnification, chondroblasts of the cellular perichondrium are evident, and it is clear that the matrix has two major components, the darker territorial matrix and the lighter interterritorial matrix. Surrounding each lacuna is the narrow, pericellular capsule. Young hyaline cartilage can grow interstitially, displaying the presence of cell nests (see Fig. 7.4, *arrow*, CP, TM, IM, *red rim*, *boxed area*).

Elastic cartilage is usually labeled as such; it is very similar to hyaline cartilage except for the large amount of elastic fibers in its matrix and in its perichondrium (Fig. 7.5, *arrow*, P). At medium magnification, it is easier to differentiate between the fibrous and cellular layers of the perichondrium. The elastic fibers criss-cross both in the perichondrium and in the matrix. Some of the lacunae appear to be empty because the chondrocyte shrunk during slide preparation (Fig. 7.6, FP, CP, EF, L, *arrows*).

Fibrocartilage is best seen in the intervertebral disc, where its chondrocytes appear to form more or less parallel rows of chondrocytes. Thick parallel bundles of type I collagen fibers separate rows of chondrocytes from each other (see Fig. 7.7, C, *arrows*). Most of the time, fibrocartilage has no perichondrium.

BONE

Decalcified compact bone is evident in the low magnification of a rib, which displays its four lamellar systems. Just deep to the periosteum is the thin outer circumferential lamellae and surrounding the marrow cavity is the inner circumferential lamellar system. Much of the thickness of the rib is formed by the osteons and interstitial lamellar system. Each osteon has a central canal, known as the haversian canal. Volkmann canals connect neighboring haversian canals (see Fig. 7.8, FP, OCL, ICL, *boxed area*, IL, HC, VC; also, see Fig. 7.17). At a high magnification, osteocytes are evident in their lacunae. The cementing line surrounding each osteon is clearly observable and the linings of the haversian canal are well defined as osteoprogenitor cells and osteoblasts. The leader line for the osteon is in the lumen of a blood vessel that occupies much of the haversian canal (see Fig. 7.9, Oc, L, Cl, Op, Os). Osteoblasts and an osteoclast with its numerous nuclei are demonstrated in microscope slides of intramembranous bone formation (see Fig. 7.10, Ob, Oc).

Ground bone (*nondecalcified bone*) should be compared to its decalcified counterpart that was just examined. Cells are not present in ground bone, but its lamellar systems are well defined. At the outer periphery, where the periosteum would be, the outer circumferential lamellae are noted; as before, the substance of the bone is composed of numerous osteons and occasional interstitial lamellae. Haversian and Volkmann canals may also be identified with ease. The lacunae that are occupied by osteocytes in living bone are filled with bone dust in ground bone (see Fig. 7.15, OCL, boxed area, IL, HC, VC, *arrows*). At high magnification, the haversian canal is noted to be surrounded by several concentric lamellae of bone. The bone dust–filled lacunae and the canaliculi are well defined (see Fig. 7.16, C, L, *arrows*).

Intramembranous bone formation is best observed in a slide of a pig embryo's head. Bone formation takes place in highly vascularized mesenchymal connective tissue that condenses to form the future periosteum, and small trabeculae of bone begin to form. As bone is added to these trabeculae, osteon formation becomes evident. Osteoblast and osteocytes in their lacunae are easily noted (see Fig. 7.19, BV, MCT, P, T, *boxed area*, *arrowhead*, *arrows*). At higher magnifications and at a little more developed region, the developing osteons are quite evident and the osteocytes (in their lacunae) and osteoblasts along the trabeculae are clearly seen (see Fig. 7.20, Os, *arrowheads*, *arrows*).

Endochondral bone formation takes place in a cartilage model. As the bone forms around the midriff of the cartilage model, the perichondrium becomes a periosteum and the subperiosteal bone collar, with osteocytes in their lacunae, continues to elongate toward the two epiphyses. Bone is also being deposited on chunks of calcified cartilage within the core of the cartilage template, forming a cartilage-calcified bone complex (Fig. 7.23, P, b, *arrows*). At a higher magnification, the periosteum and the subperiosteal bone collar with osteocytes in their lacunae are noted to be remodeled on their bone marrow aspect by osteoclasts. The vascularity of the future bone marrow is also evident by the rich presence of blood vessels. Calcified bone and calcified cartilage coexist for a period of time, to be resorbed at a later stage. Osteoblasts are continuing to manufacture bone (see Fig. 7.24, P, PC, Oc, BM, BV, B, C, Ob). At high magnification, the osteoclasts, whose numerous nuclei are clearly evident, are seen to be carving out a Howship lacuna on the trabecular surface. Mesenchymal cells are in close vicinity to the trabecula of bone. An osteoblast, almost completely surrounded by the bone matrix it deposited, is on its way to becoming an osteocyte (see Fig. 7.25, Ocl, *arrowheads*, *arrows*, Fi, T, FOc).

8 Muscle

Muscle cells are specialized for contraction that permits movement. Organisms harness the contraction of muscle cells and the arrangement of the extracellular components of muscle to permit locomotion, constriction, pumping, and other propulsive movements.

Muscle cells are called ***striated*** or ***smooth*** muscle depending on the respective presence or absence of a regularly repeated arrangement of myofibrillar contractile proteins, the myofilaments. **Striated** muscle cells display characteristic alternations of light and dark cross-bands, which are absent in smooth muscle. There are two types of striated muscle: **skeletal muscle**, accounting for most of the voluntary muscle mass of the body and approximately 40% of the total body weight, and involuntary **cardiac muscle**, limited almost exclusively to the heart. The bulk of **smooth muscle** is located in the walls of blood vessels, the walls of viscera, and in the dermis of the skin.

Unique terminology is often used to describe the components of muscle cells. Thus, muscle cell membrane is referred to as ***sarcolemma***, the cytoplasm as ***sarcoplasm***, the smooth endoplasmic reticulum (SER) as ***sarcoplasmic reticulum***, and the mitochondria are occasionally known as ***sarcosomes***. Because they are much longer than they are wide, muscle cells frequently are called ***muscle fibers***; however, unlike collagen and elastic fibers, they are living entities.

All three muscle types are derived from mesoderm. Cardiac muscle originates in splanchnopleuric mesoderm, most smooth muscle is derived from splanchnic and somatic mesoderm, and most skeletal muscles originate from somatic mesoderm.

Skeletal Muscle

Skeletal muscle is composed of long, cylindrical, multinucleated cells that undergo voluntary contraction to facilitate movement of the body or its parts.

During embryonic development, several hundred **myoblasts**, precursors of skeletal muscle fibers, line up end to end, fusing to form long multinucleated cells known as ***myotubes***. These newly formed myotubes manufacture cytoplasmic constituents, as well as the contractile elements of muscle, called ***myofibrils***. Myofibrils are composed of specific arrays of **myofilaments**, the proteins responsible for the contractile capability of the cell.

Muscle fibers are arranged parallel to one another, with their intervening intercellular spaces housing parallel arrays of **continuous capillaries**. Each skeletal muscle fiber is long, cylindrical, multinucleated, and striated. The diameters of the fibers vary, ranging from 10 μm to 100 μm, although hypertrophied fibers may exceed the latter amount (Figs. 8.1 and 8.2). The relative strength of a muscle fiber directly depends on its diameter, whereas the strength of the entire muscle is a function of the number and thickness of its component fibers.

When stained with hematoxylin and eosin (H&E), skeletal muscle appears pink to red because of its rich vascular supply as well as the presence of **myoglobin pigments**—oxygen-transporting proteins that resemble, but are smaller than, hemoglobin. Depending on the fiber diameter, quantity of myoglobin, number of mitochondria, extensiveness of the SER, concentration of various enzymes, and rate of contraction, the muscle fiber may be classified as **red**, **white**, or **intermediate** (Table 8.1). Usually, a muscle, such as the biceps, contains all three types of muscle fibers in relatively constant proportions that are characteristic of that particular muscle. In chickens, for instance, thigh muscles are predominantly red, and breast muscles are predominantly white. The innervation of the muscle fiber appears to be the factor that determines fiber type. If the innervation is experimentally switched, the fiber accommodates itself to its altered nerve supply.

CONNECTIVE TISSUE INVESTMENTS

The connective tissue investments of skeletal muscle are the epimysium, perimysium, and endomysium.

The entire muscle is surrounded by **epimysium**—a dense, irregular collagenous connective tissue. **Perimysium**, a less dense collagenous connective tissue derived from epimysium, surrounds bundles (**fascicles**) of muscle fibers. **Endomysium**, composed of reticular fibers and an **external lamina** (basal lamina), surrounds each muscle cell (Fig. 8.3). Because these connective tissue elements are interconnected, contractile forces exerted by individual muscle cells are transferred to them. Tendons and aponeuroses, which connect muscle to bone and to other tissues, are continuous with the connective tissue encasements of muscle and, therefore, act in harnessing the contractile forces for motion.

Light Microscopy

Light microscopy of skeletal muscle fibers displays long, cylindrical, multinucleated cells whose numerous nuclei are peripherally located.

Skeletal muscle fibers are multinucleated cells, with their numerous nuclei peripherally located just beneath the cell membrane (see Figs. 8.1 to 8.3). Each cell is surrounded by endomysium, whose fine reticular fibers intermingle with those of neighboring muscle cells (Figs. 8.4 to 8.6). Small **satellite cells** (**myogenic stem cells**), which have a single nucleus and act as regenerative cells, are located in shallow depressions on the muscle cell's

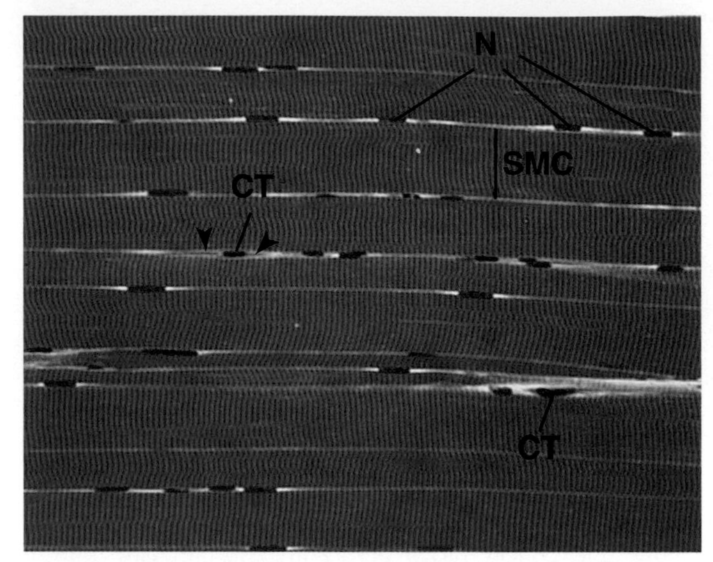

Fig. 8.1 Low-magnification photomicrograph of a longitudinal section of skeletal muscle. Observe that the nuclei (N) are located at the periphery of but within the skeletal muscle cell (SMC), whereas connective tissue cells (CT) are located between skeletal muscle fibers. *Arrowheads* indicate the cytoplasm of a connective tissue cell. (×270)

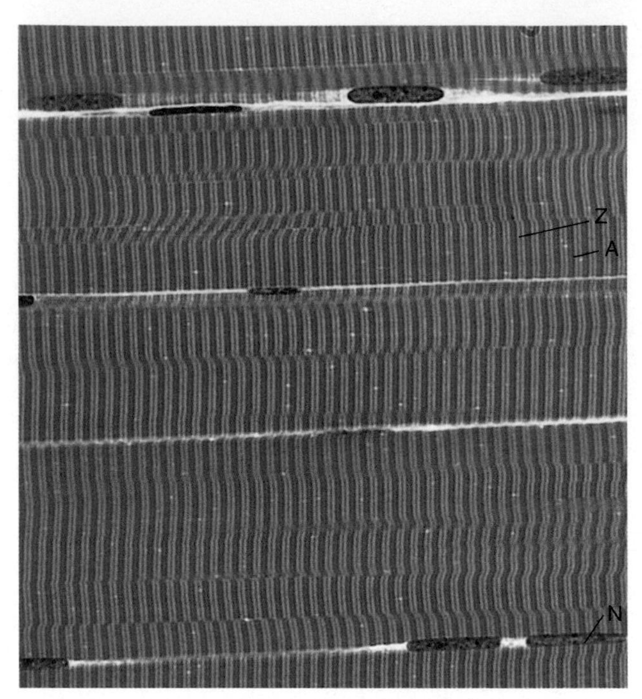

Fig. 8.2 Photomicrograph of a longitudinal section of skeletal muscle. Note the peripherally located nuclei as well as the very fine connective tissue elements between individual muscle fibers. (×540)

surface, sharing the muscle fiber's external lamina. The chromatin network of the satellite cell nucleus is denser and coarser than that of the muscle fiber.

Most of the skeletal muscle cell sarcoplasm is composed of longitudinal arrays of cylindrical **myofibrils**, each 1 to 2 µm in diameter (Fig. 8.7). Therefore, each cell has a number of closely packed myofibrils that extend the entire length of the cell and are aligned precisely with each other. This strictly ordered parallel arrangement of the myofibrils is responsible for the cross-striations of light and dark banding that are characteristic of skeletal muscle viewed in longitudinal section (see Figs. 8.1 and 8.2).

The dark bands are known as ***A bands*** (**A**nisotropic with polarized light), and the light bands are known as ***I bands*** (**I**sotropic with polarized light). The center of each A band is occupied by a pale area, the **H band**, which is bisected by a thin **M line** (**M bridge**). Each I band is bisected by a thin dark line, the **Z disk** (**Z line**). The region of the myofibril between two successive Z disks, known as a ***sarcomere***, is 2.5 µm in length and is considered to be the contractile unit of skeletal muscle fibers (Fig. 8.8; see also Fig. 8.7).

During muscle contraction, the various transverse bands become characteristically altered. The I band becomes narrower, the H band and M line are no longer evident, and adjacent Z disks move closer together (approaching the interface between the A and I bands), but the width of the A bands remains unaltered.

Fine Structure of Skeletal Muscle Fibers

Studies with the electron microscopy have revealed the functional and morphological significance of skeletal muscle structural components and the alterations of the various transverse bands when the skeletal muscle fiber contracts. The following description is based on **mammalian** skeletal muscle.

T Tubules and Sarcoplasmic Reticulum

T tubules and sarcoplasmic reticulum are essential components involved in skeletal muscle contraction.

TABLE 8.1 Types of Skeletal Muscle Fibers[a]

Characteristics	Red Muscle Fibers	White Muscle Fibers
Vascularization	Rich vascular supply	Poorer vascular supply
Innervation	Smaller nerve fibers	Larger nerve fibers
Fiber diameter	Smaller	Larger
Contraction	Slow but repetitive; not easily fatigued; weaker contraction	Fast but easily fatigued; stronger contraction
Sarcoplasmic reticulum	Not extensive	Extensive
Mitochondria	Numerous	Few
Myoglobin	Rich	Poor
Enzymes	Rich in oxidative enzymes; poor in adenosine triphosphatase	Poor in oxidative enzymes; rich in phosphorylases and adenosine triphosphatase

[a]Intermediate muscle fibers have characteristics between red and white fibers.

A distinguishing feature of the skeletal muscle membrane is that it is continued within the skeletal muscle fiber as numerous long, tubular invaginations, known as ***T tubules*** (***transverse tubules***; see Fig. 8.8) that pass transversely across the muscle cell and lie specifically in the plane of the junction of the A and I bands. Therefore, each sarcomere possesses two sets of T tubules, one at each interface of the A and I bands. These tubules branch and anastomose while remaining in a single plane. Thus, T tubules extend deep into the interior of the muscle cell and facilitate the conduction of waves of depolarization along the sarcolemma (Figs. 8.9 and 8.10).

The **sarcoplasmic reticulum**, which stores *intracellular calcium*, is maintained in close register with the A and I bands, as well as with the T tubules. The SR forms a

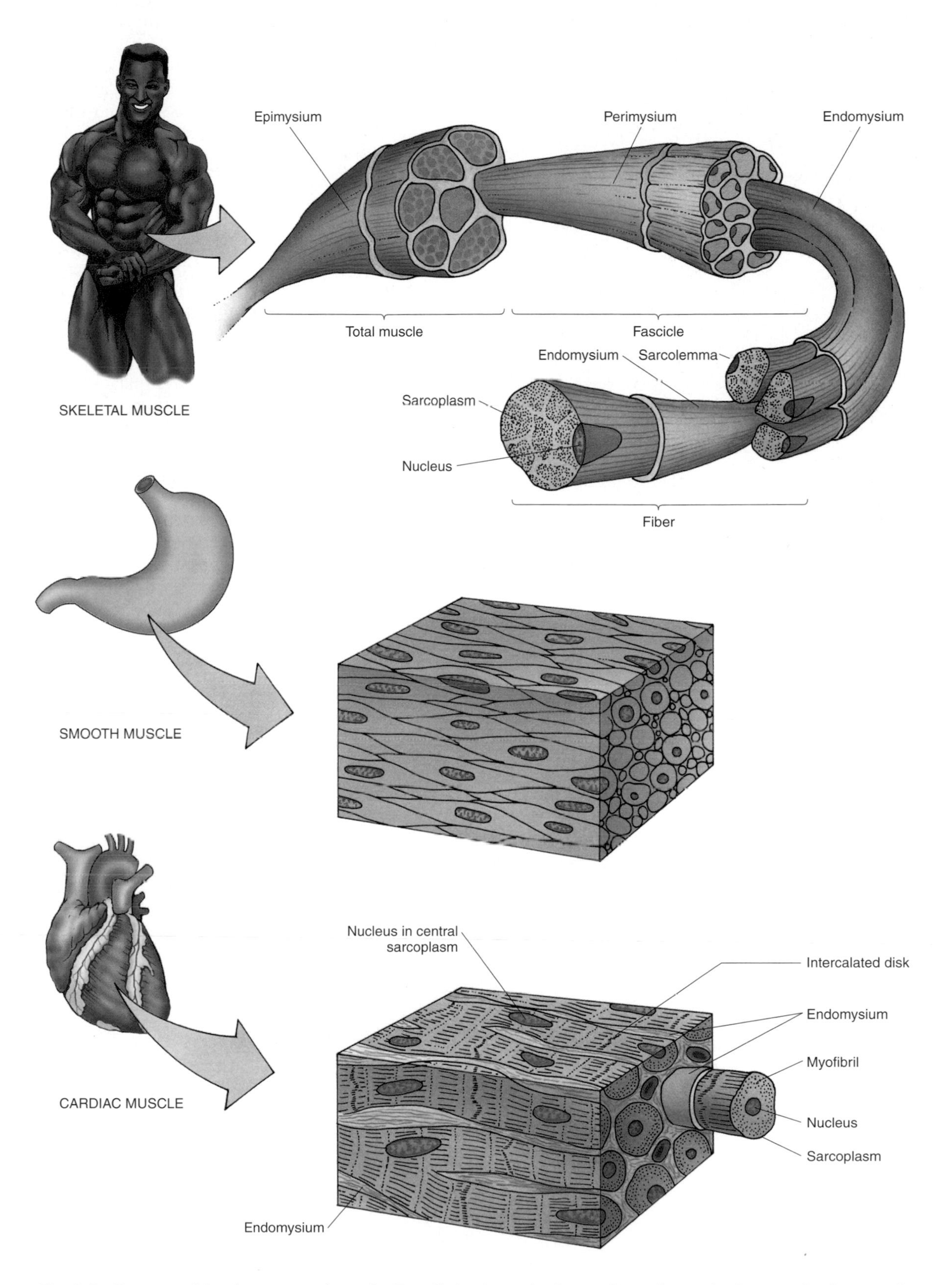

Fig. 8.3 Diagram of the three types of muscle. *Top*, Skeletal muscle. *Center*, Smooth muscle. *Bottom*, Cardiac muscle.

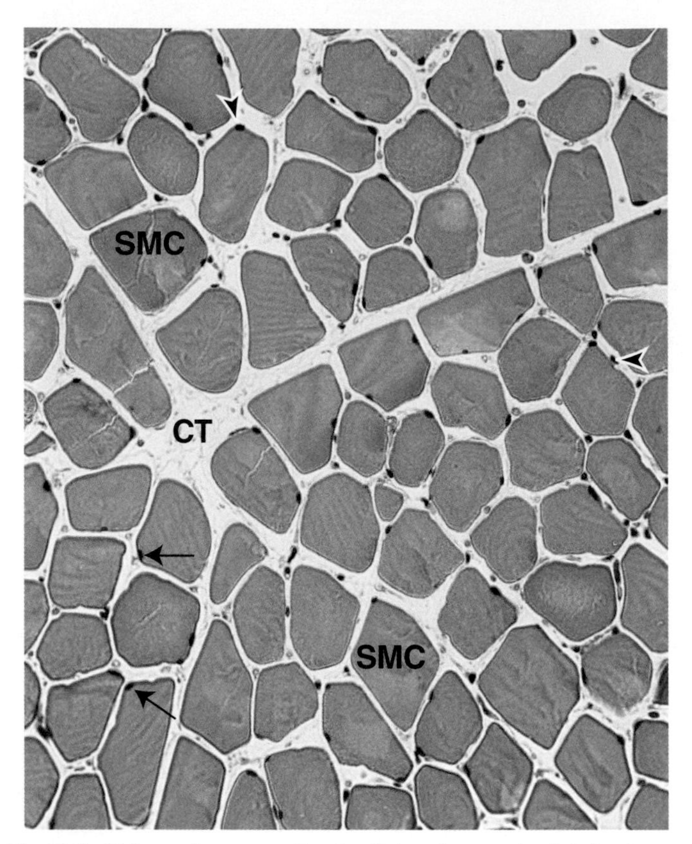

Fig. 8.4 This medium-magnification light micrograph of skeletal muscle cell (SMC) in cross-section demonstrates that the nuclei *(arrows)* are located at the periphery of the cells. (×270)

meshwork around each myofibril and displays dilated **terminal cisternae** at each A-I junction. Thus, two of these cisternae are always in close relationship with a single T tubule, forming a threefold structure known as a **triad** in which a T tubule is flanked on each side by a terminal cisterna. This arrangement permits a wave of depolarization to spread almost instantaneously from the surface of the sarcolemma throughout the cell, reaching the terminal cisternae, which possess **voltage-gated calcium release channels (junctional feet)** in their membrane.

The sarcoplasmic reticulum regulates muscle contraction through controlled sequestering (resulting in muscle relaxation) and release (resulting in muscle contraction) of calcium ions (Ca^{2+}) within the sarcoplasm. The wave of depolarization transmitted by T tubules triggers the opening of the calcium release channels of the terminal cisternae, resulting in the release of Ca^{2+} into the cytosol in the vicinity of the myofibrils.

Myofibrils are held in precise register with one another by the intermediate filaments **desmin** in the postnatal individual (and **vimentin** and some desmin in the embryo), as well as by the following desmin-associated complex of molecules. Desmin filaments bind to **plectin**, which secures these intermediate filaments to each other and to the periphery of the Z disks of neighboring myofibrils. Another protein, **αβ-crystallin**, a chaperone-like molecule, binds to desmin molecules at their union with the Z disk, ensuring that the force of muscle contraction does not damage the integrity of the desmin molecules. Desmin also has been demonstrated to bind the Z disks to the nucleus, to mitochondria, and to the actin filaments of the muscle fiber's

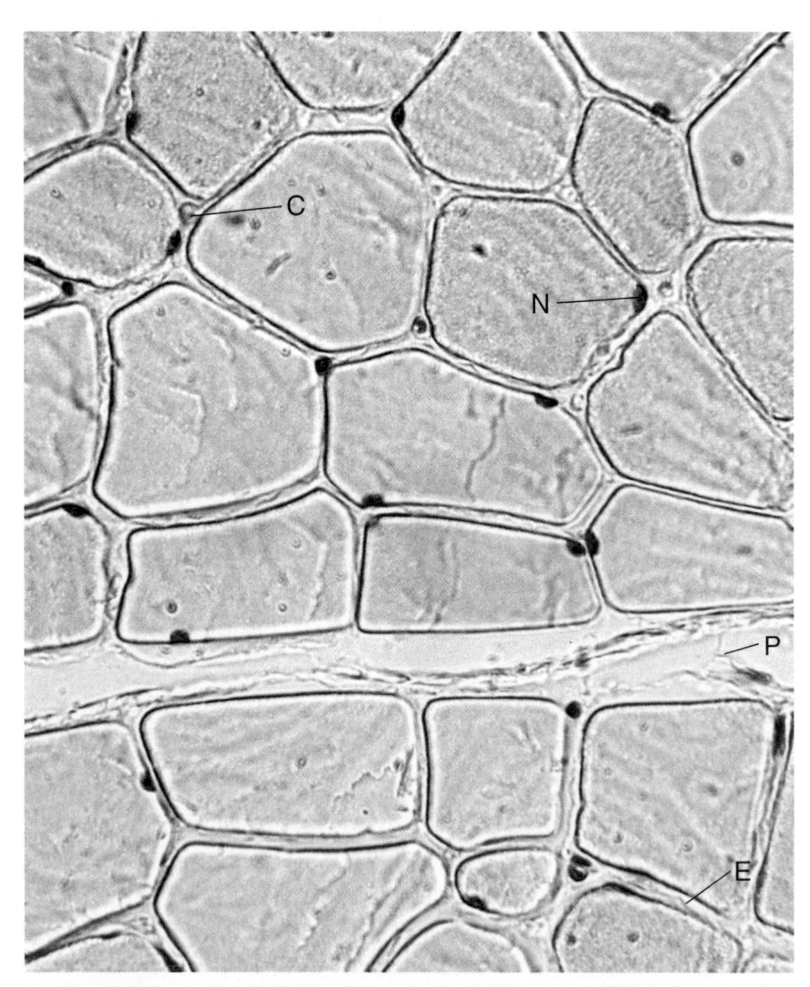

Fig. 8.5 Photomicrograph of a cross-section of skeletal muscle. Note the peripheral location of the nuclei as well as the capillary (C) located in the slender connective tissue elements of the endomysium (E). Also observe the perimysium (P) that envelops bundles of muscle fibers. (×540)

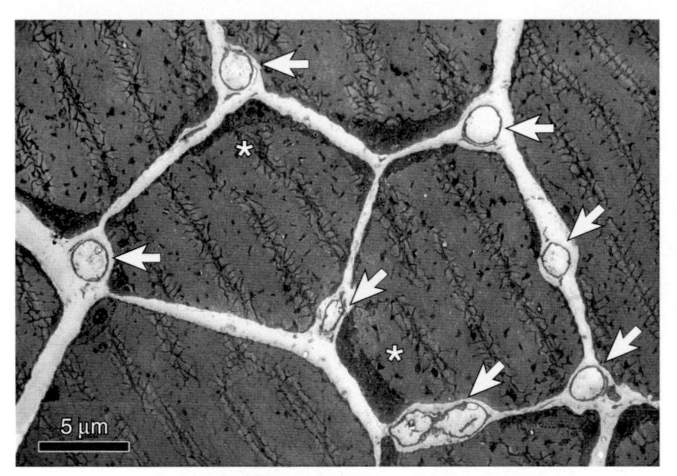

Fig. 8.6 This is a transmission electron micrograph of skeletal muscle in cross-section. Note that numerous capillaries *(arrows)* surround each skeletal muscle fiber and that clusters of mitochondria are near the capillaries *(asterisks)*. (Reprinted with permission from Baum O, Jentsch L, Odriozola A, et al. Ultrastructure of skeletal muscles in mice lacking muscle-specific VEGF expression. *Anat Rec*. 2017;300:2239-2249.)

cytoskeleton. Therefore, desmin filaments appear to be responsible for maintaining the architectural integrity of the muscle fiber.

The peripheral-most bundles of myofibrils located just adjacent to the sarcolemma are tethered by desmin filaments to specific locations on the cytoplasmic aspect of the sarcolemma, known as ***costameres***. These costameres are rich in an intricate group of sarcolemmal integral and associated proteins known as ***dystrophin-associated glycoprotein complex***, composed of **dystrophin, dystroglycan complex, sarcoglycan complex, dystrobrevin, syntrophin,** and a number of other proteins believed to be of lesser importance.

- **Dystrophin** is a very long, slim protein whose one end is attached to the actin filaments of the cytoskeleton just adjacent to the sarcolemma. The other end is attached to dystrobrevins, to the β subunit of the dystroglycan molecule, and to syntrophins. Dystrophin is believed to protect the sarcolemma from being injured during muscle contraction.

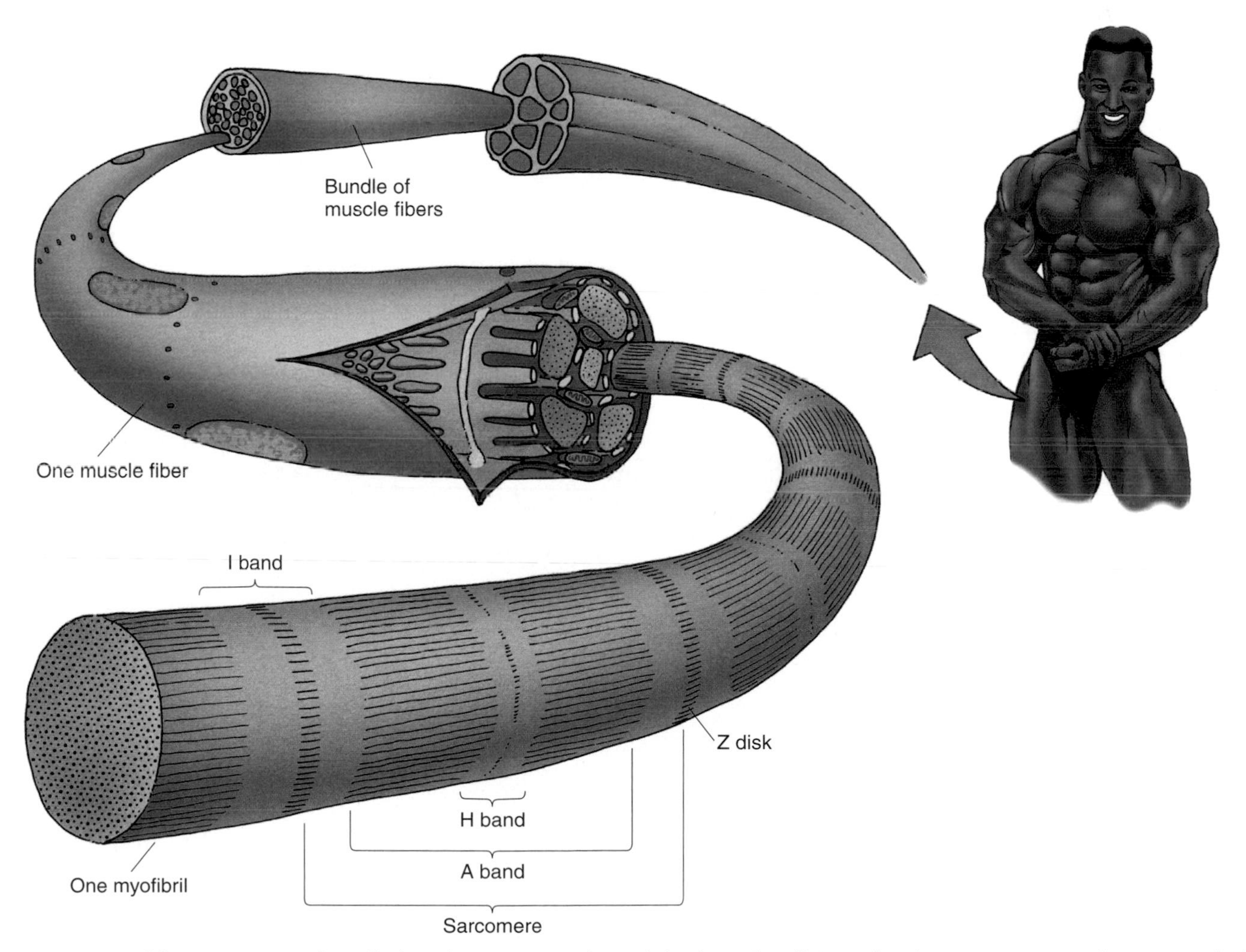

Fig. 8.7 Diagram of the organization of myofibrils and sarcomeres within a skeletal muscle cell. Note that the entire gross muscle is surrounded by a thick connective tissue investment, known as the *epimysium*, which provides finer connective tissue elements (the perimysium) that surround bundles of skeletal muscle fibers. Individual muscle cells are surrounded by still finer connective tissue elements, the endomysium. Individual skeletal muscle fibers possess a sarcolemma that has tubular invaginations, the T tubules that course through the sarcoplasm, and are flanked by terminal cisternae of the sarcoplasmic reticulum. The contractile elements of the skeletal muscle fiber are organized into discrete cylindrical units, known as *myofibrils*. Each myofibril is composed of thousands of sarcomeres.

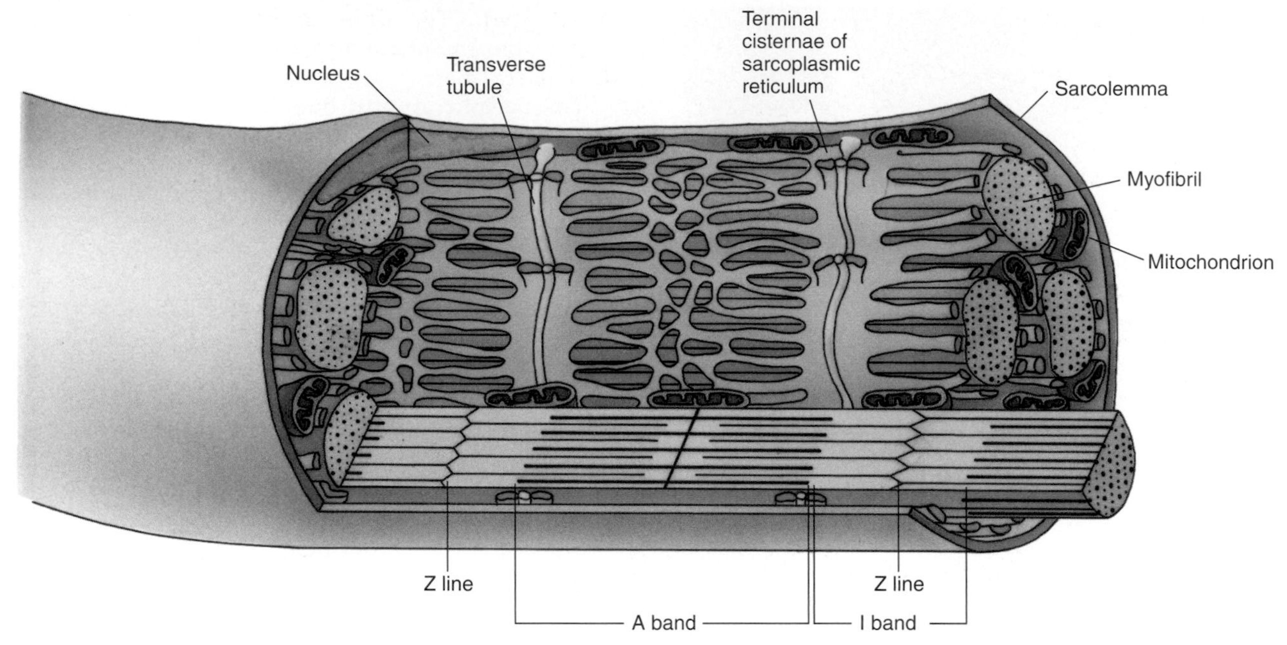

Fig. 8.8 Diagram of the organization of triads and sarcomeres of skeletal muscle. Note that, in skeletal muscle, the triad is always located at the junction of the A and I bands, permitting the quick release of calcium ions from the terminal cisternae of the sarcoplasmic reticulum just in the region where the interaction of the thick and thin filaments can produce efficient sarcomere shortening. Observe the presence of mitochondria around the periphery of the myofibrils.

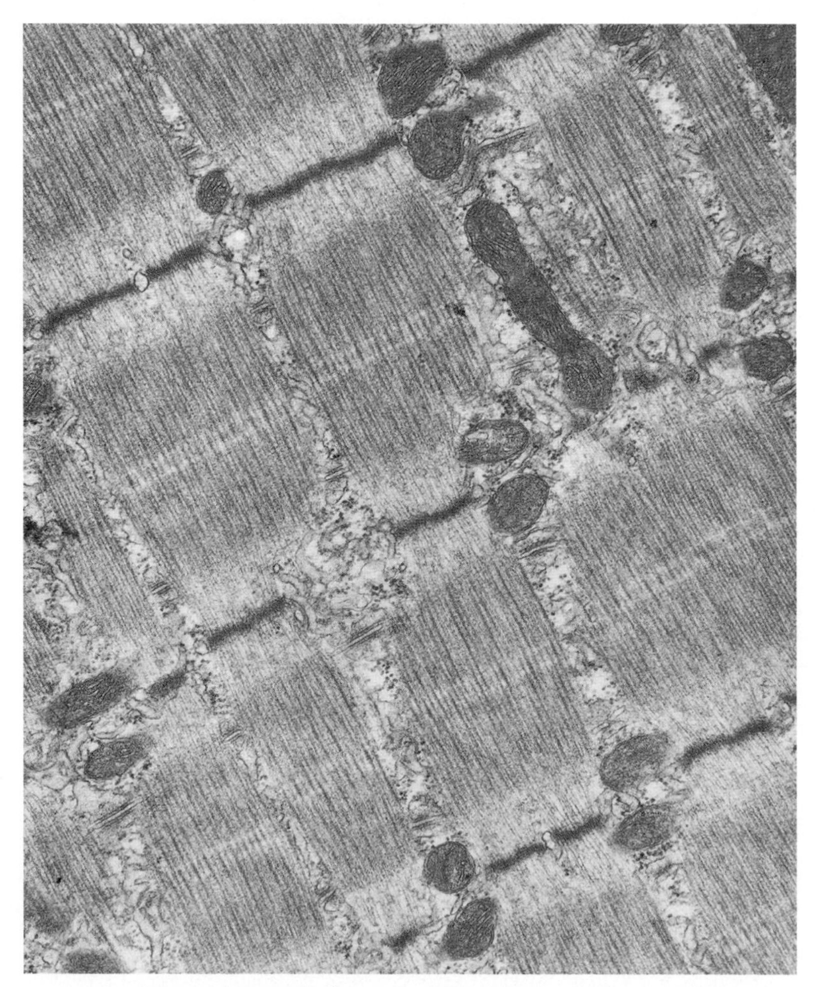

Fig. 8.9 Electron micrograph of a longitudinal section of rat skeletal muscle (×19,330). (Courtesy Dr. J. Strum.)

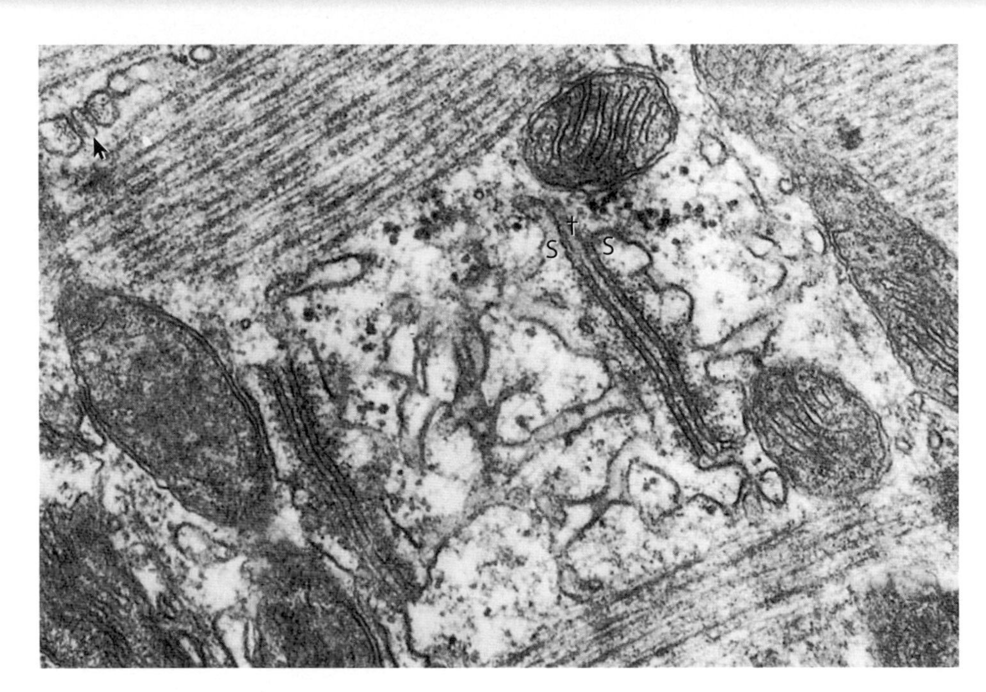

Fig. 8.10 Electron micrograph of triads and sarcoplasmic reticulum in skeletal muscle (×57,847). The *arrow* represents a cross-section of T tubule flanked by terminal cisternae. s, Terminal cisternae of the sarcoplasmic reticulum; t, T tubule. (From Leeson TS, Leeson CR, Papparo AA. *Text/Atlas of Histology*. Philadelphia: WB Saunders; 1988.)

- **The dystroglycan complex** is a glycoprotein composed of an extracellular **alpha subunit** and a transmembrane **beta subunit.** The intracellular moiety of the beta subunit binds to dystrophin, whereas the extracellular moiety binds to its alpha subunit. In turn, the alpha subunit binds to **laminin** of the **external lamina.**
- **The sarcoglycan complex** is composed of five transmembrane proteins (α, β, γ, δ, and ε) that bind to both the alpha and beta subunits of the dystroglycan, thereby reinforcing the skeletal muscle cell membrane.
- **Dystrobrevin** is a small, rod-shaped intracellular protein that binds to both dystrophin and to syntrophin, thereby providing support to dystrophin.
- **Syntrophin** binds to dystrobrevin and to dystrophin, providing further support to the costameres. Additionally, syntrophin forms bonds with the enzyme **nitric oxide synthase.** During muscle contraction, it facilitates the formation of nitric oxide, a vasodilator that increases the diameter of regional blood vessels, increasing blood flow to the area.

Deep to the sarcolemma and interspersed between and among myofibrils are numerous elongated mitochondria, with many highly interdigitating cristae. The mitochondria may either parallel the longitudinal axis of the myofibril or wrap around the myofibril. Moreover, numerous mitochondria are located just deep to the sarcoplasm.

Clinical Correlations

The term muscular dystrophy describes a series of genetic conditions resulting in escalating weakness of skeletal muscles that begins in childhood and becomes progressively worse. Although there are at least nine different forms of muscular dystrophy, over 50% of patients suffer from ***Duchenne muscular dystrophy (DMD)****, which affects male children almost exclusively. DMD, an X-lined recessive disorder (2 per 10,000 births), is first noticed when the child is about 4 years of age, and the condition deteriorates very rapidly. Muscle cells become damaged because of the paucity, and at times complete absence, of dystrophin molecules that, in a normal individual, protect the integrity of the sarcolemma during muscle contraction. The lack of this molecule results in damage to the skeletal muscle cell membrane, with an eventual death of muscle fibers. The dead muscle cells are replaced with fat cells and the gross muscle appears to be rather robust, when, in fact, it is less able to function. These affected children soon lose their ability to stand up and walk; eventually, they become wheel chair-bound. Unfortunately, there is no cure, and the average life span of these patients is around 25 years of age. However, with the administration of corticosteroids, physical therapy, and ventilator treatments, that may be extended to the early 40s. Death is usually caused by the inability to breathe, owing to dysfunctional muscles of respiration. It is hoped that gene therapy, especially genome editing using the CRISPR/Cas9 editing tool, may be able to cure this genetic disease.*

Structural Organization of Myofibrils

Myofibrils are composed of interdigitating thick and thin myofilaments.

Electron microscopy reveals the same banding as noted by light microscopy but also demonstrates the presence of parallel, interdigitating, rod-like **thick filaments** (**thick myofilaments**) and **thin filaments** (**thin myofilaments**). The **thick filaments** (15 nm in diameter and 1.5 μm long) are composed of **myosin II** and associated proteins. The **thin filaments** (7 nm in diameter and 1 μm long) are composed primarily of **F-actin** and associated proteins. The detailed structures of the thick and thin filaments are presented in this section.

The **plus ends** of *thin* filaments originate at the Z disk and project toward the center of the two adjacent sarcomeres, pointing in opposite directions. Hence, a single sarcomere has two groups of parallel arrays of thin filaments, each attached to one Z disk, with all of the filaments in each group pointing toward the middle of the sarcomere (Fig. 8.11). *Thick* filaments also form parallel arrays, interdigitating with the thin filaments in a specific fashion.

In a relaxed skeletal muscle fiber, the thick filaments do not extend the entire length of the sarcomere, and the thin filaments projecting from the two Z disks of the sarcomere do not meet in the midline. Therefore, there are regions of each sarcomere, on either side of each Z disk, where only thin filaments are present. These adjacent portions of two successive sarcomeres correspond to the I band noted by light microscopy. For instance, the region of each sarcomere that encompasses the entire length of the thick filaments is the A band and the zone in the middle of the A band, which is devoid of thin filaments, is the H band. As noted earlier, the H band is bisected by the M line, which consists of **myomesin, C protein, creatine kinase**, and other as yet poorly characterized proteins that interconnect thick filaments to maintain their specific lattice arrangement.

During contraction, individual thick and thin filaments do not shorten. Instead, the two Z disks are brought closer together as the thin filaments slide past the thick filaments (Huxley's **sliding filament theory**), effectively reducing the widths of the I and H bands without influencing the width of the A band.

Each thick filament is surrounded equidistantly by six thin filaments. Cross-sections through the region of overlapping thin and thick filaments display a hexagonal pattern, with thin filaments for the apices of each hexagon, the center of which is occupied by a thick filament (Figs. 8.11 and 8.12). Thick filaments are separated from each other by a distance of 40 to 50 nm, whereas the distance between thick and thin filaments is only 15 to 20 nm. Five proteins—titin, α-actinin, Cap Z, nebulin, and tropomodulin—are responsible for maintaining the precise structural organization of myofibrils.

Thick filaments are positioned precisely within the sarcomere, with the assistance of **titin**, a large, linear, elastic protein. Two titin molecules extend from each half of a thick filament to the adjacent Z disk; thus, four titin molecules anchor each thick filament between the two Z disks of each sarcomere.

Thin filaments are held in register by the rod-shaped protein **α-actinin**, a component of the Z disk that can bind thin filaments in parallel arrays, as well as by an additional component protein of the Z disk, known as ***Cap Z***. This protein also prevents the addition or subtraction of G actin molecules to or from the thin filament, thus maintaining its precise length. In addition, two molecules of the long, inelastic protein, **nebulin**, are wrapped around the entire length of each thin filament, further anchoring it in the Z disk and ensuring the maintenance of the specific spatial relationship of the thin filaments. Moreover, nebulin acts as a "ruler" that maintains the precise length of the thin filament. It is assisted in this function by the protein **tropomodulin**, a cap on the minus end of the thin filament that, similarly to Cap Z, prevents the addition or the deletion of G actin molecules to or from the thin filament (see Fig. 8.11).

Table 8.2 presents the proteins that constitute myofilaments and that keep them correctly positioned within myofibrils.

Thick Filaments.

Thick filaments are composed of myosin II molecules aligned end to end.

Every thick filament consists of 200 to 300 **myosin II** molecules. Each myosin II molecule (150 nm long; 2-3 nm in diameter) is composed of two **heavy chains** and two pairs of **light chains**.

The *heavy chains* resemble two golf clubs, whose rod-like polypeptide chains are wrapped around each other in an α-helix. The heavy chains can be cleaved by the enzyme trypsin into

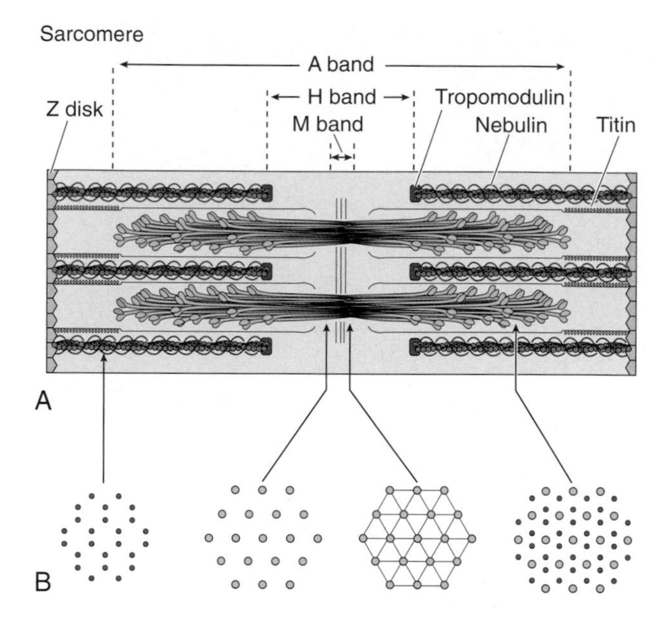

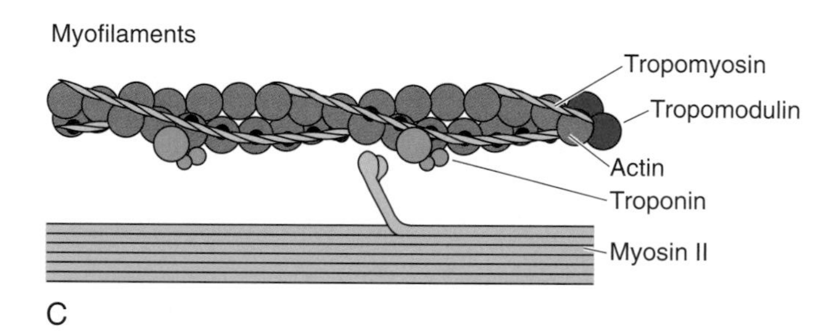

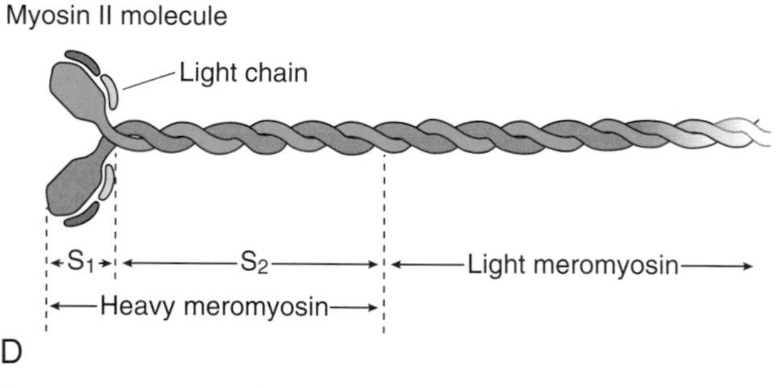

Fig. 8.11 Diagram of a sarcomere and its components. (A) Sarcomere. The myosin molecules are arranged in an antiparallel fashion so that their heads are projecting from each end of the thick filament. Each thick filament is anchored in position by four titin molecules that extend from the Z disk to the center of the thick filament at the M line. Additionally, each thin filament is fixed in place by nebulin molecules that extend from the Z disk to the distal end of the thin filament. (B) Cross-sectional profiles of sarcomere at indicated regions. Each thick filament is surrounded equidistally by six thin filaments so that there are always two thin filaments between neighboring thick filaments. (C) Thick and thin filaments. Each thin filament is composed of two chains of F actins; each F actin is composed of numerous G actin molecules assembled head to toe. Each groove of a thin filament is occupied by linear proteins, tropomyosin, that are positioned in such a fashion that they block the myosin-binding site of each G actin molecule. Additionally, the tripartite molecule, troponin, is associated with each tropomyosin molecule. When the troponin C moiety of troponin binds calcium, the conformational change in the troponin molecule pushes the tropomyosin deeper into the groove, unmasking the myosin-binding site of the G actin and permitting muscle contraction to occur. (D) Myosin molecule. Each myosin molecule is composed of two light chains and two heavy chains. The heavy chains can be cleaved by trypsin into light and heavy meromyosin, and each heavy meromyosin can be cleaved by papain into S_1 and S_2 fragments.

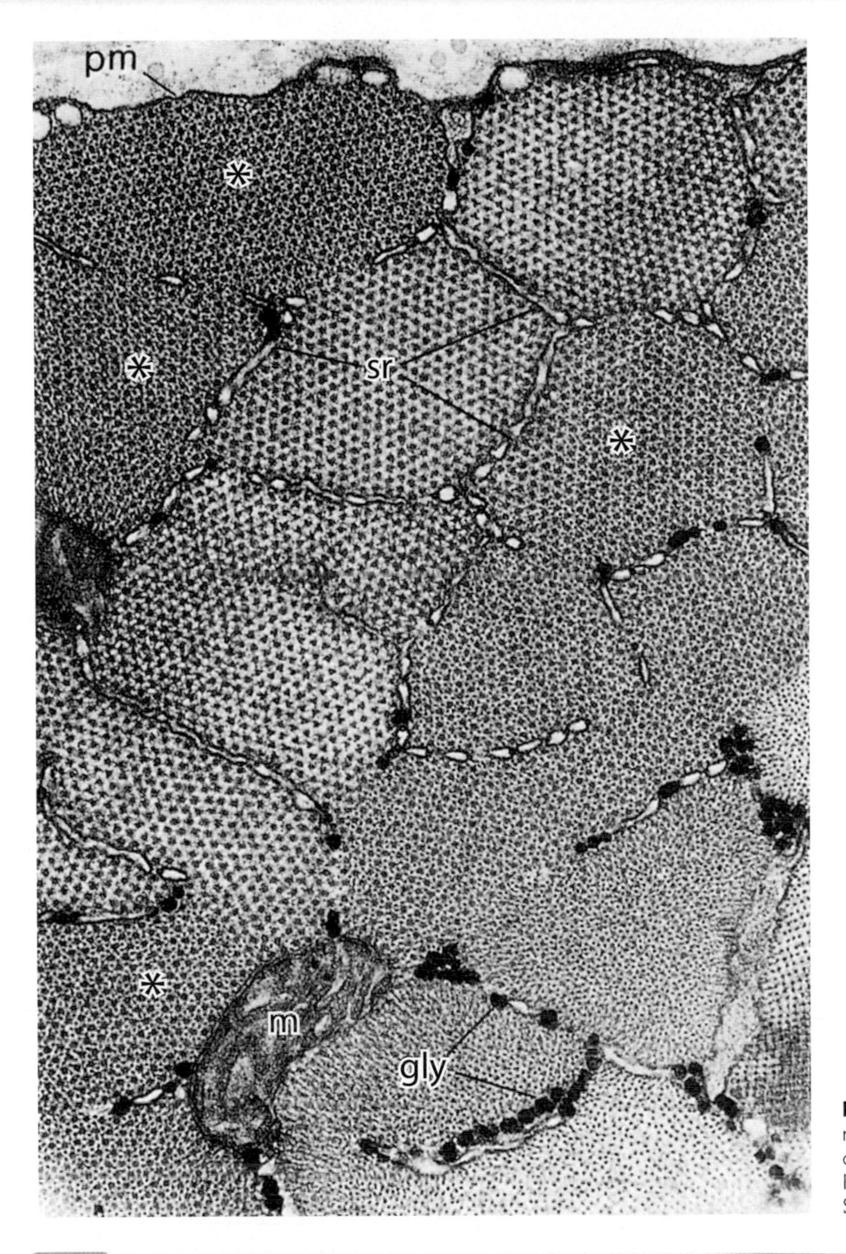

Fig. 8.12 Cross-section of skeletal muscle fiber. *Asterisks* represent thick and thin filaments. gly, Glycogen; m, mitochondria; pm, plasma membrane. (Courtesy Dr. C. Peracchia; from Hopkins CR. *Structure and Function of Cells*. Philadelphia: WB Saunders; 1978.)

TABLE 8.2 Proteins Associated with Skeletal Muscle

Protein	Molecular Weight (kD)	Subunits and Their Molecular Weight	Function
Myosin II	510	2 heavy chains, 222 kD each; 2 pairs light chains, 18 kD and 22 kD	Major protein of thick filament; its interaction with actin hydrolyzes ATP and produces contraction
Myomesin	185	None	Cross-links thick filaments that are next to each other at the M line
Titin	2500	None	Forms an elastic lattice that anchors thick filaments to Z disks
C protein	140	None	Binds to thick filaments at the M line
G actin	42	None	Polymerizes to form thin filaments of F actin; interaction of G actin with myosin II assists in hydrolyzing ATP, resulting in contraction
Tropomyosin	64	2 chains, 32 kD each	Occupies grooves of the thin filaments
Troponin	78	TnC, 18 kD TnT, 30 kD TnI, 30 kD	Binds calcium Binds to tropomyosin Binds to actin, inhibiting actin-myosin interaction
α-Actinin	190	2 units, each 95 kD	Anchors plus ends of thin filaments to Z disk
Nebulin	600	None	Z disk protein that may assist α-actinin anchor thin filaments to Z disk
Cap Z			Forms part of the Z disk and caps the plus end of the thin filament
Tropomodulin	43 kD		Caps the minus end of the thin filament

ATP, Adenosine triphosphate.

- **Light meromyosin**: A rod-like tail composed of most of the two rod-like polypeptide chains wrapped around each other
- **Heavy meromyosin**: Two globular heads with the attendant short proximal portions of the two rod-like polypeptide chains wrapped around each other

The light meromyosin functions in the proper assembly of the molecules into the bipolar thick filament. Heavy meromyosin can be cleaved by the enzyme papain into two globular (**S_1**) moieties and a short, helical, rod-like segment (**S_2**; see Fig. 8.11). The S_1 subfragment binds **adenosine triphosphate (ATP)** and functions in the formation of cross-bridges between the thick and thin myofilaments.

Light chains (not to be confused with light meromyosin) are of two types; one of each type is associated with each S_1 subfragment of the myosin II molecule. For each heavy chain, therefore, there are two light chains. Thus, a ***myosin II molecule is composed of two heavy chains and four light chains.***

Myosin II molecules are closely packed; they are lined up in a parallel but staggered manner, spaced at regular intervals, arranged head to tail, so that the middle of each thick filament is composed solely of tail regions (*light meromyosin*), whereas the two ends of the thick filament consist of both heads and tails (*heavy meromyosin*). The spatial orientation of the myosin II molecules permits the heavy meromyosin portion to project from the thick filament at a 60-degree angle relative to neighboring heavy meromyosin, so that head regions are always in register with thin filaments (remember that each thick filament is surrounded, equidistantly, by six thin filaments).

Each myosin II molecule appears to have two flexible regions, one at the junction of the heavy meromyosin with the light meromyosin and the other at the junction of the S_1 and S_2 subfragments. The flexible region between the heavy and light meromyosins permits each myosin II molecule to contact the thin filament, forming a cross-bridge between itself and the actin filament. As discussed later, the flexible region between the S_1 and S_2 subfragments enables the myosin II molecule to drag the thin filament incrementally toward the middle of the sarcomere.

Thin Filaments.

Thin filaments are composed of two chains of F-actin filaments wrapped around each other in association with tropomyosin and troponin.

The major component of each thin filament is **F-actin**, a polymer of globular **G-actin** units, wrapped around each other in a tight helix (36-nm periodicity) resembling two strands of pearls (see Fig. 8.11). All G-actin molecules polymerize in the same spatial orientation, imparting a distinct polarity to the filament.

The **plus end** of each filament is bound to the Z disk by α-actinin; the **minus end** extends toward the center of the sarcomere. Both plus and minus ends of the actin filament are capped; the plus end is capped by **Cap Z**, whereas the minus end is capped by **tropomodulin**. These two caps greatly impede the addition or the deletion of G actin monomers to or from the F actin filament, permitting its constant length to be maintained. Moreover, each G-actin molecule of the F actin chain possesses an **active site**, where the head region (S_1 subfragment) of myosin II can attach.

Running along the length of the F-actin double-stranded helix are two shallow grooves. Pencil-shaped **tropomyosin molecules**, about 40 nm long, polymerize to form head-to-tail filaments that occupy the shallow grooves of the double-stranded actin helix. Bound tropomyosin masks the active sites on the actin molecules by partially overlapping them.

Approximately 25 to 30 nm from the beginning of each tropomyosin molecule is a single **troponin molecule**, composed of three globular polypeptides: **TnT** binds the entire troponin molecule to tropomyosin; **TnC** has a great affinity for calcium; and **TnI** binds to actin, preventing the interaction between actin and myosin II. Binding of calcium by **TnC** induces a conformational shift in tropomyosin, exposing the previously blocked active sites on the actin filament so that myosin II molecules can flex, forming the cross-bridges, and so that the S_1 moieties (myosin heads) can bind to the active site on the actin molecule (see the next section).

Muscle Contraction and Relaxation

Muscle contraction obeys the all-or-none law and is followed by muscle relaxation.

Contraction effectively reduces the resting length of the muscle fiber by an amount that is equal to the sum of all shortenings that occur in all sarcomeres of that particular muscle cell. The process of contraction, usually triggered by **neural impulses**, obeys the **all-or-none law** in that a single muscle fiber either contracts or does not contract as a result of stimulation. The stimulus is transferred at the **neuromuscular junction (synapse)**.

The strength of contraction of a gross anatomical muscle, such as the biceps, is a function of the number of muscle cells that undergo contraction. Based on past experience, the brain determines how many muscle cells have to contract to lift a particular object. For example, if a glass of water is to be picked up, much fewer muscle fibers will be directed to contract than if a 5-gallon container filled with water is to be picked up.

The following sequence of events leads to contraction in skeletal muscle after depolarization of the sarcolemma:

1. An impulse, generated along the sarcolemma, is transmitted into the interior of the fiber via the T tubules. The membrane of the T tubules possesses **voltage-sensitive dihydropyridine (DHP) receptors** whose conformation is altered. Because these DHP receptors are in contact with the **Ca^{2+}-release channels (ryanodine receptors)** of the terminal cisternae of the sarcoplasmic reticulum, the altered conformation in the DHP receptors causes the Ca^{2+}-release channels to open.
2. Calcium ions leave the terminal cisternae through the open **calcium release channels**, enter the cytosol, and bind to the TnC subunit of troponin, altering its conformation.
3. Conformational change in troponin shifts the position of tropomyosin deeper into the groove of the thin filament, unmasking the active site (myosin binding site) on the actin molecule.
4. ATP bound to the S_1 subfragment of myosin II is hydrolyzed, but both adenosine diphosphate (ADP) and inorganic phosphate (P_i) remain attached to the S_1 subfragment, which twists so that the complex can bind to the active site on actin (Fig. 8.13).

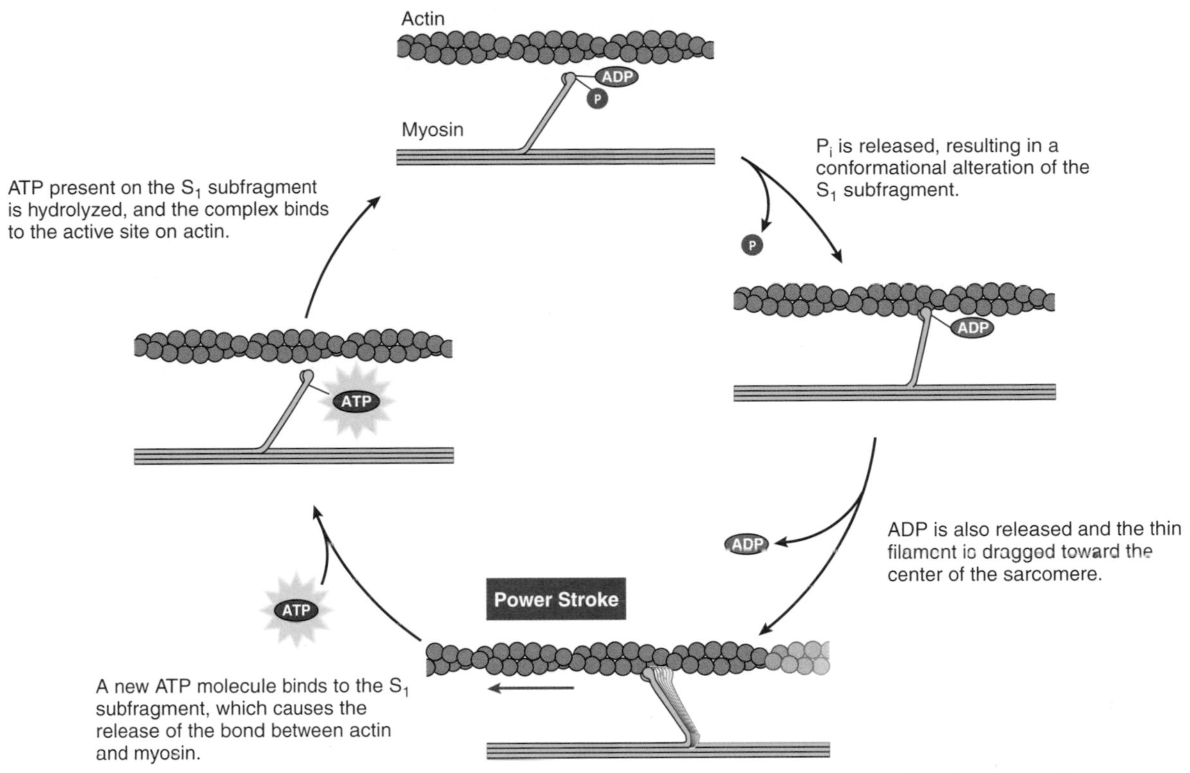

Fig. 8.13 Diagram of the role of adenosine triphosphate (ATP) in muscle contraction. ADP, Adenosine diphosphate; P and P_i, inorganic phosphate; S_1 subfragment, fragment of myosin. (Modified from Alberts B, Bray D, Lewis J, et al. *Molecular Biology of the Cell*. New York: Garland Publishing; 1994.)

5. Inorganic phosphate is released, resulting not only in a greater bond strength between the actin and myosin II but also causing a conformational alteration of the S_1 subfragment.
6. ADP is also released from the S_1 subfragment of myosin II, and the thin filament is dragged toward the center of the sarcomere ("power stroke"). Each power stroke moves the thin filament a distance of approximately 5 nm toward the center of the sarcomere.
7. The binding of a new ATP molecule to the S_1 subfragment results in the release of the bond between actin and myosin II.

The attachment and release cycles must be repeated approximately 200 times for contraction to be completed. Each attachment and release cycle requires ATP for the conversion of chemical energy into motion.

Clinical Correlations

Shortly after death. the joints become immoveable. This stiffening of the joints is referred to as **rigor mortis**; *depending on the ambient temperature, it may last as long as 3 days. Because the dead cells are unable to manufacture ATP, the dissociation of the thick and thin filaments cannot occur, and the myosin heads remain bound to the active site of the actin molecule until the muscle begins to decompose. The time of death may be estimated by the state of rigor mortis, when correlated with a record of the ambient temperature fluctuations. The facial muscles are the first to undergo rigor mortis and maximum rigor occurs 12 to 24 hours after death.*

As long as the cytosolic calcium concentration is high enough, actin filaments remain in the active state and contraction cycles continue. Once the stimulating impulses cease, however, muscle relaxation occurs, involving a reversal of the steps that led to contraction.

First, **calcium pumps** in the membrane of the sarcoplasmic reticulum actively drive Ca^{2+} ions back into the terminal cisternae, where the ions are bound by the protein **calsequestrin**. This reduces the levels of Ca^{2+} in the cytosol, causing TnC to lose its bound Ca^{2+} and to return to its original conformation, permitting tropomyosin to resume its original location in the groove of the thin filament and, once again, mask the active site on the actin molecule, preventing the interaction of actin and myosin II.

Energy Sources for Muscle Contraction

Energy sources for muscle contraction are the phosphagen energy system, glycolysis, and aerobic energy system.

The process of muscle contraction requires a great deal of energy; therefore, skeletal muscle cells maintain a high concentration of the energy-rich compounds ATP and **creatine phosphate** (**phosphocreatine**). Because both ATP and creatine phosphate contain high-energy phosphate bonds, they constitute the **phosphagen energy system,** which can provide enough energy for about a total of 9 seconds of maximum muscle activity (3 seconds for ATP and 6 seconds for creatine phosphate).

Additional energy can be derived from the breakdown of glycogen to glucose and the consequent anaerobic metabolism of glucose (**glycolysis**), which results in the formation and buildup of lactic acid. This is known as the ***glycogen–lactic acid system***. This system provides about 90 to 100 seconds of energy at almost maximal muscle activity.

The third system, known as the ***aerobic energy system***, uses the normal sources for the manufacture of ATP. The aerobic system does not support maximal muscle activity, but it can sustain normal muscle activity indefinitely if the dietary intake is maintained and the nutrients persist.

The three metabolic systems of skeletal muscle are harnessed to supply the energy requirements of the muscle according to their activity modalities. During bursts of muscle contraction, the ADP that is generated is rephosphorylated by two means: (1) **glycolysis**, leading to accumulation of lactic acid, and (2) transfer of high-energy phosphate from creatine phosphate (phosphagen system) catalyzed by **phosphocreatine kinase**. During prolonged but normal muscle activity, however, the aerobic system of energy production is employed.

Clinical Correlations

*The nodal regulator **peroxisome proliferator-activated receptor γ coactivator 1α (PCG-1α)** is a well-known regulator not only of mitochondrial self-replication and energy utilization but also of the activity of a number of transcription factors. PCG-1α expression is increased in skeletal muscle after exercise, which not only is a mood enhancer but also relieves stress-related depression. Studies have demonstrated that PCG-1α expression elevates levels of **kynurenine aminotransferase** within skeletal muscle cells; this enzyme converts **kynurenine** into its acidic form, **kynurenic acid**. When kynurenine is released from skeletal muscle cells, it enters the bloodstream and is able to cross the blood–brain barrier. It has been reported that elevated levels of kynurenine in the brain has been associated with depression. However, kynurenic acid cannot cross the blood–brain barrier; consequently, after exercise, there is a decrease in kynurenine levels in the brain. Interestingly, diabetes and obesity also cause depression. Both diabetic and obese mice display reduced levels of PCG-1α in skeletal muscle cells, suggesting that this nodal regulator may have an important function in alleviating depression.*

MYOTENDINOUS JUNCTIONS

The junction of the muscle cell with the tendon of the muscle is known as the myotendinous junction. It is here that the skeletal muscle cell becomes tapered and highly fluted and collagen fibers of the tendon penetrate deep into these infoldings and most probably become continuous with the reticular fibers of the endomysium. Within the cell, the myofilaments are anchored to the internal aspect of the sarcolemma so that the force of contraction is transmitted directly to the collagen fibers of the tendon.

INNERVATION OF SKELETAL MUSCLE

Skeletal muscle cells and the single motoneuron that innervates them constitute a motor unit.

Each skeletal muscle receives **motor**, **sensory**, and autonomic innervation. The motor nerve functions in eliciting contraction, the sensory fibers pass to muscle spindles and Golgi tendon organs (see section on muscle spindles and Golgi tendon organs in this chapter), and autonomic fibers supply the vascular elements of skeletal muscle. The specificity of motor innervation is

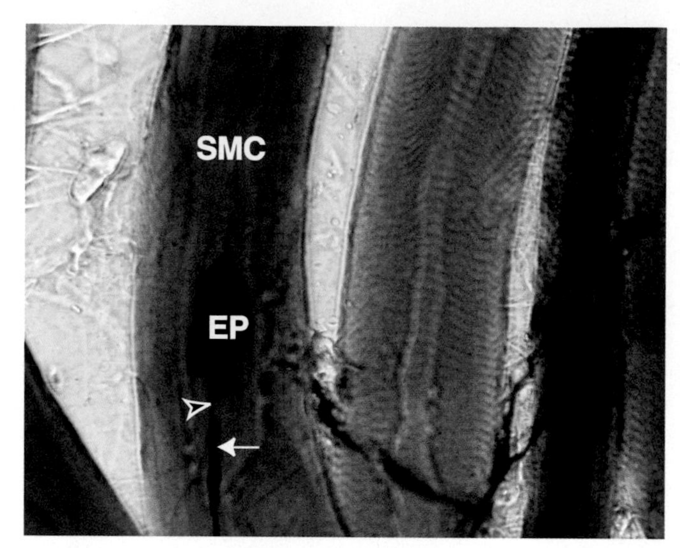

Fig. 8.14 This is a high-magnification image of an axon terminal (EP) forming a junction, the myoneural junction, with a skeletal muscle cell (SMC). Observe that the axon is myelinated *(arrow)* but loses its myelin sheath *(arrowhead)* just before it reaches the end plate *(axon terminal)*. (×540)

a function of the muscle innervated. If the muscle acts fastidiously, as do some muscles of the eye, a single motoneuron may be responsible for as few as 5 to 10 skeletal muscle cells, whereas a muscle located in the abdominal wall may have as many as 1000 muscle fibers under the control of a single motoneuron. Each motoneuron and the muscle fibers it controls form a **motor unit**. The muscle fibers of a *single* motor unit contract in unison and follow the **all-or-none law** of muscle contraction.

Impulse Transmission at the Neuromuscular Junction

Impulse transmission from the motoneuron to the skeletal muscle fiber occurs at the neuromuscular junction.

Motor fibers are **myelinated axons** of **α-motoneurons** that pass in the connective tissue compartments of the muscle. The axon arborizes, eventually losing its myelin sheath (but not its Schwann cells). The terminus of each arborized twig becomes dilated and overlies the cell membrane of individual skeletal muscle cells. Each of these nerve–muscle junctions, known as a ***neuromuscular junction*** (**myoneural junction**), is composed of an *axon terminal*, a *synaptic cleft*, and the *modified muscle cell membrane* (known specifically as the ***postsynaptic membrane*** or ***motor end plate***; Figs. 8.14 to 8.17).

The **sarcolemma at the postsynaptic membrane** is modified, forming a trough-like structure, known as the ***primary synaptic cleft***, occupied by the **axon terminal**. Opening into the primary synaptic clefts are numerous tubular invaginations known as ***junctional folds*** (**secondary synaptic clefts**), a further modification of the sarcolemma. Both the primary synaptic cleft and junctional folds are lined by a basal lamina–like **external lamina**, manufactured by the skeletal muscle cell. The sarcoplasm in the vicinity of the secondary synaptic cleft is rich in glycogen, nuclei, ribosomes, and mitochondria.

The **axon terminal** is covered by Schwann cells on its entire surface except on its **presynaptic membrane**, the surface facing the postsynaptic membrane. The axon terminal houses mitochondria, SER, and as many as 300,000 **synaptic vesicles** (each

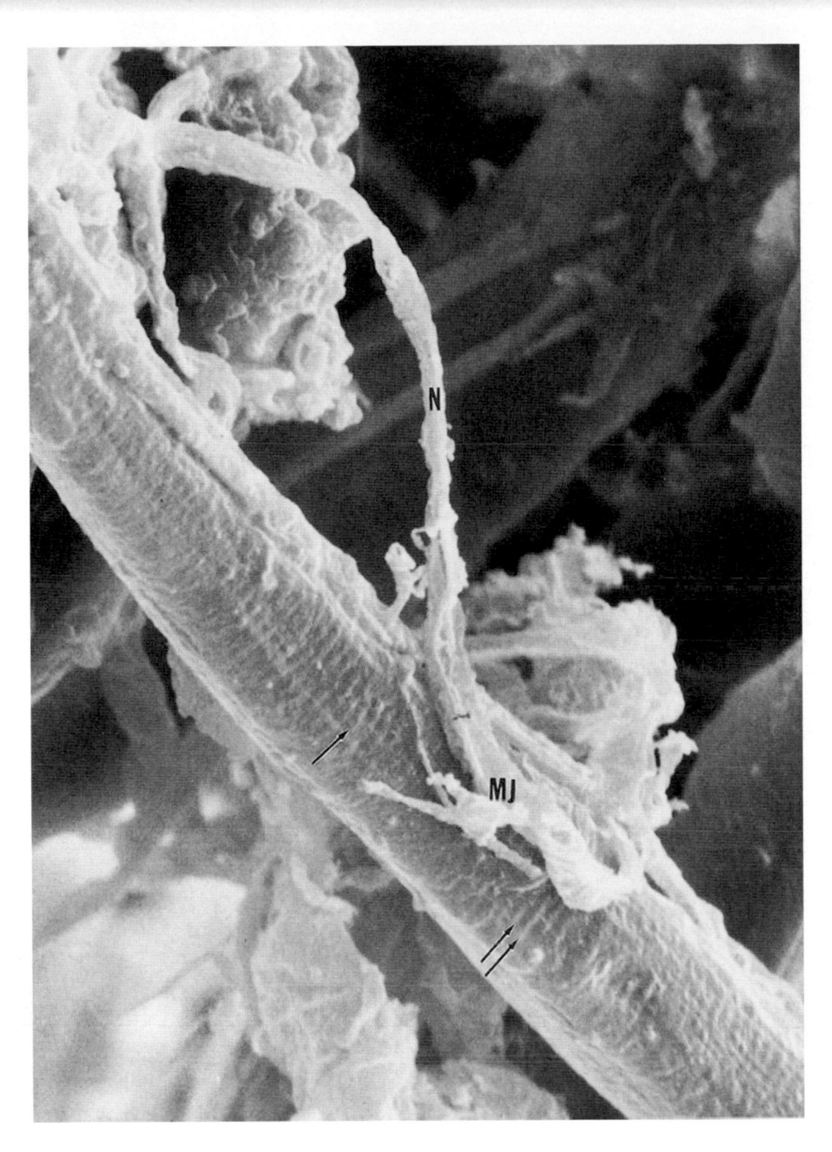

Fig. 8.15 Scanning electron micrograph of a neuromuscular junction from the tongue of a cat (×2315). *Arrows* indicate striations. MJ, Neuromuscular junction; N, nerve fiber. (Courtesy Dr. L Litke.)

40-50 nm in diameter) containing the neurotransmitter **acetylcholine**. The function of the neuromuscular junction is to transmit a stimulus from the nerve fiber to the muscle cell.

Stimulus transmission across a synaptic cleft involves the following sequence of events (Fig. 8.18):

1. When an action potential propagated along the axon arrives at the axon terminal, it depolarizes its membrane and opens the **voltage-gated calcium channels** that are located in the vicinity of linearly arranged structures known as ***dense bars.***
2. The influx of calcium ions into the axon terminal results in the fusion of about 120 synaptic vesicles for each nerve impulse with the axon terminal's membrane (**presynaptic membrane**) along specific regions of the presynaptic membrane, known as ***active sites***, adjoining the dense bars. The fusion of the vesicles with the presynaptic membrane is followed by exocytosis of a **quantum** (10,000-20,000 molecules) of the neurotransmitter **acetylcholine** (along with proteoglycans and ATP) into the primary synaptic cleft.
3. Acetylcholine then diffuses across the synaptic cleft and binds to **acetylcholine receptors** in the muscle cell membrane (**postsynaptic membrane**). These receptors, located in the vicinity of the presynaptic active sites, are **transmitter-gated sodium ion channels**, which open in response to the binding of acetylcholine. The resulting sodium ion influx leads to **depolarization** of the muscle cell membrane and creation of an **action potential** of the sarcolemma (see Chapter 9).
4. The impulse generated spreads quickly throughout the muscle fiber via the system of T tubules (see earlier section on muscle contraction and relaxation), initiating muscle contraction.

To prevent a single stimulus from eliciting multiple responses, **acetylcholinesterase**, an enzyme located in the external lamina lining the primary and secondary synaptic clefts, degrades acetylcholine into **acetate** and **choline**, permitting the reestablishment of the **resting potential**. Degradation is so rapid that all of the released acetylcholine is cleaved within a few hundred milliseconds.

Choline is transported back into the axon terminal by a **sodium-choline symport protein** powered by the sodium concentration gradient. Within the axon terminal, the acetylcholine is synthesized from activated acetate (produced in mitochondria) and the recycled choline, a reaction catalyzed by **choline acetyl transferase**. The newly formed acetylcholine is transported, through the use of an antiport system powered by a proton concentration gradient, into newly formed synaptic vesicles.

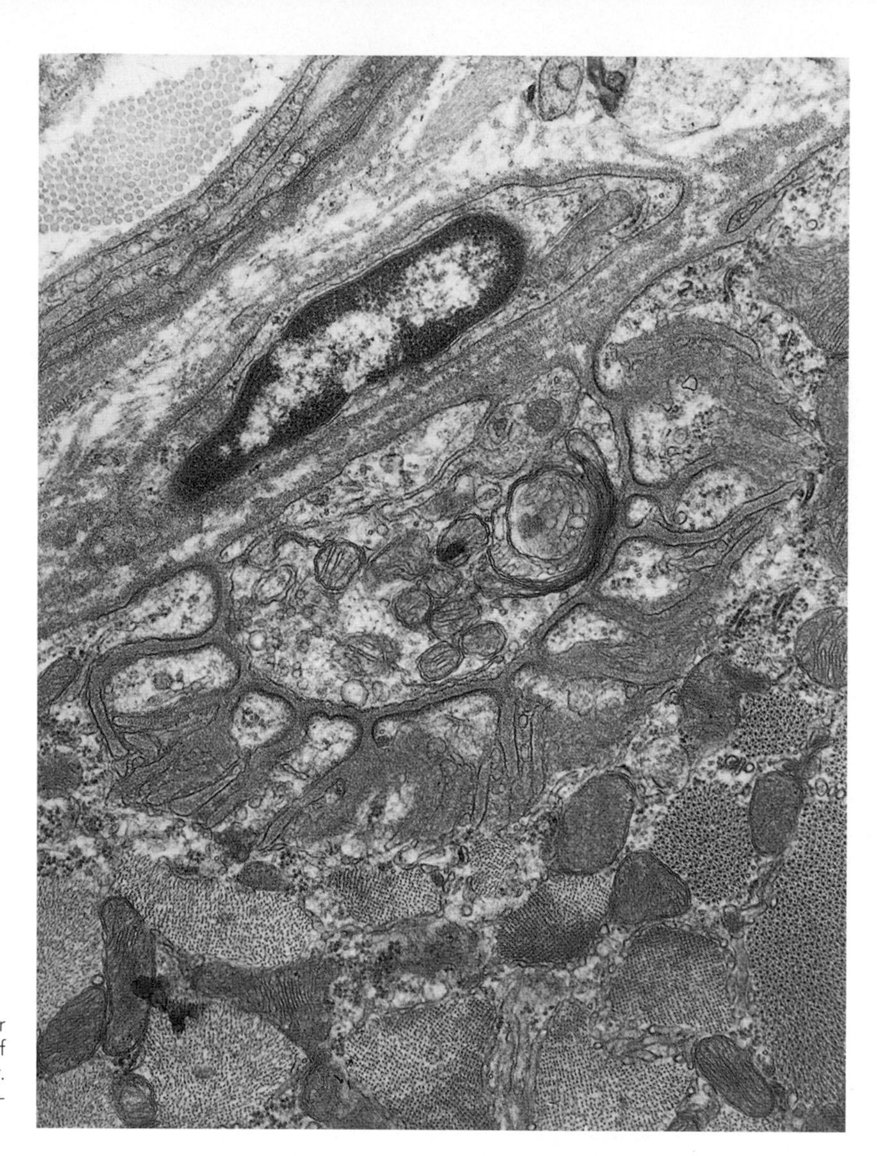

Fig. 8.16 Electron micrograph of a mouse neuromuscular junction. (From Feczko D, Klueber KM. Cytoarchitecture of muscle in a genetic model of murine diabetes. *Am J Anat.* 1988;182:224-240. Reprinted with permission from Wiley-Liss, Inc., a subsidiary of John Wiley & Sons, Inc.)

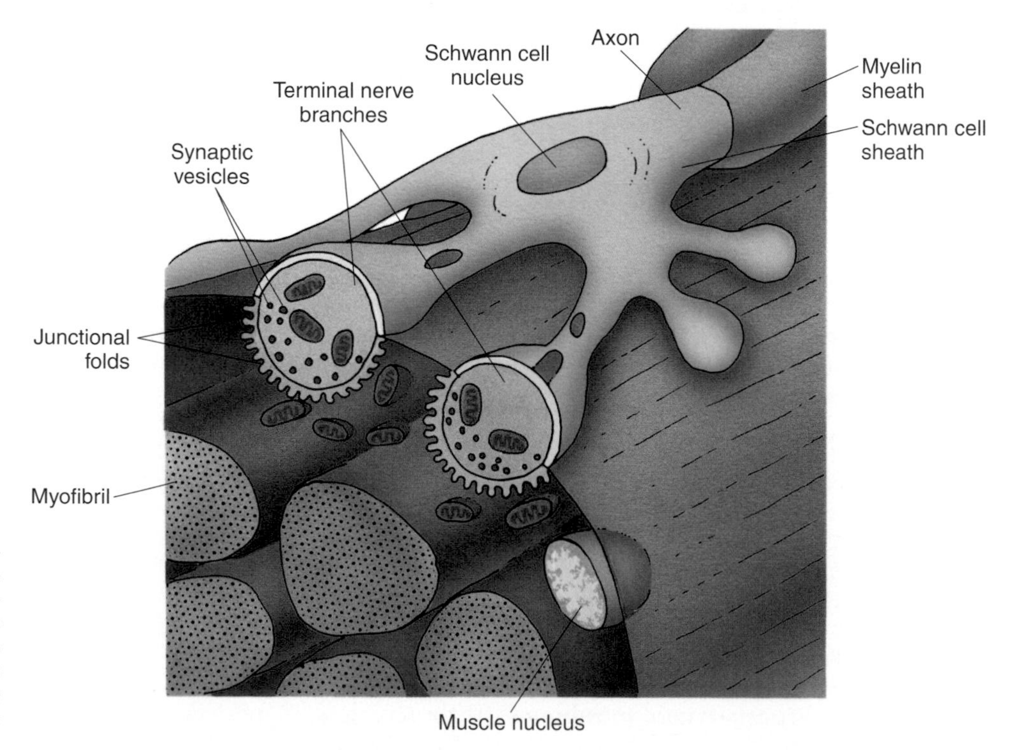

Fig. 8.17 Schematic diagram of the neuromuscular junction. Note that the myelin sheath *(yellow)* stops as the axon arborizes over the skeletal muscle fiber, but the Schwann cell sheath *(green)* continues to insulate the nerve fiber. The terminal nerve branches expand to form axon terminals that overlie the motor end plates of individual muscle fibers.

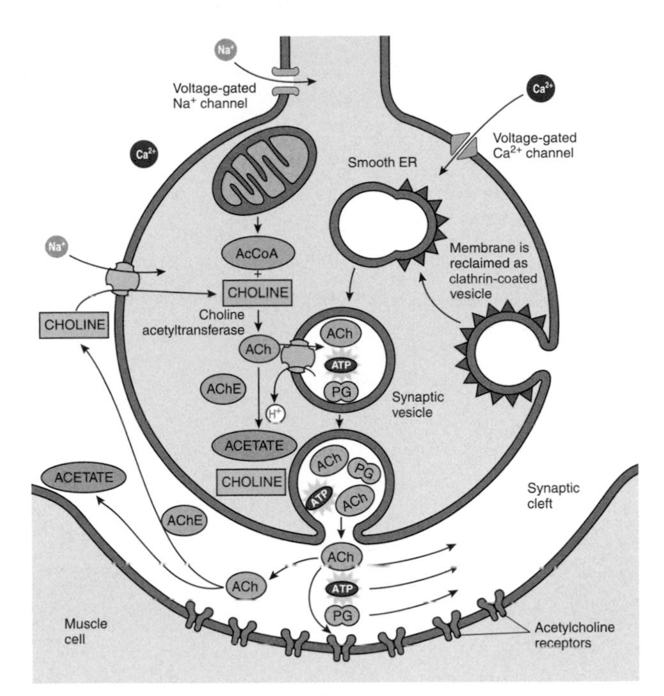

Fig. 8.18 Schematic diagram of the events occurring at the neuromuscular junction during the release of acetylcholine. AcCoA, Acetyl CoA; Ach, acetylcholine; AchE, acetylcholinesterase; ATP, adenosine triphosphate; Ca^{2+}, calcium ion; H^+, hydrogen ion; Na^+, sodium ion; PG, proteoglycan. (Modified from Katzung BG. *Basic and Clinical Pharmacology*. 4th ed. East Norwalk, CT: Appleton & Lange; 1989.)

In addition to recycling of choline, the synaptic vesicle membrane is recycled to conserve the surface area of the presynaptic membrane. This membrane recycling is accomplished by the formation of **clathrin-coated endocytotic vesicles**, which become the newly formed synaptic vesicles.

Clinical Correlations

Myasthenia gravis is an autoimmune disease in which autoantibodies attach to acetylcholine receptors, blocking their availability to acetylcholine. Receptors thus inactivated are endocytosed and replaced by new receptors, which are also inactivated by the autoantibodies. Thus, the number of locations for the initiation of muscle depolarization is reduced, and the skeletal muscles (including the diaphragm) weaken gradually. Certain ***neurotoxins****, such as the bungarotoxin of some poisonous snakes, also bind to acetylcholine receptors, causing paralysis and eventual death, owing to respiratory compromise.*

Botulism is usually caused by ingestion of improperly preserved canned foods. The toxin, produced by the microbe Clostridium botulinum*, interferes with the release of acetylcholine, with resultant muscle paralysis and, without treatment, death.*

When ***botulinum toxin type A*** *is injected into particular muscles, it inhibits the contraction of that muscle. For cosmetic purposes, the procerus and corrugator muscles are usually injected with Botox, diminishing the frown lines that the contraction of those facial muscles otherwise produce and, by eradicating the "wrinkles," make the face appear smoother and younger looking. It is interesting to note that, in 2012, almost 6 million Botox injections were performed in the United States for cosmetic purposes. The effect of the injections lasts for less than 3 months, and many patients repeat the procedure two to three times per year. There appear to be no serious side effects, although, if injected into the wrong muscles, ptosis (drooping) of the eyelids could persist for several months. Occasionally, individuals may have headaches; cold-like symptoms; nausea; and muscle weakness, pain, and inflammation in the area of the injection for as long as 4 months.*

MUSCLE SPINDLES AND GOLGI TENDON ORGANS

Muscle spindles and Golgi tendon organs are sensory receptors that monitor muscle contraction.

The neural control of muscle function requires not only the capability of inducing or inhibiting muscle contraction but also the ability to monitor the status of the muscle and its tendon during muscle activity. This monitoring is performed by two types of sensory receptors: **muscle spindles**, which provide feedback about the changes in muscle length, as well as the rate of alteration in muscle length; and **Golgi tendon organs**, which monitor the tension, as well as the rate at which the tension is being produced during movement.

The sensory feedback from these two sensory structures is generally processed at unconscious levels, within the spinal cord. The information also reaches the cerebellum and even the cerebral cortex so that the person may sense muscle position.

Muscle Spindles

Muscle spindles continuously monitor the length and changes in length of the muscle.

When a skeletal muscle is stretched, it normally undergoes reflex contraction, known as the **stretch reflex**. This proprioceptive response is initiated by the **muscle spindle**, an encapsulated sensory receptor located among, and in parallel with, the muscle cells (Fig. 8.19).

Each muscle spindle is composed of 8 to 10 modified skeletal muscle cells called ***intrafusal fibers***, surrounded by a fluid-containing **periaxial space**, which, in turn, is enclosed by a connective tissue **capsule** that is continuous with the collagen fibers of the perimysium and endomysium. The skeletal muscle fibers surrounding the muscle spindle are unremarkable and are called ***extrafusal fibers***.

Intrafusal fibers are of two types: **nuclear bag fibers** and the more numerous, thinner **nuclear chain fibers**. Furthermore, there are two categories of nuclear bag fibers: **static** and **dynamic**. The nuclei of both types of fibers occupy the centers of the cells; their myofibrils are located on either side of the nuclear region, limiting contraction to the polar regions of these spindle-shaped cells. The central regions of the intrafusal fibers do not contract. The nuclei are gathered together in the nuclear bag fibers, whereas they are aligned in a single row in nuclear chain fibers.

Within a specific muscle spindle, a single, myelinated, large, sensory nerve fiber (**group Ia**) wraps spirally around the

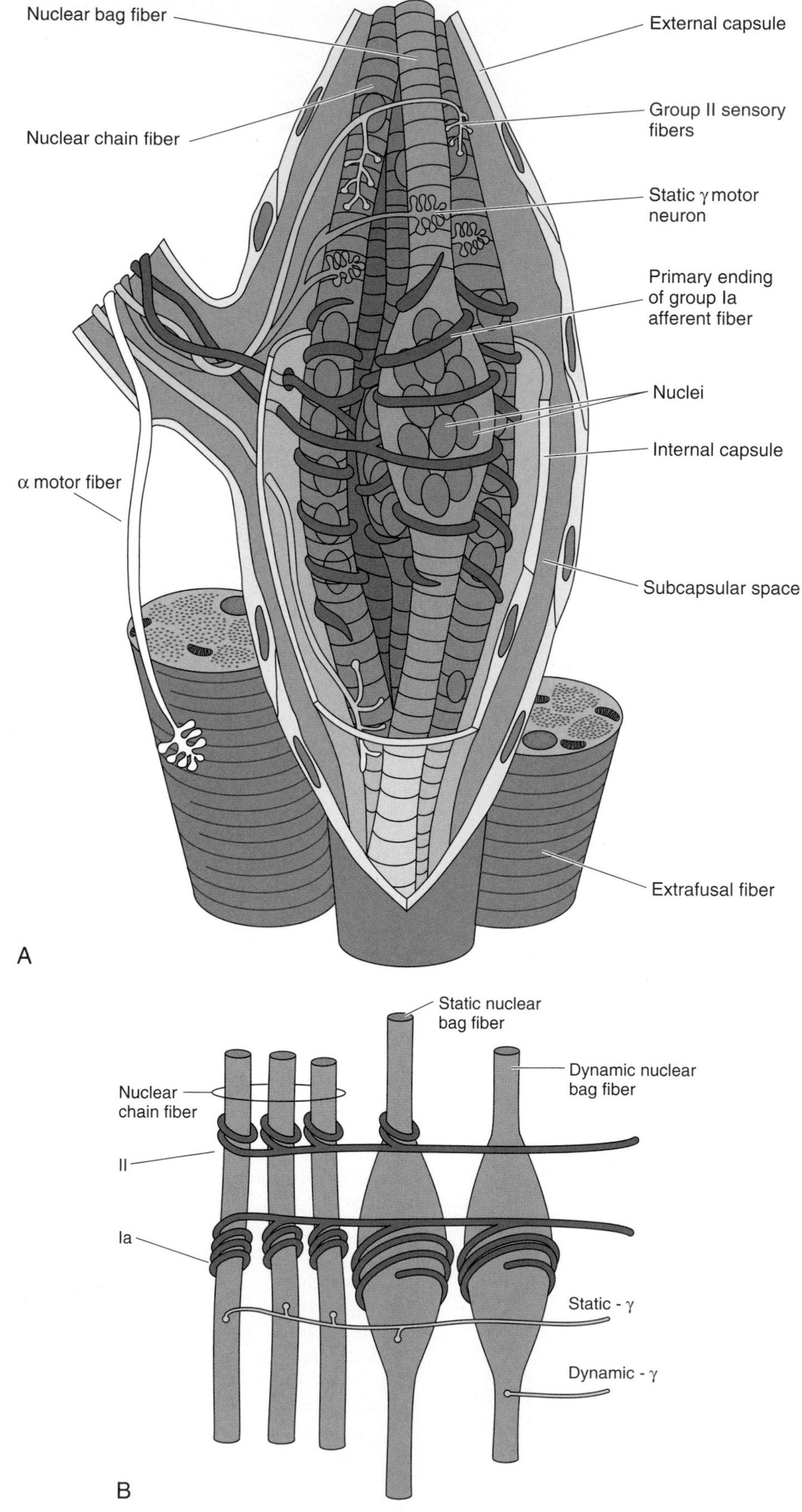

Fig. 8.19 (A) Schematic diagram of a muscle spindle. (B) The various fiber types of the muscle spindle and their innervation are presented in a spread-out fashion. Ia, Group Ia sensory fiber; II, group II sensory fiber. (A, Modified from Krstic RV. *Die Gewebe des Menschen und der Saugertiere.* Berlin: Springer-Verlag; 1978. B, Modified from Hulliger M. The mammalian muscle spindle and its central control. *Rev Physiol Biochem Pharmacol.* 1984;101:1-110.)

nuclear regions of each of the three types of intrafusal fibers, forming the **primary sensory endings** (also known as ***dynamic*** and ***Ia*** sensory endings). Additionally, **secondary sensory nerve endings** (also known as ***static*** and ***II*** sensory nerve endings) are formed by **group II** nerve fibers, which wrap around every nuclear chain fiber, as well as around the static nuclear bag fibers (see Fig. 8.19B).

The contractile regions of the intrafusal fibers receive two types of γ-motoneurons. Dynamic nuclear bag fibers are innervated by a **dynamic γ-motoneuron**, whereas all nuclear chain fibers, as well as all of the static nuclear bag fibers, are innervated by a **static γ-motoneuron** (see Fig. 8.19B).

The extrafusal fibers receive their normal nerve fibers, which are the large, rapidly conducting axons of **α-efferent neurons** (**motoneurons**).

As a muscle is stretched, the intrafusal muscle fibers of its muscle spindle are also stretched, causing the primary (group Ia, dynamic) and secondary (group II, static) sensory nerve fibers to initiate an action potential; with increased stretching, these nerve fibers accelerate their rate of firing. Both group Ia and group II fibers respond to a stretching of the muscle at a *constant rate* (**static response**). Only group Ia fibers, however, respond to a *change in the rate* (**phasic response**) at which stretching occurs, thus furnishing information concerning both the rapidity of movement and unanticipated stretching of the muscle.

Firing of the γ-motoneurons causes the polar regions of the intrafusal fibers to contract. When this occurs, the noncontractile regions of the intrafusal fibers are stretched from both directions, resulting in activation of the primary and secondary sensory nerve endings. Modulation of γ-motoneuron activity sensitizes the muscle spindle so that it can react even to a small degree of muscle stretching, as follows:

- Firing of dynamic γ-motoneurons primes the dynamic nerve endings but not the static nerve endings (because their firing does not cause contraction of the static nuclear bag fibers).
- Firing of static γ-motoneurons increases the continuous, steady response of both group Ia and group II sensory fibers (because both fibers form sensory nerve endings on static nuclear bag and all nuclear chain intrafusal fibers). However, the dynamic sensory fiber response decreases (because static γ-motoneurons do not innervate dynamic nuclear bag fibers).

Thus, modulation of the γ-motoneuron activity gives the nervous system the ability to adjust the sensitivity of the muscle spindle.

Clinical Correlations

*The **simple reflex arc**, such as the knee jerk, is an example of the function of muscle spindles. Tapping on the patellar tendon results in a sudden stretching of the muscle (and of the muscle spindles). The primary and secondary nerve endings are stimulated, relaying the stimulus to the **α-motoneurons of the spinal cord, resulting in muscle contraction**. Therefore, when a muscle is overstretched either too much or for too long a period of time, the muscle spindle reacts by stimulating muscle contraction to oppose the stretching.*

Golgi Tendon Organs (Neurotendinous Spindles)

Golgi tendon organs (neurotendinous spindles) monitor the intensity of muscle contraction.

Golgi tendon organs, also called **neurotendinous spindles**, are cylindrical structures about 1 mm in length and 0.1 mm in diameter. They are located at the juncture of a muscle, with its tendon, and are positioned in series with the muscle fibers. Golgi tendon organs are composed of **wavy collagen fibers** and the nonmyelinated continuation of a single **type Ib axon** that ramifies as free nerve endings in the interstices between the collagen fibers. Muscle contraction places tensile forces on the tendon's collagen fibers, straightening them, with a consequent compression and firing of the entwined nerve endings. The rate of firing is directly related to the amount of tension placed on the tendon.

Strenuous contraction of a muscle can generate a great amount of force that may damage not only the muscle but also its tendon and the bone to which it is attached. **Golgi tendon organs** provide an inhibitory feedback to the **α-efferent neurons** (**motoneurons**) of the muscle, resulting in relaxation of the contracting tendon's muscle and protection to all three elements. Thus, the Golgi tendon organs monitor the force of muscle contraction, whereas muscle spindles monitor the stretching of the muscle in which they are located. These two sensory organs act in concert to integrate spinal reflex systems.

Clinical Correlations

The ability of people to touch their nose in absolute darkness is due to the integrative activities of muscle spindles and, possibly, to Golgi tendon organs. These structures provide not only feedback about the amount of tension placed on the muscle and tendon but also input to the cerebellum and cerebral cortex, supplying information about the body's position in three-dimensional space. This ability is referred to as proprioception.

Cardiac Muscle

Cardiac muscle is nonvoluntary striated muscle limited to the heart and the proximal portions of the pulmonary veins.

Cardiac muscle (**heart muscle**), a nonvoluntary striated muscle, is located only in the heart and in that portion of the pulmonary veins where they join the heart. Cardiac muscle is derived from a strictly defined mass of splanchnic mesenchyme, the **myoepicardial mantle**, whose cells give rise to the **epicardium** and **myocardium**.

The adult myocardium consists of an anastomosing network of branching cardiac muscle cells arranged in layers (**laminae**). Laminae are separated from one another by slender connective tissue sheets that convey blood vessels, nerves, and the conducting system of the heart. Capillaries derived from these vessels invade the intercellular connective tissue, forming a rich, dense network of capillary beds surrounding every cardiac muscle cell, explaining the ability of these cells to use aerobic respiration for almost 90% of their energy supply.

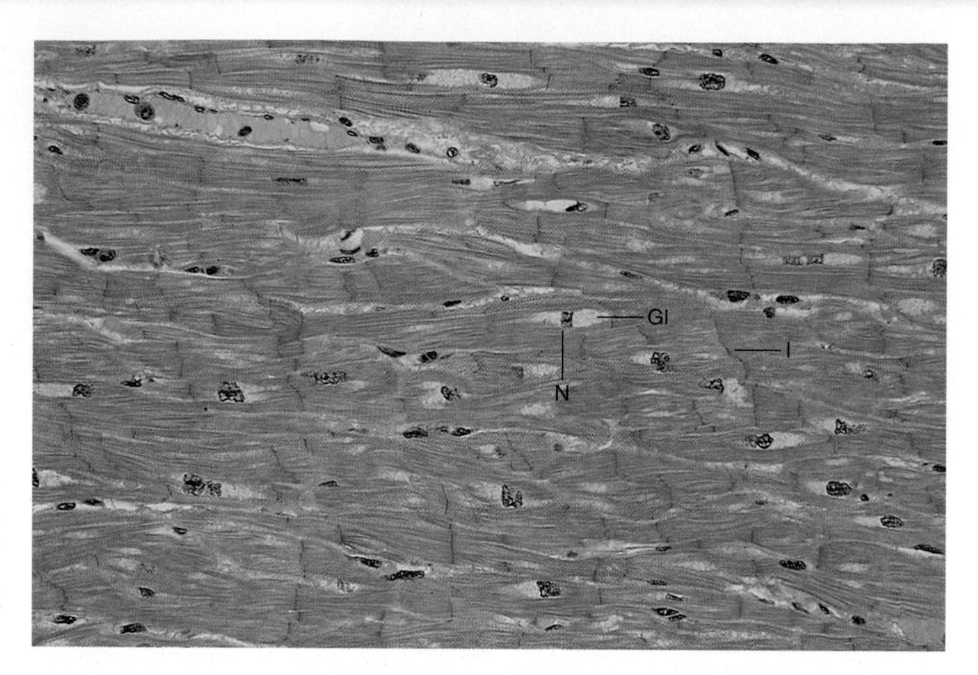

Fig. 8.20 Cardiac muscle cells in longitudinal section displaying their characteristic branching patterns and glycogen deposits (Gl). The branching of the cardiac muscle fibers, central location of the nuclei (N), and presence of intercalated disks (I) are identifying characteristics of cardiac muscle. (×270)

Cardiac muscle differs from skeletal and smooth muscles in that it possesses an **inherent rhythmicity** as well as the ability to **contract spontaneously**. A system of modified cardiac muscle cells has been adapted to ensure the coordination of its contractile actions. This specialized system, as well as the associated autonomic nerve supply, is discussed in Chapter 11.

Clinical Correlations

Cardiac amyloidosis *is a specific disease in which nonbranching, insoluble,* ***amyloid protein*** *forms clumps and accumulates in and causes expansion of the extracellular space between and among cardiac muscle cells. Although there are a number of amyloid proteins, most of the ones involved in cardiac amyloidosis originate from the light chains of antibodies and from transthyretin (TTR). TTR is the carrier protein that transports thyroxine (the thyroid hormone T_4) and retinol (vitamin A). There are three types of cardiac amyloidosis: light chain, familial, and senile, depending on the type of amyloid proteins present. The most frequently studied is* ***light chain cardiac amyloidosis****, in which the amyloid protein is derived from immunoglobulin lambda light chains produced in large quantities by clones of defective plasma cells. This condition starts relatively late in life, around 60 years of age, and affects more males than females. As these misfolded proteins accumulate in the extracellular space, they enlarge regions of the heart and interfere with normal cardiac function. The prognosis is not especially bad if it is detected early, proper therapeutic measures are engaged, and the treatment is able to reduce the number of defective plasma cell clones. However, in most cases, the patient succumbs to heart failure.* ***Familial cardiac amyloidosis*** *is due to mutations in the TRR gene, although other proteins may also be involved.* ***Senile cardiac amyloidosis*** *is also believed to be caused by a mutation in the TRR gene, but it is accompanied by carpal tunnel syndrome in men in their 70s or older.*

CARDIAC MUSCLE CELLS

Although the resting lengths of individual cardiac muscle cells vary, they are 15 μm in diameter and 80 μm long, on average. Each cell possesses a single large, oval, centrally placed nucleus, although two nuclei are occasionally present (Figs. 8.20 to 8.23).

Intercalated Disks

Cardiac muscle cells form highly specialized end-to-end junctions, referred to as *intercalated disks* (Figs. 8.24 to 8.26; see Fig. 8.21). The cell membranes involved in these junctions approximate each other so that, in most areas, they are separated by a space of less than 15 to 20 nm.

The **transverse portions** of intercalated disks have an abundance of fasciae adherentes and desmosomes and their **lateral portions** are rich in gap junctions (see Figs. 8.24 and 8.26). On the cytoplasmic aspect of the sarcolemma of intercalated disks, **thin myofilaments** attach to the fasciae adherentes, which are thus analogous to Z disks. Gap junctions are also present in regions where cardiac muscle cells lying side by side come in close contact with each other. Gap junctions facilitate synchronized contractions of cardiac muscle cells, which consequently form a **functional syncytium**.

Organelles

The extracellular fluid is the primary calcium source for cardiac muscle contraction.

The bandings of cardiac muscle fibers are identical with those of skeletal muscle, including alternating I and A bands. Each sarcomere possesses the same substructure as its skeletal muscle counterpart; therefore, the mode and mechanism of contraction are virtually identical in the two striated muscles. However, in

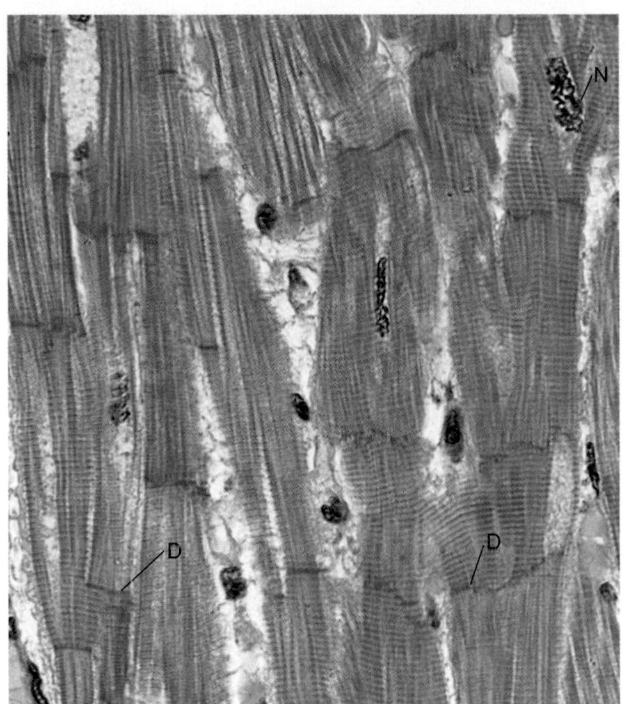

Fig. 8.21 Photomicrograph of cardiac muscle in longitudinal section. Note the nucleus (N) and presence of intercalated disks (D), regions where the cardiac muscle cells form desmosomes, fasciae adherents, and gap junctions with each other. (×540)

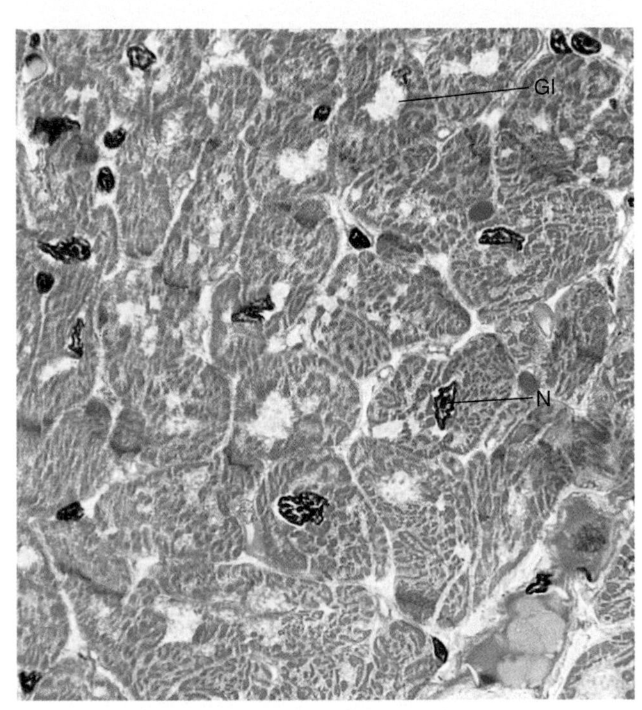

Fig. 8.23 Photomicrograph of cardiac muscle in cross-section. The nucleus (N) is centrally located and, at each pole of the nucleus, the glycogen deposits (Gl) have been extracted during the histological preparation. (×540)

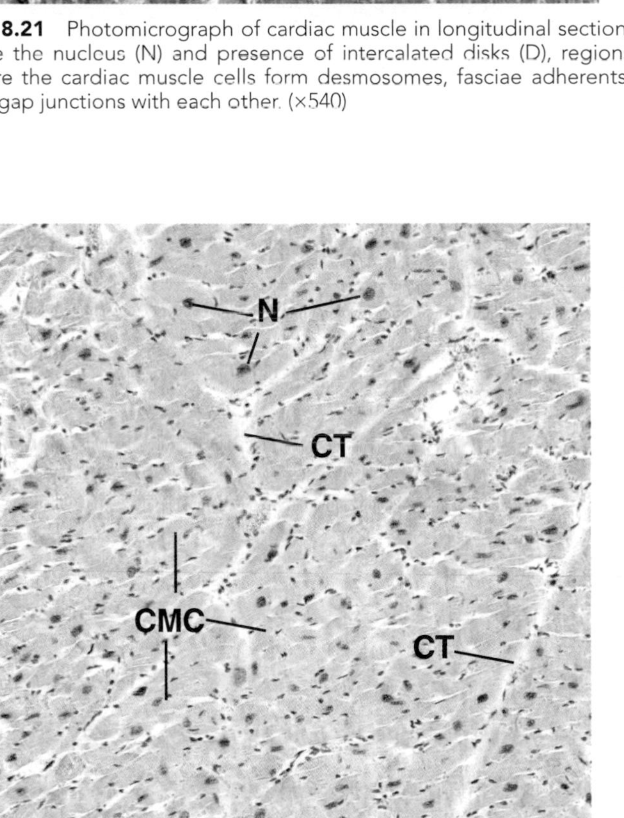

Fig. 8.22 This low-magnification photomicrograph of cardiac muscle cross-section demonstrates that each cardiac muscle cell has a centrally placed nucleus and that the muscle fiber bundles are surrounded by connective tissue septa (CT) in which smaller nuclei of endothelial cells and fibroblasts are clearly evident. (×132)

skeletal muscle, the **nebulin molecules** extend along the entire length of the thin filament all the way to the H zone, whereas, in cardiac muscle, the nebulin extends only about 20% of the length of the thin filament, far short of the H zone. There are several other major differences involving the sarcoplasmic reticulum, arrangement of T tubules, Ca^{2+} supply of cardiac muscle, ion channels of the plasmalemma, and duration of the action potential.

The sarcoplasmic reticulum of cardiac muscle is sparse and it does not form terminal cisternae; instead, there are small terminals of sarcoplasmic reticulum that possess **ryanodine receptors** and are referred to as ***corbular sarcoplasmic reticulum***. These structures approximate the T tubules but do not normally form a triad, as in skeletal muscle. Rather, the association is usually limited to two partners, resulting in a **dyad**. Unlike in skeletal muscle, where the triads are located at the A-I interfaces, the dyads in cardiac muscle cells are located in the vicinity of the Z disk. The T tubules of cardiac muscle cells are almost 2.5 times the diameter of those in skeletal muscle and, unlike in skeletal muscle fibers, they are lined by an **external lamina**.

The sparsity of the sarcoplasmic reticulum prevents it from storing enough calcium to accomplish a forceful contraction. Therefore, additional sources of calcium are necessary, which is provided by T tubules that open into the extracellular space and have relatively large lumina. Extracellular calcium flows through the T tubules and can enter cardiac muscle cells at the time of depolarization. Additionally, the negatively charged external lamina coating of the T tubule stores calcium for instantaneous release. An additional method whereby calcium can enter the cardiac muscle cells is through the large **calcium-sodium channels** described next.

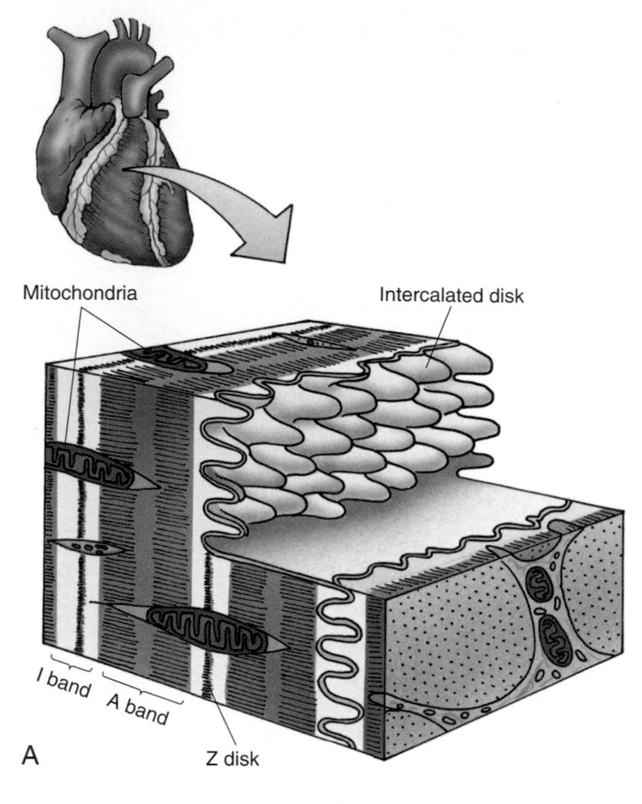

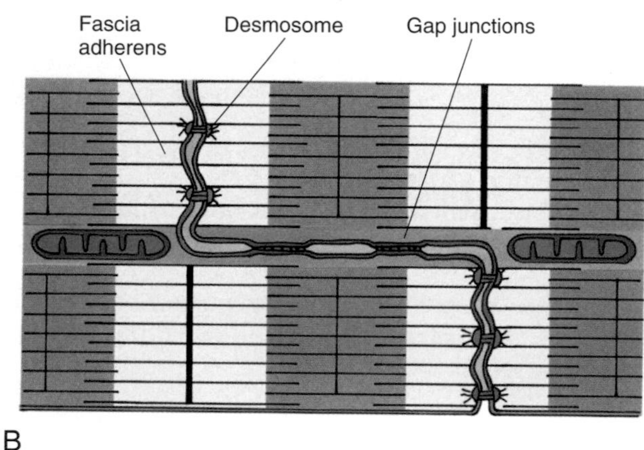

Fig. 8.24 Schematic diagram of cardiac muscle. (A) Three-dimensional view of the intercalated disk. (B) Two-dimensional view of the intercalated disk with a display of adhering and communicating junctions. The transverse portions of the intercalated disk act as a Z disk, and thin filaments are embedded in them.

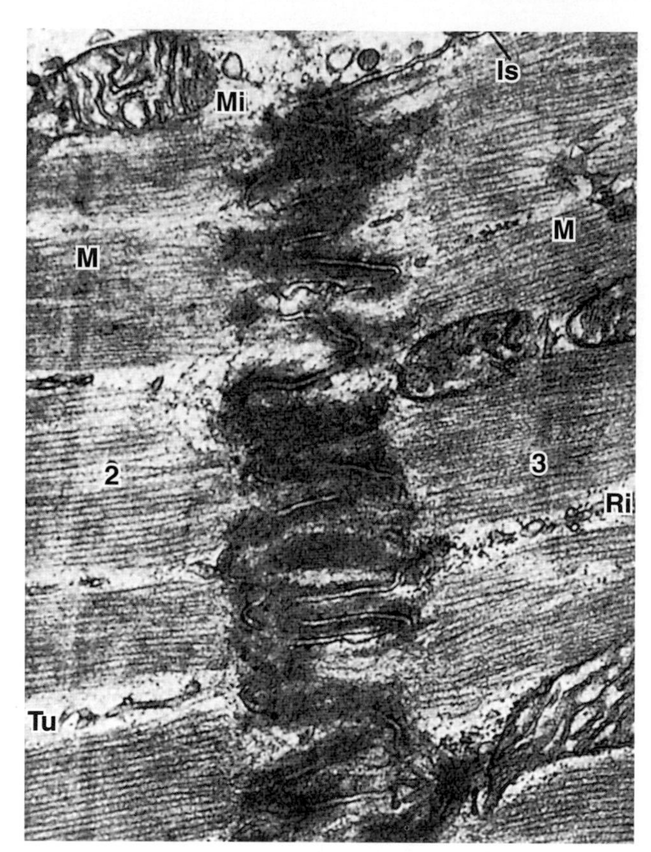

Fig. 8.25 Electron micrograph of an intercalated disk from a steer heart (×29,622). Is, Intercellular space; M, M-line; Mi, mitochondrion; Ri, ribosomes; Tu, sarcoplasmic reticulum. Numbers 2 and 3 denote the two cells, one on either side of the intercalated disk. (From Rhodin JAG. *An Atlas of Ultrastructure*. Philadelphia: WB Saunders; 1963.)

Cardiac muscle cell membranes possess, in addition to fast sodium channels, **calcium-sodium channels (slow sodium channels)**. Although these channels are slow to open initially, they remain open for a considerable period of time (several tenths of a second). During this time, a remarkable number of sodium and calcium ions can enter the cardiac muscle cell cytoplasm, increasing the calcium ion concentration supplied by the T tubule and the sarcoplasmic reticulum. Egress of potassium ions from cardiac muscle cells is impeded, resulting in a protracted action potential. When contraction is over, the calcium ions are returned to the sarcoplasmic reticulum. This process is controlled by **phospholamban**, an integral protein in the sarcoplasmic reticulum of cardiac muscle that is the principal target for phosphorylation by cyclic adenosine monophosphate **(cAMP)-dependent protein kinase**. When phospholamban is *not phosphorylated*, it inhibits the **calcium pump** of the sarcoplasmic reticulum, and *calcium ions cannot return into the sarcoplasmic reticulum*. However, when *phospholamban is phosphorylated* by cAMP-dependent protein kinase, its conformation alters and permits the **calcium pumps** of the sarcoplasmic reticulum to *open*, and calcium can leave the cytosol and enter the sarcoplasmic reticulum, causing *relaxation of the cardiac muscle cell*. Therefore, *phospholamban regulates relaxation of cardiac muscle and, in that fashion, is responsible for regulating* ***diastole***.

Almost half of the volume of the cardiac muscle cell is occupied by mitochondria, attesting to its great energy consumption. During basal heart rate, triglycerides form approximately 60% of the energy supply of the heart, and only about 40% is derived from glycogen. Because the oxygen requirement of cardiac muscle cells is high, they contain an abundant supply of the oxygen-binding molecule myoglobin.

Muscle cells of the atria are somewhat smaller than those of the ventricles. These cells house granules (especially in the right atrium) containing **atrial natriuretic peptide (ANP)** and cardiac muscle cells of ventricles house granules containing **B-type natriuretic peptide (BNP)**, substances that function to lower blood pressure (Fig. 8.27). These peptides act by decreasing the capabilities of renal tubules to resorb (conserve) sodium and water and also by interfering with vasoconstriction, thus further decreasing blood pressure. There is also a C-type natriuretic peptide that is manufactured by endothelial cells of

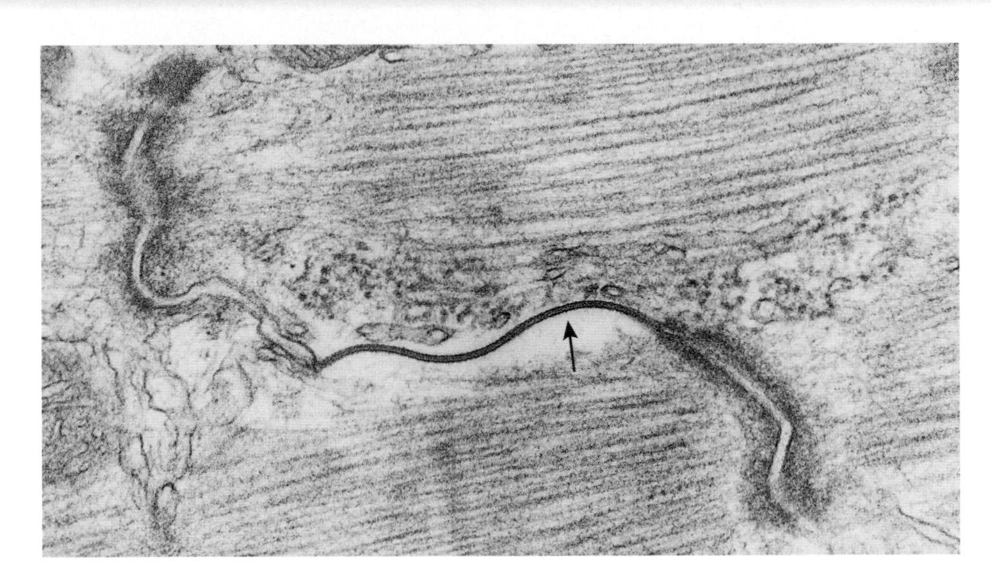

Fig. 8.26 Intercalated disk from the atrium of a mouse heart (×57,810). The *arrow* points to gap junctions. (From Forbes MS, Sperelakis N. Intercalated disks of mammalian heart: a review of structure and function. *Tissue Cell*. 1985;17:605.)

cardiac blood vessels but, unlike ANP and BNP, it acts to reduce blood pressure in an indirect fashion.

Clinical Correlations

1. *During **cardiac hypertrophy**, the number of myocardial fibers is not increased. Instead, the cardiac muscle cells become longer and larger in diameter. Damage to the heart results in limited regeneration of muscle tissue; however, most dead muscle cells are replaced by fibrous connective tissue.*
2. *Lack of Ca^{2+} in the extracellular compartment results in cessation of cardiac muscle contraction within 1 minute, whereas skeletal muscle fibers can continue to contract for several hours.*
3. *Although a small amount of energy production may be achieved by anaerobic metabolism (up to 10% during hypoxia), totally anaerobic conditions cannot sustain ventricular contraction.*

Smooth Muscle

The cells of the third type of muscle exhibit no striations; therefore, they are referred to as ***smooth muscle***. Additionally, smooth muscle cells do not possess a system of T tubules. Smooth muscle is found in the walls of hollow viscera (e.g., the gastrointestinal tract, some of the reproductive tract, and the urinary tract), walls of blood vessels, larger ducts of compound glands, respiratory passages, and small bundles within the dermis of skin. Smooth muscle is not under voluntary control; it is regulated by the autonomic nervous system, hormones (such as bradykinins), and local physiological conditions. Hence, smooth muscle is also referred to as ***involuntary muscle***.

There are two types of smooth muscle:

- Cells of **multiunit smooth muscle** can contract independently of one another, because each muscle cell has its own nerve supply.
- Cell membranes of **unitary** (**single-unit**, **visceral**) **smooth muscle** form **gap junctions** with those of contiguous smooth muscle cells, and nerve fibers form synapses with only a few of the muscle fibers. Thus, cells of unitary smooth muscle cannot contract independently of one another.

*In addition to its contractile functions, some smooth muscle is capable of exogenous **protein synthesis**.* Among the substances manufactured by smooth muscle cells for extracellular utilization are collagen, elastin, glycosaminoglycans, proteoglycans, and growth factors.

LIGHT MICROSCOPY OF SMOOTH MUSCLE FIBERS

Light microscopy reveals that smooth muscle fibers are short, spindle shaped cells with a centrally placed nucleus.

Smooth muscle fibers are **fusiform**, elongated cells whose average length is about 0.2 mm, with a diameter of 5 to 6 μm at its thickest region. The cells taper at both ends, and the expanded central portion contains an oval nucleus, housing two or more nucleoli (Figs. 8.28 and 8.29; see Fig. 8.3).

The cytoplasm of smooth muscle fibers appears unremarkable when stained with H&E; but when stained with iron hematoxylin, the cytoplasmic aspect of the sarcolemma displays the presence of **dense bodies**. Using the same stain, the smooth muscle cell cytoplasm displays thin, longitudinal striations, which represent conglomerates of **myofilaments**.

Although smooth muscle cells may occur as individual cells, they usually form sheets of various thicknesses. The smooth muscle cells are arranged, in these sheets, to form a continuous network in which the tapered portions fit almost precisely into existing spaces between the expanded regions of neighboring cells (see Fig. 8.3). In cross-section, outlines of various diameters may be noted, some containing nuclei, some not (Figs. 8.30 to 8.32). Cross-sections without nuclei represent the tapered ends of smooth muscle cells as they interdigitate with the other smooth muscle fibers.

Sheets of smooth muscle cells are frequently arranged in two layers oriented perpendicular to each other, as in the digestive and urinary systems. This arrangement permits waves of peristalsis to be established.

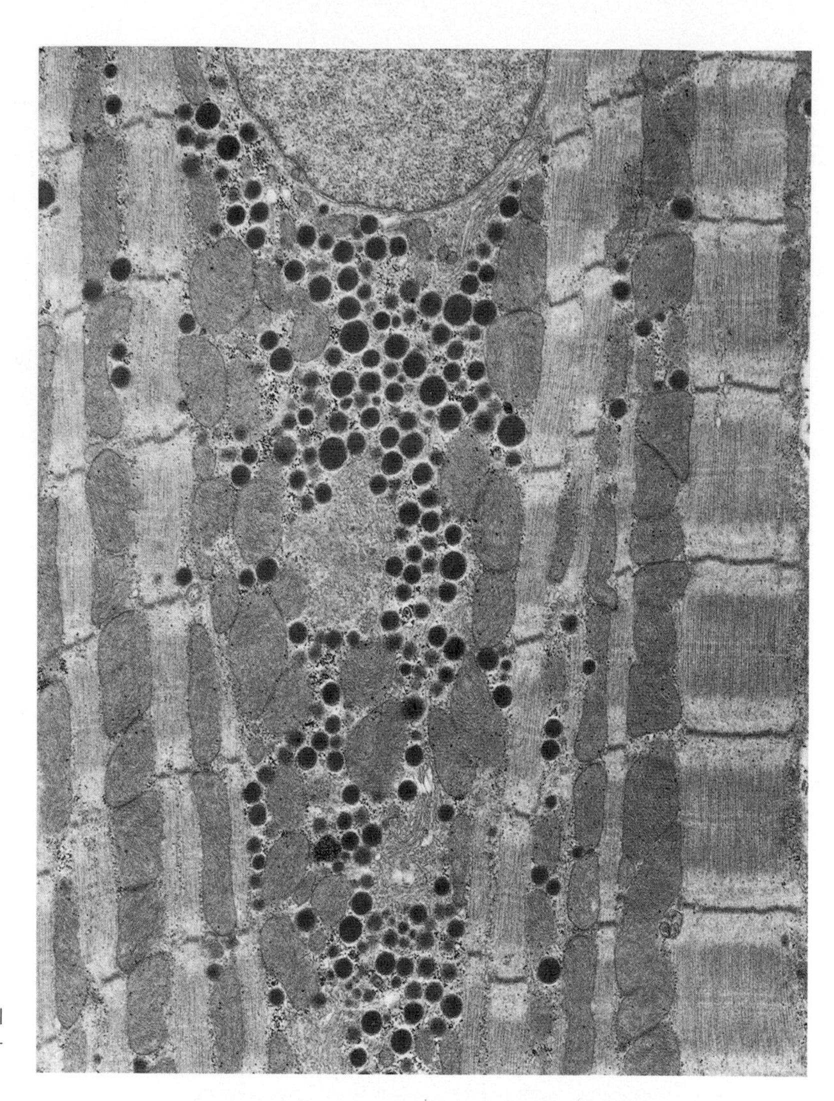

Fig. 8.27 Electron micrograph of a rat atrial muscle cell (×14,174). Observe the secretory granules containing atrial natriuretic peptide. (Courtesy Dr. Stephen C. Pang.)

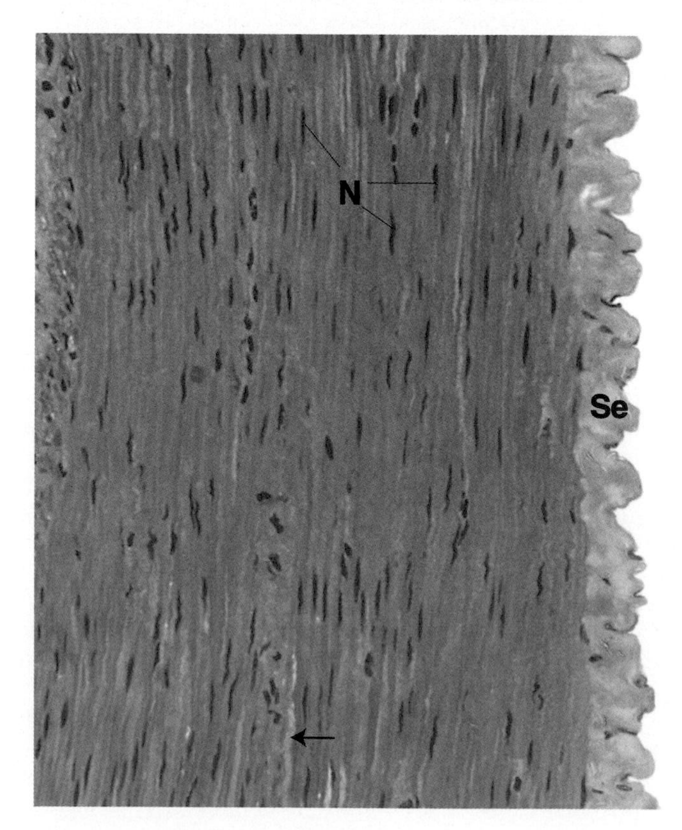

Fig. 8.28 This low-magnification photomicrograph of a longitudinal section of smooth muscle is from the muscularis externa of a monkey duodenum. Observe the serosa (Se) covering the smooth muscle layer whose nuclei (N) are elongated. Slender connective tissue strands *(arrow)* carry vascular and neural elements to the smooth muscle cells. (×132)

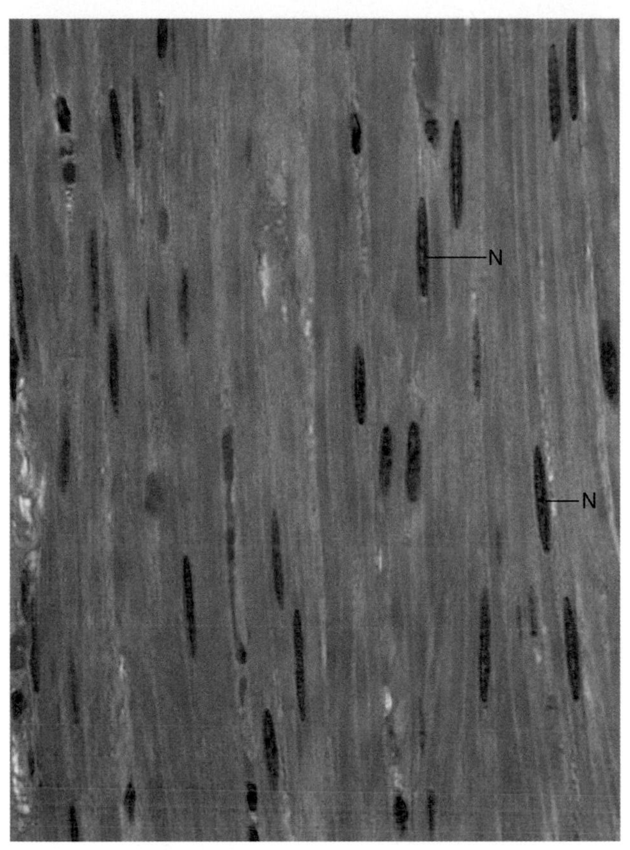

Fig. 8.29 Photomicrograph of smooth muscle in longitudinal section. Note that the nuclei (N) are located in the midline of the cell but off center so that they are closer to one lateral cell membrane than to the other. Observe that the nuclei are not corkscrew shaped, indicating that the muscle is not undergoing contraction. (×540)

During muscle contraction, the nucleus assumes a characteristic corkscrew appearance as a result of the method of smooth muscle contraction (Fig. 8.33).

Clinical Correlations

***Leiomyoma**, a benign tumor of smooth muscle cells, usually occurs in vascular channels or the alimentary canal. Most commonly, it affects the small intestine and esophagus of 30- to 60-year-old adults, where it presents as small lumps of smooth muscle cells. When this condition is present in the alimentary canal, it is usually treated by electrocautery or surgery.*

Leiomyosarcoma (LMS) is an infrequent malignant tumor of smooth muscle cells that occurs in 1/10,000 people in the United States, in a larger proportion of women than men. There are various types of LMS depending on their location—there can be cutaneous, uterine, gastrointestinal, and vascular leiomyosarcomas. The tumors are usually larger than and not nearly as hard as leiomyomas, and their histology may display necrotic and hemorrhagic regions. If caught early, surgical excision is the preferred method of treatment, followed by chemotherapy. If surgical treatment is delayed, metastasis may occur even 10 to 15 years subsequent to the excision of the primary tumor. Therefore, prognosis for long-term survival of leiomyosarcoma patients is not very favorable.

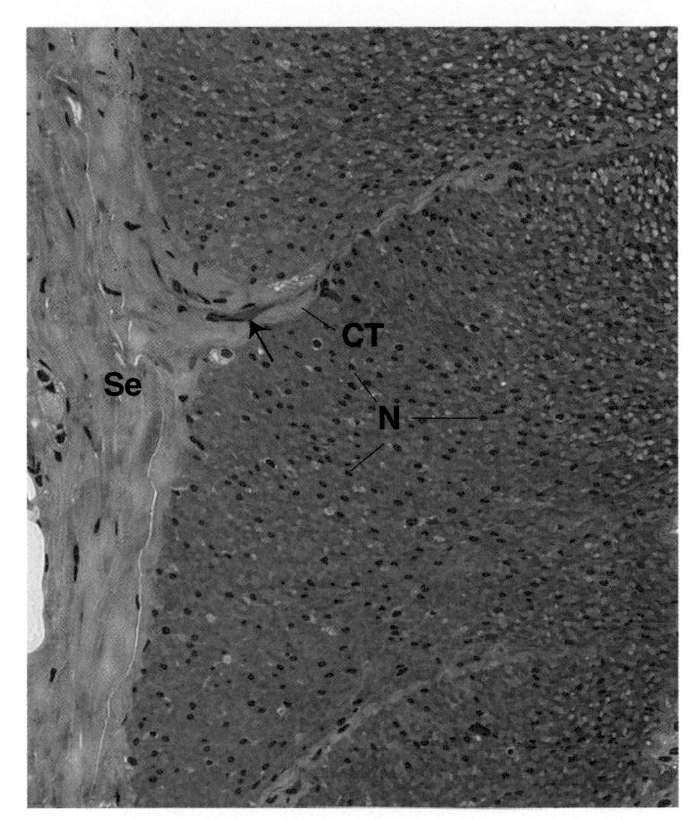

Fig. 8.30 Low-magnification photomicrograph of the muscularis externa of a monkey duodenum displaying a cross-section of smooth muscle cells. Observe that the serosa (Se) sends connective tissue septa (CT) conveying nerve fibers and blood vessels *(arrow)* to the smooth muscle cells, whose nuclei (N) appear as dark dots scattered throughout the muscle tissue. (×132)

FINE STRUCTURE OF SMOOTH MUSCLE

Transmission electron microscopy demonstrates the presence of organelles at either pole of the nucleus and displays the external lamina surrounding the muscle cell.

The regions adjacent to the two poles of the nucleus house much of the organelles, including the Golgi apparatus, rough and smooth endoplasmic reticulum, numerous mitochondria, inclusions such as glycogen. and an extensive array of interweaving thin filaments 7 nm in diameter and thick filaments 15 nm in diameter (Figs. 8.34 and 8.35A and 8.35B). The thin filaments are composed of F actin, caldesmon, tropomyosin, and calponin. Caldesmon, in concert with tropomyosin, blocks the active site of G-actin. Calponin is a protein that inhibits myosin ATPase, similar to troponin in striated muscle. The thick filaments are composed of the same myosin II as present in striated muscle.

Myofilaments of smooth muscle are not arranged in the paracrystalline fashion of striated muscle, nor is the organization of the thick filaments the same. Instead, the myosin II molecules are lined up so that the **heavy meromyosin heads** (S_1) project from the thick filaments throughout the length of the filament, with the two ends lacking heavy meromyosin. The middle of the filament, unlike that of striated muscle, also possesses heavy meromyosin, thus resulting in the availability of a larger surface area for the interaction of actin with myosin II and permitting **contractions of long duration**. Unlike in skeletal muscle, instead of 6 thin filaments, approximately 15 thin

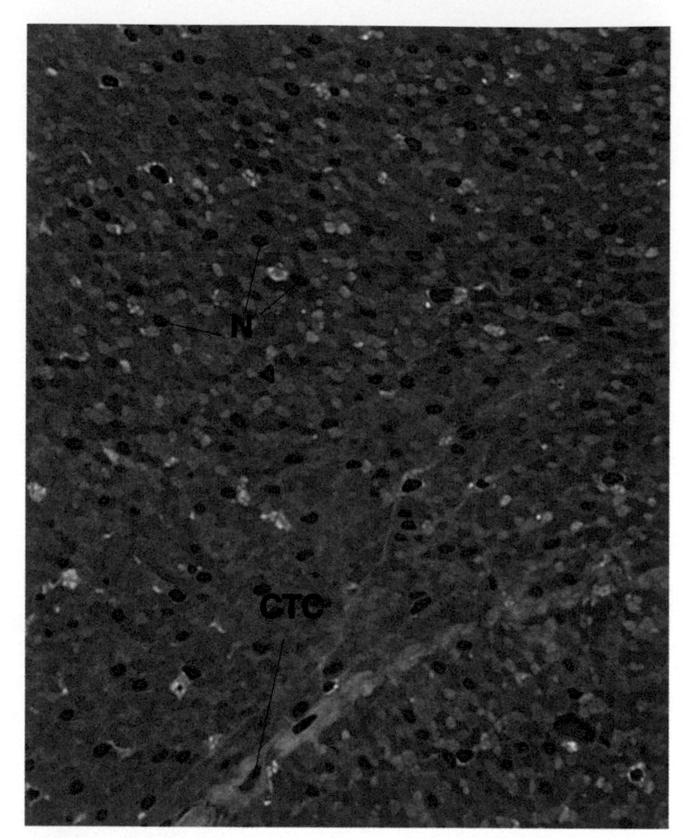

Fig. 8.31 Medium-magnification photomicrograph of the muscularis externa of a monkey duodenum displaying cross-section of smooth muscle cells. Note that the connective tissue elements house capillaries (CTC) that supply blood flow to the smooth muscle cells, whose nuclei (N) occupy the center of the smooth muscle fibers. (×270)

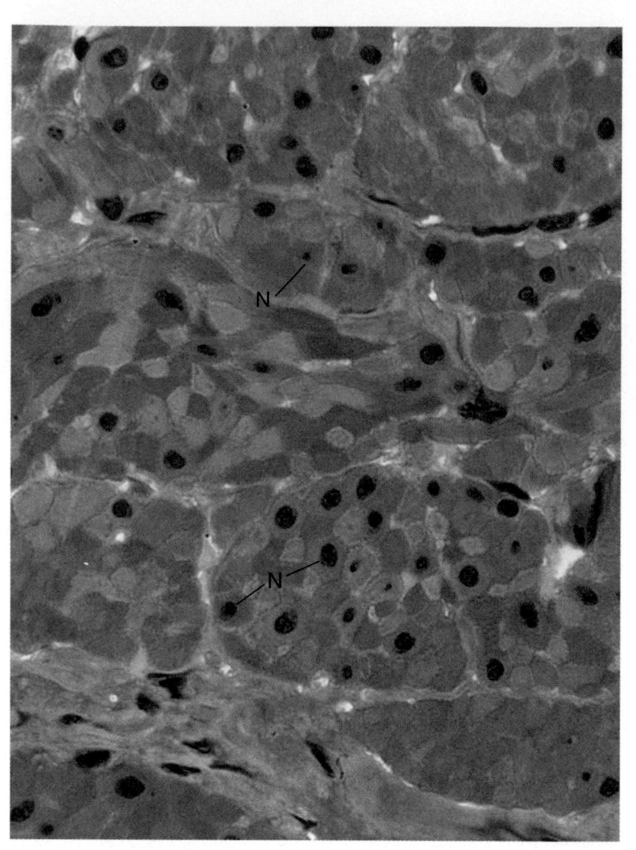

Fig. 8.32 Photomicrograph of smooth muscle in cross-section. Observe that the nuclei (N) are of various diameters, indicating that they are spindle shaped and that they have been sectioned at various regions along their length. Also, knowing that the nucleus of the cell is located at its center and that the cell is much longer than the nucleus, it is reasonable to expect that there will be many smooth muscle cells in the field that do not display their nuclei because they have been sectioned along regions of the cell that are away from the center. (×540)

filaments surround each thick filament. When smooth muscle is in its relaxed state, the myosin II molecules are unable to contact the thin filaments because their light meromyosin moieties are folded over and are bound to their own heavy meromyosin component, effectively masking that region of the heavy meromyosin that would bind to the **active site** of the actin molecules (Figs. 8.36 and 8.37).

The all-or-none law for striated muscle contraction does not apply to smooth muscle. The entire cell, or only a portion of the cell, may contract at a given instant even though the method of contraction is believed to follow the sliding filament theory of contraction.

The contractile forces are harnessed intracellularly by a system of intermediate filaments, which consist of **vimentin** and **desmin** in unitary smooth muscle (visceral smooth muscle) and **desmin** (only) in multiunit smooth muscle (nonvisceral smooth muscle). These intermediate filaments, as well as thin filaments, insert into **dense bodies**, formed of **α-actinin** and other Z disk–associated proteins. Dense bodies may be located in the cytoplasm or associated with the cytoplasmic aspect of the smooth muscle sarcolemma. They are believed to resemble Z disks in function and, in three dimensions, may even be more extensive than formerly assumed in that they form interconnected branching networks that extend throughout the cytoplasm. The force of contraction is relayed, through the association of myofilaments with dense bodies, to the intermediate filaments, which act to twist and shorten the cell along its longitudinal axis.

Associated with the cell membrane domains are structures known as ***caveolae***, small endocytotic vesicles that act, among

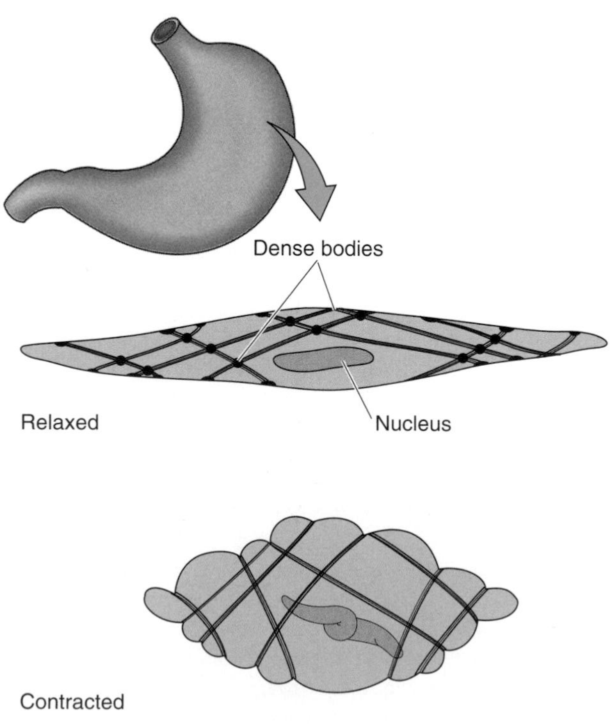

Fig. 8.33 Schematic diagram of a relaxed smooth muscle cell and a contracted smooth muscle cell. Note that, in a contracted smooth muscle cell, the nucleus appears to be corkscrew shaped.

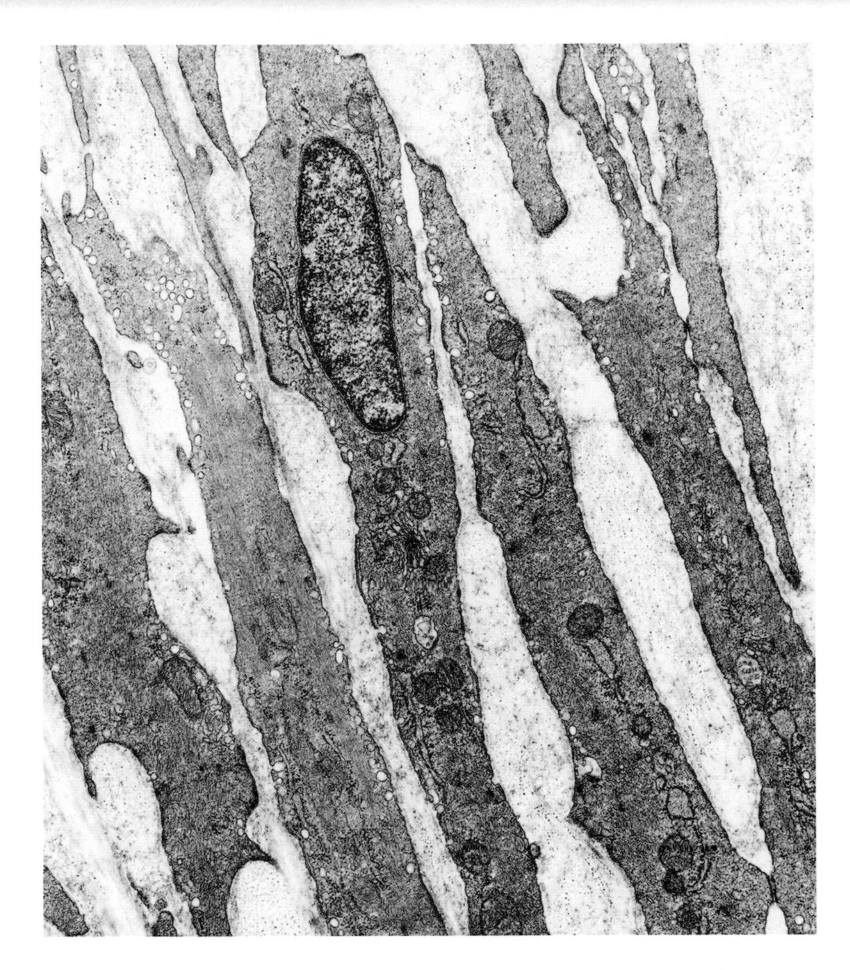

Fig. 8.34 Electron micrograph of smooth muscle cells. (Courtesy Dr. J. Strum.)

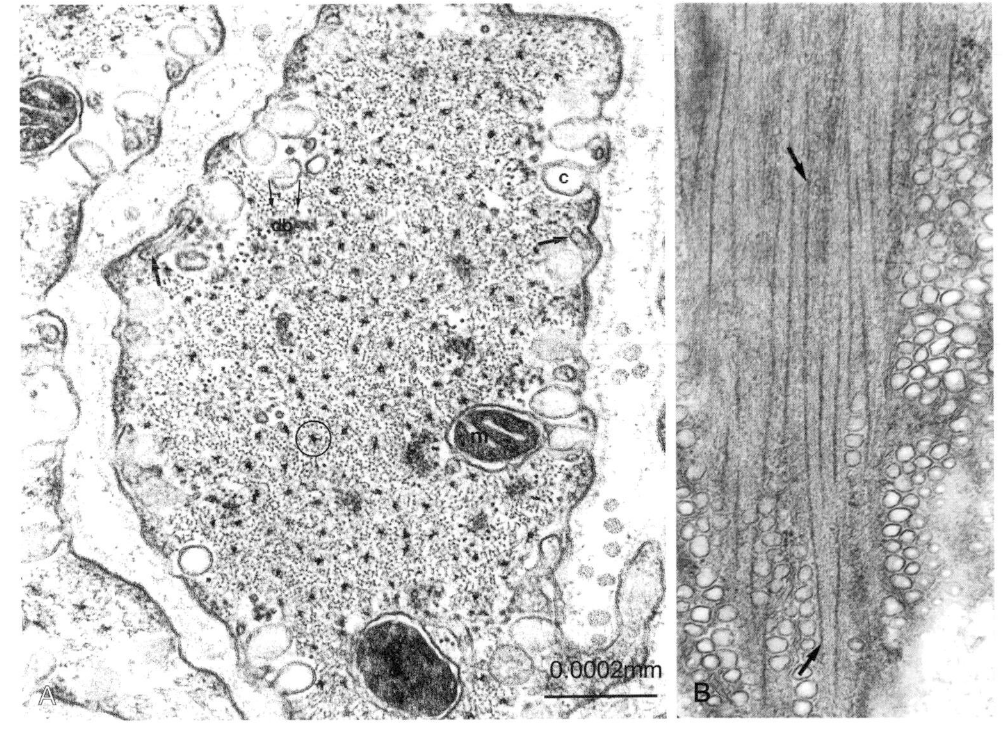

Fig. 8.35 (A) An electron micrograph of a transverse section of a smooth muscle cell in rabbit vas deferens showing a regular array of thick myosin filaments surrounded by actin filaments *(circle)*, intermediate filaments associated with dense bodies *(small arrows)*, elements of sarcoplasmic reticulum forming surface couplings with the plasma membrane *(single arrow)*, flask-shaped caveolae at the plasma membrane (c) and mitochondria (m). (Courtesy Dr. Avril V. Somlyo.) (B) An electron micrograph of a longitudinal section near the surface of smooth muscle cells in the rabbit portal mesenteric vein. A 2.3-μm long myosin filament (each end marked by *arrows*) is completely included in the section (×50,000). (From Somlyo AV. Smooth muscle myosin filament controversy, once again? *J Physiol.* 2015 Jan 15;593(2):473-475.)

other functions, as T tubules of skeletal and cardiac muscle in regulating the cytosolic-free calcium ion concentration.

Each smooth muscle cell is surrounded by an **external lamina**, which invariably separates the sarcolemmae of contiguous muscle cells from each other (see Fig. 8.34). Embedded in the external lamina are numerous **reticular fibers**, which appear to envelop individual smooth muscle cells and function in harnessing the force of contraction.

Control of Smooth Muscle Contraction

Smooth muscle cells contract slower and for a longer duration than do skeletal muscle fibers.

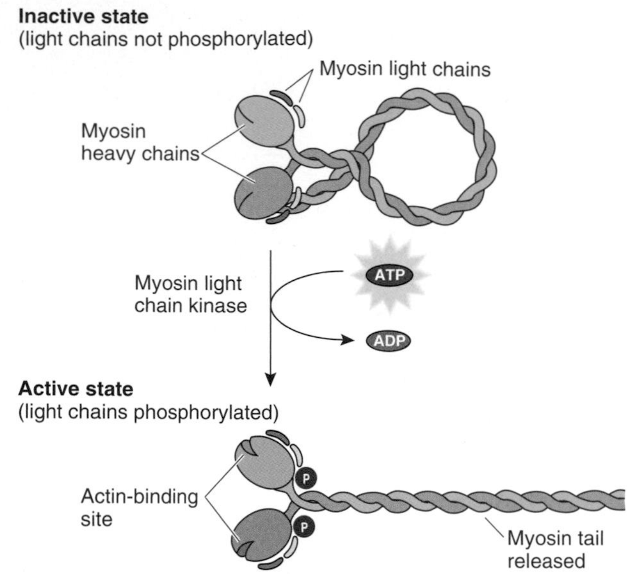

Fig. 8.36 Schematic diagram of activation of a myosin molecule of smooth muscle. ADP, Adenosine diphosphate; ATP, adenosine triphosphate; P, myosin light chain bound phosphate. (Modified from Alberts B, Bray D, Lewis J, et al. *Molecular Biology of the Cell*. New York: Garland Publishing; 1994. Reprinted with permission from Taylor & Francis, Inc./Routledge, Inc.)

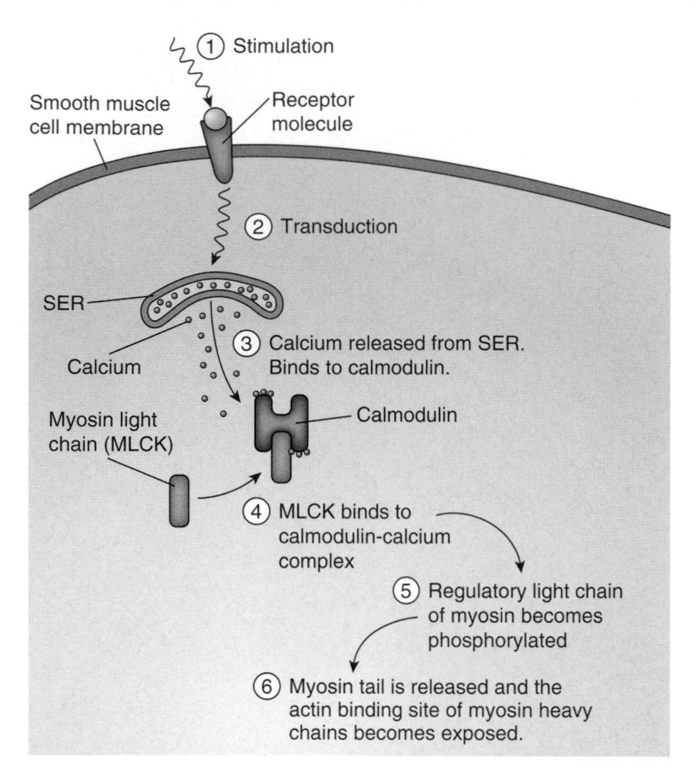

Fig. 8.37 Artist rendering of the steps leading to the phosphorylation of the regulatory light chain that permits the activation of the myosin molecule (see Fig. 8.36).

Although the regulation of contraction in smooth muscle depends on Ca^{2+}, the control mechanism differs from that encountered in striated muscle because smooth muscle thin filaments are devoid of troponin. Additionally, myosin II molecules of relaxed smooth muscle cells assume a different configuration in that their actin binding site is masked by their light meromyosin moiety and their light chains are different from those of striated muscle.

Contraction of smooth muscle fibers proceeds as follows (see Figs. 8.36 and 8.37):

1. Calcium ions, released from the sarcoplasmic reticulum and brought into the cell by caveolae, bind to **calmodulin** (a regulatory protein ubiquitous in living organisms), altering its conformation.
2. The calmodulin-Ca ion complex binds to **myosin light chain kinase** (**MLCK**), which phosphorylates the **regulatory light chain** of the myosin molecule.
3. The phosphorylated regulatory light chain permits the myosin molecule to unfold and interact with other unfolded myosin molecules to assemble, forming a temporary thick filament.
4. The protein **caldesmon**, in concert with tropomyosin, conceals the **active site** of the G actin molecules of the thin filament. However, in the presence of free calcium ions, caldesmon alters its conformation, revealing the active site of G actin molecules. Also, in the presence of calcium ions, another molecule, **calponin**, becomes phosphorylated and loses its ability to inhibit muscle contraction.
5. The phosphorylated light chain permits the interaction between actin and the S_1 subfragment of myosin II that results in contraction.
6. Because both phosphorylation and the attachment-detachment of the myosin cross-bridges occur slowly, the process of smooth muscle contraction takes longer than skeletal or cardiac muscle contraction. ATP hydrolysis also occurs much more slowly, and the myosin heads remain attached to the thin filaments for a longer time in smooth muscle than in striated muscles. Thus, smooth muscle contraction not only is *prolonged* but also requires *less energy*.
7. Smooth muscle cell contraction continues until the cytoplasmic calcium level is decreased, which results in the dissociation of the **calmodulin–calcium complex**, causing inactivation of myosin light chain kinase. The subsequent **dephosphorylation of myosin light chain**, catalyzed by the enzyme **myosin phosphatase**, brings about **masking** of the myosin's actin binding site and subsequent **relaxation** of the muscle.

INNERVATION OF SMOOTH MUSCLE

There are two types of smooth muscle innervations: multiunit and unitary.

Neuromuscular junctions in smooth muscle are not as specifically organized as those in skeletal muscle. The synapses may vary from 15 to 100 nm in width. The neural component of the synapse is the **en passant** type, which occurs as axonal swellings that contain **synaptic vesicles**, housing either **norepinephrine** for sympathetic innervation or **acetylcholine** for parasympathetic innervation.

In certain cases, every cell of a smooth muscle receives individual innervation, as in the iris and the vas deferens; smooth muscle innervated in this fashion is referred to as ***multiunit***. In other muscle cells, such as those of the gastrointestinal tract and uterus, only a few muscle cells have neuromuscular junctions. Innervation in this fashion is referred to as ***unitary*** (***single-unit*** or ***visceral smooth muscles***), and impulse conduction occurs via **nexus** (**gap junctions**) formed between neighboring smooth muscle cells. *Visceral smooth muscle may also be regulated by humoral or microenvironmental factors,*

TABLE 8.3 Comparison of the Three Types of Muscle

Feature	Skeletal Muscle	Cardiac Muscle	Smooth Muscle
Sarcomeres and myofibrils	Yes	Yes	No
Nuclei	Multinucleated; peripherally located	One (or two); centrally located	One; centrally located
Sarcoplasmic reticulum	Well developed with terminal cisterns	Poorly defined; some small terminals	Some smooth endoplasmic reticulum
T tubules	Yes; small, involved in triad formation	Yes; large, involved in dyad formation	No
Cell junctions	No	Intercalated disks	Nexus (gap junctions)
Contraction	Voluntary; all-or-none	Involuntary; rhythmic and spontaneous	Involuntary; slow and forceful; not all-or-none
Calcium control	Calsequestrin in terminal cisternae	Calcium from extracellular sources and the sarcoplasmic reticulum	Calcium from extracellular sources (via caveolae) and the sarcoplasmic/endoplasmic reticulum
Calcium binding	Troponin C	Troponin C	Calmodulin
Regeneration	Yes, via satellite cells	Very limited, perhaps 1% per year	Yes
Mitosis	No	No	Yes
Nerve fibers	Somatic motor	Autonomic	Autonomic
Connective tissue	Epimysium, perimysium, and endomysium	Connective tissue sheaths and endomysium	Connective tissue sheaths and endomysium
Distinctive features	Long; cylinder-shaped; many peripheral nuclei	Branched cells; intercalated disks; one or two nuclei	Fusiform cells with no striations; single nucleus

such as oxytocin in the uterus or stretching of the muscle fibers in the intestines.

Still other smooth muscles of the body are of an **intermediate** type, in which 30% to 60% of the cells receive individual innervation.

Table 8.3 summarizes the similarities and differences among skeletal, cardiac, and smooth muscles.

Regeneration of Muscle

- Although **skeletal muscle** cells do not have the capability of mitotic activity, the tissue can regenerate because of the presence of satellite cells (myogenic stem cells). In the adult skeletal muscle cell, approximately 95% of the nuclei evident by light microscopy belong to the muscle cell, whereas about 5% of the nuclei belong to satellite cells. There are two types of satellite cells, those that are not in the process of forming muscle cells, said to be in the **quiescent state**, and those that are in the process of cell division and forming muscle cells, said to be in the **activated state.** It has been shown that satellite cells express the homeobox gene **Pax7** and a number of myogenic regulatory factors, especially **MyoD**, **Myf5**, and **myogenin.** Most satellite cells are in the quiescent state until they are exposed to a number of local factors, which cause them to become activated. When the skeletal muscle cell is injured by physical or chemical insults or due to disease process, the satellite cells become activated and proliferate. Most of the newly formed cells are destined to repair the damage, but a small percentage of the newly formed cells replenish the satellite cell population. In response to muscle cell injury, both Pax7 and MyoD become expressed in satellite cells, causing them to leave the quiescent and enter the active stage and undergo proliferation; these proliferating cells become known as ***myoblasts*** (***myogenic precursor cells***). The protein myogenic factor Myf5 accumulates in the myoblast cytoplasm and triggers these cells to embark on the sequence of actions, leading to myogenesis. Therefore, the myoblasts line up end to end and, under the influence of myogenin, fuse to form **myotubes** and synthesize the organelles and myofilaments that result in the genesis of a mature skeletal muscle cell.
- Under certain other conditions, such as "muscle building," activated satellite cells may fuse with existing muscle cells, increasing muscle mass during skeletal muscle **hypertrophy.** Skeletal muscle cells regulate their number and size by the secretion of a member of the transforming growth factor- β (TGF-β) superfamily of extracellular signaling molecules, **myostatin** (**growth differentiation factor 8**). Certain mutant mice whose skeletal muscle fibers cannot produce myostatin have enormous muscles with many more cells whose muscle cells are much larger than those of normal mice.
- **Cardiac muscle** is capable of a very limited degree of regeneration, as was demonstrated in individuals who were exposed to atmospheric ^{14}C prior to termination of above ground nuclear testing. In these individuals, a very small percent of their cardiac muscle cells had ^{14}C, indicating that these cells were formed postnatally. In fact, approximately 1% of their cardiac muscle cells were regenerated per year. However, this amount of regeneration is not enough to repair major damage to the heart. Instead, following damage, such as a myocardial infarct, **fibroblasts** invade the damaged region, undergo cell division, and form fibrous connective tissue (scar tissue) to repair the damage.
- **Smooth muscle cells** retain their mitotic capability to form more smooth muscle cells. This ability is especially evident in the pregnant uterus, where the muscular wall becomes thicker both by hypertrophy of individual cells and by hyperplasia derived from mitotic activity of the smooth muscle cells. Small defects subsequent to injury may result in the formation of new smooth muscle cells. These new cells may be derived via mitotic activity of existing smooth muscle cells, as in the gastrointestinal and urinary tracts, or from differentiation of relatively undifferentiated **pericytes** accompanying some blood vessels.

Myoepithelial Cells and Myofibroblasts

Certain cells associated with glandular secretory units possess contractile capabilities. These **myoepithelial cells** are modified to assist in the delivery of the secretory products into the ducts of the gland. Myoepithelial cells are flattened and possess long processes that wrap around the glandular units (see Chapter 5, Figs. 5.26 and 5.27). Myoepithelial cells contain both actin and myosin as well as intermediate filaments and peripheral and cytoplasmic densities necessary to harness the interactions between actin and myosin. Mechanisms and control of contraction in myoepithelial cells resemble, but are not identical to, those in smooth muscle.

In lactating mammary glands, myoepithelial cells contract upon the release of **oxytocin**; in the lacrimal gland, they contract because of the action of **acetylcholine**.

Myofibroblasts resemble fibroblasts but have abundant actin and myosin. They can contract and are especially evident during wound contraction, as they bring the edges of a wound closer to each other.

Pathological Considerations

See Figs. 8.38 through 8.40.

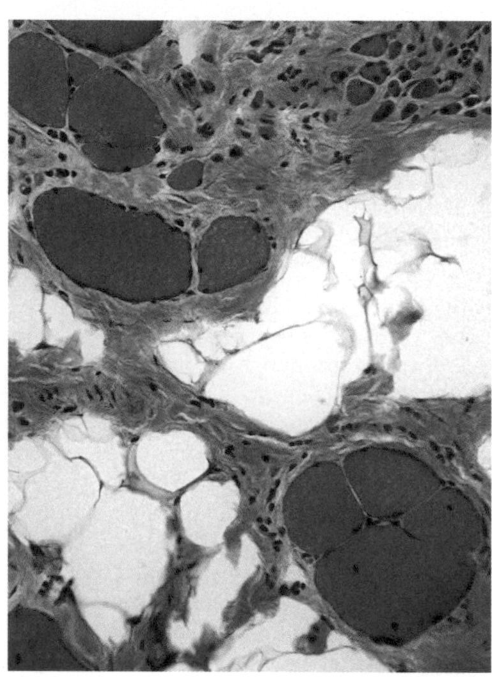

Fig. 8.38 Photomicrograph of a 9-year-old male child with Duchenne muscular dystrophy. Observe that the muscle fibers are of various diameters with greatly enlarged fibrotic endomysia. Additionally, many of the muscle cells have been replaced by fatty infiltrates. (Reprinted with permission from Kumar V, Abbas AK, Aster JC. *Robbins and Cotran Pathologic Basis of Disease*. 9th ed. Philadelphia: Elsevier; 2015:1243.)

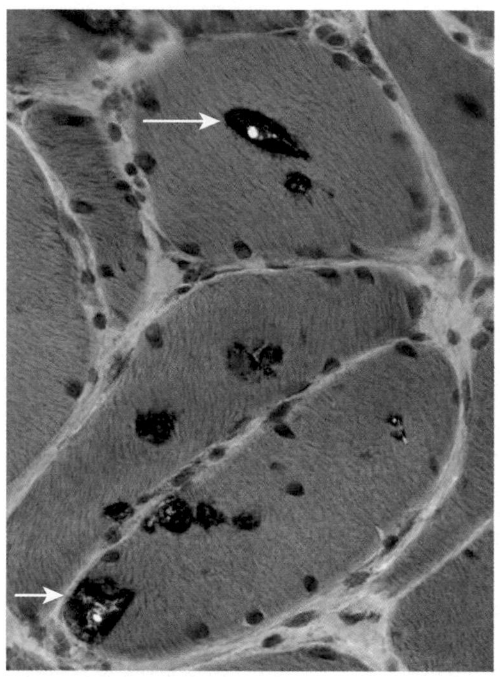

Fig. 8.39 Photomicrograph displaying a condition known as *inclusion body myositis*, a poorly understood disease that may be a process of inflammation or degenerative condition with associated inflammation. Note the presence of "rimmed" vacuoles, cytoplasmic inclusions with reddish granular rimming *(arrows)*. (Reprinted with permission from Kumar V, Abbas AK, Aster JC. *Robbins and Cotran Pathologic Basis of Disease*. 9th ed. Philadelphia: Elsevier; 2015:1240.)

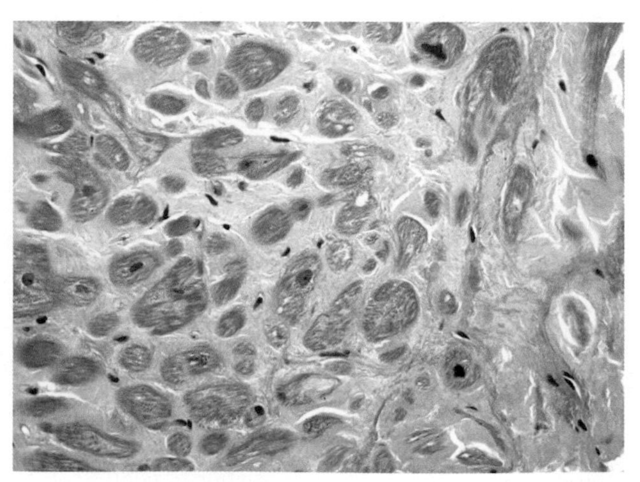

Fig. 8.40 Photomicrograph of a heart muscle displaying cardiac amyloidosis. This disease is characterized by the presence of amyloid protein deposition in the extracellular spaces surrounding cardiac muscle cells. Note the amorphous pink amyloid deposited around the cardiac muscle cells. (Reprinted with permission from Kumar V, Abbas AK, Aster JC. *Robbins and Cotran Pathologic Basis of Disease*. 9th ed. Philadelphia: Elsevier; 2015:573.)

Histology Laboratory Instructions: Muscle

Skeletal Muscle

Skeletal muscle at low magnification displays the connective tissue elements, such as epimysium or perimysium. Viewing the longitudinal section at low magnification, the long fibers with their numerous small, peripherally placed nuclei should be evident. At medium magnification, the long muscle fibers, their peripherally placed nuclei, and their cross-striations are clearly identifiable, as are the connective tissue elements of the endomysium (see Fig. 8.1, SMC, N, CT). Viewed at high magnification, the nuclei of the skeletal muscle cells can be distinguished from the darker, narrower nuclei of the connective tissue cells. The cross-striations are distinguishable and can be identified as to some of their components—Z disk in the middle of the I band and the A band. Myofibrils are also evident within the skeletal muscle cells (see Fig. 8.2, N, Z, A).

Viewed in cross-section, the low magnification of skeletal muscle can display fascicles of muscle cells surrounded by the perimysium. Each skeletal muscle cell is irregularly shaped, and a few nuclei should be visible at the periphery of the cell. At medium magnification, the perimysium and endomysium are clearly evident, and the nuclei of the skeletal muscle cells are evident at the periphery of the skeletal muscle cells (see Fig. 8.4, CT, *arrows,* SMC). At high magnification, both the perimysium and endomysium are well defined, as are the nuclei and capillaries traveling in the endomysium (see Fig. 8.5, P, E, N, C).

Cardiac Muscle

Cardiac muscle viewed in longitudinal section at low magnification displays a disarrayed image that somewhat resembles an uncombed head of hair. The nuclei of cardiac muscle appear to be in the center of the cells but there are smaller, denser nuclei that are located in between the cells. At medium magnification, the apparent disarray is resolved as the branching of the skeletal muscle cells. Clear areas at the poles of the cardiac muscle nuclei are occupied by organelles and glycogen deposits. Intercalated disks are clearly evident (see Fig. 8.20, N, Gl, I). At high magnification, the branching of the cardiac muscle cells and the nuclei of the cardiac muscle fibers are easy to recognize, as are the intercalated disks. Although not labeled, a number of capillaries may be noted in the connective tissue between cardiac muscle fibers (see Fig. 8.21, N, D).

Low magnification of cardiac muscle in cross-section displays not only the centrally placed nuclei of cardiac muscle cells but also the rich connective tissue elements that invest cardiac muscle (see Fig. 8.22, N, CMC, CT). At high magnification, the cross-section of cardiac muscle fibers displays the centrally placed nucleus of each cell and the myofibrils (not labeled) as well as the clear areas at the poles of the nuclei that are occupied by organelles and glycogen deposit. Also not labeled are capillaries in the connective tissue (see Fig. 8.23, N, Gl).

Smooth Muscle

Smooth muscle may best be seen in cross-sections of the small intestine, such as the duodenum, where both longitudinal and cross-sections are clearly identifiable. Viewing the longitudinal section at low magnification, the elongated nucleus of each smooth muscle cell is easy to recognize. Observe that some of the nuclei are corkscrew shaped, indicating that the cell is undergoing contraction. Although smooth muscle cells are very closely packed, connective tissue elements are clearly present. The duodenum is covered by a very slippery serosa that permits digestive movements to occur with very little friction (see Fig. 8.28, N, *arrow,* Se). Viewed at high magnification, the nuclei of the smooth muscle cells are seen to be centrally located along the length of the muscle fiber but are placed closer to one side of the cell (see Fig. 8.29, N).

Cross-section of smooth muscle may display the presence of connective tissue elements that convey blood vessels and nerve fibers from the serosa into the substance of the smooth muscle layer. The centrally placed nuclei appear as small dark dots (see Fig. 8.30, *arrow,* CT, Se, N). At medium magnification, capillaries conveyed by the connective tissue elements and nuclei of the smooth muscle cells are clearly evident (see Fig. 8.31, CTC, N). At high magnification, the nuclei appear to vary in size, indicating that they are spindle shaped and are sectioned at various regions along their length. Also, knowing that a smooth muscle cell is much longer than its nucleus, it is expected that many of the cells display the absence of a nucleus (see Fig. 8.32, N).

9 Nervous Tissue

The human nervous system is composed of perhaps a trillion neurons, each with a large number of interconnections. Some of these neurons possess **receptors** that are specialized for receiving different types of stimuli (e.g., mechanical, chemical, thermal), which are transduced into nerve impulses that may eventually arrive at specified nerve centers. These impulses are then transmitted to other neurons for processing and are conveyed to higher centers, where these sensations are registered and/or motor responses are initiated.

Anatomically, the nervous system is organized into the **central nervous system** (**CNS**), brain and spinal cord, and the **peripheral nervous system** (**PNS**), cranial nerves, spinal nerves, and their corresponding ganglia. It should be understood that the CNS and PNS are connected to each other.

Functionally, the PNS is divided into a **sensory** (**afferent**) **component**, which receives information and transmits impulses to the CNS for processing, and a **motor** (**efferent**) **component**, which originates in the CNS and transmits impulses to effector organs throughout the body.

The motor component has two subdivisions: the **somatic system** (**voluntary system**) where impulses originating in the CNS are transmitted directly, via a single neuron, to *skeletal muscles*; and the **autonomic system** (**involuntary system**), where impulses from the CNS first are transmitted to an **autonomic ganglion** via one neuron and a second neuron originating in the autonomic ganglion then transmits the impulses to *smooth muscles*, *cardiac muscles*, or *glands*.

In addition to neurons, nervous tissue contains numerous other cells, collectively called **neuroglial cells**, which, instead of receiving or transmitting impulses, support and assist neurons in various ways.

Development of Nervous Tissue

The nervous system develops from the ectoderm of the embryo in response to signaling molecules from the notochord.

During the early life of the embryo, the notochord releases signaling molecules inducing the overlying ectoderm to form **neuroepithelium**, which thickens, at first in a uniform fashion, to form the **neural plate**. Later, as the margins of this plate become thicker, the plate buckles, forming the **neural groove** whose edges continue to grow toward each other and fuse, forming the **neural tube**. The rostral (anterior) end of this tube develops into the brain; the remaining (caudal) portion of the neural tube forms the spinal cord. The wall of the neural tube gives rise to neurons, neuroglia, ependyma, and the choroid plexus.

Cells at the lateral margins of the neural plate remain separate from the neural tube, develop into **neural crest cells**, and early in development migrate away from the neural tube, where they form various derivatives (Box 9.1).

Clinical Correlations

Abnormal organogenesis of the CNS results in various types of congenital malformations. ***Spina bifida*** *is a defective closure of the spinal column. In severe cases, the spinal cord and meninges may protrude through the unfused areas.* ***Spina bifida anterior*** *is a defective closure of the vertebrae. Severe cases may be associated with defective development of the viscera of the thorax and abdomen.*

Anencephaly *is failure of the developmental anterior neuropore to close, with a poorly formed brain and absence of the cranial vault. It is usually not compatible with life.*

Epilepsy *may result from abnormal migration of cortical cells, which disrupts normal interneuronal functioning.*

Hirschsprung disease*, also known as* ***congenital megacolon****, is caused by failure of the neural crest cells to invade the wall of the gut. The wall lacks the* ***Auerbach plexus****, a portion of the parasympathetic system innervating the distal end of the colon. Absence of the plexus leads to dilatation and hypertrophy of the colon.*

Phenylketonuria (PKU) *is a hereditary condition in which the newborn child's liver is unable to manufacture the enzyme* ***phenylalanine hydroxylase*** *and, therefore, cannot metabolize the essential amino acid phenylalanine. Unless the child is provided with a phenylalanine-free diet, the baby will have mental retardation, seizures, and other intellectual problems. In most developed countries, all newborns are tested for PKU; if present, the mother is placed on a special diet during the period of breastfeeding. It is recommended that the affected individual adhere to a phenylalanine-free diet for life.*

BOX 9.1 DERIVATIVES OF NEURAL CREST CELLS

Most of the sensory components of the peripheral nervous system
Sensory neurons of cranial and spinal sensory ganglia (dorsal root ganglia)
Autonomic ganglia and the postganglionic autonomic neurons originating in them
Much of the mesenchyme of the anterior head and neck
Melanocytes of the skin and oral mucosa
Odontoblasts (cells responsible for production of dentin)
Chromaffin cells of the adrenal medulla
Cells of the arachnoid and pia mater
Satellite cells of peripheral ganglia
Schwann cells

Cells of the Nervous System

Cells of the nervous system are classified into two categories: neurons and neuroglia.

Neurons and neuroglia are the two categories of cells constituting the nervous system. **Neurons** perform the receptive,

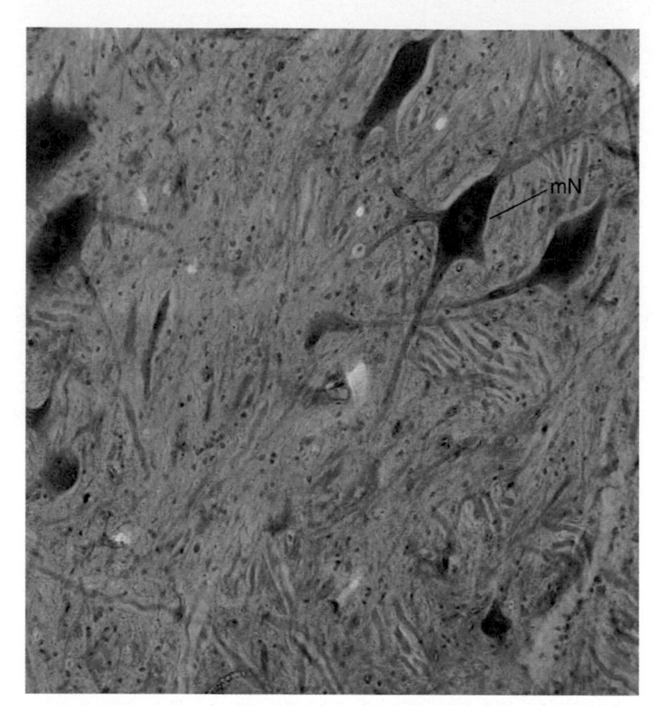

Fig. 9.1 Light micrograph of the gray matter of the spinal cord (×270). Observe the multipolar neuron (mN) cell bodies and their processes.

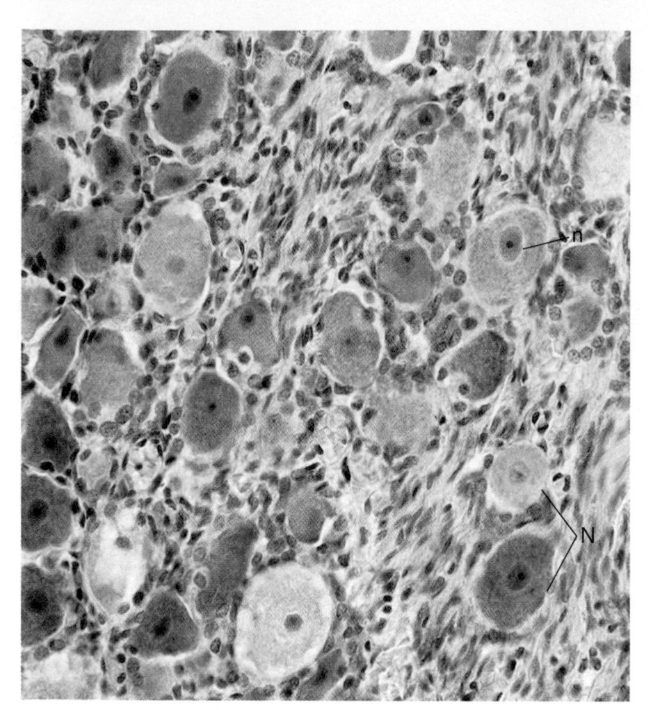

Fig. 9.2 Light micrograph of a sensory ganglion (×270). Observe the large neuronal cell bodies (N) with singular nucleoli (n).

integrative, and motor functions of the nervous system. **Neuroglial cells** support, protect, and assist neurons in performing their functions.

THE STRUCTURE AND FUNCTION OF NEURONS

Neurons are composed of a cell body, dendrites, and an axon.

Neurons, among the smallest and the largest cells in the body (ranging in diameter from 5 to 150 μm), receive and transmit nerve impulses to and from the CNS. Most neurons are composed of three distinct elements: a **cell body**, **multiple dendrites**, and a **single axon**. The **cell body** of a neuron, also known as the ***perikaryon*** or ***soma***, is the central portion of the cell, housing the nucleus and perinuclear cytoplasm. Neuron cell bodies in the CNS are usually polygonal in shape (Fig. 9.1), with slightly concave surfaces between the many cell processes, whereas neurons in the dorsal root ganglion (a sensory ganglion of the PNS) have a spherical cell body from which only one process exits (Fig. 9.2).

Projecting from the cell body are one or more **dendrites**, processes that are specialized for receiving stimuli from sensory cells, axons, and other neurons (Fig. 9.3). Frequently, they are arborized so that they can simultaneously receive multiple stimuli from many other neurons. Nerve impulses received by the dendrites are then transmitted toward the soma.

Each neuron possesses only one **axon**, a process that conducts impulses away from the soma to other neurons, muscles, or glands, but it may also receive stimuli from other neurons, which may modify its behavior. Most axons arborize and, usually, each branch has terminal dilatations known as ***axon terminals*** (***end bulbs, terminal boutons***) at or near its end. These axon terminals approach other cells to form a **synapse**, a submicroscopic gap between the axon and the plasma membrane of the target cell where impulses can be transmitted.

Neurons are classified according to their shape and the arrangement of their processes (Fig. 9.4).

Neuronal Cell Body (Soma, Perikaryon)

The cell body is the region of the neuron containing the large pale-staining nucleus and perinuclear cytoplasm.

Although the cell body is the most conspicuous region of the neuron, the largest volume of the neuron's cytoplasm is located in its dendrites and axons. The large, mostly spherical to ovoid **nucleus** is centrally located in the soma. It contains finely dispersed chromatin, indicative of a rich synthetic activity, although smaller neurons may present some condensed, inactive heterochromatin. A well-defined nucleolus is also common.

The **cytoplasm** of the cell body has abundant rough endoplasmic reticulum (RER) with many cisternae in parallel arrays, a characteristic especially prominent in large motor neurons. Polyribosomes are also scattered throughout the cytoplasm. When stained with basic dyes, these stacked RER cisternae and polyribosomes appear as clumps of basophilic material, called ***Nissl bodies***, with light microscopy. RER is also present in the dendritic region of the neuron, but is absent at the **axon hillock**, the region of the cell body where the axon arises.

Most neurons have abundant SER throughout the cell body; this reticulum extends into the dendrites and the axon, forming **hypolemmal cisternae** directly beneath the plasmalemma. These hypolemmal cisternae are continuous with the RER in the cell body and weave between the Nissl bodies on their way into the dendrites and axon. Although it is unclear how they function, it is known that hypolemmal cisternae sequester calcium and contain protein.

A prominent juxtanuclear **Golgi complex** is present in the soma, composed of several closely associated cisternae exhibiting dilated peripheries, characteristic of protein-secreting cells. The Golgi complex is also responsible for the packaging of neurotransmitter substances or the enzymes essential for their production in the axon.

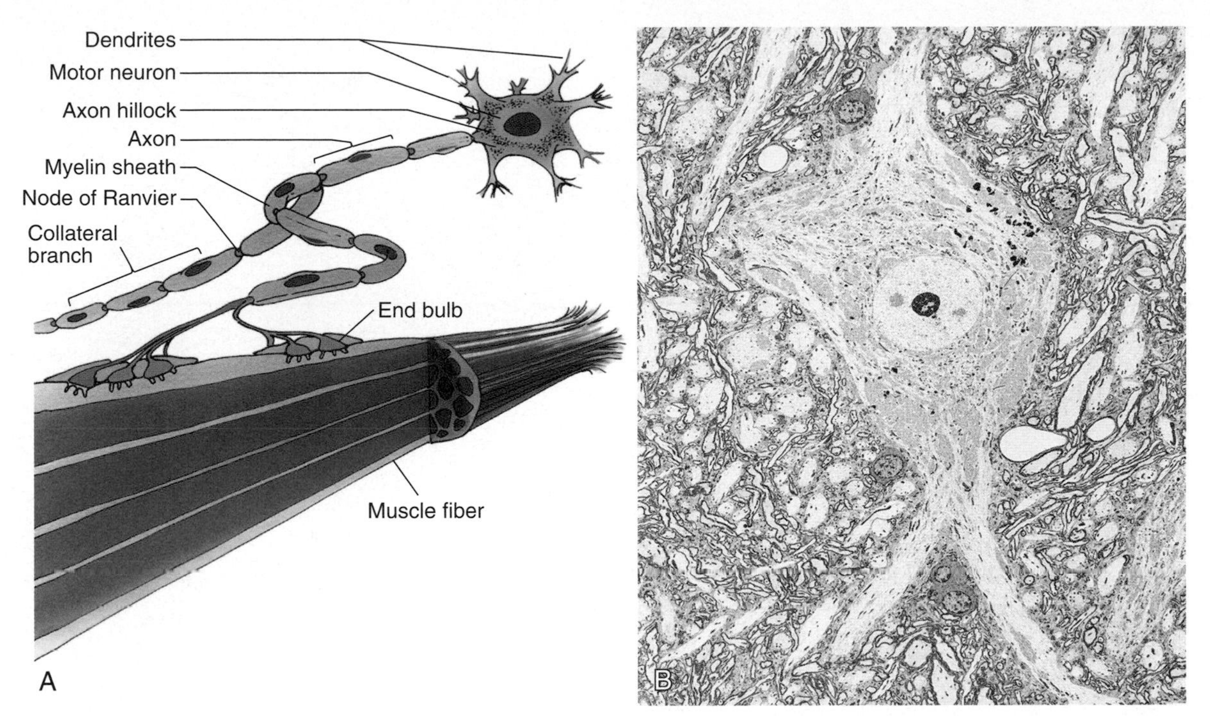

Fig. 9.3 Motoneuron. (A) Diagram of a typical motor neuron. (B) Electron micrograph of a ventral horn neuron with several of its dendrites (×1300). (From Ling EA, Wen CY, Shieh JY, et al. Neuroglial response to neuron injury: a study using intraneural injection of *Ricinus communis* agglutinin-60. *J Anat*. 1989;164:201-213. Reprinted with the permission of Cambridge University Press.)

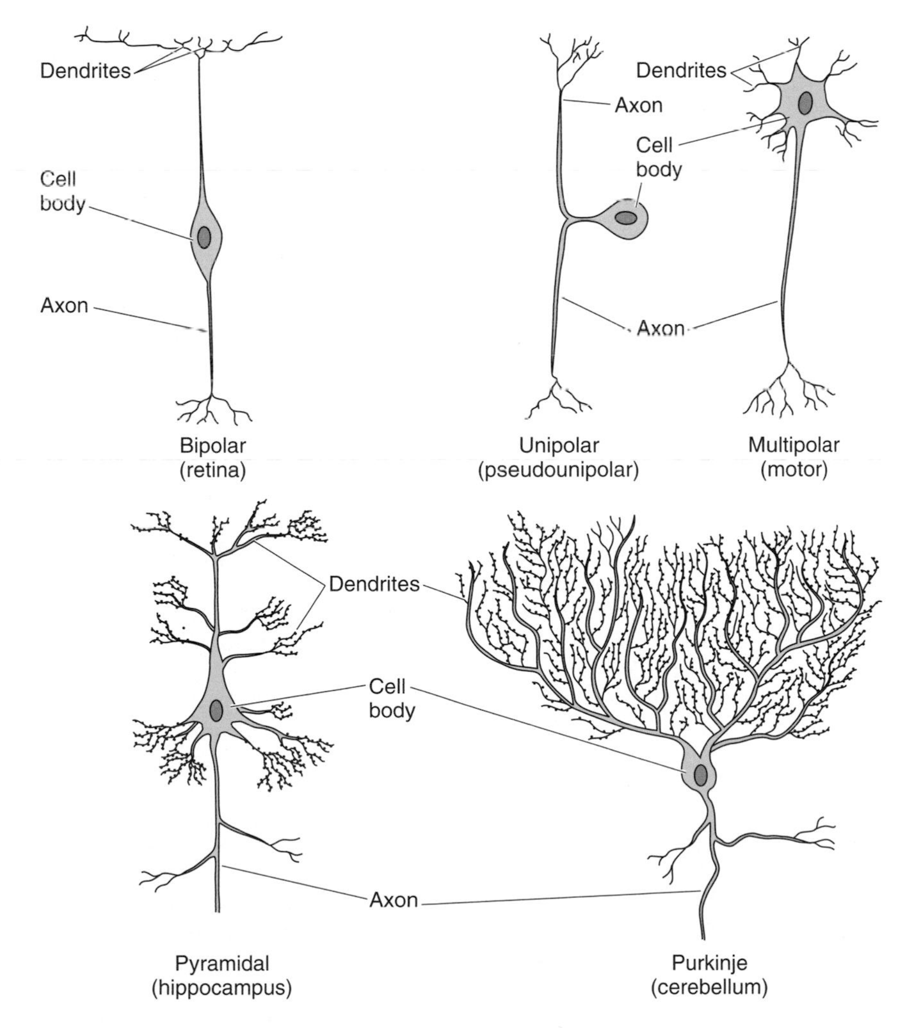

Fig. 9.4 Diagram of the various types of neurons.

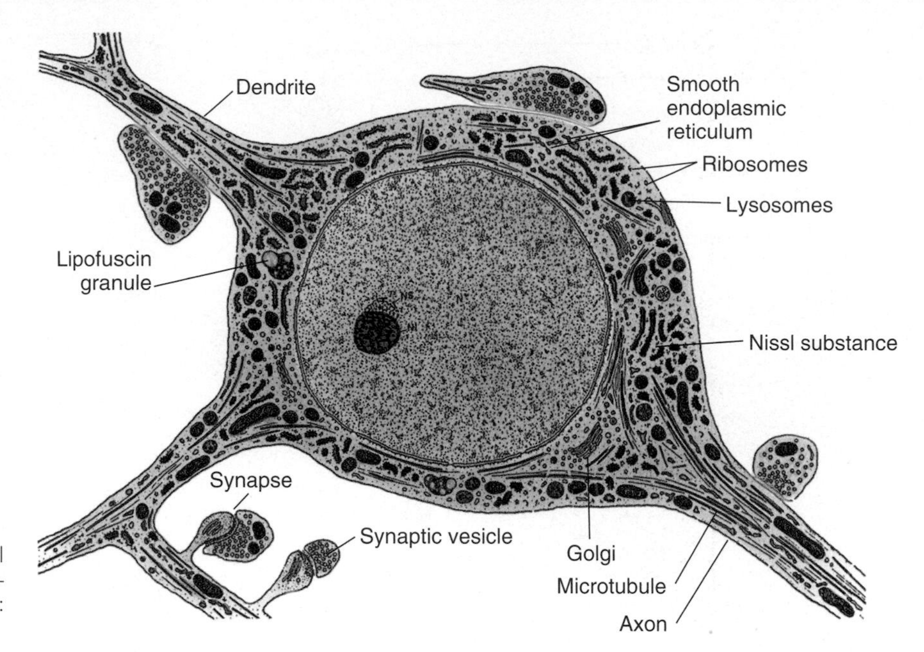

Fig. 9.5 Diagram of the ultrastructure of a neuronal cell body. (From Lentz TL. *Cell Fine Structure: An Atlas of Drawings of Whole-Cell Structure*. Philadelphia: WB Saunders; 1971.)

The soma, dendrites, and axon are well endowed with **mitochondria**, but mitochondria are most abundant at the axon terminals. Generally, these mitochondria are more slender than those in other cells and, occasionally, their cristae are oriented longitudinally rather than transversely. Mitochondria of neurons are in constant motion along microtubules in the cytoplasm.

Most adult neurons display only one **centriole**, which is associated with a basal body of a primary cilium.

Inclusions

Inclusions located in neuronal cell bodies are nonliving substances, such as melanin and lipofuscin pigments as well as lipid droplets.

Dark-brown to black **melanin granules** are located in some neurons in certain regions of the CNS (e.g., mostly in the substantia nigra and locus ceruleus) and in the sympathetic ganglia of the PNS. The function of these granules in these various locations is unknown. However, dihydroxyphenylalanine, or methyldopa, the precursor of this pigment, is also the precursor of the neurotransmitters dopamine and noradrenaline. Therefore, it has been suggested that melanin may accumulate as a by-product of the synthesis of these neurotransmitters.

Lipofuscin, an irregularly shaped, yellowish-brown pigment granule, is more prevalent in neurons of older adults and is thought to be the remnant of lysosomal enzymatic activity. Lipofuscin granules increase with advancing age and may even crowd the organelles and nucleus to one side in the cell, possibly affecting cellular function. Iron-containing pigments also may be observed in certain neurons of the CNS and may accumulate with age.

Lipid droplets sometimes are observed in the neuronal cytoplasm and may be either the result of faulty metabolism or they may function as energy reserves.

Secretory granules are present in neurosecretory cells; many contain signaling molecules.

Cytoskeletal Components

When prepared by silver impregnation for visualization with light microscopy, the neuronal cytoskeleton exhibits **neurofibrils** (up to 2 μm in diameter) coursing through the cytoplasm of the soma and extending into the processes. Electron microscopic studies reveal three different filamentous structures: **microtubules** (24 nm in diameter), **neurofilaments** (intermediate filaments 10 nm in diameter), and **microfilaments** (6 nm in diameter). The neurofibrils observed with light microscopy possibly represent clumped bundles of neurofilaments, a suggestion supported by the fact that neurofilaments are stained by silver nitrate. **Microfilaments** (actin filaments) are associated with the plasma membrane. The microtubules of neurons are identical to those of other cells, except that the **microtubule-associated protein-2 (MAP-2)** is located in somatic and dendritic cytoplasm, whereas **MAP-3** is present in the axon only.

Dendrites

Dendrites receive stimuli from other nerve cells.

Dendrites—and, in some neurons, the cell body and the proximal end of the axon—are elaborations of the receptive plasma membrane. Most neurons have a number of dendrites, each of which arises from the cell body, usually as a single, short trunk that arborizes into increasingly smaller branches, where the specific dendrite branching pattern is characteristic of each particular type of neuron. The base of the dendrite arises from the cell body and contains the usual complement of organelles, especially mitochondria, but with the notable absence of Golgi complexes (Fig. 9.5). Neurofilaments of dendrites are reduced to small bundles or single filaments, which may be cross-linked to microtubules. The branching of dendrites, which results in numerous synaptic terminals, permits a neuron to receive and integrate multiple—perhaps, as in Purkinje cells of the cerebellum, for instance—even hundreds of thousands of impulses. Small bulges, known as **spines**, located on the surfaces of some dendrites permit them to form synapses with processes of other neurons. The number of these spines diminishes with age and poor nutrition, and they may exhibit structural changes in persons with trisomy 13 and trisomy 21 (Down syndrome) and other anomalous conditions. Dendrites sometimes contain vesicles and are able to transmit impulses to other dendrites.

Axons

Axons transmit impulses to other neurons or effector cells, namely, muscle and glands.

The **axon** arises from the cell body at the axon hillock, a pyramid-shaped region of the soma devoid of ribosomes and usually located on the opposite side of the soma from the dendrites, as a single thin process, usually extending for much longer distances from the cell body than do the dendrites. In some instances, axons of motoneurons may be 1 m or even more in length. Axon thickness varies with the type of neuron, being relatively constant for a particular neuron. Thickness is directly related to conduction velocity so that the thicker the diameter, the faster the conduction velocity. Axons may possess branches, known as **collateral branches**, which arise at right angles from the axonal trunk (see Fig. 9.3A). As the axon terminates, it may ramify, forming many small branches (**terminal arbor**).

The portion of the axon from its origin at the axon hillock to the beginning of the myelin sheath is called the ***initial segment***. Deep to the **axolemma** (plasmalemma of the axon) of the initial segment, when viewed with the electron microscope, a thin, electron-dense layer is visible whose function is not known but resembles the layer located at the nodes of Ranvier (see section on astrocytes). This area of the neuron lacks RER and ribosomes but houses abundant microtubules and neurofilaments that are believed to facilitate the regulation of the axon's diameter. In some neurons, the number of neurofilaments may increase threefold in the initial segment, whereas the number of microtubules increases only slightly. It is in this initial segment, also referred to as the ***spike trigger zone***, where excitatory and inhibitory impulses are summed to determine whether propagation of an action potential is to occur (see section on generation and conduction of nerve impulses).

The axoplasm (the cytoplasm within the axon) contains short profiles of SER, many microtubules, and remarkably long, thin mitochondria. The axon lacks RER and polyribosomes; therefore, it relies on the soma for its maintenance. Microtubules are grouped in small bundles at the origin of the axon and in the initial segment. Distally, however, they become arranged as uniformly spaced, single microtubules interspersed with neurofilaments.

The plasmalemma of certain neuroglial cells forms a **myelin sheath** around some axons, ***myelinated axons***, in both the CNS and the PNS (Figs. 9.6 and 9.7), whereas axons lacking myelin sheaths are called ***unmyelinated axons*** (Fig. 9.8). Nerve impulses are conducted much faster along myelinated axons than along unmyelinated axons. In the live individual, the myelin sheath imparts a white, glistening appearance to the axon. It is the presence of myelin that permits the subdivision of the CNS into **white matter** and **gray matter**.

In addition to impulse conduction, an important function of the axon is **axonal transport** of material between the soma and axon terminals. In **anterograde transport**, the direction of transport is from the cell body to the axon terminal; in **retrograde transport**, the direction of transport is from the axon terminal to the cell body. Axonal transport is as crucial to **trophic relationships** within the axon as it is between neurons and muscles or glands. If these relationships are interrupted, the target cells atrophy.

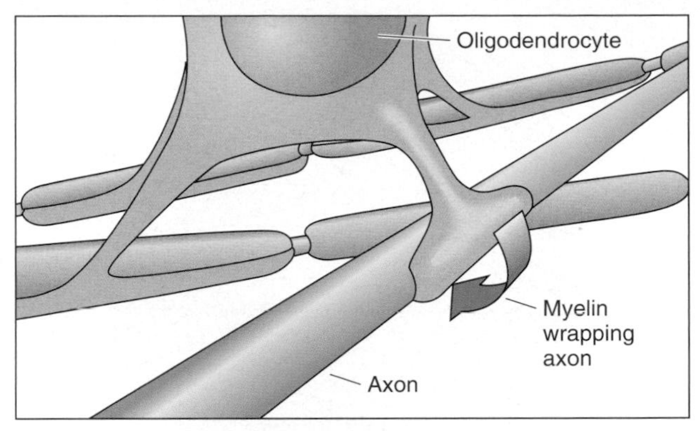

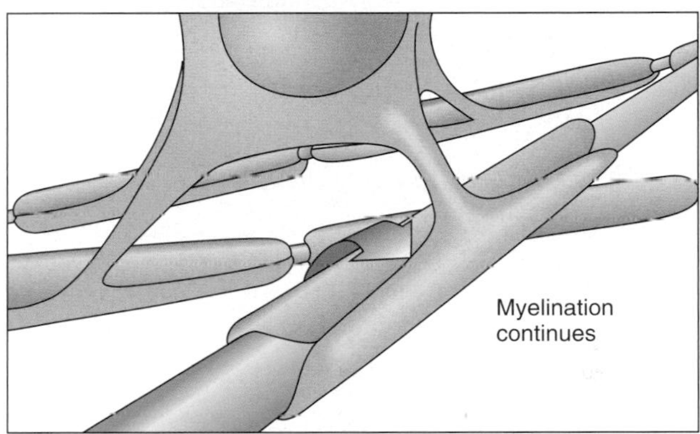

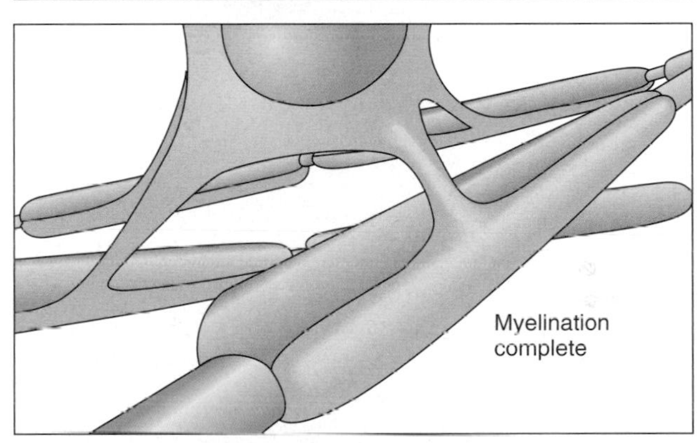

Fig. 9.6 Schematic diagram of the process of myelination in the central nervous system. Unlike the Schwann cell of the peripheral nervous system, each oligodendroglion is capable of myelinating several axons.

The velocity of axonal transport may be fast, intermediate, or slow. The most rapid transport (up to 400 mm/day) takes place in anterograde transport of organelles, which move more rapidly in the cytosol. In retrograde transport, the fastest speed is about 200 mm/day, with the slowest being only about 0.2 mm/day. Axonal transport speeds between these two extremes are considered intermediate.

- **Anterograde transport** is used in the translocation of organelles and vesicles, as well as of macromolecules, such as actin, myosin, and clathrin, and some of the enzymes necessary for neurotransmitter synthesis at the axon terminals.
- **Retrograde transport** returns material such as subunits of microtubules and neurofilaments, soluble enzymes, en-

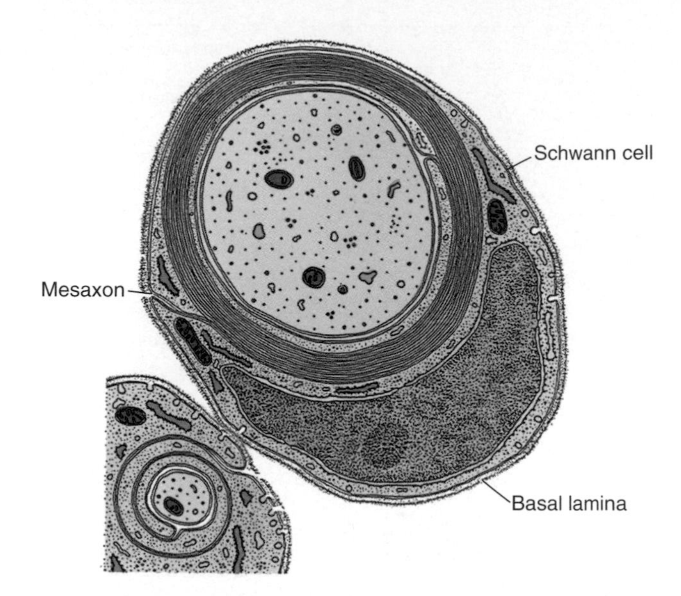

Fig. 9.7 Diagram of the fine structure of a myelinated nerve fiber and its Schwann cell. (From Lentz TL. *Cell Fine Structure: An Atlas of Drawings of Whole-Cell Structure*. Philadelphia: WB Saunders; 1971.)

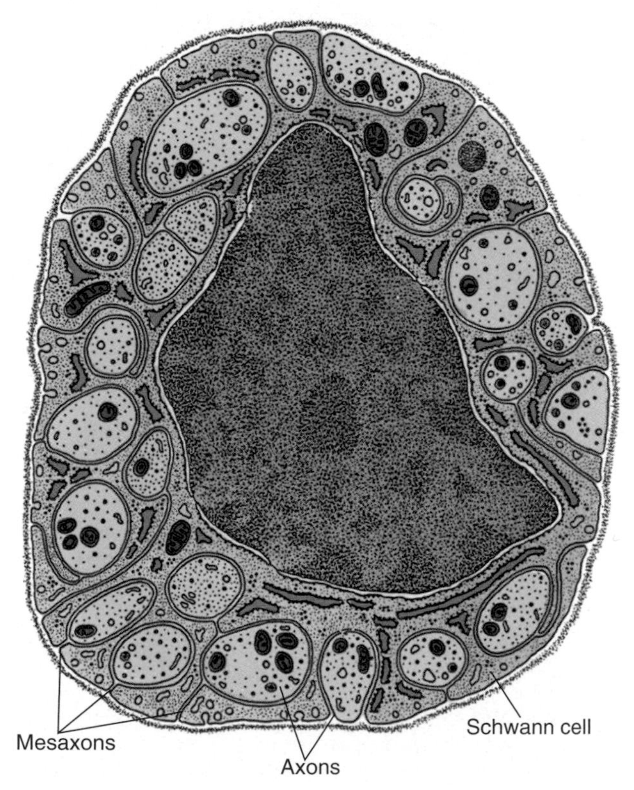

Fig. 9.8 Diagram of the fine structure of an unmyelinated nerve fiber. (From Lentz TL. *Cell Fine Structure: An Atlas of Drawings of Whole-Cell Structure*. Philadelphia: WB Saunders; 1971.)

docytosed substances (e.g., viruses and toxins), and small molecules and proteins destined for degradation, from the axon to the cell body.

- **Axonal transport** not only distributes materials for nerve conduction and neurotransmitter synthesis but also serves to provide and ensure general maintenance of the axon cytoskeleton.

Clinical Correlations

Retrograde axonal transport *is used by certain viruses (e.g., herpes simplex and rabies virus) to spread from one neuron to the next in a chain of neurons. It is also the method whereby toxins (e.g., tetanus) are transported from the periphery into the CNS.*

Since the 1970s, much has been learned about the nature and functioning of the neuron through study of the mechanism of axonal retrograde transport, with the use of the enzyme ***horseradish peroxidase****. In fact, it has become one of the most used techniques in the study of retrograde transport. When this enzyme is injected into the axon terminal, it can be detected later by histochemical techniques that mark its pathway to the cell body. In studying anterograde axonal transport, researchers inject radiolabeled amino acids into the cell body and then later determine the radioactivity at the axon terminals using autoradiography.*

Microtubules are important to fast anterograde transport because they exhibit a polarity, with their plus ends directed toward the axon terminal. **Tubulin dimers**, reaching the axoplasm via anterograde transport, are assembled onto the microtubules at their plus ends and depolymerized at their minus ends. Anterograde transport uses **kinesin**, a microtubule-associated protein, because one end attaches to a vesicle and the other end interacts in a cyclical fashion with a microtubule, permitting the kinesin to transport the vesicle at a speed of about 3 mm/sec. Retrograde transport uses **dynein**, another microtubule-associated protein, which is responsible for moving vesicles along the microtubules.

Clinical Correlations

Although ***neurological tumors*** *account for about 50% of intracranial lesions, tumors of neurons of the CNS are rare. Most intracranial tumors originate from neuroglial cells (e.g., the* ***benign oligodendrogliomas*** *and the fatal* **malignant astrocytomas***). Tumors that arise from cells of connective tissue associated with nervous tissue (e.g.,* **benign fibroma** *or* **malignant sarcoma***) are connective tissue tumors and are not related to the nervous system. Tumors of neurons in the PNS may be extremely malignant (e.g.,* **neuroblastoma** *in the suprarenal gland, which attacks mostly infants and young children).*

Morphological Classification of Neurons (see Fig. 9.4)

Neurons are classified morphologically into three major types, according to their shape and the arrangement of their processes.

The major types of neurons are as follows:

- **Bipolar neurons** possess two processes emanating from the soma, a single dendrite and a single axon. Bipolar neurons are located in the vestibular and cochlear ganglia and in the olfactory epithelium of the nasal cavity.
- **Unipolar neurons** (also known as ***pseudounipolar neurons***) possess only one process emanating from the cell body, but this process divides into a central branch and a peripheral branch. The central branch enters the CNS and

the peripheral branch proceeds to its destination in the body. Both central and peripheral branches resemble an axon and can propagate nerve impulses. The terminal aspect of the peripheral branch arborizes and displays small dendritic ends, indicating its receptor function. Unipolar neurons develop from embryonic bipolar neurons whose processes migrate toward each other during development and fuse, forming a single process that subsequently bifurcates into the central and peripheral processes just described. During impulse transmission, the impulse passes from the end of the peripheral process to the central process without necessarily involving the cell body. Unipolar neurons are located in the dorsal root ganglia of the spinal cord and in the sensory ganglia of the cranial nerves.

- **Multipolar neurons**, the most common neuron type, possess various arrangements of several dendrites emanating from the soma, as well as a single axon. Multipolar neurons are present throughout the nervous system, most of which are motoneurons (in older terminology, they were called *motor neurons*). Some multipolar neurons are named according to the morphology of their somata (e.g., pyramidal cells) or after the scientist who first described them (e.g., Purkinje cells).

Functional Classification of Neurons

Neurons are classified according to their function into three types: sensory neuron, motoneuron, and interneuron.

- **Sensory neurons** (**afferent = toward the CNS**) receive sensory input at their dendritic terminals and conduct impulses to the CNS for processing. Those located in the periphery of the body monitor changes in the external environment; those within the body monitor the internal environment.
- **Motoneurons** (**efferent = away from the CNS**) originate in the CNS and conduct their impulses to muscles, glands, and other neurons.
- **Interneurons** (**intercalated neurons**), located completely in the CNS, function as interconnectors or integrators that establish networks of neuronal circuits between sensory and motoneurons and other interneurons. With evolution, the number of neurons in the human nervous system has grown enormously, but the greatest increase has involved the interneurons, which are responsible for the complex functioning of the body.

NEUROGLIAL CELLS

Neuroglial cells function not only in the physical and metabolic support of neurons but also in regulatory capacities.

Neuroglia not only provide metabolic and mechanical support as well as protection for neurons (Fig. 9.9) but they also have a role in the regulation of neuronal propagation of impulses. It has been estimated that there may be as many as 10 times more neuroglial cells than neurons in the nervous system. Neuroglial cells undergo mitosis, whereas neurons possess a more limited capability of cell division. Although neuroglial cells form gap junctions with other neuroglial cells, they do not react to or propagate nerve impulses, although they assist neurons in the performance of their neural transmission by

- Keeping a check on synapses
- Regulating the flow of **cerebrospinal fluid** (**CSF**) through the substance of the brain

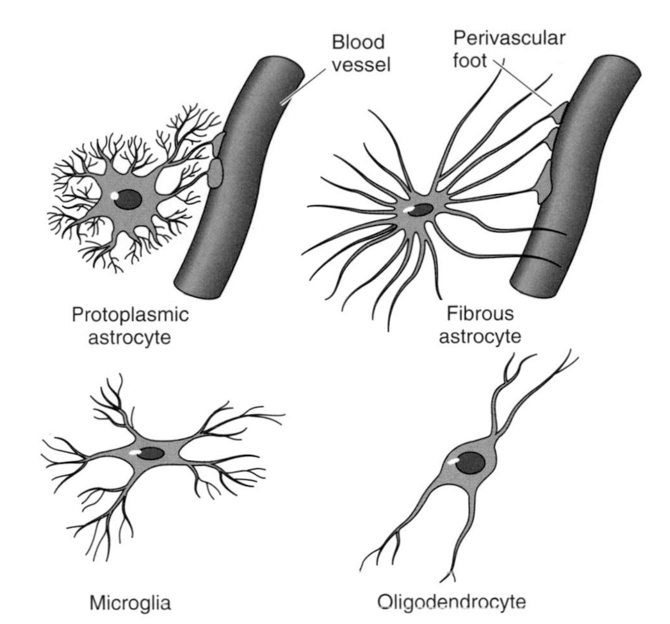

Fig. 9.9 Diagram of the various types of neuroglial cells (not drawn to scale).

- Scavenging neurotransmitters released by the axon terminals of neurons
- Releasing **gliotransmitter** substances such as adenosine triphosphate (ATP) and glutamic acid into the region of the synapse that may regulate processes that occur there

Neuroglial cells that reside exclusively in the CNS include astrocytes, oligodendrocytes, microglia (microglial cells), and ependymal cells. Schwann cells, although located in the PNS, are also considered to be neuroglial cells.

Astrocytes

Astrocytes provide structural and metabolic support to neurons and act as scavengers of ions and neurotransmitters that neurons release into the extracellular space.

Astrocytes are the largest of the neuroglial cells and exist as two distinct types: (1) protoplasmic astrocytes in the gray matter of the CNS and (2) fibrous astrocytes, present mainly in the white matter of the CNS. It is difficult to distinguish the two types of astrocytes in light micrographs, which has led some to suggest that they may be the same cells functioning in different environments. Electron micrographs display distinct cytoplasmic bundles of 8- to 11-nm intermediate filaments composed of **glial fibrillar acidic protein**, which is unique to astrocytes.

Protoplasmic astrocytes are stellate-shaped cells displaying abundant cytoplasm, a large nucleus, and many short branching processes (Figs. 9.10 and 9.11). The tips of some processes end as **pedicels** (**vascular feet**) that come into contact with blood vessels. Other astrocytes lie adjacent to blood vessels, with their cell bodies contacting the vessel wall. Still other protoplasmic astrocytes near the brain or surface of the spinal cord exhibit pedicel-tipped processes that contact the pia mater, forming the **pia-glial membrane**. Protoplasmic astrocytes also function in regulating the flow of CSF through the substance of the brain (see the section on CSF). Some smaller protoplasmic astrocytes located adjacent to neuronal cell bodies are a form of satellite cells.

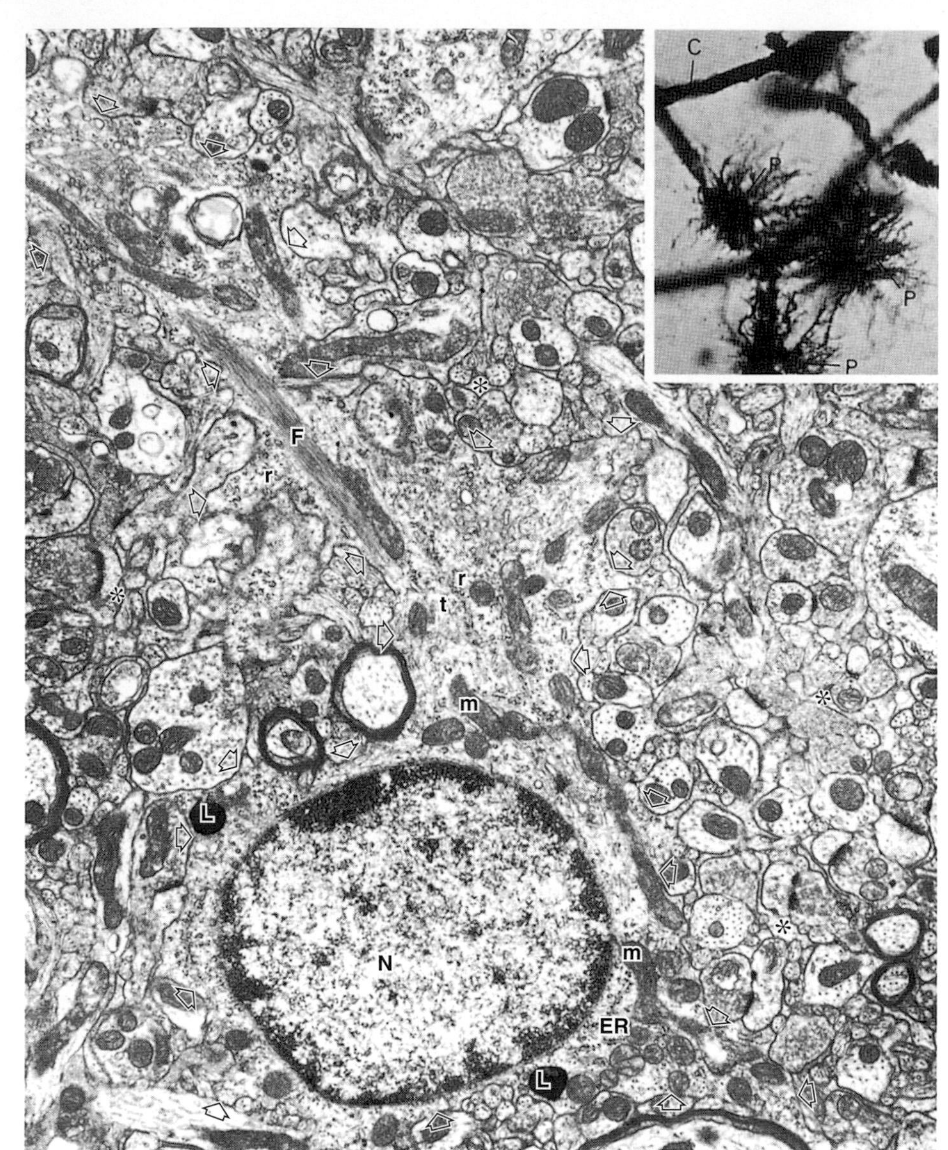

Fig. 9.10 Electron micrograph of protoplasmic astrocyte (×11,400). Observe the nucleus (N), filaments (F), mitochondria (m), microtubules (t), free ribosomes (r), and granular reticulum (ER). Two lysosomes (L) are also identified in the processes of the neuroglia. Note the irregular cell boundary, indicated by *arrowheads*. *Asterisks* indicate processes of other neuroglial cells of the neuropil. (From Peters A, Palay SL, Webster HF. *The Fine Structure of the Nervous System*. Philadelphia: WB Saunders; 1976.)
Inset, Light micrograph of three highly branched protoplasmic astrocytes (P) surrounding capillaries (C). (From Leeson TS, Leeson CR, Paparo AA. *Text/Atlas of Histology*. Philadelphia: WB Saunders; 1988.)

Fibrous astrocytes possess a euchromatic cytoplasm containing only a few organelles, free ribosomes, and glycogen, and they are surrounded by their own basal lamina (Fig. 9.12). The processes of these cells are long, mostly unbranched, and closely associated with the pia mater and blood vessels but are separated from these structures by their basal lamina.

Astrocytes function in removing ions, neurotransmitters, and remnants of neuronal metabolism—such as potassium ions (K^+), glutamate, and γ-aminobutyric acid (GABA)—accumulated in the microenvironment of the neurons, especially at the nodes of Ranvier, where they provide a cover for the axon. These cells also contribute to energy metabolism within the cerebral cortex by releasing glucose from their stored glycogen when induced by the neurotransmitters norepinephrine and vasoactive intestinal peptide (VIP). Astrocytes located at the periphery of the CNS form a continuous layer over the blood vessels and may assist in maintaining the **blood–brain barrier**. Astrocytes are also recruited to damaged areas of the CNS, where they form cellular scar tissue (**glial scar**).

Oligodendrocytes

Oligodendrocytes function in electrical insulation and in myelin production in the CNS.

Oligodendrocytes, the darkest-staining neuroglial cells, are located in both the gray and the white matter of the CNS. They resemble astrocytes but are smaller and contain fewer processes, with sparse branching. Their dense cytoplasm contains a relatively small nucleus, abundant RER, many free ribosomes, mitochondria, and a conspicuous Golgi complex, as well as microtubules, but mostly in the perinuclear zone and processes (Fig. 9.13). There are two types of oligodendrocytes, interfascicular and satellite.

Interfascicular oligodendrocytes, located in rows beside bundles of axons, manufacture and maintain **myelin** about the axons in the CNS, serving to insulate them (see Figs. 9.6 and 9.14). Unlike Schwann cells of the PNS, oligodendrocytes may have as many as 50 processes, each of which wraps a small region (**internode**) of a single axon with segments of myelin. During active myelin synthesis, interfascicular oligodendrocytes have a

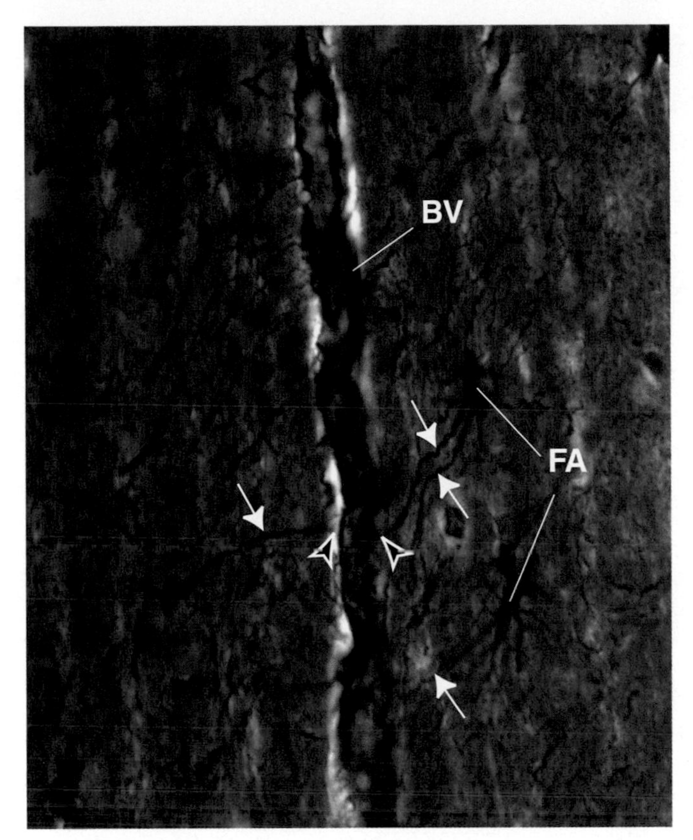

Fig. 9.11 This high-magnification photomicrograph of silver-stained human cerebral cortex displays a blood vessel (BV) flanked by numerous stellate-shaped protoplasmic astrocytes (FA) whose several short processes *(arrows)* approach the vessel wall and end there as pedicels *(arrowhead)*. (×540)

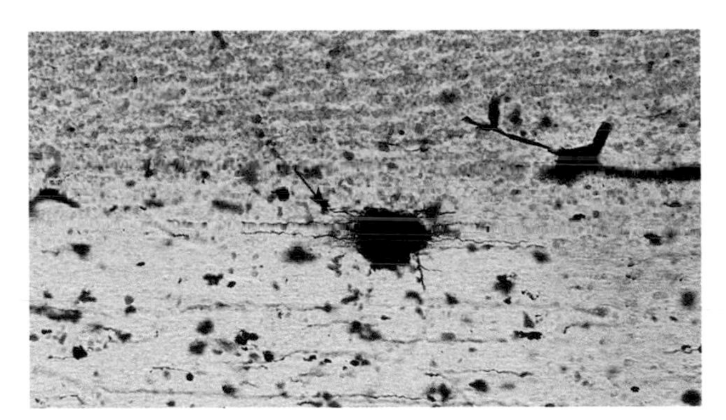

Fig. 9.12 Light micrograph of a fibrous astrocyte *(arrow)* in the human cerebellum (×132).

very high metabolic rate because they can produce as much as 300 times their weight in myelin on a daily basis. Subsequent to completion of myelinization of all of the internodes under their control, these cells maintain responsibility over the metabolic fate of the myelin that they produced.

Satellite oligodendrocytes are closely applied to cell bodies of large neurons of gray matter. Their function is not understood completely, but they appear to monitor the extracellular fluid around neuronal cell bodies and, according to some investigators, they may act in a reserve capacity. In addition, if the need arises, they may migrate into the white matter to replenish interfascicular oligodendrocytes.

Clinical Correlations

Progressive multifocal leukoencephalopathy *is a terminal but rare viral disease caused by a* ***polyoma virus (JC virus)*** *that attacks oligodendrocytes and causes demyelinization of axons, especially in the occipital and parietal lobes of the brain. Although JC virus is present in almost half of the adult population in the United States, it is benign until the patient becomes immunosuppressed and immunodeficient.*

Multiple sclerosis (MS)*, a relatively common disease affecting more that 2.5 million people throughout the world (approximately 1 million in the United States), is 1.5 to 2 times more common in females than in males. The disease is first diagnosed when the individual is between 15 and 45 years of age. Initially, patients complain about vision problems, difficulties of walking due to balance loss, and tingling sensations in the fingers and toes. These problems are the result of the principal pathological feature of MS: demyelination of axons in the CNS (optic nerve; cerebellum; and white matter of the cerebrum, spinal cord, and cranial and spinal nerves). The characteristic features of MS are episodes of random, multifocal inflammation and edema, followed by periods of remission that may last for several months to decades. Each episode may further jeopardize the patient's vitality. Any single episode of demyelination may cause deterioration or malignancy of the affected nerves and may lead to death in a matter of months. It was believed that demyelination was due to an immune reaction in which T lymphocytes attacked and destroyed the myelin sheath covering the axons. More recent studies demonstrated that oligodendrogliopathy is the primary cause of MS and the T cell reaction was a secondary response that exacerbated myelin destruction. However, if a drug is administered that either prevents B cells from presenting specific autoantigens to T cells or inhibits T cells from entering the CNS, the degree of oligodendrogliopathy can be diminished and the patient's MS can be alleviated to a certain extent. Unfortunately, current drugs are unable to do more than decrease the relapses; they cannot cure the disease. Another avenue that is being explored is the effect that intestinal microbial flora has on MS patients. It has been demonstrated that MS patients have much higher levels of Acinetobacter and Akkermansia and much lower levels of Parabacteroides than those of their healthy counterparts. When intestinal bacteria of MS patients were transferred to the intestines of mice that had an MS-like disease, the condition of the mice deteriorated by a significant degree. When the same mice received intestinal flora of healthy patients, they remained healthy. Studies are underway to explore the effects of intestinal microbiomes on MS.*

Microglial Cells

Microglia are members of the mononuclear phagocyte system.

Microglial cells, small dark-staining cells that faintly resemble oligodendrocytes, display very little cytoplasm, an oval to triangular nucleus, and irregular short processes with numerous small spines. These cells are phagocytes that originate in the bone marrow and are part of the mononuclear phagocytic

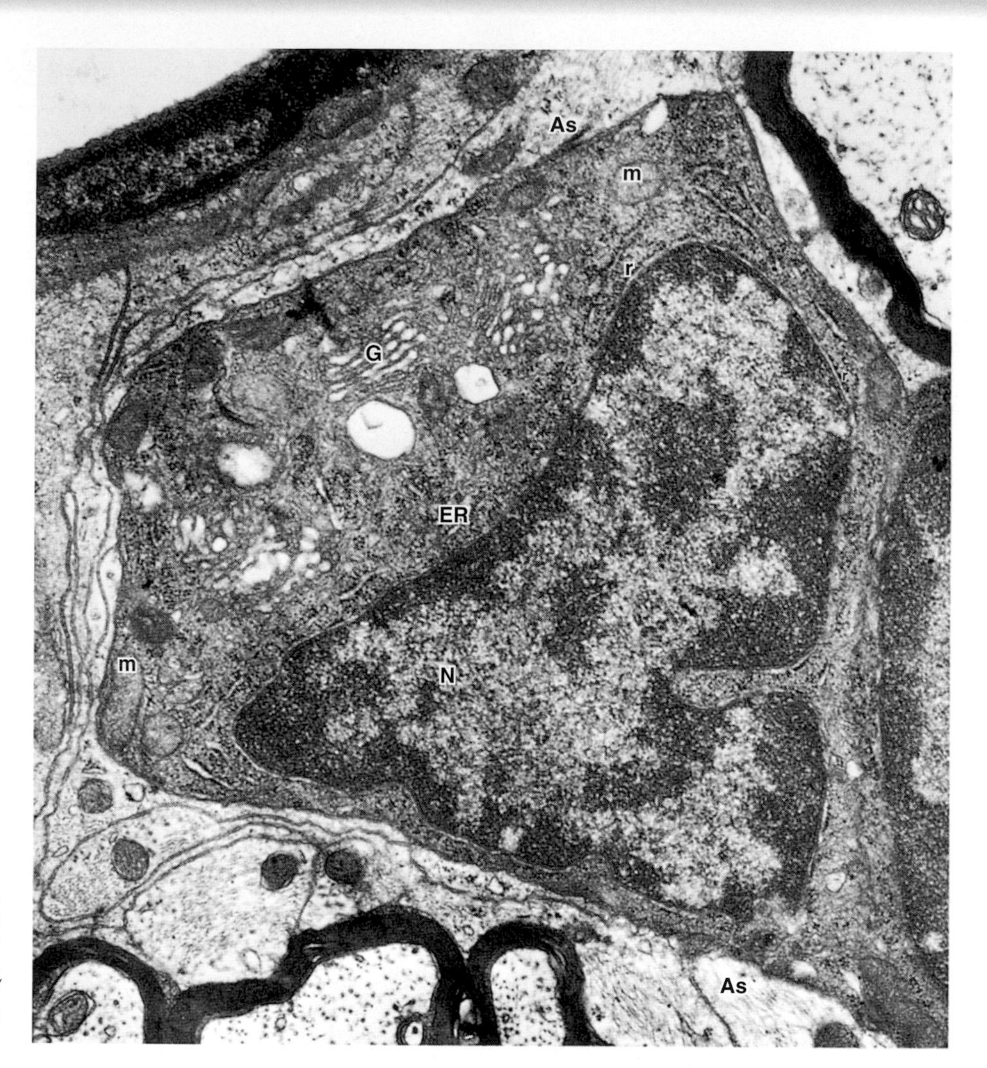

Fig. 9.13 Electron micrograph of an oligodendrocyte (×2,925). Note the nucleus (N), endoplasmic reticulum (ER), Golgi apparatus (G), and mitochondria (m). Processes of fibrous astrocytes (As) contact the oligodendrocyte. (From Leeson TS, Leeson CR, Paparo AA. *Text/Atlas of Histology*. Philadelphia: WB Saunders; 1988.)

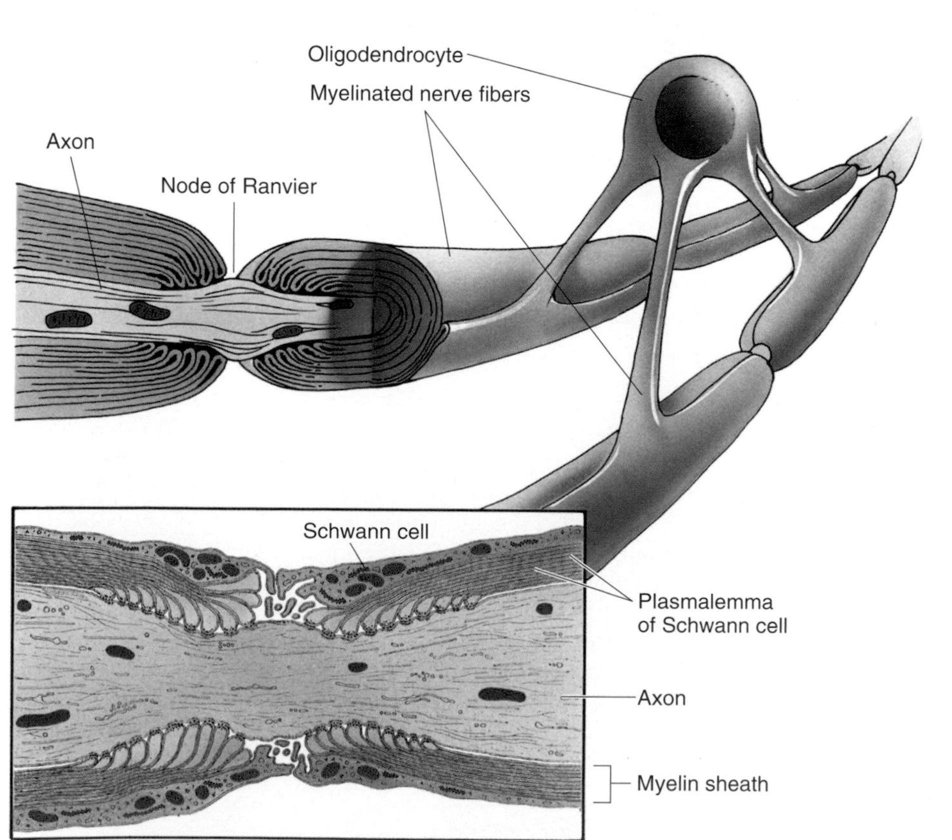

Fig. 9.14 Diagrammatic representation of the myelin structure at the nodes of Ranvier of axons in the central nervous system and peripheral nervous system *(inset)*.

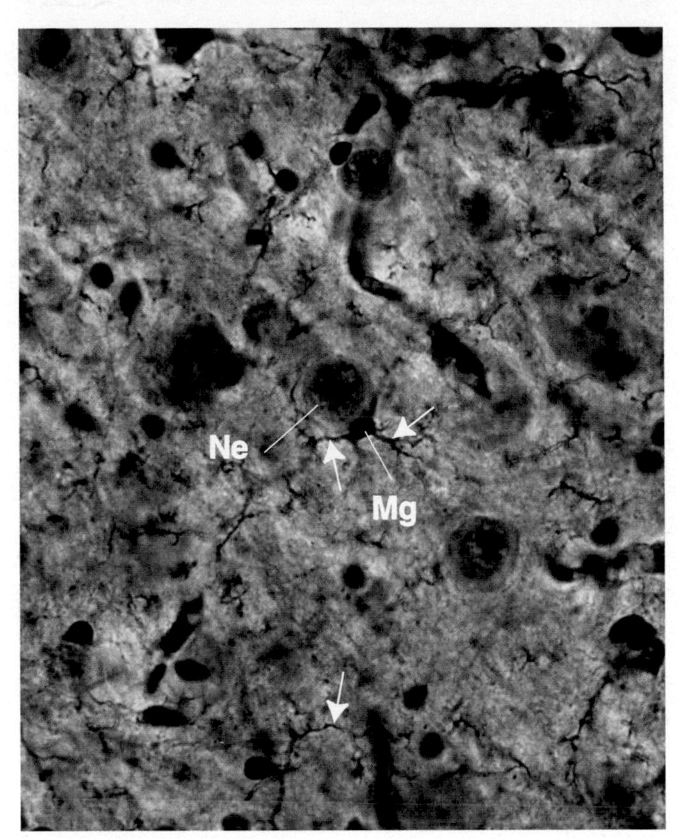

Fig. 9.15 This high-magnification photomicrograph of silver-stained human cerebral cortex displays neuronal cell bodies (Ne) flanked by microglia (Mg) whose several short processes *(arrows)* radiate in all directions (×540).

cell population whose function is clearing debris and damaged structures in the CNS. Microglial cells also protect the nervous system from viruses, microorganisms, and tumor formation. When activated by the presence of pathogens or damaged neurons in their vicinity, they secrete the cytokine interferon-γ that activates other microglia. These cells also release signaling molecules to recruit T lymphocytes into the CNS and then present epitopes to them, acting as antigen presenting cells. Microglia also recognize **complement-associated proteins C1q** and **C3** and destroy synapses that present this protein. This is especially true in the developing brain, where neurons form a large number of synapses, many of which are unnecessary and are marked by C1q and/or C3.

Clinical Correlations

1. *Large populations of microglial cells are present in the brains of patients with Acquired immunodeficiency syndrome (AIDS) and human immunodeficiency virus 1 (HIV-1). Although HIV-1 does not attack neurons, it does attack microglial cells, which then secrete neurotoxic cytokines.*
2. *The complement-associated protein C1q appears to build up at synapses as the individual ages, which results in activation of microglia and subsequent destruction of these synapses. It is possible that, after enough synapses belonging to a specific neuron are destroyed, the neuron itself may undergo degeneration.*

Ependymal Cells

Ependymal cells (ependymocytes), low columnar to cuboidal epithelial cells lining the ventricles of the brain and central canal of the spinal cord, are derived from embryonic neuroepithelium. Their cytoplasm contains abundant mitochondria and bundles of intermediate filaments. In some regions, they possess cilia that facilitate the movement of the CSF.

Where the neural tissue is thin, ependymal cells form an **internal limiting membrane** lining the ventricle and an **external limiting membrane** located beneath the pia. Modifications of some of the ependymal cells in the ventricles of the brain participate in the formation of the **choroid plexus**, which is responsible for secreting and maintaining the chemical composition of the CSF.

Tanycytes, specialized ependymal cells, extend processes into the hypothalamus, where they terminate near blood vessels and neurosecretory cells. It is believed that tanycytes transport CSF to these neurosecretory cells and, possibly under control from the anterior lobe of the pituitary, may respond to changes in hormone levels in the CSF by discharging secretory products into capillaries of the median eminence.

Schwann Cells

Schwann cells form both myelinated and unmyelinated coverings over axons of the PNS.

Unlike other neuroglial cells, **Schwann cells** are located in the peripheral nervous system, where they envelop axons, forming either myelinated or unmyelinated coverings. Axons of the PNS that have myelin wrapped around them are referred to as ***myelinated nerves***.

Electron microscopy has revealed that myelin is the plasmalemma of individual Schwann cells organized into a sheath that is wrapped several times around a small segment of the axon. Where adjoining Schwann cells form adjoining myelin segments, the axolemma is exposed. These exposed regions are called ***nodes of Ranvier*** (Fig. 9.14); the region between adjacent nodes is known as an **internode**, ranging in length from 200 to 1000 μm. Light microscopy has revealed several cone-shaped, oblique clefts in the myelin sheath of each internodal segment called ***clefts*** (***incisures***) **of Schmidt-Lanterman**, which, viewed with the electron microscope, are Schwann cell cytoplasm trapped within the lamellae of myelin.

A large number of nodes of Ranvier are present along each axon and each node of Ranvier is richly endowed with **voltage-gated** Na^+ **ion channels**. This feature permits an impulse transmission known as ***saltatory conduction***. However, internodes have few, if any, of these channels (see section on generation and conduction of nerve impulses).

The external aspect of Schwann cells is covered by a basal lamina that dips into the nodes of Ranvier. Thus, each Schwann cell is covered by a basal lamina, as is the exposed axon at the node of Ranvier. After nerve injury, the regenerating nerve is guided by the basal lamina to its proper location.

As the membrane spirals around the axon, it produces a series of spiraling, wide, dense lines alternating with narrower, spiraling less dense lines separated from each other by 12 nm. The wider line (3 nm in width) is the ***major dense line***, which represents the fused *cytoplasmic surfaces* of the Schwann cell plasma membrane. The narrower **intraperiod line** represents the apposing *outer leaflets* of the Schwann cell plasma

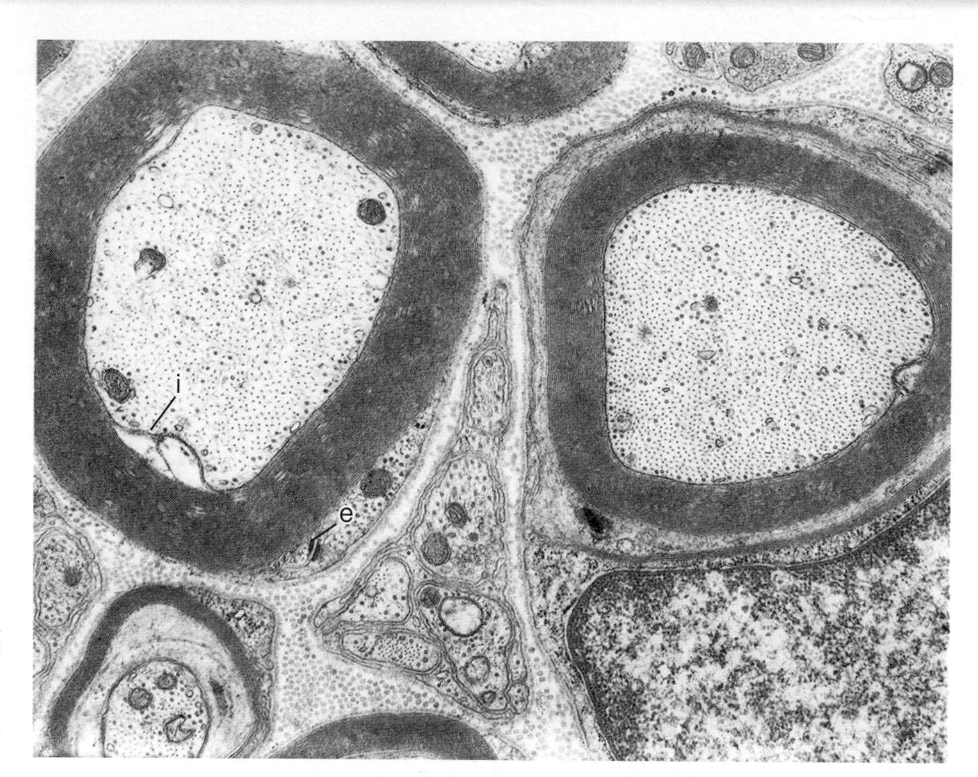

Fig. 9.16 Electron micrograph of a myelinated peripheral nerve. Note the internal (i) and external (e) mesaxons, as well as the Schwann cell cytoplasm and nucleus. (From Jennes L, Traurig HH, Conn PM. *Atlas of the Human Brain.* Philadelphia: Lippincott-Raven; 1995.)

membrane. High-resolution electron microscopy has revealed small gaps within the intraperiod line between spiraled layers of the myelin sheath, called ***intraperiod gaps***. These gaps probably provide access for small molecules to reach the axon. The region of the intraperiod line that is in intimate contact with the axon is known as the ***internal mesaxon***. Its outermost aspect, which is in contact with the body of the Schwann cell, is the **external mesaxon** (see Figs. 9.7 and 9.16).

The process of **myelination**, whereby the Schwann cell located in the PNS (or oligodendrocyte located in the CNS) concentrically wraps its membrane around the axon to form the myelin sheath, is unclear. It is believed to begin when a Schwann cell envelops an axon and in some fashion wraps its membrane around the axon. The wrapping may continue for more than 50 turns. During this process, the cytoplasm is squeezed back into the body of the Schwann cell, bringing the cytoplasmic surfaces of the membranes in contact with each other, forming the major dense line that spirals through the myelin sheath. A single Schwann cell can myelinate only one internode of a single axon (in the PNS only); oligodendrocytes can myelinate an internode of as many as 50 axons (in the CNS only).

Nerves are not myelinated simultaneously during development. Indeed, the onset and completion of myelination vary considerably in different areas of the nervous system. This variation appears to be correlated with function. For example, motonerves are nearly completely myelinated at birth, whereas sensory roots are not myelinated for several months thereafter. Some CNS nerve tracts and commissural axons are not fully myelinated until several years after birth.

Some axons in the PNS are not wrapped with the many layers of myelin typical of myelinated axons. These unmyelinated axons are surrounded by a single layer of Schwann cell plasma membrane and cytoplasm of the Schwann cell (see Fig. 9.8). Although a single Schwann cell can myelinate one axon only, several unmyelinated axons may be enveloped by a single Schwann cell.

Clinical Correlations

Radiation therapy *can lead to demyelination of the brain or spinal cord when these structures are in the radiation field during therapy. Toxic agents, such as those used in* ***chemotherapy*** *for cancer, may also lead to demyelination, resulting in neurological problems.*

Guillain-Barré syndrome *is an immune disorder that produces inflammation and rapid demyelination within the peripheral nerves and the motor nerves arising from the ventral roots. This disease is associated with recent gastrointestinal infection, especially with Campylobacter jejuni. Interestingly, some of the Campylobacter lipopolysaccharide contains ganglioside-like epitopes that resemble some of the lipids present in myelin, which then elicits an autoimmune response resulting in axonal demyelination. A symptom of this disease is muscle weakness in the extremities, reaching a high point within just a few weeks, followed by a more serious condition of demyelination of the nerves serving the diaphragm, making breathing difficult at first and eventually impossible. Early recognition of the condition followed by physical therapy, respiratory therapy, and autoimmune globulin treatments results in possibly complete reversal of the condition.*

Generation and Conduction of Nerve Impulses*

Nerve impulses are generated in the spike trigger zone of the neuron and are conducted along the axon to the axon terminal.

* Although negatively charged proteins within the cytoplasm of the neuron do not cross the cell membrane, they do affect the behavior of the various charged species. However, their role in the generation and conduction of nerve impulses is not described here. The interested reader is referred to textbooks of physiology or neuroscience for an in-depth explanation of these phenomena.

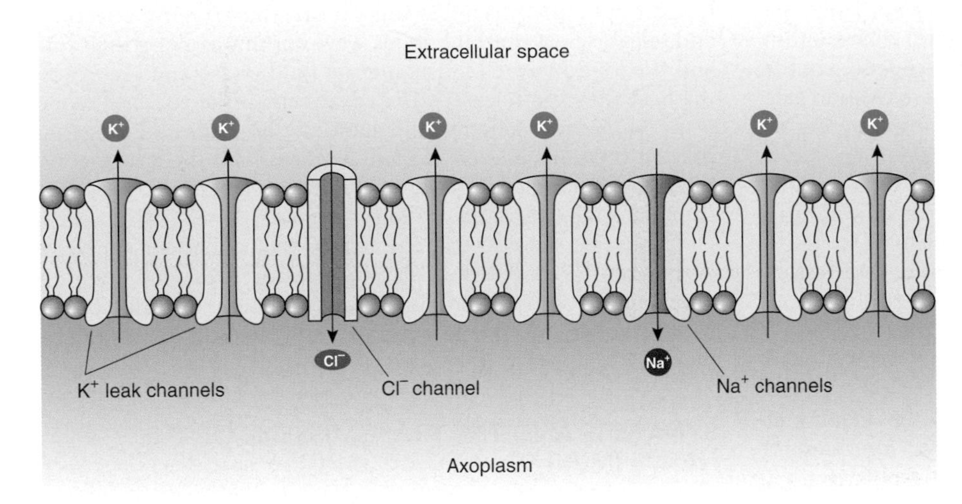

Fig. 9.17 Schematic diagram of the establishment of the resting potential in a typical neuron. Observe that the potassium ion (K^+) leak channels outnumber the sodium ion (Na^+) and calcium ion (Cl^-) channels. Consequently, more K^+ can leave the cell than Na^+ or Cl^- can enter. Because there are more positive ions outside than inside of the cell, the outside is more positive than the inside, establishing a potential difference across the membrane. Ion channels and ion pumps not directly responsible for the establishment of resting membrane potential are not shown.

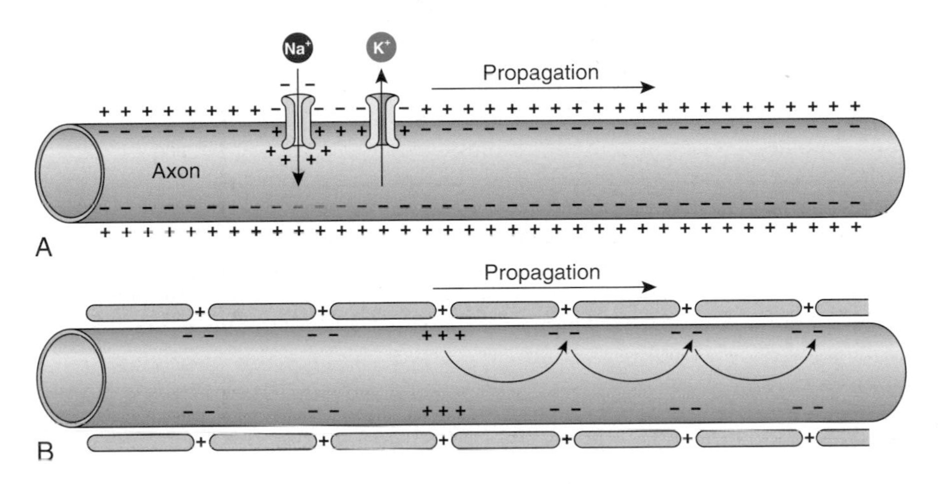

Fig. 9.18 Schematic diagram of the propagation of the action potential in an unmyelinated (A) and myelinated (B) axon (see text).

Nerve impulses are electrical signals that are most readily generated at an area of the axon hillock, the ***spike trigger zone*** that is exceptionally rich in voltage-gated sodium channels; as the result of **membrane depolarization**, impulses are conducted along the length of the axon to its axon terminal. Transmission of impulses from the terminals of one neuron to another neuron, a muscle cell, or a gland occurs at synapses (see section on synapses and the transmission of the nerve impulse).

Neurons and other cells are electrically **polarized** with a **resting potential** of about −70 mV (this simply means that the cytoplasm adjacent to the neuronal cell membrane is *less positive* than the extracellular fluid bathing the external aspect of the neuron's plasmalemma) across the plasma membrane, although in smaller muscle cells and small nerve fibers, this differential may be as low as −40 to −60 mV. This potential arises because of the difference between ion concentrations inside and outside the cell. In mammalian cells, the concentration of potassium (K^+) ions is much higher inside than outside of the cell, whereas the concentration of sodium ions (Na^+) and chloride ions (Cl^-) is much higher outside than inside the cell.

K^+ ion **leak channels** in the plasmalemma permit a relatively free flow of K^+ ions out of a cell down its concentration gradient (Fig. 9.17). Although the K^+ ion leak channel allows Na^+ ions to enter the cell, the ratio of potassium to sodium is 100 : 1 so that many more K^+ ions leave the cell than Na^+ ions enter. Thus, a small net positive charge accumulates on the outside of the plasma membrane. Although maintenance of the resting potential depends primarily on K^+ ion leak channels, **Na^+-K^+ ion pumps** in the plasma membrane assist by actively pumping Na^+ ions out of the cell and K^+ ions into the cell. For every three sodium ions pumped out, two potassium ions enter the cell, making just a slight contribution to the potential difference between the two sides of the membrane.

In most cells, the potential across the plasma membrane is generally constant. In neurons and muscle cells, however, the membrane potential can undergo controlled changes, making these cells capable of conducting an electrical signal, as follows:

1. Stimulation of a neuron causes opening of **voltage-gated Na^+ ion channels** in a small region of the membrane, leading to an influx of Na^+ ions into the cell at that site (Fig. 9.18). Thus, the overabundance of Na^+ ions inside the cell causes a **reversal of the resting potential** (i.e., the cytoplasmic aspect of the plasma membrane becomes positive relative to its extracytoplasmic aspect), and the membrane is said to be **depolarized.**
2. Depolarization inactivates those particular Na^+ ion channels for 1 to 2 msec, a condition known as the ***refractory period.*** This is a time during which those particular Na^+ ion channels are inactive, meaning that they cannot open or close, preventing Na^+ ions from traversing them. The ability to prevent Na^+ ions from going through the ion channel is because these channels have two gates, an extracytoplasmic gate (**activation gate**) that opens as a result of the depolarization of the cell membrane and remains

open as long as the membrane is depolarized. However, an intracytoplasmic gate (**inactivation gate**) closes within a few ten-thousandths of a second after the opening of the activation gate. Therefore, even though the activation gate remains open, Na^+ ions are prevented from entering or leaving the cell by the closed inactivation gate.

3. During the refractory period, **voltage-gated K^+ ion channels** open (note that these are different from the **K^+ ion leak channels** described earlier), permitting K^+ ions to leave the cell and enter the extracellular fluid, thus restoring the resting membrane potential. However, there may be a brief period of **hyperpolarization.**
4. Once the resting potential is restored, the voltage-gated K^+ ion channels close, and the refractory period is ended with the closing of the activation gate and the opening of the inactivation gate of the voltage-gated Na^+ ion channel.

The cycle of membrane depolarization, hyperpolarization, and return to the resting membrane potential is called the **action potential**, an all-or-none response that can occur at rates of 1000 times/sec. The membrane depolarization that occurs with the opening of voltage-gated Na^+ ion channels at one point on an axon spreads passively for a short distance and triggers the opening of adjacent channels, resulting in the generation of another action potential. In this manner, the **wave of depolarization**, or **impulse**, is conducted along the axon. In vivo, an impulse is conducted in only one direction, from the site of initial depolarization to the axon terminal, known as **orthodromic spread**. The inactivation of the Na^+ ion channels during the refractory periods prevents retrograde propagation, known as **antidromic spread**, of the depolarization wave. In an **unmyelinated axon**, the impulse travels slowly because it involves sodium channels that are adjacent to each other. In myelinated fiber, the impulse travels much faster because it jumps, known as ***saltatory conduction***, from one node of Ranvier to the adjacent node of Ranvier, without having to involve the membrane of the internodes. As stated earlier, the nodes of Ranvier are richly supplied by **voltage-gated Na^+ ion channels**, whereas the internodes possess very few, if any, of these channels.

Clinical Correlations

The terminals of the peripheral processes of sensory neurons that are designed to transmit pain sensations possess a very specific type of Na^+ channels, known as $Na_V1.7$. When the terminus of one of these nerve fibers is stimulated, the $Na_V1.7$ channels open, permit the movement of Na^+ ions into the cell, and thereby initiate the propagation of a nerve impulse. The discovery of these channels provided an explosion of research to find drugs and anesthetics directed specifically toward these channels to provide pain relief and anesthesia without affecting all other sodium channels of the region.

AN ALTERNATIVE THEORY OF GENERATION AND CONDUCTION OF NERVE IMPULSES

A mechanical, rather than electrical, generation and conduction of nerve impulses has been proposed for a number of years. Known as the **soliton theory**, it suggests that instead of a wave of electrical depolarization, a shock wave passes along the length of the axon. As this wave progresses, it causes a physical transformation of the lipid bilayer from a fluid phase into a liquid crystalline phase. As this occurs, the axolemma widens and releases heat until the shock wave continues along the axon and the lipid bilayer returns into its fluid phase and reabsorbs the heat that was released. The advantage of the soliton theory is that it provides a better explanation of how anesthetic agents prevent the transmission of pain impulses. This theory suggests that anesthetic agents prevent the fluid phase of the lipid bilayer from entering the liquid crystalline phase.

It must be stressed that the soliton theory has not received even tentative support from most researchers studying the propagation of nerve impulses, even though the membrane phase changes and the heat release and reabsorption aspects of the theory appear to have been verified.

SYNAPSES AND THE TRANSMISSION OF THE NERVE IMPULSE

Synapses are the sites of impulse transmission between the presynaptic and postsynaptic cells.

Synapses are the sites where nerve impulses are transmitted from a presynaptic cell (a neuron) to a postsynaptic cell (another neuron, muscle cell, or cell of a gland). Synapses thus permit neurons to communicate with each other and with effector cells (muscles and glands). Impulse transmission at synapses can occur electrically or chemically.

Although **electrical synapses** are uncommon in mammals, they are present in the brain stem, retina, and cerebral cortex. Electrical synapses are usually represented by gap junctions that permit free movement of small ions from one cell to another, resulting in a flow of current. Impulse transmission is much faster across electrical synapses than across chemical synapses.

Chemical synapses are the most common mode of interneuronal communication. The **presynaptic membrane** releases one or more **neurotransmitters** into the **synaptic cleft**, a small (20- to 30-nm) gap, located between the presynaptic membrane of the first cell and the **postsynaptic membrane** of the second cell (Fig. 9.19). The neurotransmitter diffuses across the synaptic cleft to **gated ion-channel receptors** on the postsynaptic membrane. Binding of the neurotransmitter to these receptors initiates the opening of ion channels, which permits the passage of certain ions through the postsynaptic membrane and reverses its membrane potential. *Neurotransmitters do not accomplish the reaction events at the postsynaptic membrane; they merely activate the response.*

When the stimulus at a synapse results in depolarization of the postsynaptic membrane to a threshold value that initiates an action potential, it is called an ***excitatory postsynaptic potential***. A stimulus at the synapse that results in maintaining or increasing the membrane potential, ***hyperpolarizing*** it, is called an ***inhibitory postsynaptic potential***.

Various types of synaptic contacts between neurons have been observed, the most common of which are: **axodendritic synapse** (between an axon and a dendrite), **axosomatic synapse** (between an axon and a soma), **axoaxonic synapse** (between two axons), and **dendrodendritic synapse** (between two dendrites; Figs. 9.19, 9.20, and 9.21).

Synaptic Morphology

Terminals of axons vary according to the type of synaptic contact. Often, the axon forms a bulbous expansion at its terminal end called a ***bouton terminal***. Other forms of synaptic contacts

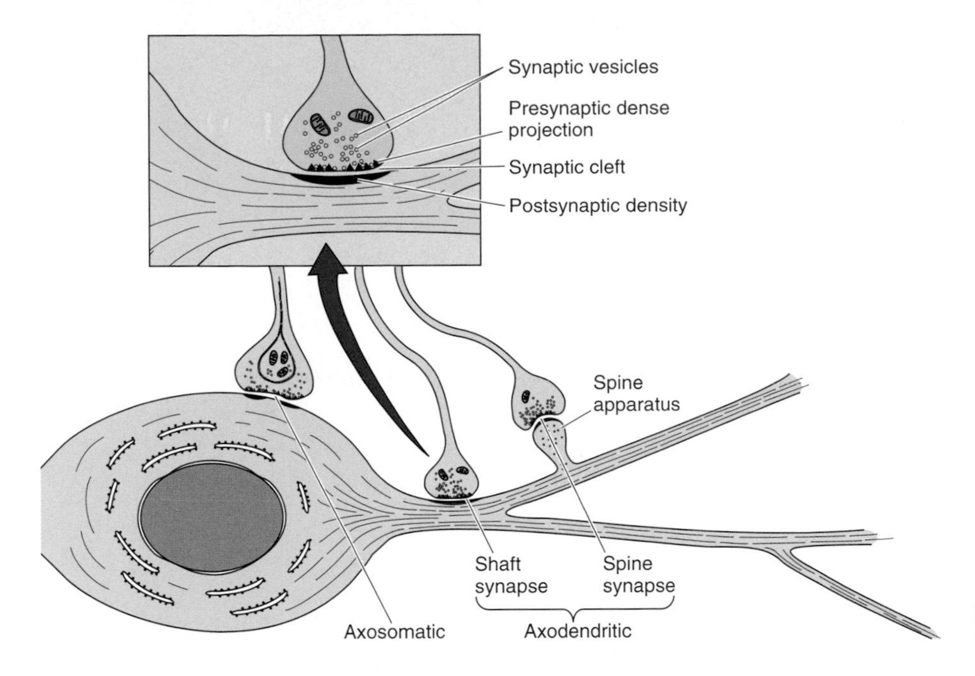

Fig. 9.19 Schematic diagram of the various types of synapses.

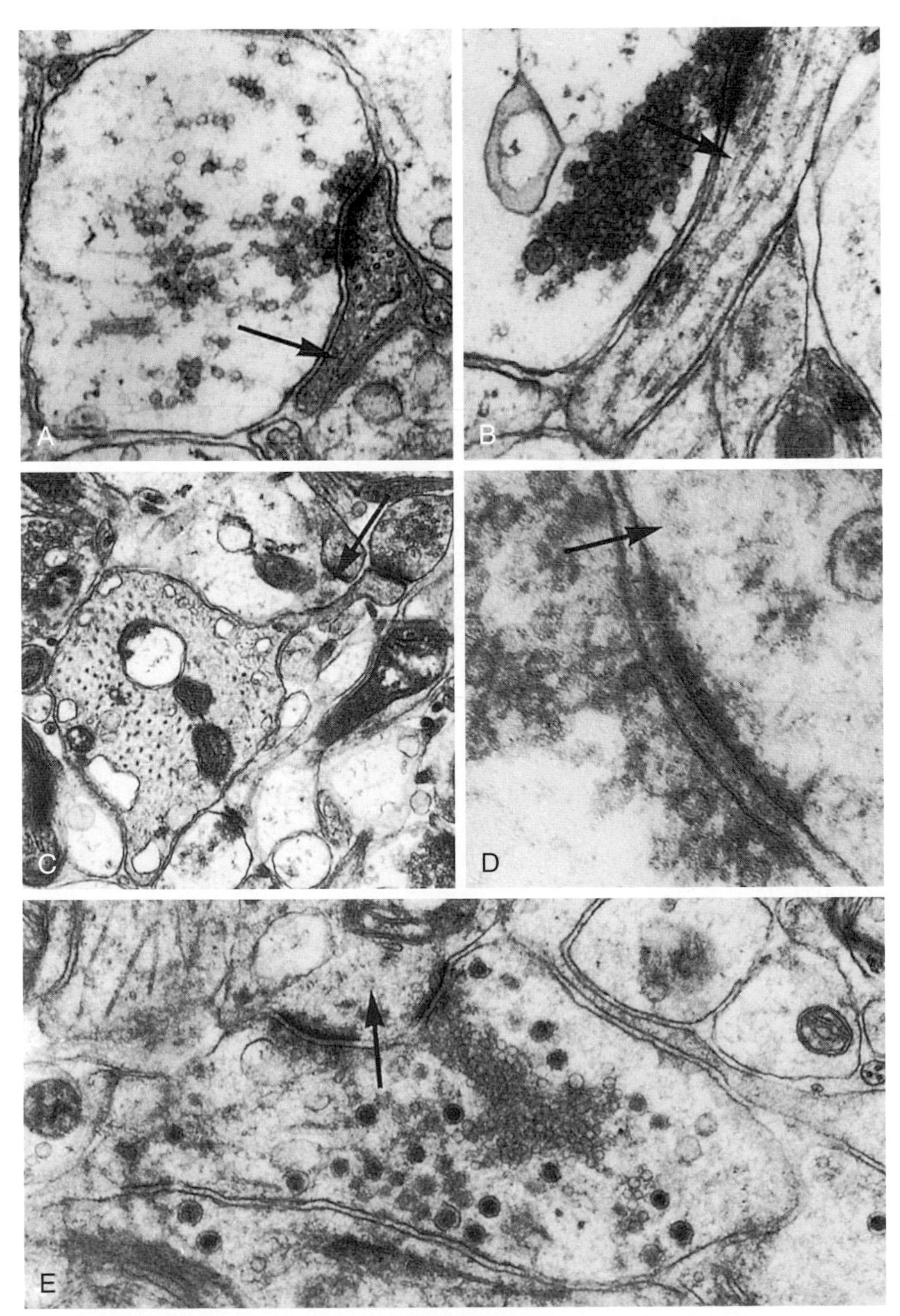

Fig. 9.20 Electron micrographs of synapses. The *arrow* indicates transmission direction. (A) Axodendritic synapse. Presynaptic vesicles are located to the left (×37,600). (B) Axodendritic synapse. Note neurotubules in dendrite (×43,420). (C) Dendrite in cross-section. Note the synapse (×18,800). (D) Axodendritic synapse. Note presynaptic vesicle fusing with the axolemma (×76,000). (E) Axon terminal with clear synaptic vesicles and dense-cored vesicles (×31,000). (From Leeson TS, Leeson CR, Paparo AA. *Text/Atlas of Histology*. Philadelphia: WB Saunders; 1988.)

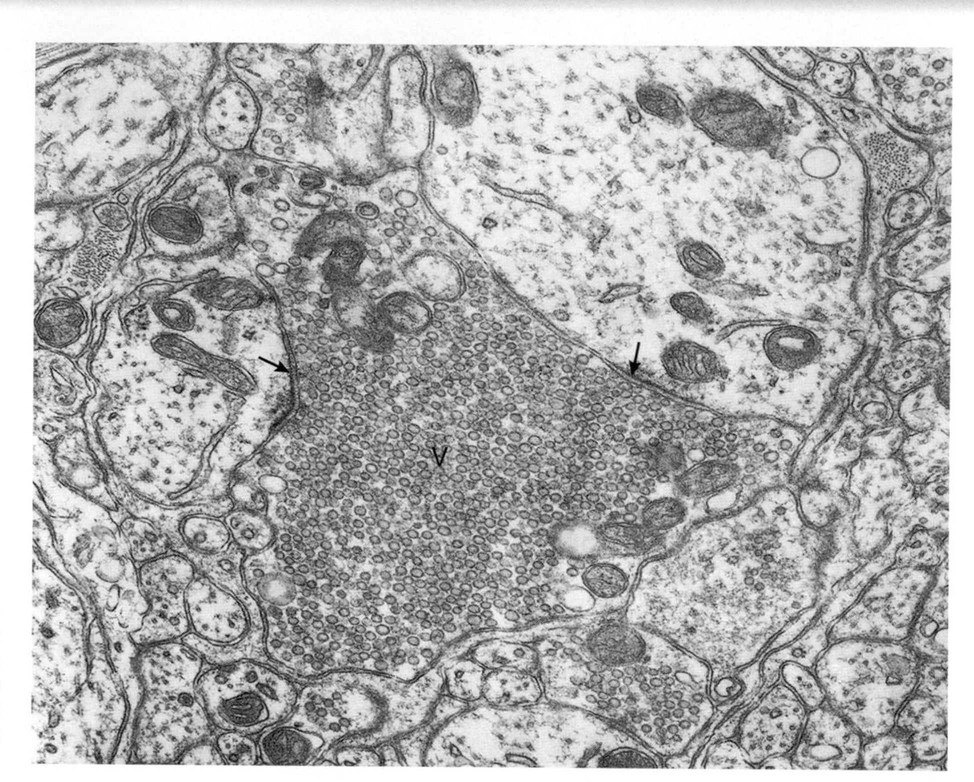

Fig. 9.21 Electron micrograph of an axodendritic synapse. Observe the numerous synaptic vesicles (v) within the axon terminal synapsing with dendrites and the synaptic clefts at these sites *(arrows)*. (From Jennes L, Traurig HH, Conn PM. *Atlas of the Human Brain.* Philadelphia: Lippincott-Raven, 1995.)

in axons are derived from swellings along the axon called ***boutons en passage***, where each bouton may serve as a synaptic site.

The cytoplasm at the **presynaptic membrane** contains mitochondria, a few elements of smooth endoplasmic reticulum (SER), and an abundance of synaptic vesicles assembled around the presynaptic membrane (Fig. 9.21). **Synaptic vesicles** are spherical structures (40–60 nm in diameter) filled with neurotransmitter substance that usually was manufactured and packaged near the axon terminal. Peptide neurotransmitters, however, are manufactured and packaged in the cell body and are transported to the axon terminal via anterograde transport. Enzymes located in the axoplasm protect neurotransmitters from degradation.

Also located on the cytoplasmic aspect of the presynaptic membrane are cone-shaped densities that project from the membrane into the cytoplasm. They appear to be associated with many of the synaptic vesicles, forming the **active site** of the synapse. The contents of synaptic vesicles associated with the active site are released at stimulation. Other synaptic vesicles, forming a reserve pool, adhere to actin microfilaments at a slight distance from the active site but migrate there once the active sites are unoccupied. **Cell adhesion molecules** are known to play an additional role in this process as signaling molecules at both the presynaptic and postsynaptic aspects of the synapse.

Synapsin-I, a small protein that forms a complex with the vesicle surface, probably assists in the clustering of synaptic vesicles that are held in reserve. When synapsin-I is phosphorylated, these synaptic vesicles become free to move to the active site in preparation for release of the neurotransmitter; dephosphorylation of synapsin-I reverses the process.

Synapsin-II and another small protein (**rab3a**) control association of the vesicles with actin microfilaments. Docking of the synaptic vesicles with the presynaptic membrane is under control of two additional synaptic vesicle proteins: **synaptotagmin** and **synaptophysin**. When an action potential reaches the presynaptic membrane, it initiates opening of the **voltage-gated calcium ion (Ca^{2+}) channels**, permitting Ca^{2+} to enter. This Ca^{2+} ion influx causes synaptic vesicles, under the influence of **SNARE (SNAP receptor)** proteins (including **synaptobrevin, syntaxin,** and **soluble *N*-ethylmaleimide–sensitive–fusion protein attachment protein-25 [SNAP-25]**) to fuse with the presynaptic membrane, exocytosing their stored neurotransmitter material into the synaptic cleft.

Excess membrane is recaptured via **clathrin-mediated endocytosis**. Recycling of synaptic vesicles involves interactions between synaptotagmin and **vesicle coat protein AP-2**. The endocytic vesicle fuses with the SER, where new membrane is continuously recycled.

Clinical Correlations

The microorganism **Clostridium botulinum** *produces a protease known as* ***neurotoxin B*** *that specifically cleaves the synaptic* ***vesicle fusion proteins*** *synaptobrevin, syntaxin, and SNAP-25. The toxin is lethal in very small quantities and can be ingested in food from damaged cans or from food that was handled improperly. Neurotoxin B selectively blocks synaptic vesicle fusion with the presynaptic membrane of myoneural junctions, preventing the exocytosis of the neurotransmitter acetylcholine without affecting any other aspect of nerve function. The absence of acetylcholine release results in flaccid paralysis of skeletal muscles. If this condition is not recognized early and antitoxins are not administered, the affected individual will succumb to respiratory failure and death.*

The **postsynaptic membrane**, a thickened portion of the plasma membrane of the postsynaptic cell, contains **neurotransmitter receptors**. Binding of the neurotransmitter to its receptors initiates **depolarization** (an excitatory response) or **hyperpolarization** (an inhibitory response) of the postsynaptic membrane. Neuroglia have been shown to increase synaptogenesis, synaptic efficacy, and action-potential firing.

The relative thicknesses and densities of the presynaptic and postsynaptic membranes, coupled with the width of the synaptic cleft, generally correlate with the nature of the response. A thick postganglionic density and a 30-nm synaptic cleft constitutes an **asymmetric synapse**, which is usually the site of **excitatory responses**. A thin postsynaptic density and a 20-nm synaptic cleft constitutes a **symmetric synapse**, which is usually the site of **inhibitory responses**.

Neurotransmitters and Neuromodulators

Neurotransmitters and neuromodulators are signaling molecules that are released at the presynaptic membranes and activate receptors on postsynaptic membranes.

Cells of the nervous system communicate mostly by the release of signaling molecules. The released molecules contact receptor molecules protruding from the plasmalemma of the target cell, eliciting a response from the target cell. These signaling molecules were called ***neurotransmitters***. However, such molecules may act on two types of receptors: (1) those directly associated with ion channels and (2) those associated with G proteins or receptor kinases, which activate a second messenger. Therefore, signaling molecules that act as "first messenger systems" (i.e., act on receptors directly associated with ion channels) are now referred to as ***neurotransmitters***. Signaling molecules that invoke the "second messenger system" are referred to as ***neuromodulators*** or ***neurohormones***. Because neurotransmitters act directly, the entire process is fast, lasting usually less than 1 msec. Events using neuromodulators are much slower and may last as long as a few minutes.

There are perhaps 100 known neurotransmitters (and neuromodulators) represented by the following four groups:

- Small-molecule transmitters
- Neuropeptides
- Gases
- Other

Small-molecule transmitters are of three major types:

- Acetylcholine (the only one in this group that is not an amino acid derivative)
- Amino acids: glutamate, aspartate, glycine, and GABA
- Biogenic amines (monoamines)—serotonin; and the three catecholamines—dopamine, **norepinephrine** (noradrenaline), and epinephrine (adrenaline)

Neuropeptides, many of which are neuromodulators, form a large group. They include the following:

- Opioid peptides: enkephalins and endorphins
- Gastrointestinal peptides produced by cells of the diffuse neuroendocrine system: substance P, neurotensin, and VIP
- Hypothalamic-releasing hormones: thyrotropin-releasing hormone and somatostatin
- Hormones: stored in and released from the neurohypoph ysis (antidiuretic hormone and oxytocin)

Certain **gases** act as neuromodulators. They are as follows:

- Nitric oxide (NO)
- Carbon monoxide (CO)

The **other category** of neurotransmitters includes the following:

- Anandamide, 2-arachidonylglycerol, and virodhamine, all of which bind to cannabinoid receptors
- Adenosine triphosphate, which binds to both P2X and P2Y receptors
- Adenosine, which binds to P1 receptors (adenosine receptors)

The most common neurotransmitters are listed inTable 9.1.

Clinical Correlations

1. ***Huntington disease (HD)*** *is a hereditary condition with an onset at about the third or fourth decade of life that currently afflicts approximately 30,000 people in the United States but genetic testing may show that there is another 200,000 individuals who may inherit the condition. It begins as involuntary jerking movements that progress to severe distortions, dementia, and motor dysfunction. The condition is thought to be related to loss of cells producing* ***GABA****, an inhibitory neurotransmitter. Most patients die within 20 years of the initial signs of the disease. The cause of HD appears to be a mutated Huntingtin gene, which interferes with the normal formation of nucleoporins that constitute the nuclear pore complexes, resulting in malfunctioning of transport between the nucleus and the cytoplasm. Although it is not known why, but neurons that are usually affected by this mutation reside in the cerebral cortex, striatum, and basal nuclei (basal ganglia). The malfunctioning of the nucleocytoplasmic transport through the nuclear pore complex eventually causes these cells to die, resulting in Huntington disease and the death of the individual.*
2. ***Parkinson disease****, a crippling disease related to the absence of* ***dopamine*** *due to degeneration of the dopamine-producing cells in the substantia nigra of the brain, is characterized by muscular rigidity, constant tremor, bradykinesia (slow movement), and, finally, a mask-like face and difficult voluntary movement. Histopathological studies of patients who died of Parkinson disease consistently demonstrated the presence of Lewy bodies, vesicles containing neurofilaments, tau protein, and α-synuclein, in the dopaminergic soma, suggesting that the presence of these bodies are indicative of Parkinson disease. Apparently, the immune system views α-synuclein as an antigen and plasma cells manufacture antibodies against it, causing the death of these dopaminergic cells. The current treatment, although not a cure, consists of the administration of L-dopa (levodopa) and carbidopa, which provides a temporary relief of the motor abnormalities, although the neurons in the affected area continue to die. There are other treatment modalities available, but none that offer a cure.*

TABLE 9.1 **Properties of the Major Neurotransmitters**

Neurotransmitter/Excite or Inhibit	Precursor	Enzyme	Location in Nervous System	Miscellaneous
Acetylcholine/excitatory	Acetyl CoA and choline	Choline acetyltransferase	Myoneural junction; autonomic nervous system; striatum	Removed by the enzyme acetylcholinesterase; cholinergic neurons degenerate in Alzheimer disease
Glutamate/excitatory	Glutamine	Glutaminase	Most excitatory neurons of the CNS	Glutamate-glutamine cycle; excitotoxicity
GABA/inhibitory	Glutamate	Glutamic acid decarboxylase	Mostly local circuit interneurons	Decreased GABA synthesis in vitamin B_6 deficiency
Glycine/inhibitory	Serine	Serine hydroxymethyltransferase	Neurons of the spinal cord	Activity blocked by strychnine
Dopamine/excitatory	Tyrosine (L-dopa)	Tyrosine hydroxylase	Neurons of the substantia nigra, arcuate nucleus, and tegmentum	Associated with parkinsonism; inhibition of prolactin release; schizophrenia
Norepinephrine (noradrenalin)/excitatory	Tyrosine (dopamine)	dopamine β--hydroxylase	Postganglionic sympathetic neurons; locus ceruleus	Associated with mood and mood disorders (mania, depression, anxiety, and panic)
Epinephrine/excitatory	Norepinephrine	Phenylethanolamine-N-methyltransferase	Rostral medulla	Not commonly present in the CNS
Serotonin (5-hydroxy-tryptamine)/excitatory	Tryptophan	Tryptophan-5-hydroxylase	Pineal body; raphe nuclei of midbrain, medulla, pons	Associated with sleep modulation; arousal, cognitive behaviors
Substance P/excitatory	Amino acids	Protein synthesis	Dorsal root and trigeminal ganglia (C and A δ fibers)	Composed of 11 amino acids; associated with transmission of pain
Somatostatin/inhibitory	Amino acids	Protein synthesis	Amygdala, small ganglion cells, and the hypothalamus	Also known as somatotropin release-inhibiting factor
α endorphin/ inhibitory	Amino acids	Protein synthesis	Hypothalamus; nucleus solitarius?	Least numerous of the opioid neurotransmitter-containing cells; function in pain suppression
Enkephalins/inhibitory	Amino acids	Protein synthesis	Raphe nucleus; striatum; limbic system; cerebral cortex	More numerous than α-endorphin- and enkephalin-containing cells; function in pain suppression
Dynorphin/inhibitory	Amino acids	Protein synthesis	Hypothalamus; amygdala; limbic system	More numerous than α-endorphin containing cells; function in pain suppression
ATP/excitatory	ADP	Oxidative phosphorylation; glycolysis	Motoneurons of spinal cord; autonomic ganglia	Also co-released with numerous neurotransmitters
Nitric oxide (NO)/inhibitory	L-arginine	NO synthase	Cerebellum; hippocampus; olfactory bulb	Smooth muscle relaxant thus strong vasodilator

Acetyl CoA, Acetyl coenzyme A; *ADP,* adenosine diphosphate; *ATP,* adenosine triphosphate; *CNS,* central nervous system; *GABA,* γ-aminobutyric acid.

Several principles appear to describe the functioning of neurotransmitters. First, a specific neurotransmitter may elicit different actions under varied circumstances. Second, the nature of the postsynaptic receptors determines the effect of a neurotransmitter on postsynaptic cells. Synaptic communication commonly involves multiple neurotransmitters. Additionally, there is mounting evidence for **volume transmission** as a method of communication between brain cells. According to this concept, chemical and electrical "neurotransmitters," believed to exist in the extracellular fluid–filled spaces between brain cells, activate groups or fields of cells that contain appropriate receptors rather than activating individual cells. Whereas synaptic communication is fast-acting, volume transmission is thought to be slow and may be related to such conditions as autonomic function, alertness, awareness, changes in brain patterns during sleep, sensitivity to pain, and moods.

Peripheral Nervous System

The PNS includes the peripheral nerves and nerve cell bodies located outside of the CNS.

PERIPHERAL NERVES

Peripheral nerves are bundles of nerve fibers (axons) located outside of the CNS, surrounded by several investments of connective tissue sheaths (Figs. 9.22 through 9.25). These bundles **(fascicles)** may be observed with the unaided eye; those that are myelinated appear white because of the presence of myelin. Usually, each bundle of nerve fibers, regardless of size, has both sensory and motor components, and are considered to be **mixed nerves**. There are, however, some nerves that are purely **sensory** and some nerves that are purely **motor**.

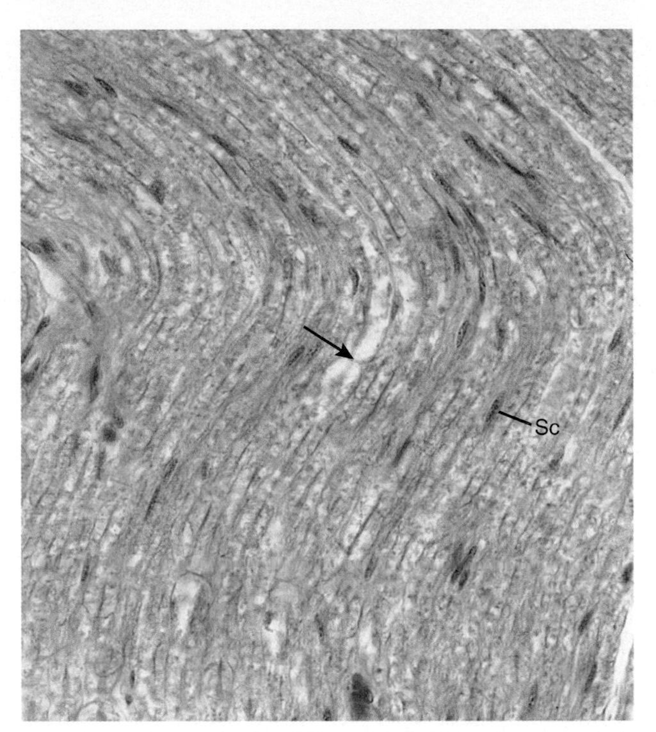

Fig. 9.22 Light micrograph of a longitudinal section of a peripheral nerve (×270). Myelin and nodes of Ranvier *(arrow)*, as well as the lightly stained oval nuclei of Schwann cells (Sc), may be observed.

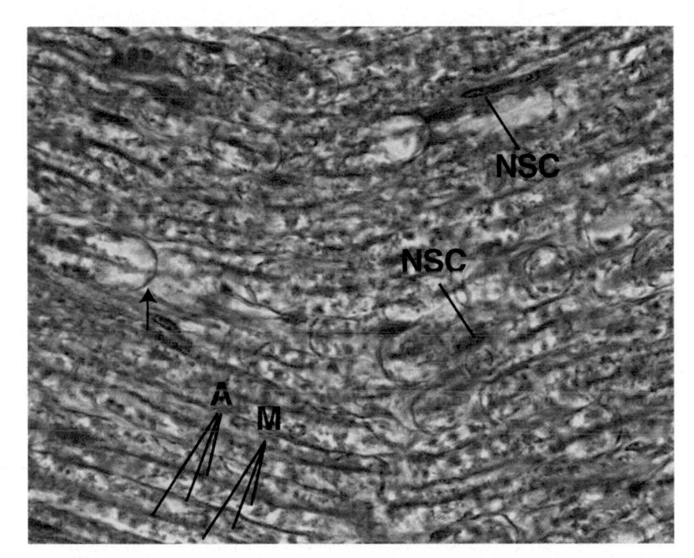

Fig. 9.23 A high-magnification light micrograph of a longitudinal section of a peripheral nerve. Note the numerous axons (A) covered with myelin (M) and the nuclei of Schwann cells (NSC). The arrow points to a node of Ranvier. (×540)

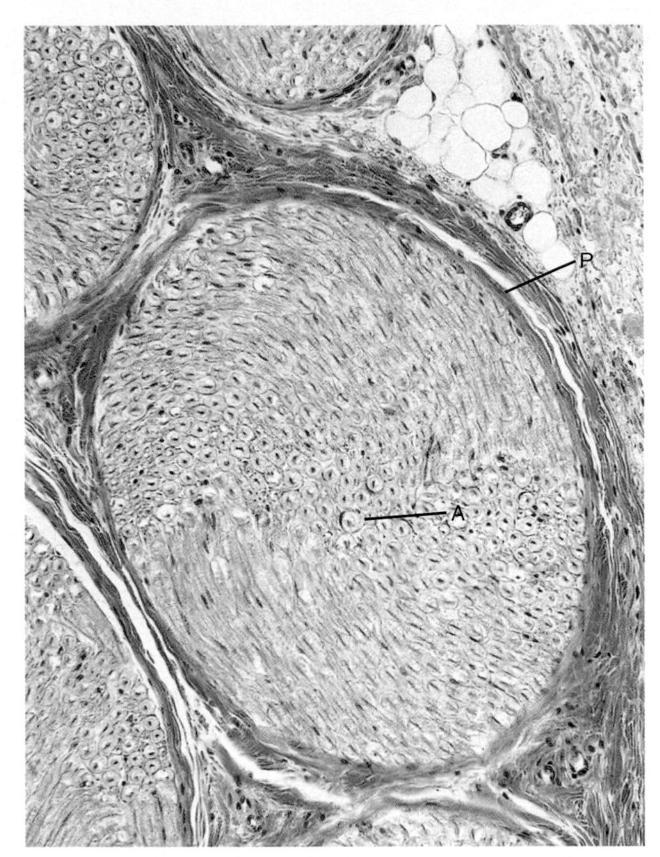

Fig. 9.24 Light micrograph of a cross-section of a peripheral nerve (×132). Observe the axons (A) and the perineurium (P) surrounding the fascicle.

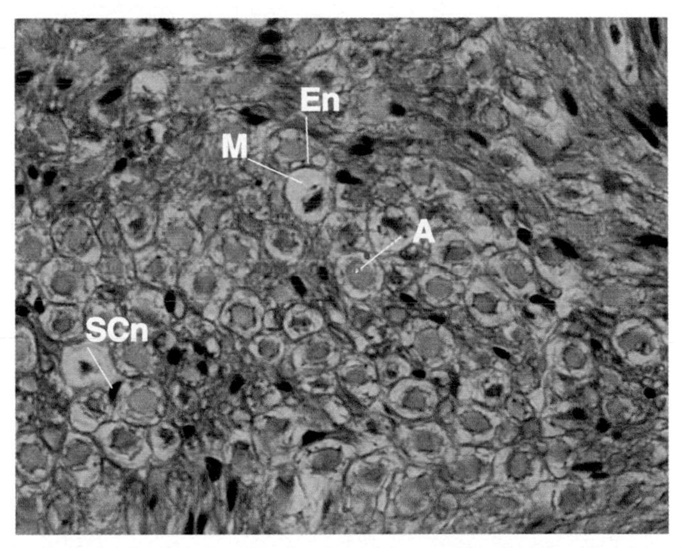

Fig. 9.25 A high-magnification light micrograph of a cross-section of a peripheral nerve. Note the endoneurium encircling each myelinated (M) axon (A). Several Schwann cell nuclei (SCn) are also evident. (×540)

Connective Tissue Investments

Connective tissue investments of peripheral nerves include the epineurium, perineurium, and endoneurium.

Epineurium is the outermost layer of the three connective tissue investments covering nerves (Fig. 9.26). The epineurium is composed of dense, irregular, collagenous connective tissue containing some thick elastic fibers that completely cover the entire spinal or cranial nerve. Collagen fibers within the sheath are aligned and oriented in such a fashion as to prevent damage by overstretching of the nerve bundle. The epineurium is thickest where it is continuous with the dura covering the CNS at the spinal cord or brain, where the spinal or cranial nerves originate, respectively. The epineurium becomes progressively thinner as the nerves branch into smaller nerve components, eventually disappearing.

Perineurium, the middle layer of connective tissue investments, covers each bundle of nerve fibers (fascicle) within the nerve. The perineurium is composed of dense connective tissue but is thinner than the epineurium. Its inner surface is lined by several layers of **epithelioid cells** joined to one another by **zonulae**

occludentes and surrounded by a basal lamina that isolates the neural environment, in that fashion creating a **blood–nerve barrier**. Between the layers of epithelioid cells are sparse collagen fibers oriented longitudinally and intertwined with a few elastic fibers. The thickness of the perineurium is progressively reduced to a sheet of flattened cells as the fascicle diminishes in diameter.

Endoneurium, the innermost layer of the three connective tissue investments of a nerve, surrounds individual nerve fibers (**axons**) and is composed of a loose connective tissue composed of a thin layer of reticular fibers (produced by the underlying Schwann cells), scattered fibroblasts, fixed macrophages, capillaries, and perivascular mast cells bathed in extracellular fluid. The endoneurium is in contact with the basal lamina of the Schwann cells. Thus, the endoneurium is a compartment that is completely isolated from the perineurium and Schwann cells. This isolation is an important factor in regulation of the microenvironment of the nerve fiber. Near the distal terminus of the axon, the endoneurium is reduced to a scant amount of reticular fibers surrounding the basal lamina of the Schwann cells.

Functional Classification of Nerves

Functionally, nerve fibers are classified as either sensory (afferent), motor (efferent), or both sensory and motor (mixed).

Nerve fibers are segregated functionally into sensory (**afferent**) fibers, motor (**efferent**) fibers, or mixed fibers. Sensory nerve fibers carry input from the cutaneous areas of the body, as well as from the viscera, back to the CNS for processing. Motor nerve fibers originate in the CNS and carry motor impulses to the effector organs. The sensory roots and motor roots of the spinal nerve unite to form **mixed peripheral nerves**, the **spinal nerves**, which carry both sensory and motor fibers.

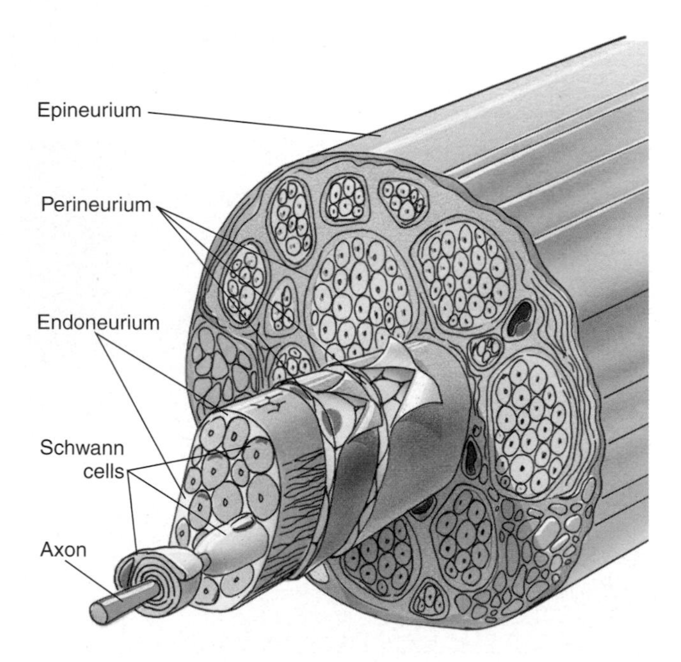

Fig. 9.26 Diagram of the structure of a nerve bundle.

Conduction Velocity

The **conduction velocity** of peripheral nerve fibers depends on the extent of their myelination. In myelinated nerves, it is only at the nodes of Ranvier that ions can cross the axonal plasma membrane, initiating depolarization for two reasons:

1. Voltage-gated Na^+ channels of the axon plasmalemma are clustered mostly at the nodes of Ranvier.
2. The myelin sheath covering the internodes prevents the outward movement of the excess Na^+ in the axoplasm associated with the action potential.

Therefore, the excess positive ions can diffuse only through the axoplasm to the next node, triggering depolarization there. As indicated earlier, the action potential "jumps" from node to node, a process called ***saltatory conduction*** (see Fig. 9.18B).

Unmyelinated nerve fibers are surrounded by a single layer of Schwann cell plasma membrane and cytoplasm, which provides little insulation. Moreover, voltage-gated Na^+ channels are distributed along the entire length of the axon plasma membrane. Therefore, impulse propagation in unmyelinated fibers occurs by **continuous conduction**, which is slower and requires more energy than the saltatory conduction occurring in myelinated fibers.

As demonstrated in Table 9.2, peripheral nerve fibers are classified into three major groups according to their conduction velocity. In thin unmyelinated fibers, the conduction velocity ranges from about 0.5 to 2 m/sec, whereas, in heavily myelinated fibers, it ranges from 15 to 120 m/sec.

The sensory components of the PNS are presented in various chapters throughout this text related to function.

Somatic Motor and Autonomic Nervous Systems

Functionally, the motor component is divided into the somatic and autonomic nervous systems.

The motor component of the nervous system is divided functionally into the somatic nervous system and the autonomic nervous system. The **somatic nervous system** provides motor impulses to the skeletal muscles, whereas the **autonomic nervous system** provides motor impulses to smooth muscles of the viscera, cardiac muscle of the heart, and secretory cells of the exocrine and endocrine glands, helping maintain homeostasis.

TABLE 9.2 Classification of Peripheral Nerve Fibers

Fiber Group	Diameter (μm)	Conduction Velocity (m/sec)	Function
Type A fibers—heavily myelinated	1–20	15–120	High-velocity fibers: acute pain, temperature, touch, pressure, proprioception, somatic efferent fibers
Type B fibers—less heavily myelinated	1–3	3–15	Moderate-velocity fibers: visceral afferents, preganglionic autonomics
Type C fibers—unmyelinated	0.5–1.5	0.5–2	Slow-velocity fibers: postganglionic autonomics, chronic pain

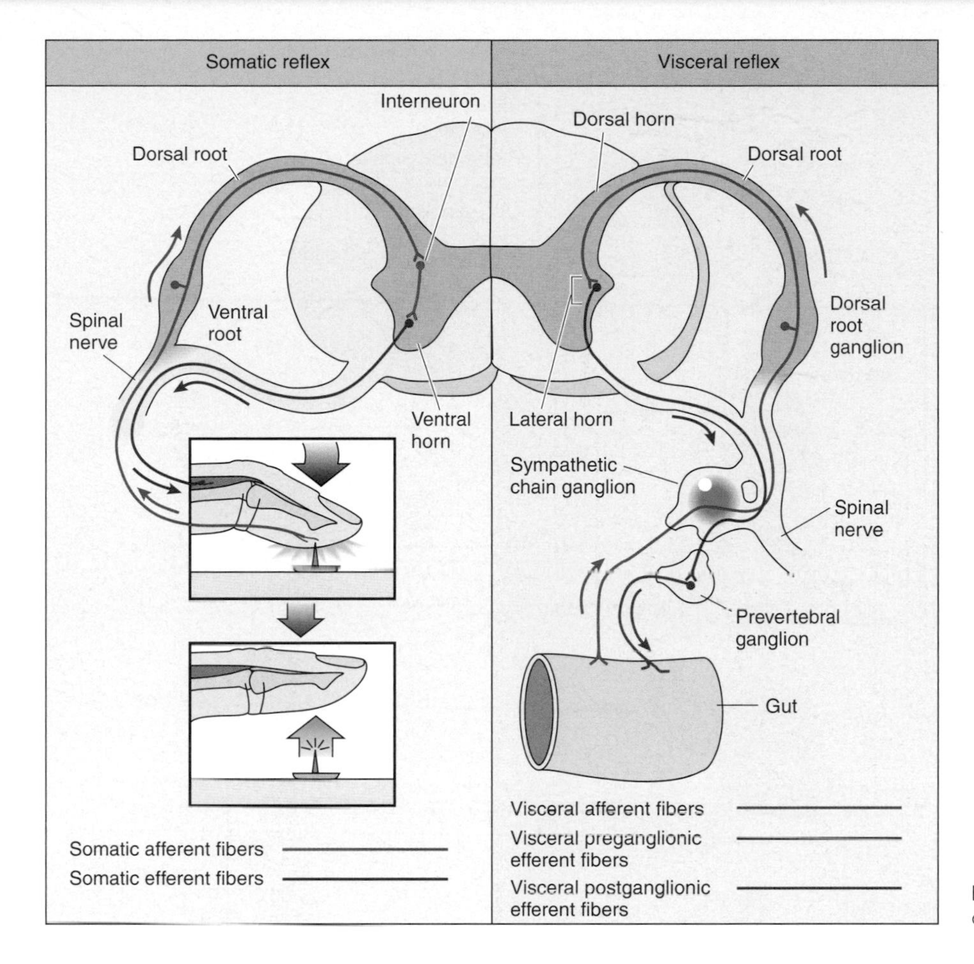

Fig. 9.27 Diagram comparing somatic and visceral reflexes.

MOTOR COMPONENT OF THE SOMATIC NERVOUS SYSTEM

Motor innervation to skeletal muscles is provided by somatic nerves.

Skeletal muscles receive motor nerve impulses conducted to them by spinal and selected cranial nerves of the somatic nervous system; these are basically under ***voluntary control***. The cell bodies of these nerve fibers originate in the CNS. The cranial nerves containing **somatic efferent components** are cranial nerves III, IV, VI, and XII (*excluding those nerves supplying muscles of branchiomeric rather than mesodermal origin*). Most of the 31 pairs of spinal nerves contain somatic efferent components to skeletal muscles.

Cell bodies of neurons of the somatic nervous system originate in motor nuclei of the cranial nerves embedded within the brain or in motor nuclei embedded in the ventral horn of the spinal cord. These neurons are multipolar, and their axons leave the brain or spinal cord and travel to the skeletal muscle via the cranial nerves or spinal nerves (Fig. 9.27). They synapse with the skeletal muscle at the motor end plate (see Chapter 8).

AUTONOMIC NERVOUS SYSTEM

Autonomic nerves provide motor innervation to smooth muscle and cardiac muscle and supply secretomotor innervation to glands.

The **autonomic (involuntary, visceral) nervous system** is generally defined as a motor system. Although agreement on this point is not universal, it is regarded as a motor system in this discussion. The autonomic nervous system controls the viscera of the body by supplying the **general visceral efferent** (**visceral motor**) fibers to smooth muscle, cardiac muscle, and secretory cells of glands.

In contrast to the somatic system, in which *one neuron*, originating in the CNS, acts directly on the effector organ, the autonomic nervous system possesses *two neurons* between the CNS and the effector organ. The soma of the first neurons in the chain are located in the CNS; their axons, known as the **preganglionic fibers** (**axons**), are usually myelinated. These enter an **autonomic ganglion**, located outside of the CNS, and synapse on multipolar cell bodies of **postganglionic neurons**. Axons of these neurons, known as **postganglionic fibers**, are usually unmyelinated but they are always enveloped by Schwann cells, and exit the ganglion to terminate on the **effector organ** (smooth muscle, cardiac muscle, or secretory cells of gland).

Postganglionic synapses of the autonomic nervous system arborize and the neurotransmitter substance diffuses out for some distance to the effector cells, thus contributing to more prolonged and widespread effects than do synapses in the somatic system. Smooth muscle cells stimulated by the neurotransmitter substance stimulate adjacent smooth muscle cells to contract by relaying the information via gap junctions.

The autonomic nervous system is subdivided into three functionally different divisions (Fig. 9.28), as detailed in the next sections.

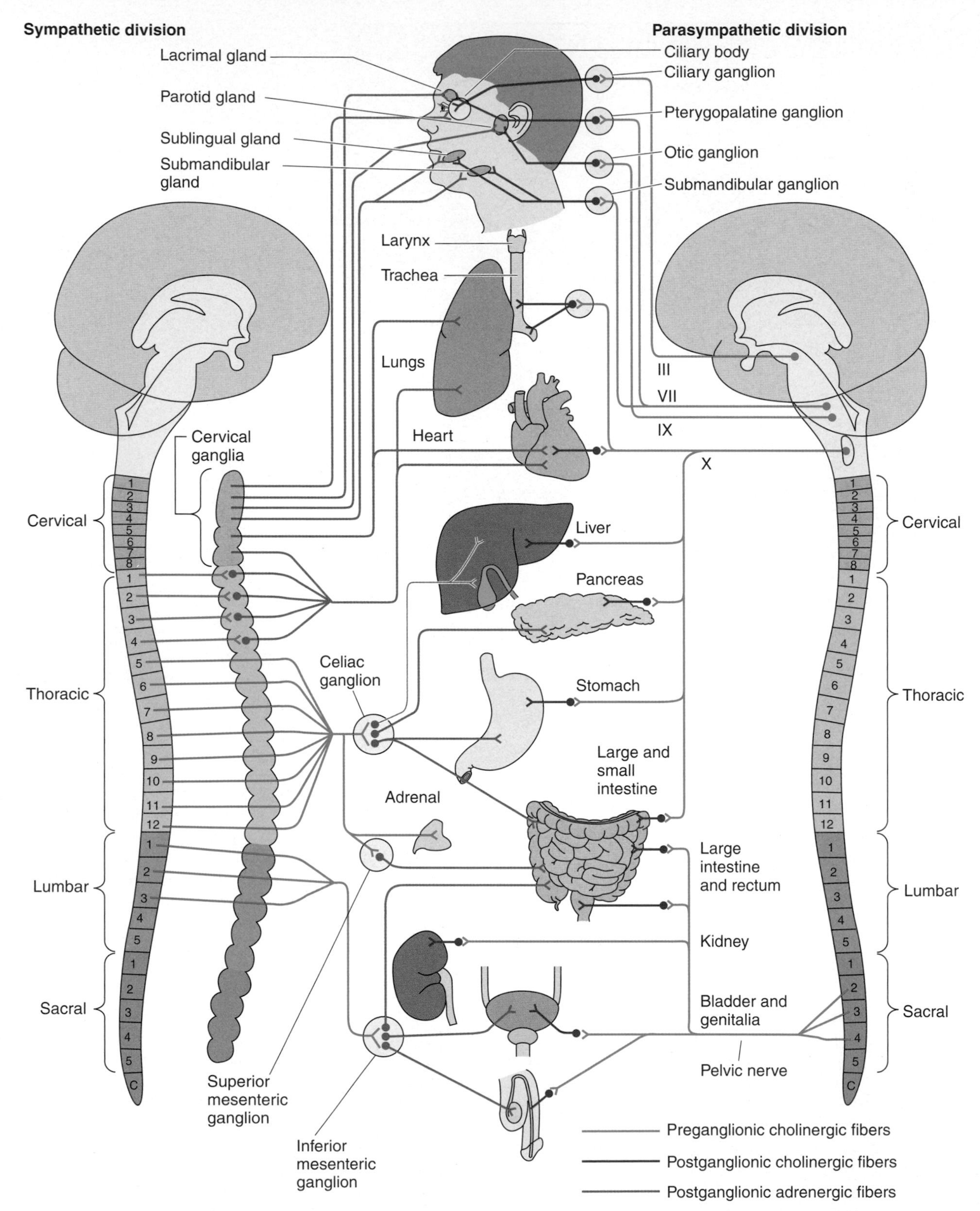

Fig. 9.28 Schematic diagram of the autonomic nervous system. *Left,* Sympathetic division. *Right,* Parasympathetic division.

Sympathetic Nervous System

The effect of the sympathetic nervous system is to prepare the body for "flight or fight or faint."

The sympathetic nervous system originates in the spinal cord from segments of the thoracic spinal cord and upper lumbar spinal cord (T1–L2). Thus, the sympathetic nervous system is sometimes called the ***thoracolumbar outflow*** (see Fig. 9.28). Cell bodies of preganglionic neurons are small, spindle-shaped cells that originate in the lateral horn of the spinal cord; their axons exit the cord via the ventral roots to join the spinal nerve. After a short distance, the fibers leave the peripheral nerve via

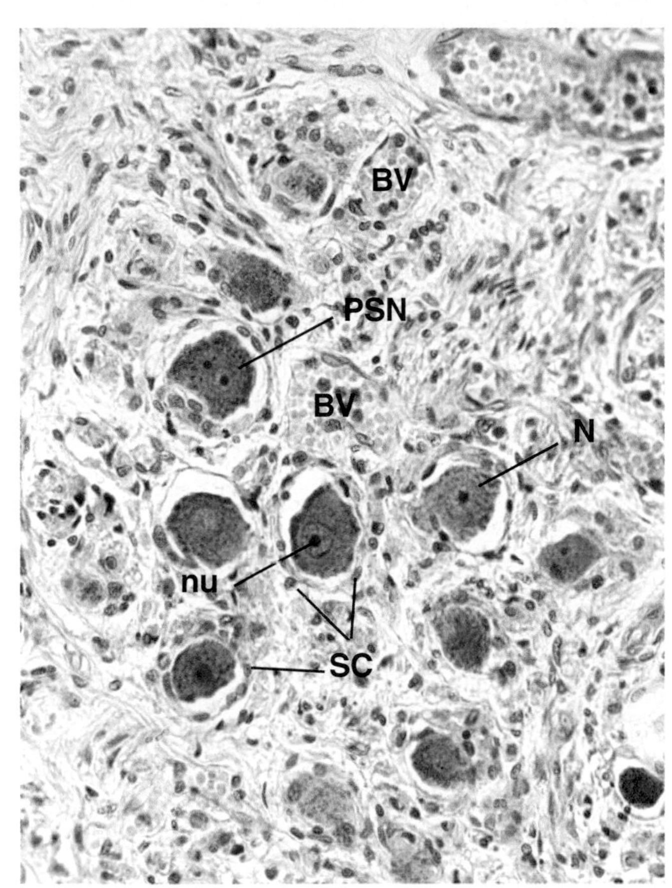

Fig. 9.29 This medium-magnification photomicrograph of a sympathetic ganglion displays numerous soma of postganglionic sympathetic neurons (PSN) whose large nuclei (N) and distinct nucleoli (nu) are clearly evident. Observe that these ganglia are highly vascular, as evidenced by the blood vessels (BV) scattered among the neuron cell bodies. Each soma is surrounded by small more or less flat supporting cells (SC). (×270)

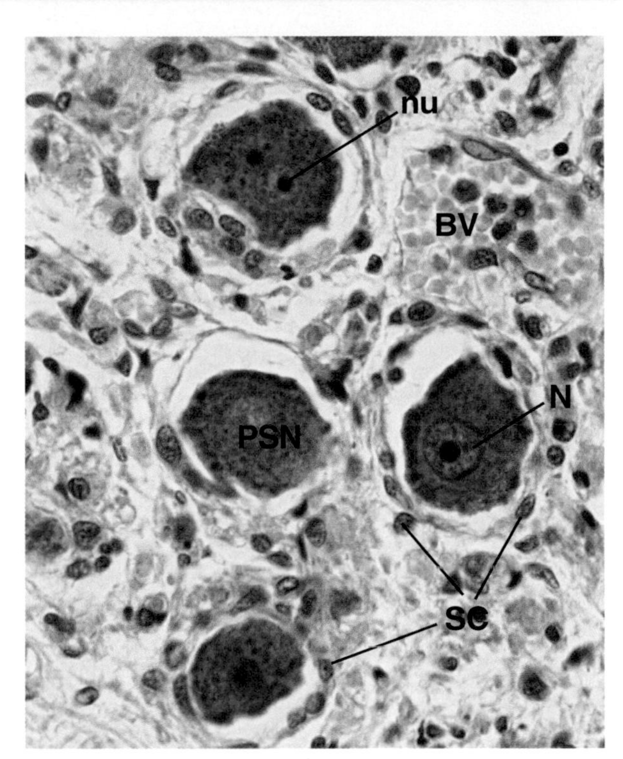

Fig. 9.30 This high-magnification photomicrograph of a sympathetic ganglion displays the soma of four postganglionic sympathetic neurons (PSN) whose large nuclei (N) and distinct nucleoli (nu) are clearly evident. Observe that these ganglia are highly vascular, as evidenced by the blood vessels (BV) scattered among the neuron cell bodies. Each soma is surrounded by small more or less flat supporting cells (SC). (×540)

white rami communicantes to enter one of the paravertebral chain ganglia, a collection of nerve cell bodies outside the central nervous system. There are two types of ganglia: those that belong to the autonomic nervous system and those that belong to the somatic nervous system (to be described later in this chapter).

Typically, the preganglionic neuron either synapses on a cell body of one of the multipolar postganglionic neurons residing in the ganglion associated with that spinal cord segment or ascends or descends in the sympathetic trunk to synapse on a cell in another of the chain ganglia. Certain preganglionic fibers do not synapse in the chain ganglia, however, instead pass through to enter the abdominal cavity as splanchnic nerves. Here, they seek collateral ganglia located along the abdominal aorta for synapsing on cell bodies of postganglionic fibers residing there.

Axons of postganglionic neurons housed in the chain ganglia (Figs. 9.29 and 9.30) exit the ganglia via gray rami communicantes to reenter the peripheral nerve for distribution to effector organs in the periphery (i.e., sweat glands, blood vessels, dilator pupillae muscles, cardiac muscle, bronchial tree, salivary glands, and arrector muscles of hair).

Axons of postganglionic neurons housed in the collateral ganglia exit the ganglia and accompany the myriad blood vessels to the viscera, where they synapse on the effector organs (i.e., blood vessels and the smooth muscles and glands of the viscera).

Essentially, the sympathetic nervous system prepares the body to fight an attacker or flee from an attacker by increasing respiration, blood pressure, heart rate, and blood flow to the skeletal muscles, dilating pupils of the eye, and generally slowing down visceral function. In the case of a catastrophic event, it causes the individual to freeze (or faint) to simulate death in hopes of stopping the attack.

Parasympathetic Nervous System

The effect of the parasympathetic nervous system is to prepare the body to "rest or digest."

The **parasympathetic nervous system** originates in the brain and sacral segments of the spinal cord (S2–S4); thus, the parasympathetic system is called the ***craniosacral outflow*** (see Fig. 9.28). Cell bodies of **preganglionic parasympathetic neurons** originating in the brain lie in the **visceromotor nuclei** of the four cranial nerves that carry visceral motor components (cranial nerves III, VII, IX, and X).

Axons of **preganglionic parasympathetic fibers** of cranial nerves III, VII, and IX seek **parasympathetic (terminal) ganglia** located outside the brain case, where they synapse on cell bodies of **postganglionic parasympathetic neurons** housed in the ganglia. Axons of these nerves, the **postganglionic parasympathetic nerves**, usually join branches of cranial nerve V to the effector organs they serve, including salivary glands and mucous glands; postganglionic parasympathetic fibers destined for the ciliary muscles and the sphincter pupillae muscles of the eye join branches of cranial nerve III (Fig. 9.31). Axons of

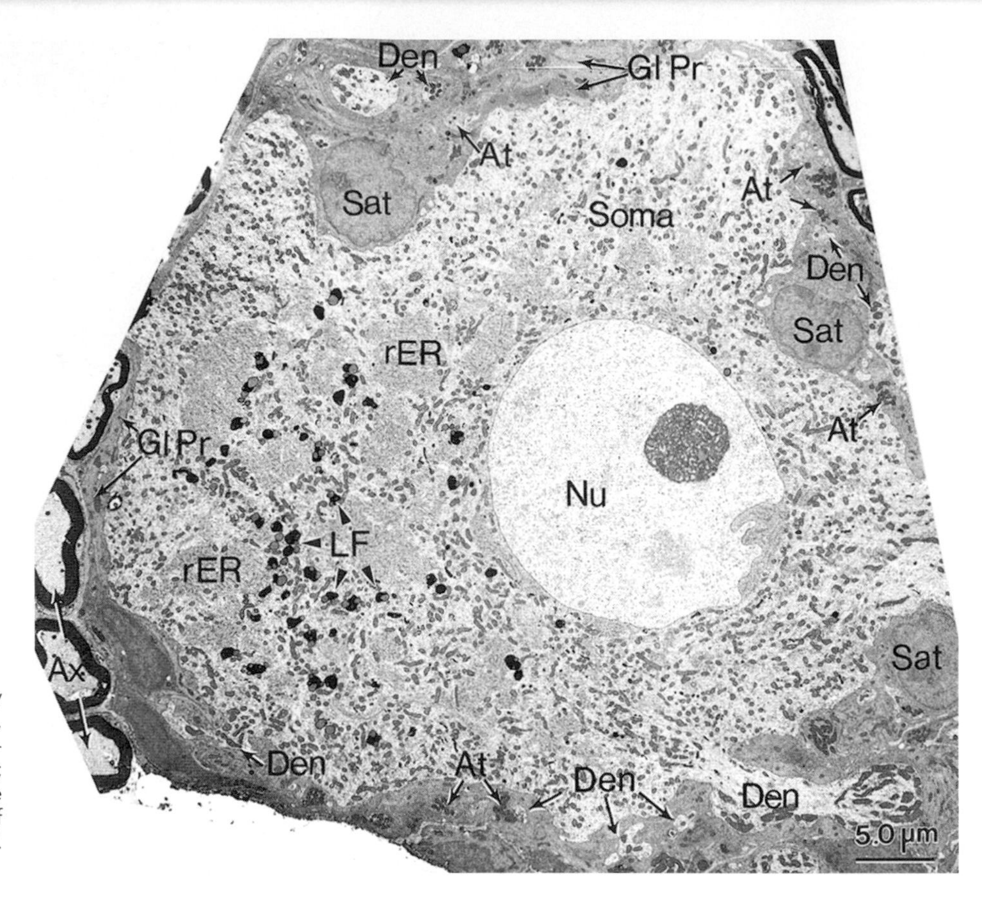

Fig. 9.31 Electron micrograph of the ciliary ganglion. At, Axon terminal; Ax, axon; Den, dendrite; GIPr, gastric inhibitory peptide receptor; LF, lipofuscin granules; Nu, nucleus; rER, rough endoplasmic reticulum; Sat, satellite cells. (From May PJ, Warren S. Ultrastructure of the macaque ciliary ganglion. *J Neurocytol.* 1993;22:1073–1095.)

preganglionic parasympathetic fibers in cranial nerve X travel to the thorax and abdomen before synapsing in the terminal ganglia within the respective viscera.

*Axons of **postganglionic parasympathetic nerves** synapse on cells of glands, smooth muscles, and cardiac muscle.*

Cell bodies of **preganglionic parasympathetic nerves** originating in segments of the sacral spinal cord are located in the lateral segment of the ventral horn and leave via the ventral root with the sacral nerves. From here, the axons project to the enteric nervous system, specifically to ganglia located in plexuses in the walls of the gastrointestinal tract.

Axons of other **postganglionic neurons** synapse on the effector organs in the viscera of the lower abdominal wall and the pelvis.

GENERALIZED COMPARISON OF THE SYMPATHETIC AND PARASYMPATHETIC NERVOUS SYSTEMS

The **parasympathetic nervous system** tends to be functionally antagonistic to the sympathetic system in that it decreases respiration, blood pressure, and heart rate; reduces blood flow to skeletal muscles; constricts the pupils; and generally increases the actions and functions of the visceral system. Thus, the parasympathetic nervous system brings about homeostasis, whereas the sympathetic nervous system prepares the body for "flight or fight or freeze (faint)." The sympathetic nervous system is broadly considered to function in **vasoconstriction**, whereas the parasympathetic nervous system is broadly considered to be **secretomotor** in function. Because the visceral components of the body receive innervation from both divisions of the autonomic nervous system, these two systems are balanced in health.

Acetylcholine is the neurotransmitter at all synapses between preganglionic and postganglionic fibers and between parasympathetic postganglionic endings and effector organs. **Norepinephrine** and **epinephrine** are the neurotransmitters at synapses between postganglionic sympathetic fibers and effector organs. However, sweat glands and arrector pili muscles that elevate the hair follicles of skin are the exceptions to this rule because the postganglionic sympathetic fibers to these structures release **acetylcholine** rather than the expected epinephrine or norepinephrine.

Generally, preganglionic fibers of the sympathetic system are short and postganglionic fibers are long. In contrast, preganglionic fibers of the parasympathetic system are long, whereas postganglionic fibers are short.

Enteric Nervous System

The function of the enteric nervous system is to control the digestive processes of the gastrointestinal tract.

The enteric nervous system has two components, those that belong only to the **enteric nervous system**, the intrinsic components, and those that belong to the sympathetic and parasympathetic nervous systems, the **extrinsic components**.

The **intrinsic components** are derived from neural crest material and are located completely within the wall of the alimentary canal. The neurons of the enteric nervous system project to two sets of ganglia, known as the **Meissner submucosal plexus** and **Auerbach myenteric plexus**. It has been estimated that the total number of neurons intrinsic to the enteric nervous system is equal to or greater than the number of neurons located in the entire spinal cord.

- **Auerbach myenteric plexus** functions in the localized aspects of the digestive tract, such as eliciting secretions from the glands of the mucosa and contractions of the smooth

muscle cells of the muscularis mucosae. This plexus is located between the inner circular and outer longitudinal layers of the muscularis externa of the digestive tract.
- **Meissner submucosal plexus** functions in the overall process of digestion—namely, peristalsis—which is the movement of food along the length of the alimentary canal. This plexus is located at the junction of the submucosa with the inner circular layer of the muscularis externa.
- There is a constant communication between the Auerbach and Meissner plexuses to ensure that the process of digestion progresses in the proper fashion.

Although the enteric nervous system can act independently in controlling the digestive process, the **extrinsic components** of the enteric nervous system—namely, the **sympathetic nerve fibers** derived from the splanchnic nerves and the **parasympathetic nerve fibers** carried by cranial nerve X (the vagus nerve)—impinge on and modulate the activities of the intrinsic components of the enteric nervous system. The former decreases and the latter increases the rate of peristalsis. The process of digestion is described in Chapters 17 and 18.

SENSORY GANGLIA OF THE SOMATIC NERVOUS SYSTEM

Sensory ganglia house cell bodies of sensory neurons.

Sensory ganglia are associated with ***cranial nerves*** V, VII, IX, and X and with ***each of the spinal nerves*** originating from the spinal cord. A sensory ganglion of a cranial nerve appears as a swelling of the nerve either inside the cranial vault or at its exit. Ganglia are usually identified with specific names that relate to the nerves. Sensory ganglia of the spinal nerves are called **dorsal root ganglia**; they house unipolar (pseudounipolar) cell bodies of the sensory nerves enveloped by cuboidal **capsule cells**. These capsule cells are then surrounded by a connective tissue capsule composed of **satellite cells** and collagen. The endoneurium of each axon becomes continuous with the connective tissue surrounding the ganglia. Peripheral processes of the neurons possess specialized receptors at their terminals to transduce various types of stimuli from the internal and external environments. Central processes pass from the ganglion to the brain within the cranial nerves or to the spinal cord within the spinal nerves, where they terminate on other neurons for processing (Figs. 9.32 and 9.33)

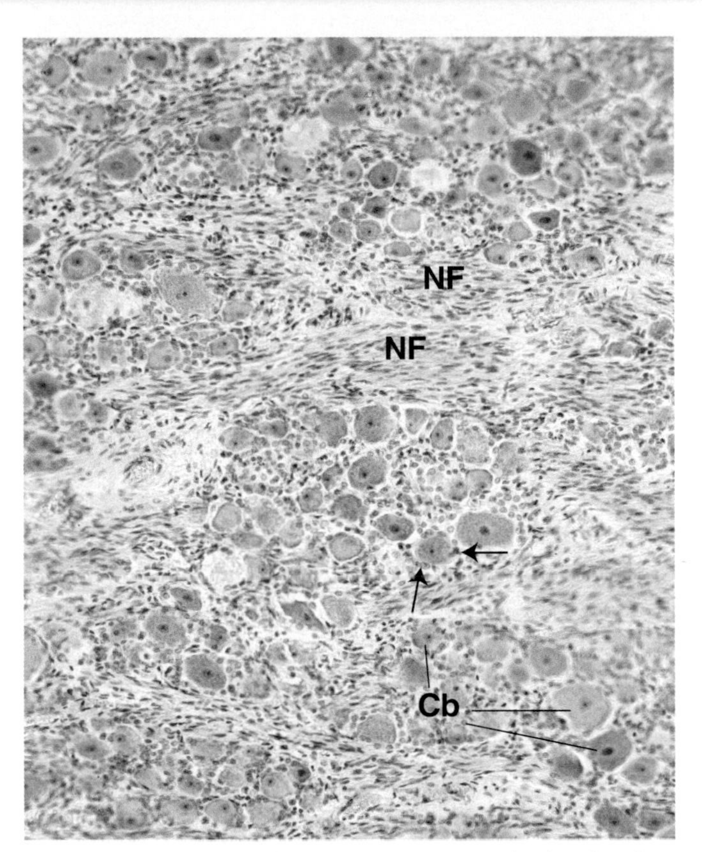

Fig. 9.32 This low-magnification photomicrograph of a dorsal root ganglion displays numerous cell bodies of unipolar neurons (Cb) whose large nuclei and prominent nucleoli are clearly evident. The central and peripheral processes of these unipolar neurons are gathered as collections of nerve fibers (NF). Observe that each cell body is surrounded by small cuboidal cells, known as capsule cells *(arrows)*. (×132)

Central Nervous System

The **central nervous system**, composed of the brain and spinal cord, consists of white matter and gray matter without intervening connective tissue elements; therefore, the CNS has the consistency of a semi-firm gel.

White matter is composed mostly of myelinated nerve fibers, along with some unmyelinated nerve fibers and neuroglial cells; its white color results from the abundance of myelin surrounding the axons. **Gray matter** consists of aggregations of neuronal cell bodies, dendrites, and unmyelinated portions of axons, as well as neuroglial cells; the absence of myelin causes these regions to appear gray in live tissue.

Axons, dendrites, and neuroglial processes form a tangled network of neural tissue called the ***neuropil*** (Fig. 9.34). In certain regions, aggregations of neuron cell bodies embedded in white matter are called ***nuclei***. Their counterparts in the PNS are called *ganglia*—an exception to this rule was the basal ganglia, a group of nerve cell bodies housed in the white matter of the brain. However, recently, the basal ganglia was renamed the *basal nuclei* to adhere to convention.

Gray matter in the brain is located at the periphery (**cortex**) of the cerebrum and cerebellum and also forms the deeper positioned basal nuclei, whereas the white matter lies deep to the cortex and surrounds the basal nuclei. The reverse is true in the spinal cord; white matter is located in the periphery of the spinal cord, whereas gray matter lies deep in the spinal cord, where it forms an H shape in cross-section. A small **central canal**, lined by **ependymal cells** and representing the lumen of the original neural tube, lies in the center of the crossbar of the H. The upper vertical bars of the H represent the **dorsal horns** of the spinal cord, which receive central processes of the sensory neurons whose cell bodies lie outside the central nervous system, in the **dorsal root ganglion**. Another group of neurons—called **interneurons** (**internuncial neurons** or **intercalated neurons**), located in the dorsal horns—form networks of communication for integration between sensory and motor neurons. These cells constitute the vast majority of the neurons of the body. The lower vertical bars of the H represent the **ventral horns** of the spinal cord, which house cell bodies of large multipolar motor neurons whose axons exit the spinal cord via the ventral roots of the spinal nerves.

MENINGES

The three connective tissue coverings of the brain and spinal cord are the **meninges**. The outermost layer of the meninges is the **dura mater**, the intermediate layer is the **arachnoid**, and the innermost or intimate layer of the meninges is the **pia mater** (Fig. 9.35).

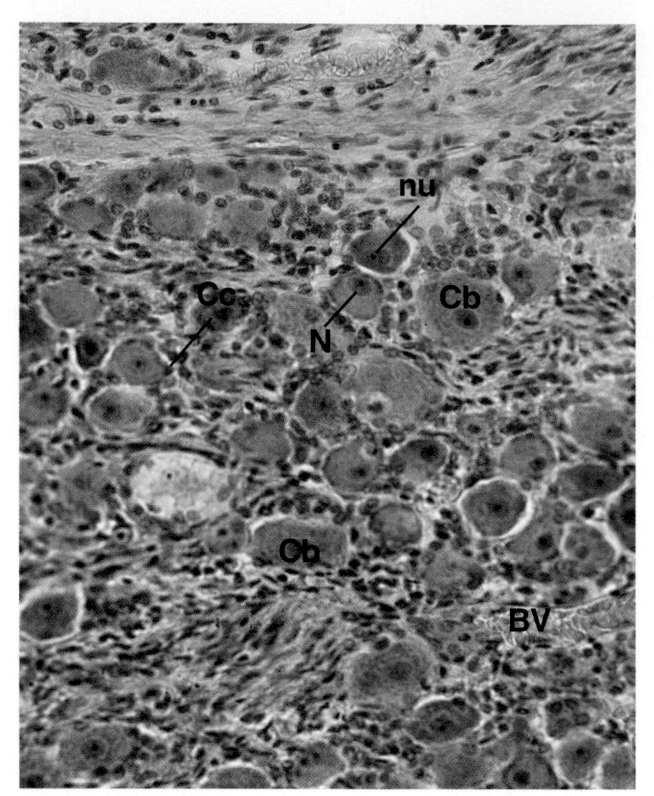

Fig. 9.33 This medium-magnification photomicrograph of a dorsal root ganglion displays its rich vascular supply (BV) that serves the numerous cell bodies of unipolar neurons (Cb) whose large nuclei (N) and prominent nucleoli (nu) are clearly evident. Note that each cell body is surrounded by small cuboidal cells, known as capsule cells (Cc). (×270)

Dura Mater

The dura mater, the outermost layer of the meninges, is composed of a dense collagenous connective tissue.

The **dura mater** covering the brain is a very tough, dense, collagenous connective tissue composed of two layers that are closely apposed in the adult. The **periosteal dura mater**, the outer layer, is composed of osteoprogenitor cells, fibroblasts, and organized bundles of collagen fibers that are loosely attached to the inner surface of the skull, except at the sutures and base of the skull, where the attachment is firm. As the name implies, periosteal dura mater serves as the periosteum of the inner surface of the skull and, as such, it is well vascularized. The periosteal dura mater of the cranium stops at the foramen ovale rather than continuing into the vertebral canal.

The inner layer of the dura, the **meningeal dura mater**, is composed of fibroblasts displaying dark-staining cytoplasm, elongated processes, ovoid nuclei, and sheet-like layers of fine collagen fibers. This layer also contains small blood vessels and nerve fibers.

A layer of cells internal to the meningeal dura, called the **border cell layer**, is composed of flattened fibroblasts exhibiting long processes that are occasionally attached to one another by desmosomes and gap junctions. Collagen fibers are lacking in this layer; in their place, an extracellular, amorphous, flocculent material (believed to be composed of a proteoglycan) surrounds the fibroblasts and extends into the interface between this layer and the meningeal dura.

The **spinal dura mater**, a continuation *only* of the meningeal layer of the cranial dura, does not adhere to the walls of the vertebral canal. Rather, it forms a continuous tube from the foramen magnum to the second segment of the sacrum and

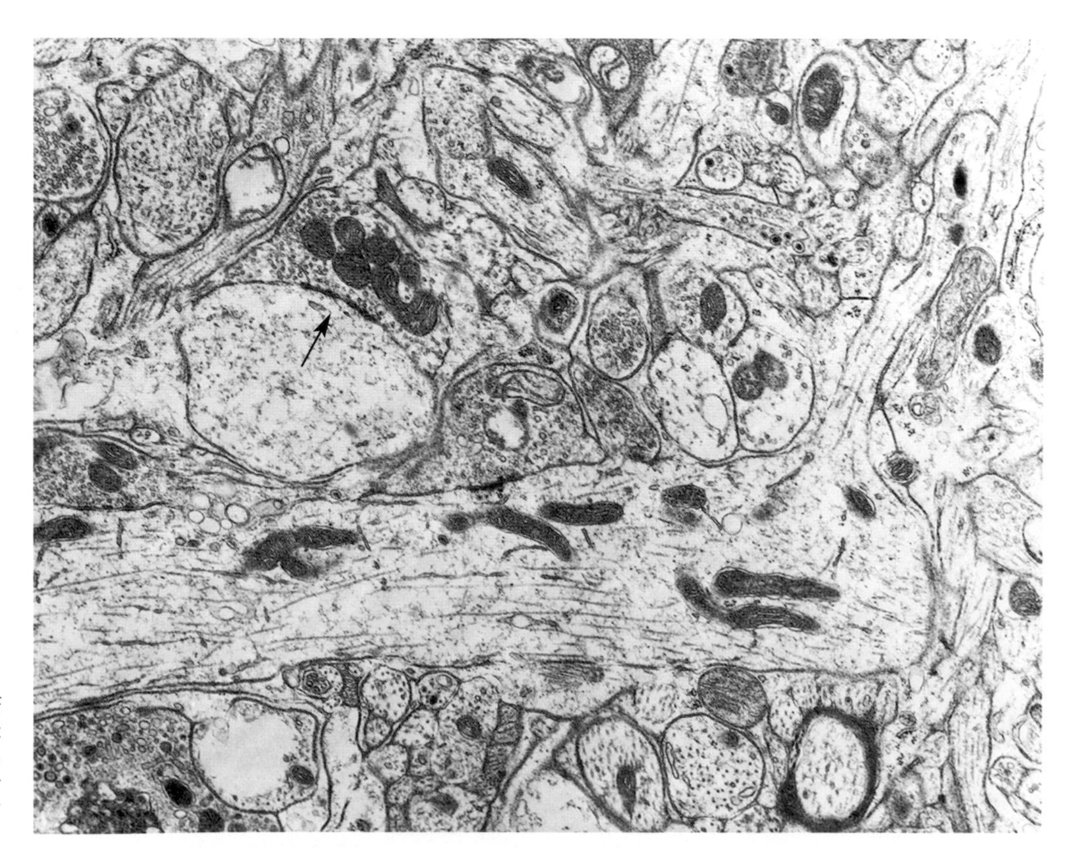

Fig. 9.34 Electron micrograph of axodendritic synapses *(arrow)* that form the neuropil. (From Jennes L, Traurig HH, Conn PM. *Atlas of the Human Brain*. Philadelphia: Lippincott-Raven; 1995.)

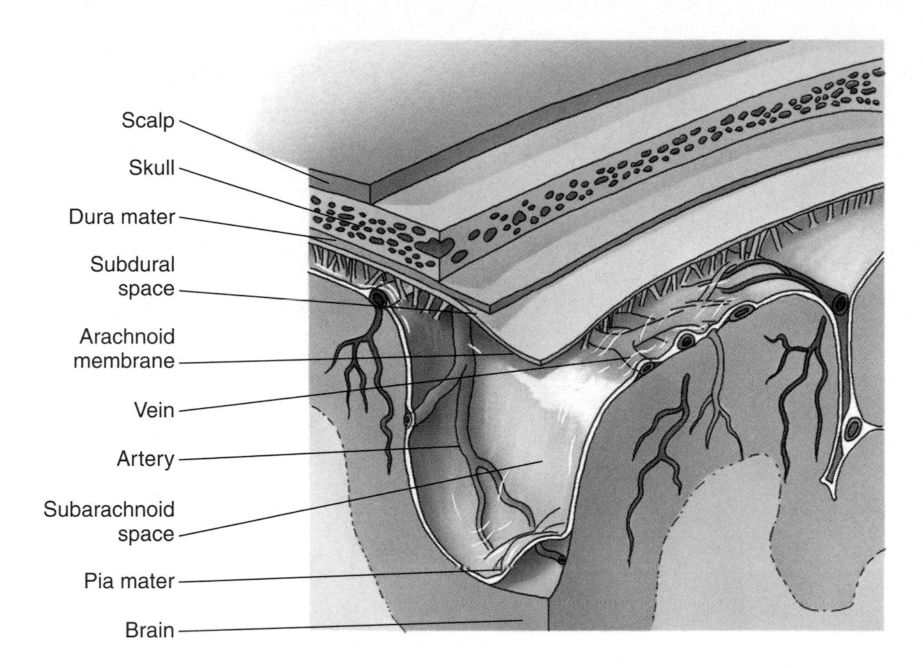

Fig. 9.35 Diagram of the skull and the layers of the meninges covering the brain.

is pierced by the spinal nerves. The **epidural space**, the space between the dura and the bony walls of the vertebral canal, is filled with epidural fat and a venous plexus.

Arachnoid

The arachnoid is the intermediate layer of the meninges.

The **arachnoid** layer of the meninges is avascular, that is, it does not have a vascular supply of its own, even though blood vessels course through it. This intermediate layer of the meninges consists of fibroblasts, collagen, and some elastic fibers. The fibroblasts form gap junctions and desmosomes with one another. The arachnoid is composed of two regions. The first is a flat, sheet-like membrane in contact with the dura. The interface between the dura and arachnoid, the **subdural space**, is considered a potential space because it appears only as the aftermath of injury resulting in subdural hemorrhage, when blood forces these two layers apart. The second is a deeper, gossamer-like region composed of loosely arranged **arachnoid trabecular cells** (modified fibroblasts), along with a few collagen fibers, which form trabeculae that contact the underlying pia mater. These arachnoid trabeculae span the **subarachnoid space**, the space between the sheet-like portion of the arachnoid and the pia. The arachnoid trabecular cells have long processes that attach to one another via desmosomes and communicate with one another by gap junctions.

Blood vessels from the dura pierce the arachnoid on their way to the vascular pia mater. However, these vessels are isolated both from the arachnoid and from the subarachnoid space by a close investment of arachnoid-derived, modified fibroblasts. In certain regions, the arachnoid extends through the dura to form **arachnoid villi**, which protrude into the spaces connected to the lumina of the **dural venous sinuses**. These specialized structures of the arachnoid function in transporting CSF from the subarachnoid space into the dural venous sinuses that eventually drain into the venous system. In later life, the villi enlarge and become sites for calcium deposits.

The interface between the arachnoid mater and pia mater is difficult to distinguish; therefore, the two layers are often called the ***pia-arachnoid***, with both surfaces being covered by a thin layer of squamous **epithelioid cells** composed of modified fibroblasts.

Pia Mater

The pia mater, the innermost, highly vascular layer of the meninges, is in close contact with the brain.

The **pia mater** is the innermost layer of the meninges and is intimately associated with the brain tissue, following closely all of its contours. The pia mater does not quite come into contact with the neural tissue, however, because a thin layer of neuroglial processes is always interposed between them.

The pia mater is composed of a thin layer of flattened, modified fibroblasts that resemble arachnoid trabecular cells. Blood vessels, abundant in this layer, are surrounded by **pial cells** interspersed with macrophages, mast cells, and lymphocytes. Fine collagenous and elastic fibers lie between the pia and neural tissue.

Blood vessels penetrate the neural tissues and are covered by pia mater until they form the **continuous capillaries** characteristic of the CNS. **End-feet of astrocytes**, known as ***pedicels***, rather than pia mater, cover capillaries within the neural tissue.

Clinical Correlations

1. ***Meningiomas*** *are slow-growing tumors of the meninges that are usually benign and produce clinical effects by compressing the brain and increasing intracranial pressure.*
2. ***Meningitis****, an inflammation of the meninges, is caused by bacteria or viruses invading the CSF. Bacterial meningitis, much more hazardous than viral meningitis, is easily spread and could be a very dangerous condition leading to brain damage, hearing loss, learning disability, and death, if untreated. The most common organisms*

Clinical Correlations—cont'd

involved in younger people are Neisseria meningitides and Streptococcus pneumoniae. In pregnant women, older individuals, and immunocompromised people, it is Listeria monocytogenes. The most telling symptoms of bacterial meningitis include stiff neck, headache, pain upon exposure to bright light, nausea, vomiting, fever, heavy drowsiness, and confusion. The symptoms develop very quickly, in less than 24 hours. Diagnosis is based on spinal fluid culture to determine the bacterial species involved, followed by treating with a specific antibiotic. Bacterial meningitis can be spread by the exchange of respiratory and throat secretions. Presently, in the United States, all children 4 years of age or younger have been vaccinated for the most common form of bacterial meningitis. Viral meningitis is more common than its bacterial form; usually, it is not serious and can resolve itself without treatment. However, it is important that affected individuals be seen by their physicians. A much less common form is fungal meningitis, but this is almost only present in immunocompromised patients.

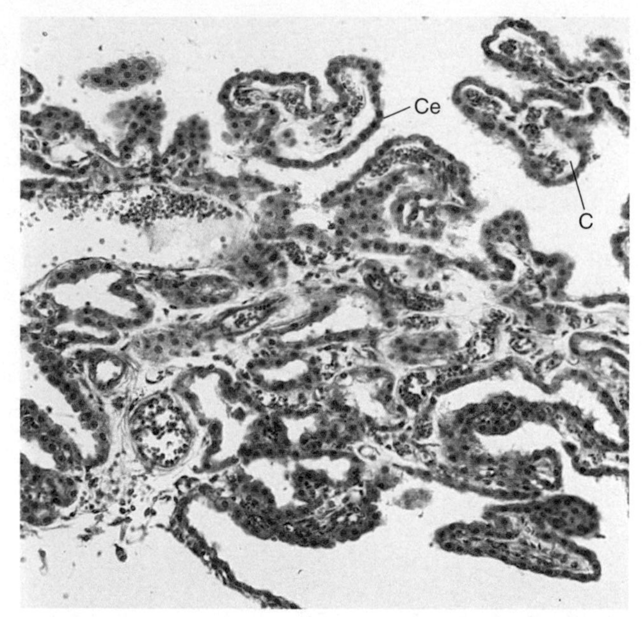

Fig. 9.36 Light micrograph of the choroid plexus (×270). Observe capillaries (c) and the simple cuboidal epithelium of the choroid plexus (Ce).

BLOOD–BRAIN BARRIER

Endothelial cells of CNS capillaries form a barrier known as the blood–brain barrier that prevents the free passage of selective blood-borne substances into the neural tissue.

The neural tissues of the CNS are protected from contacting blood-borne substances by a highly selective barrier known as the **blood–brain barrier**. This barrier is established by the **fasciae occludentes** formed between contiguous endothelial cells lining the **continuous capillaries** that traverse and supply the cells of the CNS. These tight junctions block the paracellular route (the flow of materials between cells). Additionally, these endothelial cells have relatively few pinocytotic vesicles, and vesicular traffic is almost completely restricted to **receptor-mediated transport** out of and into capillaries. Certain substances, however—such as oxygen, water, and carbon dioxide—can easily penetrate the blood–brain barrier, mostly owing to the presence of **aquaporins** located in endothelial cell membrane. Other small molecules, such as lipid-soluble materials and certain drugs, can also cross the blood–brain barrier. Molecules such as glucose, amino acids, certain vitamins, and nucleosides are transferred across the blood–brain barrier by specific carrier proteins, many via facilitated diffusion. Ions are also transported across the blood–brain barrier through carrier proteins via active transport. The energy requirement for this process is provided by the presence of large numbers of mitochondria within the endothelial cell cytoplasm.

Capillaries of the CNS are invested by well-defined basal laminae, which, in turn, are almost completely surrounded by the end-feet of numerous astrocytes, collectively called the ***perivascular glia limitans***. It is believed that these astrocytes help convey metabolites from blood vessels to neurons. Additionally, astrocytes remove excess K^+ and neurotransmitters from the neuron's environment, maintaining the neurochemical balance of the CNS extracellular milieu.

The blood–brain barrier (capillary endothelium), end-feet of protoplasmic astrocytes contacting the blood vessels of the brain, pericytes, and neurons that adjoin the blood vessels of the brain form what is now referred to as the ***neurovascular unit***. These components of the neurovascular unit interact with each other to maintain the integrity of the blood–brain barrier, as well as to control the movement of molecules across this barrier.

Clinical Correlations

1. *Because the blood–brain barrier is very selective, antibiotics, some therapeutic drugs, and certain neurotransmitters (e.g., dopamine) cannot penetrate it. Perfusion of a hypertonic solution of* ***mannitol*** *dehydrates the endothelial lining, causing these cells to shrink and thereby transiently relaxing the tight junctions of the capillary endothelial cells, permitting the movement of therapeutic drugs across the blood–brain barrier. Therapeutic drugs can also be bound to antibodies developed against* ***transferrin receptors*** *in the endothelial cells of the capillaries, permitting their transport across the blood–brain barrier and into the CNS.*
2. *In some diseases of the CNS (e.g., stroke, infection, tumors), the integrity of the blood–brain barrier is compromised, resulting in the accumulation of toxins and extraneous metabolites in the extracellular environment.*

CHOROID PLEXUS

The choroid plexus, composed of folds of pia mater within the ventricles of the brain, produces the CSF.

Folds of pia mater housing an abundance of fenestrated capillaries and invested by the simple cuboidal (ependymal) lining extend into the lateral, third, and fourth ventricles of the brain, forming the **choroid plexus** (Fig. 9.36). The choroid plexus produces **CSF**, which fills the ventricles of the brain and central canal of the spinal cord. As it circulates through the subarachnoid space, the CSF bathes the CNS. Although more than half of the CSF is produced by the choroid plexus, there is evidence that parenchyma in several other regions of the brain produce a substantial amount of CSF, which diffuses through the ependymal lining to enter the ventricles.

Cerebrospinal Fluid

CSF bathes, nourishes, and protects the brain and spinal cord.

CSF is produced at the rate of about 14 to 36 mL/h, replacing its total volume about four to five times daily. CSF circulates through the ventricles of the brain, the subarachnoid space, the perivascular space, and the central canal of the spinal cord. CSF is low in protein but rich in sodium, potassium, and chloride ions. It is clear and has a low density. Consisting of about 90% water and ions, it may also contain a few desquamated cells and occasional lymphocytes.

CSF is important to the metabolic activity of the CNS because brain metabolites diffuse into the CSF as it passes through the subarachnoid space. It also serves as a liquid cushion for protection of the CNS. CSF is able to flow by diffusion, and much of it is reabsorbed through the thin cells of the arachnoid villi in the superior sagittal venous sinus, from where the CSF is eventually returned to the bloodstream. However, some of it makes its way into the extracellular spaces of the brain tissue itself by occupying the **perivascular spaces** of small blood vessels that penetrate the brain tissue. It has been shown that the total water content in the CNS is housed in four separate compartments. A little less than 70% is intracellularly located, about 10% is in blood vessels, approximately 10% is CSF in the perivascular spaces, and the remaining 10% or so is CSF in the extracellular spaces (interstitial spaces). The movement of CSF from the perivascular spaces of the arterial side of the vasculature to the extracellular spaces occurs through aquaporin 4 (AQP4) channels located in the end-foot processes of the perivascular astrocytes. As the CSF continues to pass through the perivascular end-feet, the fluid pressure drives the CSF into the extracellular spaces. When it reaches perivascular end-feet of astrocytes covering small venules, it passes through the AQP4 channels of the astrocyte end-feet to enter the venous channel's perivascular space and from there into the venous vessel itself to be taken away into the venous outflow. This pathway for the flow of CSF through the interstitial spaces of the brain has been named the "**glial-associated lymphatic pathway**" or "**glymphatic pathway**."

Recently, it was discovered that the flow of CSF through the brain tissue increases while the individual is asleep. It appears that, during sleep, protoplasmic astrocytes shrink, thereby increasing the interstitial spaces in the gray matter by at least 50%. Due to this enlargement, the flow rate and flow volume of the CSF are greatly increased through the gray matter. It is believed that this rapid flow and increased volume permit a more efficient "flushing" of the interstitial spaces, thus removing waste products and excess ions and neurotransmitter substances from the microenvironment of the neurons and their synapses. It is now proposed that this cleansing of the interstitial spaces of the CNS is the reason why almost all members of the animal kingdom have to sleep. Once the individual awakens, the protoplasmic astrocytes become swollen, decreasing the interstitial spaces and limiting the rate and volume of CSF perfusion of the interstitial spaces of the CNS.

Clinical Correlations

Because CSF is constantly being produced, any decrease in absorption of the fluid by the arachnoid villi or blockage within the ventricles of the brain causes swelling in the brain tissue. This condition, called ***hydrocephalus****, leads to enlargement of the head in fetuses and neonates, impairment of mental and muscular functions, and death if left untreated.*

TABLE 9.3 Comparison Between Serum and Cerebrospinal Fluid

Constituent	Serum	Cerebrospinal Fluid
White blood cells (cells/mL)	0	0–5
Protein (g/L)	60–80	Negligible
Glucose (mmol/L)	4.0–5.5	2.1–4.0
Na^+ (mmol/L)	135–150	135–150
K^+ (mmol/L)	4.0–5.1	2.8–3.2
Cl^- (mmol/L)	100–105	115–130
Ca^{2+} (mmol/L)	2.1–2.5	1.0–1.4
Mg^{2+} (mmol/L)	0.7–1.0	0.8–1.3
pH	7.4	7.3

Blood–Cerebrospinal Fluid Barrier

The chemical stability of the CSF is maintained by the blood–CSF barrier, which is composed of zonulae occludentes between the cells of the simple cuboidal epithelium. These tight junctions impede the movement of substances between cells, compelling the substances to take the transcellular route. The production of CSF thus depends on facilitated and active transport across the simple cuboidal epithelium, resulting in differences in composition between the CSF and plasma (Table 9.3).

CEREBRAL CORTEX

The cerebral cortex is responsible for learning, memory, sensory integration, information analysis, and initiation of motor responses.

Gray matter at the periphery of the cerebral hemispheres is folded into many **gyri** and **sulci** called the ***cerebral cortex***. This portion of the brain is responsible for learning, memory, information analysis, initiation of motor response, and integration of sensory signals.

The cerebral cortex is divided into six layers, each of which exhibits a specific combination of neuronal types unique to the particular layer. The most superficial layer lies just deep to the pia mater (Fig. 9.37); the sixth, or deepest, layer of the cortex is bordered by white matter of the cerebrum. The six layers and their components are as follows:

1. The **molecular layer** is composed mostly of nerve terminals originating in other areas of the brain, **horizontal cells**, and neuroglia.
2. The **external granular layer** contains mostly **granule** (stellate) **cells** and neuroglial cells.
3. The **external pyramidal layer** contains neuroglial cells and large **pyramidal cells**, which become increasingly larger from the external to the internal border of this layer.
4. The **internal granular layer** is a thin layer characterized by closely arranged, small **granule** (stellate) **cells**, **pyramidal cells**, and neuroglia. This layer has the greatest cell density of the cerebral cortex.
5. The **internal pyramidal layer** contains the largest **pyramidal cells** and neuroglia. This layer has the lowest cell density of the cerebral cortex.
6. The **multiform layer** consists of cells of various shapes (**Martinotti cells**) and neuroglia.

Clinical Correlations

Dementia

Dementia *is a cluster of symptoms characterized by reversible or irreversible deterioration of an individual's memory and intellectual capacity that interferes with that person's capacity to execute routine daily functions.* ***Reversible dementia*** *can be due to issues such as drug interactions, thyroid malfunction, or dehydration and, once corrected, the symptoms disappear.* ***Irreversible dementia*** *is a progressive disease whose progress can be retarded but cannot be reversed.*

Alzheimer Disease

Approximately 80% of irreversible dementia cases fall in the category of ***Alzheimer disease****. Because this is a progressive disease, the Alzheimer's Association divides it into seven overlapping phases. In* ***phase 1****, the individual's behavior is indistinguishable from normal behavior; however, a positron emission tomography (PET) scan can diagnose the beginning of this disease.* ***Phase 2*** *is not very different, although occasional inability of the person to remember common words or lack of memory regarding where the individual placed certain objects occurs with increased frequency.* ***Phase 3*** *is when the problem becomes apparent to close family members and friends; the affected individual repeatedly asks the same question, forgets names, cannot remember recently acquired information, and has difficulty in making plans. During* ***phase 4****, the patient often loses the ability to remember the date or day of the week and cannot perform tasks previously performed on a routine basis. During* ***phase 5****, the patient's condition continues to deteriorate and the patient cannot remember personal information, such as home address, telephone number, and information that was just provided. At this point, the patient begins to be unable to live independently. During* ***phase 6****, the patient can still recognize faces but cannot recall an individual's name or who that person is (e.g., wife, grandchild, child). By the time* ***phase 7*** *is reached, patients have to be fed, dressed, and assisted in walking and sitting because they are unable to perform any of these functions for themselves.*

The cause of Alzheimer disease is unknown but it is accompanied by a decrease in the number of synapses and neurons in the cerebral cortex and the accumulation of tau proteins in the neuronal cytoplasm and amyloid beta proteins that form plaques in the extracellular spaces (interstitial spaces). It appears that increasing accumulation of tau proteins in the neuronal cytoplasm initially has a deleterious effect on the neuron's ability to function and eventually results in the death of the neuron, whereas the amyloid beta plaque deposits elicit an inflammatory response. Recent studies have demonstrated that, thanks to the glymphatic system, the increased CSF flow clears a large fraction of the amyloid beta plaque from the extracellular spaces while the individual is asleep, suggesting that a proper-length sleep cycle may retard the progression of Alzheimer disease.

Additional evidence suggests that approximately 20% of all Alzheimer cases are correlated with the presence of APOE4, a gene that codes for the synthesis of apolipoprotein E. Within the CNS, apolipoprotein hinders the insulin receptors of neurons from binding insulin, diminishing the neuron's ability to endocytose glucose, the principal energy source of neurons. The reduction in glucose endocytosis causes reduced functioning and eventually the death of the affected neurons. Because the problem is related to insulin use, it has been suggested that Alzheimer disease could be considered to be a different version of diabetes, called ***type 3 diabetes****. Phase 2 clinical studies using insulin sprays administered nasally in Alzheimer patients have demonstrated a slowing of the progression of the disease in these patients. Further studies are required before any definitive conclusions can be reached.*

CEREBELLAR CORTEX

The cerebellar cortex is responsible for balance, equilibrium, muscle tone, and muscle coordination.

The layer of gray matter located in the periphery of the cerebellum is called the ***cerebellar cortex*** (Fig. 9.38). This portion of the brain is responsible for maintaining balance and equilibrium, muscle tone, and coordination of skeletal muscles. Histologically, the cerebellar cortex is divided into three layers:

1. The **molecular layer** lies directly below the pia mater and contains superficially located stellate cells, dendrites of **Purkinje cells**, basket cells, and unmyelinated axons from the granular layer.
2. The **Purkinje cell layer** houses the large, flask-shaped Purkinje cells, which are present in the cerebellum only (Figs. 9.38 and 9.39). Their arborized dendrites project into the molecular layer, and their myelinated axons project into the white matter. Each Purkinje cell receives hundreds of thousands of excitatory and inhibitory synapses that it must integrate to form the proper response. The Purkinje cell is the only cell of the cerebellar cortex that sends information to the outside, and it is always an **inhibitory output** using GABA as the neurotransmitter.
3. The **granular layer** (the deepest layer) consists of small granule cells and **glomeruli** (**cerebellar islands**). Glomeruli are regions of the cerebellar cortex where synapses are taking place between axons entering the cerebellum and the granule cells.

Nerve Regeneration in the Peripheral Nervous System

If a peripheral nerve fiber is injured or transected, the neuron attempts to repair the damage, regenerate the process, and restore function by initiating a series of structural and metabolic events, collectively called the ***axon reaction***. The reactions to the trauma are characteristically localized in three regions of the neuron: (1) at the site of damage (**local changes**), (2) distal to the site of damage (**anterograde changes**), and (3) proximal to the site of damage (**retrograde changes**). Some of the changes occur simultaneously, whereas others may occur weeks or months apart. The following description of nerve regeneration assumes that the cut ends remain near each other; otherwise, regeneration is unsuccessful (Fig. 9.40).

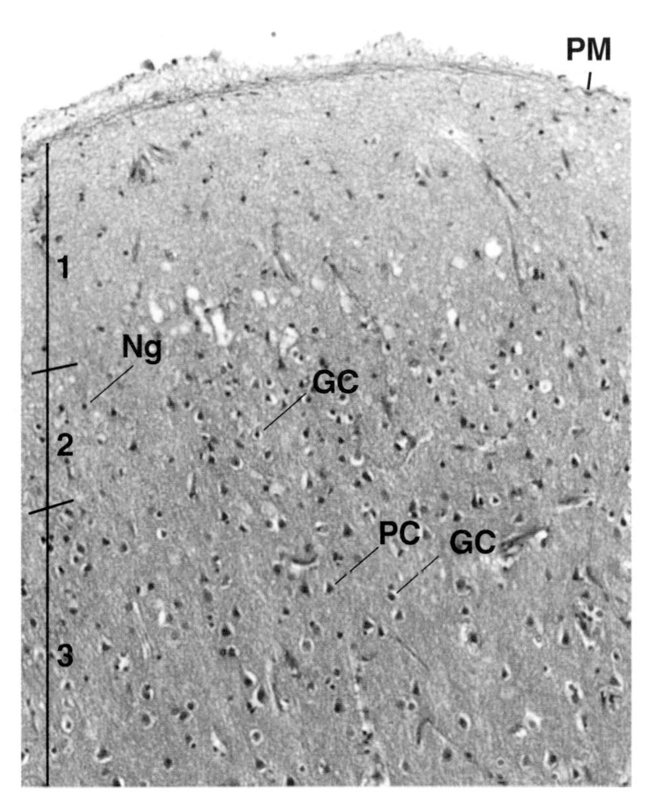

Fig. 9.37 This low magnification photomicrograph of the cerebral cortex displays its outermost three layers, as well as its vascular pia mater (PM) that supplies capillaries that serve the neural tissues. Observe that the extent of the subpial layer, the molecular layer, also known as *layer 1*, is easily recognized because of the sparsity of the neurons. The external granular layer, also known as *layer 2*, has numerous granule cells (GC) and neuroglia (Ng), whereas the third layer, the external pyramidal layer, is characterized by the presence of pyramidal cells (PC), granule cells (GC), and many neuroglia. (×132).

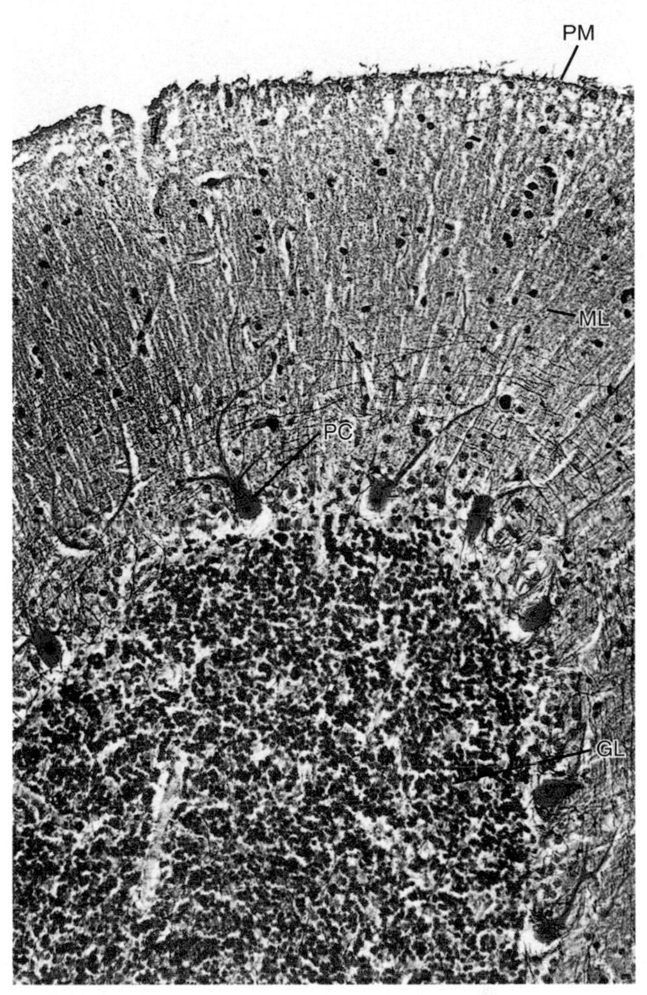

Fig. 9.38 Light micrograph of the cerebellum showing its layers (×132). Molecular layer (ML), granular layer (GL) the prominent Purkinje cells of the Purkinje cell layer (PC); the pia mater (PM) covers the molecular layer.

LOCAL REACTION

Local reaction to injury involves repair and removal of debris.

The severed ends of the axon retract away from each other, and the cut membrane of each stump fuses to cover the open end, preventing loss of axoplasm. Each severed end begins to expand as material delivered by axoplasmic flow accumulates and the cytoskeleton of the axon begins to disintegrate. The Schwann cells in the damaged region stop manufacturing myelin and produce cytokines that promote Schwann cell mitosis. These newly formed cells, along with the few resident macrophages, begin to phagocytose the damaged myelin, along with the disintegrating axonal cytoskeleton. Damage to the nerve fiber disrupts the blood–nerve barrier, causing macrophages and fibroblasts to infiltrate the damaged area, secrete cytokines and growth factors, and up-regulate the expression of their receptors. Macrophages invade the basal lamina and, to a certain, limited extent assisted by Schwann cells, phagocytose the debris.

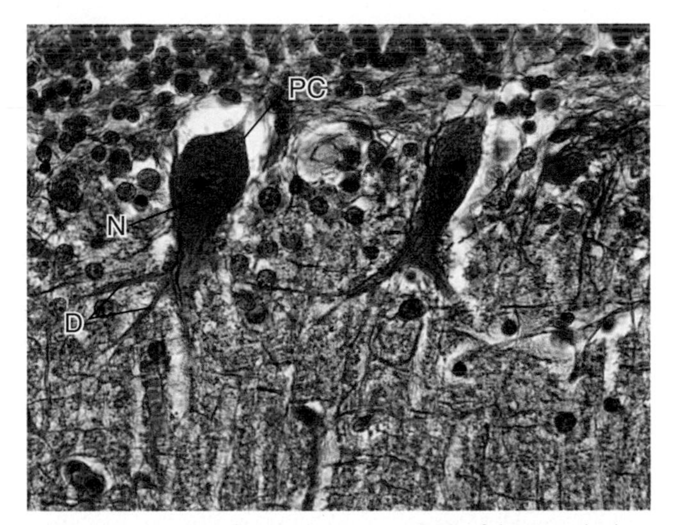

Fig. 9.39 Higher magnification light micrograph of the granular layer of the cerebellum illustrating Purkinje cells of the Purkinje cell layer. The multipolar Purkinje cells (PC) display a nucleus (N) and a dendritic tree (D). Please note that this figure is upside down compared with Fig. 9.29 (×540).

ANTEROGRADE REACTION

The portion of the axon that is distal to an injury undergoes degeneration and is phagocytosed.

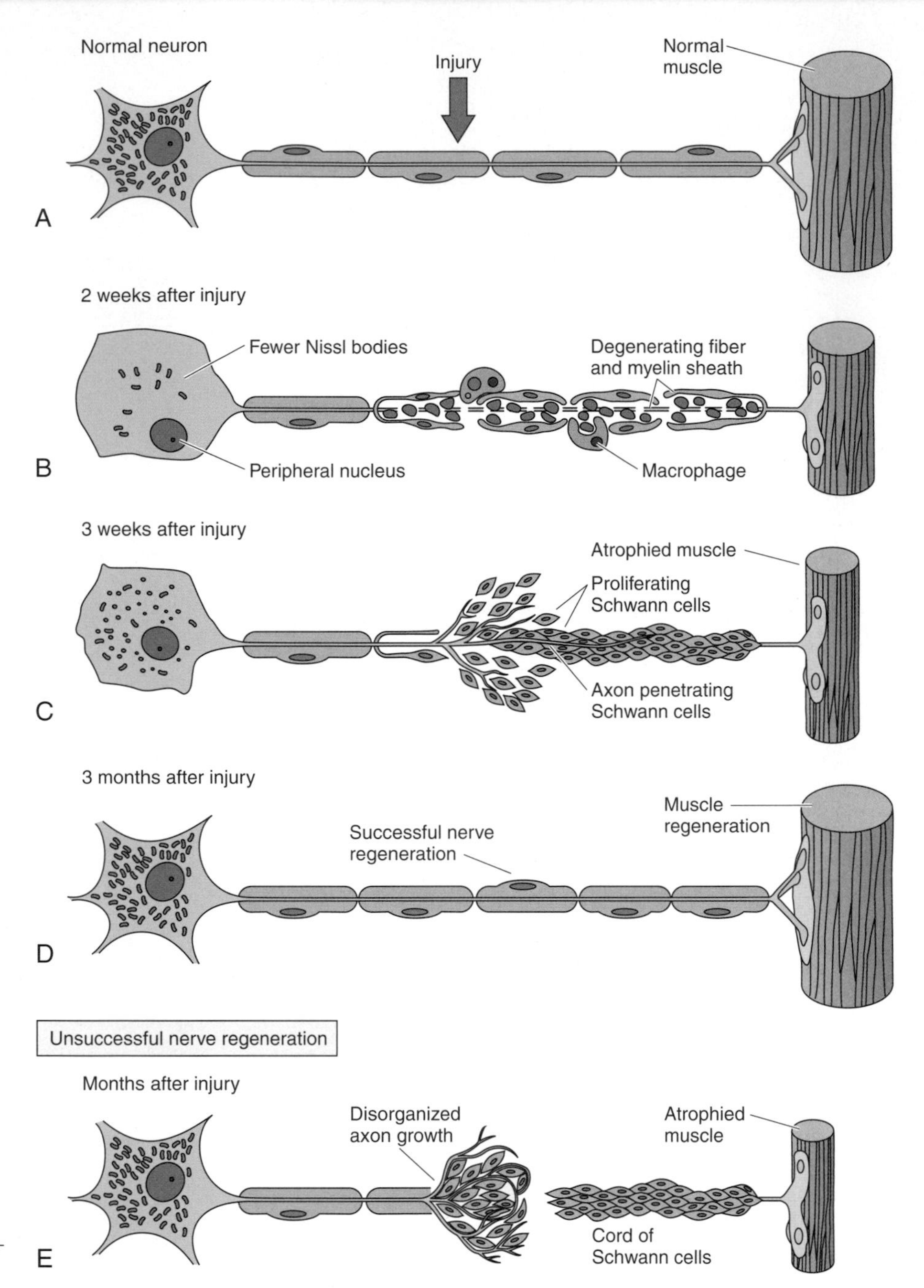

Fig. 9.40 Schematic diagram of nerve regeneration.

The axon undergoes anterograde changes as follows:

1. The axon terminal becomes hypertrophied and degenerates within 1 week; as a result, contact with the postsynaptic membrane is terminated. Schwann cells proliferate and phagocytose the remnants of the axon terminal, and the newly formed Schwann cells occupy the synaptic space.
2. The distal portion of the axon undergoes **Wallerian degeneration** (**orthograde degeneration**), whereby distal to the lesion, the axon and the myelin disintegrate, Schwann cells dedifferentiate, and myelin synthesis is discontinued. Moreover, macrophages—and, to a certain extent, Schwann cells—continue to phagocytose the disintegrated remnants.
3. Schwann cells proliferate, forming a cylinder of Schwann cells (**Schwann tubes**) enclosed by the original basal lamina of the endoneurium.

RETROGRADE REACTION AND REGENERATION

The proximal portion of the injured axon undergoes degeneration followed by sprouting of a new axon whose growth is directed by Schwann cells.

The portion of the axon proximal to the damage undergoes the following changes:

1. The perikaryon of the damaged neuron becomes hypertrophied, its Nissl bodies disperse, and its nucleus is displaced. These events, called ***chromatolysis***, may last several months. Meanwhile, the soma is actively producing free ribosomes and synthesizing proteins and various macromolecules, including ribonucleic acid (RNA). During this time, the proximal axon stump and surrounding myelin sheath degenerate as far proximally as the nearest collateral axon.

2. Numerous "sprouts" of axon emerge from the proximal axon stump, enter the endoneurium, and are guided by the Schwann cells to their target cell. For regeneration to occur, the Schwann cells, macrophages, and fibroblasts, as well as the basal lamina, must be present. These cells manufacture growth factors and cytokines and upregulate the expression for the receptors of these signaling molecules.
3. These sprouts are guided by the Schwann cells that redifferentiate and either begin to manufacture myelin around the growing axon or, in nonmyelinated axons, form a Schwann cell sheath. The one sprout that reaches the target cell first forms a synapse, whereas the other sprouts degenerate. The process of regeneration proceeds at about 3 to 4 mm/day.

TRANSNEURONAL DEGENERATION

The nerve cell has a **trophic influence** on the cells it contacts. If the neuron dies, sometimes its target cells atrophy and degenerate, or other cells targeting that particular neuron also atrophy and degenerate. This process, called ***transneuronal degeneration***, may thus be anterograde or retrograde but occurs only infrequently.

Nerve Regeneration in the Central Nervous System

Regeneration in the CNS is much less likely than in the PNS because connective tissue sheaths are absent in the CNS. Injured cells within the CNS are phagocytosed by **microglia**, and the space liberated by the phagocytosis becomes occupied by proliferation of glial cells, which form a cell mass called a **glial scar**. It is believed that the glial cell masses hinder the process of repair. Thus, generally, neuronal damage within the CNS appears to be irreparable.

Although neurons do not divide readily, there is evidence that there are neural stem cells within the adult mammalian and human brain that, when provided the proper stimulus, could be activated to replace lost or injured neurons. Some of these cells have the capacity to produce glial cells and others are able to differentiate into neurons. It has been shown that these neural stem cells exhibit multipotential ability to differentiate into the cells of the tissue into which they were introduced.

Clinical Correlations

It has been shown recently that reducing additional cell damage or cell death within 1 hour of spinal cord injury increases the survivability of neurons in the vicinity of the lesion. This information—coupled with results of recent investigations concerning growth factors, applications of embryonic neural stem cells, reducing neuron growth inhibitors, applying axon grafts, and grafting axons directly into the gray matter of the spinal cord—are providing promising results for the future in spinal cord therapy.

NEURONAL PLASTICITY (NEUROPLASTICITY, BRAIN PLASTICITY)

Neuronal plasticity is the ability of neural pathways and synapses to alter their original function adapting to various factors, such as damage, behavior, or changes in the individual's environment. Such plasticity is evident during development because the neurons that are present in excess or not making correct connections must be destroyed. However, it has been shown in adult mammals that after injury, neuronal circuits may be reestablished from the growth of neuronal processes located some distance away from the lesion that are able to provide at least some functional recovery. Regeneration of this sort relies on growth factors called ***neurotrophins*** produced by neurons, glial cells, Schwann cells, and certain target cells. Evidence for neuronal plasticity in humans may be observed in stroke victims as well as in victims of other neurological injuries.

Pathological Considerations

See Figs. 9.41 to 9.43.

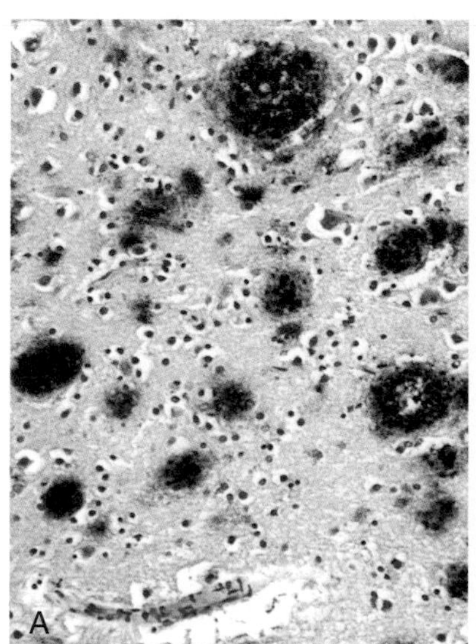

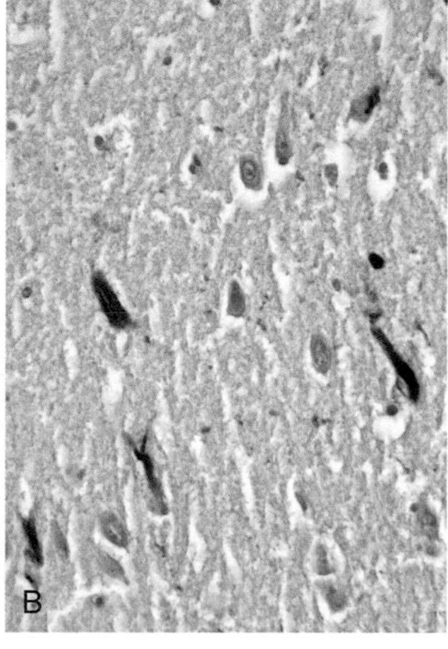

Fig. 9.41 The brains of individuals with Alzheimer disease display the presence of amyloid β accumulations that may be well demonstrated by the application of histochemical staining techniques *(left photomicrograph)*. Additionally, neurofibrillary tangles, composed of cytoskeletal elements—especially microtubule-associated protein tau—are also present and can be demonstrated by immunocytochemistry *(right photomicrograph)*. (Reprinted with permission from Young B, Stewart W, O'Dowd G. *Wheater's Basic Pathology: A Text, Atlas and Review of Histopathology*. 5th ed. Oxford: Churchill Livingstone/Elsevier Limited; 2011:302.)

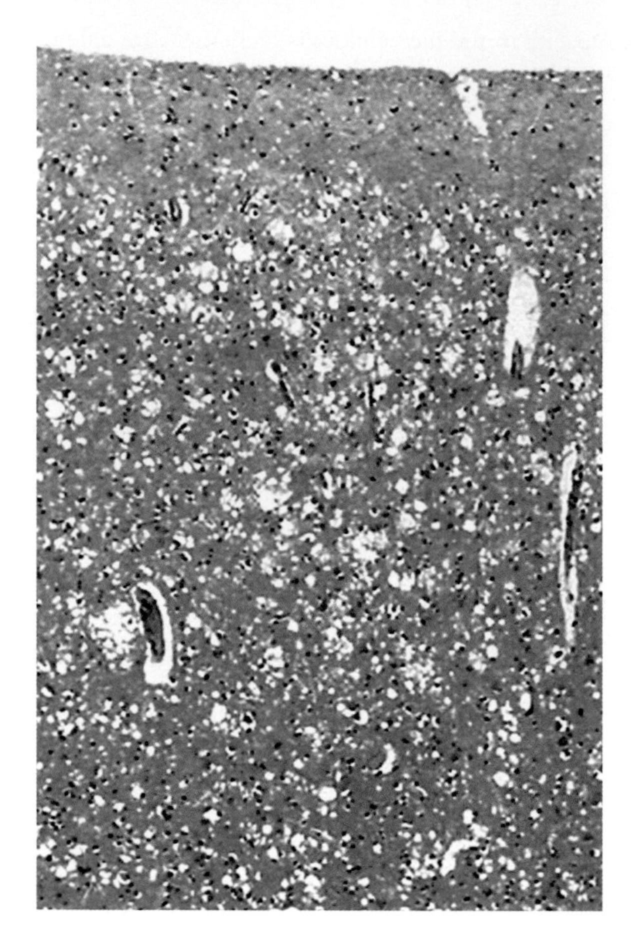

Fig. 9.42 The brains of individuals with prion diseases display the presence of spongiform changes as evidenced in the sponge-like appearance of the cerebral cortex in this photomicrograph. (Reprinted with permission from Young B, Stewart W, O'Dowd G. *Wheater's Basic Pathology: A Text, Atlas and Review of Histopathology*. 5th ed. Oxford: Churchill Livingstone/Elsevier Limited; 2011:304.)

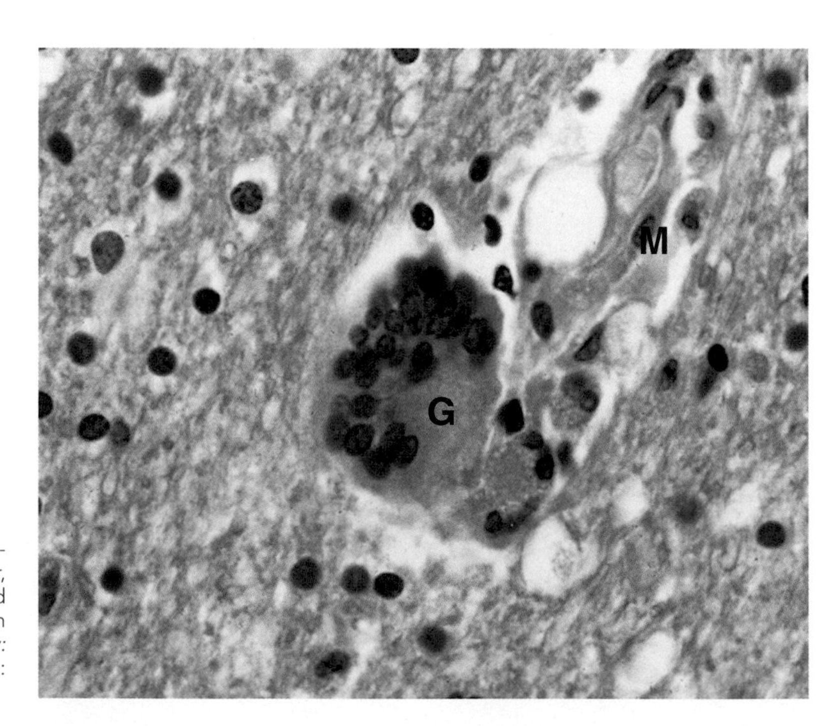

Fig. 9.43 The brains of individuals with HIV-induced encephalitis display the presence of inflammation in the white matter, as evidenced by the presence of mononuclear cells (M) and multinucleated giant cells (G). (Reprinted with permission from Young B, Stewart W, O'Dowd G. *Wheater's Basic Pathology: A Text, Atlas and Review of Histopathology*. 5th ed. Oxford: Churchill Livingstone/Elsevier Limited; 2011:306.)

Histology Laboratory Instructions: Nervous Tissue

Neurons and Neuroglia

The best example of a *multipolar neuron* is located in the ventral horn of the spinal cord. The large, more or less diamond-shaped cells with their numerous dendrites and a single axon are clearly evident. The small cells, only whose nuclei are visible, are neuroglia (see Fig. 9.1, mN). Very good examples of *unipolar neurons* (previously called *pseudounipolar neurons*) are best seen in the dorsal root ganglia, where they appear as large circular cells with large round nuclei and usually a single large nucleolus. The unipolar neurons are surrounded by cuboidal-shaped capsule cells (see Fig. 9.2, N, n). Other neuroglial cells may be seen in the silver-stained cerebral cortex. Look for stellate-shaped *protoplasmic astrocytes* whose several short processes extend toward and contact blood vessels with their pedicels (see Fig. 9.11, FA, *arrows,* BV, *arrowhead*). Small *microglia* with their short processes are also clearly visible surrounding neurons in the cerebellum (see Fig. 9.15, Mg, *arrows,* Ne). *Fibrous astrocytes*, visible in the Bielschowsky stained cerebellum, are recognizable as dark smudges with long, unbranched processes (see Fig. 9.12, *arrows*).

Peripheral Nerves

Longitudinal sections of peripheral nerves superficially resemble longitudinal sections of tendons. However, on close observation, it is evident that nerves have a wave-like appearance. The oval nuclei of Schwann cells are much lighter-stained than fibroblast nuclei of tendons. Observe also the myelin sheath and the occasional node of Ranvier (see Fig. 9.22, Sc, *arrow*). At high magnification, the granular-appearing myelin surrounds the axons that appear as thin lines. Numerous Schwann cell nuclei are visible, as are a number of nodes of Ranvier (see Fig. 9.23, M, A, NSC, *arrow*). *Cross-sections of peripheral nerves*, at low magnification, are seen to be segmented into fascicles, where each fascicle is surrounded by its own perineurium. Within the perineurium are numerous myelinated axons partially ensconced by the nuclei of Schwann cells (Fig. 9.24, P, A). At high magnification, the endoneurium is evident as a fine line surrounding the myelin sheath of the axon; Schwann cell nuclei are also clearly evident (see Fig. 9.25, En, M, A, SCn).

Sympathetic Ganglia

Sympathetic ganglia are quite vascular and house multipolar postganglionic sympathetic neurons, motor neurons, of the autonomic nervous system. These irregularly shaped neurons possess large round nuclei, each with a prominent nucleolus, and are surrounded by flat, supporting cells (see Figs. 9.29 and 9.30, BV, PSN, N, nu, SC).

Dorsal Root Ganglia

Dorsal root ganglia are sensory ganglia that house the soma of the unipolar (pseudounipolar) neurons. Each soma has a large nucleus and nucleolus and is surrounded by small cuboidal-shaped capsule cells. The central and peripheral processes of these unipolar cells are gathered into nerve fiber bundles. The presence of numerous blood vessels indicates that dorsal root ganglia have a rich vascular supply. (see Figs. 9.32 and 9.33, Cb, N, nu, Cc, NF, BV).

Choroid Plexus

The *choroid plexus* is a fold of pia mater housing an abundance of fenestrated capillaries invested by a simple cuboidal, ependymal epithelium (see Fig. 9.36, C, Ce).

Cerebral Cortex

The *cerebral cortex*, covered by pia mater, is composed of six layers, each of which exhibits a specific combination of neuronal types unique to that particular layer. The layer directly deep to the pia mater is the first layer, the molecular layer, which has very few neurons and the nuclei present belong to the neuroglia. The second layer, the external granular layer, displays the presence of granule cells and neuroglia. The third layer, the external pyramidal layer, is characterized by the presence of pyramidal cells, granule cells, and neuroglia. Note that the nuclei of granule cells are larger than those of neuroglia. The fourth, fifth, and sixth layers are not represented in this photomicrograph (see Fig. 9.37, PM, GC, Ng, PC, GC).

Cerebellar Cortex

The *cerebellar cortex* has three layers that are well presented in a low-magnification photomicrograph. The external surface of the cerebellar cortex is covered by the vascular pia mater, deep to which is the molecular layer. The second layer is only a single cell in thickness, which is the Purkinje layer composed of Purkinje cells. The deepest layer of the cortex is the granular layer. The molecular layer is sparsely populated by cell bodies; the nuclei represent basket cells. The Purkinje cell layer houses the large cell bodies of Purkinje cells and the granular layer is tightly packed with the soma of the granule cells (see Fig. 9.38, PM, ML, PC, GL). High magnification of the Purkinje cell layer of the cerebral cortex displays two large Purkinje cells with their round nuclei and well-defined nucleoli, as well as their highly developed dendritic tree entering the molecular layer (see Fig. 9.39, PC, N, D).

10 Blood and Hemopoiesis

Blood, a specialized connective tissue, is a bright- to dark-red, viscous, slightly alkaline fluid (pH 7.4) that accounts for approximately 7% of the total body weight with a total volume of approximately 5 L in an average adult. It is composed of formed elements—**red blood cells (RBCs; erythrocytes)**, **white blood cells (WBCs; leukocytes)**, and **platelets**—suspended in a fluid component (the extracellular matrix), known as ***plasma*** (Figs. 10.1 and 10.2).

Because blood circulates throughout the body within the confines of the circulatory system, it is an ideal vehicle for the transport of materials. The primary functions of blood include conveying nutrients from the gastrointestinal system to all of the cells of the body and, subsequently, delivering the waste products of these cells to specific organs for elimination. Numerous other metabolites, cellular products (e.g., hormones and other signaling molecules), and electrolytes are also ferried by the bloodstream to their final destinations. Oxygen (O_2) is carried by hemoglobin within erythrocytes from the lungs for distribution to the cells of the organism and carbon dioxide (CO_2) is conveyed both by hemoglobin and by the fluid component of plasma (as bicarbonate ion, HCO_3^-, as well as in its free form) for elimination by the lungs.

Blood also helps regulate body temperature and aids in maintaining the acid–base and osmotic balance of the body fluids. Finally, blood acts as a pathway for migration of WBCs between various connective tissue compartments of the body.

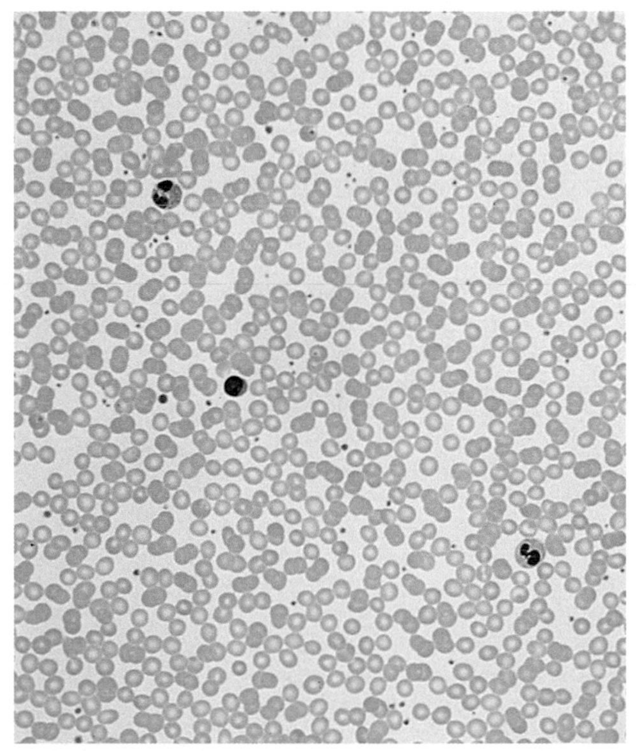

Fig. 10.1 Photomicrograph of circulating blood. Note the abundance of erythrocytes, as well as the three leukocytes. Also, observe the presence of numerous platelets that appear as small dots interspersed among the erythrocytes. (×270)

The fluid state of blood necessitates the presence of a protective mechanism, **coagulation** (**clotting**), to stop its flow in case of damage to the vascular tree. The process of coagulation is mediated by platelets and blood-borne factors that transform blood from a liquid to a gel state.

When blood is removed from the body and placed in a test tube, clotting occurs unless the tube is coated by an anticoagulant such as heparin. Upon centrifugation of liquid blood, the formed elements settle to the bottom of the tube as a red precipitate (44%) covered by a thin translucent layer, the **buffy coat** (1%), and the fluid plasma remains on top as the supernatant (55%). The red precipitate is composed of RBCs, and the total RBC volume is known as the ***hematocrit***, whereas the buffy coat consists of WBCs and platelets.

The finite life span of blood cells requires their constant renewal to maintain a steady circulating population. This process of blood cell formation from established blood cell precursors is called ***hemopoiesis*** (also referred to as *hematopoiesis*).

Blood

Blood is composed of a fluid component (plasma) and formed elements, consisting of the various types of blood cells, as well as platelets.

Light microscopy identifying circulating blood cells relies on either the Wright or Giemsa modifications of the original Romanovsky technique of using a mixture of methylene blue and eosin. Methylene blue stains acidic cellular components blue, and eosin stains alkaline components pink. Still other components are colored a reddish blue by binding to **azures**, substances formed when methylene blue is oxidized.

PLASMA

Plasma is a yellowish fluid in which cells, platelets, organic compounds, and electrolytes are suspended and/or dissolved.

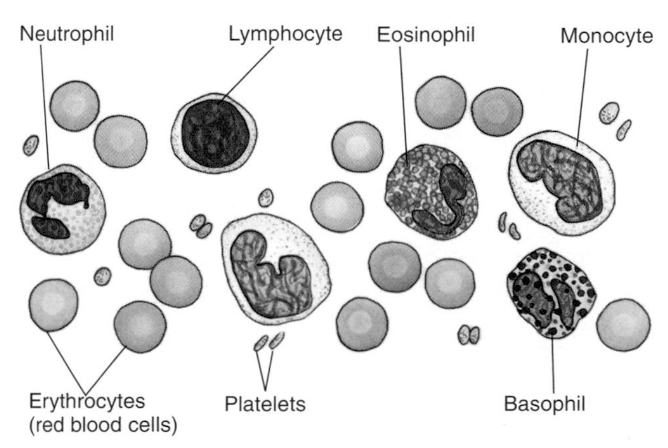

Fig. 10.2 Diagram of cells and platelets of circulating blood.

TABLE 10.1 Proteins of Plasma

Protein	Size	Source	Function
Albumin	60,000–69,000 Da	Liver	Maintains colloid osmotic pressure and transports certain insoluble metabolites
Globulins α- and β-Globulins	80,000–1 × 10⁶ Da	Liver	Transport metal ions, protein-bound lipids, and lipid-soluble vitamins
γ-Globulin		Plasma cells	Antibodies of immune defense
CLOTTING PROTEINS			
(e.g., prothrombin, fibrinogen, accelerator globulin)	Varied	Liver	Formation of fibrin threads
Complement proteins C1 through C9	Varied	Liver	Destruction of microorganisms and initiation of inflammation
PLASMA LIPOPROTEINS			
Chylomicrons	100–500 μm	Intestinal epithelial cells	Transport of triglycerides to liver
Very low-density lipoprotein (VLDL)	25–70 nm	Liver	Transport of triglycerides from liver to body cells
Low-density lipoprotein (LDL)	3 × 10⁶ Da	Liver	Transport of cholesterol from liver to body cells

During coagulation, some of the organic and inorganic components of **plasma** become integrated into the clot. The remaining straw-colored fluid, which no longer has the clot-forming components dissolved or suspended in it, is known as ***serum***.

Plasma is composed of approximately 90% water, 9% protein, and 1% inorganic salts, ions, nitrogenous compounds, nutrients, and gases. The types, origins, and functions of the **blood proteins** are listed in Table 10.1. Capillaries and small venules are leaky and allow plasma to enter the connective tissue spaces, where it is known as **extracellular fluid**, whose composition of electrolytes and small molecules is similar to that in plasma. However, the concentration of proteins in extracellular fluid is much lower than that in plasma because not even small proteins, such as albumin, can escape the endothelial lining of a capillary or that of a venule.

Clinical Correlations

***Albumin**, one of the proteins in plasma, is chiefly responsible for the establishment of blood's **colloid osmotic pressure**, the force that maintains normal blood volume by opposing the movement of fluid from the capillaries and venules into the interstitial spaces.*

FORMED ELEMENTS

RBCs, WBCs, and platelets constitute the formed elements of blood.

Erythrocytes

Erythrocytes (RBCs) are the smallest and most numerous cells of blood; they have no nuclei and are responsible for the transport of oxygen and carbon dioxide to and from the tissues of the body.

Each **erythrocyte** (**RBC**) resembles a biconcave-shaped disk that is 7.5 μm in diameter, 2.0 μm thick at its widest region, and less than 1 μm thick at its center. When stained with Giemsa or Wright stains, erythrocytes display a salmon-pink color (Figs. 10.3 and 10.4). This shape provides the cell with a large surface area relative to its volume, enhancing its capability for gaseous exchange. Although precursor cells of the erythrocyte possess nuclei and organelles during their development and maturation, they expel them prior to entering the circulation. Thus, mature, circulating erythrocytes have neither nuclei nor organelles, but they do have soluble enzymes in their cytosol. Within the erythrocyte, the enzyme **carbonic anhydrase** facilitates the formation of carbonic acid from CO_2 and water. This acid dissociates to form bicarbonate (HCO_3^-) and hydrogen (H^+). It is as bicarbonate that most of the CO_2 is ferried to the lungs for exhalation. The ability of bicarbonate to cross the erythrocyte cell membrane is mediated by the integral membrane protein **band 3**, a coupled anion transporter that exchanges intracellular bicarbonate for extracellular Cl^-; this exchange is known as the ***chloride shift***. Additional enzymes include those of the **glycolytic pathway** (**Embden-Meyerhoff pathway**) as well as enzymes that are responsible for the **pentose monophosphate shunt** (**hexose monophosphate shunt**) for the production of the high-energy molecule **reduced nicotinamide adenine dinucleotide phosphate (NADPH)**, a reducing agent. The pentose monophosphate shunt does not require the presence of oxygen and is the chief method whereby the erythrocyte produces adenosine triphosphate (ATP), necessary for its energy requirement.

Clinical Correlations

1. *During its 120-day life, each erythrocyte negotiates the entire circulatory system at least 100,000 times and, therefore, must pass through innumerable capillaries whose lumen is smaller than the cell's diameter. To navigate through such small-bore vessels, the erythrocyte undergoes deformations of its shape and becomes subject to tremendous shear forces. It is the erythrocyte cell membrane and the underlying cytoskeleton that contribute to the ability of the RBC to maintain its structural and functional integrity. As erythrocytes reach their 120-day life span, they become fragile and display on their surface a group of oligosaccharides that act as signals for macrophages of the liver, bone marrow, and spleen to destroy these old RBCs.*
2. *Males have more erythrocytes per unit volume of blood than do females (5×10^6 vs. 4.5×10^6 per mm^3), and members of both sexes living at higher altitudes have correspondingly more RBCs than residents living at lower altitudes.*

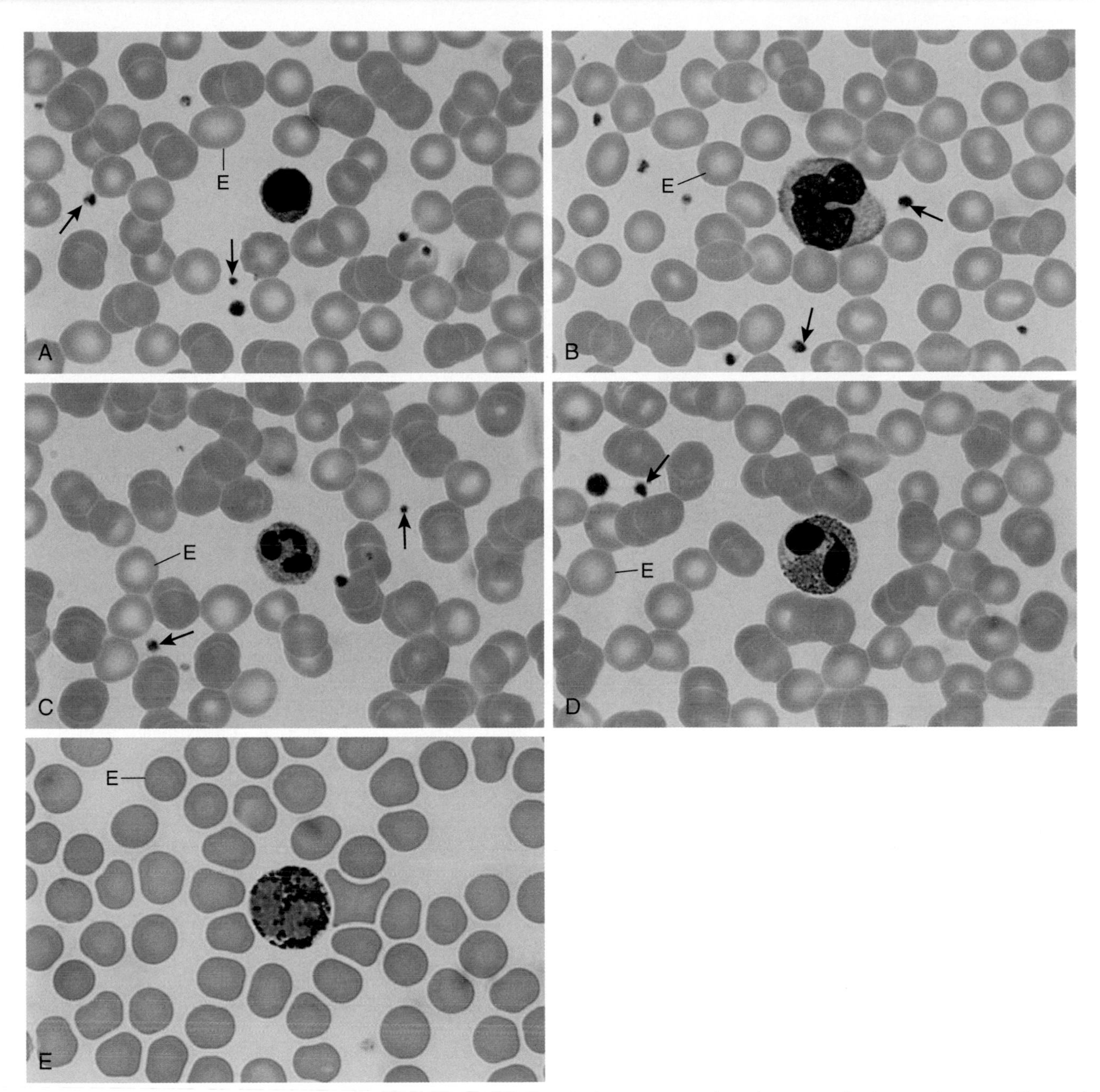

Fig. 10.3 Photomicrograph of cells and platelets of circulating blood. Each photomicrograph in this series displays erythrocytes (E), platelets *(arrows)*, and a single white blood cell. (A) Lymphocyte. (B) Monocyte. (C) Neutrophil. (D) Eosinophil. (E) Basophil. (×1325)

Hemoglobin

Hemoglobin is a large protein composed of four polypeptide chains, each of which is covalently bound to a heme group.

Erythrocytes are packed with **hemoglobin**, a large tetrameric protein (68,000 Da) composed of four polypeptide chains, each of which is covalently bound to an iron-containing **heme**. The iron is protected from oxidation by the globin chain even though oxygen can bind to it. The globin moiety of hemoglobin releases CO_2 in regions of high oxygen concentration, such as in the lungs, and O_2 binds to the iron of each heme. However, in oxygen-poor regions, as in body tissues, hemoglobin releases O_2 and binds CO_2. This property of hemoglobin makes it ideal for the conveyance of respiratory gases. Hemoglobin carrying O_2 is known as ***oxyhemoglobin***, and hemoglobin carrying CO_2 is called ***carbaminohemoglobin*** (or ***carbamylhemoglobin***).

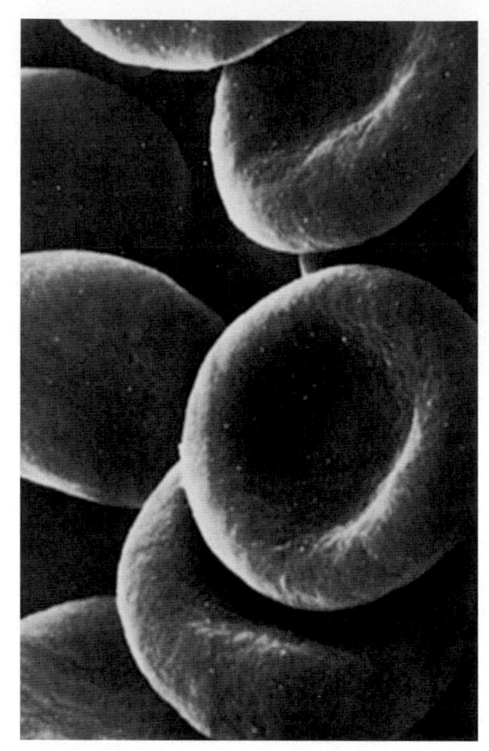

Fig. 10.4 Scanning electron micrograph of circulating red blood cells displaying their biconcave disk shape (×5,850). (From Leeson TS, Leeson CR, Paparo AA. *Text/Atlas of Histology*. Philadelphia: WB Saunders; 1988.)

Clinical Correlations

1. ***Hypoxic tissues** release 2,3-diphosphoglyceride, a carbohydrate that facilitates the release of oxygen from the erythrocyte. Hemoglobin also binds NO, a neurotransmitter substance that causes dilation of blood vessels, permitting RBCs to release more oxygen and pick up more CO_2 within the tissues of the body.*
2. ***Carbon monoxide (CO)** has a much greater affinity, about 250-fold, than O_2 for the heme portion of hemoglobin, and when CO binds to the iron of the heme, the hemoglobin molecule is transformed to its (R-) Hb form and increases its affinity to oxygen so that it cannot be released to the tissues, even in hypoxic regions. People who are trapped in areas of poor ventilation with a running gasoline-powered engine or in a building on fire frequently succumb to CO poisoning. Many such victims, especially those who are fair-skinned, instead of being cyanotic (with a bluish pallor) present with healthy-looking, cherry-red skin because of the color of the CO-hemoglobin complex (carbon monoxyhemoglobin) even though they are dead.*

On the basis of the amino acid sequences, there are four normal human polypeptide chains of hemoglobin, designated α, β, γ, and δ. The principal hemoglobin of the fetus, **fetal hemoglobin (HbF)**, composed of two alpha chains and two gamma chains, is replaced shortly after birth by **adult hemoglobin (HbA)**. There are two types of normal HbAs, **HbA1** ($\alpha_2\beta_2$) and the much rarer form, **HbA2** ($\alpha_2\delta_2$). In an adult, approximately 96% of the hemoglobin is HbA_1, 2% is HbA_2, and the remaining 2% is HbF.

Clinical Correlations

1. *Several hereditary diseases result from defects in the genes encoding the hemoglobin polypeptide chains. Diseases referred to as thalassemia are marked by decreased synthesis of one or more hemoglobin chains. In β-thalassemia, synthesis of the β-chains is impaired. In the homozygous form of this disease, which is most prevalent among persons of Mediterranean descent, HbA is missing and high levels of HbF persist after birth. In the past couple of years, gene therapy has demonstrated great success in treating this condition. Inactivated lentivirus was used to infect the patients' own immature stem cells retrieved from their bone marrow with the normal globin gene in vitro. Then, the patients underwent chemotherapy to destroy their mutated stem cells, and the genetically modified stem cells were introduced. The modified stem cells migrated to the bone marrow and started producing normal hemoglobin. The clinical trial consisted of 22 patients, nine of whom had a severe case of thalassemia. Of these patients, three no longer required transfusions and six required 74% fewer transfusions than prior to treatment. The remaining 13 patients who had milder cases of thalassemia no longer required transfusions. Clinical trials are currently progressing to verify and extend the results.*
2. ***Sickle cell anemia** is the result of a point mutation at a single locus of the β-chain (valine is incorporated into the sequence instead of glutamate), forming the abnormal hemoglobin HbS. When the oxygen tension is reduced (e.g., during strenuous exercise), HbS changes shape, producing abnormal-shaped (crescent-shaped) erythrocytes that are less pliant, more fragile, and more prone to hemolysis than normal cells. Sickle cell anemia is prevalent in the black population, especially in those whose ancestors lived in regions of Africa where malaria is endemic. In the United States, about 1 of 600 newborn African-American babies is stricken with this condition. Individuals with sickle cell anemia are more resistant to **malaria**, a disease caused by a parasite, than people whose hemoglobin is not mutated. It was believed that sickle-shaped erythrocytes were more resistant to the entry of the parasite Plasmodium falciparum, the most fatal of the five Plasmodium species that cause malaria. However, it has been reported recently that the erythrocytes of individuals with sickle cell anemia manufacture an increased amount of the enzyme heme oxygenase-1. This enzyme produces CO, a gas that not only protects hemoglobin from degradation, but also limits the toxic ability of P. falciparum, thus providing more time for the individual's immune system to fight the parasitic invasion.*
3. ***Hemoglobin A1c (HbA1c** or **A1c)** is a glycated hemoglobin that forms when plasma glucose levels are elevated and glucose molecules attach to the N-terminus of hemoglobin's beta chain. This is a nonreversible reaction, so, once attached, the hemoglobin molecules do not lose their glucose. If the plasma glucose levels remain elevated, glycated hemoglobin levels also increase; therefore, a measure of A1c levels is indicative of the blood sugar concentrations for the previous 2 to 3 months. The normal glycated hemoglobin level in adults is approximately 4% to 5.6%. Individuals with diabetes have higher A1c levels because their blood sugar concentrations are usually greater than those of individuals without diabetes. For a patient with diabetes, an A1c level below 7% is considered to be very good, indicating a good control of blood glucose levels. A1c levels higher than 7% is worrisome because the higher the level, the greater the probability of acquiring diabetes-related conditions.*

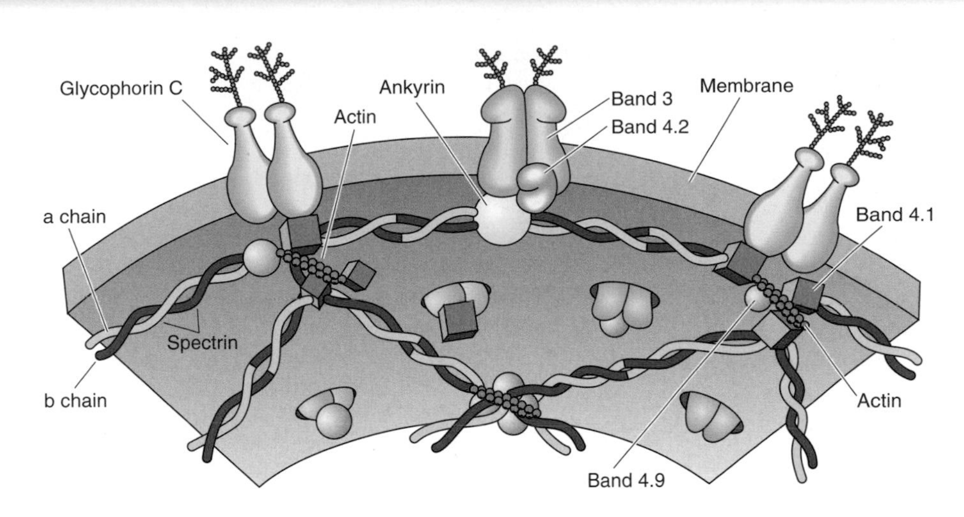

Fig. 10.5 Diagram of the cytoskeleton and integral proteins of the erythrocyte plasmalemma. Spectrin forms a hexagonal latticework that is anchored to the erythrocyte plasma membrane by band 4.1 and band 3 proteins as well as by ankyrin.

Erythrocyte Cell Membrane

The cell membrane of the erythrocyte and the underlying cytoskeleton are highly pliable and can withstand great shear forces.

The RBC plasma membrane, a typical lipid bilayer, is composed of about 50% protein, 40% lipids, and 10% carbohydrates. Most of the proteins are transmembrane proteins, principally **glycophorin A** (as well as lesser quantities of glycophorins B, C, and D), **ion channels** (calcium-dependent potassium channels and Na^+-K^+ ATP), and the anion transporter **band 3 protein**, which transports Cl^- and HCO^-_3. It also acts as an anchoring site for **ankyrin**, band 4.1 protein, hemoglobin, and glycolytic enzymes (Fig. 10.5). The RBC membrane also possesses the peripheral proteins: spectrin, ankyrin, band 4.1 protein, and actin. **Band 4.1 protein** acts as an anchoring site for spectrin, band 3 protein, and glycophorins. Thus, ankyrin, band 3 protein, and band 4.1 protein anchor the cytoskeleton—a hexagonal lattice composed chiefly of **spectrin tetramers**, **actin**, and **adducin**—to the cytoplasmic aspect of the RBC plasmalemma (see Chapter 2). This subplasmalemmal cytoskeleton helps maintain the biconcave disk shape of the erythrocyte.

Clinical Correlations

1. *Defects in the cytoskeletal components of erythrocytes result in various conditions marked by abnormally shaped cells.* ***Hereditary spherocytosis****, for instance, is caused by synthesis of an abnormal spectrin, band 3 protein, and protein 4.2. RBCs of patients with this condition are more fragile and transport less oxygen compared with normal erythrocytes. Moreover, these spherocytes are preferentially destroyed in the spleen, leading to anemia.*
2. *Deficiency of glycophorin C is responsible for* ***elliptocytic RBCs*** *without the resultant hemolytic anemia. These cells are unstable and fragile and are less capable of deformation than normal erythrocytes.*

The extracellular surface of the RBC plasmalemma has specific inherited carbohydrate chains that act as antigens and determine the blood group of an individual for the purposes of blood transfusion. The most notable of these are the **A**, **B**, and **H antigens**, which determine the four primary blood groups, **A**, **B**, **AB**, and **O**, in which H antigen determines the O blood type

TABLE 10.2 ABO Blood Group System

Blood Group	Antigens Present	Miscellaneous
A	Antigen A	
B	Antigen B	
AB	Antigens A and B	Universal acceptor
O	H antigen only but neither antigen A nor B	Universal donor

(Table 10.2 and Fig. 10.6). People who lack either the A or B antigen, or both, have antibodies against the missing antigen in their blood; if they undergo transfusion with blood containing the missing antigen, the donor erythrocytes are attacked by the recipien's serum antibodies and are eventually lysed. Because type O blood has neither A nor B antigen, everyone can receive type O blood, making type O people "universal donors," and because type AB individuals have no antibodies against A, B, or H antigens, they can accept blood from anyone, therefore, they are "universal acceptors."

Clinical Correlations

1. *It is interesting to note that the carbohydrate chains of the A and B blood groups are identical, with the exception of their terminal sugar molecules and that people possessing the O blood group also have the same carbohydrate chains but do not have the terminal sugar molecule present in the A or B blood types (i.e., they have one fewer member in their carbohydrate group than A or B antigens). The addition of the terminal sugar group of A and B antigens each requires a specific enzyme, and neither of these two enzymes is present in individuals with the O blood group. For the type A blood group, the enzyme A-transferase (N-acetylgalactosamine transferase) adds a terminal N-acetylgalactosamine to the type H antigen. In the type B blood group, the enzyme terminal B-transferase (galactose transferase) adds a terminal galactose to the type H antigen. In blood type AB, both enzymes are present and form both type A and type B. In blood type O, neither enzyme is present; therefore, neither galactose nor N-acetylgalactosamine is added to the H antigen.*

Clinical Correlations—cont'd

2. *Recent reports have demonstrated that individuals with the AB blood group have a greater prevalence of impaired cognitive function related to aging than individuals possessing other blood groups. The reason for this occurrence is not as yet understood.*
3. *In an experiment, a group of volunteers drank water containing E. coli isolated from a patient with diarrhea. Of the volunteers whose blood type was A or AB, 81% had diarrhea whereas only 50% of type O and Type B volunteers had diarrhea. These blood type antigens are present also on the cells lining the intestines. Apparently, the E. coli are more likely to attach to the type A antigen than to type H or type B antigens. Once attached, they release their toxin, which causes diarrhea.*

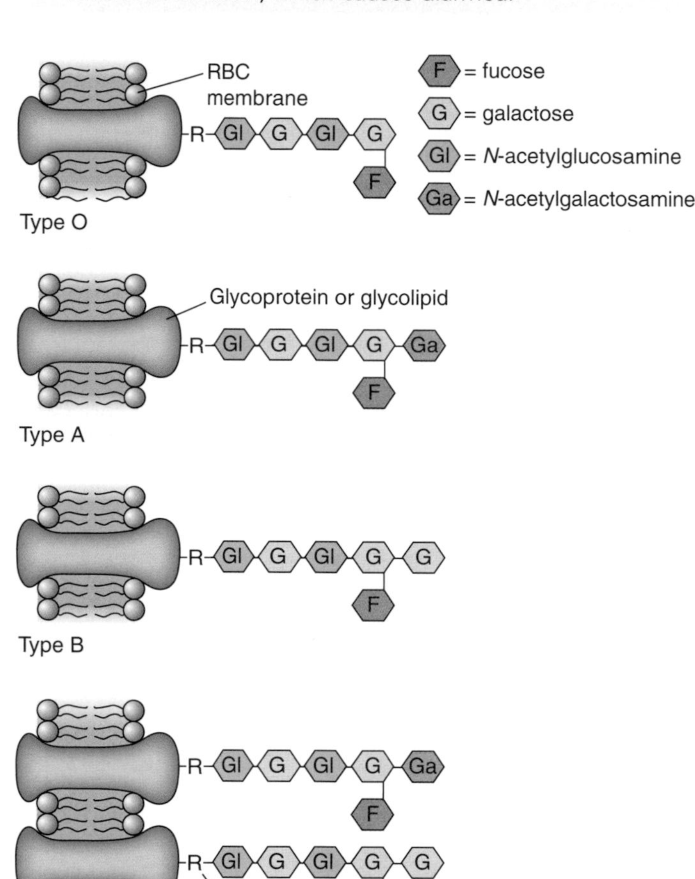

Fig. 10.6 The ABO blood group antigens are polysaccharide chains that are affixed on the extracellular aspect of the erythrocyte plasma membrane. The polysaccharide chains are identical to each other with the exception of the terminal sugar molecule. Type O individuals have fucose as their only terminal sugar molecule (type H antigen); type A individuals have fucose and N-acetylgalactosamine sugars (type A antigen) as their terminal sugar molecules; type B individuals have fucose and galactose sugars (type B antigen) as their terminal sugar molecules; and type AB individuals have both type A and type B antigen on their cell membrane.

Another important blood group, the **Rh** group, is so named because it was first identified in rhesus monkeys. This complex group comprises almost 50 antigens, although many are relatively rare. One of the Rh antigens, **D antigen** (**Rh factor**), is so common in the human population that the erythrocytes of 85% of Americans have D antigen on their surface; these individuals are thus said to be **Rh positive** (**Rh+**). The remaining 15% of the population does not have the antigen and is said to be **Rh negative** (**Rh−**).

Clinical Correlations

When an Rh^- pregnant woman delivers her first Rh^+ baby, enough of the baby's blood is likely to enter her circulation to induce the formation of anti-Rh antibodies in the mother. Because the first antibody to be produced is immunoglobulin M (IgM), it is too large to be able to cross the placental barrier (see Chapter 12 on the lymphoid [immune] system). During a subsequent pregnancy with an Rh^+ fetus, the new fetus's RBCs enter the mother's bloodstream. This second exposure elicits the formation of IgG antibodies, which are smaller and are able to cross the placental barrier. These antibodies attack the erythrocytes of the fetus, causing erythroblastosis fetalis, a condition that may be fatal to the newborn. Prenatal and postnatal transfusions of the fetus are necessary to prevent brain damage and death of the newborn unless the mother has been treated with anti-D globulin (RhoGAM) before or shortly after the birth of the first Rh^+ baby. The anti-D globulin complexes with D antigen, preventing the mother's immune system from recognizing it as an antigenic molecule. Therefore, the mother's immune system does not produce antibodies that would otherwise attack the fetus's erythrocytes, preventing the occurrence of erythroblastosis fetalis.

Leukocytes

Leukocytes are white blood cells that are classified into two major categories: granulocytes and agranulocytes.

The number of **leukocytes** (**WBCs**) is much smaller than that of RBCs. In fact, in a healthy adult, there are only 6500 to 10,000 WBCs per mm^3 of blood. Unlike erythrocytes, leukocytes do not function within the bloodstream but rather use it as a means of traveling from one region of the body to another. When leukocytes reach their destination, they leave the bloodstream by migrating between the endothelial cells of the blood vessels (**diapedesis**), enter the connective tissue spaces, and perform their function. Within the bloodstream as well as in smears, leukocytes are round; in connective tissue, they are pleomorphic. They generally defend the body against foreign substances.

WBCs are classified into two groups:

- Granulocytes, which have specific granules in their cytoplasm
- Agranulocytes, which lack specific granules in their cytoplasm

Both granulocytes and agranulocytes possess nonspecific (**azurophilic**) granules, now known to be **lysosomes**.

There are three types of granulocytes, differentiated according to the color of their specific granules after application of Romanovsky-type stains: neutrophils, eosinophils, and basophils. There are two types of agranulocytes: lymphocytes and monocytes. The differential leukocyte count and various properties of the leukocytes are detailed in Table 10.3.

Neutrophils

Neutrophils compose most of the white blood cell population; they are avid phagocytes, destroying bacteria that invade connective tissue spaces.

TABLE 10.3 Leukocytes

	GRANULOCYTES			AGRANULOCYTES	
Features	**Neutrophils**	**Eosinophils**	**Basophils**	**Lymphocytes**	**Monocytes**
Number/mm^3	3500–7000	150–400	50–100	1500–2500	200–800
% of WBCs	60–70%	2–4%	<1%	20–25%	3–8%
Diameter (µm)					
Section	8–9	9–11	7–8	7–8	10–12
Smear	9–12	10–14	8–10	8–10	12–15
Nucleus	3–4 lobes	2 lobes (sausage shaped)	S shaped	Round	Kidney shaped
Specific granules	0.1 µm, light pink[a]	1–1.5 µm, dark pink[a]	0.5 µm, blue/black[a]	None	None
Contents of specific granules	Type IV collagenase, phospholipase A_2, lactoferrin, lysozyme, phagocytin, alkaline phosphatase, vitamin B_{12}–binding protein	Aryl sulfatase, histaminase, β-glucuronidase, acid phosphatase, phospholipase, major basic protein, eosinophil cationic protein, neurotoxin, ribonuclease, cathepsin, peroxidase	Histamine, heparin, eosinophil chemotactic factor, neutrophil chemotactic factor, peroxidase, neutral proteases, chondroitin sulfate	None	None
Surface markers	Fc receptors, platelet-activating factor receptor, leukotriene B_4 receptor, leukocyte cell adhesion molecule-1	IgE receptors, eosinophil chemotactic factor receptor	IgE receptors	*T cells:* T-cell receptors, CD molecules, IL receptors *B cells:* Surface immunoglobulins	Class II HLA, Fc receptors
Life span	< 1 wk	< 2 wk	1–2 y (in murines)	A few months to several years	A few days in blood, several months in connective tissue
Function	Phagocytosis and destruction of bacteria	Phagocytosis of antigen–antibody complex; destruction of parasites	Similar to mast cells to mediate inflammatory responses	*T cells:* Cell-mediated immune response *B cells:* Humorally mediated immune response	Differentiate into macrophage: phagocytosis, presentation of antigens

[a]Using Romanovsky-type stains (or their modifications).
CD, Cluster of differentiation; *HLA,* human leukocyte antigen; *IgE,* immunoglobulin E; *IL,* interleukin; *WBC,* white blood cell.

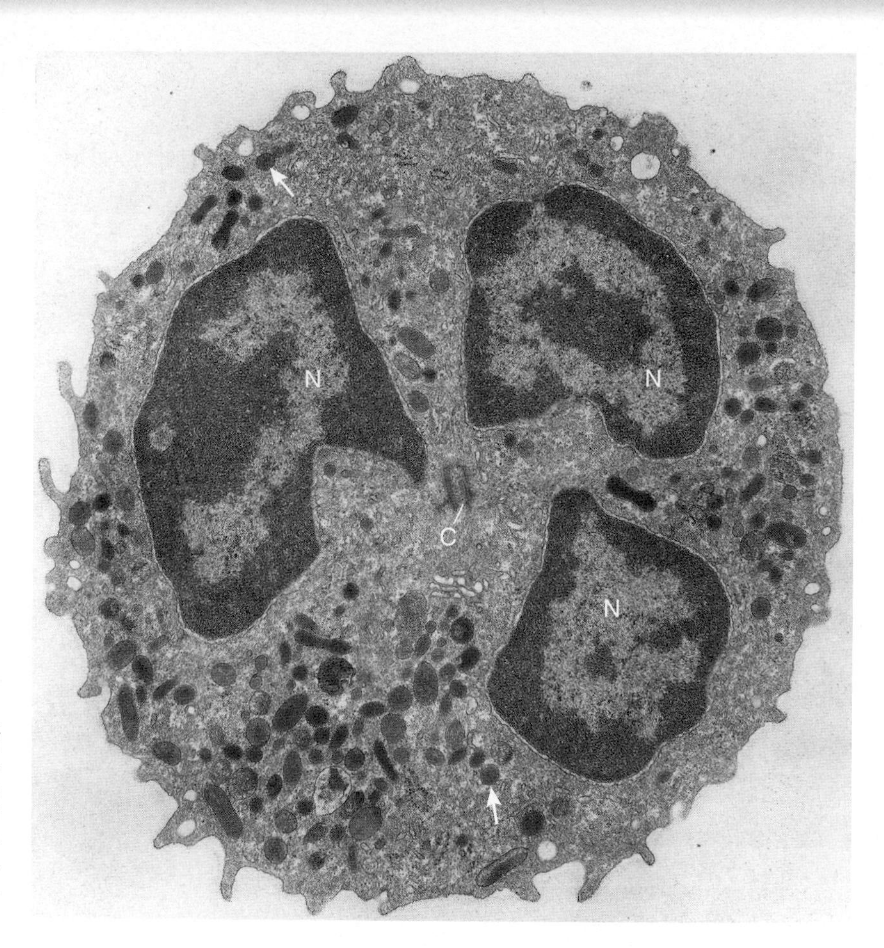

Fig. 10.7 Electron micrograph of a human neutrophil. Note the three lobes of the nucleus (N), the presence of granules *(arrows)* throughout the cytoplasm, and the centrally located centriole (C). Although it appears as if there were three distinct nuclei in this image, they are lobes of the same nucleus, and the connections are merely outside of the present field of view. (From Zucker-Franklin D, Greaves, M.F., Grossi, C.E. et al, eds. *Atlas of Blood Cells.* Vol 1. Milan: Edi Ermes; 1981.)

Neutrophils (polymorphonuclear leukocytes, polys) are granulocytes and are the most numerous of the WBCs, constituting 60% to 70% of the total leukocyte population. In blood smears, neutrophils are 9 to 12 μm in diameter and have a multilobed nucleus (see Figs. 10.2 and 10.3). The lobes, joined by slender connections, increase in number as the cell ages. In females, the nucleus presents a characteristic small appendage, the "**drumstick**" (***Barr body*** or ***sex chromosome***), which contains the condensed, inactive second X chromosome; it is not evident in every cell. The neutrophil plasmalemma possesses complement receptors, as well as Fc receptors for IgG. They are among the first defensive cells to appear in *acute* bacterial infections.

Neutrophil Granules

Neutrophils possess specific, azurophilic, and tertiary granules.

Three types of granules are present in the cytoplasm of neutrophils: small specific granules (0.1 μm in diameter), larger azurophilic granules (0.5 μm in diameter), and tertiary granules.

Specific granules contain enzymes and pharmacological agents that aid the neutrophil in performing its antimicrobial functions (see Table 10.3). In electron micrographs, these granules appear to be somewhat oblong (Fig. 10.7).

Azurophilic granules are lysosomes that house acid hydrolases, myeloperoxidase (MPO), the antibacterial agent lysozyme, bactericidal permeability–increasing protein, cathepsin G (an enzyme that may contribute to the destruction and degradation of pathogens phagocytosed by these cells), elastase, and nonspecific collagenase.

Tertiary granules contain gelatinase and cathepsins, as well as glycoproteins that are inserted into the plasmalemma.

Neutrophil Functions

Neutrophils phagocytose and destroy bacteria by using the contents of their various granules.

Neutrophils interact with chemotactic agents to migrate to sites invaded by microorganisms. They accomplish this by entering postcapillary venules in the region of inflammation and adhering to the various **selectin molecules** located on the luminal cell membranes of the endothelial cells of these vessels by use of their **selectin receptors**. The interaction between the neutrophil's selectin receptors and the selectins of the endothelial cells causes the neutrophils to roll slowly along the vessel's endothelial lining. As the neutrophils are slowing their migrations, **interleukin-1 (IL-1)** and **tumor necrosis factor (TNF)** induce the endothelial cells to express **intercellular adhesion molecule type 1 (ICAM-1)**, to which the **integrin molecules** of neutrophils avidly bind.

When binding occurs, the neutrophils stop migrating in preparation for their passage through the endothelium of the postcapillary venule to enter the connective tissue compartment (Fig. 10.8). Once there, they destroy the microorganisms by phagocytosis and by the release of hydrolytic enzymes (and **respiratory burst**). In addition, by manufacturing and releasing **leukotrienes**, neutrophils assist in the initiation of the inflammatory process. The sequence of events is as follows:

1. The binding of neutrophil chemotactic factor (NCF), released by mast cells and basophils to NCF receptors of the neutrophil's plasmalemma, facilitates the release of the contents of tertiary granules into the extracellular matrix.

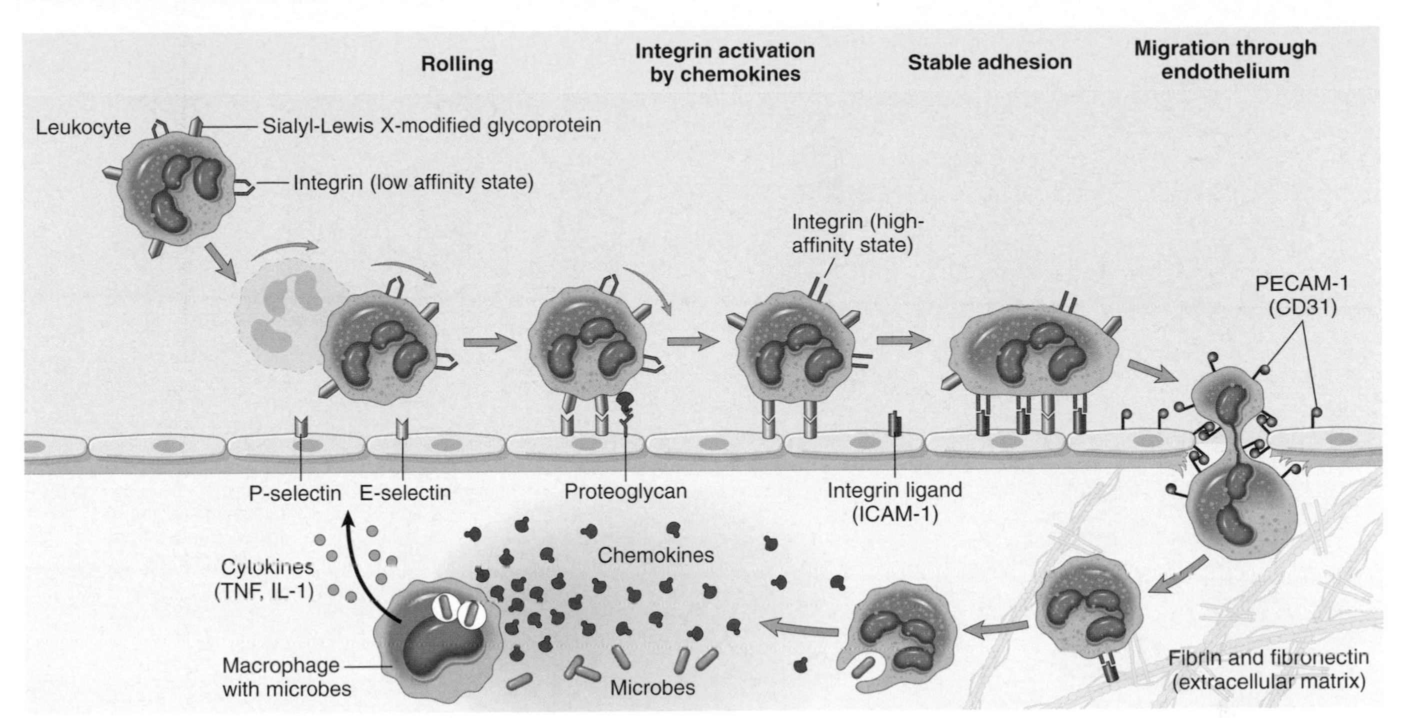

Fig. 10.8 Diagram demonstrating the multistep process of migration of neutrophils across the endothelial lining of blood vessels. (borrowed from Kumar, V, Abbas, A.K., and Aster, J.C. : Robbins and Cotran Pathologic Basis of Disease, 9th ed. Figure 3-4 P. 75, Elsevier 2015.)

2. Gelatinase and cathepsins degrade the basal lamina, facilitating neutrophil migration. Glycoproteins present in the tertiary granules become inserted in the cell membrane and aid the process of phagocytosis.
3. The contents of the specific granules are also released into the extracellular matrix, where they attack the invading microorganisms and aid neutrophil migration.
4. Microorganisms, phagocytosed by neutrophils, become enclosed in phagosomes (Fig. 10.9A,B). Enzymes and pharmacological agents of the azurophilic granules are usually released into the lumina of these intracellular vesicles, where they destroy the ingested microorganisms. Because of their phagocytic functions, neutrophils are also known as *microphages* to distinguish them from the larger phagocytic cells, the macrophages.
5. Bacteria are killed not only by the action of enzymes but also by the formation of reactive oxygen compounds within the phagosomes of neutrophils. These are superoxide (O_2^-), formed by the action of NADPH oxidase on O_2 in a respiratory burst; hydrogen peroxide, formed by the action of superoxide dismutase on superoxide; and hypochlorous acid, formed by the interaction of MPO and chloride ions with hydrogen peroxide (see Figs. 10.9C,D).
6. Frequently, the contents of the azurophilic granules are released into the extracellular matrix, causing tissue damage, but usually catalase and glutathione peroxidase limit the tissue injury by degrading hydrogen peroxide.
7. Once neutrophils perform their function of killing microorganisms, they also die, resulting in the formation of pus (the accumulation of dead leukocytes, bacteria, and extracellular fluid).
8. Not only do neutrophils destroy bacteria, but they also synthesize leukotrienes from arachidonic acids in their cell membranes. These newly formed leukotrienes aid in the initiation of the inflammatory process.

Clinical Correlations

1. *Children with hereditary deficiency of NADPH oxidase are subject to persistent bacterial infections because their neutrophils cannot form a respiratory burst response to the bacterial challenge. Their neutrophils cannot generate superoxide, hydrogen peroxide, or hypochlorous acid during phagocytosis of bacteria.*
2. *Individuals suffering from neutropenia, low levels of neutrophils in circulating blood, have problems fighting bacterial infections. This condition may be acute, lasting less than 3 months, or chronic, lasting more than 3 months. Neutropenia may be mild (1000–1500 neutrophils per mm^3 of blood), moderate (500–1000 neutrophils per mm^3 of blood), or severe (less than 500 neutrophils per mm^3 of blood). The causes of neutropenia may be decreased neutrophil production by the bone marrow or excess neutrophil destruction outside the bone marrow.*

Eosinophils

Eosinophils phagocytose antigen–antibody complexes and kill parasitic invaders.

Eosinophils are granulocytes that constitute less than 4% of the total WBC population. They are round cells in suspension and in blood smear (10–14 µm in diameter) but they may be pleomorphic during their migration through connective tissue. They have a sausage-shaped, bilobed nucleus in which the two lobes are linked by a thin connecting strand (see Figs. 10.2 and 10.3) and their cell membrane has receptors for IgG, IgE, and complement. Electron micrographs display a small, centrally located Golgi apparatus, a limited amount of rough endoplasmic reticulum (RER), and only a few mitochondria that are usually located in the vicinity of the centrioles near the cytocenter. Eosinophils are produced in the bone marrow, and **interleukin-5 (IL-5)** causes proliferation of their precursors and their

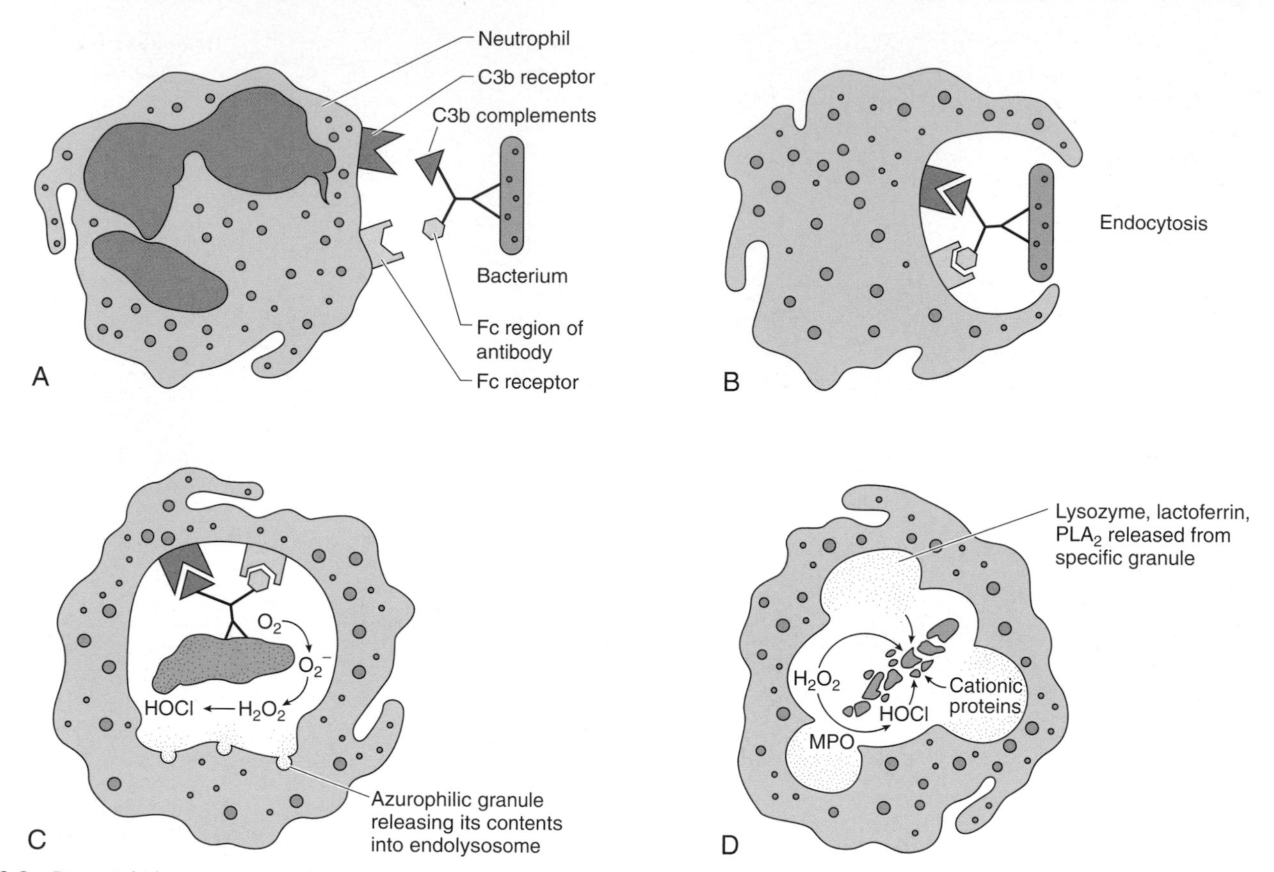

Fig. 10.9 Bacterial phagocytosis and destruction by a neutrophil. These actions are dependent on the ability of the neutrophil to recognize the bacterium via the presence of complement and/or antibody attached to the microorganism. H_2O_2, Hydrogen peroxide; HOCl, hypochlorous acid; MPO, myeloperoxidase; O_2^-, superoxide.

differentiation into mature cells. In the absence of IL-5, basophils develop instead of eosinophils.

Eosinophil Granules

The specific granules of eosinophils possess an externum and an internum.

Eosinophils possess specific granules and azurophilic granules. Specific granules are oblong (1.0–1.5 µm in length, < 1.0 µm in width) and stain deep pink with Giemsa and Wright stains. Electron micrographs demonstrate that *specific granules* have a crystal-like, electron-dense center, the **internum**, surrounded by a less electron-dense **externum** (Fig. 10.10). The internum houses **major basic protein, eosinophilic cationic protein**, and **eosinophil-derived neurotoxin**, the first two of which are highly efficacious agents in combating parasites. The externum houses the enzymes listed in Table 10.3.

The nonspecific azurophilic granules are lysosomes (0.5 µm in diameter) containing hydrolytic enzymes similar to those found in neutrophils. These enzymes function both in the destruction of parasitic worms and in the hydrolysis of antigen–antibody complexes internalized by eosinophils.

Eosinophil Functions

Eosinophils assist in the elimination of antibody–antigen complexes and in the destruction of parasitic worms.

The binding of histamine, leukotrienes, and eosinophil chemotactic factor (released by mast cells, basophils, and neutrophils) to eosinophil cell membrane receptors induces the migration of these cells to the site of allergic reaction, inflammatory reaction, or parasitic worm invasion. Eosinophils degranulate their major basic protein or eosinophil cationic protein on the surface of the parasitic worms, killing them by forming pores in their pellicles, thus facilitating access of agents such as superoxides and hydrogen peroxide to the parasite cell membrane and cytoplasm.

Eosinophils also release substances that inactivate the pharmacological initiators of the inflammatory response, such as histamine and leukotriene C. Additionally, they engulf antigen–antibody complexes that pass into the eosinophil's endosomal compartment for eventual degradation. The ribonucleases in the azurophilic granules of eosinophils combat viral pathogens. Moreover, eosinophils participate in the degradation of fibrin.

Clinical Correlations

Connective tissue cells in the vicinity of antigen–antibody complexes release the pharmacological agents histamine and IL-5, causing increased formation and release of eosinophils from the bone marrow. In contrast, elevation of blood corticosteroid levels depresses the number of eosinophils in circulation.

Basophils

Basophils are similar to mast cells in function even though they originate from different precursors in the bone marrow.

Basophils are granulocytes that constitute less than 1% of the total leukocyte population. They are round cells in suspension

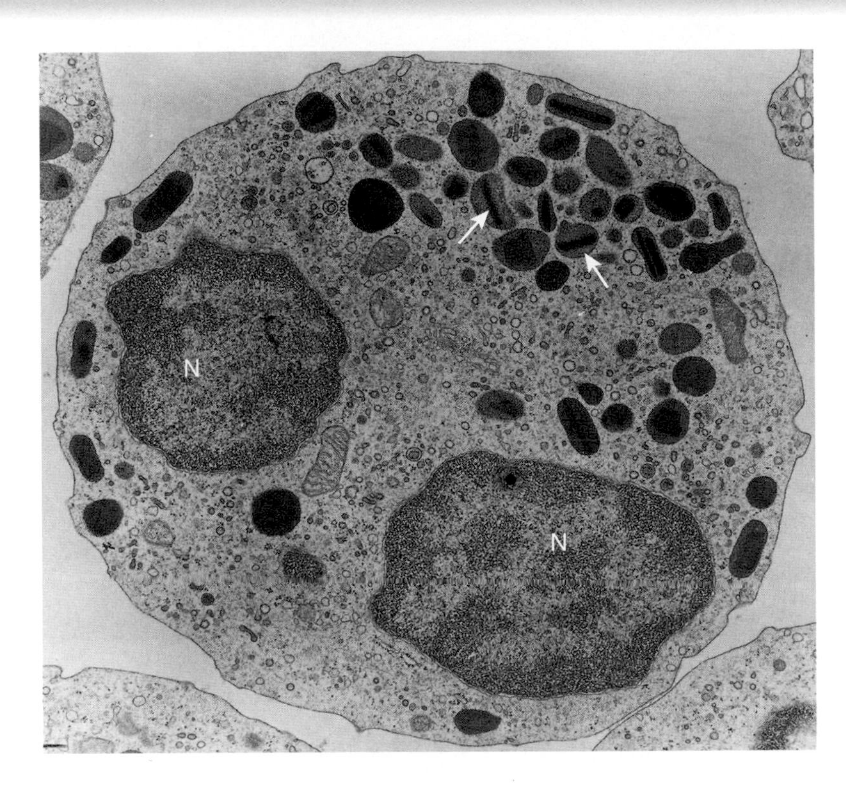

Fig. 10.10 Electron micrograph of a human eosinophil. Note the electron-dense internum *(arrows)* of the eosinophilic granules and the two lobes of the nucleus (N). (From Zucker-Franklin D. Eosinophil function and disorders. *Adv Intern Med.* 1974;19:1–25.)

but may be pleomorphic during migration through connective tissue. They are 8 to 10 μm in diameter (in blood smears) and have an **S**-shaped nucleus, which is commonly masked by the large specific granules present in the cytoplasm (see Figs. 10.2 and 10.3). Electron micrographs demonstrate the presence of the small Golgi apparatus, few mitochondria, extensive RER, and occasional glycogen deposits. Basophils have a number of surface receptors on their plasmalemma, including **immunoglobulin E (IgE) receptors (FcεRI)**. Basophils originate in the bone marrow but can be formed only in the absence of IL-5.

Basophil Granules

Basophils possess specific and azurophilic granules.

The **specific granules** of basophils stain dark blue to black with Giemsa and Wright stains. They are approximately 0.5 μm in diameter and frequently press against the periphery of the cell, creating the basophil's characteristic "roughened" perimeter, as seen by light microscopy. These granules contain heparin, histamine, eosinophil chemotactic factor, neutrophil chemotactic factor, neutral proteases, chondroitin sulfate, and peroxidase (see Table 10.3). The nonspecific **azurophilic granules** are lysosomes, which contain enzymes similar to those of neutrophils.

Basophil Functions

Basophils function as initiators of the inflammatory process.

In response to the presence of some antigens in certain individuals, plasma cells manufacture and release a particular class of immunoglobulin, IgE. The Fc portions of the IgE molecules become attached to the **FcεRI** receptors of basophils and mast cells without any apparent effect. However, the next time the same antigens enter the body, they bind to the IgE molecules on the surface of these cells. Although mast cells and basophils appear to have similar functions (see Chapter 6), they are different cells and they originate from different precursors in the bone marrow.

Clinical Correlations

In certain hyperallergic individuals, a second exposure to the same allergen may result in an intense generalized response. A large number of basophils (and mast cells) degranulate, resulting in widespread vasodilation and sweeping reduction in blood volume (because of vessel leakiness). Thus, the person goes into circulatory shock. The smooth muscles of the bronchial tree constrict, causing respiratory insufficiency. The combined effect is a life-threatening condition known as anaphylactic shock.

Monocytes

Monocytes, the largest of the circulating blood cells, are agranulocytes; they enter the connective tissue spaces, where they are known as macrophages.

Monocytes, the largest of the circulating blood cells (12–15 μm in diameter in blood smears), are agranulocytes constituting 3% to 8% of the leukocyte population. They have a large, acentric, kidney-shaped nucleus that frequently has a "moth-eaten," soap-bubbly appearance and whose lobe-like extensions appear to overlap one another. The chromatin network is coarse but not overly dense, and typically two nucleoli are present, although they are not always evident in smears. The cytoplasm is bluish gray and has numerous azurophilic granules (lysosomes) and occasional vacuole-like spaces (see Figs. 10.2 and 10.3).

Electron micrographs display both heterochromatin and euchromatin in the kidney-shaped nucleus, as well as the two nucleoli. The Golgi apparatus is usually near the indentation of the nucleus. The cytoplasm contains deposits of glycogen granules, a few profiles of RER, some mitochondria, free ribosomes, and numerous lysosomes. The periphery of the cell displays microtubules, microfilaments, pinocytotic vesicles, and filopodia.

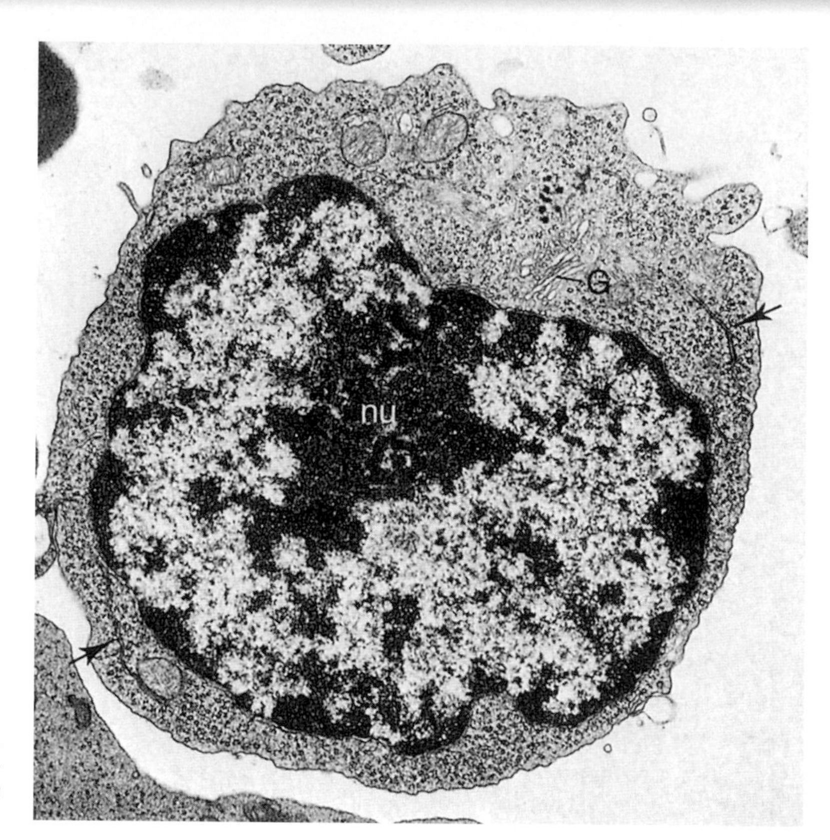

Fig. 10.11 Electron micrograph of a lymphocyte (×14,173). *Arrows* point to the rough endoplasmic reticulum. G, Golgi apparatus; nu, nucleus. (From Hopkins CR. *Structure and Function of Cells*. Philadelphia: WB Saunders; 1978.)

Monocytes stay in circulation for only a few days; they then migrate through the endothelium of venules and capillaries into the connective tissue, where they differentiate into **macrophages** or **dendritic cells**. An introduction to the properties and functions of macrophages follows here (see Chapter 12 for more details).

Function of Macrophages

Macrophages phagocytose unwanted particulate matter, produce cytokines that are required for the inflammatory and immune responses, and present epitopes to T lymphocytes.

Macrophages are avid phagocytes and, as members of the mononuclear phagocyte system, they phagocytose and destroy dead and defunct cells (e.g., senescent erythrocytes) as well as antigens and foreign particulate matter (e.g., bacteria). The destruction occurs within the phagosomes through both enzymatic digestion and the formation of superoxide, hydrogen peroxide, and hypochlorous acid. These cells produce cytokines that activate the inflammatory response, as well as the proliferation and maturation of other cells.

Moreover, certain macrophages and dendritic cells are antigen-presenting cells that phagocytose antigens and present the most antigenic fragments of these macromolecules, known as *epitopes*, in conjunction with the integral proteins, class II human leukocyte antigen (**class II HLA**), also known as *major histocompatibility complex antigens* (MHC II), to immunocompetent T lymphocytes.

In response to large foreign particulate matter, macrophages can fuse with one another, forming foreign-body giant cells that are large enough to phagocytose the large foreign particle.

Lymphocytes

Lymphocytes are agranulocytes that form the second largest population of white blood cells.

Lymphocytes are agranulocytes that constitute 20% to 25% of the total circulating leukocyte population. They are round cells in blood smears, but they may be pleomorphic as they migrate through connective tissue. Lymphocytes are somewhat larger than erythrocytes, 8 to 10 μm in diameter (in blood smears), and have a slightly indented, round nucleus that occupies most of the cell. The nucleus is dense, rich in heterochromatin, and somewhat acentrically located. The peripherally situated cytoplasm stains light blue and houses azurophilic granules. On the basis of size, lymphocytes may be described as small (8–10 μm in diameter), medium (12–15 μm in diameter), or large (15–18 μm in diameter), although the latter two are much less numerous (see Figs. 10.2 and 10.3).

Electron micrographs of lymphocytes display a scant amount of peripheral cytoplasm housing a few mitochondria, a small Golgi apparatus, and a few profiles of RER. A small number of lysosomes, representing azurophilic granules (0.5 μm in diameter), and an abundant supply of ribosomes are also evident (Fig. 10.11).

Lymphocytes are discussed in greater detail in Chapter 12; an introduction to their properties and functions follows here.

Types of Lymphocytes

There are three types of lymphocytes: T lymphocytes, B lymphocytes, and null cells.

Lymphocytes are subdivided into three functional categories: **B lymphocytes (B cells)**, **T lymphocytes (T cells)**, and **null cells**. Although they are indistinguishable from each other morphologically, they may be recognized immunocytochemically by the differences in their cell membrane surface markers (see Table 10.3). Approximately 80% of the circulating lymphocytes are T cells, about 15% are B cells, and the rest are null cells. Their life spans also differ widely: some T cells may live for years, whereas some B cells may die within a few months.

Functions of B and T Cells

In very general terms, B cells are responsible for the humorally mediated immune system, whereas T cells are responsible for the cellularly mediated immune system.

Lymphocytes have no function in the bloodstream, but in the connective tissue, these cells are responsible for the proper functioning of the immune system. To be immunologically competent, immature lymphocytes migrate to specific body compartments to mature and to express specific surface markers and receptors. Lymphocytes destined to be B cells enter as yet unidentified regions of the **bone marrow**, whereas lymphocytes destined to be T cells migrate to the cortex of the **thymus**. Once they have become immunologically competent, lymphocytes leave their respective sites of maturation, enter the lymphoid system, and undergo mitosis, each forming a group of identical cells known as a ***clone***. All members of a particular clone can recognize and respond to the same antigen.

After stimulation by a specific antigen, both B and T cells proliferate and differentiate into two subpopulations:

- Memory cells (whether B memory cells or T memory cells) do not participate in the immune response but rather remain as part of the clone with an "immunological memory," ready to undergo cell division and their progeny mount a response against a subsequent exposure to a particular antigen or foreign substance.
- Effector cells are classified as B cells and T cells (and their subtypes) and are detailed in the following section.

Effector Cells

Effector cells are immunocompetent lymphocytes that can perform their immune functions, that is, eliminating antigens, foreign cells, and virally altered cells.

B cells are responsible for the **humorally mediated immune system**; that is, they differentiate into **plasma cells**, which produce **antibodies** against **antigens**. T cells are responsible for the **cellularly mediated immune system**. Some T cells differentiate into **cytotoxic T cells (T killer cells)** and **natural killer T cells (NKT cells)**, which make physical contact with **foreign** or **virally altered cells** and kill them. In addition, certain T cells are responsible for the initiation and development **(T helper cells)** or for the suppression (**regulatory T cells** [**T reg cells**], formerly known as *T suppressor cells*) of most humorally and cellularly mediated immune responses. They accomplish this by releasing signaling molecules known as ***cytokines*** (***lymphokines***) that elicit specific responses from other cells of the immune system (see Chapter 12).

Null Cells. **Null cells** are composed of two distinct populations:

- Circulating stem cells, which give rise to all of the formed elements of blood
- Natural killer (NK) cells, which can kill some foreign and virally altered cells on their own, without the influence of the thymus or T cells

Clinical Correlations

Lymphomas are cancers of lymphocytes (although some authors also consider noncancerous tumors of lymphocytes under the same heading). Even though there are various subcategories of lymphomas, historically, they were subdivided into two major types, Hodgkin disease (Hodgkin lymphoma) and non Hodgkin disease (non-Hodgkin lymphoma). The former accounted for 25% of all lymphomas and the latter for about 75% of all lymphomas. The general symptoms include swollen lymph nodes without accompanying pain, tiredness, itchiness, night sweat, elevated temperature, generalized malaise, and unexplained loss of weight.

1. *Hodgkin disease occurs in two age groups: individuals in their late teens and early 30s and people in their mid-50s to early 60s. In both groups, it usually originates in and spreads from lymph node to lymph node. As the disease progresses, it spreads to the liver, spleen, bone marrow, and intestines. Histopathology of the affected organs presents with characteristically large, modified B cells (30–60 μm in diameter), known as Reed-Sternberg cells, with two distinctive nuclei that are mirror images of one another.*
2. *Non-Hodgkin disease occurs mostly in middle-aged and older individuals. The cancer is mostly of B-cell origin, although in approximately 10% of cases, T cells give rise to the malignancy. The cancer originates in lymph nodes in 75% of cases, whereas in 25% of cases the disease originates in other regions of the body, such as the brain, intestines, stomach, and even the thyroid gland. Classically, non-Hodgkin disease may be of low-grade malignancy that takes years to develop or high-grade malignancy that develops over a period of weeks or months.*

Platelets

Platelets (thrombocytes) are small, disk-shaped, nonnucleated cell fragments derived from megakaryocytes in the bone marrow.

Platelets are about 2 to 4 μm in diameter in blood smears (see Figs. 10.2 and 10.3). In light micrographs, they display a peripheral clear region, the **hyalomere**, and a central darker region, the **granulomere**. The platelet plasmalemma has numerous receptor molecules, as well as a relatively thick (15–20 nm) **glycocalyx** composed of glycoproteins, glycosaminoglycans, coagulation factors, and the extracellular moiety of the transmembrane glycoprotein Ib. There are between 250,000 and 400,000 platelets per mm^3 of blood, each with a life span of less than 14 days.

Platelet Tubules and Granules

Platelets possess three types of granules (alpha, delta, and lambda) as well as two tubular systems (dense and surface opening).

Electron micrographs of platelets display 10 to 15 microtubules arranged parallel to each other and forming a ring within the hyalomere. The microtubules assist platelets in maintaining their discoid morphology. Associated with this bundle of microtubules are actin and myosin monomers, which can rapidly assemble to form a contractile apparatus.

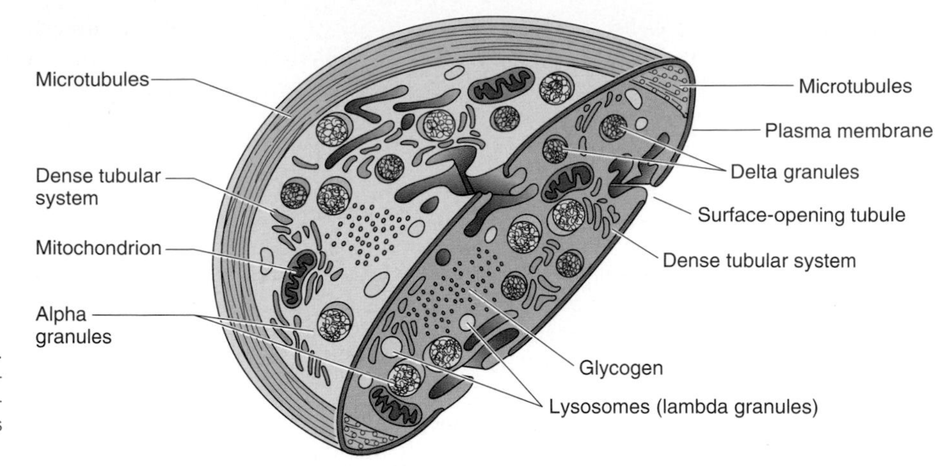

Fig. 10.12 Diagram of platelet ultrastructure. Note that the periphery of the platelet is occupied by actin filaments that encircle the platelet and maintain the discoid morphology of this structure.

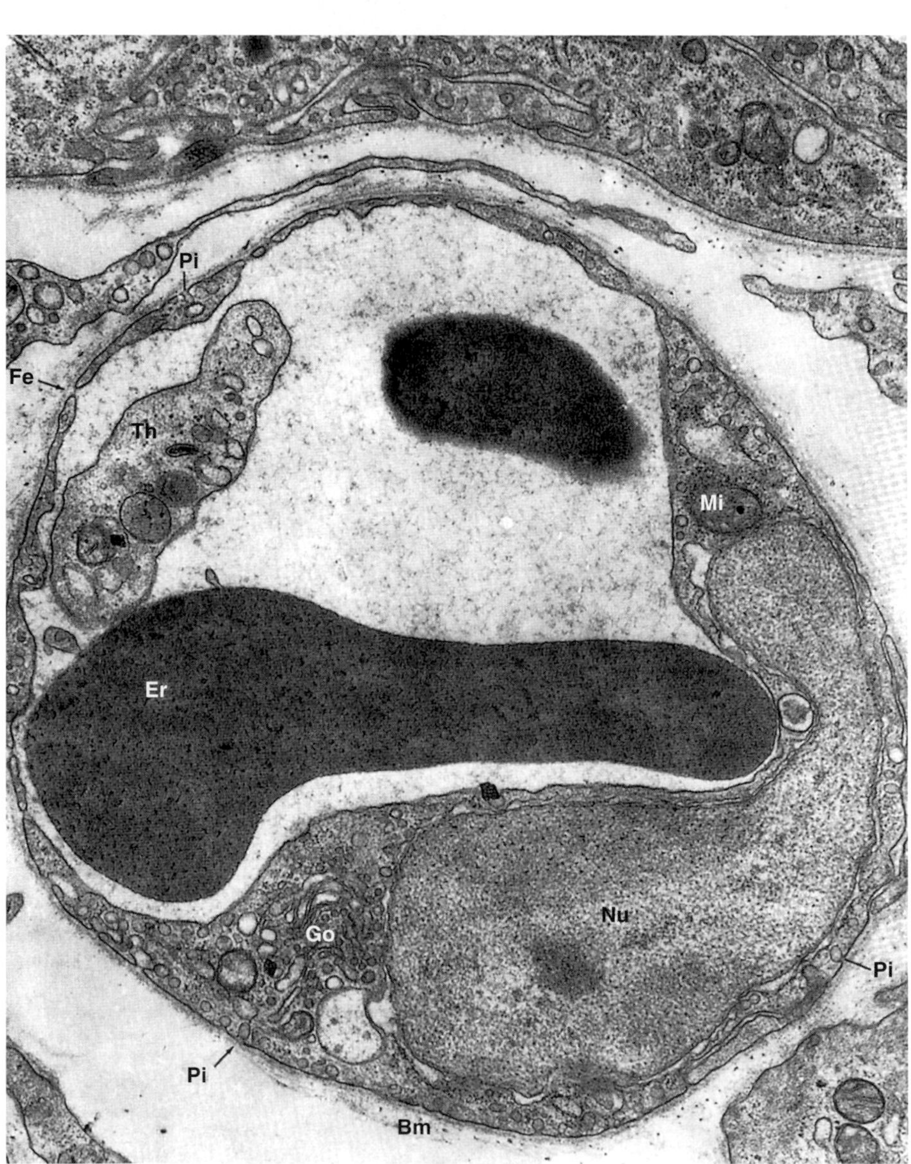

Fig. 10.13 Electron micrograph of a platelet and two erythrocytes in the gastric mucosa capillary (×22,100). Bm, Basal lamina; Er, erythrocyte; Fe, fenestra; Go, Golgi apparatus; Nu, nucleus of the capillary; Pi, pinocytotic vesicles; Th, platelet. (From Rhodin JAG. *An Atlas of Ultrastructure*. Philadelphia: WB Saunders; 1963.)

There are two tubular systems in the hyalomere, the surface-opening (connecting) and the dense tubular systems (Figs. 10.12 and 10.13). The surface-opening system is coiled, forming a labyrinthine complex within the platelet. Because this system communicates with the outside, the luminal aspect of this tubular system is a continuation of the outer surface of the platelet, thus increasing the platelet surface area by a factor of seven or eight.

Electron microscopy displays the presence of a small number of mitochondria, glycogen deposits, peroxisomes, and three

TABLE 10.4 Platelet Tubules and Granules

Structure (Size)	Location	Contents	Function
Surface-opening tubule system	Hyalomere		Expedites rapid uptake and release of molecules from activated platelets
Dense tubular system	Hyalomere		Probably sequesters calcium ions to prevent platelet "stickiness"
α-Granules (300–500 nm)	Granulomere	Fibrinogen, platelet-derived growth factor, platelet thromboplastin, thrombospondin, coagulation factors	Contained factors facilitate vessel repair, platelet aggregation, and coagulation of blood
δ-Granules (dense bodies; 250–300 nm)	Granulomere	Calcium, ADP, ATP, serotonin, histamine, pyrophosphatase	Contained factors facilitate platelet aggregation and adhesion, as well as vasoconstriction
λ-Granules (lysosomes; 200–250 nm)	Granulomere	Hydrolytic enzymes	Contained enzymes aid clot resorption

ADP, Adenosine diphosphate; *ATP*, adenosine triphosphate.

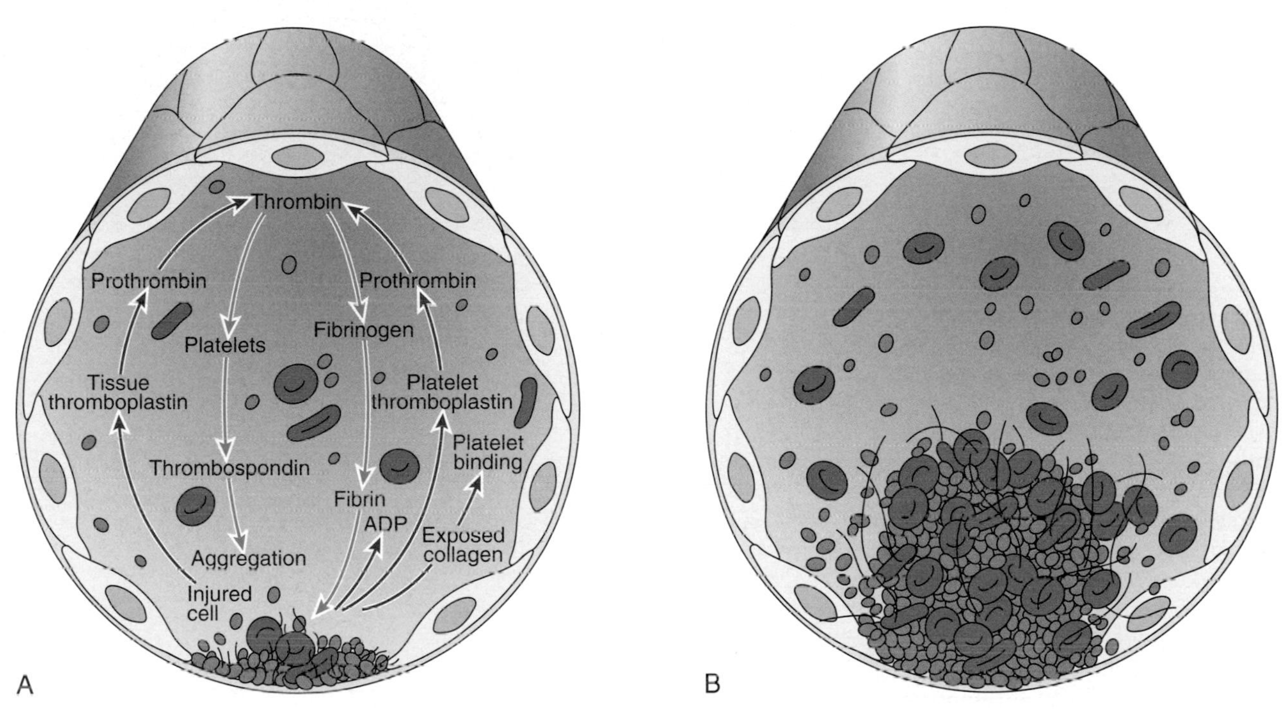

Fig. 10.14 Schematic diagram of clot formation. (A) Injury to the endothelial lining releases various clotting factors and ceases the release of inhibitors of clotting. (B) The increase in the size of the clot plugs the defect in the vessel wall and stops the loss of blood. ADP, Adenosine diphosphate. (From Fawcett DW. *Bloom and Fawcett's A Textbook of Histology*. 12th ed. New York: Chapman and Hall; 1994.)

types of granules: **alpha-granules (α-granules)**, **delta granules (δ-granules)**, and **lambda-granules (λ-granules**, lysosomes) in the granulomere. The tubules and granules, as well as their contents and functions, are listed in Table 10.4. The granulomere also houses a system of enzymes that permits platelets to catabolize glycogen, consume oxygen, and generate ATP.

Platelet Function

Platelets function in limiting hemorrhage to the endothelial lining of the blood vessel in case of injury.

If the endothelial lining of a blood vessel is disrupted and platelets come in contact with subendothelial collagen fibers, they become **activated**, release the contents of their granules, adhere to the damaged region of the vessel wall (**platelet adhesion**), and adhere to each other (**platelet aggregation**). They also participate in **clot retraction** and **clot removal**. Interactions of tissue factors, plasma-borne factors, and platelet-derived factors form a blood clot (Figs. 10.14 and 10.15). Although the mechanism of platelet aggregation, adhesion, and blood clotting is beyond the scope of histology, some of its salient features are as follows:

1. Normally, the intact endothelium produces prostacyclins and nitric oxide (NO), which inhibit platelet aggregation. It also blocks coagulation because thrombomodulin and heparin-like molecules, two membrane-associated molecules, inactivate specific coagulation factors.
2. Injured endothelial cells do not produce or express inhibitors of coagulation and platelet aggregation; also, they release von Willebrand factor (vWF), tissue factor (also known as *thromboplastin*), and endothelin, a powerful vasoconstrictor that reduces the loss of blood.
3. The glycoprotein Ib molecules of platelet membranes avidly adhere to vWF, which then adheres to the exposed

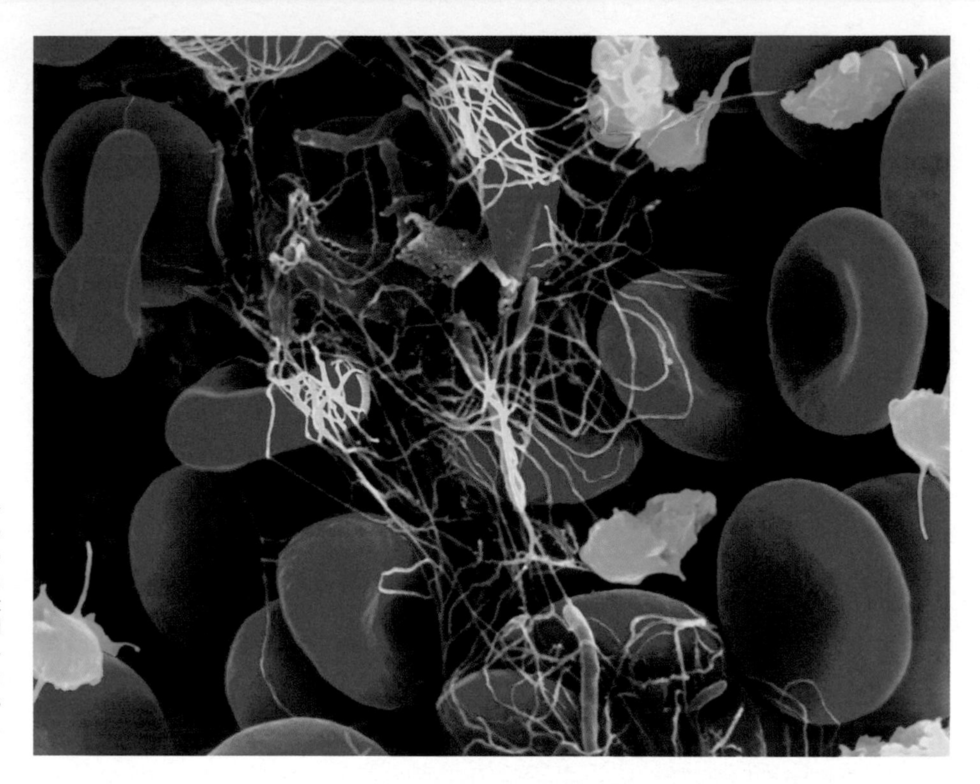

Fig. 10.15 This close-up view of a clot forming in human blood shows beautifully how the different blood components are crammed into the plasma. (The scanning electron micrograph has been colored to emphasize the different structures.) Red blood cells *(red)* are entangled with the fibrin *(yellow)* that makes up the scaffolding of the clot. The platelets *(blue)*, which initiate clotting, are fragments of larger cells (megakaryocytes). (Courtesy Dennis Kunkel, PhD.)

collagen fibers of the vessel wall. This contact between vWF and the glycoprotein Ib induces the platelets to release the contents of their granules and adhere to one another. These three events are collectively called *platelet activation.*

4. The release of some of their granular contents—especially calcium ions, adenosine diphosphate, and thrombospondin—makes glycocalyx of the platelets "sticky," causing circulating platelets to adhere to the collagen-bound platelets and to degranulate.
5. Arachidonic acid, formed in the activated platelet plasmalemma, is converted to thromboxane A_2, a potent vasoconstrictor and avid platelet activator.
6. The aggregated platelets act as a plug, blocking hemorrhage, and the platelets maintain their contact with each other by exposing additional integrin molecules, glycoproteins IIb/IIIa, whose extracellular moieties make firm bonds with those of adjacent platelets, eventually forming the rather weak primary hemostatic plug. Less than a half an hour after its formation, enough fibrinogen, a normal constituent of blood, contacts the primary hemostatic plug that its adhering platelets are induced to contract, forming a dense, stable secondary hemostatic plug that is fixed to the site of injury by the fibrin filaments resulting from the coagulation process. To prevent the formation of an overly large secondary hemostatic plug, the endothelial cells release prostacyclins and NO. As this is occurring, the adhering platelets express platelet factor 3 on their plasmalemma, providing the necessary phospholipid surface for the proper assembly of the coagulation factors (especially of thrombin).
7. As part of the complex cascade of reactions involving the various coagulation factors, tissue factor and platelet thromboplastin both act on circulating prothrombin, converting it into thrombin. Thrombin is an enzyme that facilitates platelet aggregation. In the presence of calcium (Ca^{2+}), it also converts fibrinogen to fibrin. The mechanism of blood coagulation is described in the next section.
8. The fibrin monomers thus produced polymerize and form a fibrin reticulum that attaches to the secondary hemostatic plug, establishing a reticulum of clot, entangling additional platelets, erythrocytes, and leukocytes into a stable, gelatinous blood clot (thrombus). The erythrocytes facilitate platelet activation, whereas neutrophils and endothelial cells limit both platelet activation and thrombus size.
9. Approximately 1 hour after clot formation, actin and myosin monomers form thin and thick filaments, which interact by using ATP as their energy source. As a result, the clot contracts to about half its previous size, pulling the cut edges of the damaged vessel closer together and minimizing blood loss.
10. When the vessel is repaired, the endothelial cells release tissue plasminogen activators and urokinase-type plasminogen activator, which convert circulating plasminogen to plasmin, the enzyme that initiates lysis of the thrombus, a process that is assisted by the hydrolytic enzymes of λ-granules.

Clinical Correlations

1. *In a patient with a* ***thromboembolism****, the most common type of embolism, clots break free and circulate in the bloodstream until they reach a vessel whose lumen is too small to accommodate them. If a clot is large enough to occlude the bifurcation of the pulmonary artery (saddle embolus), it can result in sudden, unexpected death. If a clot obstructs branches of the coronary artery, a myocardial infarct may occur.*
2. *Several types of* ***coagulation disorders*** *that result in excessive bleeding have been identified. The disorder may be acquired (as in vitamin K deficiency) or hereditary (as in hemophilia) or may be caused by low levels of blood platelets (thrombocytopenia). Vitamin K is required by the liver as a cofactor in the synthesis of the clotting factors VII, IX, and X and prothrombin. Absence of or reduced levels of these factors results in partial or complete dysfunction of the clotting process.*
3. *In patients with* ***thrombocytopenia****, the blood level of platelets is decreased. The condition becomes serious when the platelet level is below 50,000/mm^3. Although bleeding is common in these patients, the bleeding is generalized and occurs from small vessels, resulting in purplish splotches on the skin. This condition is believed to be an autoimmune disease, in which antibodies are formed to one's own platelets, and these antibodies destroy the platelets.*

Blood Coagulation Cascade. The **coagulation of blood** (**blood clotting**) involves the interactions of a number of factors that circulate in the blood, but it also requires the presence of phospholipid complexes on the plasma membranes of activated platelets and calcium ions (factor IV). Coagulation occurs by way of two pathways (Table 10.5), the **tissue factor pathway** (**extrinsic pathway**) and **contact activation pathway** (**intrinsic pathway**). The final few steps of the two pathways are identical and, therefore, are referred to as the ***common pathway***. It is important to note that the tissue factor pathway is the *principal coagulation pathway* and that the contact activation pathway is of secondary importance.

- The **tissue factor** (**extrinsic**) **pathway** is a rapid-onset pathway that occurs within seconds subsequent to an injury of a blood vessel if, *in addition* to the endothelium, the wall of the vessel is damaged. Connective tissue cells exposed to blood and endothelial cells release **tissue factor** (**factor III**, also known as ***tissue thromboplastin***).
- **The contact activation** (**intrinsic**) **pathway** is a **slow-onset** pathway that occurs minutes after the endothelium (*but not the vessel wall*) is injured. Because the endothelium is damaged, collagens of the vessel wall are contacted by **factor XII** (**Hageman factor**), which initiates blood coagulation.
- The **common pathway** is where the two other pathways converge and **fibrin monomers** are formed. These monomers join to produce the fibrin reticulum that attach to the secondary hemostatic plug and form the reticulum of the clot.

Clinical Correlations

1. *The most common type of hemophilia is caused by* ***factor VIII deficiency (classic hemophilia)****, a recessive hereditary trait transmitted by mothers to their male children. Because the trait is carried on the X chromosomes, girls would not be affected unless both parents had deficient X chromosomes. Affected persons are likely to bleed after trauma, usually involving damage to larger vessels.*
2. ***Gray platelet syndrome*** *(also known as* ***alpha granule deficiency****) is caused by a lack or deficiency in the number of α-granules in the platelets. This autosomal recessive mutation results in thrombocytopenia with enlarged platelets with reduced granulomeres. Individuals with this syndrome present with increased bleeding disorders and myelofibrosis (increased collagen deposits in the bone marrow that reduces available space for hemopoiesis) due to the release of α-granule enzymes into the bone marrow during platelet formation by megakaryocytes.*

Bone Marrow

Bone marrow, a gelatinous, vascular connective tissue located in the marrow cavity, is richly endowed with cells that are responsible for hemopoiesis.

The medullary cavity of long bones and the interstices between trabeculae of spongy bones house the soft, gelatinous, highly vascular and cellular tissue known as ***bone marrow***, which constitutes almost 5% of the total body weight and is isolated from bone by the endosteum. It is responsible for the formation of blood cells (**hemopoiesis**) and their delivery into the circulatory system, performing this function from the fifth month of prenatal life until the person dies. Bone marrow also provides a microenvironment for much of the maturation process of B lymphocytes and for the initial maturation of T lymphocytes.

The marrow of the newborn is called ***red marrow*** because of the great number of erythrocytes being produced there. By age 20 years, however, the diaphyses of long bones house only **yellow marrow** because of the accumulation of large quantities of fat and the absence of hemopoiesis in the shafts of these bones. However, flat bones, short bones, irregular bones, and the epiphyses of long bones of the adult continue to house red marrow.

The vascular supply of bone marrow in long bones is derived from the nutrient arteries that pierce the diaphysis via the nutrient foramina, tunnels leading from the outside surface of bone into the medullary cavity. These arteries enter the marrow cavity and give rise to a number of small, peripherally located vessels that provide numerous branches both centrally, to the marrow, and peripherally, to the cortical bone. The centrally directed branches of the bone marrow deliver their blood to the extensive network of large venous spaces known as ***sinusoids*** (45–80 μm in diameter). The sinusoids drain into a **central longitudinal vein**, which is drained by veins leaving the bone via the nutrient canal.

It is interesting that the veins of bone marrow are *smaller* than those of the arteries, establishing high hydrostatic pressure

TABLE 10.5 Diagram of the Blood Coagulation Pathways

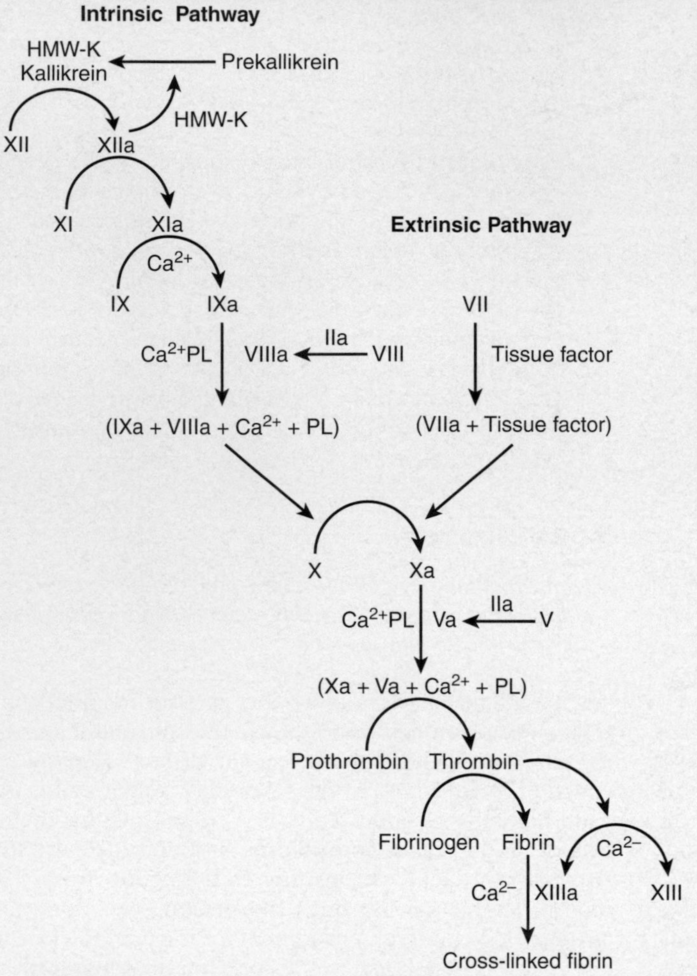

Intrinsic Pathway

HMW-K
Kallikrein ← Prekallikrein
HMW-K
XII → XIIa
XI → XIa
Ca^{2+}
IX → IXa
Ca^{2+}PL VIIIa ← IIa VIII
(IXa + VIIIa + Ca^{2+} + PL)

Extrinsic Pathway

VII
Tissue factor
(VIIa + Tissue factor)

X → Xa
Ca^{2+}PL Va ← IIa V
(Xa + Va + Ca^{2+} + PL)
Prothrombin → Thrombin
Fibrinogen → Fibrin
Ca^{2-}
Ca^{2-} XIIIa XIII
Cross-linked fibrin

Coagulation

Number	Common Name
I	Fibrinogen
Ia	Fibrin
II	Prothrombin
IIa	Thrombin
III	Tissue factor
IV	Ca^{2+} ions
V	Proaccelerin (labile factor)
Va	Accelerin
VII	Proconvertin (stable factor)
VIIa	Convertin
VIII	Antihemophilic factor A
IX	Christmas factor
X	Stuart-Prower factor
XI	Plasma thromboplastin antecedent
XIa	Plasma thromboplastin
XII	Hageman factor
XIII	Fibrin stabilizing factor (HMWK)

Contact Activation Pathway (Intrinsic Pathway)

1. High-molecular-weight kininogen (HMW-K) in concert with factor XII activates prekallikrein to form kallikrein.

2. Kallikrein and HMW-K activate factor XII to form factor XIIa.

3. Factor XIIa converts factor XI to factor XIa.

4. Factor XIa, in the presence of Ca^{2+} ions, converts factor IX to factor IXa.

5. Factor IXa, in the presence of Ca^{2+} ions and platelet phospholipids (PL) activate factor X to become factor Xa.

Tissue Factor Pathway (Extrinsic Pathway)

6. When the extrinsic pathway is activated, endothelial cells, and some connective tissue cells release tissue factor, which activates factor VII to factor VIIa.

7. Factor VIIa in concert with tissue factor and in the presence of Ca^{2+} ions activates factor X to factor Xa.

Common Pathway

8. The common pathway starts with the activation of factor X to factor Xa.

9. Factor Xa, in concert with factor Va in the presence of Ca^{2+} ions and platelet membrane phospholipids form a prothrombinase complex that converts prothrombin (factor II) to thrombin (factor IIa).

10. Thrombin converts fibrinogen (factor I) to fibrin monomers (factor Ia).

11. Factor XIIIa, in the presence of Ca^{2+} ions, facilitates the cross linking of fibrin monomers to form a fibrin plug.

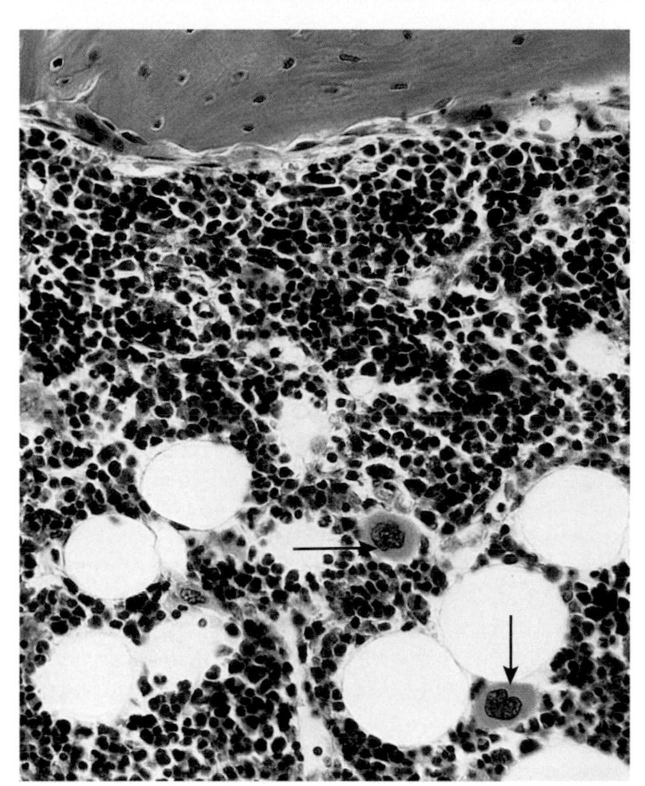

Fig. 10.16 Photomicrograph of human bone marrow displaying two megakaryocytes *(arrows)*. Observe that marrow has a much greater population of nucleated cells than does peripheral blood. Also note the presence of adventitial reticular cells that resemble adipocytes. At the top of the photomicrograph, the decalcified bone with osteocytes located in lacunae is evident. (×270)

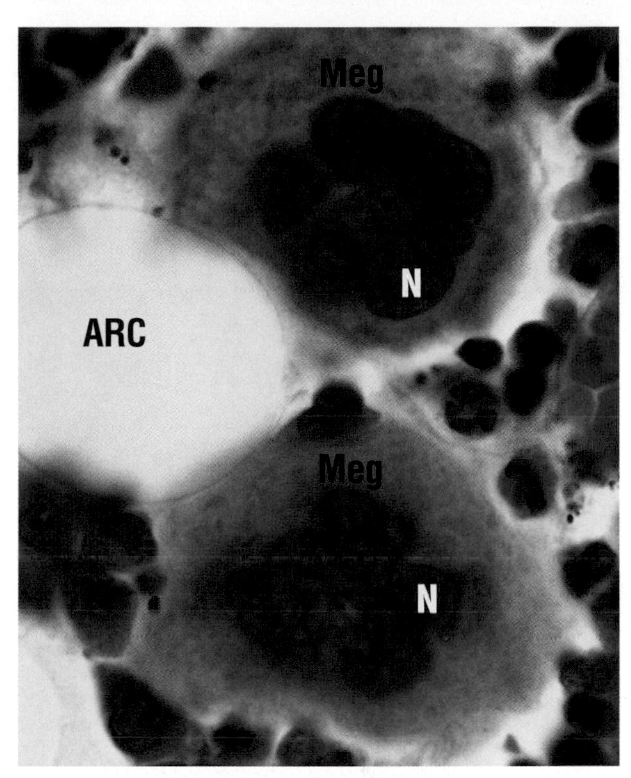

Fig. 10.17 This is a very high magnification of two megakaryocytes (Meg) displaying their large nuclei (N) that underwent endomitosis. Observe that the adventitial reticular cell (ARC) resembles a fat cell. The small cells at the periphery are precursors of leukocytes and erythrocytes. (×1325).

within the sinusoids, and this increased pressure maintains their patency. The veins, arteries, and sinusoids form the **vascular compartment**, and the intervening spaces are filled with pleomorphic clusters of hemopoietic cells that merge, forming the **hemopoietic compartment** (Figs. 10.16 and 10.17).

The sinusoids are lined by endothelial cells and are surrounded by slender threads of **reticular fibers** and a large number of **adventitial reticular cells**. Processes of adventitial reticular cells touch the sparse basement membrane of the endothelial cells, covering a large portion of the sinusoidal surface. Additional processes of these cells are directed away from the sinusoids and are in contact with similar processes of other adventitial reticular cells, forming a three-dimensional network surrounding discrete clusters of hemopoietic cells known as ***hemopoietic cords*** (***hemopoietic islands***, which are composed of blood cells in various stages of maturation as well as **macrophages**). These cells not only destroy the extruded nuclei of erythrocyte precursors, malformed cells, and excess cytoplasm but also regulate the differentiation of hemopoietic cell differentiation and maturation. In addition, they deliver iron to developing erythroblasts, to be used in the synthesis of the heme portion of hemoglobin. Frequently, processes of macrophages penetrate the spaces between endothelial cells to enter the sinusoidal lumina.

As adventitial reticular cells accumulate fat in their cytoplasm, they begin to resemble adipose cells. The volume occupied by these very large cells reduces the size of the hemopoietic compartment, transforming the red marrow to yellow marrow.

Clinical Correlations

In certain leukemias or in severe bleeding, adventitial reticular cells may lose their lipids and decrease in size, transforming yellow marrow to red marrow, making more space available for hemopoiesis.

PRENATAL HEMOPOIESIS

Prenatally, hemopoiesis is subdivided into four phases: mesoblastic, hepatic, splenic, and myeloid.

Blood cell formation begins 2 weeks after conception (**mesoblastic phase**) in the mesoderm of the yolk sac, where mesenchymal cells aggregate, forming clusters known as ***blood islands***. The peripheral cells of these islands form the vessel wall, and the remaining cells become **erythroblasts**, which differentiate into nucleated **erythrocytes** containing HbF. It is only around the time of birth that the erythrocytes house HbA_1, and HbA_2 as well as a very small amount of HbF.

The mesoblastic phase begins to be replaced by the **hepatic phase** by the sixth week of gestation. The circulating erythrocytes still have nuclei, and nonerythroid progenitors appear by the eighth week of gestation. The **splenic phase** begins during the second trimester; both hepatic and splenic phases continue until the end of gestation.

Hemopoiesis in the bone marrow (**myeloid phase**) begins by the end of the second trimester. As the skeletal system continues to develop, the bone marrow assumes an increasing role in blood cell formation. Although the liver and spleen are not active in hemopoiesis postnatally, they can revert to forming new blood cells if the need arises.

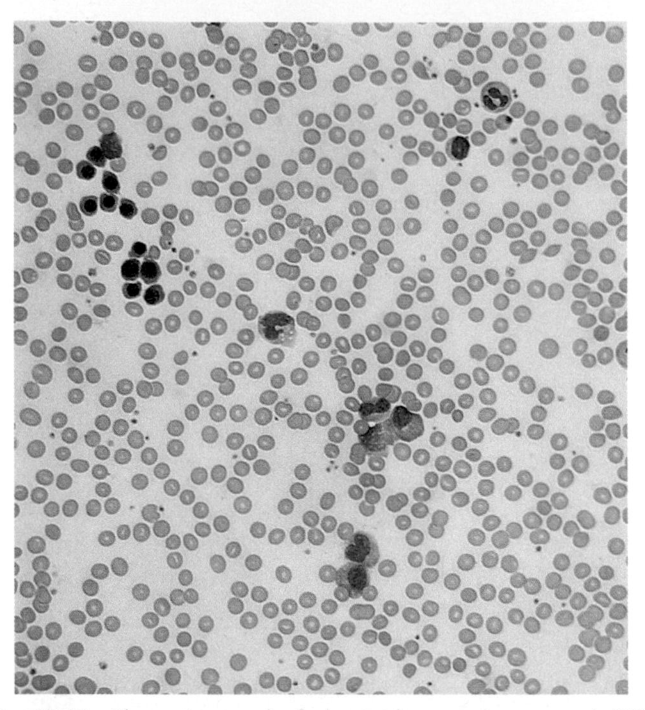

Fig. 10.18 Photomicrograph of a human bone marrow smear (×270).

POSTNATAL HEMOPOIESIS

Postnatal hemopoiesis occurs almost exclusively in bone marrow.

Because all blood cells have a finite life span, they must be replaced continuously. This replacement is accomplished by hemopoiesis, starting from a common population of stem cells within the bone marrow (Fig. 10.18). On a daily basis, more than 10^{11} blood cells are produced in the marrow to replace cells that leave the bloodstream, die, or are destroyed. During hemopoiesis, stem cells undergo multiple cell divisions and differentiate through several intermediate stages, eventually giving rise to the mature blood cells. Table 10.6 outlines the numerous intermediate cells in the formation of each type of mature blood cell. The entire process is regulated by various growth factors and cytokines that act at different steps to control the type of cells formed and their rate of formation.

Stem Cells, Progenitor Cells, and Precursor Cells

The least differentiated of the cells responsible for the formation of the formed elements of blood are stem cells; stem cells give rise to progenitor cells that differentiate into precursor cells.

TABLE 10.6 Cells of Hemopoiesis[a]

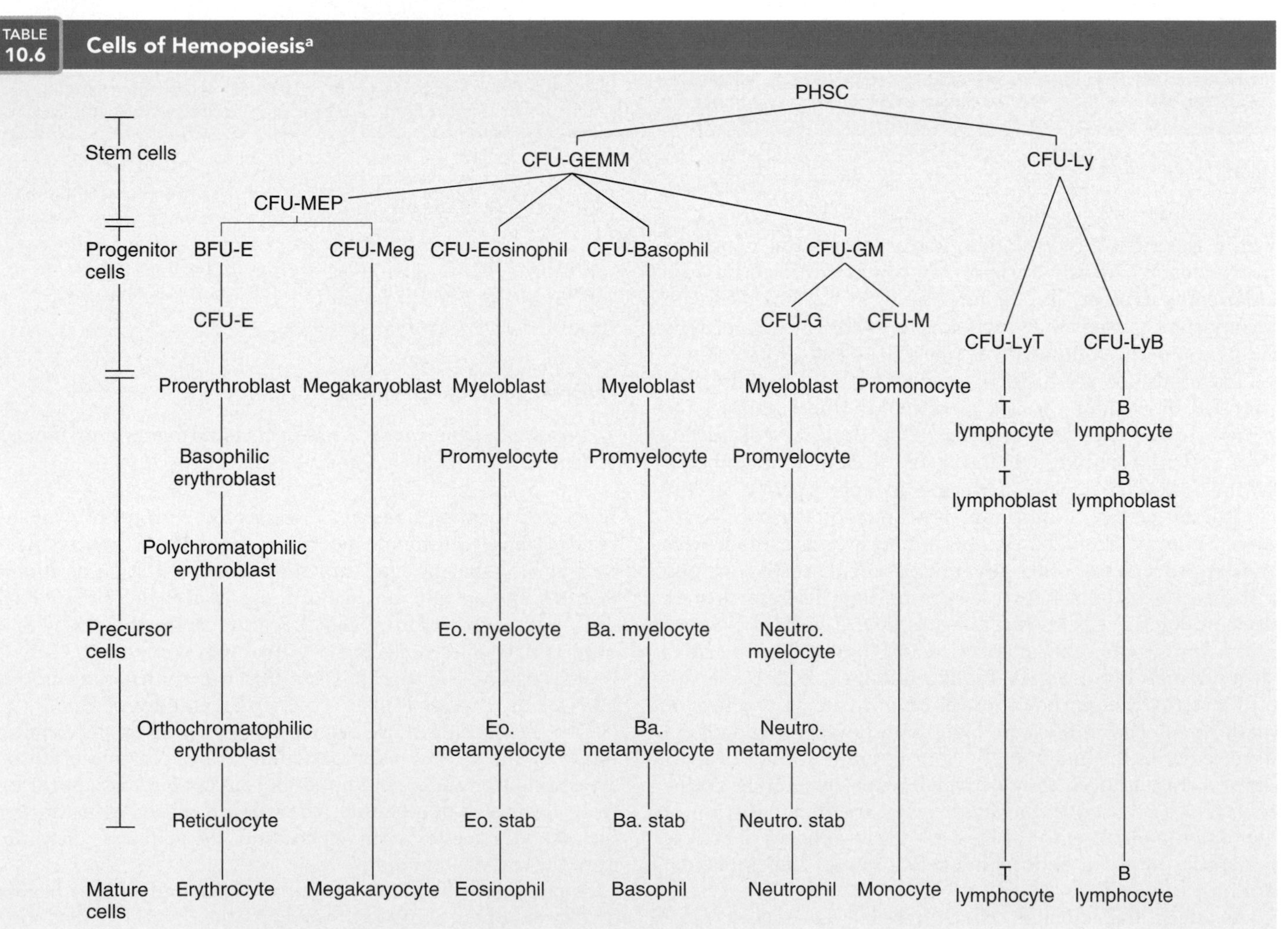

[a]Note that the lineage of NK cells, mast cells, and dendritic cells are not included in this table.

Modified from Gartner LP, Hiatt JL, Strum J. *Histology.* Baltimore: Williams & Wilkins; 1988.

Ba., Basophil; *BFU,* burst-forming unit (*E,* erythrocyte); *CFU,* colony-forming unit (*E,* erythrocyte); Eo., eosinophil; *G,* granulocyte; GEMM, granulocyte, erythrocyte, monocyte, megakaryocyte; *GM,* granulocyte-monocyte; *Ly,* lymphocyte; *Meg,* megakaryoblasts; *MEP,* megakaryocytic-erythroid progenitor; *Neutro.*, neutrophil; *PHSC,* pluripotential hemopoietic stem cell.

All blood cells arise from **pluripotential hemopoietic stem cells (PHSCs;** also known as ***hemopoietic stem cells*** [***HSC***]), which account for about 0.01% of the nucleated cell population of bone marrow. They are usually amitotic but may undergo bursts of cell division, giving rise to more PHSCs, as well as to two types of **multipotential hemopoietic stem cells (MHSCs),** also known as ***multipotent progenitors***. The two populations of MHSCs are **colony-forming unit–lymphocyte (CFU-Ly),** also known as ***common lymphoid progenitors*** (***CLP***), and **CFU-GEMM (colony-forming unit-granulocyte, erythrocyte, monocyte, megakaryocyte),** also known as ***common myeloid progenitors*** (***CMP***). These two populations of MHSCs are responsible for the formation of a series of **progenitor cells** (also known as ***committed precursors***), each of which gives rise to one specific type of the various types of blood cells and platelets.

- CFU-GEMM cells (common myeloid progenitors) are predecessors of the myeloid cell lines (erythrocytes, granulocytes, monocytes, dendritic cell, mast cells, and platelets).
- CFU-Ly (common lymphoid progenitors) are predecessors of the lymphoid cell lines (T cells, B cells, NK cells, and, perhaps, dendritic cells).

Both PHSCs and MHSCs resemble lymphocytes and constitute a small fraction of the null-cell population of circulating blood.

Stem cells are commonly in the G_0 stage of the cell cycle but can be driven into the G_1 stage by various growth factors and cytokines. Early stem cells may be recognized because they express the specific marker molecules CD34, CD59, CD133, Thy1, and c-*kit* on their plasma membranes. **Homeobox genes** may be active in the differentiation of the early stages of hemopoietic cells, specifically *Hox1* in the myeloid (*but not* MEP) cell lines and certain members of *Hox2* group in the MEP (but not granulocytic or monocyte) cell lines.

- CD34 assists in attaching the cell to the extracellular matrix as well as to stromal cells of bone marrow.
- CD59 inhibits complement from forming the membrane attack complex (discussed in Chapter 12).
- CD133 appears to assist in the organization of the three-dimensional morphology of the cell membrane; in that fashion, it may assist the function of CD59.
- Thy1 also appears to assist CD34 in its function of attaching the cell to the extracellular matrix, as well as to stromal cells of bone marrow.
- The c-kit is the membrane-bound receptor for stem cell factor (also known as *steel factor* or *c-kit ligand*, discussed later).

Progenitor cells also resemble small lymphocytes but are **unipotential** (i.e., committed to forming a single cell line, such as eosinophils). Their mitotic activity and differentiation are controlled by specific hemopoietic factors. These cells have only limited capacity for self-renewal.

Precursor cells arise from progenitor cells, are incapable of self-renewal, and *have specific morphological characteristics that permit them to be recognized as the first cell of a particular cell line*. Precursor cells undergo cell division and differentiation, eventually giving rise to a clone of mature cells. As cell maturation and differentiation proceed, succeeding cells become smaller, their nucleoli disappear, their chromatin network becomes denser, and the morphological characteristics of their cytoplasm approximate those of the mature cells (Fig. 10.19).

Clinical Correlations

1. *Patients who require bone marrow transplants after therapeutic procedures (e.g., irradiation or chemotherapy) must be matched for the major histocompatibility complex (MHC, discussed in Chapter 12) of the donor. Unless an identical twin is available for the transplantation, grafting failure is common. This can be circumvented by freezing the patient's own bone marrow in liquid nitrogen and reintroducing it (in an autologous transplant) to the patient after treatment with irradiation or chemotherapy. Because the number of stem cells per unit volume of bone marrow is relatively small, large volumes of marrow have to be harvested from the patient. Newer procedures that permit the isolation of pluripotential hemopoietic stem cells by the use of monoclonal antibodies against the CD34 molecule, which is expressed only by these cells, permit the use of small volumes of bone marrow enriched in PHSCs. These procedures are being investigated clinically, involving patients with various types of malignancies.*
2. *Perhaps in the relatively near future, people with hereditary blood cell disorders (e.g., sickle cell anemia) may be treated by the use of genetically engineered stem cells using the CRSPR/Cas 9 system. Pluripotential hemopoietic stem cells isolated from the patient may be transfected with the normal gene (e.g., for hemoglobin) and reintroduced as an autologous transplant. These genetically engineered cells bearing the normal gene would proliferate, and their progeny would produce normal blood cells. Although the patient would still produce some defective cells, it is hoped that enough normal cells would be produced to minimize the hereditary defect.*

Hemopoietic Growth Factors (Colony-Stimulating Factors)

Hemopoiesis is regulated by a number of cytokines and growth factors, such as interleukins, colony-stimulating factors, macrophage-inhibitory protein-α, and steel factor.

Hemopoiesis is regulated by numerous growth factors, mostly glycoproteins, produced by various cell types. Each factor acts on specific stem cells, progenitor cells, and precursor cells, generally inducing rapid mitosis, differentiation, or both (Table 10.7). Some of these growth factors also promote the functioning of mature blood cells.

Three routes are used to deliver growth factors to their target cells: (1) transport via the bloodstream (as endocrine hormones), (2) secretion by stromal cells of the bone marrow near the hemopoietic cells (as paracrine hormones), and (3) direct cell–cell contact (as surface signaling molecules).

Certain growth factors—principally, stem cell factor (also known as *steel factor* or *c-kit ligand*), GM-CSF, PU.1 transcription factor, IL-1, IL-3, IL-6, and IL-7—stimulate proliferation of pluripotential and multipotential stem cells, thus maintaining their populations. Additional cytokines—granulocyte colony-stimulating factor (G-CSF), monocyte colony-stimulating factor (M-CSF), IL-2, IL-5, IL-6, IL-11, IL-12, macrophage-inhibitory protein-α (MIP-α), thrombopoietin, and erythropoietin—are believed to be responsible for the mobilization and differentiation of these cells into unipotential progenitor cells.

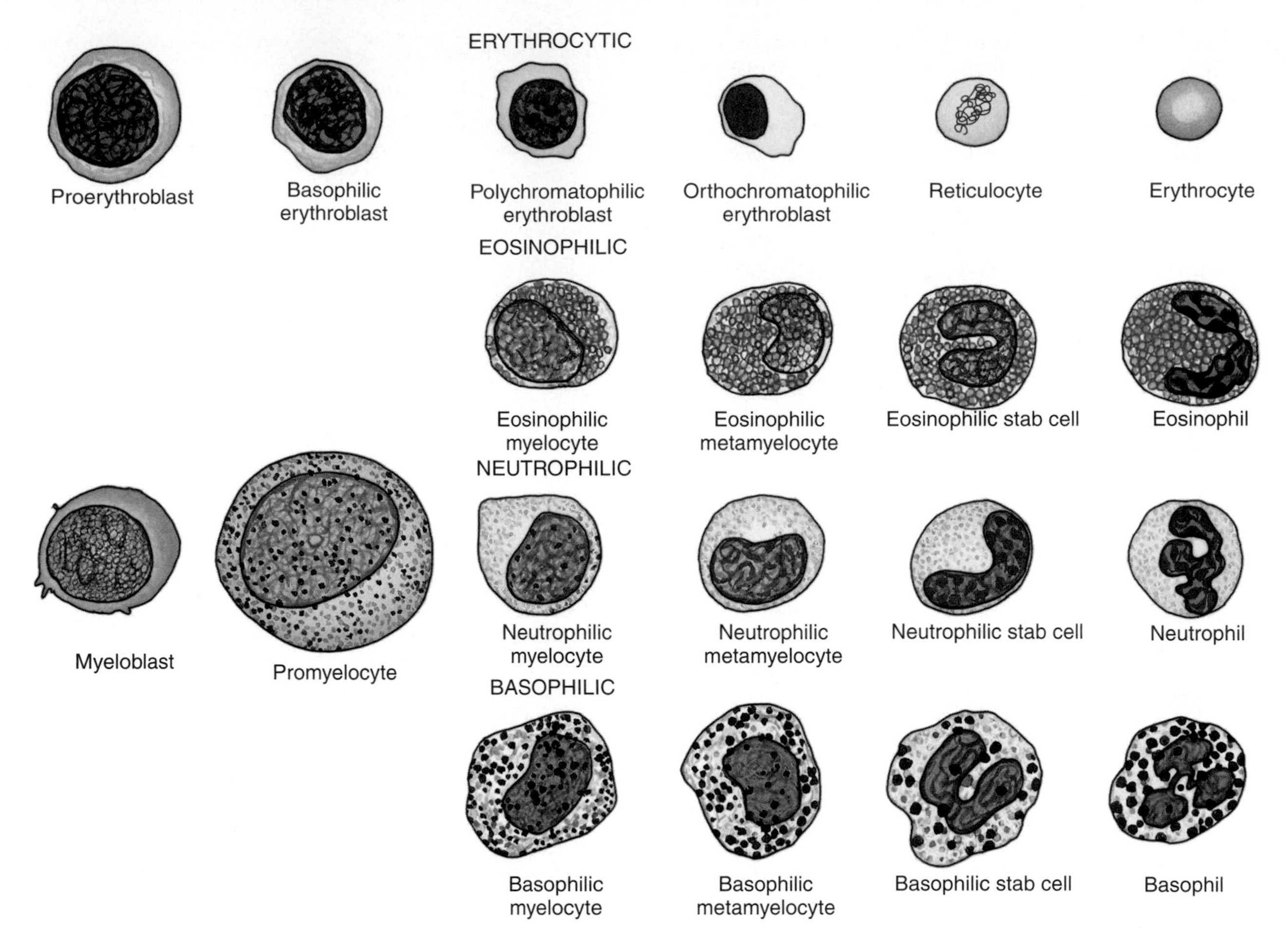

Fig. 10.19 Schematic diagram of precursor cells in formation of erythrocytes and granulocytes. The myeloblast and promyelocyte intermediaries in the formation of eosinophils, neutrophils, and basophils are indistinguishable for the three cell types.

TABLE 10.7 Hemopoietic Growth Factors

Factors	Principal Action	Site of Origin
Stem cell factor (steel factor, c-kit ligand)	Stimulates proliferation of pluripotential and multipotential stem cells and the formation of mast cells	Stromal cells of bone marrow
GM-CSF	Promotes CFU-GM mitosis and differentiation; facilitates granulocyte activity	T cells; endothelial cells
G-CSF	Promotes CFU-G mitosis and differentiation; facilitates neutrophil activity	Macrophages; endothelial cells
M-CSF	Promotes CFU-M mitosis and differentiation	Macrophages; endothelial cells
IL-1	In conjunction with IL-3 and IL-6, it promotes proliferation of PHSC, CFU-GEMM, and CFU-Ly; suppresses erythroid precursors	Monocytes; macrophages, endothelial cells
IL-2	Stimulates activated T- and B-cell mitosis; induces differentiation of NK cells	Activated T cells
IL-3	In conjunction with IL-1 and IL-6, it promotes proliferation of PHSC, CFU-GEMM, and CFU-Ly as well as all unipotential precursors (except for LyB and LyT); also promotes formation of BFU-E	Activated T and B cells
IL-4	Stimulates T- and B-cell activation and development of mast cells and basophils; also promotes formation of BFU-E	Activated T cells
IL-5	Promotes CFU-Eo mitosis and activates eosinophils	T cells
IL-6	In conjunction with IL-1 and IL-3, it promotes proliferation of PHSC, CFU-GEMM, and CFU-Ly; also facilitates CTL and B-cell differentiation	Monocytes and fibroblasts
IL-7	Promotes differentiation of CFU-LyB; CFU-LyT, and enhances differentiation of NK cells	Stromal cells

TABLE 10.7 Hemopoietic Growth Factors—cont'd

Factors	Principal Action	Site of Origin
IL-8	Induces neutrophil migration and degranulation	Leukocytes, endothelial cells, and smooth muscle cells
IL-9	Induces mast cell activation and proliferation; modulates IgE production; promotes T helper cell proliferation	T helper cells
IL-10	Inhibits cytokine production by macrophages, T cells, and NK cells; facilitates CTL differentiation and proliferation of B cells and mast cells	Macrophages and T cells
IL-12	Stimulates NK cells; enhances CTL and NK cell function	Macrophages
IL-15	Stimulates NK cell maturation	Macrophages
γ-Interferons	Activate B cells and monocytes; enhance CTL differentiation; augment the expression of class II HLA	T cells and NK cells
Erythropoietin	Induces CFU-E differentiation; BFU-E mitosis	Endothelial cells of the peritubular capillary network of kidney; hepatocytes
Thrombopoietin	Proliferation and differentiation of CFU-Meg and megakaryoblasts	Hepatocytes and liver sinusoidal lining cells; kidney proximal tubule cells, and stromal cells of bone marrow
GATA3 transcription factor	Differentiation of B and T lymphocytes	Expressed in the relevant cells
Ikaros family of transmission factors	Differentiation of B and T lymphocytes	Expressed in the relevant cells
Pax5 transcription factor	B lymphocyte maturation	Expressed in the relevant cells
PU.1 transcription factor	Development of granulocytes, macrophage and B lymphocytes	Expressed in the relevant cells

BFU-E, Burst forming unit–erythrocyte; *CFU-E*, colony forming unit–erythrocyte; *CSF*, colony-stimulating factor; *CTL*, cytotoxic T cell; *Eo*, eosinophil; *G*, granulocyte; *GEMM*, granulocyte, erythrocyte, monocyte, megakaryocyte; *GM*, granulocyte-monocyte; *HLA*, human leukocyte antigen; *IL*, interleukin; *Ly*, lymphocyte; *M*, monocyte; *NK*, natural killer; *PHSC*, pluripotential hemopoietic stem cell.

Colony-stimulating factors (**CSFs**) are also responsible for the stimulation of cell division and for the differentiation of unipotential cells of the granulocytic and monocytic series. **Erythropoietin** activates cells of the erythrocytic series, whereas **thrombopoietin** stimulates platelet production.

Steel factor (**stem cell factor**), which acts on pluripotential, multipotential, and unipotential stem cells, is produced by stromal cells of the bone marrow and is inserted into their own cell membranes. Stem cells must come in contact with these stromal cells before they can become mitotically active. It is believed that hemopoiesis cannot occur without the presence of cells that express stem cell factors, which is why postnatal blood cell formation is restricted to the bone marrow (and liver and spleen, if necessary).

Hemopoietic cells are programmed to undergo **apoptosis** unless they come into contact with growth factors. Such dying cells display clumping of the chromatin in their shrunken nuclei and a dense, granular-appearing cytoplasm. On their cell surface, they express specific macromolecules that are recognized by receptors of the macrophage plasma membrane. These phagocytic cells engulf and destroy the apoptotic cells.

It has been suggested that there are factors responsible for the release of mature (and almost mature) blood cells from the marrow. These proposed factors have not yet been characterized completely, but they most probably include ILs, CSF, and steel factor.

Erythropoiesis

Erythropoiesis, the formation of red blood cells, is under the control of several cytokines: steel factor, interleukin-3, interleukin-4, and erythropoietin.

The process of **erythropoiesis**, RBC formation, generates 2.5 $\times 10^{11}$ erythrocytes every day. In order to produce such a tremendous number of cells, two types of unipotential progenitor cells arise from the **colony forming unit-megakaryocytic erythroid progenitor** (**CFU-MEP**): the **burst-forming units–erythrocyte (BFU-E)** and **colony-forming units–erythrocyte (CFU-E)**.

If the circulating RBC level is low, the kidney produces a high concentration of **erythropoietin**, which, in the presence of IL-3, IL-4, and stem cell factor, induces CFU-MEP to differentiate into BFU-E. These cells undergo a "burst" of mitotic activity, forming a large number of CFU-E. Interestingly, this transformation requires the loss of IL-3 receptors.

CFU-E requires a low concentration of erythropoietin not only to survive but also to form the first recognizable erythrocyte precursor, the **proerythroblast** (Fig. 10.20; see Fig. 10.19). The proerythroblasts and their progeny (Figs. 10.21 to 10.23) form spherical clusters around macrophages (**nurse cells**), which phagocytose extruded nuclei and excess or deformed erythrocytes. Nurse cells may also provide growth factors to assist erythropoiesis. The properties of the cells in the erythropoietic series are presented in Table 10.8.

Clinical Correlations

1. ***Iron deficiency anemia***, *the most common form of anemia resulting from nutritional deficiency, affects about 10% of the United States population. Although the cause may be low dietary intake of iron, that is usually not the case in the United States; instead, it is caused by either malabsorption or chronic blood loss. The erythrocytes of an iron-deficient person are smaller than usual; the patient presents a whitish pallor, and the nails appear spoon shaped with accentuated longitudinal ridges. The patient complains of generalized weakness, constant tiredness, and lack of energy.*
2. ***Polycythemia vera (PCV)*** *is a rare type of neoplasm that results in the overproduction of erythrocytes in the bone marrow. More men than women are affected and most patients are older than 60 years of age. The increased number of erythrocytes causes reduced fluidity of the blood with a consequential sluggish blood flow, formation of thrombi, stroke, myocardial infarct, enlarged liver, and deep venous thrombosis. Most commonly, the presence of erythromelalgia, (sporadic blood clots that preferentially block small blood vessels, with resultant swelling of the hands and feet accompanied by a burning sensation) may occur. Additionally, almost half the patients experience generalized itching and less than a quarter of the patients present with inflammatory arthritis of their big toe (gout). Almost all patients with Add PCV have a mutation in their JAK2 kinase gene that greatly increases the sensitivity of CFU-MEP to erythropoietin, resulting in the overproduction of BFU-E and CFU-E. At the same time, erythropoietin production by the kidney is reduced and a low concentration of erythropoietin is required not only for the survival of CFU-E cells but also for their transformation into proerythroblasts, the first recognizable erythrocyte precursor. If untreated, PCV can be terminal; however, a variety of treatments are available that alleviate the symptoms and greatly increase not only the life span but also the quality of life of the patient. These treatment modalities include phlebotomy, whereby blood is removed from the patient at regular intervals to reduce hematocrit to normal levels, accompanied by administration of low-dose aspirin (81 mg) to reduce problems with blood clots. More aggressive treatments include chemotherapy, such as hydroxyurea, busulfan, and ruxolitinib.*

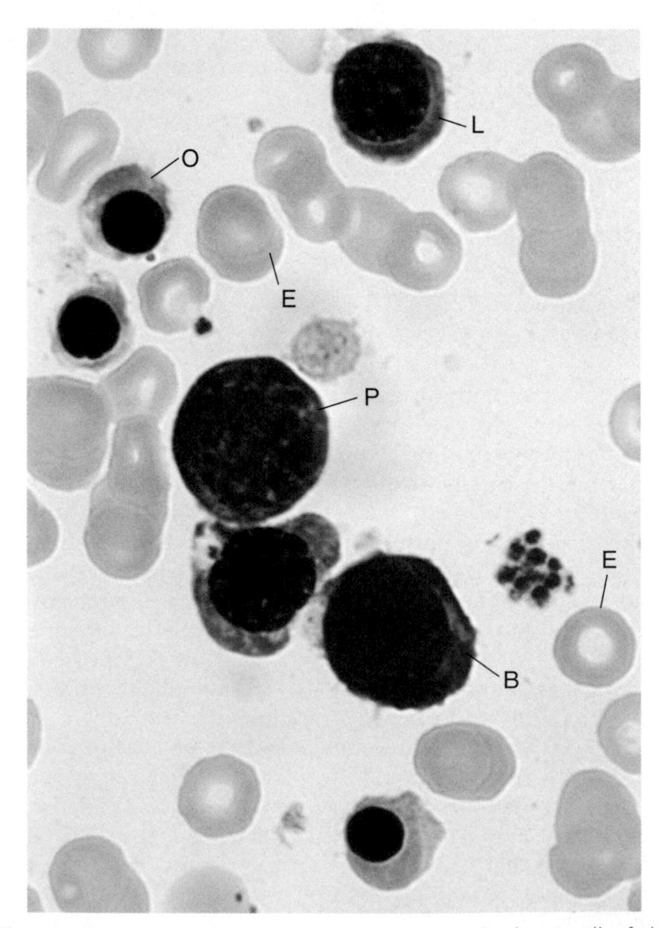

Fig. 10.20 Photomicrograph of bone marrow displaying all of the stages of red blood cell formation, except for reticulocytes. B, Basophilic erythroblast; E, erythrocyte; L, polychromatophilic erythroblast; O, orthochromatophilic erythroblast; P, proerythroblast. (×1325).

Granulocytopoiesis

Granulocytopoiesis—the formation of the granulocytes neutrophils, eosinophils, and basophils, and mast cells—is under the influence of several cytokines, including stem cell factor, G-CSF and GM-CSF, PU.1 transcription factor, as well as IL-3, IL-5, IL-6, IL-8, and TNF-α.

Although the granulocytic series is usually discussed under a single heading, as it is here, the three types of granulocytes are actually derived from their own unipotential (or bipotential, as with neutrophils) stem cells (see Table 10.6). Each of these stem cells is a descendant of the pluripotential stem cell CFU-GEMM. Thus, CFU-Eo, of the eosinophil lineage, and CFU-Ba, of the basophil lineage, each undergo cell division, giving rise to the precursor cell, or **myeloblast**. Neutrophils originate from the bipotential stem cell, **CFU-GM**, whose mitosis produces two unipotential stem cells, **CFU-G** (of the neutrophil line) and **CFU-M**, responsible for the monocyte lineage. Similar to CFU-Ba and CFU-Eo, CFU-G divides to give rise to myeloblasts.

The proliferation and differentiation of these stem cells are under the influence of G-CSF, IL-3, and GM-CSF. Therefore, these three factors facilitate the development of neutrophils, basophils, and eosinophils. In turn, PU.1 transcription factor, TNF-α, IL-3, IL-6, and IL-8 are cofactors necessary for the synthesis and release of G-CSF and GM-CSF. In addition, if IL-5 is present, it drives the differentiation toward the formation of eosinophils. In the absence of IL-5, basophils form. **Myeloblasts** (Fig. 10.24; see also Fig. 10.19) are precursors of all three types of granulocytes and, histologically, they cannot be differentiated from one another. It is not known whether a single myeloblast can produce all three types of granulocytes or whether there is a specific myeloblast for each type of granulocyte. Myeloblasts undergo mitosis, giving rise to promyelocytes, which, in turn,

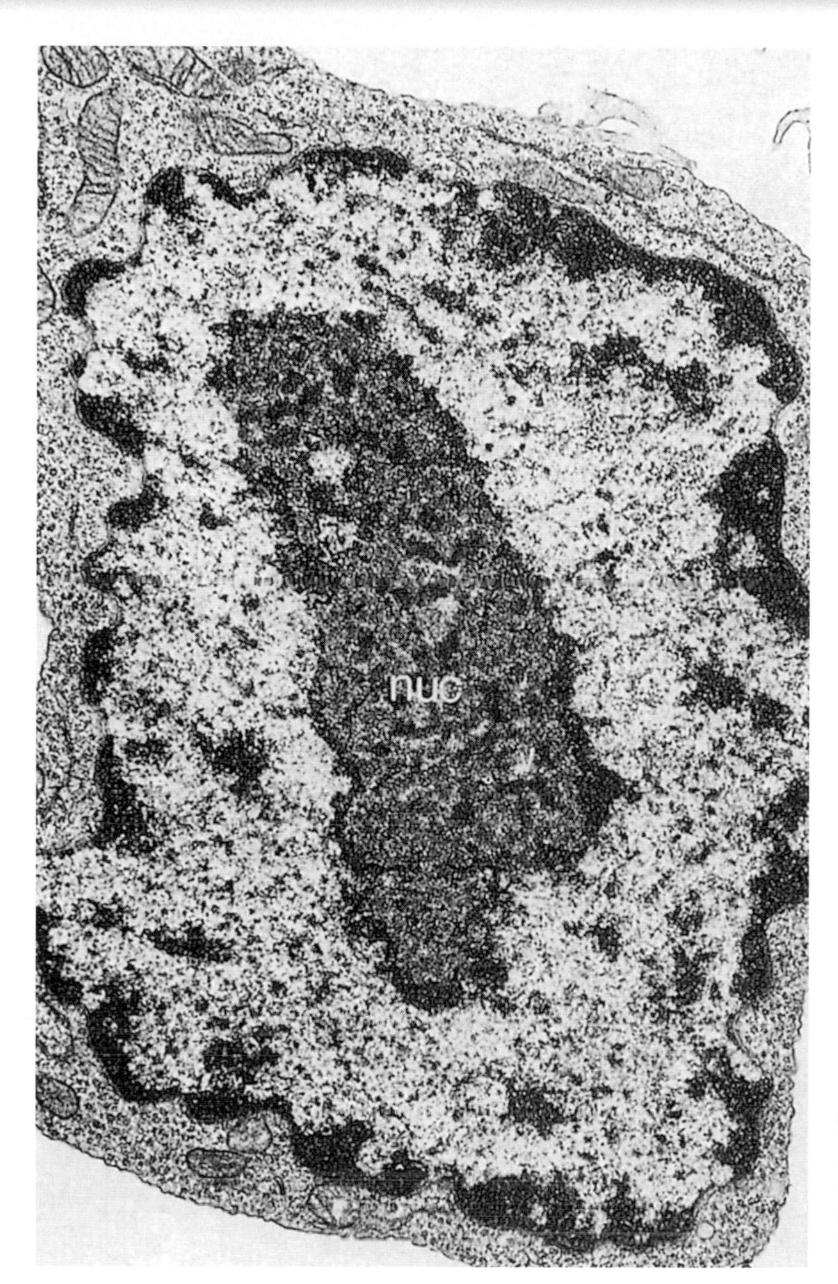

Fig. 10.21 Electron micrograph of a procrythroblast, displaying its nucleus as well as the perinuclear cytoplasm. Note that the nucleoplasm is relatively smooth in appearance and that the cytoplasm is rich in mitochondria and free ribosomes, indicating that the cell is active in protein synthesis (×14,000). nuc, Nucleolus. (From Hopkins CR. *Structure and Function of Cells.* Philadelphia: WB Saunders; 1978.)

divide to form myelocytes. It is at the myelocyte step that specific granules are present and the three granulocyte lines may be recognized histologically. Each day, the average adult produces approximately 800,000 neutrophils, 170,000 eosinophils, and 60,000 basophils.

Table 10.9 details the neutrophil lineage. The eosinophil and basophil lineages appear to be identical to the neutrophil lineage except for the differences in their specific granules (Figs. 10.25 to 10.27; see Fig. 10.24). **Mast cells** also arise from myeloblasts but require **stem cell factor** for their differentiation.

Newly formed neutrophils leave the hemopoietic cords by *piercing* the endothelial cells lining the sinusoids rather than by *migrating* between them. Once neutrophils enter the circulatory system, they **marginate**; that is, they adhere to the endothelial cells of the blood vessels and remain there until they are needed. The process of margination requires the sequential expression of various transmembrane adhesion molecules and integrins by the neutrophils as well as specific surface receptor molecules by the endothelial cells, the description of which is beyond the scope of this textbook. Because of the process of margination, there are always many more neutrophils in the circulatory system than in the circulating blood.

Clinical Correlations

Acute myeloblastic leukemia *results from uncontrolled mitosis of a transformed stem cell whose progeny do not differentiate into the mature cell. The cells involved may be the CFU-GM, CFU-Eo, or CFU-Ba, whose differentiation stops at the myeloblast stage. The disease affects young adults between 15 and 40 years of age. It is treated by intensive chemotherapy and, more recently, by bone marrow transplantation.*

Monocytopoiesis

Monocytes share their bipotential cells with neutrophils. CFU-GM undergoes mitosis and gives rise to CFU-G and **CFU-M** (**monoblasts**). The progeny of CFU-M are **promonocytes**, large

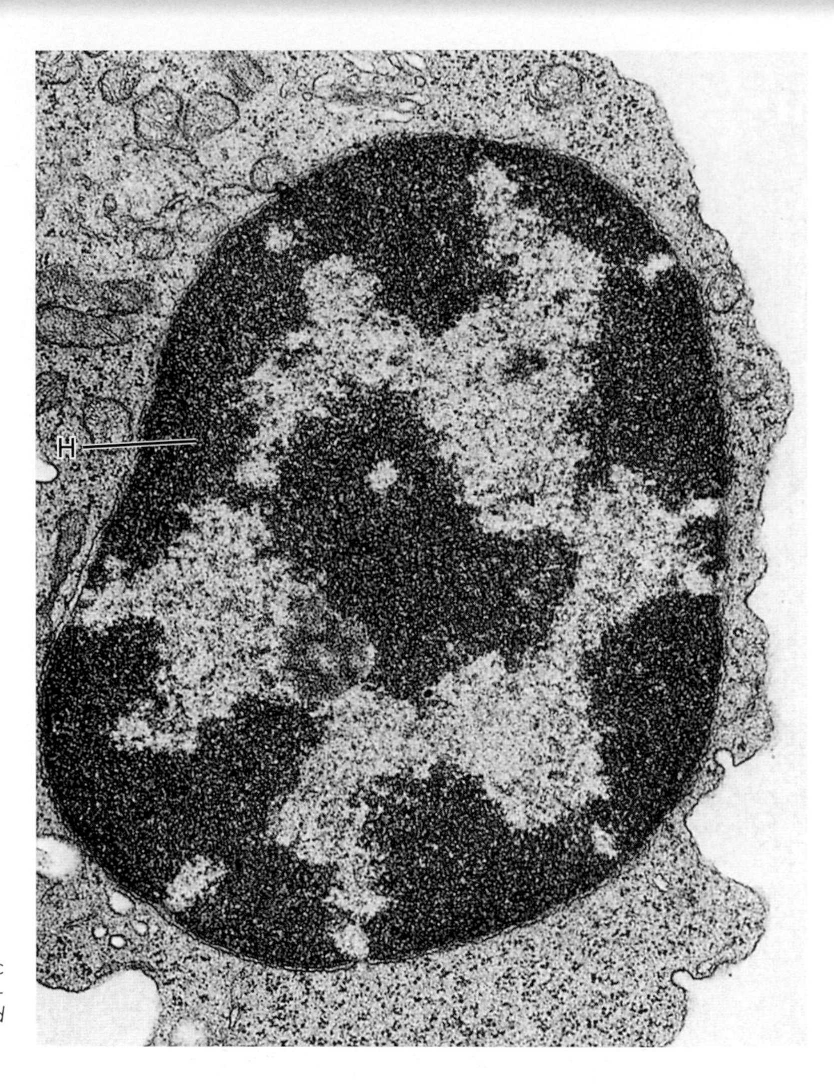

Fig. 10.22 Electron micrograph of an orthochromatophilic erythroblast. Observe that the nucleus possesses a lot of heterochromatin (H) (×21,300). (From Hopkins CR. *Structure and Function of Cells*. Philadelphia: WB Saunders; 1978.)

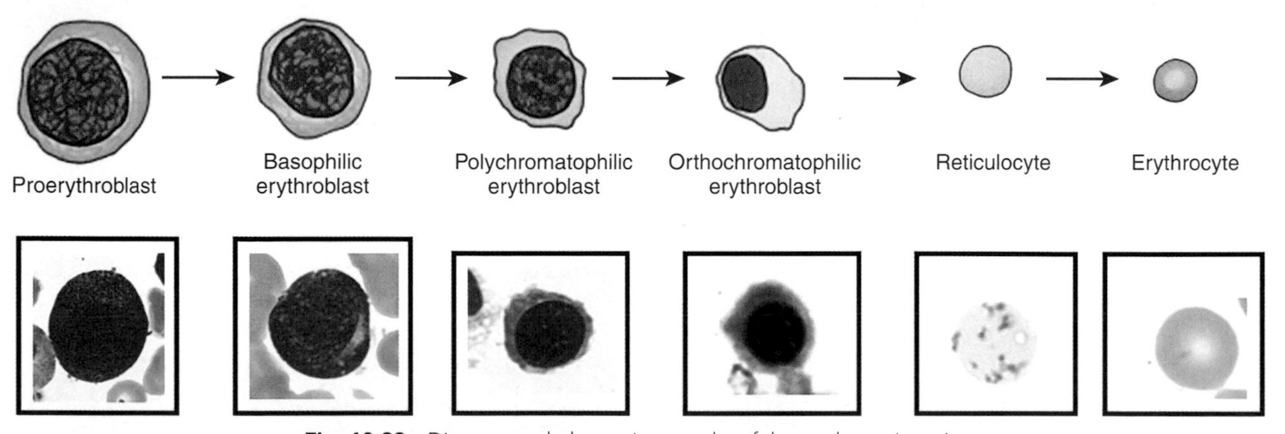

Fig. 10.23 Diagram and photomicrographs of the erythrocytic series.

cells (16–18 μm in diameter) that have a kidney-shaped, acentrically located nucleus. The cytoplasm of promonocytes is bluish and houses numerous azurophilic granules.

Electron micrographs of promonocytes disclose a well-developed Golgi apparatus, abundant RER, and numerous mitochondria. The azurophilic granules are lysosomes, about 0.5 μm in diameter. Every day, the average adult forms more than 10^{10} monocytes, most of which enter the circulation. Within a day or two, the newly formed monocytes enter the connective tissue spaces of the body and differentiate into **macrophages**, **monocyte-derived dendritic cells**, **osteoclasts**, and **microglia**.

Platelet Formation

The formation of platelets is under the control of thrombopoietin, which induces the development and proliferation of giant cells known as megakaryoblasts.

CFU-MEP gives rise to the unipotential platelet progenitor, **CFU-Meg**, which forms a very large cell, the **megakaryoblast**

TABLE 10.8 Cells of the Erythropoietic Series

Cell	Size (μm)	Nucleus[a] and Mitosis	Nucleoli	Cytoplasm[a]	Electron Micrographs
Proerythroblast	14–19	Round, burgundy-red; chromatin network: fine; mitosis	3–5	Gray-blue, peripheral clumping	Scant RER; many polysomes, few mitochondria; ferritin
Basophilic erythroblast	12–17	Same as above but chromatin network is coarser; mitosis	1–2?	Similar to above but slight pinkish background	Similar to above but some hemoglobin is present
Polychromatophilic erythroblast	12–15	Round and densely staining; very coarse chromatin network; mitosis	None	Yellowish-pink in bluish background	Similar to above but more hemoglobin is present
Orthochromatophilic erythroblast	8–12	Small, round, dense; eccentric or is being extruded; no mitosis	None	Pink in a slight bluish background	Few mitochondria and polysomes; much hemoglobin
Reticulocyte	7–8	None	None	Similar to mature RBC but when stained with cresyl blue, display bluish reticulum in pink cytoplasm	Clusters of ribosomes; cell is filled with hemoglobin
Erythrocyte	7.5	None	None	Pink cytoplasm	Only hemoglobin

[a]Colors as appear using Romanovsky-type stains (or their modifications).
RBC, Red blood cell; RER, rough endoplasmic reticulum.

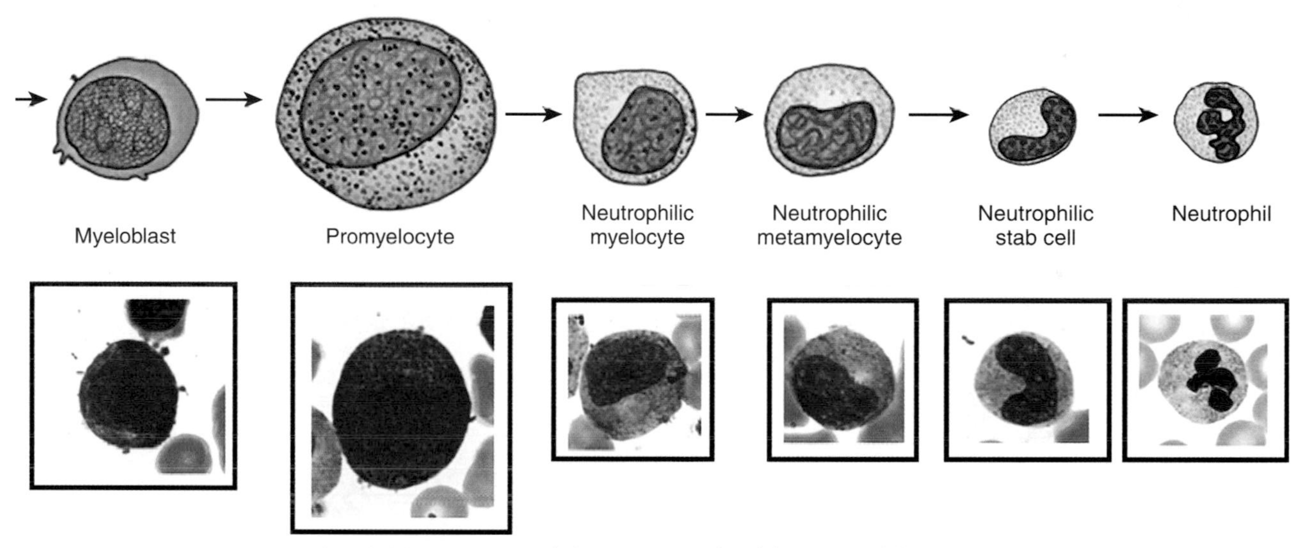

Fig. 10.24 Diagram and photomicrographs of the neutrophilic series.

(25–40 μm in diameter), whose single nucleus has several lobes. These cells undergo **endomitosis**, whereby the cell does not divide. Instead, it becomes larger and the nucleus becomes polyploid, as much as 64 N. The bluish cytoplasm accumulates azurophilic granules. These cells are stimulated to differentiate and proliferate by thrombopoietin.

Megakaryoblasts differentiate into **megakaryocytes** (see Figs. 10.16 and 10.17), which are large cells (40–100 μm in diameter), each with a single lobulated nucleus. Electron micrographs of megakaryocytes display a well-developed Golgi apparatus, numerous mitochondria, abundant RER, and many lysosomes (Fig. 10.28).

Megakaryocytes are located next to sinusoids, into which they protrude their cytoplasmic processes. These cytoplasmic processes fragment along complex, narrow invaginations of the plasmalemma, known as ***demarcation channels***, into clusters of **proplatelets**. Shortly after the proplatelets are released, they disperse into individual platelets. Each megakaryocyte can form several thousand platelets. The remaining cytoplasm and nucleus of the megakaryocyte degenerate and are phagocytosed by macrophages.

Lymphopoiesis

Pluripotential hemopoietic stem cells give rise to the myeloid series of cells via CFU-GEMM, as well as to the lymphoid series of cells via CFU-Ly.

The multipotential stem cell **CFU-Ly** divides in the bone marrow to form the two unipotential progenitor cells, CFU-LyB, CFU-LyT, as well as CFU-NK cells, none of which are immunocompetent. The differentiation of CFU-Ly to CFU-LyB and CFU-LyT requires the expression of **zinc finger proteins**: the **Ikaros family of transcription factors** as well as the expression of a moderate level of **PU.1 transcription factor**.

TABLE 10.9 Cells of the Neutrophilic Series

Cell	Size (μm)	Nucleus[a] and Mitosis	Nucleoli	Cytoplasm[a]	Granules	Electron Micrographs
Myeloblast	12–14	Round, reddish-blue; chromatin network: fine; mitosis	2–3	Blue clumps in a pale-blue background; cytoplasmic blebs at cell periphery	None	RER, small Golgi, many mitochondria and polysomes
Promyelocyte	16–24	Round to oval, reddish blue; chromatin network: coarse; mitosis	1–2	Bluish cytoplasm; no cytoplasmic blebs at cell periphery	Azurophilic granules	RER, large Golgi, many mitochondria, numerous lysosomes (0.5 μm in diameter)
Neutrophilic myelocyte	10–12	Flattened, acentric; chromatin network: coarse; mitosis	0–1	Pale-blue cytoplasm	Azurophilic and specific granules	RER, large Golgi, numerous mitochondria, lysosomes (0.5 μm) and specific granules (0.1 μm)
Neutrophilic metamyelocyte	10–12	Kidney shaped, dense; chromatin network: coarse; no mitosis	None	Pale-blue cytoplasm	Azurophilic and specific granules	Organelle population is reduced, but granules are as above
Neutrophilic band (stab; juvenile)	9–12	Horseshoe shaped; chromatin network: very coarse; no mitosis	None	Pale-blue cytoplasm	Azurophilic and specific granules	Same as above
Neutrophil	9–12	Multilobed; chromatin network: very coarse; no mitosis	None	Pale bluish-pink	Azurophilic and specific granules	Same as above

[a]Colors as appear using Romanovsky-type stains (or their modifications).
RER, Rough endoplasmic reticulum.

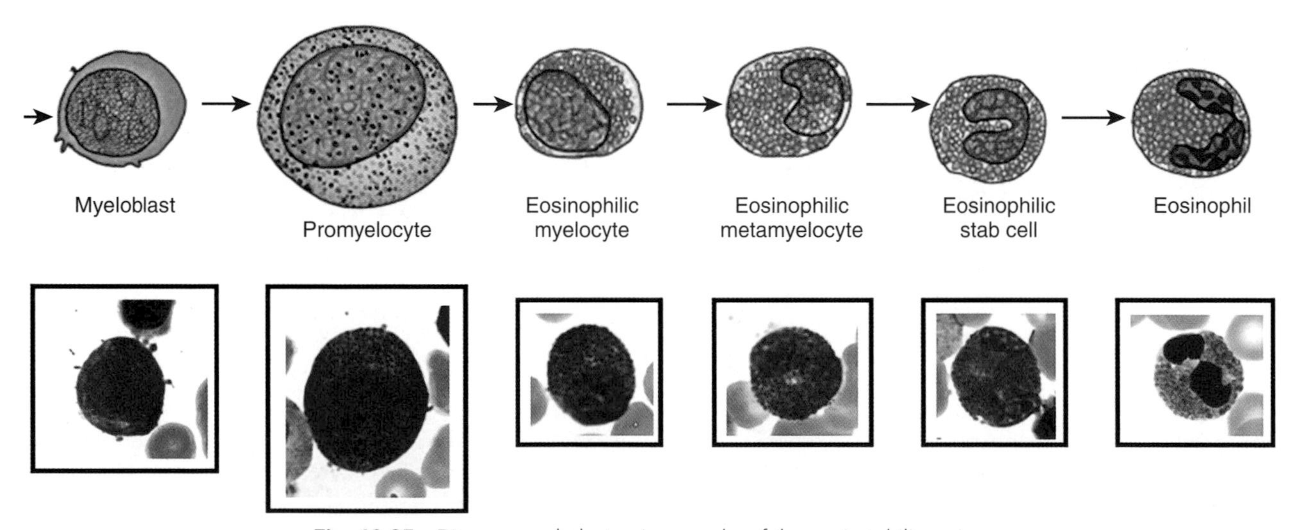

Fig. 10.25 Diagram and photomicrographs of the eosinophilic series.

In birds, **CFU-LyB** migrates to a diverticulum attached to the gut, known as the ***bursa of Fabricius*** (thus, the name *B cell*). Here, CFU-LyB divides several times, giving rise to ***immunocompetent B lymphocytes*** expressing specific surface markers, including antibodies. A similar event occurs in mammals; however, in the absence of a bursa, this development of immunocompetence occurs in a bursa-equivalent location in the bone marrow. The process of B cell maturation is partially controlled by **IL-7** and **Pax5 transcription factor**.

CFU-LyT cells undergo mitosis, forming ***immunoincompetent T cells***, which travel to the cortex of the thymus, where they proliferate, mature, and begin to express cell surface markers. As these surface markers appear on the T-cell plasmalemma (e.g., T-cell receptors and clusters of differentiation markers), the cells become ***immunocompetent T lymphocytes***. Most of these newly formed T cells are destroyed in the thymus and are phagocytosed by resident macrophages. The process of T-cell maturation is partially controlled by **IL-7** and **GATA3 transcription factor**.

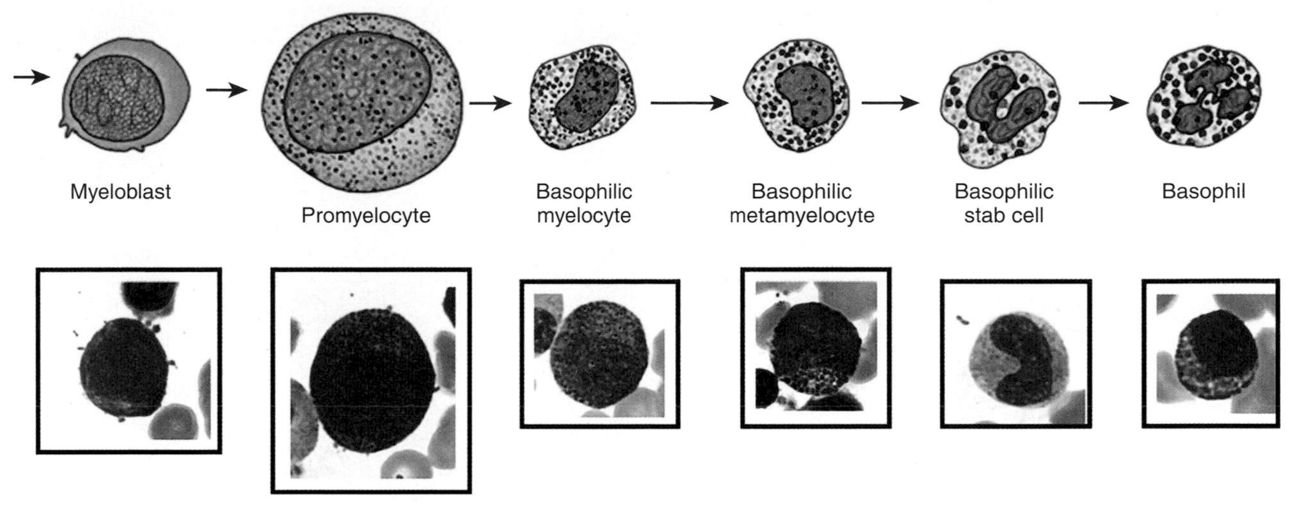

Fig. 10.26 Diagram and photomicrographs of the basophilic series.

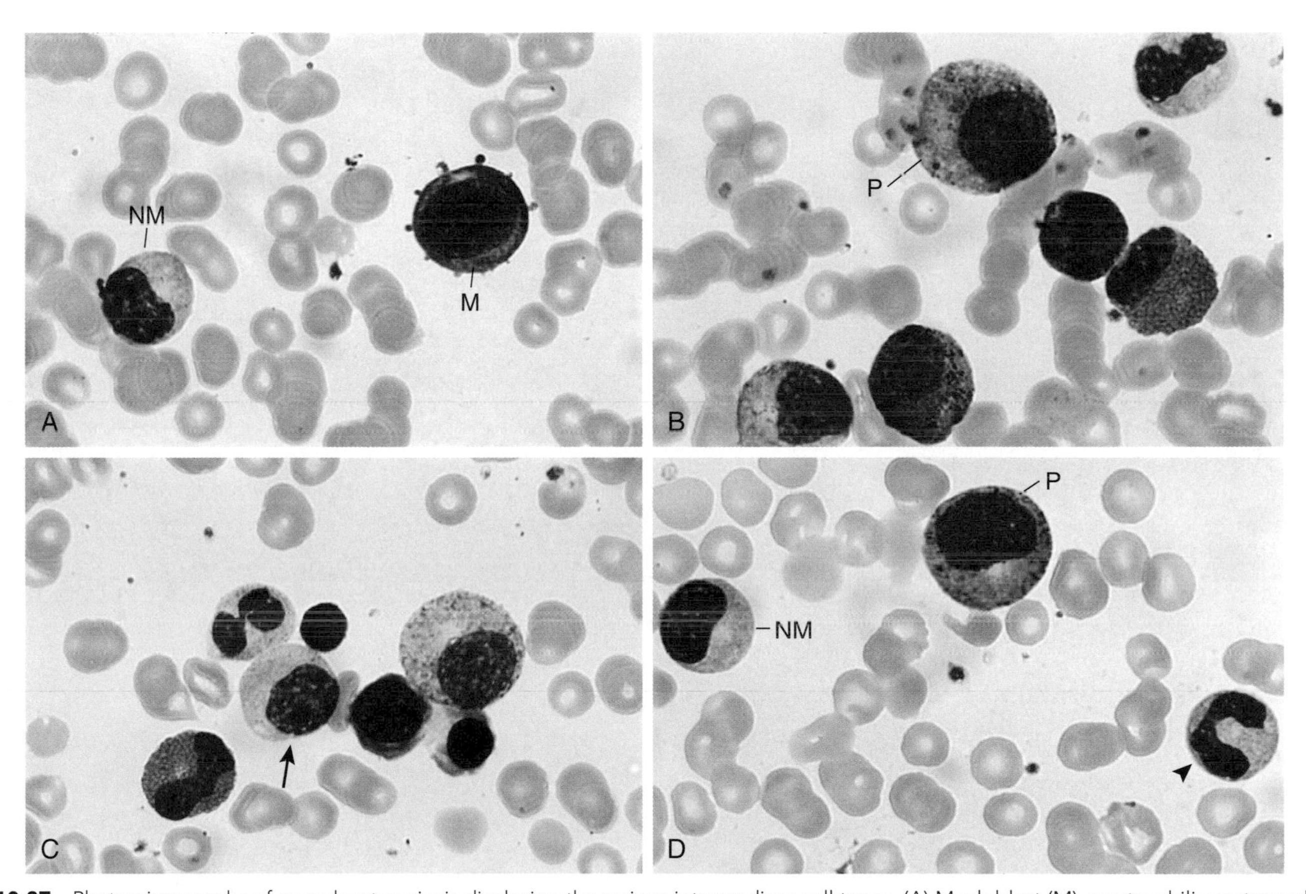

Fig. 10.27 Photomicrographs of granulocytopoiesis displaying the various intermediary cell types. (A) Myeloblast (M), neutrophilic metamyelocyte (NM). (B) Promyelocyte (P). (C) Neutrophilic myelocyte *(arrow)*. (D) Neutrophilic metamyelocyte (NM), neutrophilic stab cell *(arrowhead)*, promyelocyte (P). (×1234)

Both B lymphocytes and T lymphocytes proceed to lymphoid organs (e.g., the spleen and lymph nodes), where they form clones of immunocompetent T and B cells in well-defined regions of these organs. It has also been demonstrated that the differentiation of both B cells and T cells, as well as their activation, relies on the presence of specific micro-ribonucleic acids.

NK cells also migrate to a yet unknown region of the bone marrow where they will become immunocompetent. The process of NK cell maturation is partially controlled by IL-12 and **IL-15**.

The lymphocytic series is discussed in more detail in Chapter 12.

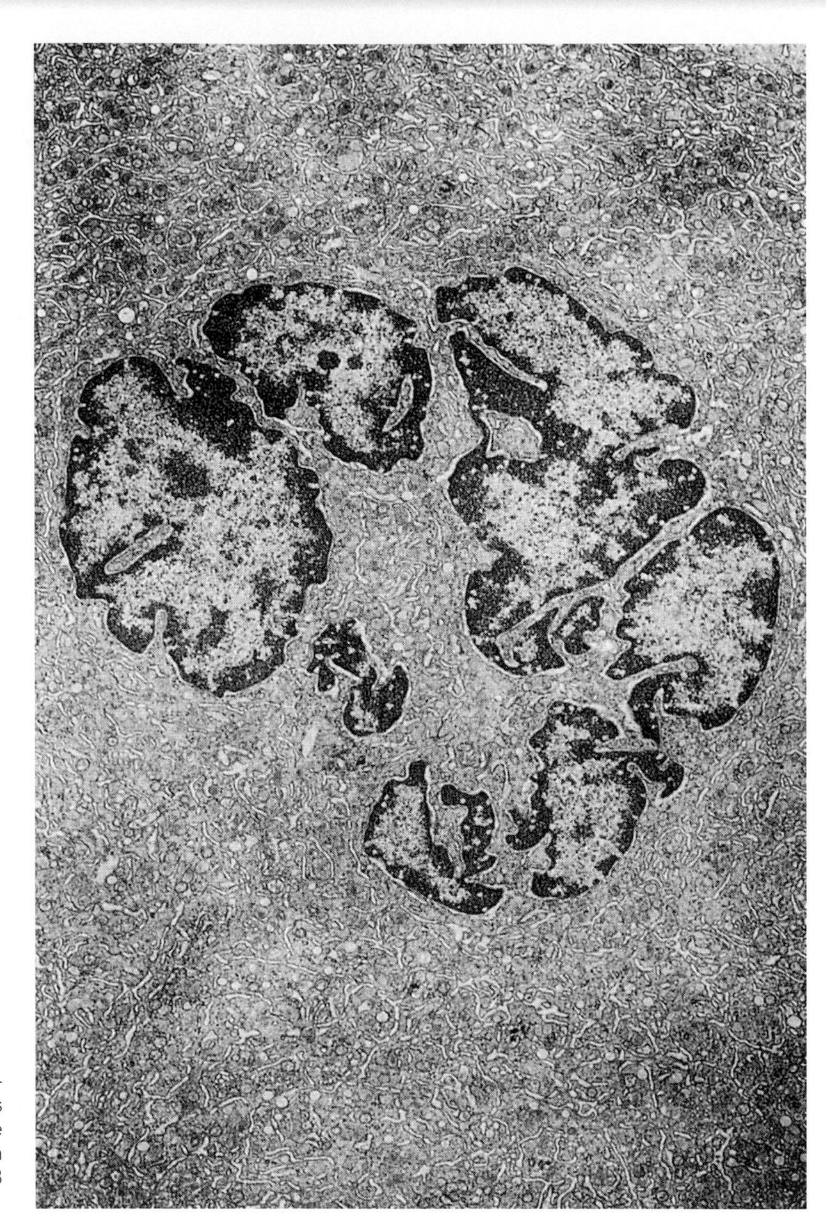

Fig. 10.28 Electron micrograph of a megakaryocyte displaying segmentation in the formation of platelets. Although this cell possesses a single nucleus, it is lobulated, which gives the appearance of the cell possessing several nuclei (×3166). (From Hopkins CR. *Structure and Function of Cells*. Philadelphia: WB Saunders; 1978.)

Pathological Considerations

See Figs. 10.29 through 10.31.

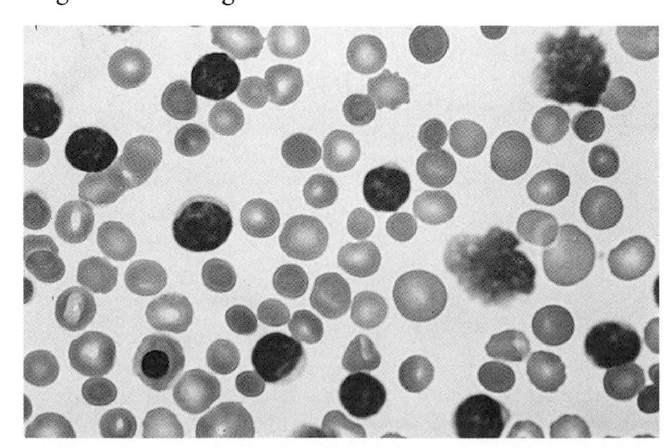

Fig. 10.29 Photomicrograph of a peripheral bloodstream of an individual with chronic lymphocytic leukemia. Note the presence of numerous lymphocytes, as well as the characteristic "smudge cells," which are dead tumor cells in the *upper right* corner and in the *middle right* of the field. (Reprinted with permission from Kumar V, Abbas AK, Aster JC. *Robbins and Cotran Pathologic Basis of Disease*. 9th ed. Philadelphia: Elsevier; 2015:594.)

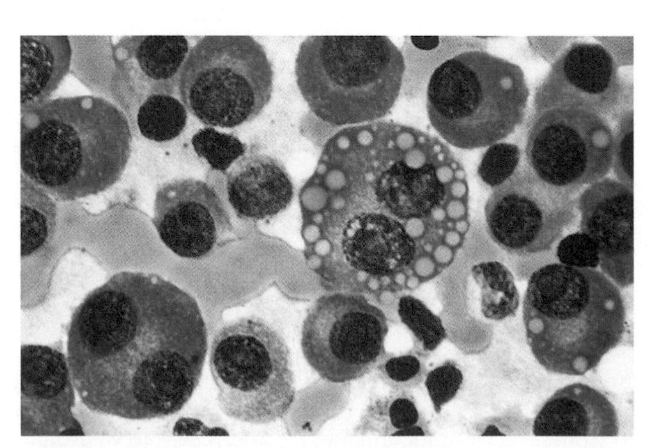

Fig. 10.30 Photomicrograph of a bone marrow aspirate of an individual with multiple myeloma. Note the presence of numerous mast cells, some with more than one nucleus, housing very large nucleoli. The cytoplasmic granules are filled with immunoglobulin. (Reprinted with permission from Kumar V, Abbas AK, Aster JC. *Robbins and Cotran Pathologic Basis of Disease*. 9th ed. Philadelphia: Elsevier; 2015:600.)

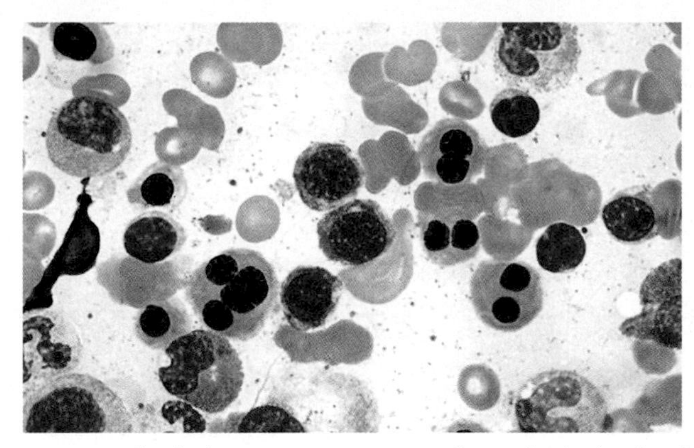

Fig. 10.31 Photomicrograph of a bone marrow aspirate of an individual with a form of myelodysplasia. Observe that some of the erythrocytic precursors possess two or more nuclei, some of which are multilobed. (Reprinted with permission from Kumar V, Abbas AK, Aster JC. *Robbins and Cotran Pathologic Basis of Disease*. 9th ed. Philadelphia: Elsevier; 2015:615.)

Histology Laboratory Instructions: Blood and Hemopoiesis

Formed Elements of Blood

The best way of identifying cells of the blood is by viewing a blood smear stained with Wright or Giemsa modification of the Romanovsky-type stain. All of the following cells (and platelets) are clearly identified in Fig. 10.3 A–E.

Erythrocytes are small biconcave disks whose diameter is about 7 µm. These are the most numerous cells on the microscope slide; they have no nuclei, and are salmon-pink. Because their center is thinner than their periphery, the center may look as though there is a hole in it.

Lymphocytes are a little larger in diameter than erythrocytes; they are approximately 8 to 10 µm in diameter. Most of the cell is taken up by the dark-blue, acentric nucleus with a coarse chromatin network. The narrow, pale-blue peripherally placed cytoplasm is wider at one pole of the nucleus. Azurophilic granules may be visible in the cytoplasm.

Monocytes are the largest of the blood cells, 12 to 15 µm in diameter. The kidney-shaped, acentrically located nucleus looks "moth-eaten," with a coarse chromatin network. Lobes of the nucleus appear to overlap each other. The cytoplasm is bluish-gray and sports numerous azurophilic granules.

Neutrophils are larger than lymphocytes but smaller than monocytes; they are 9 to 12 µm in diameter. They possess a dark-blue, multilobed nucleus with a coarse chromatin network. The cytoplasm is pink and has a slightly granular appearance due to its three types of granules: specific, tertiary, and azurophilic.

Eosinophils are somewhat larger than neutrophils (10 to 14 µm in diameter) and have a dark-blue bilobed nucleus with a coarse chromatin network. These cells have very prominent, numerous, large, round, dark-pink specific granules that are easily recognizable. Their azurophilic granules are not easy to find because the cytoplasm is packed with the specific granules.

Basophils are the least numerous of the blood cells; therefore, they may not be found easily. They are 8 to 10 µm in diameter; their large specific granules are dark blue and press on the cell membrane, giving it a rough, angular appearance. The S-shaped nucleus may be hidden by the large number of specific granules.

Platelets are small cell fragments. They are approximately 2 to 4 µm in diameter and they are relatively easy to spot because there are so many of them. They appear to have a nucleus, but that darker area is the granulomere housing their three types of granules surrounded by a lighter area, known as the ***hyalomere***, which contains their two tubular systems and their peripherally located microtubules.

Cells of Red Bone Marrow

The best way of identifying cells of red bone marrow is by viewing a bone marrow smear stained with Wright or Giemsa modification of the Romanovsky-type stain. Look for those cells that can be recognized histologically (i.e., do not try to identify any of the CFU cells, T lymphocytes, or B lymphocytes). Also, realize that nucleoli are not stained dark, as in H&E sections, but rather are a light gray that is initially difficult to distinguish.

Erythrocytic Series (Figs. 10.20 and 10.23)

Proerythroblasts are large, round cells with a wine-red nucleus containing a fine chromatin network with three to four pale-gray nucleoli. The centrally placed nucleus occupies most of the cell with a rim of dark-blue clumps in a grayish-colored cytoplasm.

Basophilic erythroblasts are similar to proerythroblasts but are somewhat smaller. The chromatin network of the round nuclei of these cells are somewhat coarse in appearance and have only one or two pale nucleoli. The nucleus is much smaller and occupies less of the cytoplasm, which sports a smaller amount of bluish clumps in a pale-gray background.

Polychromatophilic erythroblasts are smaller than the basophilic erythroblasts; their nuclei appear dark with a condensed, coarse chromatin network and possess no nucleoli. The cytoplasm is pale pink with a hint of blue.

Orthochromatophilic erythroblasts are approximately the same size as the polychromatophilic erythroblasts, but their nuclei are dark and very condensed. Frequently, they are seen to be extruded from the cell. Their cytoplasm is similar to that of mature erythrocytes but with a hint of blue.

Reticulocytes have to be stained with supravital dyes to be recognized. They possess a centrally located blue-green reticulum; otherwise, they have the same characteristics as mature erythrocytes. They possess no nuclei.

Granulocytic Series

Only the neutrophilic series will be described because the eosinophilic and basophilic series are identical, with the exception of their specific granules and the shape of their nuclei (Fig. 10.24. The eosinophilic series are shown in Fig. 10.25 and the Basophilic series in Fig. 10.26).

Myeloblasts are very similar to proerythroblasts, but myeloblast nuclei are a little smaller and have a little less wine-red coloration; they possess two or three pale-gray nucleoli. Their cytoplasm is simi-

Continued

Histology Laboratory Instructions: Blood and Hemopoiesis—cont'd

lar to those of proerythroblasts; however, they frequently possess cytoplasmic blebs protruding from their periphery.

Promyelocytes are much larger than myeloblasts and their reddish-blue nuclei have a somewhat coarser chromatin network. An occasional nucleolus or two is also present. The cytoplasm of these cells possesses a bluish coloration and numerous azurophilic granules are present.

Neutrophilic myelocytes are smaller than promyelocytes and can be recognized to belong to the neutrophil line due to the presence of their specific granules in addition to their azurophilic granules. The nucleus is located acentrically, resembles a half moon in appearance, and has a somewhat coarse chromatin network. A clear region, representing the Golgi complex, is nestled close to the flattened region of the nucleus.

A neutrophilic metamyelocyte is approximately the same size as a neutrophil. Its dense, dark nucleus has no nucleoli but it is indented and resembles the shape of a kidney. The indentation houses the Golgi complex, which is recognizable as a clear area in the cytoplasm.

A neutrophilic stab cell (band cell) resembles a mature neutrophil except for the nucleus, which has no lobes and is less dense and its chromatin network is less coarse in appearance.

Platelet Formation

Platelet formation is best seen in an H&E stained section of red bone marrow because megakaryocytes are too large to survive the technique of making a bone marrow smear.

Megakaryoblasts are among the largest cells of bone marrow. These cells undergo endomitosis so that their nuclei are polyploid and can be as much as 64-ploid. They have a bluish cytoplasm with many azurophilic granules.

Megakaryocytes may be considerably larger than megakaryoblasts and their nuclei are more lobulated. Usually, megakaryocytes are located near the sinusoids of bone marrow; if one sees a fortuitous section, then cytoplasmic processes of the megakaryocyte are visible extending into the sinusoid. These cytoplasmic processes fragment along demarcation channels into clusters of proplatelets which eventually disperse into individual platelets.

11 Circulatory System

The circulatory system is composed of two separate but related components: the cardiovascular system and the lymphatic vascular system. The function of the **cardiovascular system** is to carry blood in both directions between the heart and the tissues. The function of the **lymphatic vascular system** is to collect **lymph**, the excess extracellular fluid (tissue fluid), and to deliver it back to the cardiovascular system. Thus, the lymphatic system provides one-way transport, whereas the cardiovascular system provides two-way circulation.

Cardiovascular System

The cardiovascular system is composed of two circuits: the pulmonary circuit to the lungs and the systemic circuit to the tissues of the body.

The **cardiovascular system** is composed of the **heart**, a muscular organ that pumps the blood into two separated circuits: the **pulmonary circuit**, which carries blood to and from the lungs, and the **systemic circuit**, which distributes blood to and from all of the organs and tissues of the rest of the body. The vessels of the cardiovascular system are of three major components: **arteries**, that transport blood away from the heart by branching into vessels of increasingly smaller diameters, eventually to capillaries, to supply all regions of the body with blood; **capillaries**, which are thin-walled vessels with the smallest diameter, forming capillary beds, where gases, nutrients, metabolic wastes, hormones, and signaling substances are interchanged or passed between the blood and the tissues of the body to sustain normal metabolic activities; and **veins**, which drain capillary beds and form increasingly larger vessels, returning blood to the heart.

GENERAL STRUCTURE OF BLOOD VESSELS

Arteries generally have thicker walls and are smaller in diameter than their venous counterparts.

Most blood vessels have several features that are structurally similar, although it is the dissimilarities that form the bases for classifying the vessels into different identifiable groups. Generally, arteries have thicker walls and are smaller in diameter than are the corresponding veins. Moreover, in histological sections, arteries are round and usually have no blood in their lumina, whereas veins are flattened and frequently contain blood in their lumina.

Vessel Tunics

Walls of blood vessels are composed of three layers: the tunica intima, tunica media, and tunica adventitia.

Three separate concentric layers of tissue, or **tunics**, make up the wall of the typical blood vessel (Fig. 11.1). The innermost layer, the **tunica intima**, is composed of a single layer of flattened, squamous endothelial cells, which form a tube lining the lumen of the vessel, and the underlying subendothelial connective tissue. The intermediate layer, the **tunica media**, is composed mostly of smooth muscle cells helically oriented around the lumen. The outermost layer, the **tunica adventitia**, is composed mainly of fibroelastic connective tissue whose fibers are arranged longitudinally.

Tunica Intima

The tunica intima is composed of a simple squamous epithelium, known as the endothelium, and the subendothelial connective tissue, including the internal elastic lamina.

The endothelial cells (simple squamous epithelium) lining the lumen of the blood vessel rest on a basal lamina. These flattened cells are elongated into a sheet such that their long axis is more or less parallel to the long axis of the vessel, which nearly permits each endothelial cell to surround the lumen of a small-caliber vessel. In larger-bore vessels, many individual endothelial cells are required to line the circumference of the lumen. Endothelial cells not only provide an exceptionally smooth surface to reduce frictional forces acting on the flow of blood but they also have additional functions (Table 11.1), such as:

- Secreting collagen (types II, IV, and V), laminin, endothelin, nitric oxide (NO), von Willebrand factor (vWF), tissue factor, and P-selectin

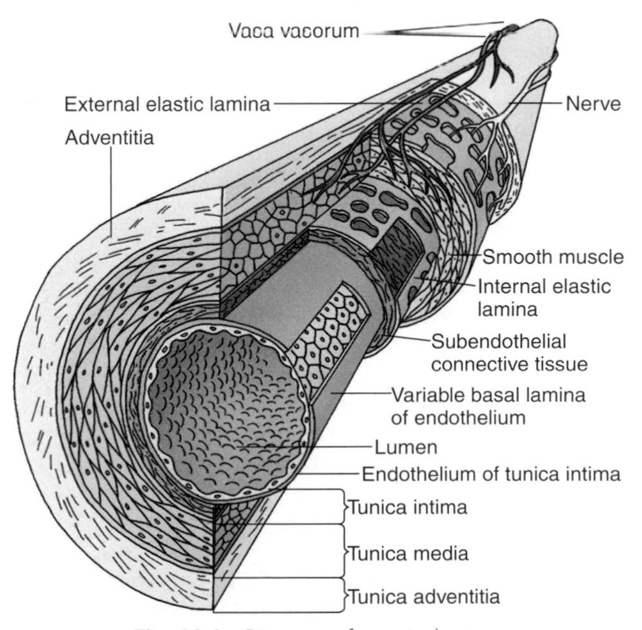

Fig. 11.1 Diagram of a typical artery.

TABLE 11.1 **Functions of Endothelial Cells**

Function	Regions of the vascular tree	Miscellaneous
Selective permeability	Capillaries and postcapillary venules	Semipermeable barrier that permits movement of certain small molecules across the cell membrane and has receptor-mediated transport for others.
Migration of white blood cells	Postcapillary (high endothelial venules)	Receptor molecules facilitate the migration of white blood cells into the connective tissue spaces.
Inhibition of clot formation	Throughout the vascular system	Anticoagulants are produced by the intact endothelial cells that maintain blood in a fluid state.
Promotion of clot formation	Throughout the vascular system	Damaged endothelial cells release von Willebrand factor and tissue factor to facilitate blood clot formation and reduce blood loss from the vessel.
Localized regulation of blood pressure	Throughout the vascular system	Injured endothelial cells release powerful vasoconstrictors such as endothelins, prostaglandins, and thromboxane A_2 to reduce blood loss from the vessel.
Systemic regulation of blood pressure	Although all blood vessels are affected, it is vasoconstriction of *arterioles* that have the greatest effect on blood pressure.	Angiotensin I, a mild vasoconstrictor, is converted to angiotensin II by ACE (angiotensin-converting enzyme) located on the luminal plasmalemmae of capillary endothelia. Angiotensin II is a potent vasoconstrictor that reduces the diameter of blood vessels, resulting in increased blood pressure.
Formation of new blood vessels	Occur throughout the vascular system	Damaged blood vessels are repaired during wound healing; also forms new blood vessels that invade and supply nutrients to growing tumors.

- Cleaving **angiotensin I** to generate **angiotensin II** (see discussion later in this chapter on the regulation of arterial blood pressure) by their membrane-bound enzyme, **angiotensin-converting enzyme** (**ACE**); inactivating bradykinin, serotonin, prostaglandins, thrombin, and norepinephrine by additional membrane-bound enzymes; and binding **lipoprotein lipase**, the enzyme that degrades lipoprotein triglycerides into glycerol and fatty acids

Loose connective tissue, the **subendothelial layer**, lies deep to the endothelial cells. The deepest component of the subendothelial connective tissue layer is the **internal elastic lamina**, which is especially well developed in muscular arteries. The internal elastic lamina is composed of a fenestrated sheet of **elastin**, whose fenestrations permit the diffusion of substances from the lumen into the deeper regions of the arterial wall to nourish the cells there.

Tunica Media

The tunica media, usually the thickest layer of the vessel wall, is composed of helically disposed layers of smooth muscle and the external elastic lamina, when present.

The tunica media is the thickest layer of the vessel, composed mostly of helically arranged smooth muscle cells. Interspersed within the layers of smooth muscle cells are some elastic fibers, type III collagen, and proteoglycans. The fibrous elements form lamellae within the ground substance and is secreted by smooth muscle cells. Larger muscular arteries have an **external elastic lamina**, which is more delicate than the internal elastic lamina and separates the tunica media from the tunica adventitia. Small vessels, such as capillaries and postcapillary venules, do not have a tunica media; it is replaced by **pericytes** (see discussion later in this chapter on capillaries).

Tunica Adventitia

The tunica adventitia, the outermost layer of the vessel wall, blends into the surrounding connective tissue.

Covering the vessels on their outside surface is the **tunica adventitia**, composed of a dense, irregular, collagenous connective tissue consisting mostly of fibroblasts, types I and III collagen fibers, and longitudinally oriented elastic fibers. This layer becomes continuous with the connective tissue elements surrounding the vessel.

Vasa Vasorum

Vasa vasorum (vessels of the vessel) furnish the muscular walls of blood vessels with a blood supply.

The thickness and muscularity of larger vessels prevent the cells composing the tunics from being nourished by diffusion from the lumen of the vessel. The deeper cells of the tunica media and tunica adventitia are nourished by the **vasa vasorum** (**vessels of the vessel**), small arteries that enter the vessel walls and branch profusely to serve the cells located primarily in the tunica media and tunica adventitia. Compared with arteries, veins have more cells that cannot be supplied with oxygen and nutrients by diffusion because venous blood contains less oxygen and nutrients than arterial blood. For this reason, the vasa vasorum are more prevalent in the walls of veins than in the walls of arteries.

Nerve Supply to Vessels

Sympathetic nerves supply vasomotor innervation to the smooth muscles of the tunica media.

A network of **vasomotor nerves** of the sympathetic component of the autonomic nervous system supplies smooth muscle cells of blood vessels. These unmyelinated, postganglionic sympathetic nerves are responsible for **vasoconstriction** of the vessel walls. Because the nerves seldom enter the tunica media of the vessel, they do not synapse directly on the smooth muscle cells. Instead, they release the neurotransmitter **norepinephrine**, which diffuses into the media and acts on smooth muscle cells nearby. These impulses are propagated throughout all of the smooth muscle cells via their gap junctions, orchestrating contractions of the entire smooth muscle cell layer and thus reducing the diameter of the vessel lumen.

TABLE 11.2 Characteristics of Various Types of Arteries

Artery	Tunica Intima	Tunica Media	Tunica Adventitia
Elastic arteries (conducting; e.g., aorta) Diameter: greater than 10 mm	Endothelium with Weibel-Palade bodies, basal lamina, subendothelial layer, incomplete internal elastic lamina	40–70 fenestrated elastic membranes, smooth muscle cells interspersed between elastic membranes, thin external elastic lamina, vasa vasorum in outer half	Thin layer of fibroelastic connective tissue, vasa vasorum, lymphatic vessels, nerve fibers
Muscular arteries (distributing, e.g., femoral artery) Diameter: 1–10 mm	Endothelium with Weibel-Palade bodies, basal lamina, subendothelial layer, thick internal elastic lamina	Up to 40 layers of smooth muscle cells, thick external elastic lamina	Thin layer of fibroelastic connective tissue; vasa vasorum not very prominent; lymphatic vessels, nerve fibers
Arterioles (are not named) Diameter: 10 to 100 μm	Endothelium with Weibel-Palade bodies; basal lamina, subendothelial layer not very prominent; some elastic fibers instead of a defined internal elastic lamina	One or two layers of smooth muscle cells	Loose connective tissue, nerve fibers
Metarterioles (are not named) Diameter: ~8 μm	Endothelium, basal lamina	Smooth muscle cells form precapillary sphincter	Sparse, loose connective tissue

Arteries are more heavily endowed with vasomotor nerves than the veins are, but veins also receive vasomotor nerve endings in the tunica adventitia. The arteries supplying skeletal muscles of the body receive cholinergic (parasympathetic) nerves to bring about vasodilation that reduces the velocity of blood flow, permitting a greater exchange of gases.

ARTERIES

Arteries are blood vessels that carry blood away from the heart.

Arteries are efferent vessels that transport blood away from the heart to the capillary beds. The two major arteries that arise from the right and left ventricles of the heart are the **pulmonary trunk**, which branches, shortly after exiting the right ventricle of the heart, into right and left pulmonary arteries that enter the lungs for distribution (see Chapter 15) and the **aorta**, which exits the left ventricle of the heart and gives rise to the coronary arteries that supply the heart muscle. The aorta then courses in an obliquely posterior arch to descend in the thoracic cavity, where it sends branches to the body wall and viscera; it then enters the abdominal cavity, where it also sends branches to the body wall and viscera. The abdominal aorta terminates by bifurcating into the right and left common iliac arteries in the pelvis. The major branches of the aorta continue to arborize, forming large numbers of increasingly smaller arteries, which continues until the vessel walls contain a single layer of endothelial cells. The resulting vessels, called ***capillaries***, are the smallest functional vascular elements of the cardiovascular system.

Classification of Arteries

Arteries are of three types: elastic arteries (conducting arteries), muscular arteries (distributing arteries), and arterioles.

Arteries are classified into three major types based on their relative size, morphological characteristics, or both (Table 11.2): the largest are the elastic (conducting) arteries, followed by the muscular (distributing) arteries, and the smallest are the arterioles.

Because the vessels decrease in diameter in a continuous fashion, there are gradual changes in morphological characteristics in going from one type to another. Therefore, some vessels having characteristics of two categories cannot be assigned to a specific category with certainty.

Elastic Arteries

Concentric layers of elastic membranes, known as fenestrated membranes, occupy much of the tunica media.

The aorta and the branches originating from the aortic arch (the common carotid artery and the subclavian artery), the common iliac arteries, and the pulmonary trunk are **elastic (conducting) arteries** (Fig. 11.2). The walls of these vessels may be yellow in the fresh state because of the abundance of elastin.

The **tunica intima** of the elastic arteries is composed of an endothelium that is supported by a narrow layer of underlying subendothelial connective tissue containing a few fibroblasts, occasional smooth muscle cells, and collagen fibers. Thin laminae of elastic fibers, the **internal elastic lamina**, are also present (Fig. 11.3)

The endothelial cells of the elastic arteries are 10 to 15 μm wide and 25 to 50 μm long; their long axes are oriented parallel to the longitudinal axis of the vessel. These cells are connected mostly by occluding junctions. Their plasma membranes form small endocytic and exocytotic vesicles, which probably transport water, macromolecules, and electrolytes. Occasional blunt processes may extend from the plasma membrane through the internal elastic lamina to form gap junctions with smooth muscle cells located in the subendothelial connective tissue. The endothelial cells house **Weibel-Palade bodies (W-P bodies)**, membrane-bound inclusions, 0.1 μm in diameter and 3 μm long. W-P bodies have a dense matrix in which tubular elements are embedded. These tubular elements contain the glycoprotein **von Willebrand factor (vWF)**, as well as **tissue factor** and **P-selectin**. The vWF facilitates the coagulation of platelets during clot formation and is manufactured by most endothelial cells but is stored in arteries only. Tissue factor enhances the process of coagulation, and P-selectin induces leukocytes to leave the bloodstream, to enter the connective tissue spaces, and to function in the immune process.

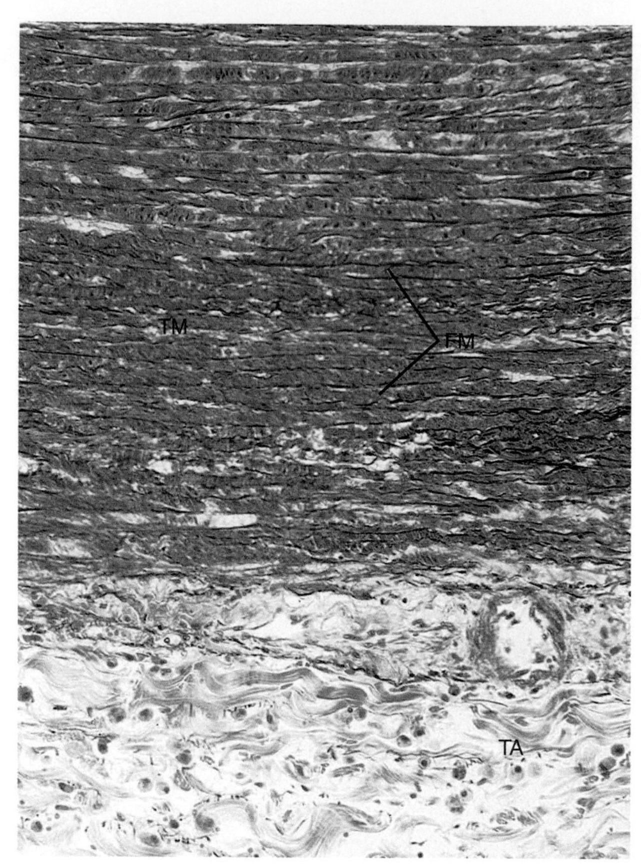

Fig. 11.2 Light micrograph of an elastic artery (×132). Observe the fenestrated membranes (FM), tunica media (TM), and tunica adventitia (TA). The tunica intima is not shown.

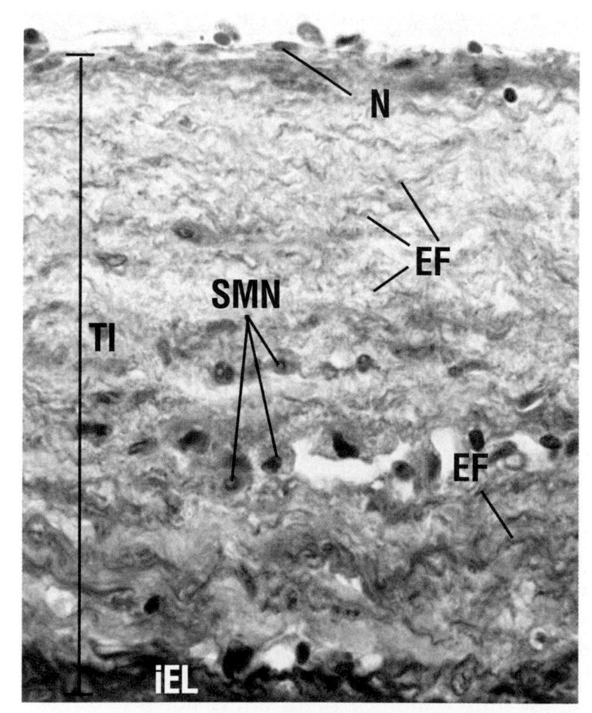

Fig. 11.3 Light micrograph of the tunica intima (TI) of the human aorta. Note the nuclei (N) of the endothelial cells as well as those of the occasional smooth muscle cells (SMN). Although there is no definite internal elastic lamina, there are many elastic fibers spread throughout the subepithelial connective tissue. (×540)

Clinical Correlations

Patients with **von Willebrand disease**, *an inherited disorder that results in impaired adhesion of platelets, have prolonged coagulation times and excessive bleeding at an injury site.*

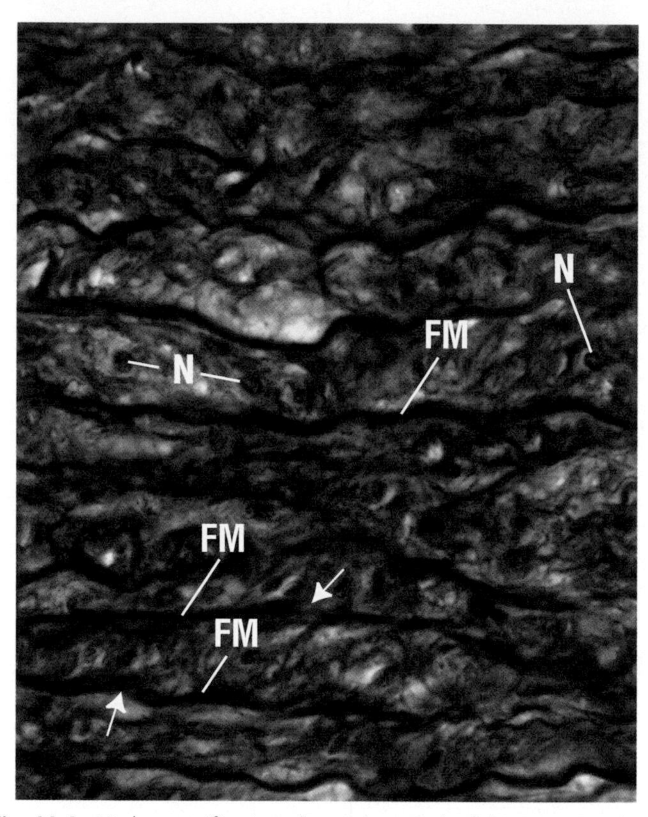

Fig. 11.4 High-magnification photomicrograph of the tunica media of the aorta. Note the nuclei of the smooth muscle cells throughout this layer of the wall of the aorta. The thick fenestrated membranes (FM) have openings in them, known as fenestrae *(arrows)*, which permit the diffusion of extracellular fluid carrying oxygen, carbon dioxide, nutrients, and cellular waste products. (×450)

The **tunica media** of the elastic arteries consists of many fenestrated lamellae of elastin, known as the ***fenestrated membranes***, alternating with circularly oriented layers of smooth muscle cells. There are approximately 40 lamellae of fenestrated membranes in newborns and 70 in adults. These fenestrated membranes also increase in thickness because of the continued deposition of elastin on their surfaces; smooth muscle cells are less abundant in elastic arteries than in most muscular arteries. The extracellular matrix, secreted by the smooth muscle cells, is composed mostly of chondroitin sulfate, collagen, and reticular and elastic fibers (see Figs. 11.2 and Fig. 11.4). An **external elastic lamina** is also present in the tunica media.

The **tunica adventitia** of elastic arteries is relatively thin and is composed of loose fibroelastic connective tissue housing some fibroblasts (see Fig. 11.2). Vasa vasorum also are abundant throughout the adventitia. Capillary beds arise from the vasa vasorum and extend to the tissues of the tunica media, where they supply the connective tissue and smooth muscle cells with oxygen and nutrients. Fenestrations in the elastic laminae permit some diffusion of oxygen and nutrients to the cells in the tunica media from the blood flowing through the lumen, although most of the nourishment is derived from branches of the vasa vasorum.

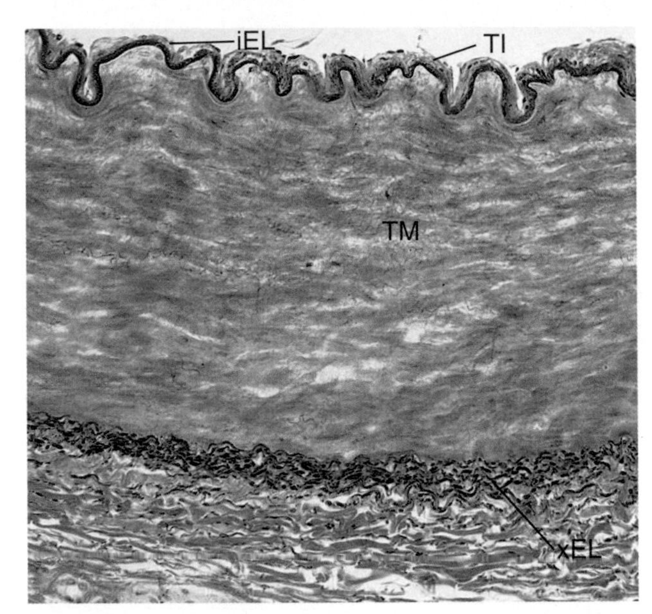

Fig. 11.5 Light micrograph of a muscular artery (×132). Note the tunica adventitia, internal (iEL) and external (xEL) elastic laminae within the thick tunica media (TM). TI, Tunica intima.

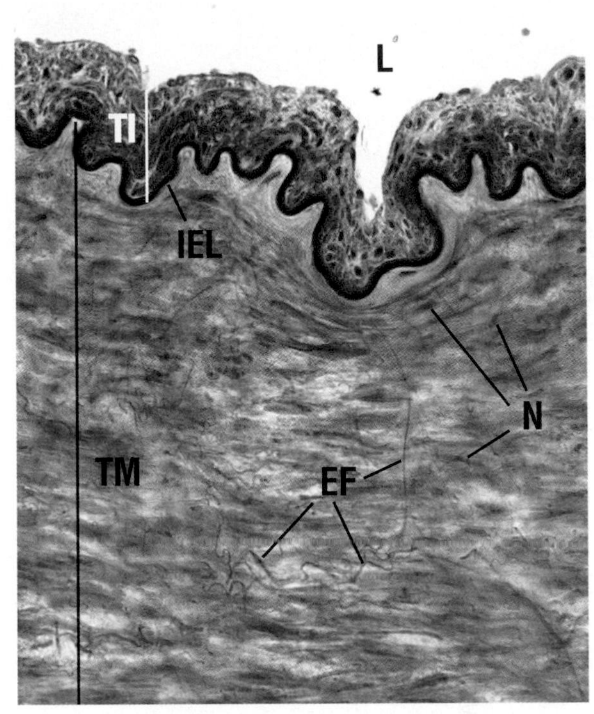

Fig. 11.6 Medium-magnification photomicrograph of the tunica intima (TI) and tunica media (TM) of a muscular artery. The lumen is lined by endothelial cells and deep to the subendothelial connective tissue is the internal elastic lamina (IEL). Nuclei (N) of smooth muscle cells are evident in the tunica media, as are the curly elastic fibers (EF). (×270)

Muscular Arteries

Muscular arteries are characterized by a thick tunica media that is composed mostly of smooth muscle cells.

Muscular (distributing) arteries include most vessels arising from the aorta, except for the major trunks originating from the arch of the aorta and the terminal bifurcation of the abdominal aorta, which are identified as elastic arteries. Indeed, most of the named arteries, even those with a diameter of only slightly greater than 1 mm, are classified as muscular arteries. The identifying characteristic of muscular arteries is a relatively thick tunica media composed mostly of layers of smooth muscle cells (Fig. 11.5).

The **tunica intima** in the muscular arteries is thinner than that in the elastic arteries, but the subendothelial layer contains a few smooth muscle cells. Also, in contrast with that of elastic arteries, the **internal elastic lamina** of the muscular arteries is prominent and displays an undulating surface, to which the endothelium conforms (Figs. 11.5 to 11.7). Occasionally, the internal elastic lamina is duplicated; this is called ***bifid internal elastic lamina***. The endothelial cells have processes that pass through fenestrations within the internal elastic lamina and make gap junctions with smooth muscle cells of the tunica media that are near the interface with the tunica intima. It is believed that these gap junctions may couple metabolically the endothelium and smooth muscle cells.

The **tunica media** of the muscular arteries is composed predominantly of smooth muscle cells that are helically oriented in the region where the tunica media interfaces with the tunica intima (Fig. 11.8). However, a few bundles of smooth muscle fibers are arranged longitudinally in the tunica adventitia. Large muscular arteries may have as many as 40 layers of helically arranged smooth muscle cells; the number of cell layers decreases as the diameter of the artery diminishes so that small muscular arteries have only three or four layers of smooth muscle cells in their tunica media.

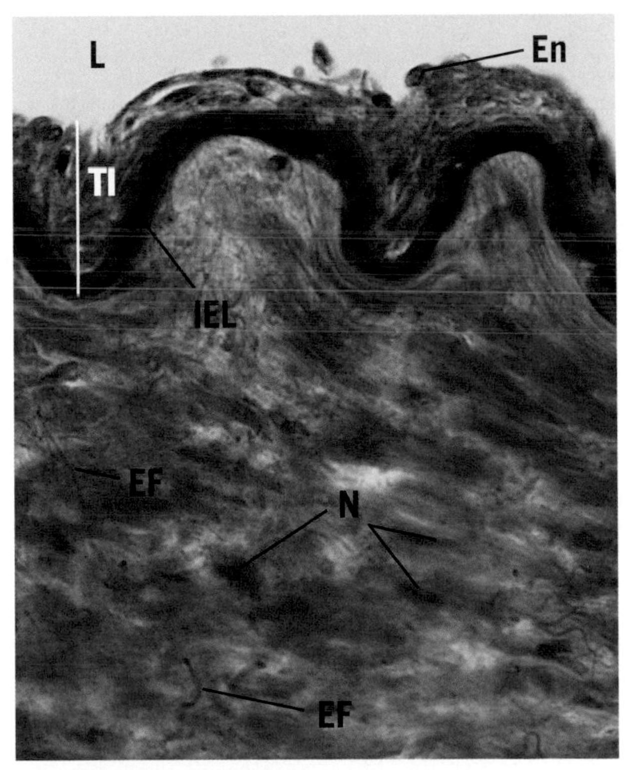

Fig. 11.7 High-magnification photomicrograph of the tunica intima (TI) and a portion of the tunica media (TM) of a muscular artery. The lumen is lined by endothelial cells (En) and deep to the subendothelial connective tissue is the internal elastic lamina (IEL). Nuclei (N) of smooth muscle cells are evident in the tunica media as are the curly elastic fibers (EF). (×540)

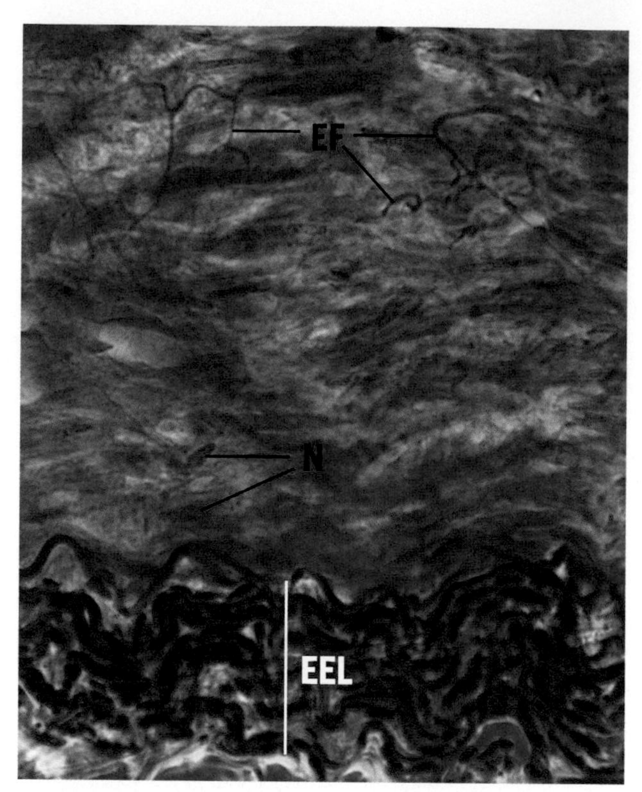

Fig. 11.8 High-magnification photomicrograph of the tunica media of a muscular artery. Note the nuclei (N) of the smooth muscle cells, as well as the curly elastic fibers (EF) distributed throughout the tunica media. The external elastic lamina (EEL) of the tunica media lies against the tunica adventitia. (×450)

Each smooth muscle cell is enveloped by an **external lamina** (similar to a **basal lamina**), although smooth muscle cell processes extend through intervals in the external lamina to form gap junctions with other smooth muscle cells, ensuring coordinated contractions within the tunica media. Interspersed within the layers of smooth muscle cells are elastic fibers, type III collagen fibers, and chondroitin sulfate, all secreted by the smooth muscle cells. Type III collagen fibers (30 nm in diameter) are located in bundles within the extracellular spaces.

An **external elastic lamina** is identifiable in histological sections of larger muscular arteries as several layers of thin elastic sheets; in electron micrographs, these sheets display fenestrations.

The **tunica adventitia** of the muscular arteries consists of elastic fibers, collagen fibers (60–100 nm in diameter), and ground substance composed mostly of dermatan sulfate and heparan sulfate. This extracellular matrix is produced by fibroblasts in the adventitia. The collagen and elastic fibers are oriented longitudinally and blend into the surrounding connective tissues. Located at the outer regions of the adventitia are vasa vasorum and unmyelinated nerve endings. Neurotransmitter released at the nerve endings diffuses through fenestrations in the external elastic lamina into the tunica media to depolarize some of the superficial smooth muscle cells. Depolarization is propagated to all of the muscle cells of the tunica media via gap junctions.

Clinical Correlations

1. *Aneurysm, a sac-like dilation of the wall of an artery (or less often of a vein), results from weakness in the vessel wall and is usually age related. The aneurysm occurs in regions of the vessel wall where—frequently as a result of atherosclerosis, Marfan syndrome, syphilis, and Ehlers-Danlos syndrome—elastic fibers are displaced by collagen fibers. The abdominal aorta is the most common vessel with this type of aneurysm. When discovered, the ballooned area can be repaired, but if it is not discovered and it ruptures, there is rapid massive blood loss that may result in the death of the individual.*
2. *Artery location dictates the thickness of the various tunics. For example, the thickness of the tunica media in the arteries of the leg is greater than those of the upper extremity. This is in response to the continued pressure on the blood column in the vessel resulting from gravitational forces. Moreover, the coronary arteries, serving the heart, are high-pressure arteries and, as such, have a thick tunica media. Conversely, arteries in the pulmonary circulation are under low pressure; thus, the tunica media in these vessels are thinner.*

Arterioles

Arteries with a diameter of less than 0.1 mm are considered to be arterioles.

Arterioles, the terminal branches of arteries, regulate blood flow into metarterioles and capillary beds. In histological sections, the width of the wall of an arteriole is approximately equal to the diameter of its lumen (Fig. 11.9). Deep to the endothelium of the **tunica intima** is a thin layer of connective tissue consisting of type III collagen and a sparse amount of elastic fibers embedded in ground substance. Larger arterioles also display a thin, fenestrated **internal elastic lamina**, which is absent in small and terminal arterioles (Fig. 11.10). In large arterioles, the **tunica media** is composed of a two or three layers of smooth muscle cell layer, whereas in small arterioles there is only a single layer of smooth muscle cells that completely encircles the endothelial cells (Fig. 11.11). Arterioles do not have an external elastic lamina. The **tunica adventitia** of arterioles is scant and is represented by fibroelastic connective tissue housing a few fibroblasts.

Arteries that supply blood to capillary beds are called ***metarterioles***. They are approximately 8 μm in diameter and differ structurally from arterioles in that their smooth muscle layer is not continuous. Rather, the individual muscle cells (known as **precapillary sphincters**) are spaced apart, and each encircles the endothelium of a capillary arising from the metarteriole. It is believed that this arrangement permits these smooth muscle cells to function as a sphincter upon contraction, thus controlling blood flow into the capillary bed.

Clinical Correlations

Almost 10% of US adults suffer from gastroesophageal reflux disease and are prescribed proton pump inhibitors (PPIs), which inhibit the ability of parietal cells of the stomach to produce hydrochloric acid. Unfortunately, chronic, long-term use of these drugs—some of which are available without prescription—have been demonstrated to cause damage to endothelial cells in vitro. Apparently, PPIs not only inhibit parietal cells from producing HCl but also interfere with the acidity of lysosomes of endothelial cells, resulting in the inability of lysosomes to destroy intracellular debris and, thereby, reducing the smoothness of the luminal surface of the endothelial cells. It is suggested that the roughened lining of blood vessels cause platelets and blood cells to adhere to the endothelium, initiating the beginning of arteriosclerosis. Because this work was an in vitro study, further research is needed to see if it can be replicated in vivo.

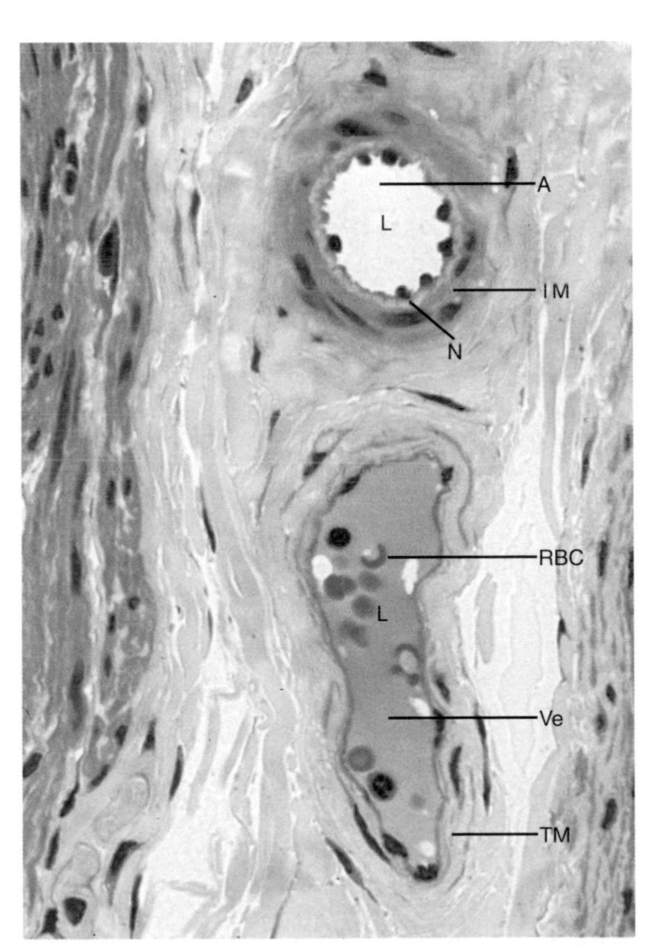

Fig. 11.9 Light micrograph of an arteriole and a venule containing blood cells (×540). The arteriole (A) is well defined, with a thick tunica media (TM). Nuclei of endothelial cells bulge into the lumen (L). The venule (Ve) is poorly defined, with a large, poorly defined lumen containing red blood cells (RBC). The tunica media of the venule is not as robust as that in the arteriole.

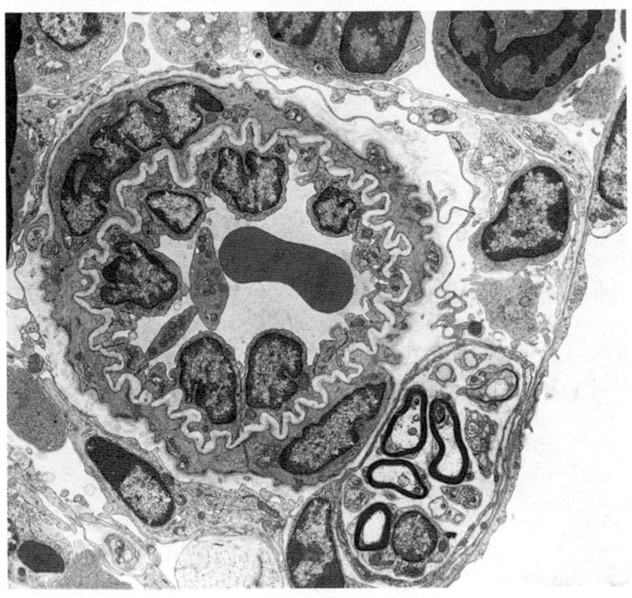

Fig. 11.10 Electron micrograph of an arteriole. (From Yamazaki K, Allen TD. Ultrastructural morphometric study of efferent nerve terminals on murine bone marrow stromal cells, and the recognition of a novel anatomical unit: the "neuro-reticular complex." *Am J Anat.* 1990;187:261–276. Reprinted with permission from Wiley-Liss, Inc., a subsidiary of John Wiley & Sons, Inc.)

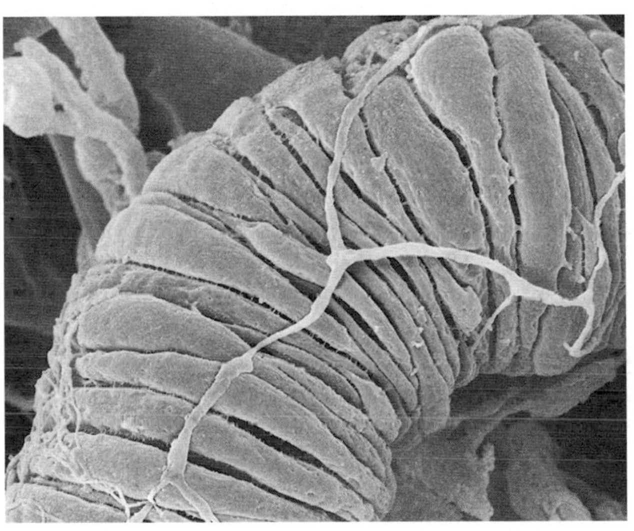

Fig. 11.11 Scanning electron micrograph of an arteriole illustrating its compact layer of smooth muscle and its attendant nerve fibers (×4200). (From Fujiwara T, Uehara Y. The cytoarchitecture of the wall and innervation pattern of the microvessels in the rat mammary gland: a scanning electron microscopic observation. *Am J Anat.* 1984;170:39–54. Reprinted with permission from Wiley-Liss, Inc., a subsidiary of John Wiley & Sons, Inc.)

Specialized Sensory Structures in Arteries

Specialized sensory structures in the arteries include the carotid sinus, carotid body, and aortic bodies.

Three types of specialized sensory structures are located in the major arteries of the body: **carotid sinuses**, **carotid bodies**, and **aortic bodies**. Nerve endings in these structures monitor blood pressure and blood composition, providing essential inputs to the brain for controlling heartbeat, respiration, and blood pressure.

Carotid Sinus

The carotid sinus is a baroreceptor located in the wall of the internal carotid artery just distal to the bifurcation of the common carotid artery.

The carotid sinus, located within the wall of the internal carotid artery, is a baroreceptor—that is, it perceives changes in blood pressure. At this site, the adventitia of this vessel is relatively thicker and is richly endowed with sensory nerve endings from the glossopharyngeal nerve (cranial nerve IX). In contrast, the tunica media is relatively thin, permitting it to be distended during increases in blood pressure, which stimulates the nerve endings. The afferent impulses, received at the vasomotor center in the brain, trigger adjustments in vasoconstriction, resulting in maintenance of proper blood pressure. Additional small baroreceptors are located in the aorta and in some of the larger vessels.

Clinical Correlations

The Joint National Committee on Prevention, Detection, Evaluation, and Treatment of High Blood Pressure (JNC), in releasing its comprehensive guidelines on blood pressure-related risks of cardiovascular disease in 2017, modified its previous guidelines concerning the categories of blood pressure.

Category of Blood Pressure	Systolic (mm Hg)	Diastolic (mm Hg)
Normal	< 120	< 80
Elevated	120–129	< 80
Hypertension Stage 1	130–139	80–89
Hypertension Stage 2	≥ 140	≥ 90

Under the earlier guideline, when hypertension was considered to be 140/80, there were 74 million hypertensive adults in the United States; under the current guideline, there are 105 million hypertensive adults. It is estimated that if patients adhere to the current guidelines, the lives of approximately 330,000 patients will be saved annually. Additionally, approximately 600,000 patients will avoid strokes, myocardial infarcts, atrial fibrillation, kidney disease, and other consequences of cardiovascular disease. In order to comply with the new guidelines, 11 million more US adults will have to be placed on antihypertensive medications, but the new guidelines also emphasize that patients should consider life style changes. These include losing weight, reducing alcohol and salt consumption, increasing potassium intake, increasing the amount of exercise, and going on a DASH (dietary approaches to stop hypertension) diet . DASH suggests a decreased consumption of meat, saturated and trans fats, and increasing the amount of fish, poultry, fruits, vegetables, and whole-grain foods.

Carotid Body

The carotid body functions as a chemoreceptor monitoring changes in oxygen and carbon dioxide levels, as well as hydrogen ion concentration.

The ***carotid body***, located at the bifurcation of the common carotid artery, is a small oval structure that possesses specialized chemoreceptor nerve endings responsible for monitoring blood H^+ concentration, as well as changes in oxygen and carbon dioxide levels. This structure, 3 to 5 mm in diameter, is composed of multiple clusters of pale-staining cells embedded in connective tissue. Using electron microscopy, two types of parenchymal cells have been identified in the carotid body: **glomus (type I) cells** and **sheath (type II) cells.**

Glomus cells are distinguished by the presence of dense-cored vesicles, 60 to 200 nm in diameter, that resemble vesicles located in the chromaffin cells of the suprarenal medulla. Cell processes also contain longitudinally oriented microtubules, more dense-cored vesicles, and a few small electron-lucent vesicles. These processes contact other glomus cells and capillary endothelial cells.

Sheath cells are more complex and have long processes that almost completely ensheath the processes of the glomus cells. The nuclei of these cells are irregular and contain more heterochromatin compared with the round nuclei of glomus cells; moreover, sheath cells contain no dense-cored vesicles. As nerve terminals enter clusters of glomus cells, they lose their Schwann cells and become covered by the sheath cells in much the same way as glial cells would ensheath fibers in the central nervous system (CNS).

Carotid bodies contain catecholamines (as do the cells of the suprarenal medulla and paraganglia), but whether they produce hormones is unclear. The glossopharyngeal and vagus nerves supply the carotid body with numerous afferent fibers. In some of the synapses, the glomus cells appear to function as presynaptic cell bodies, but the specific relationships are as yet not understood.

Aortic Bodies

Aortic bodies, located at the arch of the aorta and between the left common carotid artery and the left subclavian artery, resemble that of the carotid bodies. Therefore, they are assumed to be chemoreceptors.

Regulation of Arterial Blood Pressure

Arterial blood pressure is regulated by the vasomotor center in the brain.

The heart, which serves as the cardiovascular pump, rests between each stroke, propelling a pressurized burst of blood that enters the elastic arteries, then moves into the muscular arteries and arterioles, and, finally, into capillaries. The **vasomotor center** in the brain controls the state of contraction of the vessel walls (**vasomotor tone**) by a combination of vasoconstriction and vasodilation. **Vasodilation** is a function of the parasympathetic nervous system. **Vasoconstriction** is accomplished via vasomotor nerves of the sympathetic nervous system, as well as by endothelins 1, 2, and 3; angiotensin II; and, in cases of major blood loss, antidiuretic hormone (vasopressin).

Vasodilation occurs when acetylcholine released from the parasympathetic nerve terminals in the vessel walls initiates release of **nitric oxide (NO)** from the endothelium. The NO diffuses into the smooth muscle cells, where it activates the cyclic guanosine monophosphate system, resulting in relaxation of the muscle cells, thus dilating the vessel lumen.

Vasomotor-induced **vasoconstriction** occurs when the sympathetic fibers release norepinephrine, which reaches some of the smooth muscle cells of the tunica media, causing them to undergo contraction. Since not every smooth muscle cell has its own nerve supply, the contraction stimulus is transmitted from smooth muscle cells to other smooth muscle cells via gap junctions.

Clinical Correlations

Localized vasoconstriction occurs when the epithelial lining of blood vessels becomes damaged. The injured endothelial cells release **endothelin**, *a large peptide composed of 21 amino acids, which binds to its receptors on smooth muscle cells, causing them to undergo contraction and reduce blood loss from the injured vessel. Damaged endothelial cells release other vasoconstrictor substances, such as prostaglandins and thromboxane* A_2.

Dehydration and severe hemorrhage induce the posterior pituitary to release **antidiuretic hormone (vasopressin)**, *another powerful vasoconstrictor.*

When *systemic blood pressure* is low, the kidneys secrete the enzyme **renin**, which cleaves **angiotensinogen** circulating in the blood, forming **angiotensin I**. This mild vasoconstrictor is converted to **angiotensin II** by **ACE (angiotensin converting enzyme)**, which is located on the luminal plasmalemmae of capillary endothelia (especially capillaries of the lungs). Angiotensin II is a potent vasoconstrictor that initiates smooth muscle contraction, thereby reducing vessel lumen diameter, resulting in increased blood pressure (see Chapter 19).

Clinical Correlations

Normal and Pathological Vascular Changes

The largest arteries continue to grow until about age 25 years, and there is progressive thickening of their walls and an increase in the number of elastic laminae. In the muscular arteries, from middle age on, deposits of collagen and proteoglycans increase in the walls, reducing their flexibility. The coronary vessels are the first to display the effects of aging, with the intima displaying the greatest age-related changes. These natural changes are not unlike the regressive changes observed in arteriosclerosis.

Arteriosclerosis

Small arteries and arterioles, especially those of the kidneys, are prone to arteriosclerosis (hardening of the arteries), displaying a hyaline or concentric thickening that is often associated with hypertension and diabetes.

Atherosclerosis

Atherosclerosis, *a forerunner to heart attack and stroke, is a very common form of arteriosclerosis. The vessels most susceptible to this condition are the coronary arteries, carotid arteries, and the major arteries of the brain. However, the renal arteries, arteries of the lower limbs, and arteries supplying the alimentary canal can also be affected. Atherosclerosis is distinguished by infiltrations of soft, noncellular lipid material (atheromas) into the tunica intima; these infiltrations can reduce the luminal diameter appreciably even by age 25 years. It is not clear whether these conditions in a young person are physiological or a manifestation of a disease process. The fibrous plaques that form in the intima of older persons, however, are pathological.*

The smooth muscle cell layer in the tunica media of a healthy person undergoes renewal, but when the endothelium is injured, platelets that accumulate at the lesion site release **platelet-derived growth factor (PDGF)**, *stimulating proliferation of smooth muscle cells. As a consequence, these cells begin to get packed with cholesterol-rich lipids, which stimulate the muscle cells to manufacture additional collagen and proteoglycans, resulting in a cycle whereby the tunica intima becomes thickened. The endothelium is then further damaged, leading to necrosis. This attracts more platelets and, finally, clotting occurs, forming a thrombus that may occlude the vessel at that site. Alternatively, if released into the general circulation, it may occlude a more vulnerable vessel (e.g., a coronary vessel or a cerebral vessel).*

The pathogenesis is still unclear, although current research theories point to the role of cholesterol, lipoproteins, and certain mitogens. A correlation between blood cholesterol levels and heart disease has been demonstrated, and it has been noted that **C-reactive protein** *(CRP), synthesized by the liver, can be used as a marker for inflammation, which appears to be a far more accurate indicator of the risk for cardiovascular disease. Statins, which have been used extensively for reducing cholesterol levels in the blood, thereby reducing the risk of heart disease, have also been shown to reduce the levels of CRP. This fact is important because there are data supporting that the response to inflammation is as critical to heart disease as are high levels of cholesterol. Thus, there appears to be a commonality between inflammation and cardiovascular disease.*

CAPILLARIES

Capillaries arise from the terminal ends of arterioles and also from metarterioles (Fig. 11.12). By branching and anastomosing, capillaries form capillary beds (capillary networks) between the arterioles and the venules.

General Structure of Capillaries

Capillaries, composed of a single layer of endothelial cells, are the smallest blood vessels.

Capillaries are the smallest of the vascular channels, approximately 50 μm in length, on average, with a diameter of 8 to 10 μm, permitting individual blood cells to traverse the entire length of the capillary. These slender, small vessels are formed by a single layer of squamous endothelial cells rolled into a tube, with the long axis of the cells paralleling the blood flow. These endothelial cells are flattened, with the attenuated ends tapering to a thickness to 0.2 μm or less, although an elliptical nucleus bulges out into the lumen of the capillary. The cytoplasm

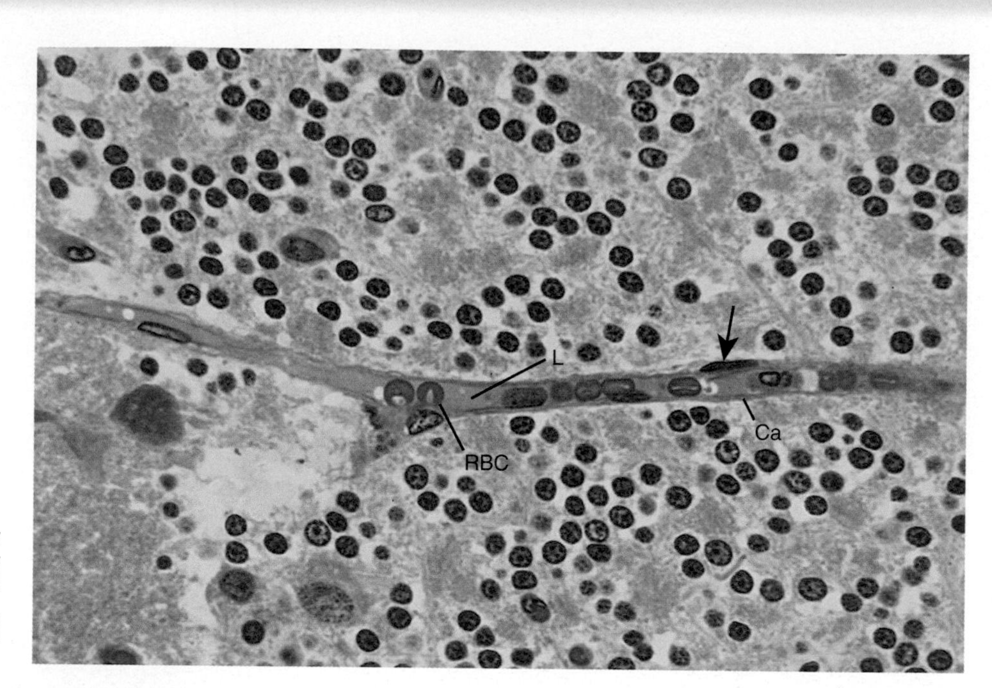

Fig. 11.12 Photomicrograph of a capillary in the monkey cerebellum (×270). A capillary (Ca) is present in the field of view and red blood cells (RBC) are evident in its lumen (L). Note the nucleus *(arrow)* of an endothelial cell bulging into the lumen.

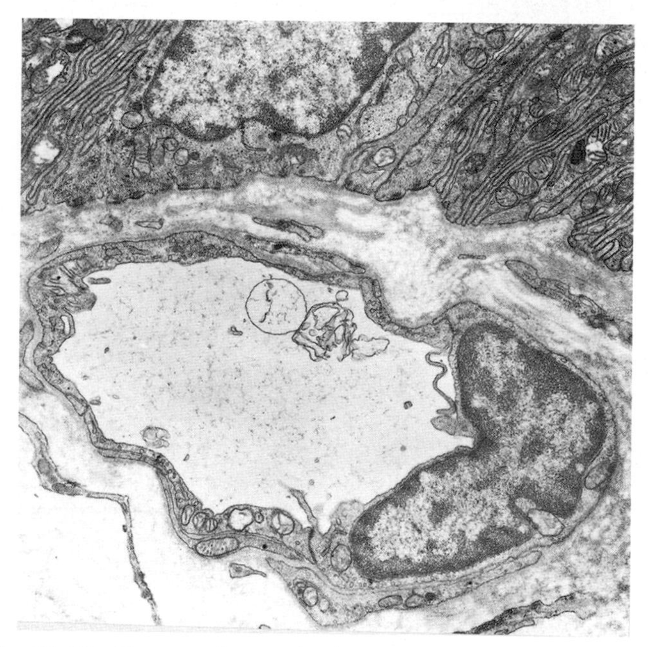

Fig. 11.13 Electron micrograph of a continuous capillary in the rat submandibular gland (×13,000). The pericyte shares the endothelial cell's basal lamina. (From Sato A, Miyoshi S. Morphometric study of the microvasculature of the main excretory duct subepithelia of the rat parotid, submandibular, and sublingual salivary glands. *Anat Rec.* 1990;226:288–294. Reprinted with permission from Wiley-Liss, Inc., a subsidiary of John Wiley & Sons, Inc.)

contains a Golgi complex, a few mitochondria, some rough endoplasmic reticulum (RER), and free ribosomes (Figs. 11.13 and 11.14). Intermediate filaments (9–11 nm), located about the perinuclear zone, are composed of **desmin** and/or **vimentin** and provide structural support to the endothelial cells.

The large number of pinocytotic vesicles associated with the endothelial cell plasmalemma is an identifying characteristic of capillaries. These vesicles may be in singular array, two single vesicles may be fused, or several vesicles may be fused, forming a transient channel across the thickness of the cell. Where the endothelial cells are the thinnest, a single array of fused vesicles may span from the adluminal plasmalemma across the cytoplasm to the abluminal plasmalemma of the endothelial cell.

Capillaries form plexuses, known as capillary beds, and several capillary beds are suspended from metarterioles. Not all of the capillary beds are open at any one time; however, increased demand of the tissue or organ supplied by the capillary beds initiates the opening of more beds, increasing blood flow to meet physiological needs. The external surfaces of the endothelial cells are surrounded by a basal lamina secreted by the endothelial cells (see Fig. 11.14). When viewed in cross-section, it is evident that the circumference of small capillaries is formed by a single endothelial cell, whereas portions of two or three endothelial cells contribute to forming the circumference of larger capillaries. At these cellular junctions, the endothelial cells tend to overlap, forming a **marginal fold** that projects into the lumen. Endothelial cells are joined together by **fasciae occludentes**, or **tight junctions**, although occasional gap junctions and desmosomes are also evident.

Pericytes, located along the outside of the capillaries and small venules, appear to be surrounding them and share the basal laminae of the endothelial cells (Figs. 11.15 and 11.16). These cells have long primary processes, which are located along the long axis of the capillary and from which secondary processes arise to wrap around the capillary, forming a few **gap junctions** with the endothelial cells. Pericytes possess a small Golgi complex, mitochondria, RER, microtubules, and filaments extending into the processes. These cells also contain tropomyosin, isomyosin, and protein kinase, which are all related to the contractile process that regulates blood flow through the capillaries. Furthermore, as discussed in Chapter 6, after injury, pericytes may undergo differentiation to become smooth muscle cells and endothelial cells in the walls of arterioles and venules.

Classification of Capillaries

Capillaries are of three types: continuous, fenestrated, and sinusoidal (Fig. 11.17); they differ in their location and structure.

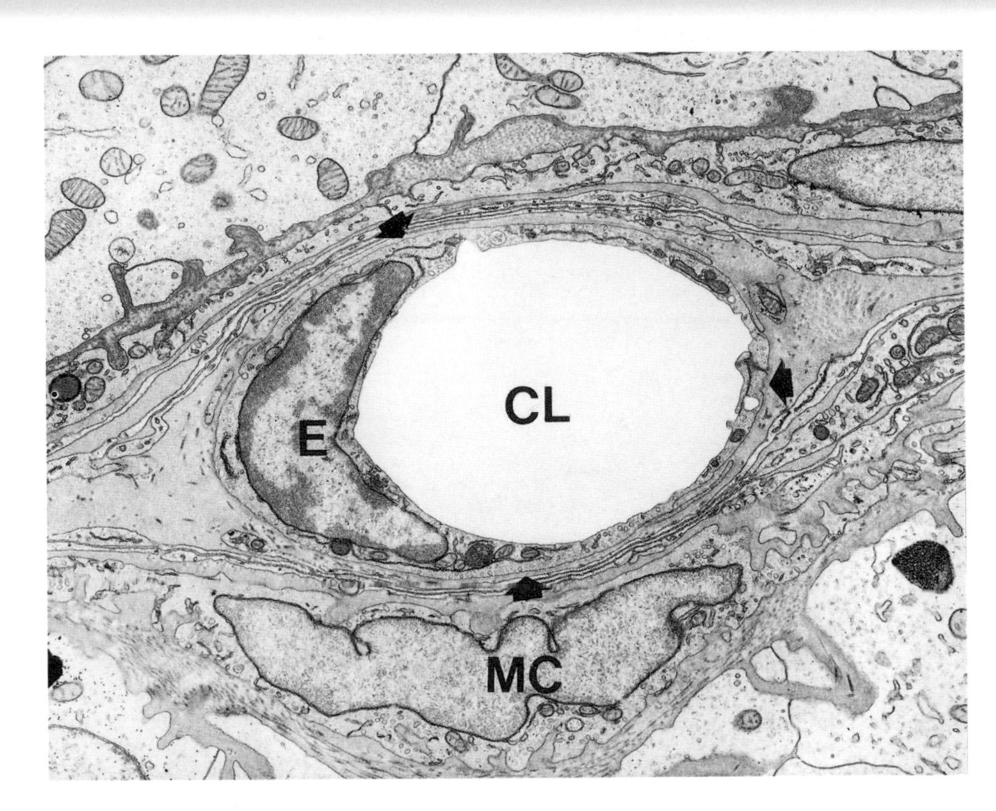

Fig. 11.14 Electron micrograph of a testicular capillary. CL, Capillary lumen; E, nucleus of endothelial cell; MC, myoid cell. *Arrows* represent the basal lamina. (From Meyerhofer A, Hikim APS, Bartke A, Russell LD. Changes in the testicular microvasculature during photoperiod-related seasonal transition from reproductive quiescence to reproductive activity in the adult golden hamster. *Anat Rec.* 1989;224:495–507. Reprinted with permission from Wiley-Liss, Inc., a subsidiary of John Wiley & Sons, Inc.)

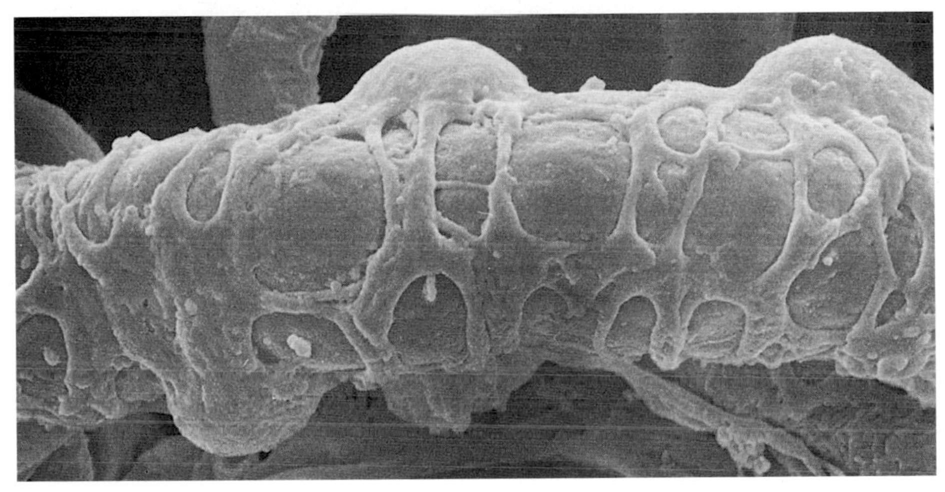

Fig. 11.15 Scanning electron micrograph of a capillary displaying pericytes on its surface (×5000). (From Fujiwara T, Uehara Y. The cytoarchitecture of the wall and innervation pattern of the microvessels in the rat mammary gland: a scanning electron microscopic observation. *Am J Anat.* 1984;170:39–54. Reprinted with permission from Wiley-Liss, Inc., a subsidiary of John Wiley & Sons, Inc.)

Continuous Capillaries (Somatic Capillaries)

Continuous capillaries (somatic capillaries) have no pores or fenestrae in their walls.

Continuous capillaries (also known as ***somatic capillaries***) are present in muscle, nervous, and connective tissues, as well as in the lungs and exocrine glands. The intercellular junctions between their endothelial cells are **fasciae occludentes**, which prevent passage of many molecules. Substances such as amino acids, glucose, nucleosides, and purines move across the capillary wall via carrier-mediated transport, as evidenced by the numerous pinocytotic vesicles associated with these types of capillaries. The cells exhibit a polarity with the transport systems, such that Na^+-K^+ adenosine triphosphatase (ATPase) is located in the adluminal cell membrane only. In the CNS, the blood–brain barrier regulation resides within the endothelial cells but is influenced by signaling molecules formed by the astrocytes associated with the capillaries. Continuous capillaries of the CNS have a much reduced number of pinocytotic vesicles.

Fenestrated Capillaries (Visceral Capillaries)

Fenestrated capillaries (visceral capillaries) possess pores (fenestrae) in their walls that are covered by pore diaphragms.

Fenestrated capillaries (also known as ***visceral capillaries***) are located in the pancreas, intestines, endocrine glands, and kidneys. They have **pores** (**fenestrae**) in their walls that are 60 to 80 nm in diameter, which are bridged by an ultrathin **pore diaphragm** (although the **renal glomerulus** is composed of fenestrated capillaries whose fenestrae lack diaphragms). When viewed after processing with platinum-carbon shadowing, the diaphragm displays eight fibrils radiating out from a central area and forming wedge-like channels, each with an opening of

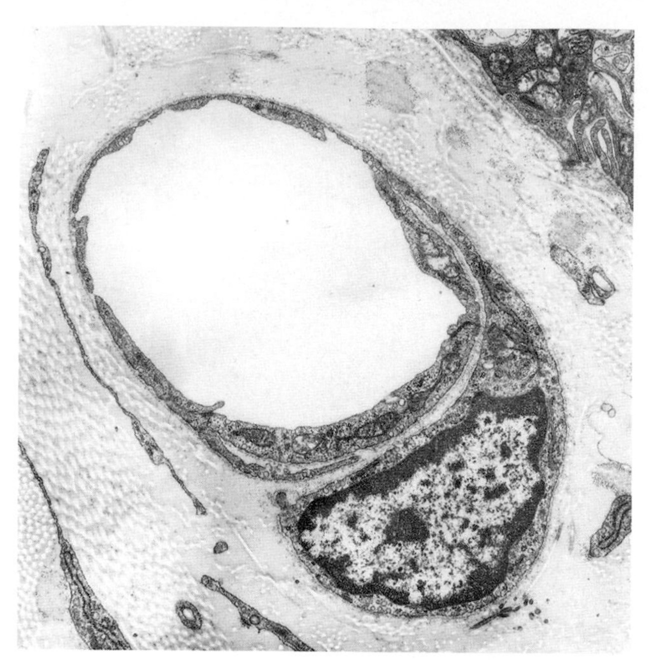

Fig. 11.16 Electron micrograph of a fenestrated capillary and its pericyte in a cross-section. Note that the capillary endothelial cells and the pericyte share the same basal lamina. (From Sato A, Miyoshi S. Morphometric study of the microvasculature of the main excretory duct subepithelia of the rat parotid, submandibular, and sublingual salivary glands. *Anat Rec.* 1990;226:288–294. Reprinted with permission from Wiley-Liss, Inc., a subsidiary of John Wiley & Sons, Inc.)

about 5.5 nm. These pore–diaphragm complexes are regularly spaced about 50 nm apart but are located in clusters; thus, most of the endothelial wall of the fenestrated capillary is without fenestrae (see Fig. 11.17B).

Sinusoidal Capillaries

Sinusoidal capillaries may possess discontinuous endothelial cells and basal lamina and contain many large fenestrae without diaphragms, enhancing exchange between blood and tissue.

The irregular blood pools or channels that conform to the shape of the structure in which they are located are vascular channels called ***sinusoids***; they are located in certain organs of the body, including the bone marrow, liver, spleen, lymphoid organs, and some endocrine glands.

Because of their location, sinusoidal capillaries have an enlarged diameter of 30 to 40 μm (see Fig. 11.17C). Not only do their endothelial cells possess many large fenestrae that lack diaphragms but the endothelial lining and its basal lamina may be discontinuous, facilitating an enhanced leakage of fluids (but not blood cells or platelets) between the blood and the tissues. In certain organs, the endothelium is thin and continuous (as in some lymphoid organs); in others, it may have continuous areas intermingled with fenestrated areas (as in endocrine glands). Macrophages may be located either in or along the outside of the sinusoidal wall.

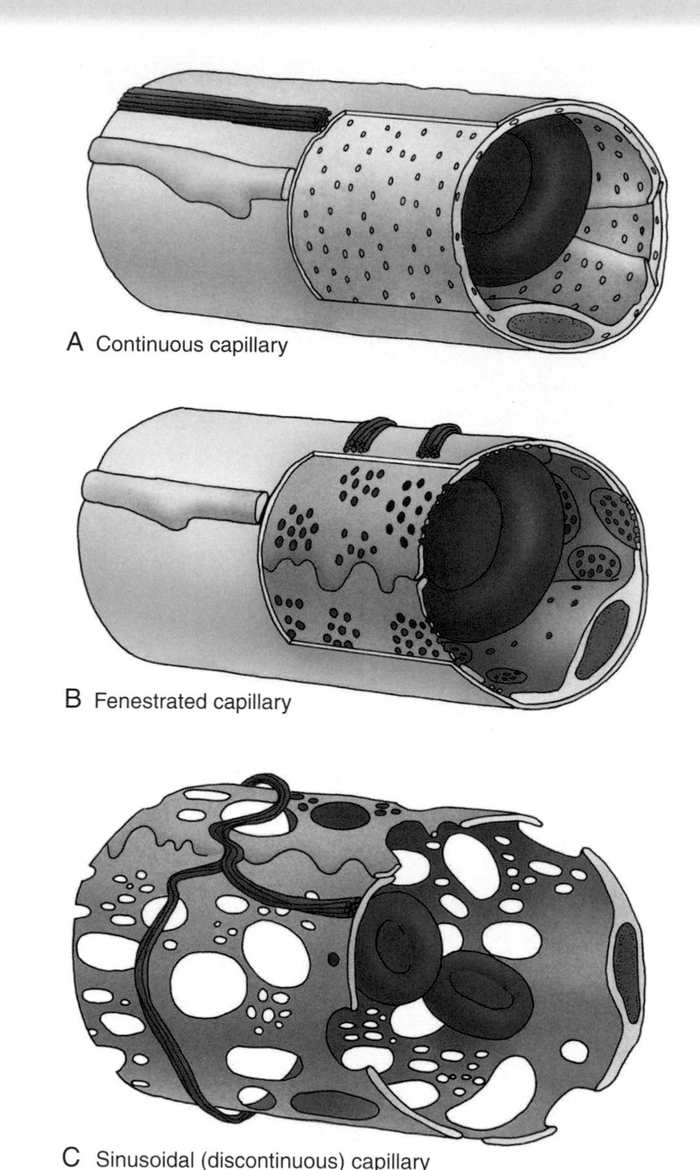

Fig. 11.17 Diagram of the three types of capillaries. (A) Continuous. (B) Fenestrated. (C) Sinusoidal.

Regulation of Blood Flow into a Capillary Bed

Arteriovenous Anastomoses (Arteriovenous Shunts)

Arteriovenous anastomoses (arteriovenous shunts) are direct vascular connections between arterioles and venules that bypass the capillary bed.

Terminals of most arterioles (**terminal arterioles**) end in capillary beds, which deliver their blood to venules for the return back to the venous side of the cardiovascular system. In many parts of the body, however, the arteriole is connected to a venous channel by a vessel that forms an **arteriovenous anastomosis (AVA, arteriovenous shunt)**. The structures of the arterial and venous ends of the AVA are similar to those of an artery and vein, respectively, whereas the intermediate segment has a thickened tunica media, and its subendothelial layer is composed of modified, longitudinally arranged smooth muscle cells.

When the AVAs are closed, the blood passes through the capillary bed; when they are open, a large amount of blood bypasses the capillary bed and flows through the AVA. These arteriovenous shunts are useful in thermoregulation and are abundant in skin. The intermediate segments of the AVAs are richly innervated with adrenergic and cholinergic nerves. Whereas most peripheral nerves are controlled somewhat by local environmental stimuli, the nerves of the AVAs are controlled by the thermoregulatory system in the brain.

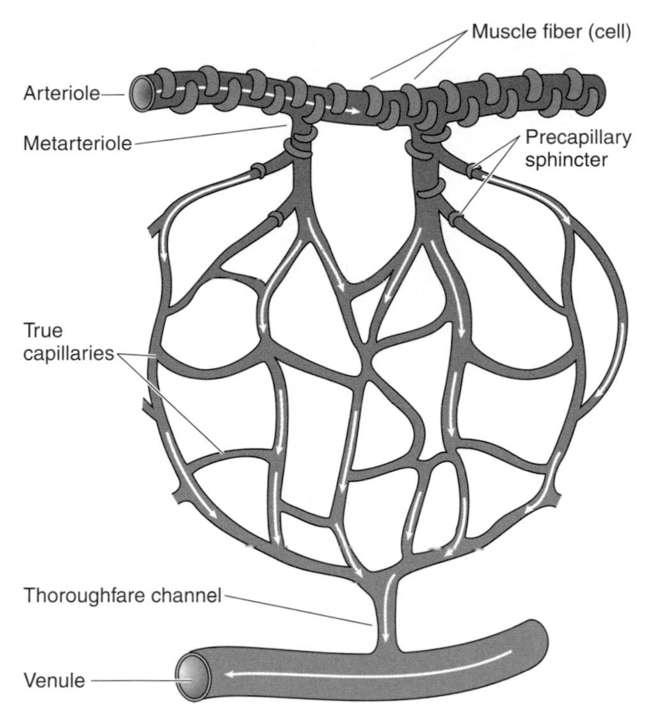

Fig. 11.18 Diagram of the control of blood flow through a capillary bed. The central channel, composed of the metarteriole on the arterial side and the thoroughfare channel on the venous side, can bypass the capillary bed by closure of the precapillary sphincters.

Glomera

Nail beds and the tips of the fingers and toes are vascularized by **glomera** (singular, **glomus**). The glomus is a small organ that receives an arteriole devoid of an elastic lamina and acquires a richly innervated smooth muscle cell layer, which surrounds the vessel lumen, thus directly controlling blood flow to the region before emptying into a venous plexus. The glomera complex is not fully understood.

Central Channel

Metarterioles form the proximal portion of a central channel, and thoroughfare channels form the distal portion of a central channel.

Blood flow from the arterial system is controlled either by **terminal arterioles** directly or by **metarterioles** (with precapillary sphincters). **Metarterioles**, the first part of a **central channel**, pass through capillary beds to deliver blood from arterioles to venules. The distal portion of the metarteriole drains into a **thoroughfare channel** that ends in a **small venule** (**postcapillary venule**). Metarterioles possess precapillary sphincters, whereas thoroughfare channels do not. If the precapillary sphincters are open, blood from the metarterioles pass into the capillary bed. The capillaries convey their blood to the thoroughfare channel and then into a small venule. If the precapillary sphincters are not open, blood bypasses the capillary bed and goes directly from the metarteriole into the thoroughfare channel and, from there, into a small venule (postcapillary venule) of the venous system (Fig. 11.18).

Histophysiology of Capillaries

Capillaries are regions where blood flow is very slow, permitting exchange of material between the circulating blood and the extravascular connective tissue.

The endothelial cells of capillaries may contain two distinct pore systems: **small pores** (~9–11 nm in diameter) and **large pores** (~50–70 nm in diameter). The small pores are believed to be discontinuities between endothelial cell junctions. The large pores are represented by fenestrae and transport vesicles. Oxygen, carbon dioxide, and glucose may diffuse or be transported across the plasmalemma, then diffuse through the cytoplasm and, finally, make their way through the abluminal plasmalemma into the extravascular space. Water and hydrophilic molecules (~1.5 nm) simply diffuse through the intercellular junctions.

Water-soluble molecules greater than 11 nm in diameter are transported from the *adluminal* plasmalemma to the *abluminal* plasmalemma by the numerous pinocytotic vesicles adjacent to the cell membrane. This process is called ***transcytosis*** (Fig. 11.19) because the material traverses the entire cell instead of remaining within the cell. In continuous capillaries, substances are taken up by open vesicles located on the *adluminal* plasmalemma. The vesicles are then transported across the cytoplasm to the *abluminal* plasmalemma, where the vesicles fuse with the cell membrane to deliver their contents into the extravascular space. This is an efficient process because the number of vesicles in these endothelial cells may exceed 1000/μm^2. It appears that they are members of a stable population of vesicles arising from the Golgi complex via a fusion–fission mechanism of renewal.

Leukocytes leave the bloodstream to enter the extravascular space by passing through the junctions via a mechanism called ***diapedesis*** (see Chapter 10, Fig. 10.8). **Histamine** and **bradykinin**, whose levels are increased during the inflammatory process, increase capillary permeability, causing excessive fluid passage into the extravascular spaces. This excess extravascular fluid causes the tissues to swell and is known as ***edema***.

Clinical Correlations

Capillaries serve a maintenance role in converting such substances as serotonin, norepinephrine, bradykinin, prostaglandins, and thrombin into inactive compounds. Additionally, enzymes on the luminal surface of endothelial cells of the capillaries in adipose tissue degrade lipoproteins into monoglycerides and fatty acids for storage within adipocytes.

VEINS

Veins are vessels that return blood to the heart.

At the discharging ends of capillaries are small venules, the beginning of the venous return, which conduct blood away from the organs and tissues and return it to the heart. These venules empty their contents into larger veins; the process continues as the vessels become still larger, and it is the largest ones that empty into the heart. Veins not only outnumber arteries but also usually have larger luminal diameters. Therefore, at any one time, almost 70% of the total blood volume is in these vessels. In histological sections, veins parallel arteries. Because venous return is a low-pressure system, the walls of veins are usually thinner and less elastic than arterial walls. Of the three layers, the tunica adventitia is usually the thickest in veins, and veins have a richer supply of vasa vasorum than do arteries. In histological sections, veins are usually collapsed and their lumina contain blood.

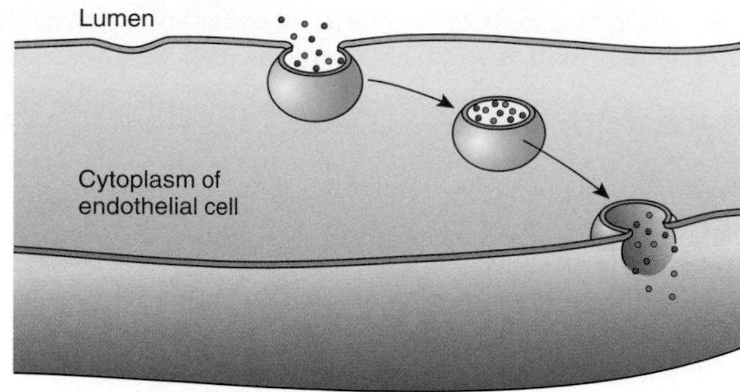

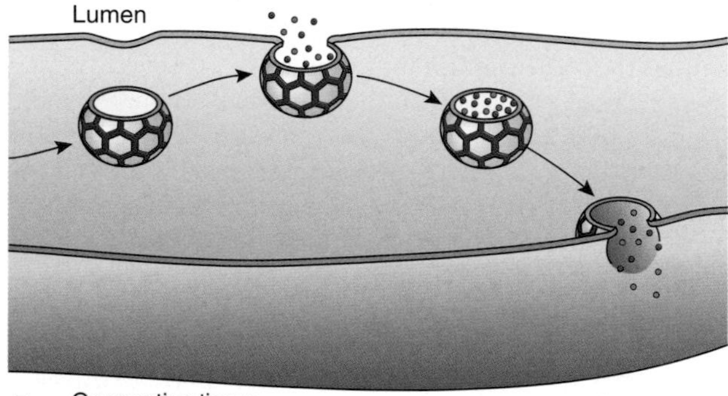

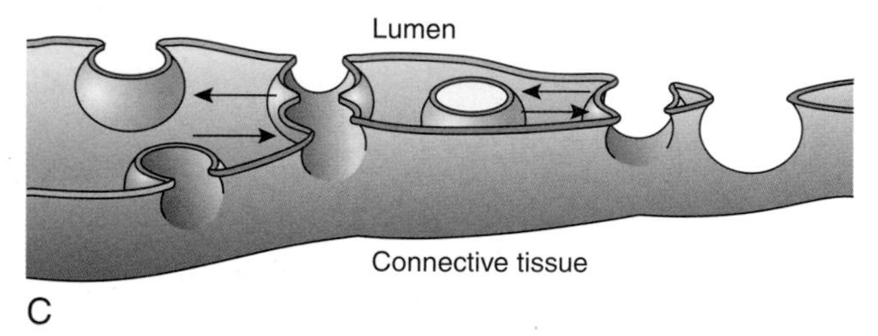

Fig. 11.19 Diagram of the various methods of transport across capillary endothelia. (A) Pinocytotic vesicles, which form on the luminal surface, traverse the endothelial cell, and their contents are released on the opposite surface into the connective tissue spaces. (B) *Trans* Golgi network–derived vesicles possessing clathrin coats and receptor molecules fuse with the luminal surface of the endothelial cells and pick up specific ligands from the capillary lumen. They then detach and traverse the endothelial cell, fuse with the membrane of the opposite surface, and release their contents into the connective tissue spaces. (C) In regions where the endothelial cells are highly attenuated, the pinocytotic (or *trans* Golgi network–derived) vesicles may fuse with each other to form transient fenestrations through the entire thickness of the endothelial cell, permitting material to travel between the lumen and the connective tissue spaces. (Modified from Simionescu N, Simionescu M. In: Ussing H, Bindslev N, Sten-Knudsen O, eds. *Water Transport Across Epithelia*. Copenhagen: Munksgaard International Publishers Ltd; 1981.)

Classification of Veins

Veins are classified into three groups on the basis of their diameter and wall thickness: small, medium, and large.

The structure of veins is not necessarily uniform, even for veins of the same size or for the same vein along its entire length. Veins are described as having the same three layers (i.e., tunicae intima, media, and adventitia) as arteries (Table 11.3). Although the muscular and elastic layers are not as well developed, the collagenous connective tissue components in veins are more pronounced than those of arteries. In certain areas of the body, where the structures housing the veins protect them from pressure (e.g., retina, meninges, placenta, penis), the veins have little or no smooth muscle in their walls; moreover, the boundaries between the tunica intima and the tunica media of most veins are not clearly distinguishable.

Venules and Small Veins.

Venules are similar to but larger than capillaries; larger venules possess smooth muscle cells instead of pericytes.

As the blood pools from the capillary bed, it is discharged into **small venules** (**postcapillary venules**), which are 15 to 20 μm in diameter. Their walls are similar to those of capillaries, with a thin endothelium surrounded by reticular fibers and pericytes (see Fig. 11.9). The pericytes of postcapillary venules form an intricate, loose network surrounding the endothelium. Pericytes are replaced by smooth muscle cells in larger venules (> 1 mm in diameter), first as scattered smooth muscle cells. Then, as venule diameter increases, the smooth muscle cells become more closely spaced, forming a continuous layer in the largest venules and small veins. Materials are exchanged between the connective tissue spaces and vessel lumina, not only in the capillaries but also in the postcapillary venules, whose walls are even more permeable. Indeed, this is the preferred location for emigration of the leukocytes from the bloodstream into the tissue spaces (Fig. 11.20). These vessels respond to pharmacological agents, such as histamine and serotonin.

The endothelial cells of venules located in certain lymphoid organs are cuboidal rather than squamous and are called ***high-endothelial venules***. These function in lymphocyte recognition and segregation by type-specific receptors on their luminal surface, ensuring that specific lymphocytes migrate into the proper regions of the lymphoid parenchyma (see Chapter 12).

TABLE 11.3 Characteristics of Veins

Type	Tunica Intima	Tunica Media	Tunica Adventitia
Large veins	Endothelium; basal lamina, valves in some; subendothelial connective tissue	Connective tissue, smooth muscle cells	Smooth muscle cells oriented in longitudinal bundles; cardiac muscle cells near their entry into the heart; collagen layers with fibroblasts
Medium and small veins	Endothelium, basal lamina; valves in some; subendothelial connective tissue	Reticular and elastic fibers, some smooth muscle cells	Collagen layers with fibroblasts
Venules	Endothelium, basal lamina (pericytes, postcapillary venules)	Sparse connective tissue and a few smooth muscle cells	Some collagen and a few fibroblasts

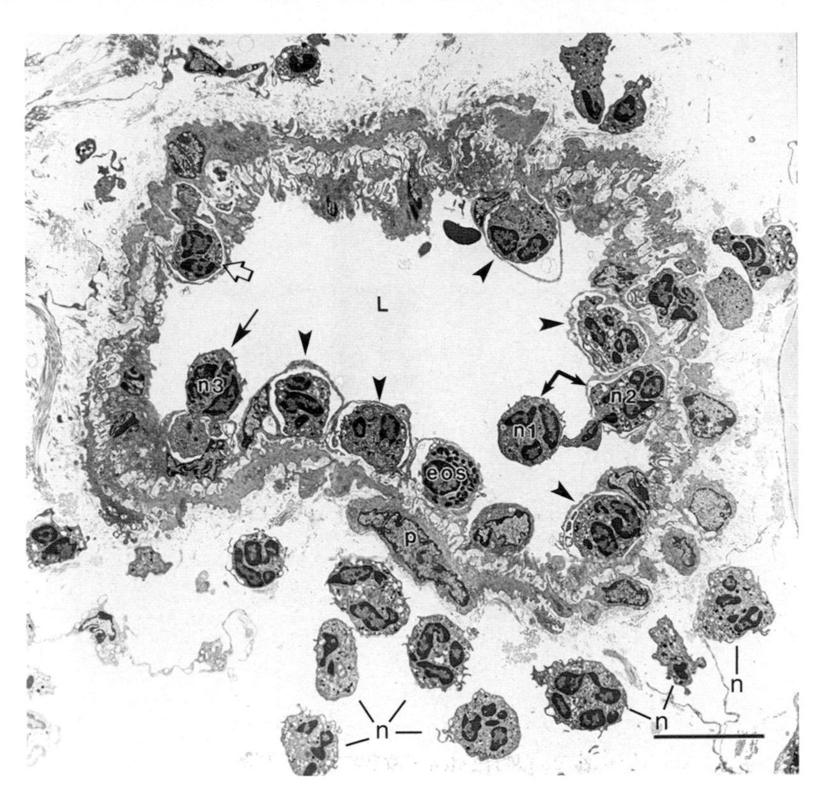

Fig. 11.20 Large venule in guinea pig skin harvested 60 minutes after intradermal injection of 10^{-5} M *N*-formyl-methionyl-leucyl-phenylalanine (*F*-MLP). Many neutrophils and a single eosinophil (eos) are captured at various stages of attachment to and extravasation across vascular endothelium and underlying pericytes (p). Two neutrophils *(single joined arrow)*, one in another lumen and another partway across the endothelium, are tethered together. Another neutrophil *(long arrow)* has projected a cytoplasmic process into an underlying endothelial cell (EC). Other neutrophils *(arrowheads)* and the eosinophil have crossed the EC barrier but remain superficial to pericytes, forming dome-like structures that bulge into the vascular lumen. Still another neutrophil *(open arrow)* that has already crossed the endothelium has extended a process into the basal lamina and indents an underlying pericyte. Other neutrophils (some indicated by *n*) have crossed both the EC and pericyte barriers and have entered the surrounding connective tissues. L, Lumen; *bar*, 10 μm. (Modified from Feng D, Nagy JA, Pyne K, et al. Neutrophils emigrate from venules by a transendothelial cell pathway in response to FMLP. *J Exp Med*. 1998;187:903–915.)

Medium Veins

Medium veins are less than 1 cm in diameter.

Medium veins are the ones draining most of the body, including most of the regions of the extremities (Fig. 11.21). Their tunica intima includes the endothelium and its basal lamina and reticular fibers. Sometimes an elastic network surrounds the endothelium, but these elastic fibers do not form laminae characteristic of an internal elastic lamina. The smooth muscle cells of the tunica media are in a loosely organized layer interwoven with collagen fibers and fibroblasts. The tunica adventitia, the thickest of the tunics, is composed of longitudinally arranged collagen bundles and elastic fibers along with a few scattered smooth muscle cells. Small and medium veins have a diameter that ranges between 1 and 9 mm.

Large Veins

Large veins return venous blood directly to the heart from the extremities, head, liver, and body wall.

Large veins include the vena cava and the pulmonary, portal, renal, internal jugular, iliac, and azygos veins. The tunica intima of the large veins is similar to that of the medium veins, except that large veins have a thick subendothelial connective tissue layer containing fibroblasts and a network of elastic fibers. Although only a few major vessels (e.g., the pulmonary veins) have a well-developed smooth muscle layer, most large veins are without a tunica media; in its place is a well-developed tunica adventitia. An exception are the superficial veins of the legs, which have a well-defined muscular wall, perhaps to resist the distention caused by gravity.

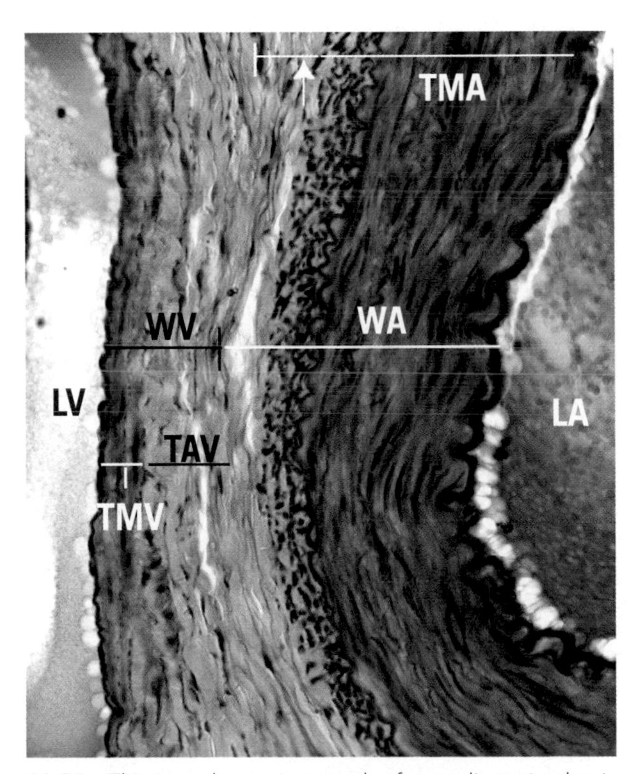

Fig. 11.21 This is a photomicrograph of a medium-sized vein and its corresponding artery. Note that the lumen of the vein (LV) is on the left and the lumen of the artery (LA) is on the right. The wall of the vein (WV) is much thinner than the wall of the artery (WA). The division between the tunica media of the artery (TMA) and the tunica adventitia of the artery is indicated by the *arrow*. The tunica adventitia of the vein (TAV) is much thicker than the tunica media of the vein (TMV). (×132)

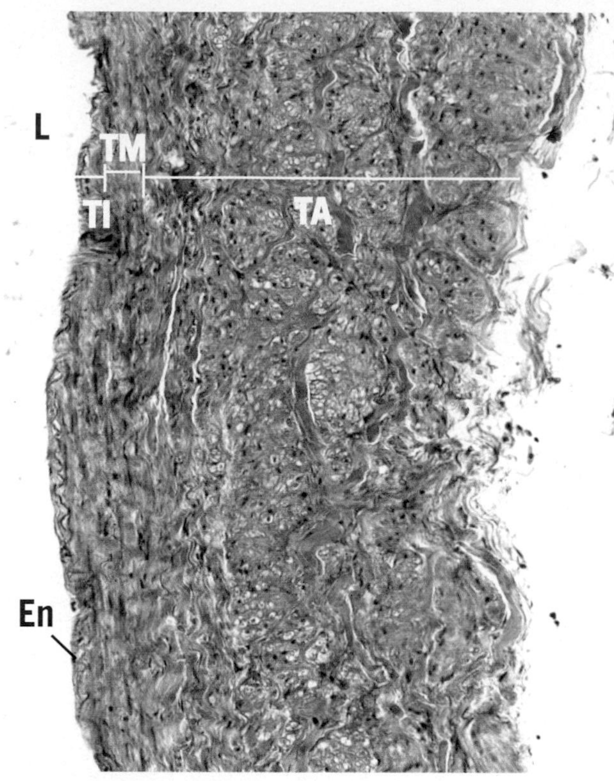

Fig. 11.22 This is a low-magnification photomicrograph of a cross-section of the human inferior vena cava. Note that the lumen (L) is lined by endothelial cells (En) of the tunica intima (TI). Observe that the tunica media (TM) is much narrower than the tunica adventitia (TA). (×132)

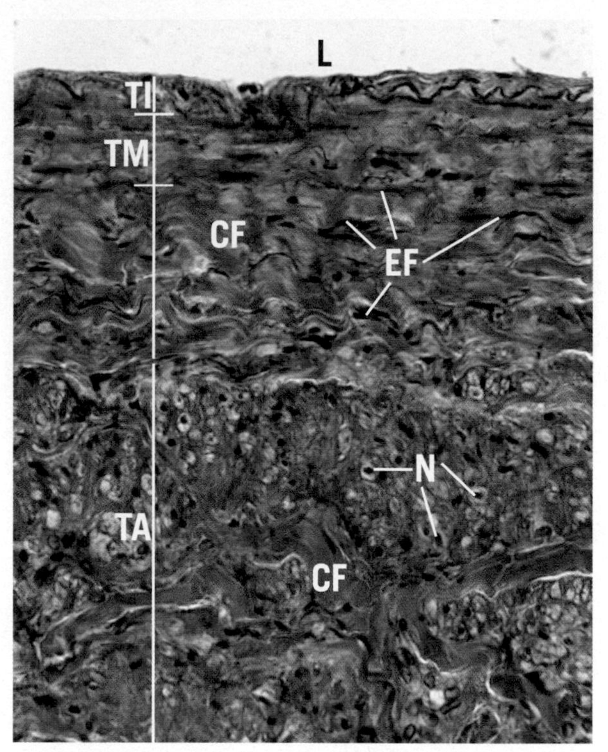

Fig. 11.23 This is a medium-power magnification of the tunica intima (TI), tunica media (TM) and part of the tunica adventitia (TA) of a cross-section of the human inferior vena cava. Note the thin tunicae intima and media. Also, observe the thick tunica adventitia, where the spirally disposed collagen fiber bundles (CF) are interspersed with thin elastic fibers. The nuclei (N) of the longitudinally oriented smooth muscle cells are compartmentalized into fascicles by bundles of collagen fibers. (×270)

The tunica adventitia of large veins contains many elastic fibers, abundant collagen fibers, and vasa vasorum. The inferior vena cava is unusual in that it has longitudinally arranged smooth muscle cells in its adventitia (Figs. 11.22 and 11.23). As the pulmonary veins and the vena cava approach the heart, their adventitia contains some cardiac muscle cells.

Valves of Veins

A venous valve is composed of two leaflets, each having a thin fold of the intima jutting out from the wall into the lumen.

Many medium-sized veins have **valves** that function to prevent the backflow of blood. These valves are especially abundant in the veins of the legs, where they act against the force of gravity. Venous valves are composed of two leaflets, each having a thin fold of the intima jutting out from the wall into the lumen. The thin leaflets are structurally reinforced by collagen and elastic fibers that are continuous with those of the vessel's wall. As blood flows to the heart, the valve cusps are deflected in the direction of the blood flow toward the heart. Backward flow of blood forces the cusps to approximate each other, thus blocking backflow.

Clinical Correlations

*Varicose veins are abnormally enlarged, tortuous veins usually affecting the superficial veins in the legs of older persons. This condition results from loss of muscle tone, degeneration of vessel walls, and valvular incompetence. Varicose veins may also occur in the lower end of the esophagus (**esophageal varices**) or at the terminus of the anal canal (**hemorrhoids**).*

HEART

The heart is a four-chambered pump of the cardiovascular system.

The muscular wall (**myocardium**) of the heart is composed of cardiac muscle (see Chapter 8). The heart consists of four chambers: two **atria**, which receive blood, and two **ventricles**, which discharge blood from the heart (Fig. 11.24) The **superior** and **inferior venae cavae** return systemic venous blood to the **right atrium** of the heart. From here, the blood passes through the **right atrioventricular valve (tricuspid valve)** into the **right ventricle**. As the ventricles contract, blood from the right ventricle is pumped out the **pulmonary trunk**, a large vessel that bifurcates into the right and left **pulmonary arteries** to deliver deoxygenated blood to the lungs for gaseous exchange. Oxygenated blood from the lungs returns to the heart via the **pulmonary veins**, which empty into the **left atrium**. From here, the blood passes through the **left atrioventricular valve** (also known as the **bicuspid valve** or **mitral valve**) to enter the **left ventricle**. Again, ventricular contraction expels the blood from the left ventricle into the aorta, from which many branches emanate to deliver blood to the tissues of the body. On a daily basis, the heart pumps approximately 2000 gallons of blood, which translates into 50 million gallons of blood in an average life span.

The atrioventricular valves prevent regurgitation of the ventricular blood back into the atria, whereas the **semilunar**

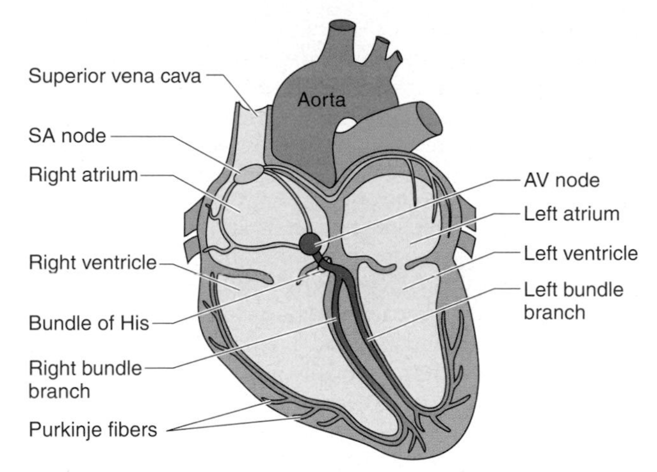

Fig. 11.24 Locations of the sinoatrial (SA) and atrioventricular (AV) nodes, Purkinje fibers, and bundle of His of the heart.

valves, located in the pulmonary trunk and the aorta near their origins, prevent backflow from these vessels into the heart.

Layers of the Heart Wall

The three layers that constitute the heart wall are the **endocardium**, **myocardium**, and **epicardium**, homologous to the tunica intima, tunica media, and the tunica adventitia, respectively, of the blood vessels.

Endocardium

The endocardium, a simple squamous epithelium and underlying subendothelial connective tissue, lines the lumen of the heart.

The **endocardium** is continuous with the tunica intima of the blood vessels entering and leaving the heart. It is composed of an **endothelium**, consisting of a simple squamous epithelium and an underlying layer of fibroelastic connective tissue with scattered fibroblasts. Lying deeper is a layer of dense connective tissue, heavily endowed with elastic fibers interspersed with smooth muscle cells. Deep to the endocardium is a **subendocardial layer** of loose connective tissue that contains small blood vessels, nerves, and Purkinje fibers from the conduction system of the heart. The subendocardial layer forms the boundary of the endocardium as it attaches to the endomysium of the cardiac muscle.

Clinical Correlations

1. *Children who have had* **rheumatic fever** *may later develop* **rheumatic heart valve disease** *as a result of scarring of the valves stemming from the rheumatic fever episode. This condition develops because the valves cannot properly close (incompetence) or open (stenosis), owing to reduced elasticity as a result of rheumatic fever. The* **bicuspid** *(***mitral***)* **valve***, followed by the* **aortic valves***, is the valve most commonly affected.*
2. *It has been demonstrated that in vivo administration of two microribonucleic acids (microRNAs), hsa-miR-590 and hsa-miR-199a, was able to cause regeneration of cardiac muscle cells subsequent to myocardial infarction in mice to the extent that these animals recovered almost completely and had stable cardiac function. It is hoped that this finding can be applied to humans in the near future.*

Myocardium

The thick middle layer of the heart (the myocardium) is composed of cardiac muscle cells.

The **myocardium**, the middle and thickest of the three layers of the heart, contains cardiac muscle cells, arranged in complex spirals around the orifices of the chambers. Certain cardiac muscle cells attach the myocardium to the fibrous cardiac skeleton, others are specialized for endocrine secretions, and still others are specialized for impulse generation or impulse conduction.

The heart rate (~70–80 beats per minute) is controlled by the **sinoatrial (SA) node (pacemaker)** located at the junction of the superior vena cava and the right atrium (see Fig. 11.24). These specialized nodal cardiac muscle cells can spontaneously depolarize 70 to 80 times per minute, creating an impulse that spreads over the atrial chamber walls by internodal pathways to the **atrioventricular node**, located in the septal wall just above the tricuspid valve. Modified cardiac muscle cells of the atrioventricular node, regulated by impulses arriving from the sinoatrial node, transmit signals to the myocardium of the atria via the **atrioventricular bundle** (**bundle of His**). Fibers from the atrioventricular bundle pass down the interventricular septum to conduct the impulse to the cardiac muscle, producing a rhythmic contraction (see Fig. 11.24). The atrioventricular bundle travels in the subendocardial connective tissue as large, modified cardiac muscle cells, forming **Purkinje fibers** (Fig. 11.25), which transmit impulses to the cardiac muscle cells located at the apex of the heart (Purkinje fibers are not be confused with the *Purkinje cells* in the cerebellar cortex). It should be noted that although the autonomic nervous system does not initiate the heartbeat, it does modulate the rate and stroke volume of the heartbeat. Stimulation of sympathetic nerves accelerates the heart rate, whereas stimulation of the parasympathetic nerves serving the heart slows the heart rate.

Specialized cardiac muscle cells, located primarily in the atrial wall and in the interventricular septum, produce **atrial natriuretic peptide which is released into the surrounding capillaries**. Cardiac muscle cells of the ventricle produce **B-type natriuretic peptide**, which is also released into the surrounding capillaries (Fig. 11.26). These peptides aid in fluid maintenance and electrolyte balance and decrease blood pressure by decreasing blood volume.

Clinical Correlations

B-type natriuretic peptide (BNP) release by the specialized cardiac muscle cells of the ventricles has been correlated with **congestive heart failure***. Indeed, the more serious the condition, the more BNP is released.*

Epicardium

The epicardium represents the homologue of the tunica adventitia in blood vessels.

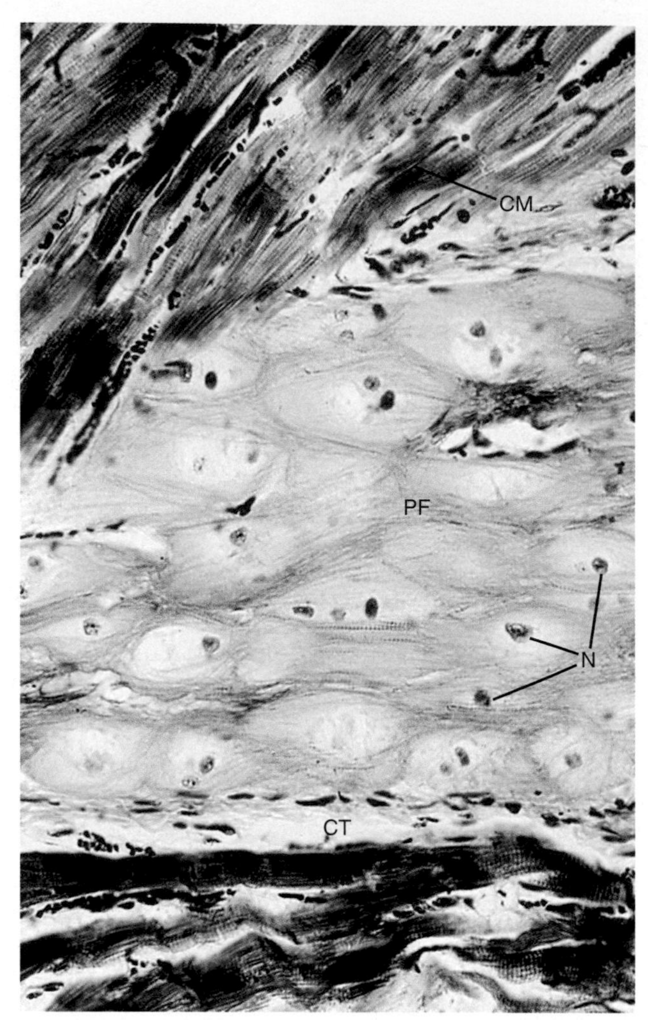

Fig. 11.25 Light micrograph of Purkinje fibers. Cardiac muscle (CM) appears very dark, whereas Purkinje fibers (PF) with their solitary nuclei (N) appear light with this stain. Slender connective tissue elements (CT) surround the Purkinje fibers. (×270)

Epicardium, the outermost layer of the heart wall, is also called the ***visceral layer of the pericardium*** (composed of a simple squamous epithelium known as a ***mesothelium*** and the underlying loose connective tissue, the **subepicardium**). The subepicardium houses the coronary vessels, nerves, and ganglia. It also is the region where fat is stored on the surface of the heart. At the roots of the vessels entering and leaving the heart, the visceral pericardium becomes continuous with the serous layer of the parietal pericardium. These two layers of the pericardium enclose the pericardial cavity, a space containing a small amount of serous fluid for lubricating the serous layer of the pericardium and the visceral pericardium, providing almost friction-free conditions for contractile movement of the heart.

Clinical Correlations

*Infection in the pericardial cavity, called **pericarditis**, severely restricts the heart from beating properly because the space is obliterated by adhesions between the epicardium and the serous layer of the pericardium.*

Cardiac Skeleton

The cardiac skeleton, composed of dense collagenous connective tissue, includes three main components:

- **Annuli fibrosi**, formed around the base of the aorta, pulmonary artery, and the atrioventricular orifices
- **Trigonum fibrosum**, formed primarily in the vicinity of the cuspal area of the aortic valve
- **Septum membranaceum**, constituting the upper portion of the interventricular septum

In addition to providing a structural framework for the heart and attachment sites for the cardiac muscle, the cardiac skeleton provides a discontinuity between the myocardia of the atria and the myocardia of the ventricles, ensuring a rhythmic and cyclic beating of the heart controlled solely by the conduction mechanism of the atrioventricular bundles.

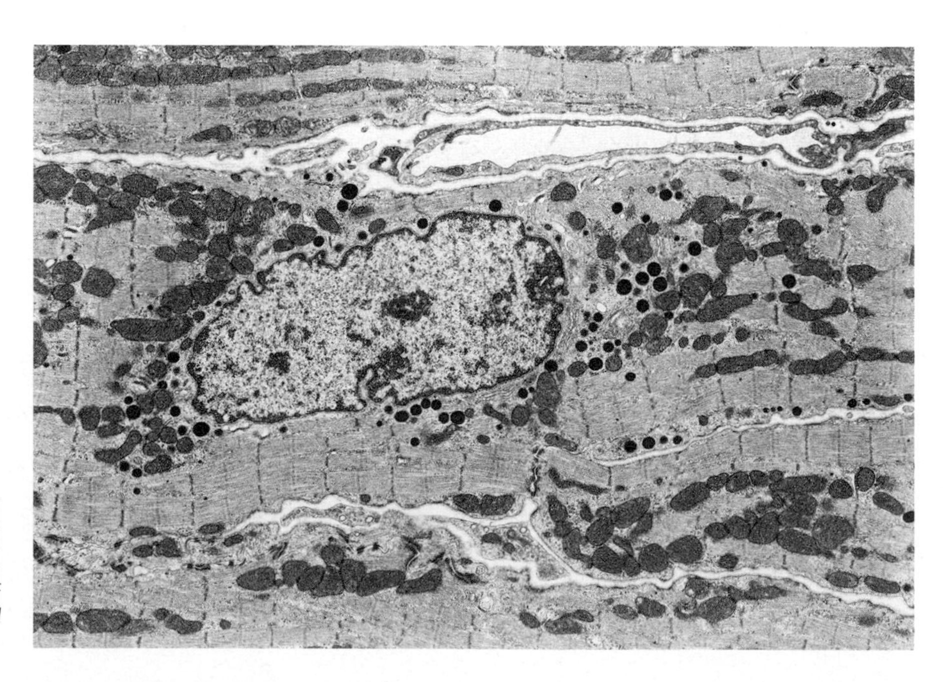

Fig. 11.26 Electron micrograph of a cardiac muscle cell containing clusters of vesicles with atrial natriuretic peptide (ANP). (From Mifune H, Suzuki S, Honda J, et al. Atrial natriuretic peptide (ANP): a study of ANP and its mRNA in cardiocytes, and of plasma ANP levels in non-obese diabetic mice. *Cell Tissue Res.* 1992;267:267–272.)

Clinical Correlations

1. *Ischemic (coronary) heart disease, especially prevalent in older persons, is related to* **atherosclerosis of the coronary vessels** *serving the myocardium. As atherosclerotic plaques reduce the lumina of the coronary vessels, the patient may experience referred pain and pressure, known as* **angina pectoris**, *from lack of oxygen. Continued narrowing results in ischemia of the heart wall, which may be fatal if untreated. Angioplasty is the current mode of initial invasive treatment for partially occluded arteries.*
2. *Prinzmetal angina (coronary vessel spasm) is a rare condition affecting about 4 people per 100,000, in which the coronary arteries undergo spasms and restrict blood flow to the heart. These spasms may occur randomly (though usually when the patient is resting) and cause angina-like chest pains. The condition is not related to coronary arterial disease or to atherosclerosis and is more common in females than in males. Smoking, cocaine use, and stress are some of the few known aggravating conditions that bring about the spasms. Orally administered calcium channel blockers and nitrates appear to prevent the spasms from occurring. Without treatment, the possibility of cardiac arrest is increased.*
3. *Atrial fibrillation is a condition of arrhythmic heartbeat involving the atria only. The erratic atrial heartbeat disrupts normal blood flow and may cause the formation of small blood clots. If these small clots enter the circulation, they can occlude smaller vessels, including those in the brain. It has been demonstrated that as many as 15% of stroke victims present with atrial fibrillation that may have been responsible for the stroke in these patients.*

Lymphatic Vascular System

The lymphatic vascular system consists of vessels that collect the excess extracellular fluid (interstitial fluid) and return it to the cardiovascular system.

The **lymphatic vascular system** is composed of a series of vessels that remove excess extracellular fluid from the extracellular tissue spaces and return it to the cardiovascular system. Lymphatic vessels are present throughout the body except in the CNS (although some investigators suggest otherwise), orbit, internal ear, epidermis, cartilage, and bone. Unlike the cardiovascular system, which contains a pump (the heart) and circulates blood in a *closed* system, the lymphatic vascular system is an *open* system in that there is no pump and no circulation of fluid.

The lymphatic vascular system begins in the tissues of the body as blind-ended **lymphatic capillaries** (Fig. 11.27), which simply act as drain fields for excess extracellular fluid. The lymphatic capillaries empty their contents, known as ***lymph***, into **lymphatic vessels**, which empty into successively larger vessels until one of the two **lymphatic ducts** is reached. From either of these ducts, the lymph is emptied into the venous portion of the cardiovascular system at the junctions of the internal jugular and the subclavian veins.

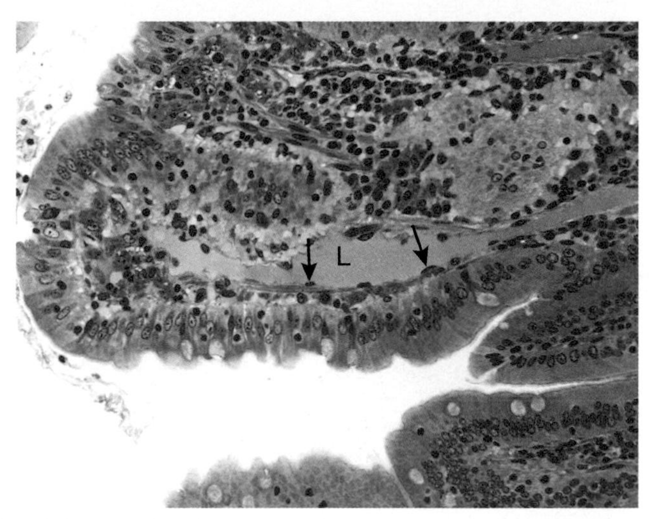

Fig. 11.27 The lymph vessel in the villus core of the small intestine is known as a *lacteal* (L). Observe the endothelial lining of the lacteal *(arrows)*. This photomicrograph is taken of the monkey duodenum. (×270)

Lymph nodes are interposed along the paths of lymphatic vessels, and lymph must pass through them to be filtered. **Afferent lymphatic vessels** deliver lymph into the lymph nodes, where lymph is distributed into labyrinthine channels (medullary sinuses) lined by an endothelium and abundant macrophages. Here, the lymph is filtered and cleared of particulate matter. Lymphocytes are added to the lymph as it leaves the lymph node via **efferent lymphatic vessels**, eventually reaching a lymphatic duct. Lymph nodes are discussed in Chapter 12.

LYMPHATIC CAPILLARIES AND VESSELS

Lymphatic capillaries are composed of a single layer of attenuated endothelial cells with an incomplete basal lamina.

The blind-ended, thin-walled **lymphatic capillaries** are composed of a single layer of attenuated endothelial cells with an incomplete basal lamina (Fig. 11.28). The endothelial cells overlap each other in places but have ample intercellular clefts that permit easy access to the lumen of the vessel. These cells do not have fenestrae and do not make tight junctions with each other. Bundles of **lymphatic anchoring filaments** (5–10 nm in diameter) terminate on the abluminal plasma membrane. It is thought that these filaments may play a role in maintaining the luminal patency of these flimsy vessels.

Small and medium lymphatic vessels are characterized by closely spaced valves. Large lymphatic vessels resemble small veins structurally, except that their lumina are larger and their walls are thinner. Large lymphatic vessels have a thin layer of elastic fibers beneath their endothelium and a sparse layer of smooth muscle cells. This smooth muscle layer is then overlaid with elastic and collagen fibers that blend with the surrounding connective tissue, much like a tunica adventitia. Although some histologists describe tunics similar to those in blood vessels, most do not concur because there are no clear

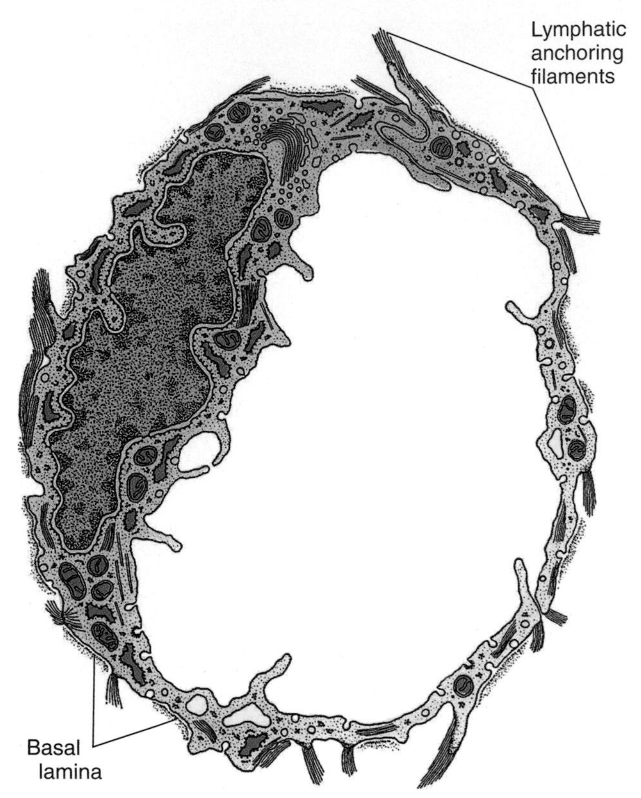

Fig. 11.28 Diagram of the ultrastructure of a lymphatic capillary. (From Lentz TL. *Cell Fine Structure: An Atlas of Drawings of Whole-Cell Structure*. Philadelphia: WB Saunders; 1971.)

boundaries between the layers and because the walls of lymph vessels are so varied.

LYMPHATIC DUCTS

Lymphatic ducts are similar to large veins; they empty their contents into the great veins of the neck.

Clinical Correlations

Malignant tumor cells (especially carcinomas) are spread throughout the body by lymphatic vessels. When the malignant cells reach a lymph node, they are slowed and multiply there, eventually leaving to metastasize to a secondary site. Therefore, in surgical removal of a cancerous growth, examination of the lymph nodes and removal of both enlarged lymph nodes in the pathway and associated lymphatic vessels are essential in preventing secondary growth of the tumor.

The **lymphatic ducts**, which are similar in structure to large veins, are the final two collecting vessels of the lymphatic vascular system. The short **right lymphatic duct** empties its contents into the venous system at the junction of the right internal jugular and right subclavian veins. The larger, the **thoracic duct**, empties its contents at the junction of the left internal jugular and left subclavian veins. The right lymphatic duct collects lymph from the upper right quadrant of the body, whereas the thoracic duct collects lymph from the remainder of the body.

The tunica intima of lymphatic ducts is composed of an endothelium and several layers of elastic and collagen fibers. At the interface with the tunica media, a layer of condensed elastic fibers resembles an internal elastic lamina. Both longitudinal and circular layers of smooth muscle are present in the media. The tunica adventitia contains longitudinally oriented smooth muscle cells and collagen fibers that blend into the surrounding connective tissue. Piercing the walls of the thoracic duct are small vessels homologous to the vasa vasorum of the arteries.

Pathological Considerations

See Figs. 11.29 through 11.32.

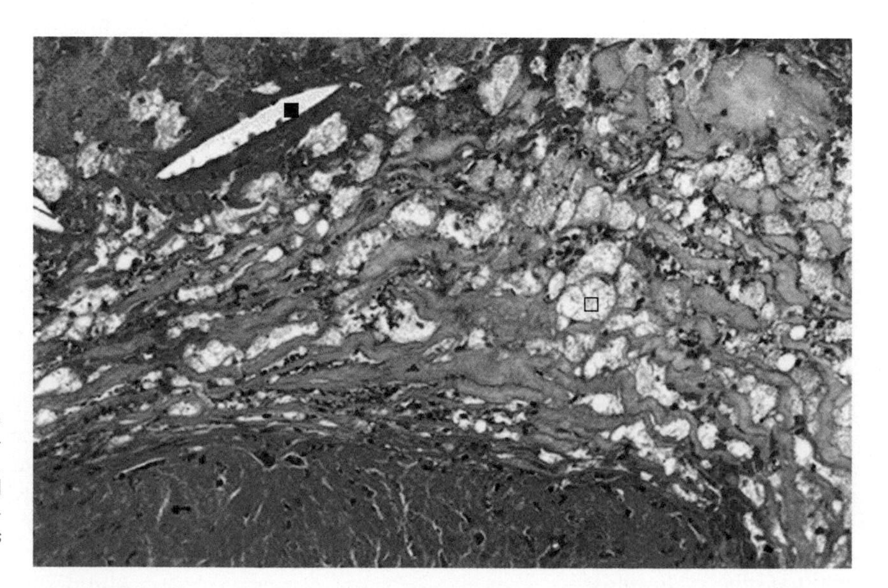

Fig. 11.29 Photomicrograph of a coronary artery with atherosclerosis. Note that there are residual smooth muscle cells in the tunica media and the atheroma overlying it. Observe the presence of fat deposits *(open square)* and cholesterol clefts *(filled square)*. (Reprinted with permission from Klatt EC. *Robbins and Cotran: Pathological Basis of Disease*. 2nd ed. Philadelphia: Elsevier; 2010:5.)

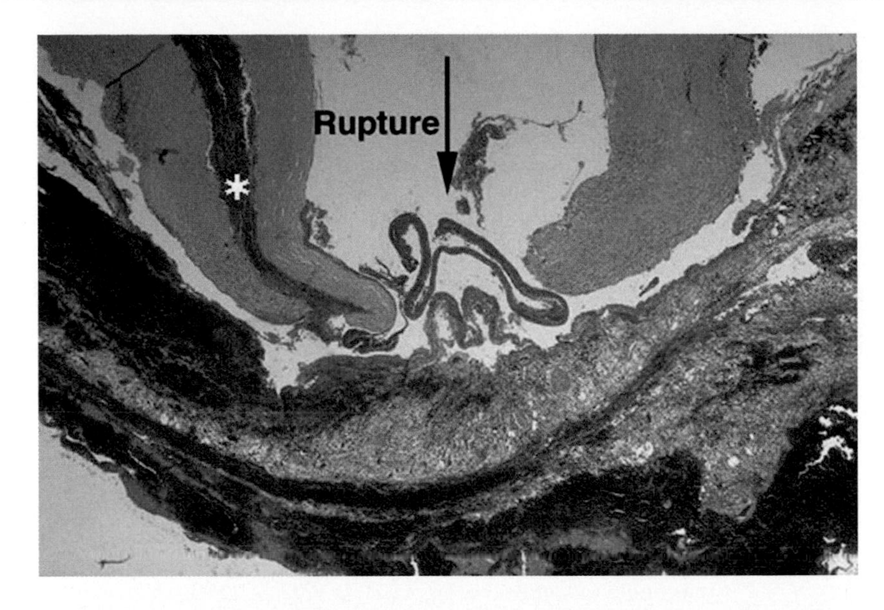

Fig. 11.30 Photomicrograph of the aorta displaying a rupture, as well as the aortic dissection along the tunica media caused by the pressure created by the escaped blood *(asterisk)*. (Reprinted with permission from Klatt EC. *Robbins and Cotran: Pathological Basis of Disease*. 2nd ed. Philadelphia: Elsevier; 2010:11.)

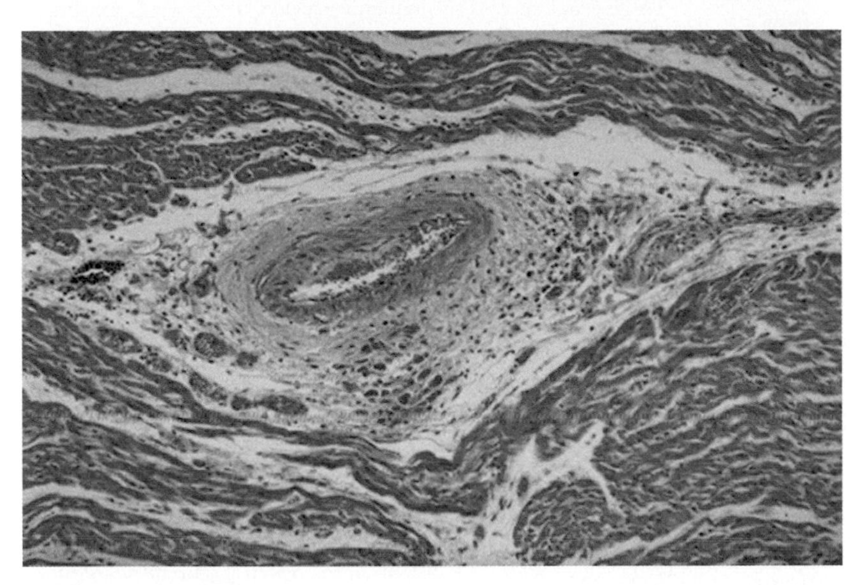

Fig. 11.31 Photomicrograph of rheumatic heart disease. Note the presence of the characteristic Aschoff nodule at the lower middle of the field, composed of mostly mononuclear inflammatory cells. (Reprinted with permission from Klatt EC. *Robbins and Cotran: Pathological Basis of Disease*. 2nd ed. Philadelphia: Elsevier; 2010:46.)

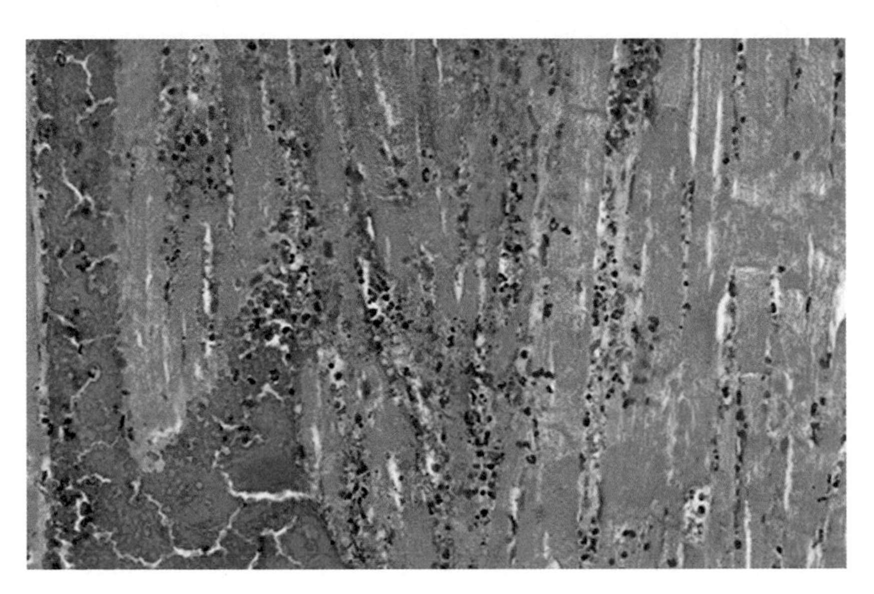

Fig. 11.32 Photomicrograph of a myocardial infarction about 3 to 4 days after the damage. Note the necrotic cardiac muscle cells as well as the acute infiltration of inflammatory cells. (Reprinted with permission from Klatt EC. *Robbins and Cotran: Pathological Basis of Disease*. 2nd ed. Philadelphia: Elsevier; 2010:41.)

Histology Laboratory Instructions: Circulatory System

The Three Tunicae of a Blood Vessel

Before studying the various types of arteries and veins, it is advisable to understand the ***three tunicae*** (three layers) that constitute the wall of a vessel. The best way of observing these is to look at the microscopic image of the cross-section of a muscular artery at a low magnification. Identify the lumen and the very thin tunica intima (composed of the endothelium, subendothelial connective tissue, and internal elastic lamina) that lines it. Proceeding away from the lumen is the tunica media—the thick, muscular region of the vessel wall that includes the external elastic lamina. The outermost region of the vessel wall is the tunica adventitia, composed of collagenous connective tissue, through which thin elastic fibers ramify. The tunica adventitia is thicker than the tunica intima but thinner than the tunica media and in larger vessels house vasa vasorum and nerve fibers (see Fig. 11.5, L, TI, iEL, TM, xEL). These three tunicae and their component parts are modified in the various types of arteries and veins, but the concept of the three layers remains constant.

Arteries

Elastic arteries, such as the aorta, display the three tunics. The tunica intima has three components, the endothelial lining, the thick subendothelial connective tissue with its smooth muscle cells and elastic fibers, and the sparse internal elastic lamina (see Fig. 11.3, TI, N, SMN, EF, iEL). The tunica media has many layers of fenestrated sheets of elastin—known as the fenestrated membranes—where the gaps, fenestrae, are clearly evident. Between the fenestrated membranes, the nuclei of the numerous smooth muscle cells are visible (see Fig. 11.4, FM, N, *arrows* indicate fenestrae). The interface between the tunica media and the tunica adventitia are plainly evident. The fenestrated membranes dominate the tunica media, whereas the tunica adventitia has only a limited number of slender elastic fibers in its collagenous connective tissue. A vasa vasorum (unlabeled) is present as a round, mostly empty structure at the bottom right near the interface of the tunica media and the tunica adventitia (see Fig. 11.2, TM, TA, FM)

Muscular arteries appear quite different from elastic arteries. Their tunic intima is very slender and its internal elastic lamina separates it from the very muscular tunica media. The external elastic lamina of the tunica media separates it from the collagenous connective tissue of the tunica adventitia (see Fig. 11.5, TI, iEL, TM, xEL). Viewed at medium magnification, the lumen of a muscular artery is seen to be lined by the endothelium, subendothelial connective tissue, and internal elastic lamina, the three components of the tunica intima. The smooth muscle fibers of the tunica media are seen to be permeated by thin elastic fibers (see Fig. 11.6, L, IEL, TI, N, TM, EF). At high magnification, the endothelial lining of the tunica intima, the internal elastic lamina, and the intervening collagenous connective tissue composing the subendothelial connective tissue are all clearly evident. Observe the thin elastic fibers and the nuclei of the smooth muscle cells (see Fig. 11.7, En, TI, IEL, EF, N). The thin elastic fibers, the nuclei of the smooth muscle cells, and the external elastic lamina of the tunica media are well represented in this high-magnification photomicrograph (see Fig. 11.8, EF, N, EEL).

Arterioles are less than 0.1 mm in diameter and the width of their walls approximate the diameter of their lumina. Their tunica media is very muscular in comparison with the size of the vessel. Usually, the lumen of an arteriole is empty of blood, unlike the lumen of their corresponding venule (Fig. 11.9, A, TM, L, Ve).

Capillaries are the smallest of the vascular channels, about 8 to 10 µm in diameter. They are present in most areas of the body but are best seen in longitudinal sections in the cerebellum. Note that capillaries are simply tubes of endothelial cells and their nuclei bulge into the lumen, which may or may not house blood cells (see Fig. 11.12, Ca, *arrow*, L, RBC)

Veins

Venules are larger than their corresponding arterioles and their lumina usually contain blood cells. Their tunica media are reduced in thickness and possess a relatively thick tunica adventitia (see Fig. 11.9, Ve, L, RBC, TM).

Medium veins have a much thinner wall than their corresponding muscular arteries and their tunica media is relatively slender, housing few smooth muscle cells. The thickest component of the medium vein is its tunica adventitia (see Fig. 11.21, WV, TMV, TAV).

Large veins, such as the human vena cava, also possess the three tunicae, with a slender tunica intima whose endothelial cells line the lumen, the thin tunica media, and their thick tunica adventitia (see Fig. 11.22, TI, En, L, TM, TA). Viewing the human vena cava at a medium magnification displays the narrow tunica intima lining the lumen of the vessel. The tunica media houses sparse circularly displayed smooth muscle cells and a few narrow elastic fibers embedded in a collagenous connective tissue. The thickest of the three tunicae is the tunica adventitia, with its outermost spirally arranged collagen fiber bundles, the large number of longitudinally disposed smooth muscle cells divided into fascicles by thick collagen fiber sheaths. Although not shown, the tunica adventitia is said to be composed of three concentric layers (see Fig. 11.23, TI, L, TM, EF, CF, TA).

Heart

The ***heart*** is a thick modified blood vessel that is composed of three layers, which are, from the lumen outward, the endocardium, myocardium, and the visceral layer of the epicardium. The endocardium consists of an endothelium that lines the ventricles and atria of the heart. Deep to the endocardium is a subendocardial layer of loose connective tissue that contains small blood vessels, nerve fibers, and Purkinje fibers whose smaller branches penetrate the myocardium, the thick layer of the heart composed mostly of cardiac muscle cells. Purkinje fibers and their branches are modified cardiac muscle cells with a centrally placed nucleus among the cardiac muscle cells of the myocardium, which are surrounded by a scant amount of connective tissue (see Fig. 11.25, PF, N, CM, CT).

Lymph Vessels

The best place to see lymph vessels is the capsule of lymph nodes, which will be described in Chapter 12, as will the lymphatic sinusoids. Lymphatic capillaries are blind-ended vessels composed of a single layer of attenuated endothelial cells with an incomplete basal lamina. The best place to see them is in the core of the villi of the small intestine, where they are known as lacteals. The endothelium lining their lumina is composed of highly attenuated cells. Their lumen houses no blood cells (see Fig. 11.27, L, *arrows*).

12

Lymphoid (Immune) System

The lymphoid system is responsible for the immunological defense of the body. Some of its component organs—**bone marrow**, **lymph nodes**, **thymus**, and **spleen**—are surrounded by connective tissue capsules, whereas its other components, members of the **diffuse lymphoid system**, are not encapsulated. The cells of the lymphoid system protect the body against foreign macromolecules, viruses, bacteria, and other invasive microorganisms, and they kill cells of the self that were virally transformed.

There are two categories of lymphoid organs: primary and secondary. **Primary lymphoid organs** (bone marrow and thymus) participate in the development of immunocompetent lymphocytes. **Secondary lymphoid organs** (lymph nodes, spleen, tonsils, and diffuse lymphoid tissue) function in trapping antigens and providing sites for the interactions of antigen-presenting cells (APCs) with immunocompetent lymphocytes, where they can mount an immune response and thereby remove the antigenic assault.

Overview of the Immune System

The immune system has two components: the innate immune system and the adaptive immune system.

The first line of defense against invading pathogens is a physical barrier—the skin and the mucosa—structures that completely cover and line the external and internal surfaces of the body. Breaching of the skin and mucosa, permitting foreign substances to attempt penetration or actually penetrate the intact barrier, activates the innate and the adaptive immune systems—the second and third lines of defense, respectively.

The complexity of the immune system prevents a complete treatment of the topic here. To make the reading of this material easier for the student, certain information is repeated in various sections of the presentation to avoid the need for cross-referencing.

The **innate immune system** (natural immune system) is *nonspecific* and is composed of (1) a system of blood-borne macromolecules (C1 to C9) known as ***complement***; (2) natural (polyreactive) antibodies present in the bloodstream; (3) **Toll-like receptors (TLRs)**, a family of integral proteins localized on either the plasmalemma or endosomal (and RER) membranes of cells; (4) groups of cells known as ***macrophages*** and ***neutrophils***, which phagocytose invaders; and (5) another group of cells, **natural killer (NK) cells**, which kill tumor cells, virally infected cells, bacteria, and parasites.

The **adaptive immune system** (**acquired immune system**) is responsible for eliminating threats from *specific* invaders. Whereas a macrophage can phagocytose most bacteria, the adaptive immune system not only reacts against one specific antigenic component of a pathogen but also its ability to react against that particular component improves with subsequent confrontations with it.

Although the two systems differ in their mode of responses, they are intimately related to one another, and each affects the other's activities.

THE INNATE IMMUNE SYSTEM

The innate immune system responds rapidly, has no immunological memory, and depends on complement and TLRs for initiating inflammatory and/or immune responses.

Although the **innate immune system** is much older than the adaptive immune system, it responds rapidly, usually within a few hours, to an antigenic invasion; it responds in a nonspecific manner; and it has no immunological memory. The critical components of the innate immune system are complement, antimicrobial peptides, cytokines, macrophages, neutrophils, NK cells, and TLRs. (Table 12.1 presents acronyms and abbreviations used in this chapter.)

Complement is a series of blood-borne proteins that attack microbes that found their way into the bloodstream. As complement proteins precipitate on the surface of these invading pathogens, they form a **membrane attack complex** (**MAC**) that damages the microbe's cell membrane. Phagocytic cells, such as neutrophils and macrophages, of the host have receptors for a specific moiety of complement (**C3b**) and the presence of C3b on the microbial surface facilitates phagocytosis of microbes by these host defense cells.

Natural (**polyreactive**) **antibodies** are formed prior to birth, even in germ-free mice by innate B cells that have not as yet been exposed to antigens and are able to bind to many different antigens. These antibodies are able to recognize and react against oxidized lipids on cells that have entered apoptosis, as well as membrane lipids present in invading microorganisms. Unlike antibodies of the adaptive immune systems, polyreactive antibodies bind with a low binding affinity.

Antimicrobial peptides, such as **defensins**, are synthesized and released by epithelial cells. They not only defend the body against Gram-negative bacteria but also are chemoattractants for immature dendritic cells and T lymphocytes.

Cytokines are signaling molecules that are released by various cells of the innate and adaptive immune systems to effect responses from their target cells. Cytokines that are released by lymphocytes are known as **lymphokines**, usually named **interleukins**, whereas cytokines that possess chemoattractant capabilities are usually referred to as **chemokines.** Those cytokines that stimulate differentiation and mitotic activity of hemopoietic cells are known as **colony-stimulating factors** (**CSFs**), whereas cytokines displaying antiviral properties are referred to as **interferons**.

TABLE 12.1 Acronyms and Abbreviations

Acronym/ Abbreviation	Meaning of Acronym/Abbreviation
ADDC	Antibody-dependent cellular cytotoxicity
AIDS	Acquired immunodeficiency syndrome
APC	Antigen-presenting cell
BALT	Bronchus-associated lymphoid tissue
B lymphocyte	Bursa-derived lymphocyte (bone marrow-derived lymphocyte)
C3b	Complement 3b
CD	Cluster of differentiation molecule (followed by an Arabic numeral)
CLIP	Class II-associated invariant protein
CSF	Colony-stimulating factor
CTL	Cytotoxic T lymphocyte (T killer cell)
Fab	Antigen binding fragment of an antibody
Fas protein	CD95 (induces apoptosis)
Fc	Crystallized fragment (constant fragment of an antibody
GALT	Gut-associated lymphoid tissue
G-CSF	Granulocyte–colony-stimulating factor
GM-CSF	Granulocyte-macrophage–colony-stimulating factor
HEV	High endothelial venules
HIV	Human immunodeficiency virus
IFN-γ	Interferon-gamma
Ig	Immunoglobulin (followed by a capital letter: A, D, E, G, or M)
IL	Interleukin (followed by an Arabic numeral)
M cell	Microfold cell
MAC	Membrane attack complex
MALT	Mucosa-associated lymphoid tissue
MHC I and MHC II	Major histocompatibility class I molecules and class II molecules
MIIC vesicle	MHC class II–enriched compartment
NK cell	Natural killer cells
PALS	Periarterial lymphatic sheath
sIgs	Surface immunoglobulins
TAP	Transporter protein (1 and 2)
TCM	Central memory T cell
TCR	T-cell receptor
TEM	Effector T memory cell
T_h cell	T helper cell (followed by an Arabic numeral)
TLRs	Toll-like receptors
T lymphocyte	Thymus-derived lymphocyte
TNF-α	Tumor necrosis factor-alpha
T reg cell	Regulatory T cell

Macrophages possess (1) receptors for the constant portions of antibodies (Fc receptors), (2) complement receptors, and (3) receptors that recognize carbohydrates that are not usually present on the surface of vertebrate cells. Macrophages are also antigen-presenting cells (APCs) because they are able to present antigens to both T and B lymphocytes. They also release CSFs and other signaling molecules that induce the formation of neutrophils and their release into the circulating blood.

Neutrophils leave the vascular system in the region of inflammation and enter the bacteria-laden connective tissue compartment, where they phagocytose and destroy bacteria. Bacterial killing is effected either in an oxygen-dependent manner, by the formation of hydrogen peroxide, hydroxyl radicals, and singlet oxygen within the phagolysosomes/endosomes, or via enzymatic digestion, using cationic proteins as well as myeloperoxidase and lysozymes.

NK cells are similar to cytotoxic T cells of the adaptive immune system. However, unlike T cells, they do not have to enter the thymus to become mature killer cells. NK cells use nonspecific markers to recognize their target cells via two different methods.

1. NK cells possess Fc receptors, recognizing the constant portion of the immunoglobulin G (IgG) antibody that acts as a signal to kill the target cell. This is known as ***antibody-dependent cellular cytotoxicity*** (***ADDC***).
2. The NK cell surface also displays transmembrane proteins known as ***killer activating receptors*** that bind to certain markers on the surface of nucleated cells. In order to control this killing process, NK cells also possess **killer inhibitory receptors** (**KIPs**) that recognize major histocompatibility (MHC) type I molecules located on the plasma membranes of all cells. The presence of MHC I molecule activates the KIPs, which prevent NK cells from killing healthy cells. The absence of MHC I molecules from the cell membrane or the presence of defective or altered MHC I molecules on the cell membrane indicates to NK cells that these are either foreign cells or virally altered self cells (target cells) that have to be destroyed.

The presence of various cytokines—such as interleukins 12, 15, and 18 (IL-12, IL-15, and IL-18) and type I interferons—enhance the cytotoxic activities of NK cells by causing them to become **effector NK cells.** IL-12 and IL-15 also induce NK cells to enter the cell cycle, thus increasing the number of effector NK cells.

Effector NK cells release perforin molecules that attach to the plasmalemmae of target cells, where they assemble to form pores. They also release granzymes that pass through these pores to enter the target cell cytoplasm, forcing them into apoptosis. Effector NK cells also release interferon gamma (IFN-γ), which recruits and activates macrophages to the area of the response. The activated macrophages destroy invading microorganisms and provide time for the adaptive immune system to control the infection.

Clinical Correlations

Major histocompatibility (MHC) I molecules, discussed later, are required to be present on cell membranes of almost every nucleated cell for cytotoxic T lymphocytes (CTLs) to recognize them as targets for destruction. However, tumor cells and cells that are infected by viruses suppress the production of MHC I molecules in order to prevent their recognition as targets for CTLs. This evasive maneuver permits them to become targets of NK cells because their killer inhibitory receptors do not become activated. In addition to MHC I molecules, MHC II molecules are located on the surface of APCs.

TLRs are highly conserved integral proteins present in the plasma and endosomal membranes of macrophages and dendritic cells of the innate immune system. Humans have been shown to possess at least 10 different TLRs (Table 12.2), each with different roles. TLRs function in pairs so that two TLR partners form a single active receptor. These may be the same TLRs (e.g., TLR4-TLR4; homodimers) or different TLRs (TLR1-TLR2; heterodimers). Some of the TLRs are present on cell membranes so that they have both *intracellular* and *extracellular moieties*, whereas other TLRs are located only

TABLE 12.2 Toll-Like Receptors, Their Locations, and Their Putative Functions

Domains	Toll-Like Receptor Pair	Located on/in Cell	Functions
Intracellular and extracellular (on cell membrane)	TLR1–TLR2	Monocytes, macrophages, dendritic cells, B cells, mast cells	Binds to bacterial lipoprotein; also binds to certain proteins of parasites
	TLR2–TLR2	Monocytes, macrophages, dendritic cells, B cells, mast cells	Binds to peptidoglycan of bacteria
	TLR2–TLR6	Monocytes, macrophages, dendritic cells, B cells, mast cells	Binds to lipoteichoic acid of gram-positive bacterial wall; also binds to zymosan, a fungally derived polysaccharide
	TLR4–TLR4	Monocytes, macrophages, mast cells, lining cells of the digestive system	Binds to LPS (lipoprotein saccharide) of Gram-negative bacteria
	TLR5–??[a]	Monocytes, macrophages, dendritic cells, mast cells, lining cells of the digestive system	Binds to flagellin of bacterial flagella
Intracellular only	TLR3–??[a]	Dendritic cells and B cells	Binds to double-stranded viral RNA (dsRNA)
	TLR7–??[a]	Monocytes, macrophages, dendritic cells, B cells	Binds to single-stranded viral RNA (ssRNA)
	TLR8–??[a]	Monocytes, macrophages, dendritic cells, mast cells	Binds to single stranded viral RNA (ssRNA)
	TLR9–??[a]	Monocytes, macrophages, dendritic cells, B cells	Binds to bacterial and viral DNA
	TLR10–??[a]	Monocytes, macrophages, B cells	Unknown

[a]Currently, TLR partner is unknown.

intracellularly on the membranes of endosomes and rough endoplasmic reticulum (RER) and possess no extracellular moieties.

TLR pairs recognize various pathogens by their specific recurring molecular signatures, known as ***pathogen-associated molecular patterns*** (***PAMPs***). TLRs located on the cell membrane distinguish PAMPs belonging to bacteria, fungi, and protozoa, whereas intracellular TLRs recognize PAMPs of pathogens that are capable of entering the cytoplasm. All TLRs (with the exception of TLR3) associate with and activate the **NF-κB (nuclear factor kappa-light chain enhancer of activated B cells)** pathway that acts through several cytosolic proteins, including MyD88, which induces an intracellular cascade of TLR-specific responses. This sequence of events results not only in the release of **cytokines** that induce systemic inflammation (**IL-1**, **IL-12**, and **tumor necrosis factor-α [TNF-α]**) but also in the activation of B and T cells in order to mount a specific *adaptive immune response*.

NF-κB is held in the inactive state by **IκB**. However, binding of the TLR to their ligands activates a kinase that phosphorylates IκB and, in turn, permits the activation of NF-κB. The activated NF-κB enters the nucleus, where it and a coactivator factor induce transcription of a target gene, resulting in an inflammatory reaction, the commencement of an **innate immune response**, and the conscription of NK cells, thereby also initiating an **adaptive immune response** (see the next section). Therefore, TLRs have the ability to modulate the immune response, suggesting that the innate immune system is not a static, one-size-fits-all type of response but is dynamic in nature and is capable of regulating both the inflammatory and immune responses equally.

Clinical Correlations

1. ***Hypoactivity*** *of TLRs can result in greater susceptibility to pathogens, whereas their* ***hyperactivity*** *may be responsible for some autoimmune diseases, such as systemic lupus erythematosus, cardiovascular diseases, and rheumatoid arthritis.*
2. *High levels of TLR4 are expressed in mice that are sleep deprived. When injected with malignant cells, the tumors that developed in sleep-deprived animals were larger, more aggressive, and grew at a more rapid rate than in mice that were permitted to sleep normally. Additionally, instead of eliminating the tumor cells, the macrophages that the sleep-deprived animals recruited to the site of the tumor elicited the development of a vascular supply that encouraged tumor growth.*

THE ADAPTIVE IMMUNE SYSTEM

The adaptive immune system responds slower than the innate immune system, has immunological memory, and depends on B and T lymphocytes to mount an immune response.

The **adaptive immune response** exhibits four distinctive properties: **specificity**, **diversity**, **memory**, and **self/nonself recognition**—that is, the ability to distinguish between structures that belong to the organism, **self**, and those that are foreign, **nonself**. Additional characteristics of the adaptive immune system include **clonal expansion**, the ability to increase the number of cells that can react to a renewed antigenic challenge, and **contraction and homeostasis**, the ability of the immune system to respond simultaneously to multiple antigenic challenges.

T lymphocytes, **B lymphocytes**, and specialized macrophages known as **antigen-presenting cells** (**APCs**) function not only in the (adaptive) immune response but also communicate with members of the innate immune system. They communicate by releasing signaling molecules (**cytokines**) in response to encounters with foreign substances called **antigens** (**anti**body **gene**rators) and also by the sporting markers on their cell membranes, such as clusters of differentiation molecules (CD molecules), T-cell receptors (TCRs), and surface immunoglobulins (sIgs).

Recognition of a substance as foreign by the immune system stimulates a complex sequence of reactions that result either in the production of **immunoglobulins** (also known as **antibodies**), which bind to the antigen, or in the induction of a **group of cells** that specialize in killing foreign cells, invading pathogens, or altered self cells (e.g., tumor cells). The immune response that depends on the formation of antibodies is called the **humoral immune response**, a function of B cells, whereas the cytotoxic response is known as the **cell-mediated immune response**, a function of T cells.

The cells that constitute the functional components of the innate and adaptive immune systems (T cells, B cells, macrophages, and their subcategory, APCs) are all formed in the bone marrow. B cells become immunocompetent in the bone marrow, whereas T cells migrate to the thymus to become immunocompetent there. Therefore, bone marrow and the thymus are called the **primary** (**central**) **lymphoid organs**. After lymphocytes become immunocompetent in the bone marrow or thymus, they migrate to the **secondary** (**peripheral**) **lymphoid organs**—diffuse lymphoid tissue (mucosa-associated lymphoid tissue [MALT]), lymph nodes, spleen, and tonsils—where they come into contact with antigens.

IMMUNOGENS AND ANTIGENS

Immunogens are molecules that always elicit an immune response; antigens are molecules to which antibodies bind but do not necessarily elicit an immune response.

A foreign structure that can elicit an immune response in a particular host is known as an **immunogen**; an **antigen** is a molecule that can react with an antibody irrespective of its ability to elicit an immune response. Although not all antigens are immunogens, in this textbook, the two terms are considered to be synonymous, and only the term *antigen* is used.

The region of the antigen that reacts with an **antibody**, or **TCR** (**T-cell receptor**), is known as its **epitope**, or antigenic determinant. Each epitope is a small portion of the antigen molecule and consists of only 8 to 12 or 15 to 22 hydrophilic amino acid or sugar residues that are accessible to the immune apparatus. Large foreign invaders such as bacteria have several epitopes, each capable of binding to a different antibody. Although the term is not frequently used, it should be mentioned that the portion of an antibody that has an affinity to epitopes is referred to as a **paratope**.

Clinical Correlations

The complexity of a foreign substance is also important in determining its antigenicity. Hence, large polymeric molecules that have relatively simple chemical compositions, such as certain human-made plastics, have minimal immunogenicity. Therefore, these substances are used in the manufacture of artificial implants (e.g., hip replacement).

CLONAL SELECTION AND EXPANSION

During embryonic development, an extremely large number of small clusters (clones) of lymphocytes are formed; each clone can recognize one specific foreign antigen (epitope).

The immune system can recognize and combat an astonishing number of different antigens because during embryonic development an enormous number ($\sim 10^{15}$) of lymphocyte **clones** are formed by rearrangement of the 400 or so genes encoding immunoglobulins or TCRs. All of the cells of a particular clone have identical surface markers and can react with a specific antigen, even though they have not yet been exposed to that antigen. The cell-surface proteins that enable lymphocytes to interact with antigens are **membrane-bound antibodies** (**B-cell receptors** or **surface immunoglobulins** [**sIgs**]) in the case of B cells and **TCRs** in the case of T cells. Although the molecular structures of antibodies and TCRs differ, they are functionally equivalent in their ability to recognize and interact with specific epitopes.

The first time an organism encounters an antigen, the adaptive immune response is slow to begin and not very robust; this response is called the **primary immune response**. Subsequent exposures to the same antigen elicit the **secondary immune response** (**anamnestic response**), which begins rapidly and is much more intense than the primary response. The increased potency of the secondary reaction is due to the process of **immunological memory**, which is inherent to the adaptive immune system. Both B and T cells are said to be **virgin cells** (**naïve cells**) before exposure to antigens. After a virgin cell comes in contact with an antigen, it proliferates to form activated cells and memory cells.

Activated cells, also known as **effector cells**, are responsible for carrying out an immune response. Effector cells derived from B cells are called **plasma cells**, which produce and release antibodies. Effector cells derived from T cells either secrete cytokines or destroy foreign cells or altered self cells.

Memory cells, similar to virgin lymphocytes, express either B-cell receptors (sIgs) or TCRs, which can interact with specific antigens. Memory cells are not directly involved in the immune response during which they are generated. However, these cells live for months or years and have a much greater affinity for antigens than do virgin lymphocytes. Moreover, formation of memory cells after first exposure to an antigen increases the size of the original clone, a process called **clonal expansion**. Because of the presence of an expanded population of memory cells with an increased affinity for the antigen, subsequent exposure to the same antigen induces a secondary immune response.

Immunological Tolerance

Macromolecules of the self are not viewed as antigens and, therefore, do not elicit an immune response.

The immune system can recognize macromolecules that belong to the self and does not attempt to mount an immune response against them (**immunological tolerance**). The mechanism of immunological tolerance depends on killing or disabling those cells that would react against the self. During embryonic development, if a lymphocyte encounters the substance to which it is designed to react, the cell is either killed (**clonal deletion**) so that this particular clone does not form or the lymphocyte is disabled (**clonal anergy**) and cannot mount an immune response, even though it is present.

Clinical Correlations

Autoimmune diseases involve a malfunction of the immune system that results in the loss of immunological tolerance. One example is Graves disease, in which the receptors for thyroid-stimulating hormone (TSH) on the follicular cells of the thyroid gland are perceived to be antigens. Antibodies formed against TSH receptors bind to these receptors and stimulate the cells to release an excess amount of thyroid hormone. Patients with Graves disease have an enlarged thyroid gland and exophthalmos (protruding eyeballs).

Immunoglobulins

Immunoglobulins are antibodies (also known as gamma globulins) that are manufactured by plasma cells; a typical immunoglobulin has one pair of heavy and one pair of light chains attached to each other by disulfide bonds.

Immunoglobulins (**antibodies, gamma globulins**) are glycoproteins that inactivate antigens (including viruses) and elicit an extracellular response against invading microorganisms. The response may involve phagocytosis in the connective tissue spaces by macrophages (or neutrophils) or the activation of the blood-borne **complement system**.

Clinical Correlations

The **complement system** *is composed of 20 plasma proteins that assemble in a specific sequence and fashion on the surface of invading microorganisms to form a* **membrane attack complex (MAC)** *that lyses the foreign cell. The key component of the complement system is protein C3. Deficiency of protein C3 predisposes a person to recurring bacterial infections.*

Immunoglobulins are manufactured in large number by plasma cells, which release them into the lymph or blood vascular system. There are five classes of antibodies (IgA, IgD, IgE, IgG, and IgM). Members of the various classes of antibodies share certain characteristics and, because IgG is the typical antibody, it will be described as a template for all classes of immunoglobulins (Table 12.3). Each IgG is a Y-shaped molecule, composed of two long identical polypeptides, known as **heavy chains** (55- to 70-kilodalton [kD]), and two shorter identical 25-kD polypeptides, the **light chains**. The four chains are bound to each other by several disulfide bonds and noncovalent bonds in such a way that the stem of the Y is composed only of heavy chains and the diverging arms consist of both light and heavy chains (Fig. 12.1).

The region in the vicinity of the disulfide bonds between the two heavy chains, the **hinge area**, is flexible and permits the arms to move away from or toward each other. The distal regions on the tips of the arms (the amino-terminal segments) are responsible for binding to the epitope; hence, each antibody molecule can bind two *identical* epitopes.

The enzyme papain cleaves the antibody molecule at its hinge areas (see Fig. 12.1), forming three fragments: one **Fc fragment** composed of the stem of the Y and containing equal parts of the two heavy chains, and two **Fab fragments**, each composed of the remaining part of one heavy chain and one entire light chain. Fc fragments are easily crystallized (hence, the *c* designation), whereas the Fab fragment is the antigen-binding region of the antibody (hence, the *ab* designation).

The amino acid sequence of the Fc fragment is mostly constant in its class; thus, the stem of an antibody has the ability to bind to Fc receptors of many different cells. The amino acid sequence of the Fab region is variable; the alterations of that sequence determine the **specificity** of the antibody molecule for its particular antigen.

Each antibody is specific against a particular epitope; thus, the Fab regions of all antibodies against that particular epitope are identical. It is believed that there are 10^6 to 10^9 different types of antibodies in a person, each specific against one particular antigen. Each type of antibody is manufactured by members of the same **clone**. Thus, there are 10^6 to 10^9 clones whose members discern and react to a particular epitope (or a small number of very similar epitopes).

As noted earlier, small amounts of immunoglobulins are made by B cells and inserted into their plasmalemmae; these are known as **sIgs** (**surface immunoglobulins**) or **B-cell receptors**; they function as antigen-receptor molecules. They are slightly different from antibodies in that they possess a membrane-binding component composed of two pairs of membrane-spanning chains, **Igβ** and **Igα**, which bind the heavy chains of the antibody molecule to the cell membrane.

Classes of Immunoglobulins

There are five classes (isotypes) of immunoglobulins in humans: IgG, IgM, IgA, IgD, and IgE.

Humans have five **isotypes** (classes) of immunoglobulins: **IgG**, the monomeric form of immunoglobulin described earlier; **IgM**, which resembles five IgG molecules bound to each other (pentameric form of immunoglobulin); **IgA**, which resembles two IgG molecules bound to each other (dimeric form of immunoglobulin); **IgD**, present in very low concentration in the blood but found on the B-cell surface as a monomeric form of immunoglobulin known as surface IgD (sIgD); and **IgE**, a monomeric form of immunoglobulin present on the surface of basophils and mast cells.

The classes of immunoglobulins are also determined by the amino acid sequences of their heavy chains. The various heavy chains are designated by the Greek letters α, δ, γ, ε, and μ and are associated with IgA, IgD, IgE, IgG, and IgM, respectively. The characteristics of the five isotypes of immunoglobulins are detailed in Table 12.3.

CELLS OF THE ADAPTIVE IMMUNE SYSTEMS

The cells of the adaptive immune system are B lymphocytes (and plasma cells), T lymphocytes, and antigen-presenting cells (macrophages and dendritic cells).

B Lymphocytes

B lymphocytes originate and become immunocompetent in the bone marrow; they are responsible for the humorally mediated immune system.

B lymphocytes, also known as ***B cells***, are small lymphocytes (see Chapter 10) that both originate and become **immunocompetent** in the bone marrow. However, in birds, in which

TABLE 12.3 Properties of Human Immunoglobulins

Class	Cytokines[a]	No. of Units[b]	Ig in Blood (%)	Crosses Placenta	Binds to Cells	Biological Characteristics
IgA	TGF-β	1 or 2	10–15	No	Temporarily to epithelial cells during secretion	Also known as *secretory antibody* because it is secreted into tears, saliva, the lumen of the gut, and the nasal cavity as dimers; individual units of the dimer are held together by J protein manufactured by plasma cells and protected from enzymatic degradation by a secretory component manufactured by the epithelial cell; combats antigens and microorganisms in the lumen of gut, nasal cavity, vagina, and conjunctival sac; secreted into milk, thus protecting neonates with passive immunity; monomeric form in bloodstream; assists eosinophils in recognizing and killing parasites
IgD		1	< 1	No	B-cell plasma membrane	Surface immunoglobulin; assists B cells in recognizing antigens for which they are specific; functions in the activation of B cells subsequent to antigenic challenge to differentiate into plasma cells
IgE	IL-4, IL-5	1	< 1	No	Mast cells and basophils	Reaginic antibody; when several membrane-bound antibodies are cross-linked by antigens, IgE facilitates degranulation of basophils and mast cells, with subsequent release of pharmacological agents, such as heparin, histamine, eosinophil and neutrophil chemotactic factors, and leukotrienes; elicits immediate hypersensitivity reactions; assists eosinophils in recognizing and killing parasites
IgG	IFN-γ, IL-4, IL-6	1	80	Yes	Macrophages and neutrophils	Crosses placenta and, thus, protects fetuses with passive immunity; secreted in milk and, thus, protects neonates with passive immunity; fixes complement cascade; functions as opsonins, that is, by coating microorganisms, facilitates their phagocytosis by macrophages and neutrophils, cells that possess Fc receptors for the Fc region of these antibodies; also participates in antibody-dependent cell-mediated cytotoxicity by activating NK cells; produced in large quantities during secondary immune responses
IgM		1 or 5	5–10	No	B cells (in monometric form)	Pentameric form is maintained by J-protein links, which bind Fc regions of each unit; activates cascade of the complement system; is the first isotype to be formed in the primary immune response

[a]Cytokines responsible for switching to this isotype.
[b]A unit is a single immunoglobulin composed of two heavy and two light chains; thus, IgA exists as both a monomer and as a dimer.
Fc, Crystallizable fragment; *IFN*, interferon; *Ig*, immunoglobulin; *IL*, interleukin; *NK*, natural killer; TGF, tumor growth factor.

B cells were first identified, they become immunocompetent is a diverticulum of the cloaca, known as the ***bursa of Fabricius*** (hence, the designation "B" cells). During the process of becoming immunocompetent, each cell goes from an immature pre–B cell stage to a **transitional B cell**, which manufactures a series of identifying immunoglobulin chains. Transitional B cells migrate to the spleen to be killed or to be permitted to develop into a **mature B cell**. Each mature B cell manufactures 50,000 to 100,000 **IgM** and **IgD** immunoglobulins and inserts these in its plasma membrane so that the epitope-binding sites of the antibodies face the extracellular space. The Fc region of the antibody is embedded in the phospholipid bilayer by the assistance of two pairs of transmembrane proteins, Igβ and Igα, whose carboxyl termini are in contact with certain intracellular protein complexes. Every member of a particular clone of B cells has antibodies that bind to the same epitope. When the surface immunoglobulin reacts with its epitope, the Igβ and Igα transduce (relay) the information to the intracellular protein

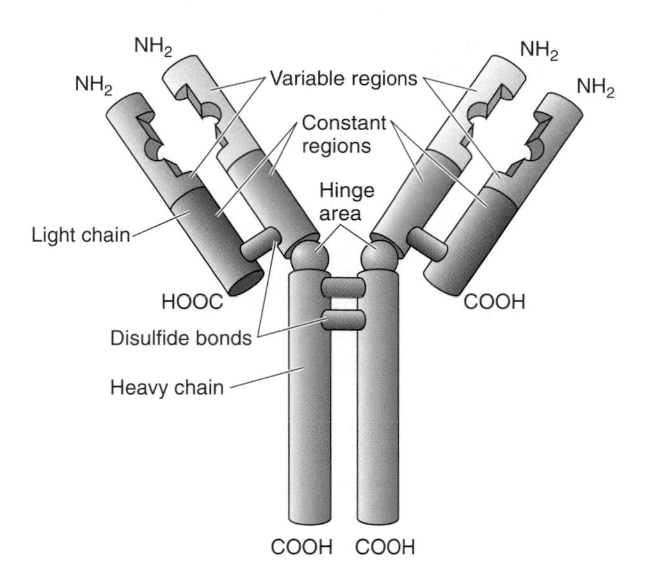

Fig. 12.1 Schematic diagram of an antibody, indicating its regions.

complex with which they are in contact, initiating a chain of events that results in **activation** of that particular B cell.

Types of B Cells

There are a number of different types of B cells: B-1 B cells, B-2 B cells, B memory cells, spleen follicular B cells, and spleen marginal zone B cells.

During the ensuing presentation of B-cell types, various T-cell types have to be mentioned even though they and their functions have not as yet been discussed. B cells are considered to be members of the APC population because they are able to complex epitopes with class II MHC molecules and present them to T_H1 cells. It is believed that they present epitopes only during an anamnestic response, not the primary immune response. When they act as APCs, not only do they synthesize and secrete IL-12, a cytokine that prompts T_H1 cells to proliferate and induce NK cells to become active, but they also differentiate into plasma cells and increase their population of B memory cells.

- **B-1 B cells** are derived from hemopoietic stem cells that develop in the fetal liver. They arise early in development of the individual and populate the mucosae of the respiratory and gastrointestinal systems, and the peritoneum. They manufacture IgM that they place on their plasmalemmae. They have a limited ability to produce antibody diversity and respond mostly to carbohydrates of the most common microorganisms without the need to interact with T cells. They constitute approximately 50% of the mucosal B cells but do not form memory B-1 B cells. They do not have CD40 molecules on their cell membranes.
- **B-2 B cells** (*referred to simply as **B cells** in this textbook*) are the most numerous of the B cell population. They possess CD40 molecules on their cell membrane with which they contact and signal T_H2 cells. In response, the T_H2 cells release signaling molecules that inhibit T_H1 cells from entering the cell cycle and prompt B cells to form plasma cells and B memory cells. The T_H2 cells release additional cytokines that allow the B cell to manufacture a different class of immunoglobulin, a process known as ***class switching (isotype switching)***. The cytokines that are released by T-helper cells depend on the type of pathogens present:
  - During parasitic worm invasion, T cells release IL-4 and IL-5; B cells differentiate into plasma cells and, after class switching, form IgE to elicit mast cell degranulation on the surface of the parasites.
  - During bacterial and viral invasions, T cells release IFN-γ and IL-6; B cells switch to forming IgG, which opsonizes bacteria, fixes complement, and stimulates NK cells to kill virally altered cells (antibody-dependent cell-mediated cytotoxicity [ADCC]).
  - During viral or bacterial invasion of mucosal surfaces, T cells release tumor growth factor-β (TGF-β), and B cells switch to IgA formation, which is secreted onto the mucosal surface.
- **B memory cells** are long-lived cells that not only increase the size of the clone that is specific against a particular antigen but also react faster and more vigorously than the cells comprising the original clone.
- **Splenic B cells** are of two types, follicular B cells and marginal zone B cells:
  - **Follicular B cells** are the most populous of the B cells of the primary and secondary follicles of the spleen. These are almost mature cells, and they express IgM, IgD, and CD21 molecules on their cell membranes. These cells are T-cell dependent, and they migrate in and out of the various lymphoid organs, where they are always located in the B cell follicles. Because they migrate, they are also known as ***recirculating B cells.***
  - **Marginal zone B cells** have a limited range of antibody diversity, are T-cell independent, and are located very close to marginal sinuses of the spleen. They can migrate to lymph nodes in humans and have the ability to react to self antigens as well as to bacterial polysaccharide antigens. They possess IgM, CD1, CD9, and CD21 molecules on their cell membranes; during an antigenic challenge, they differentiate into plasma cells that release IgM.
- **Plasma cells** are B cells that have undergone differentiation into antibody-forming cells that possess no surface antibody. All antibodies manufactured by plasma cells that are derived from a single clone of B cells manufacture the identical antibodies that are specific against one particular antigen (or to antigens that are very similar to that specific antigen). Because plasma cells release the antibodies that they manufactured into connective tissue from where the antibodies enter blood vessels or lymph vessels, B cells are responsible for the **humorally mediated immune response.**

As naïve B cells first become activated, they make IgM, which, when bound to the surface of an invading pathogen, is able to activate the complement system (**complement fixation**). IgM molecules can also bind to viruses, preventing them from contacting the cell surface, thus protecting the cells from viral invasion.

Certain antigens (e.g., polysaccharides of microbial capsules) can elicit a humoral immune response without a T-cell intermediary. These are known as ***thymic-independent antigens***. They cannot induce formation of B-memory cells and can elicit only IgM-antibody formation. However, most antigens require participation of a T-cell intermediary before they can induce a humoral immune response (see section on humoral immune response).

T Lymphocytes

T lymphocytes originate in the bone marrow and migrate to the thymus to become immunocompetent; they are responsible for the cellularly mediated immune response.

T lymphocytes (**T cells**) are also formed in the bone marrow, but they migrate to the thymic cortex, where they become immunocompetent by expressing specific molecules on their cell membranes that permit them to perform their functions. The process whereby T cells become immunocompetent is discussed later.

Although histologically T cells appear to be identical to B cells, there are important differences between them:

- T cells have TCRs rather than sIgs on their cell surfaces.
- Although TCRs belong to the immunoglobulin superfamily, they are never secreted.
- T cells, except for NKT cells, respond to protein antigens only.
- For T cells to respond to antigens, the epitopes have to be presented to them bound to MHC molecules present on the surface of APCs.
- Because of the MHC constraint, T cells are said to be MHC restricted (see the later section on MHC restriction and T cells).
- T cells perform their functions at short distances only.

T cells express **clusters of differentiation proteins** (**CD molecules** or **CD markers**) on their plasmalemmae. These accessory proteins bind to specific ligands on target cells. Although almost 300 CD molecules are known, Table 12.4 lists only those that are immediately pertinent to the subsequent discussion of cellular interactions in the immune process. The membrane-bound portion of the **TCR** associates with the membrane proteins, **CD3**, and either **CD4** or **CD8**, forming the **TCR complex**. Several other membrane proteins play roles in signal transduction and in strengthening the interaction between the TCR and an epitope, thus facilitating antigen-stimulated T-cell activation.

Similar to sIgs on B cells, **TCRs** on the plasmalemma of T cells function as antigen receptors. The **constant regions** of the TCR are membrane bound, whereas the variable **amino-terminal regions** containing the antigen-binding sites extend from the cell surface. There are two types of TCRs, depending on their protein chain compositions: **gamma** and **delta** (**γ** and **δ**), known as **γ/δ T cells**, and **alpha** and **beta** (**α** and **β**), known as **α/β T cells**. There is yet another category of T cells, known as **natural killer T cells**.

- **γ/δ T cells** form a small population. They reside mostly in the mucosa of the gastrointestinal tract, react typically to microbial pathogenic invasion, and have a very fast reaction time. Unlike their α/β counterparts, they do not form memory T cells and are not MHC restricted. It is believed that γ/δ T cells recognize microbial nonprotein antigens, and these antigens do not require APCs to present them. Although these cells become "educated" in the cortex of the thymus to become immunocompetent, they spend considerably less time there than do their α/β T-cell counterparts.
- **Natural killer T cells** (**NKT cells**) spend very little time in the thymus and possess some α/β TCRs on their surfaces that are designed to recognize lipid antigens bound to CD1 molecules (similar to class I MHC molecules) presented to them by APCs. Therefore, NKT cells are said to be CD1 restricted (rather than MHC restricted). NKT cells secrete IL-4, IL-10, and IFN-γ. It is believed that these cells kill bacteria whose cell walls are rich in lipids.
- The majority of T cells are **α/β T cells**; they have the ability to form memory T cells. Although they react much slower than their γ/δ counterparts, they are the most common T cells to respond to antigenic challenges. Maturation of these cells is described in the following section.

Maturation of α/β T Cells

Because **α/β T cells** spend a considerable amount of time in the thymus, only their maturation is presented in this textbook. While in the thymus, the α/β T cells are exposed to various signaling molecules and growth factors produced by reticular epithelial cells of the thymus that control their development into immunocompetent T cells.

1. **Progenitor T lymphocytes** formed in the bone marrow are *immunoincompetent* (i.e., they are unable to participate in an immune response). From the bone marrow, these cells travel to the medulla of the thymus, where they leave the postcapillary venule at the corticomedullary junction and enter the thymic cortex, where they are known as **thymocytes.** The thymocytes migrate to the outer region of the cortex. These thymocytes possess **Notch-1 receptors** on their surfaces; however, because they have neither CD4 nor CD8 molecules, they are referred to as **double-negative T cells.** The thymus possesses various types of epithelial reticular cells (see the section on the thymus), some of which release **signaling**

TABLE 12.4 Selected Surface Markers Involved in the Immune Process

Protein	Cell Surface	Ligand and Target Cell	Function
CD3	All T cells	None	Transduces epitope–MHC complex binding into intracellular signal, activating T cell
CD4	T-helper cells	MHC II on APCs	Coreceptor for TCR binding to epitope–MHC II complex, activation of T-helper cell
CD8	Cytotoxic T cells and T reg cells	MHC I on most nucleated cells	Coreceptor for TCR binding to epitope–MHC I complex; activation of cytotoxic T cell
CD28	T-helper cells	B7 on APCs	Assists in the activation of T-helper cells
CD40	B cells	CD40 receptor molecule expressed on activated T-helper cells	Binding of CD40 to CD40 receptor permits T-helper cell to activate B cells to proliferate into B memory cells and plasma cells

APC, Antigen-presenting cell; *MHC*, major histocompatibility complex; *TCR*, T-cell receptors.

molecules that are recognized by the Notch-1 receptors. *Double-negative T cells do not express CD3 or TCR molecules on their cell membranes.*

2. The **signaling molecules** activate Notch-1 on the surface of the double-negative cells, inducing these cells to manufacture both CD4 and CD8 molecules and place them on their plasma membranes. Because both CD4 and CD8 molecules are present on these cells, they are now referred to as **double-positive T cells**, which begin to express TCRs and CD3 molecules on their surfaces. As double-positive cells proliferate, they go through **gene rearrangement**, forming a large number of cells, each expressing a *different variable region* in their α/β TCR molecules.
3. Various *self epitope–MHC complexes* are presented to the double-positive T cells by epithelial reticular cells of the thymic cortex. Double-positive T cells that bind very weakly to self peptides presented by self MHC molecules are preserved, whereas those that make a strong bond with them are killed. Therefore, this is a *positive selection of thymocytes* because they have to demonstrate only a weak recognition to self epitope–MHC molecule complexes. An amazing 90% of double-negative T cells are killed in the thymic cortex. The reason why the killing of these cells is essential is that *only those T cells may be allowed to survive that recognize* ***only*** *foreign epitopes presented by self MHC molecules.*
4. There are two types of MHC molecules, MHC I and MHC II. The epithelial reticular cells present either *self epitope–MHC I* or *self epitope–MHC II complexes* to the double-positive T cells. The double-positive T cells that are exposed to MHC I molecules cease to express CD4 molecules on their surfaces but continue to express CD8 molecules and are referred to as **single-positive CD8 T cells** (also known as **CD 8 cells**). Similarly, the double-positive T cells that are exposed to MHC II molecules cease to express CD8 molecules on their surfaces but continue to express CD4 molecules and are referred to as **single-positive CD4 T cells** (also known as **CD 4 cells**).
5. The **single-positive T cells (I T cells)** that are not forced into apoptosis are immunocompetent; they leave the thymic cortex and migrate into the medulla of the thymus. These I T cells also possess CD45RA molecules on their cell membranes.
6. Once in the medulla, medullary epithelial reticular cells present **self epitope–MHC II** complexes to these I T cells. The I T cells that show a strong response to these complexes are also forced into apoptosis to prevent the mounting of an immune response by these cells to the self (i.e., to prevent an autoimmune response). Therefore, this is a negative selection of thymocytes because they do not recognize the epitope–MHC complex as self. But not all of these I T cells that show a strong response to the self epitope–MHC complex are forced into apoptosis. In an unknown fashion, some of these I T cells escape the "death sentence" and differentiate into **regulatory T cells (T reg cells)** that suppress an immune response (see the section on effector T cells).
7. Epithelial reticular cells of the medulla possess the capability to force those I T cells into apoptosis that would mount an immune response against **tissue-specific antigens**, such as insulin. The epithelial reticular cells are able to do this because they release **autoimmune regulator (AIRE)**, a transcription factor that permits these tissue-specific antigens to be expressed in the thymus and thus be presented to the T cells.

> **Clinical Correlations**
>
> *Mutations in the AIRE gene are responsible for the* ***autoimmune polyendocrine syndrome type 1*** *that damages various endocrine glands, as well as counters the function of* T_H17 *T cells as a result of immune intolerance. Because the thymus was unable to delete (i.e., kill) I T cells that would mount an immune response* ***against tissue-specific antigens****—such as insulin, parathormone, IL-17, and IL-22—the affected patients may suffer from autoimmune parathyroidism, hypogonadism, adrenalitis, and chronic mucocutaneous candidiasis. The patient's candidiasis is caused by the autoantibodies formed against IL-17 and IL-22, the interleukins produced by* T_H17 *T cells, the body's primary defense against fungal infections.*

8. The I T cells that remain alive use the vascular system to leave the thymic medulla and enter the various lymphoid organs located throughout the body. After they leave the thymic medulla, they are referred to as **naïve T cells.**

A TCR can recognize an epitope only if the epitope is a polypeptide (composed of amino acids) and if the epitope is bound to an **MHC complex molecule**, such as those in the plasmalemma of an APC. There are two classes of these glycoproteins: MHC class I and MHC class II molecules (although in humans they are known as HLA class I and HLA class II molecules, these terms are used only infrequently [HLA= human leukocyte antigen]). Most nucleated cells express MHC I molecules on their surfaces, whereas APCs can express both MHC I and MHC II on their plasmalemmae. The MHC molecules are unique in each individual (except for identical twins); to be activated, T cells must recognize not only the foreign epitope but also the MHC molecule as self. If a T cell recognizes the epitope but not the MHC molecule, it does not become stimulated; hence, the T cell's capacity to act against an epitope is said to be **MHC restricted**.

There are three types of T cells, some with two or more subtypes:

- Naïve T cells
- Memory T cells
- Effector T cells

Naïve T Cells

Naïve T cells possess CD45RA molecules on their cell surfaces and leave the thymus programmed as immunologically competent cells, but they must become **activated T cells** in order to be able to function. To do that, *naïve T cells have to contact their specific antigen after they leave the thymic medulla*. When a T lymphocyte becomes activated, it will undergo cell division and will form both memory T cells and effector T cells.

Memory T Cells

Memory T cells are of two types: central memory T cells and effector memory T cells. They are responsible for the immunological memory of the adaptive immune system.

Memory T cells express CD45R0 molecules on their cell membranes; they form the immunological memory of the adaptive immune system because they form a clone whose members are identical and have the capability of combating a particular antigen. These memory cells can become activated and express effector capabilities. There are two types of memory T cells: those that *express* **CR7** molecules on their surfaces and are known as **central memory T cells** (**TCM**; **CR7$^+$ cells**) and those that *do not express* CR7 molecules on their surface and are known as **effector T memory cells** (**TEM**; **CR7$^-$ cells**). **TCMs** populate and remain in the T cell–rich zones of lymph nodes (in the paracortex). They are incapable of immediate effector function; however, when they recognize the epitope presented to them by APCs, they stimulate the APCs to release IL-12. This signaling molecule binds to IL-12 receptors of TCMs and stimulates them to differentiate into **TEMs**. TEMs express receptors that permit these cells to migrate to regions of inflammation, where they have immediate effector function by proliferating and differentiating into **effector T cells**.

Effector T Cells

Effector T cells are able to respond to an immunological challenge. There are three types of effector T cells: T helper cells, cytotoxic T lymphocytes, and regulatory T cells.

Effector T cells are derived from TEMs. They are immunologically competent cells that are capable of responding to and mounting an immune response. There are three types of effector T cells: T helper cells, T killer cells (cytotoxic T lymphocytes [CTLs]), and T reg cells; T helper and T reg cells have their own cell subtypes.

T Helper Cells

There are several subtypes of T helper cells, all of which display CD4 molecules on their cell membranes. They are responsible for the recognition of foreign antigens and for mounting an immunological response against them.

T helper cells possess **CD4 molecules** (in addition to the CD3 and TCR) as their cell membrane markers. They interact with other cells of the innate and adaptive immune systems, they synthesize and release various cytokines, and they have the ability to activate cells of the cell-mediated immune system to mount a response against invading pathogens and eliminate them. T helper cells also play a major role in stimulating the humorally mediated immune system by interacting with B cells and stimulating them to differentiate into antibody-producing plasma cells. There are a number of subtypes of T helper cells: T_H0, T_H1, T_H2, T17, and $T_H\alpha\beta$. An additional subtype, the T_H3 cell, has been reclassified as the inducible T reg cell (see later discussion).

T_H0 Cells. **T_H0 cells** are precursor cells that have the capability of manufacturing and releasing a large number of cytokines. These cells can differentiate into T_H1, T_H2, T17, or $T_H\alpha\beta$ cells, depending on the signaling molecules that they receive from APCs. Then, their repertoire of cytokine release becomes limited.

T_H1 Cells. **T_H1 cells** are crucial for the control of intracellular pathogens and are also responsible for the induction of the cell-mediated immune response, as in acute allograft rejection and in the cases of multiple sclerosis. These cells secrete IFN-γ, TNF-α, and IL-2.

- IL-2 stimulates proliferation of activated T cells and B cells as well as cytotoxicity of CD8 T cells (CTLs).
- IFN-γ stimulates macrophages to become activated so that they can phagocytose pathogens, such as mycobacteria, protozoa, and fungi. This cytokine also activates cytotoxic T cells to kill altered or foreign cells.
- TNF-α stimulates activated macrophages to produce oxygen radicals in order to be able to kill the phagocytosed pathogens within their endosomes.
  - **Macrophages** release IL-12, which *induces the proliferation* of T_H1 cells and *inhibits the proliferation* of T_H2 cells; it also activates NK cells.
  - Macrophages that phagocytose bacteria express CD40 molecules on their surfaces, and T_H1 cells express CD40 ligand, whose interaction not only increases the macrophage's phagocytic capability but also induces the macrophage to release TNFα, IL-1, and IL-12.

T_H2 Cells. **T_H2 cells** elicit a response against a parasitic (IgE) or mucosal (IgA) infection. They secrete IL-4, IL-5, IL-6, IL-9, IL-10, and IL-13, and many of these interleukins facilitate the production of antibodies by plasma cells.

- IL-4 stimulates B cells to proliferate and differentiate into plasma cells and to switch from IgM production to IgG and IgE synthesis. Thus, it plays an important role in allergic reactions.
- IL-5 stimulates B cells to proliferate, differentiate into plasma cells, and to switch from IgM production to IgE synthesis.
- IL-6 stimulates B cells to proliferate, differentiate into plasma cells, and to switch from IgM production to IgG synthesis.
- IL-9 prompts T_H2 cells to proliferate and enhances mast cell activity.
- IL-10, acting in concert with IL-4, suppresses the differentiation of T_H0 cells to T_H1 cells.
- IL-13 suppresses the differentiation of T_H0 cells to T_H1 cells and enhances the functions of IL-4.

T_H17 Cells. **T_H17 cells** secrete IL-17, a cytokine that not only attracts neutrophils to the site of antigenic attack but also boosts their ability to phagocytose and destroy the bacterial pathogens. Additionally, T_H17 cells secrete IL-21 and IL-22.

- IL-21 stimulates the activities of B cells, T cells, and NK cells.
- IL-22 facilitates the inflammatory response and enhances the integrity of the epithelial barrier.

$T_H\alpha\beta$ Cells. **$T_H\alpha\beta$ cells** secrete IL-10 and IFN-ß (or IFN-ß) to provide immunity against viruses. When overly exuberant in combating autoantigens, these cells are responsible for the initiation of a type 2 hypersensitivity.

- IL-10 activates NK cells which force virally infected cells into apoptosis.

Cytotoxic T Lymphocytes.

Cytotoxic T lymphocytes (CTLs, T killer cells) display CD8 molecules on their cell membranes and are responsible for killing foreign cells, tumor cells, and virally altered cells.

CTLs (**T killer cells**) possess **CD8 molecules** (in addition to CD3 and TCRs) on their cell membranes. They recognize epitopes that are displayed on the cell membranes of foreign cells, tumor cells, and cells that have been altered by viruses (and display viral epitopes on their plasmalemmae); they then kill these cells. The epitopes on the target cell surface must be presented to the CTL by **class I MHC molecules**. The killing of these cells is performed in one of two ways: via the perforin/granzyme pathway or the Fas/FasL pathway.

Perforin/Granzyme Pathway.

- CTLs place perforins into the cell membranes of the virally altered cell.
- Perforins promote the formation of pores in the plasmalemma.
- CTLs transfer granzymes through the pores into the cytoplasms of the virally altered cell.
- Granzymes stimulate caspases to induce apoptosis, thus killing the virally altered cell.

Fas/FasL Pathway.

- CTLs express FasL, also known as *death ligand* (*CD95L*), on their cell membranes.
- Fas, also known as *CD95* (*death receptor*), on the surface of the target cell is activated.
- When Fas is activated, it stimulates an apoptotic cascade, resulting in the death of the target cell.

Subsequent to killing the target cell, the CTL can detach from it and find additional target cells, killing them in the same fashion just described.

Clinical Correlations

Cancer treatment in the past few years has been increasingly focused on modifying and using the patient's own immune system to combat the disease. In 2017, the US Food and Drug Administration approved the use of ***chimeric antigen receptor (CAR)*** *T cells in* ***diffuse large B-cell lymphomas (DLBCL)*** *and in* ***acute lymphoblastic leukemias (ALL)*** *in children and young adults whose malignancy is nonresponsive to conventional treatment. The patient's T cells, removed from their blood, are stimulated in the laboratory by cytokines to proliferate and are genetically engineered so that they synthesize specific* ***CARs*** *that recognize the patient's specific cancer cells. The T cells place these CARs on their cell membranes and then are known as* ***CAR T cells****. Prior to reintroducing the CAR T cells to the patient's vascular system, the patients are exposed to chemotherapy designed to reduce their circulating leukocytes. The subsequent lymphodepletion causes an increase in the patient's production of factors that increases leukocyte production, as well as the proliferation of the CAR T cells that have been infused into the patient. Although CAR T-cell therapy has been exceptionally successful in eliminating ALL and DLBCL, there are serious side effects that have to be resolved. A large number of clinical trials are being conducted to ameliorate the problems.*

Regulatory T Cells

Regulatory T cells (T reg cells) possess CD4 molecules on their cell membranes and function in suppressing the immune response.

T reg cells display CD4 molecules on their cell membranes and function in suppressing the immune response. Historically, the role of suppressing the immune response was ascribed to a theoretical T suppressor cell. However, it was shown that there are specific cells that suppress the immune function, and these cells were named **regulatory T cells (T reg cells)**. There are two types of T reg cells: natural (constitutive) T reg cells and inducible (adaptive) T reg cells. Both express **CD4 molecules** on their plasma membranes.

- **Natural T reg cells** (**nT reg cells**) develop in the thymus under the indirect influence of epithelial reticular cells (most probably those of Hassall corpuscles) that release **thymic stromal lymphopoietin**, a cytokine that causes dendritic cells in the vicinity to prompt naïve T cells to express CD25 and FoxP3 (forkhead family transcription factor) molecules on their plasma membrane, thus converting *naïve T cells* to **nT reg cells.** These natural T reg cells leave the thymus, and when their TCRs bind to an *APC* or *effector T cell*, they suppress the immune response by secreting IL-10 and TGF-β. Usually, the nT reg cells perform their functions once the pathogen is eliminated or if the response is against the self (autoimmune response).
- **Inducible T reg cells** (also known as **T_H3 cells**) originate outside of the thymus and are also derived from naïve T cells. They also have CD4, CD25, and FoxP3 on their cell membranes and secrete cytokines, such as IL-10 and TGF-β, which inhibit the formation of T_H1 cells, thereby suppressing the immune response.

It is possible that the two types of T reg cells have overlapping functions and that they act in concert to suppress the autoimmune response to self molecules.

Natural Killer T Cells. **NKT cells** are effector T cells that resemble NK cells but must enter the thymic cortex to become immunocompetent effector cells. They release the following cytokines: IFN-γ, IL-4, and IL-10. They are similar to NK cells in that they can be activated almost immediately. These are very unusual cells because they are able to recognize *lipid antigens* that are presented to them on the surfaces of immature dendritic cells. In order for NKT cells to recognize antigenic lipids, the lipids must be co-presented to them with **CD1 molecules**, and they recognize the antigen-CD1 complex via their TCRs (as indicated previously, CD1 molecules resemble MHC class I molecules). There are four isoforms of CD1 molecules, which are located either on the cell surface or are monitoring lysosomal and late endosomal compartments.

Major Histocompatibility Molecules

Major histocompatibility molecules present epitopes of pathogens to T cells. There are two classes of MHC molecules: MHC I and MHC II.

The prime importance of **MHC molecules** is to permit APCs and cells under viral attack (or cells already virally transformed) to present the epitopes of the invading pathogen to the **T cells**. These epitopes are short polypeptides that fit into a groove on the surface of the MHC molecule. As noted earlier, in humans, MHC molecules are also referred to as **human leukocyte antigen** (**HLA**) molecules. Therefore, there are class I HLA and class II HLA molecules that correspond to class I and class II MHC molecules.

Although there are three classes of MHC molecules, only class I and class II are discussed in this textbook because class III MHC molecules do not function in presenting epitopes.

- MHC I molecules (class I MHC molecules) function in presenting short polypeptide fragments (8–12 amino acids in length) derived from **endogenous proteins** (i.e., proteins manufactured by the cell).

- MHC II molecules (class II MHC molecules) function in presenting longer polypeptide fragments (13–25 amino acids in length) derived from **exogenous proteins** (i.e., proteins that were phagocytosed by these cells from the extracellular space).

As already indicated, almost every nucleated cell synthesizes and displays MHC I molecules, but only APCs synthesize and display MHC II molecules in addition to their MHC I molecules.

In humans, the MHC molecules are unique in each individual (except for identical twins). To be activated, T cells must recognize not only the foreign epitope but also recognize that the MHC molecule belongs to that particular individual, that is, the MHC molecule is "self." If a T cell recognizes the epitope as foreign but not the MHC molecule as self, it does not become stimulated. Hence, the T cell's capacity to act against an epitope is **MHC restricted**.

Loading Epitopes on MHC I Molecules

Epitopes derived from endogenous proteins are transported by specialized transporter proteins into the RER cisternae.

Proteins manufactured by a cell, whether they belong to the cell or to a virus or parasite that has overtaken the protein synthetic machinery of the cell, are known as ***endogenous proteins***. The quality of the proteins that the cell manufactures is controlled by **proteasomes**, which are modified to splice defective or foreign proteins into the proper-sized polypeptide fragments (8–12 amino acids in length) that fit in the groove of an MHC I molecule. These fragments, known as ***epitopes***, are transported by specialized **transporter proteins** (**TAP1** and **TAP2**) into the cisternae of the RER, where they are complexed to MHC I molecules that were manufactured on the RER surface. The **MHC I–epitope complex** is transported to the Golgi apparatus and is packaged, within the *trans*-Golgi network, into clathrin-coated vesicles for transport to and insertion into the cell membrane. In this fashion, **CTLs** can "look" at the cell surface and "see" whether the cell is producing self or nonself proteins.

Loading Epitopes on MHC II Molecules

Epitopes derived from proteins endocytosed by macrophages and APCs are loaded onto MHC II molecules within specialized intracellular compartments known as the major histocompatibility complex II compartment (MIIC).

Macrophages and other APCs endocytose proteins from their extracellular milieu by the formation of pinocytotic vesicles or phagosomes. The contents of these vesicles, known as **exogenous proteins**, are delivered into early endosomes, where they are enzymatically cleaved into polypeptide fragments. The polypeptide fragments are transported to late endosomes, where they are further cleaved to be the proper size (13–25 amino acids long) so that they can fit into the groove of the MHC II molecule.

MHC II molecules are synthesized on the RER. As they are assembled in the RER cisternae, a protein known as **CLIP** (**cl**ass II–associated **i**nvariant **p**rotein) is loaded into the groove of the MHC II molecule, preventing the accidental loading of the molecule with an endogenous epitope. The **MHC II–CLIP complex** is transported into the Golgi apparatus and is sorted into clathrin-coated vesicles within the *trans*-Golgi network for delivery to MHC class II–enriched compartments **(MIIC vesicle)**, dedicated vesicles that specialize in loading epitopes onto the MHC II molecule.

The MIIC vesicle receives not only MHC II–CLIP complex but also the epitopes from the processed antigens from late endosomes. Within the MIIC vesicle, the CLIP is enzymatically dissociated from the MHC II molecule and is replaced by an epitope. The **MHC II–epitope complex** is then transported to and inserted into the cell membrane.

In this fashion, **T-helper cells** can "look" at the cell surface and "see" whether the cell is encountering nonself proteins.

MHC Restriction and T Cells

As already noted, in order for T cells to perform their immunological function, they must be presented epitopes that are complexed with MHC molecules.

- MHC I molecules are recognized by cytotoxic T cells (which are CD8+ cells).
- MHC II molecules are recognized by T_H1 and T_H2 cells (which are CD4+ cells).
- Both MHC I and MHC II molecules are recognized by T memory cells (CD45R0 cells).

Antigen-Presenting Cells

APCs express both MHC I and MHC II molecules on their plasmalemmae, and they phagocytose, catabolize, process, and present antigens.

APCs phagocytose, catabolize, and process antigens, attach their epitopes to MHC II molecules, and present this complex to T cells. Most APCs are derived from monocytes and, therefore, belong to the mononuclear phagocyte system. APCs include **macrophages**, **dendritic cells** (e.g., Langerhans cells of the epidermis and oral mucosa), and two types of **non–monocyte-derived APCs** (B cells and those epithelial reticular cells of the thymic medulla that are responsible for elimination of naïve T cells that would recognize the self as well as those that are responsible for nT reg cell development).

Similar to T-helper cells, APCs manufacture and release **cytokines**. These signaling molecules are needed to activate target cells to perform their specific functions, not only in the immune response but also in other processes. Table 12.5 lists some of these cytokines but includes only properties that relate specifically to the immune response.

INTERACTION AMONG THE LYMPHOID CELLS

Cells of the lymphoid system interact with each other to effect an immune response. The process of interaction is regulated by recognition of surface molecules; if the molecules are not recognized, the cell is eliminated to prevent an incorrect response. If the surface molecules are recognized, the lymphocytes proliferate and differentiate. The initiation of these two responses is called ***activation***. At least two signals are required for activation:

- Recognition of the antigen (or epitope)
- Recognition of a second, costimulatory signal, which may be mediated by a cytokine or membrane-bound signaling molecule

T-Helper Cell–Mediated (T_H2 cells) Humoral Immune Response

Except for thymus-independent antigens, B cells can respond to an antigen only if instructed to do so by the T_H2 subtype of

TABLE 12.5 **Origin and Selected Functions of Some Cytokines**

Cytokine	Cell Origin	Target Cell	Function
IL-1a and IL-1b	Macrophages and epithelial cells	T cells and macrophages	Activate T cells and macrophages
IL-2	T_H1 cells	Activated T cells and activated B cells	Promotes proliferation of activated T cells and B cells
IL-4	T_H2 cells	B cells	Promotes proliferation of B cells and their maturation to plasma cells; also facilitates switch from production of IgM to IgG and IgE
IL-5	T_H2 cells	B cells	Promotes B-cell proliferation and maturation; also facilitates switch from production of IgM to IgE
IL-6	Antigen-presenting cells and T_H2 cells	T cells and activated B cells	Activates T cells; promotes B-cell maturation to IgG-producing plasma cells
IL-10	T_H2 cells	T_H1 cells	Inhibits development of T_H1 cells and inhibits them from secreting cytokines
IL-12	B cells and macrophages	NK cells and T cells	Activates NK cells and induces the formation of T_H1-like cells
IL-18	Macrophages	T_H1 cells and NK cells	Induces T_H1 cells to form and release IFN-γ; activates NK cells
IL-21	T_H17	B cells, T cells, NK cells	Stimulates the activities of B cells, T cells, and NK cells
IL-22	T_H17	Inflammatory cells; epithelial cells	Facilitates the inflammatory response and enhances the integrity of the epithelial barrier
IL-23	Macrophages	$CD8^+$ cells	Diminishes $CD8^+$ cell motility
TNF-α	Macrophage	Macrophages	Self-activates macrophages to release IL-12
	T_H1 cells	Hyperactive macrophages	Stimulates hyperactive macrophages to produce oxygen radicals, thereby facilitating bacterial killing
IFN-α	Cells under viral attack	NK cells and macrophages	Activates macrophages and NK cell
IFN-β	Cells under viral attack	NK cells and macrophages	Activates macrophages and NK cells
IFN-γ	T_H1 cells	Macrophages and T cells	Promotes cell killing by cytotoxic T cells and phagocytosis by macrophages

Ig, Immunoglobulin; *IL*, interleukin; *INF*, interferon; *NK*, natural killer; *T_H*, T-helper; *TNF*, tumor necrosis factor.

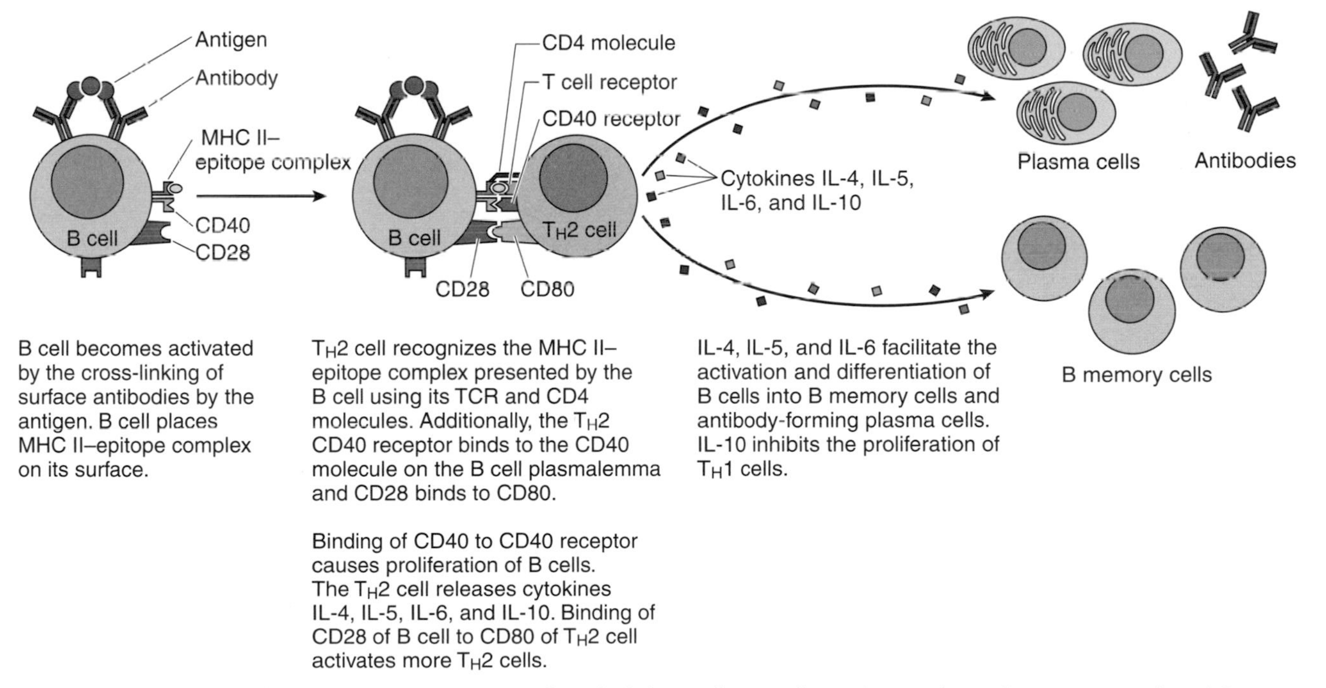

Fig. 12.2 Schematic diagram of the interaction between B cells and T-helper cell (T_H2 cell) in a thymus-dependent, antigen-induced, B-memory and plasma cell formation. CD, Cluster of differentiation; IL, interleukin; MHC, major histocompatibility complex; TCR, T-cell receptor.

T-helper cells (Fig. 12.2). When the B cell binds antigens on its sIgs, it internalizes the antigen–antibody complex, removes the epitope, attaches it to MHC II molecules, places the epitope–MHC II complex on its surface, and presents it to a T_H2 cell.

Signal 1. The T_H2 cell not only must recognize the epitope with its TCR but also must recognize the MHC II molecule with its CD4 molecule.

Signal 2. The T_H2 cell's CD40 receptor must bind to the B cell's CD40 molecule, and the T_H2 cell's CD28 has to contact the B cell's CD80 molecule.

If both signaling events are executed properly, the B cell becomes activated and rapidly proliferates. During proliferation, the T_H2 cell releases IL-4, IL-5, IL-6, and IL-10. The first three of these cytokines facilitate the differentiation of the newly

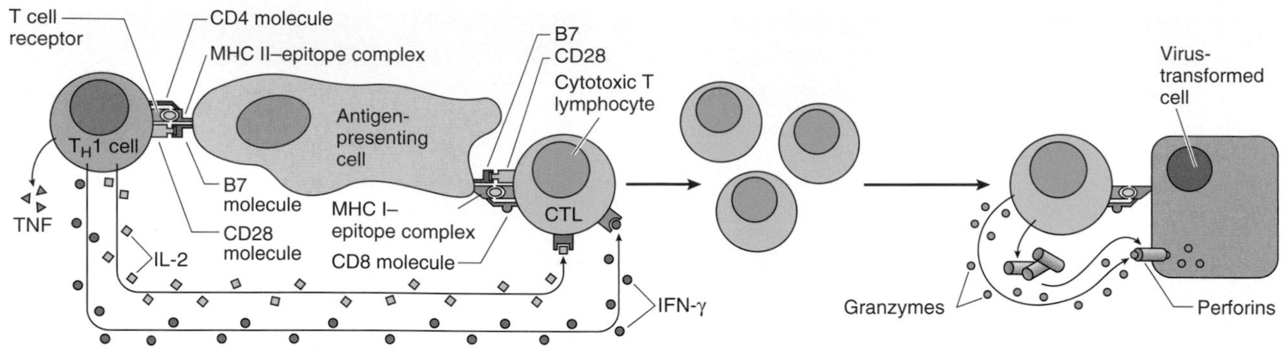

T_H1 cell TCR binds to MHC II–epitope complex of antigen-presenting cell. The CD4 molecule of the T_H1 cell recognizes MHC II. These two events cause the APC to express B7 molecules on its surface, which bind to CD28 of the T_H1 cell, causing it to release IL-2, IFN-γ, and TNF.

The same APC also has **MHC I–epitope** complex expressed on its surface that is bound by a CTL's CD8 molecule and T-cell receptor. Additionally, the CTL has CD28 molecules bound to the APC's B7 molecule. The CTL also possesses IL-2 receptors, which bind the IL-2 released by the T_H1 cell, causing the CTL to undergo proliferation, and IFN-γ causes its activation.

The newly formed CTLs attach to the MHC I–epitope complex via their TCR and CD8 molecules and secrete **perforins** and **granzymes**, killing the virus-transformed cells. Killing occurs when granzymes enter the cell through the pores established by perforins and act on the intracellular components to drive the cell into apoptosis.

Fig. 12.3 Schematic diagram of the T-helper cell (T_H1 cell) activation of cytotoxic T cells in killing virus-transformed cells. APC, Antigen-presenting cell; CD, cluster of differentiation; CTL, cytotoxic T lymphocyte; IFN-γ, interferon-gamma; MHC, major histocompatibility complex; TCR, T-cell receptor; TNF, tumor necrosis factor.

formed B cells into **B memory cells** and antibody-secreting **plasma cells**, whereas IL-10 inhibits the proliferation of T_H1 cells. The interaction of CD40 with the CD40 ligand facilitates isotype switching from IgM to IgG, and IL-4 facilitates the isotype switching to IgE.

T-Helper Cell–Mediated (T_H1) Killing of Virally Transformed Cells

In most cases, CTLs need to receive a signal from a T_H1 cell to be capable of killing virally transformed cells. Before that signal can be given, however, the T_H1 cell must be activated by an APC that offers the proper epitope (Fig. 12.3).

Signal 1. The TCR and the CD4 molecule of a T_H1 cell must recognize the epitope–MHC II complex on the surface of an APC. If this occurs, the APC expresses a molecule called ***B7*** on its surface.

Signal 2. The CD28 molecule of the T_H1 cell binds to the B7 molecule of the APC.

The T_H1 cell is now activated and releases IL-2, IFN-γ, and TNF. **IFN-γ** causes activation and proliferation of the CTL, ***if*** that CTL is bound to the same APC ***and if*** the following conditions are met:

Signal 1. The TCR and the CD8 molecule of the CTL must recognize the epitope–MHC I complex of the APC. Also, the CD28 molecule of the CTL must bind with the B7 molecule of the APC.

Signal 2. IL-2 released by the T_H1 cell binds to the IL-2 receptors of the CTL.

The CTL is now activated and rapidly proliferates. The newly formed CTLs seek out virally transformed cells by binding with their TCR and CD8 to the transformed cell's epitope–MHC I complex. Target cell killing may occur in one of the following ways:

1. Binding (in the presence of calcium) causes release of perforins, a group of glycoproteins that are closely related to the C9 fraction of the complement membrane attack complex. Perforins embed themselves into the cell membranes of the transformed cells and, by aggregating, form hydrophilic pores. These pores may become so large and so abundant that the target cell cannot maintain its cytoplasmic integrity, and the cells undergo necrosis. It should be noted that the CTL is protected from autodestruction by perforin in two ways:
   a. The CTL moves away from the target cell as the process of perforin release is taking place.
   b. Cathepsin B, a proteolytic enzyme is co-released by the vesicle that released the perforin. This enzyme remains by the CTL cell membrane and degrades perforin molecules that attempt to embed themselves into the CTL's membrane.
2. Binding (in the presence of calcium) causes the release of perforins and granzymes. Granzymes are released from the storage granules of the CTL. These enzymes enter the transformed cells via the perforin-formed pores and drive the cells into apoptosis, killing them within a few minutes.
3. Binding can also bring the CTL's Fas ligand (a transmembrane protein; a member of the tumor necrosis family, also known as *CD95L*) in contact with the target cell membrane's "death receptor," known as the *Fas receptor* (*CD95*). When a threshold number of these Fas ligands and Fas proteins bond, the clustering of the Fas proteins induces the intracellular protein cascade that leads to apoptosis.

Note that certain highly vigorous APCs can act as the first signal. In such an instance, the CTL does not require a T-helper cell intermediary but can release IL-2 and can activate itself.

Clinical Correlations

Cells use spell-checking to ensure that they have copied their DNA correctly and, if not, that they have corrected those errors during mitosis. Mutations that prevent cells from DNA mismatch repair have beneficial effects in ***PD-L1*** *and* ***PD-L2 (programmed cell death ligand-1 and programmed cell death ligand-2) blockade immunotherapy*** *against certain cancers. These immunotherapies were able to able to counter several types of solid tumors of various origins, including those arising from the pancreas and gastrointestinal tract. The tumor cells take advantage of the fact that when the cancer cells' PD-L1 binds to PD-1 receptors on CTLs' cell membranes, it inactivates the cytotoxic T cells, rendering them unable to kill the tumor cells. Pembrolizumab was developed to block the PD-1 receptors of CTLs, preventing the PD-L1 of tumor cells from contacting and binding to the PD-1 receptors. Thus, the cytotoxic T cells are able to perform their job of killing the tumor cells even if the tumor has metastasized. In some patients in the clinical study, the cancer disappeared. In other patients, the tumors shrunk, the cancerous cells disappeared, and the tumor appeared to consist of immune cells. The treatment did not work in a few patients because they developed additional mutations that affected their immune cells. There are some side effects of the immune therapy—including thyroid issues, diarrhea, and skin rashes—because some of the CTLs attacked other tissues. Even though current studies are in progress that attempt to mitigate and eliminate these side effects, in 2017, due to the efficacy of pembrolizumab, the US Food and Drug Administration approved the drug to be used in cancer patients with mismatch repair mutations.*

T_H1 Cells Assist Macrophages in Killing Bacteria

Bacteria that are phagocytosed by macrophages can readily proliferate within the phagosome (becoming infected) because macrophages cannot destroy these microorganisms unless they are activated by T_H1 cells (Fig. 12.4).

Signal 1. The TCR and CD4 molecules of the T_H1 cell must recognize the epitope–MHC II complex of the macrophage that phagocytosed the bacteria.

Signal 2. The T_H1 cell expresses IL-2 receptors on its surface and releases IL-2, which binds to the receptors, thus activating itself.

The activated T_H1 cell rapidly proliferates, and the newly formed T_H1 cells contact macrophages that are infected with bacteria.

Signal 1. The TCR and CD4 molecules of the T_H1 cell must recognize the epitope–MHC II complex of the infected macrophage, and the T cell releases IFN-γ.

Signal 2. The IFN-γ activates the macrophage, which then expresses TNF-α receptors on its surface and releases the cytokine TNF-α.

When these two factors, IFN-γ and TNF-α, bind to their receptors on macrophages, they facilitate the production of oxygen radicals by the macrophage, resulting in the killing of bacteria.

Clinical Correlations

Human immunodeficiency virus (HIV), the cause of acquired immunodeficiency syndrome (AIDS), binds to CD4 molecules of T-helper cells and injects its core into the cell. The virus incapacitates the cell, and as the virus spreads, it infects other T-helper cells, reducing their number. As a result, infected persons eventually become incapable of mounting an immune response against bacterial or viral infections. Victims succumb to secondary infections, owing to opportunistic microorganisms or to malignancies. Numerous treatment strategies have ameliorated the lethal effects of the virus; in developed countries, most HIV patients have a normal lifespan. A combination of two or more broadly neutralizing antibodies that have the ability to bind to a number of loci of various strains of HIV can overcome the virus's facility to mutate readily, preventing it from spreading and perhaps even providing therapeutic results.

Lymphoid Organs

The lymphoid organs are classified into two categories, primary and secondary:

1. **Primary (central) lymphoid organs** are responsible for the development and maturation of lymphocytes into mature, immunocompetent cells.
2. **Secondary (peripheral) lymphoid organs** are responsible for the proper environment in which immunocompetent cells can interact with each other, as well as with antigens and other cells to mount an immunological challenge against invading antigens or pathogens.

In humans, the fetal liver, prenatal and postnatal bone marrow, and thymus constitute the primary lymphoid organs. The lymph nodes, spleen, and MALT, as well as the postnatal bone marrow, constitute the secondary lymphoid organs.

THYMUS

The thymus is a primary lymphoid organ that is the site of maturation of T lymphocytes.

The thymus, situated in the superior mediastinum and extending over the great vessels of the heart, is a small encapsulated organ composed of two **lobes**. Each lobe arises separately in the third (and possibly fourth) pharyngeal pouches of the embryo. The T lymphocytes that enter the thymus to become instructed to achieve immunological competence arise from mesoderm and, after birth, in the bone marrow.

The thymus originates early in the embryo and continues to grow until puberty, when it may weigh as much as 35 to 40 g. After the first few years of life, the thymus begins to **involute** (atrophy) and becomes infiltrated by adipose cells. However, it may continue to function, even in older adults.

The capsule of the thymus, composed of dense, irregular collagenous connective tissue, sends septa into the lobes, subdividing them into incomplete **lobules** (Fig. 12.5). Each lobule is composed of a cortex and a medulla, although the medullae of adjacent lobules are confluent with each other.

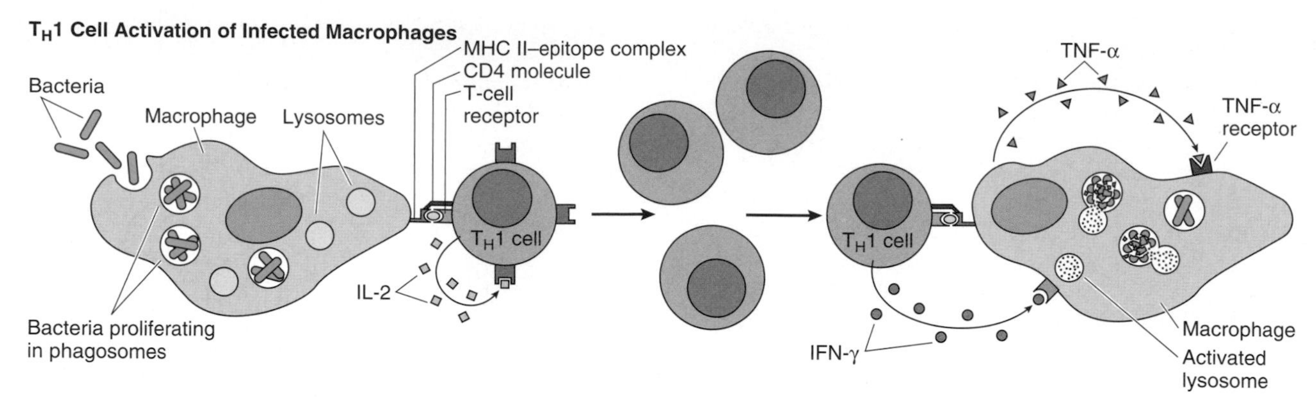

T_H1 cell's TCR and CD4 molecules recognize the MHC II–epitope complex presented by a macrophage that was infected by bacteria. The T_H1 cell becomes activated, expresses IL-2 receptors on its surface, and releases IL-2. Binding of IL-2 results in proliferation of the T_H1 cells.

The newly formed T_H1 cells contact infected macrophages (TCR and CD4 recognition of MHC II–epitope complex) and release IFN-γ. IFN-γ activates the macrophage to express TNF-α receptors on its surface, as well as to release TNF-α. Binding of IFN-γ and TNF-α on the macrophage cell membrane facilitates the production of oxygen radicals by the macrophage resulting in killing of bacteria.

Fig. 12.4 Schematic diagram of macrophage activation by T cells. CD, Cluster of differentiation; IL, interleukin; INF, interferon; TCR, T-cell receptor; TNF, tumor necrosis factor.

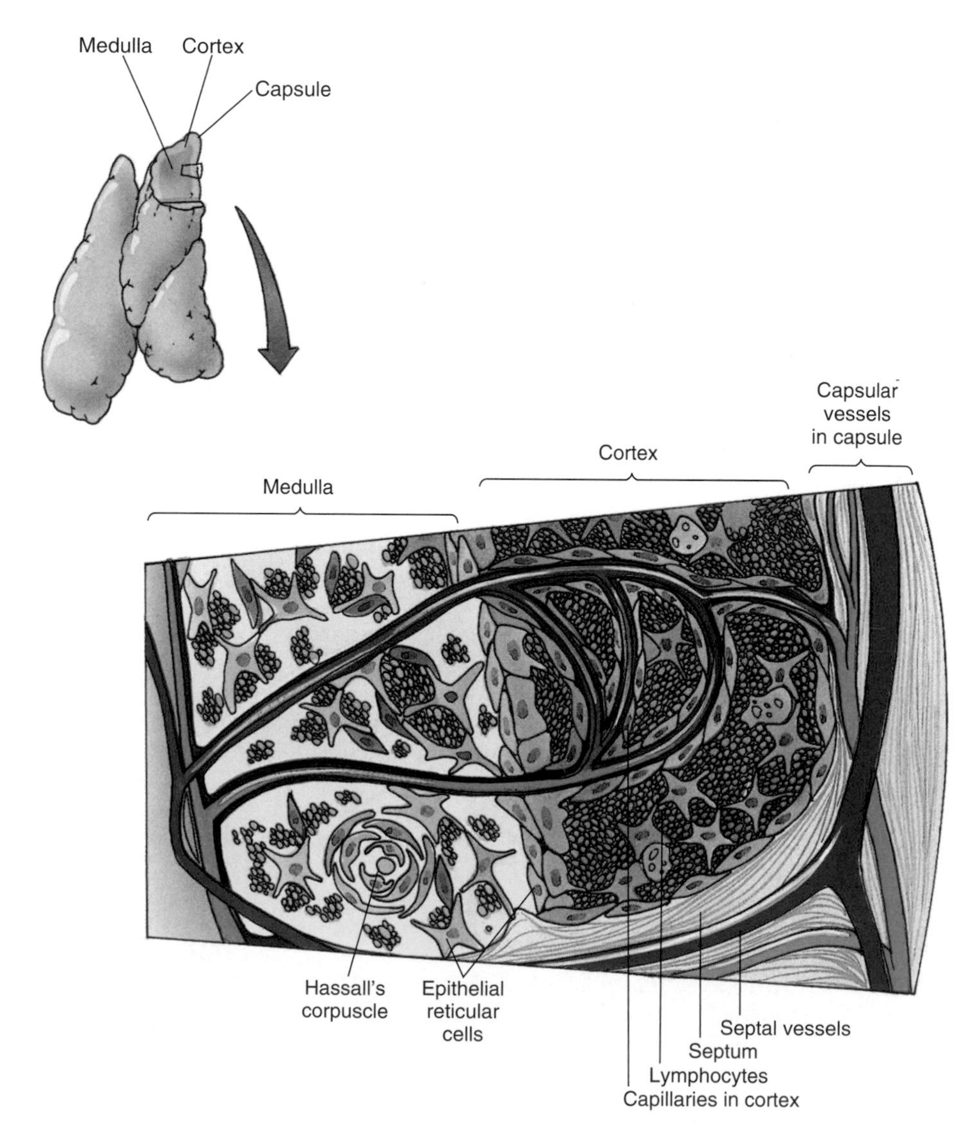

Fig. 12.5 Diagram of the thymus demonstrating its blood supply and its histological arrangement.

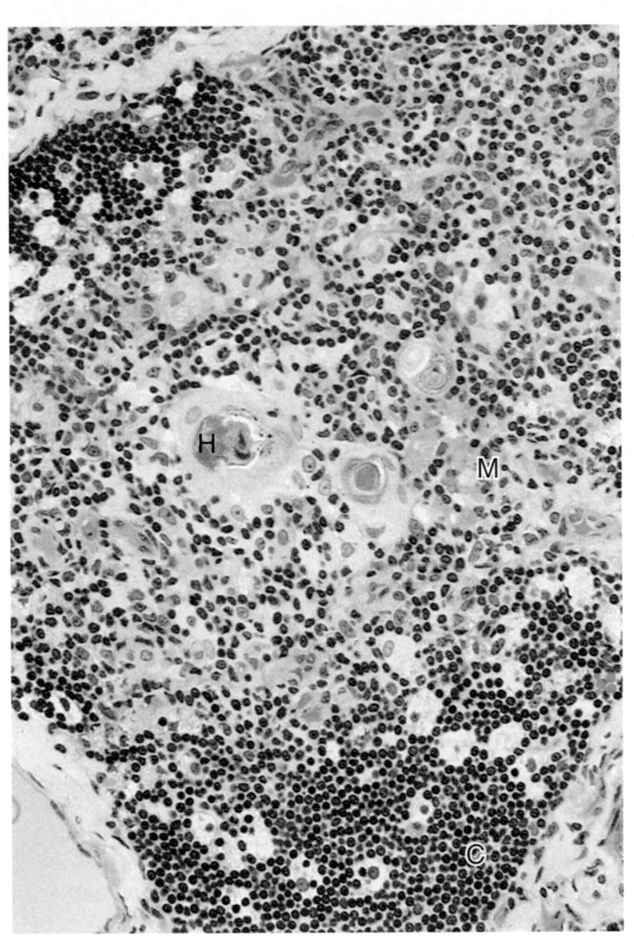

Fig. 12.6 Photomicrograph of a lobule of the thymus. The peripheral cortex (C) stains darker than the central medulla (M) that is distinguished by the presence of Hassall corpuscles (H). (×124)

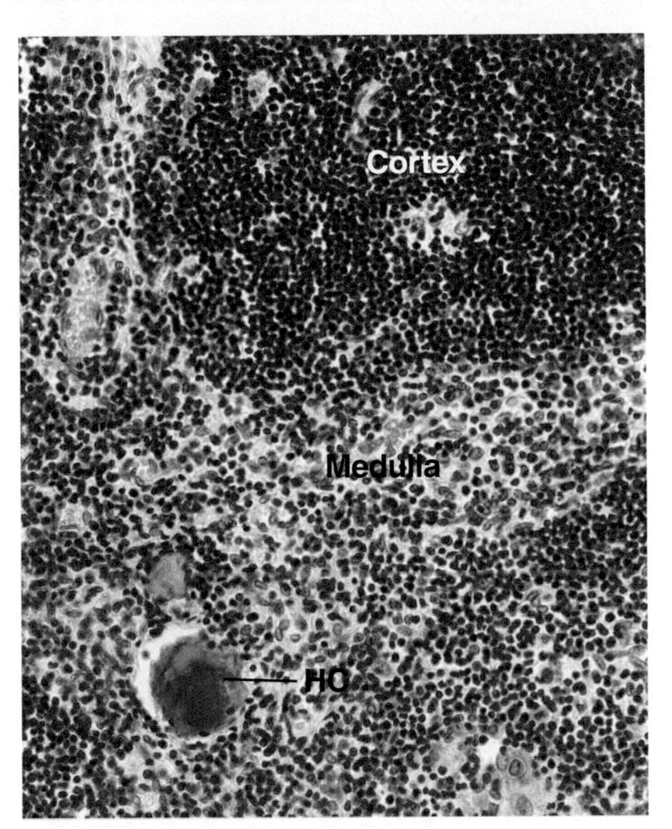

Fig. 12.7 Photomicrograph of the cortex and medulla of a thymic lobule. Note that the cortex is much darker than the medulla because of its closely packed small cells with large nuclei. The medulla is lighter because its cells are farther apart from each other. Observe the presence of a Hassall corpuscle (HC) in the medulla. (×270)

Cortex

Immunological competency of T cells, elimination of self-intolerant T lymphocytes, and MHC recognition occur in the thymic cortex.

The **cortex** of the thymus appears much darker histologically than does the medulla because of the presence of a large number of **T lymphocytes** (**thymocytes**; Figs. 12.6 to 12.8; see Fig. 12.5). Immunologically incompetent T cells leave the bone marrow and migrate to the periphery of the thymic cortex, where they undergo extensive proliferation and instruction to become immunocompetent T cells (see earlier discussion). In addition to the thymocytes, the cortex houses macrophages, dendritic cells, and **epithelial reticular cells** (**thymic epithelial cells**) (Table 12.6). It is believed that, in humans, epithelial reticular cells are derived from the endoderm of the third (and possibly fourth) pharyngeal pouch. Three types of epithelial reticular cells are present in the thymic cortex.

Type I cells separate the cortex from the connective tissue capsule and trabeculae and surround vascular elements in the cortex. These cells form occluding junctions with each other, completely isolating the thymic cortex from the remainder of the body. The nuclei of type I cells are polymorphous and have well-defined nucleoli.

Type II cells are located in the midcortex. These cells have long, wide, sheath-like processes that form desmosomal junctions with each other. Their processes form a cytoreticulum that subdivides the thymic cortex into small, lymphocyte-filled compartments. The nuclei of type II cells are large, pale structures with little heterochromatin. The cytoplasm is also pale and is richly endowed with tonofilaments.

Type III cells are located in the deep cortex and at the corticomedullary junction. The cytoplasm and the nuclei of these cells are denser than those of type I and type II epithelial reticular cells. The RER of type III cells displays dilated cisternae, which is indicative of protein synthesis. Type III epithelial reticular cells also have wide, sheath-like processes that form lymphocyte-filled compartments. These cells participate in the formation of occluding junctions with each other and with epithelial reticular cells of the medulla; this isolates the cortex from the medulla.

These three types of epithelial reticular cells completely isolate the thymic cortex and, thus, prevent developing T cells from contacting foreign antigens. Types II and III cells, as well as bone marrow–derived **interdigitating cells** (**APCs**), present **self-antigens**, **MHC I** molecules, and **MHC II** molecules to the developing T cells. Developing T lymphocytes whose TCRs recognize self proteins or whose CD4 or CD8 molecules cannot recognize the MHC I or MHC II molecules are forced into apoptosis before they can leave the cortex. It is interesting that 98% of developing T cells die in the cortex and are phagocytosed by resident macrophages, which are referred to as ***tingible body macrophages***. The surviving thymocytes enter the medulla of the thymus as I T lymphocytes (*single positive T cells*). From there (or from the corticomedullary junction), they are distributed to secondary lymphoid organs via the vascular system.

Medulla

The medulla is characterized by the presence of Hassall corpuscles; all thymocytes of the medulla are immunocompetent T cells.

The thymic **medulla** stains much lighter than the cortex because its lymphocyte population is not nearly as profuse and because it houses macrophages, dendritic cells, a small population of B cells, and a large number of endothelially derived epithelial reticular cells (see Figs. 12.5, 12.6, and 12.9). There are three types of epithelial reticular cells in the medulla (see Table 12.6).

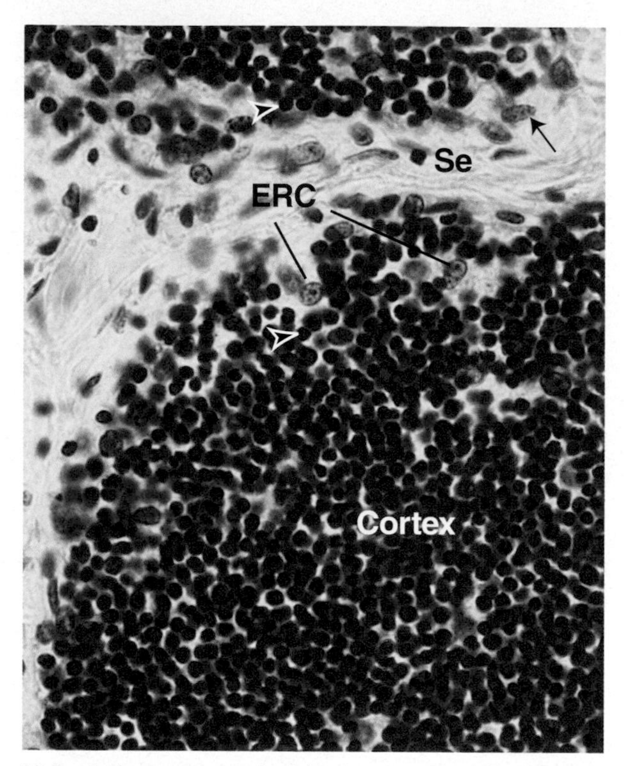

Fig. 12.8 A photomicrograph of the thymic cortex of two neighboring lobules separated from each other by a septum (Se). Note the presence of epithelial reticular cells *(arrow)* that are most probably type I epithelial reticular cells. Within the cortex, observe more epithelial reticular cells (ERC); these are type II epithelial reticular cells. The most prominent cell population of the cortex is composed of thymocytes *(arrowheads)* that are immunoincompetent T cells. (×540)

Type IV cells are found in close association with type III cells of the cortex and assist in the formation of the corticomedullary junction. The nuclei of these cells have a coarse chromatin network, and their cytoplasm is dark-staining and richly endowed with tonofilaments.

Type V cells form the cytoreticulum of the medulla. The nuclei of these cells are polymorphous, with a well-defined perinuclear chromatin network and a conspicuous nucleolus.

Type VI cells compose the most characteristic feature of the thymic medulla. These large, pale-staining cells coalesce around each other, forming whorl-shaped **thymic corpuscles** (**Hassall corpuscles**), whose numbers increase with a person's age (see Figs. 12.5, 12.6 and 12.9). Type VI cells may become highly cornified and even calcified. The function of thymic corpuscles is not understood completely, although they might be the site of T lymphocyte cell death in the medulla, and it has been demonstrated that it is the type VI epithelial reticular cells of Hassall corpuscles that manufacture thymic stromal lymphopoietin, a signaling molecule that functions in T reg cell development. It has also been suggested that once medullary epithelial reticular cells cease to express the transcription factor AIRE (autoimmune regulator), they become type VI cells and form Hassall corpuscles.

Vascular Supply

The cortical vascular supply forms a very powerful blood–thymus barrier to prevent developing T cells from contacting blood-borne macromolecules.

The thymus receives numerous small arteries, which enter the capsule and are distributed throughout the organ via the trabeculae between adjacent lobules. Branches of these vessels do not gain access to the cortex directly; instead, from the trabeculae, they enter the corticomedullary junction, where they form capillary beds that penetrate the cortex.

The capillaries of the cortex are of the **continuous** type, possess a thick basal lamina, and are invested by a sheath of type I epithelial reticular cells that form a **blood–thymus barrier**. Thus, the developing T cells of the cortex are protected from contacting

TABLE 12.6 Epithelial Reticular Cells of the Thymus and Their Function

Cell Type	Location	Function
I	Cortex	Separate the cortex from the connective tissue capsule and trabeculae and surround vascular elements in the cortex. These cells form occluding junctions with each other, completely isolating the thymic cortex from the remainder of the body and participate in the formation of the blood–thymus barrier.
II	Mid-cortex	Their processes form a cytoreticulum that subdivides the thymic cortex into small, lymphocyte-filled compartments. They express MHC I and MHC II molecules complexed with self epitopes and test developing T cells for self recognition.
III	Cortical aspect of corticomedullary junction	Participate in the formation of occluding junctions with each other and with type IV epithelial reticular cells of the medulla, isolating the cortex from the medulla. They express MHC I and MHC II molecules complexed with self epitopes and test developing T cells for self-recognition.
IV	Medullary aspect of corticomedullary junction	Participate in the formation of occluding junctions with each other and with type III epithelial reticular cells of the cortex, isolating the cortex from the medulla.
V	Medulla	Form the cytoreticulum of the medulla and provide compartment for T cells.
VI	Medulla	Form whorl-shaped thymic corpuscles (Hassall corpuscles) where, perhaps, T cells are eliminated; they also synthesize and release thymic stromal lymphopoietin, the signaling molecule that participates in the development of T reg cells.

MHC, Major histocompatibility complex.

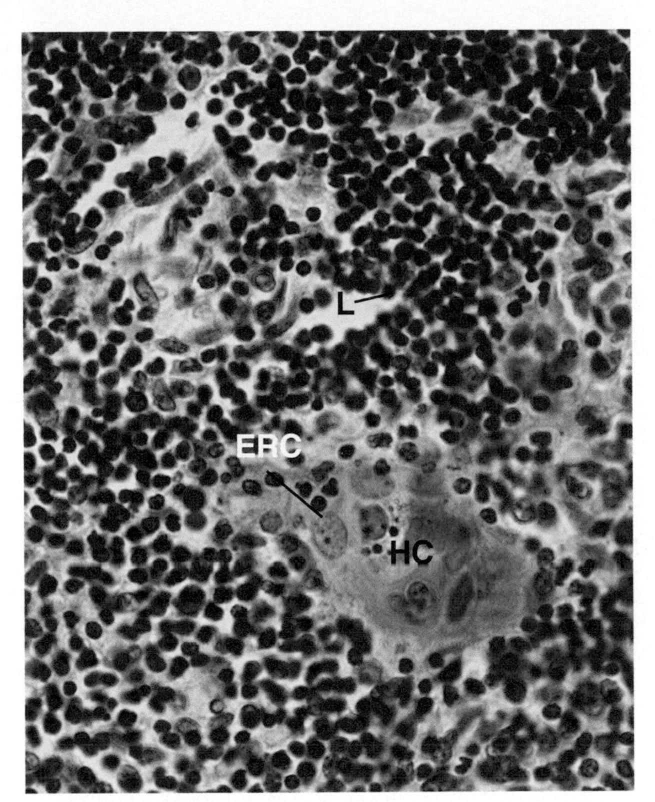

Fig. 12.9 A high-magnification photomicrograph of a Hassall corpuscle (HC) of the thymic medulla. Hassall corpuscles are composed of type VI epithelial reticular cells (ERC). Note the numerous lymphocytes (Ly) in the medulla. (×540)

blood-borne macromolecules. However, self macromolecules are permitted to cross the blood–thymus barrier (probably controlled by the epithelial reticular cells), possibly to eliminate those T cells that are programmed against self antigens. The cortical capillary network drains into small venules in the medulla.

Newly formed, immunologically incompetent T cells arriving from the bone marrow leave the vascular supply at the corticomedullary junction and migrate to the periphery of the cortex. As these cells mature, they move deeper into the cortex and enter the medulla as **single positive T cells (I T cells)** that are inactive immunocompetent cells. As they leave the thymic medulla via veins draining the thymus, they are referred to as **naïve T cells**.

Histophysiology of the Thymus

The primary function of the thymus is to instruct immunoincompetent T cells to achieve immunocompetence.

As the developing T cells proliferate extensively in the cortex, they begin to express their surface markers, and are tested for their ability to recognize **self MHC molecules** and **self epitopes**. T cells that are unable to recognize self MHC I and self MHC II molecules are destroyed by being driven into apoptosis. Additionally, T lymphocytes whose TCRs are programmed against self macromolecules are also destroyed.

The epithelial reticular cells of the thymus produce the transcription factor known as **AIRE** and the cytokine **thymic stromal lymphopoietin**. These factors facilitate dendritic cell activation as well as T-cell proliferation and maturation, such as expression of their surface markers and differentiation into T-cell subtypes. Additionally, hormones from extrathymic sources—especially the gonads and the pituitary, thyroid, and suprarenal glands—influence T-cell maturation. The most potent effects are due to (1) **adrenocorticosteroids**, which decrease T-cell numbers in the thymic cortex; (2) **thyroxin**, which stimulates the cortical epithelial reticular cells to facilitate T-cell and NK-cell activity; and (3) **somatotropin**, which promotes T-cell development in the thymic cortex.

Clinical Correlations

Congenital failure of the thymus to develop is called ***DiGeorge syndrome****. It is due to the deletion of a small portion of chromosome 22, resulting in the loss of some 3 dozen genes located near the center of this chromosome. Patients with this disease exhibit various conditions, among others: delay in development, heart defects (such as tetralogy of Fallot), hearing loss, and abnormal kidneys. They also exhibit immune disorders because they cannot produce T cells, making their cellularly mediated immune response nonfunctional. These patients subsequently die at an early age from infection. Because these patients also lack parathyroid glands, death also may be caused by tetany.*

LYMPH NODES

Lymph nodes are small, encapsulated, oval structures that are interposed in the path of lymph vessels to serve as filters for the removal of bacteria and other foreign substances from lymph.

Lymph nodes are located in various regions of the body but are most prevalent in the neck, in the axilla, in the groin, along major vessels, and in the body cavities. Their parenchyma is composed of collections of T and B lymphocytes, APCs, macrophages, dendritic cells, follicular dendritic cells, and stromal cells. These lymphoid cells react to the presence of antigens by mounting an immunological response in which macrophages phagocytose bacteria and other microorganisms that enter the lymph node by way of the lymph.

Each lymph node is a relatively small, soft structure that is less than 3 cm in diameter; they have a fibrous connective tissue capsule, usually surrounded by adipose tissue (Figs. 12.10 and 12.11). Lymph nodes have a convex surface that is perforated by **afferent lymph vessels** with **valves**, which ensure that lymph flows only in one direction, entering the substance of the node. The concave surface of the node, the **hilum**, is the site of arteries and veins entering and exiting the node. Additionally, lymph leaves the node via the **efferent lymph vessels**, also located at the hilum. The efferent lymph vessels have valves that prevent regurgitation of lymph back into the node.

Histologically, a lymph node is subdivided into three regions: cortex, paracortex, and medulla. All three regions have a rich supply of sinusoids, enlarged endothelially lined spaces through which lymph percolates.

Cortex

The cortex of the lymph node is subdivided into incomplete compartments that house B-cell–rich primary and secondary lymphoid nodules.

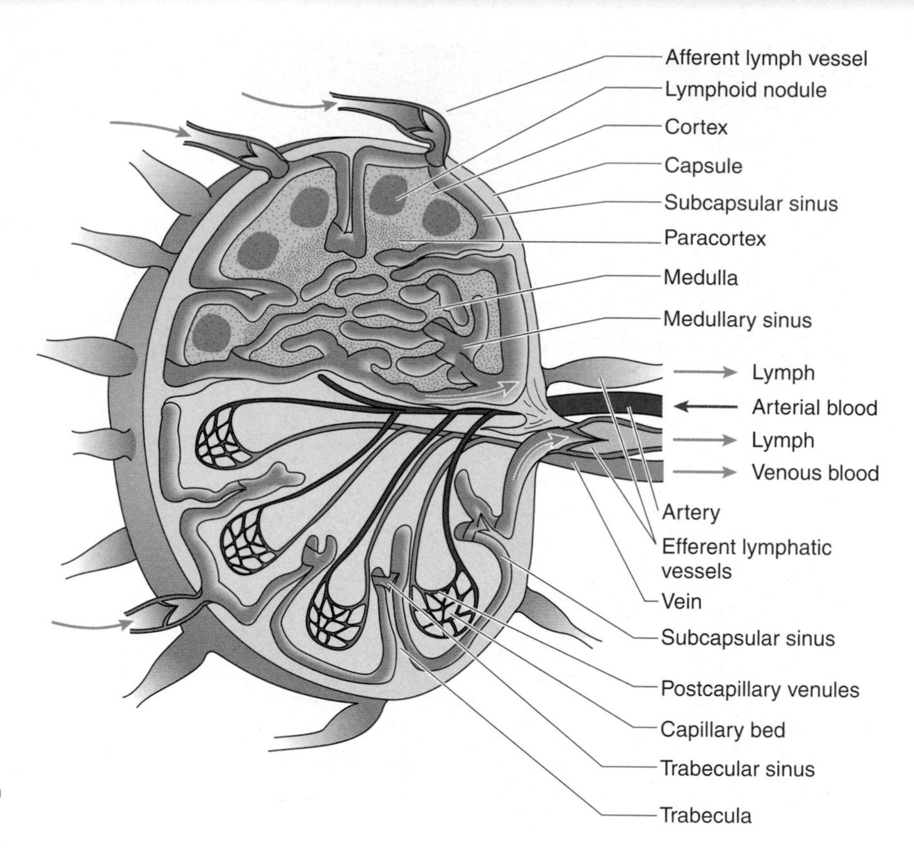

Fig. 12.10 Schematic diagram of a typical lymph node.

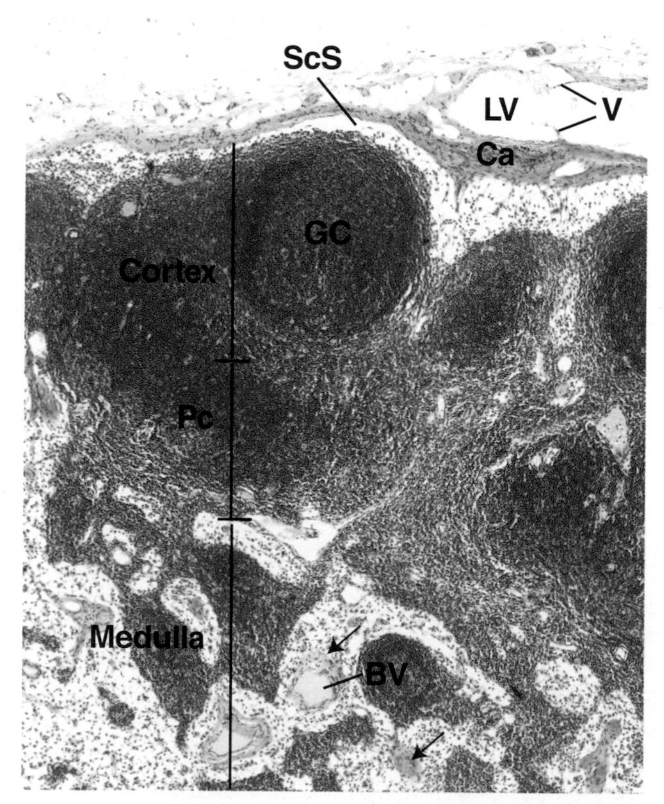

Fig. 12.11 This is a very-low-magnification photomicrograph of the capsule, cortex, paracortex (Pc), and a portion of the medulla of a lymph node. Observe the dense, irregular, collagenous capsule (Ca) with a lymph vessel (LV) whose valves (V) ensure that the lymph will enter the subcapsular sinus (ScS) of the lymph node and not reflux into the vessel. Observe that the lymph nodule has a very large germinal center (GC). The medulla is richly endowed with veins (BV) and arterioles (arrows). (×14)

The dense, irregular, collagenous connective tissue **capsule** sends **trabeculae** into the substance of the lymph node, subdividing the outer region of the **cortex** into incomplete compartments. These partitioned regions extend along the entire periphery of the node (Figs. 12.12 and 12.13; see Fig. 12.10) all the way to the vicinity of the hilum. The capsule is thickened at the hilum; as vessels enter the substance of the node, they are surrounded by a connective tissue sheath derived from the capsule. Suspended from the capsule and trabeculae is a three-dimensional network of **reticular connective tissue** that forms the architectural framework of the entire lymph node.

Clinical Correlations

In the presence of antigens or bacteria, lymphocytes of the lymph node rapidly proliferate, and the node may increase to several times its normal size, becoming hard, palpable, and painful to the touch at times.

The **afferent lymph vessels** pierce the capsule on the convex surface of the node and empty their lymph into the **subcapsular sinus**, which is located just deep to the capsule. This sinus is continuous with the **cortical sinuses** (**paratrabecular sinuses**) that parallel the trabeculae and deliver the lymph into the **medullary sinuses**, eventually to enter the **efferent lymphatic vessels.** These sinuses have a network of **stellate reticular cells,** whose processes contact those of other cells and the endothelium-like simple squamous epithelium. Collagen fibers, coated by processes of reticular cells, form a loose web in the lumina of these sinuses, reducing the velocity of flow of the lymph and creating turbulence. This provides **macrophages** attached to the stellate reticular cells the

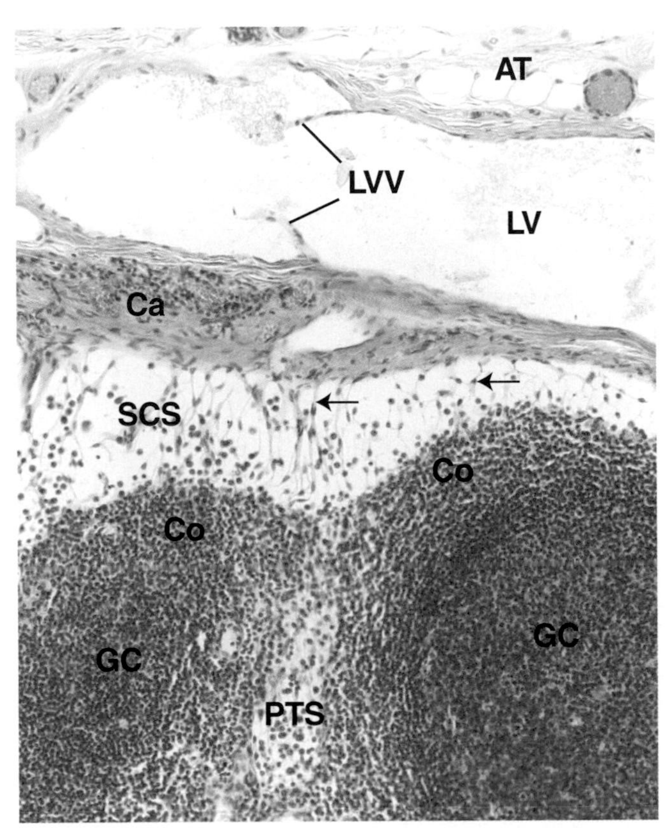

Fig. 12.12 This is a higher-magnification photomicrograph of Fig. 12.11 showing that the capsule (Ca) is surrounded by adipose tissue (AT). The valves (LVV) of the lymph vessel (LV) function to retard the back-flow of the lymph. Observe that the stellate reticular cells *(arrows)* in the subcapsular sinus (SCS) span the sinus to slow down the flow of the lymph. Paratrabecular sinuses (PTS) receive lymph from the subcapsular sinus. The corona (Co) and the germinal center (GC) of the lymph nodules are well differentiated. (×132)

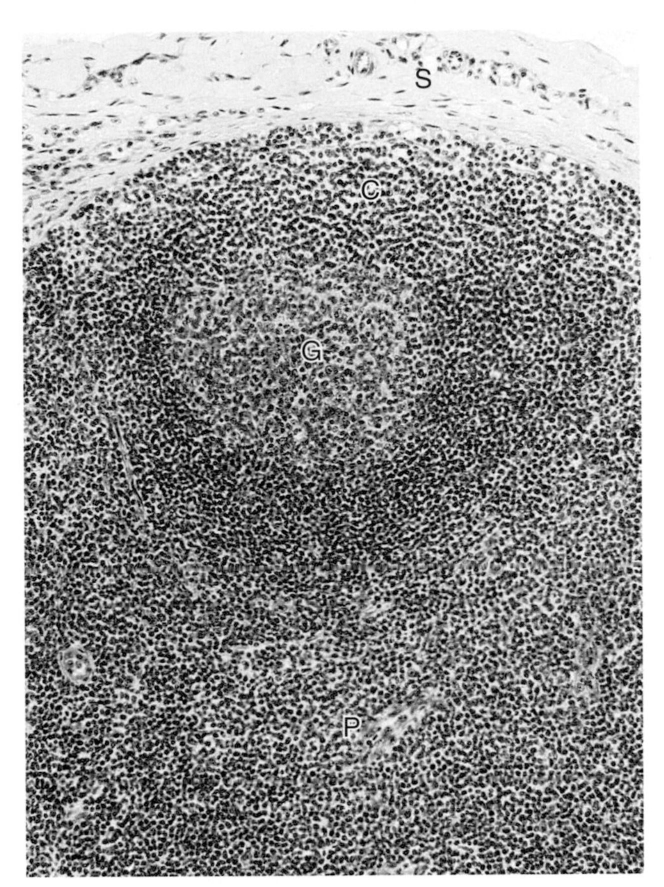

Fig. 12.13 Photomicrograph of the lymph node cortex, displaying the subcapsular sinus (S), a secondary lymphoid nodule with its corona (C), germinal center (G), and the paracortex (P). (×132)

opportunity to phagocytose foreign particulate matter. Additional channels are present that allow lymph to flow from the subcapsular sinus, as well as from the paratrabecular sinuses to **perivenular channels** that surround **high endothelial venules (HEVs)** of the paracortex. These channels are known as ***fibroblastic reticular cell conduits*** because they are formed by **fibroblastic reticular cells**. They permit rapid movement of material through the lymph node. These conduits are surrounded by dendritic cells as well as by a tightly packed population of **naïve T cells** that have entered the paracortex via the HEVs. The naïve T cells are mostly **T_H cells**, although **CTLs** are also present. The population of CTLs becomes greatly enlarged during viral pathogenesis.

Lymphoid Nodules

There are two types of lymphoid nodules: primary and secondary. Secondary lymphoid nodules have a germinal center.

The incomplete compartments within the cortex house **primary lymphoid nodules**, which are spherical aggregates of **B lymphocytes** (both virgin B cells and B memory cells) clustered around **follicular dendritic cells (FDCs)** whose processes contact those of their neighboring FDCs to form a three-dimensional web-like network. These B lymphocytes are in the process of entering or leaving the lymph node (see Figs. 12.10 to 12.13). In addition to the B cells, some T cells are also present. Frequently, the centers of the lymphoid nodules are stained paler and house **germinal centers**; these lymphoid nodules are then known as ***secondary lymphoid nodules***. Secondary lymphoid nodules form only in response to an antigenic challenge; it is believed that they are the sites of **B memory cell** and **plasma cell** generation.

The region of the lymphoid nodule peripheral to the germinal center is composed of a dense accumulation of small lymphocytes that are migrating away from their site of origin within the germinal center. This peripheral region is called the **corona (mantle)**.

Germinal centers display three zones: a dark zone, basal light zone, and apical light zone. The **dark zone** is the site of the intense proliferation of closely packed B cells (that do not possess sIgs). These cells, known as **centroblasts**, migrate into the **basal light zone**, express sIgs, switch immunoglobulin class, and develop into centrocytes. **Centrocytes** are exposed to antigen-bearing **follicular dendritic cells** and undergo hypermutation to become more proficient at forming antibodies against antigens. Cells that do not synthesize the proper sIgs are forced into apoptosis, and their remnants are destroyed by macrophages. The newly formed centrocytes that are permitted to survive enter the **apical light zone**, where they become either **B memory cells** or **plasma cells** and subsequently leave the secondary follicle.

Paracortex

The region of the lymph node between the cortex and the medulla is the paracortex. It houses mostly T cells and fibroblastic reticular cells and is the thymus-dependent zone of the lymph node.

The **paracortex** is a T cell–rich region that is located between the medulla and the follicle-rich region of the cortex (Figs. 12.11, 12.13, and 12.14). APCs (e.g., Langerhans cells from skin

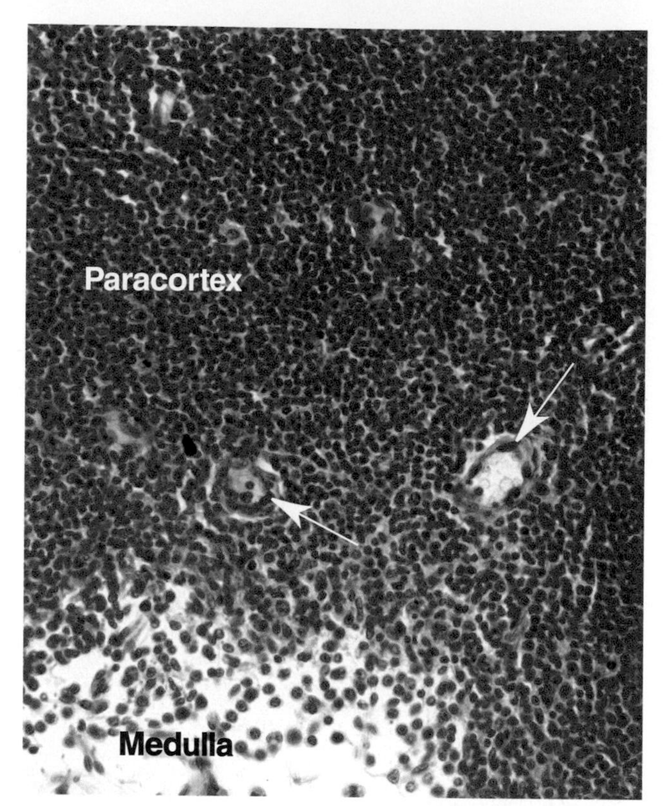

Fig. 12.14 This is a higher magnification of the paracortex of a lymph node. Observe the high endothelial vessels *(arrows)* where lymphocytes leave the circulatory system to enter the lymph node. Observe how much more cellular the paracortex is than the medulla. (×270)

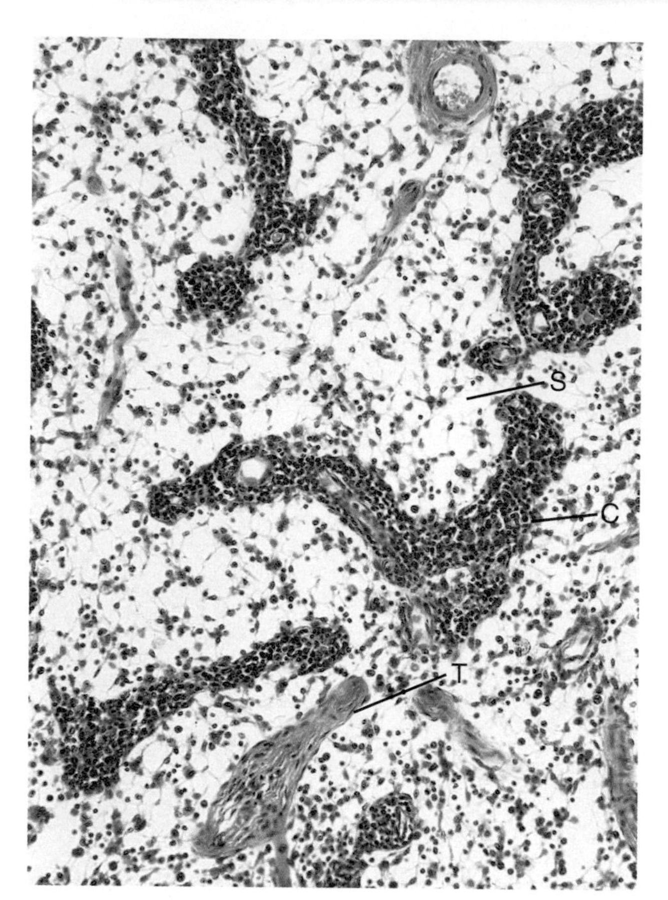

Fig. 12.15 Photomicrograph of the lymph node medulla with its medullary sinusoids (S), medullary cords (C), and trabecula (T). (×132)

or dendritic cells from the mucosa) migrate to the **paracortex** region of the lymph node to present their epitope–MHC II complex to T helper cells. If T helper cells become activated, they proliferate, increasing the width of the paracortex to such an extent that it may intrude deep into the medulla. Newly formed T cells then migrate to the medullary sinuses, leave the lymph node, and proceed to the area of antigenic activity.

HEVs (**postcapillary venules**) are located in the paracortex. Lymphocytes leave the vascular supply by migrating between the cuboidal cells of this unusual endothelium and enter the substance of the lymph node. B cells migrate to the outer cortex, whereas most T cells remain in the paracortex.

The lymphocyte plasma membrane expresses surface molecules, known as **selectins**, that aid the cell in recognizing the endothelial cells of HEVs and permit it to roll along the surface of these cells. When the lymphocyte contacts additional signaling molecules that are located on the endothelial cell plasmalemma, the selectins become activated, bind firmly to the endothelial cell, and stop the rolling action of the lymphocyte. Then, via **diapedesis**, the lymphocyte migrates between the cuboidal endothelial cells to leave the lumen of the postcapillary venule and enter the lymph node parenchyma (see Chapter 10, Fig. 10.8).

Medulla

The medulla is composed of large, tortuous lymph sinuses surrounded by lymphoid cells that are organized in clusters known as medullary cords.

The cells of the **medullary cords** (lymphocytes, plasma cells, and macrophages) are enmeshed in a network of reticular fibers and reticular cells (Figs. 12.15 and 12.16; see Fig. 12.10). The

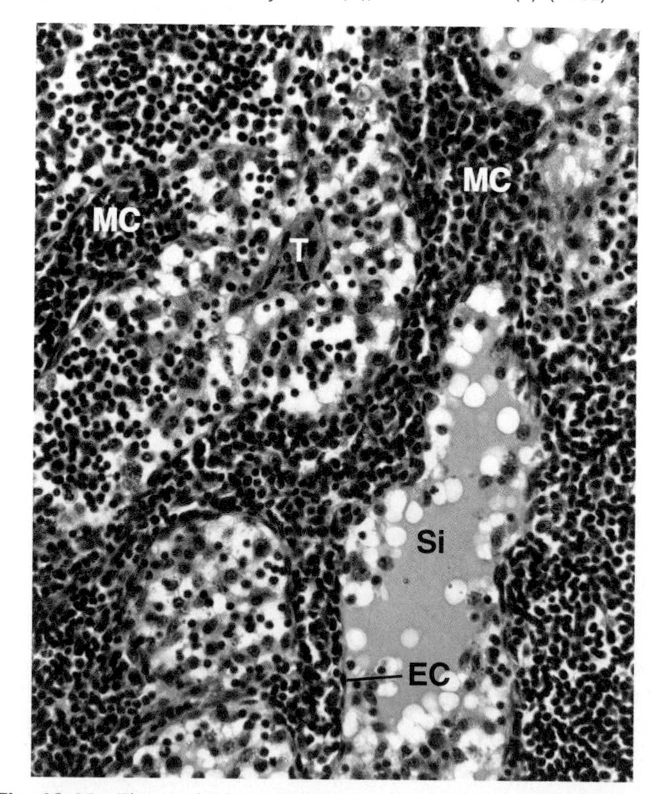

Fig. 12.16 This is a high-magnification photomicrograph of the lymph node medulla. Note that the medullary cords (MC) are composed of a large number of closely packed lymphocytes, plasma cells, and macrophages. Endothelial cells (EC) line the sinusoids (Si) and trabeculae (T) convey blood vessels in and out of the lymph node. (×540)

lymphocytes migrate from the cortex to enter the medullary sinuses from which they enter the efferent lymphatic vessels to leave the lymph node. Histological sections of the medulla also display the presence of trabeculae, arising from the thickened capsule at the hilum, conveying blood vessels into and out of the lymph node.

Vascularization of the Lymph Node

The arterial supply enters the substance of lymph nodes at the hilum. The vessels course through the medulla within trabeculae and become smaller as they repeatedly branch. Eventually, they lose their connective tissue sheath, travel within the substance of medullary cords, and contribute to the formation of the medullary capillary beds. The small branches of the arteries continue in the medullary cords until they reach the cortex. Here, they form a cortical capillary bed, which is drained by **postcapillary venules**. Blood from postcapillary venules drains into larger veins, which exit the lymph node at the hilum.

Histophysiology of Lymph Nodes

Lymph nodes filter lymph, segregate T and B cells from each other, and act as sites for antigen recognition.

Lymph nodes function in attracting B cells and T cells to their proper residence in the cortex, providing a location for combating antigens and removing foreign particulate matter from the lymph that enters the node.

In order to be able to attract B and T cells to their proper location in the cortex, stromal cells release factors known as **chemotactic chemokines for lymphocytes (CCLs)** that are specific for attracting **B cells** and **follicular dendritic cells** as well as **CCLs** that are specific for attracting **T cells** and **dendritic cells**. Both types of chemokines are released by these stromal cells, and the chemokines attach to the luminal surface of endothelial cells of **postcapillary venules** (**high endothelial cell venules; HEVs**). As the T cells and dendritic cells and B cells and follicular dendritic cells reach these chemokine-coated endothelial cells, they attach to the endothelial cells, penetrate the intercellular spaces, leave the lumen of the blood vessel, enter the stroma of the lymph node cortex, and follow their designated chemokines to the paracortex (in the case of T cells and dendritic cells) and to the lymph nodules (in the case of B cells and follicular dendritic cells). In the paracortex, certain dendritic cells and certain stromal cells express **AIRE**, a transcription factor that functions in forcing those T cells into **apoptosis** that were able to escape from the thymus even though they are anti-self.

As lymph enters the lymph node, the flow rate is reduced, which gives the macrophages that reside in (or have their processes intrude into) the sinuses more time to phagocytose foreign particulate matter. In this fashion, 99% of the unwanted substances present in lymph are removed.

Lymph nodes also function as sites of antigen recognition because APCs that contact antigens migrate to the nearest lymph node and present their epitope–MHC complex to lymphocytes. Additionally, antigens percolating through the lymph node are trapped by **follicular dendritic cells** and **B lymphocytes** that are in the lymphoid nodule or migrate into the lymphoid nodule and recognize the antigen.

If an antigen is recognized and a B cell becomes activated, that B cell migrates to a **primary lymphoid nodule** and proliferates, forming a germinal center, converting the primary lymphoid nodule into a **secondary lymphoid nodule**. The newly formed cells differentiate into B memory cells and plasma cells; they leave the cortex to enter the medulla, and form the medullary cords. About 10% of the newly formed plasma cells stay in the medulla and release antibodies into the medullary sinuses. The rest of the plasma cells enter the sinuses and go to the bone marrow, where they continue to manufacture antibodies until they die. Some B memory cells stay in the primary lymphoid nodules of the cortex, but most leave the lymph node to take up residence in other secondary lymphatic organs of the body. Therefore, if there is a second exposure to the same antigen, a large number of memory cells are available so that the body can mount a prompt and potent secondary response.

Most of the T cell immune responses depend on epitope-bearing dendritic cells that migrate into the lymph nodes, then progress to the paracortex, where they present their epitope-MHC complex to T cells. The T cells that recognize the epitope–MHC complex become activated and initiate a cell-mediated immune response.

Clinical Correlations

Lymph nodes are located along the paths of lymph vessels, forming a chain of lymph nodes so that lymph flows from one node to the next. For this reason, infection can spread, and malignant cells may metastasize through a chain of nodes to remote regions of the body.

SPLEEN

The spleen, the largest lymphoid organ in the body, is invested by a collagenous connective tissue capsule. It has a convex surface and a concave aspect, known as the hilum.

The **spleen**, the largest lymphoid organ in the body, weighs approximately 150 g in an adult and is located in the upper left quadrant of the abdominal cavity. Its dense, irregular fibroelastic connective tissue capsule, occasionally housing **smooth muscle cells**, is completely surrounded by visceral peritoneum, which provides the spleen with a very smooth surface. The spleen functions not only in the immunological capacity of antibody formation and T-cell and B-cell proliferation but also as a filter of the blood and in destroying old erythrocytes and old platelets. During fetal development, the spleen is a hemopoietic organ; if necessary, it can resume that function in an adult. Additionally, in some animals (but not in humans), the spleen also acts as a reservoir of red blood cells, which may be released into circulation as the need arises.

The spleen has a convex surface as well as a concave aspect, known as the ***hilum***. The capsule of the spleen is thickened at the hilum—it is here that arteries and their accompanying nerve fibers enter and veins and lymph vessels leave the spleen.

Clinical Correlations

A relatively common congenital anomaly is the presence of **accessory spleens (spleniculi)***, in which several small spleens are present in addition to the large spleen. These are about 1 cm in diameter (but can exceed that by a factor of 2 or 3), have an identical histology to the spleen, present no problems in a healthy individual, and occur in 10% to 15% of the population. The only problem that these accessory structures present is if the spleen has to be removed for medical purposes—as in patients who have immune thrombocytopenia purpura or hereditary spherocytosis. If the splenectomy does not include the accessory spleens, the surgery will not cure the medical condition because the accessory spleens will assume the functions of the removed spleen.*

The trabeculae, arising from the capsule, carry blood vessels into and out of the parenchyma of the spleen (Fig. 12.17). Histologically, the spleen has a three-dimensional network of **reticular fibers** and associated reticular cells. The reticular fiber network is attached to the capsule and the trabeculae, forming the architectural framework of this organ (Fig. 12.18).

The interstices of the reticular tissue network are occupied by **venous sinuses**, trabeculae conveying blood vessels, and the splenic parenchyma. The cut surface of a fresh spleen shows gray areas surrounded by red areas; the former are called ***white pulp***, and the latter are known as ***red pulp***. White pulp is composed mostly of lymphocytes, and red pulp is composed mostly of venous sinuses and the splenic cords, loose reticular connective tissue. Unlike lymph nodes, the spleen does not have a cortex or medulla or afferent lymph vessels serving it.

Central to the appreciation of the organization and function of the spleen is an understanding of its blood supply.

Vascular Supply of the Spleen

The spleen is supplied by the splenic artery and is drained by the splenic vein; both vessels enter and leave the spleen at the hilum.

The splenic artery branches repeatedly as it pierces the connective tissue capsule at the hilum of the spleen. Branches of these vessels, **trabecular arteries**, are conveyed into the substance of the spleen by trabeculae of decreasing sizes (see Fig. 12.17). When the trabecular arteries are reduced to about 0.2 mm in diameter, they leave the trabeculae. The tunica adventitia of these vessels becomes loosely organized, and they become infiltrated by a sheath of lymphocytes, the **periarterial lymphatic sheath (PALS)**. Because the vessel occupies the center of the PALS, it is called the ***central artery*** (***central arteriole***). Branches of the central artery, known as ***follicular arterioles***, serve the lymphoid nodules of the spleen.

At its termination, the central artery loses its lymphatic sheath and subdivides into several short, parallel branches, known as ***penicillar arteries***, which enter the red pulp. The penicillar arteries have three regions: (1) the **pulp arteriole**, (2) **sheathed arteriole** (a thickened region of the vessel surrounded by a sheath of macrophages, the Schweigger-Seidel sheath), and (3) **terminal arterial capillaries**.

Although it is known that the terminal arterial capillaries deliver their blood into the splenic sinuses, the method of delivery is not completely understood, which has prompted the formulation of three theories of circulation in the spleen: (1) closed circulation, (2) open circulation, and (3) a combination of the two theories.

Proponents of the **closed-circulation theory** believe that the endothelial lining of the terminal arterial capillaries is continuous with the sinus endothelium (Figs. 12.19 and 12.20). Investigators who subscribe to the **open-circulation theory** believe that the terminal arterial capillaries terminate prior to reaching the sinusoids, and blood from these vessels percolates through the red pulp into the sinuses. Still other investigators believe that some vessels connect to the sinusoids, whereas other vessels terminate as open-ended channels in the red pulp, suggesting that the spleen has both an **open** and a **closed system of circulation**.

Splenic sinuses are drained by small **veins of the pulp**, which are tributaries of increasingly larger veins that merge to form the **splenic vein**, a tributary of the **portal vein**.

White Pulp and Marginal Zone

The white pulp is composed of the periarterial lymphatic sheath, housing T cells, and lymphoid nodules, housing B cells. The marginal zone also houses B cells that are specialized to recognize thymic-independent antigens.

The structure of the **white pulp** is closely associated with the central artery. The PALS that surrounds the central artery is composed of T lymphocytes. Frequently, enclosed within the PALS are **lymphoid nodules (lymphoid follicles)**, which are composed of B cells and displace the central artery to a peripheral position. As indicated previously, follicular arterioles branch from the central artery to serve the lymphoid nodules. Lymphoid nodules may display **germinal centers**, indicative of antigenic challenge (Figs. 12.21 and 12.22). The PALS and lymphoid nodules constitute the white pulp and, as in the lymph node, the T and B cells are stationed in specific locations. Between the white pulp and the red pulp is an intermediate zone, known as the *marginal zone*, where T cells and B cells are present but occupy prescribed locations (see later discussion). In order to ensure that B cells and T cells migrate to their appropriate locations in the spleen, splenic stromal cells release B cell– and T cell–specific **chemotactic chemokines for lymphocytes (CCLs)**. Those CCLs that are specific to T cells attract them to the PALS and to T cell–rich regions of the marginal zone, whereas those CCLs that are specific to B cells attract them to the lymphoid nodules and to B cell–rich regions of the marginal zone.

The white pulp is surrounded by a **marginal zone**, approximately 100 μm in width, that separates the white pulp from the red pulp (Figs. 12.22 and 12.23). This zone is composed of plasma cells, T and B lymphocytes, two types of macrophages (MZ [marginal zone] macrophages and MZ metallophilic macrophages), and interdigitating dendritic cells. Additionally, numerous small vascular channels, **marginal sinuses**, are present in the marginal zone, especially surrounding lymphoid nodules. Slender blood vessels, radiating from the central arteriole, pass into the red pulp, recur, and deliver their blood into the marginal sinuses.

Because the spaces between the endothelial cells of these sinuses may be as wide as 2 to 3 μm, it is here that blood-borne cells, antigens, and particulate matter have their first free access

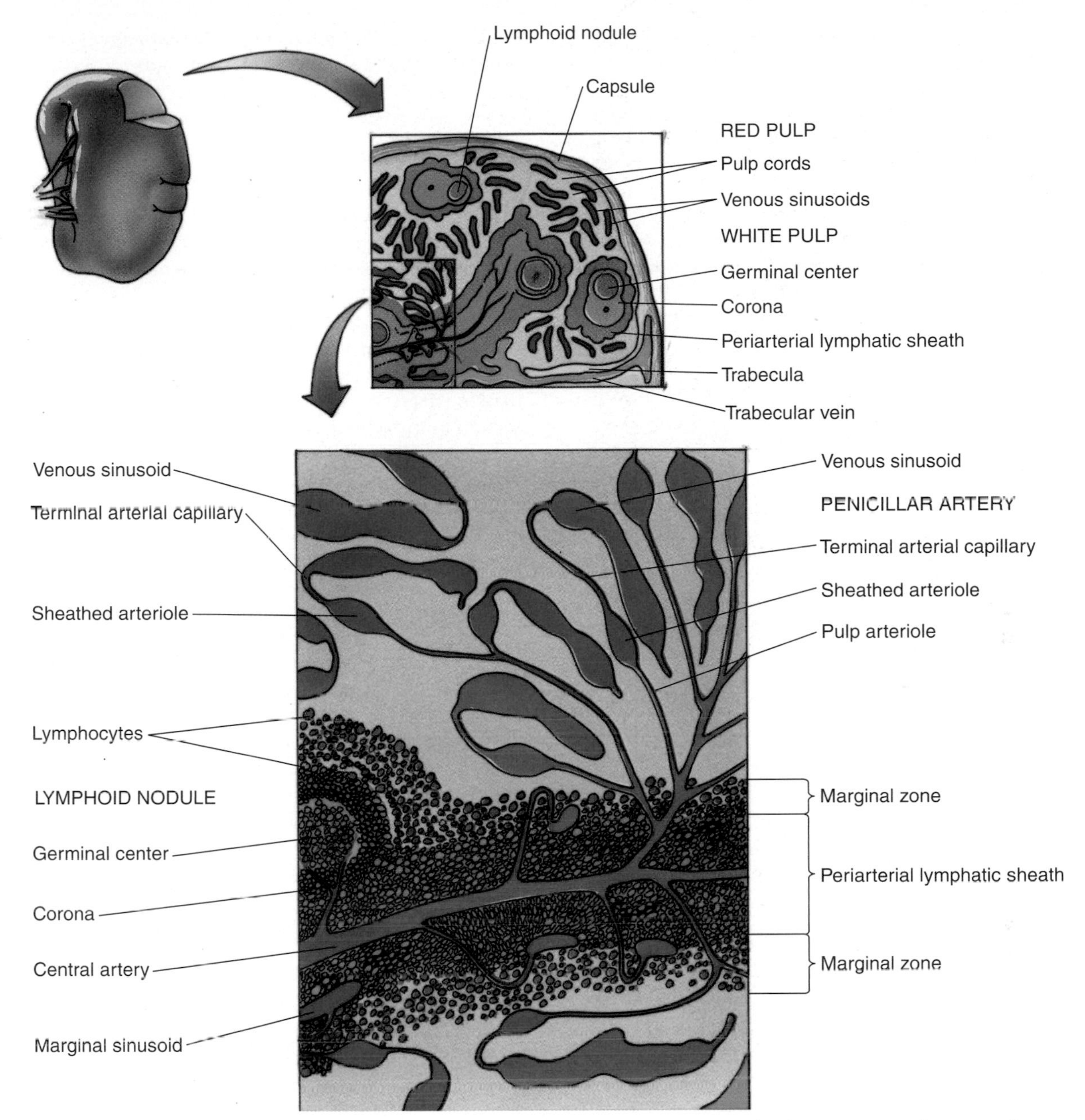

Fig. 12.17 Schematic diagram of the spleen. *Top:* Low-magnification view of white pulp and red pulp. *Bottom:* Higher-magnification view of the central arteriole and its branches.

to the parenchyma of the spleen. Thus, the following events occur at the MZ:

1. APCs sample the material traveling in blood, searching for antigens.
2. MZ macrophages attack microorganisms present in the blood and interact with B cells of the marginal zone, activating them to present epitopes to MZ T cells.
3. MZ metallophilic macrophages recognize membrane-bound oligosaccharide ligands interacting with B cells of the marginal zone, activating them to present epitopes to T cells located in the MZ, as well as to T cells located in the periarterial lymphatic sheath.
4. The circulating pool of T and B lymphocytes leaves the bloodstream to enter its preferred locations within the white pulp.
5. Lymphocytes may also come into contact with the interdigitating dendritic cells; if they recognize the epitope–MHC complex borne by these cells, the lymphocytes initiate an immune response within the white pulp.
6. B cells recognize and react to thymus-independent antigens (e.g., polysaccharides of bacterial cell walls) and are able to act on their own without the assistance of T helper cells.

Red Pulp

The red pulp of the spleen is composed of splenic sinuses and splenic cords (of Billroth).

The **red pulp** resembles a sponge in that the spaces within the sponge represent the sinuses and the sponge material among the spaces denotes the splenic cords (see Figs. 12.17, 12.23, and 12. 24).

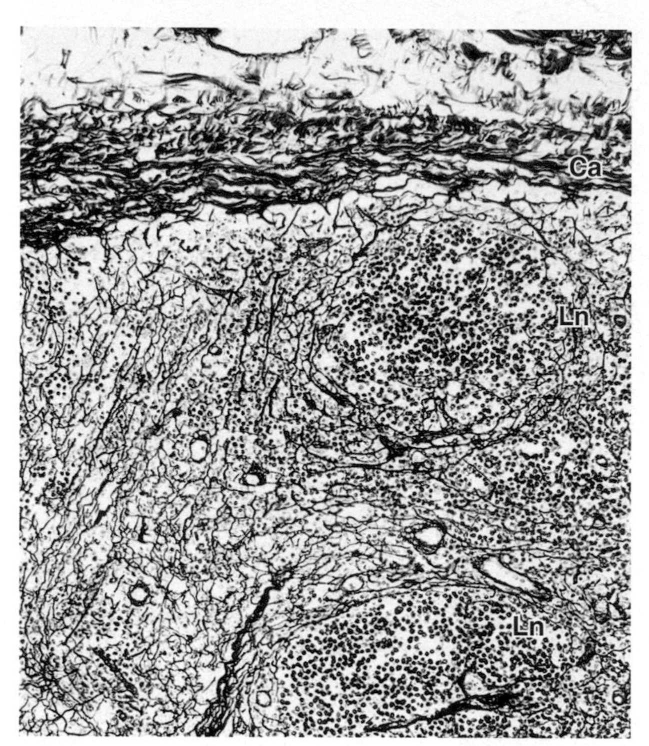

Fig. 12.18 Photomicrograph of the reticular fiber architecture of the spleen. Note the capsule (Ca) and lymphoid nodule (Ln). Silver stain (×132).

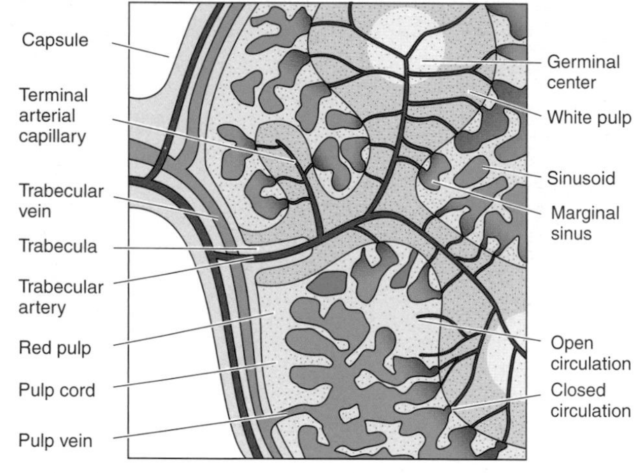

Fig. 12.19 Diagram of open and closed circulation in the spleen.

The endothelial lining of **splenic sinuses** is unusual in that its cells are fusiform in shape, resembling staves of a barrel (Fig. 12.25), and spaces 2 to 3 μm wide between adjoining cells are common. The sinuses are surrounded by reticular fibers (continuous with those of the splenic cords) that wrap around the sinuses as individual thin strands of thread. The reticular fibers are arranged perpendicular to the longitudinal axis of the sinuses and are coated by **basal lamina**. Thus, splenic sinuses have a discontinuous basal lamina.

The **splenic cords** are composed of a loose network of reticular fibers whose interstices are permeated by extravasated blood. The reticular fibers are enveloped by **stellate reticular cells**, which isolate the type III collagen fibers from blood, preventing coagulation from occurring. **Macrophages** are particularly numerous in the vicinity of the sinusoids.

Histophysiology of the Spleen

The spleen filters blood, forms lymphoid cells, eliminates or inactivates blood-borne antigens, destroys aged platelets and erythrocytes, and participates in hemopoiesis.

As blood enters the marginal sinuses of the marginal zone, it flows past a macrophage-rich area. These cells phagocytose blood-borne antigens, bacteria, and other foreign particulate matter. Material that is not eliminated in the MZ is cleared in the red pulp at the periphery of the splenic sinuses.

Lymphoid cells are formed in the white pulp in response to an antigenic challenge. B memory cells and plasma cells are formed in lymphoid nodules, whereas T cells of various subcategories are formed in the periarterial lymphatic sheaths. The newly formed B and T cells enter the marginal sinuses and migrate to the site of antigenic challenge or become part of the circulating pool of lymphocytes. Some plasma cells may stay in the MZ, manufacture antibodies, and release the immunoglobulins into the marginal sinuses. Most plasma cells, however, migrate to the bone marrow to manufacture and release their antibodies into the bone marrow sinuses.

Soluble blood-borne antigens are inactivated by the antibodies formed against them, whereas bacteria become **opsonized** and are eliminated by macrophages or neutrophils. Virus-transformed cells are killed by CTLs formed in the PALS of the white pulp.

Macrophages kill aged platelets and monitor erythrocytes as they migrate from the splenic cords between the endothelial cells into the sinuses (Fig. 12.26). Because older erythrocytes lose their flexibility (as do erythrocytes infected by the malaria parasite), they cannot penetrate the spaces between the endothelial cells and are phagocytosed by macrophages. The phagocytes also monitor the surface coats of red blood cells, which are destroyed in the following manners:

1. Old erythrocytes lose sialic acid residues from their surface macromolecules, exposing galactose moieties.
2. Galactose moieties that are exposed on erythrocyte membranes induce their phagocytosis.
3. Erythrocytes phagocytosed by macrophages are destroyed within phagosomes.
4. Hemoglobin is catabolized into its heme and globin portions.
5. The globin moiety is disassembled into its constituent amino acids, which become part of the circulating amino acid pool of the blood.
6. Iron molecules are conveyed to the bone marrow by transferrin and are used in the formation of new red blood cells.
7. Heme is converted to bilirubin and excreted by the liver in bile.
8. Macrophages also phagocytose damaged or defunct platelets and neutrophils.

During the second trimester of gestation, the spleen actively participates in **hemopoiesis**; after birth, however, blood cell formation occurs in the bone marrow only. If the necessity arises, the spleen can resume its hemopoietic function.

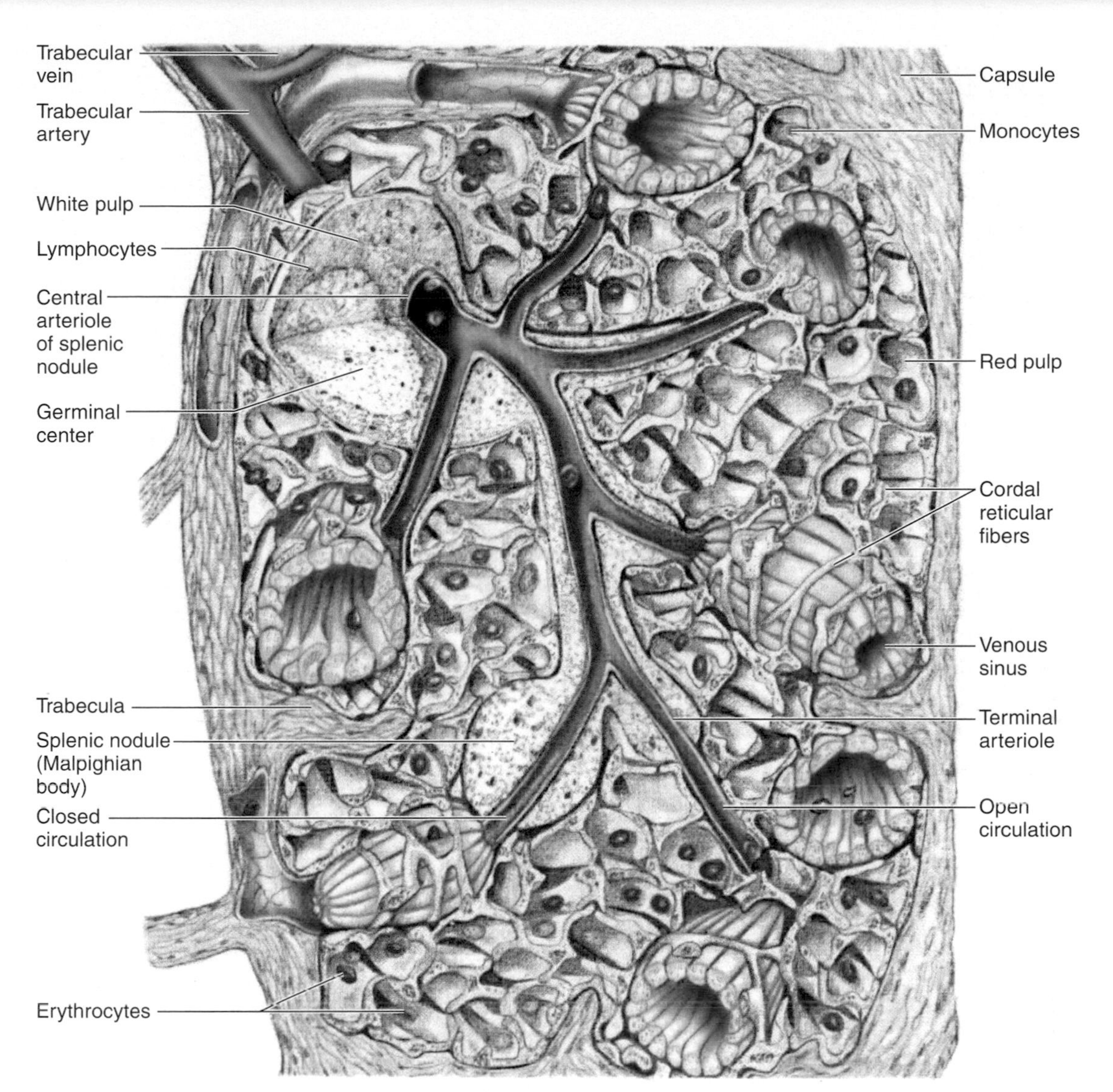

Fig. 12.20 A diagrammatic representation of a splenic lobule. The white pulp consists of nodules and aggregations of lymphocytes that surround and follow the arterial blood vessels, and the red pulp is an open mesh with sinusoids. (From Leeson TS, Leeson CR, Paparo M. *Text Atlas of Histology*. Philadelphia: WB Saunders; 1988.)

Clinical Correlations

Because the spleen is a friable (fragile) organ, major trauma to the upper left abdominal quadrant may cause rupture of the spleen. In severe cases, the spleen may be removed surgically without compromising a person's life. Aged red blood cells are then phagocytosed by macrophages of the liver and bone marrow.

MUCOSA-ASSOCIATED LYMPHOID TISSUE

MALT is composed of a nonencapsulated, localized lymphocyte infiltration and lymphoid nodules in the mucosa of the gastrointestinal, respiratory, and urinary tracts. The best examples of these accumulations are those associated with the mucosa of the gut: **gut-associated lymphoid tissue** (**GALT**), the **bronchus-associated lymphatic tissue** (**BALT**), and the **tonsils**.

Gut-Associated Lymphoid Tissue

The most prominent accumulation of GALT is located in the ileum and is known as Peyer patches.

GALT is composed of lymphoid follicles along the length of the gastrointestinal tract. Most of the lymphoid follicles are isolated from each other; in the ileum, however, they form lymphoid aggregates, known as ***Peyer patches*** (Figs. 12.27 and 12.28). The lymphoid follicles of Peyer patches are composed of B cells surrounded by a looser region of T cells and numerous APCs.

Although the ileum is lined by a simple columnar epithelium, the regions immediately adjacent to the lymphoid follicles are lined by squamous-like cells, known as ***M cells*** (***microfold cells***). It is believed that M cells capture antigens and transfer them (without first processing them into epitopes) to macrophages located in Peyer patches (see Chapter 17 for more information concerning immunity in the gastrointestinal tract).

Peyer patches have no afferent lymphatic vessels, but they do have efferent lymph drainage. They receive small arterioles that form a capillary bed, drained by HEVs. Lymphocytes destined to enter Peyer patches have homing receptors that are specific for the HEVs of GALT.

Bronchus-Associated Lymphoid Tissue

BALT is similar to Peyer patches, except that it is located in the walls of bronchi, especially in regions where bronchi and

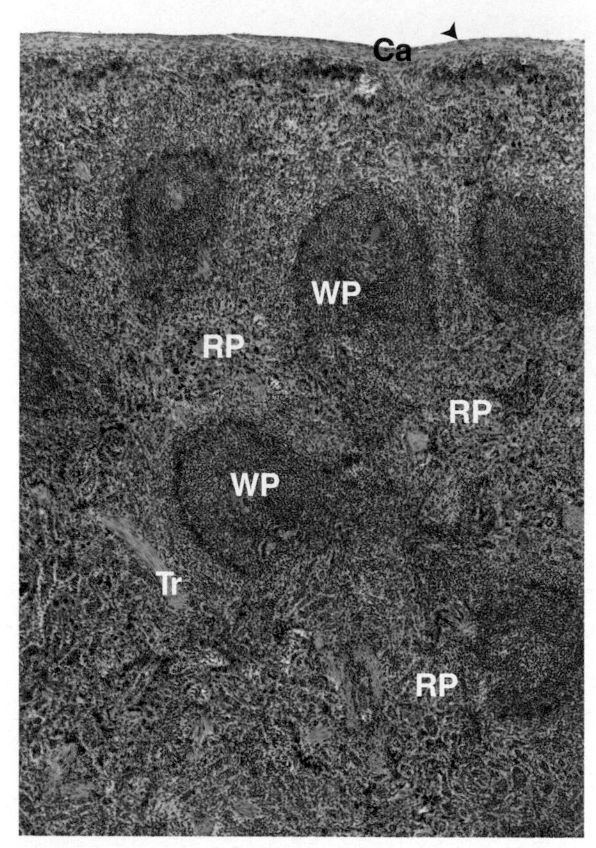

Fig. 12.21 This is a very-low-magnification photomicrograph of the spleen displaying its dense irregular collagenous connective tissue capsule (Ca) that is covered by the visceral peritoneum *(arrowhead)*. Observe the white pulp (WP) and the red pulp (RP) as well as the collagenous connective tissue trabeculae (Tr) that convey blood vessels into and out of the spleen. (×14).

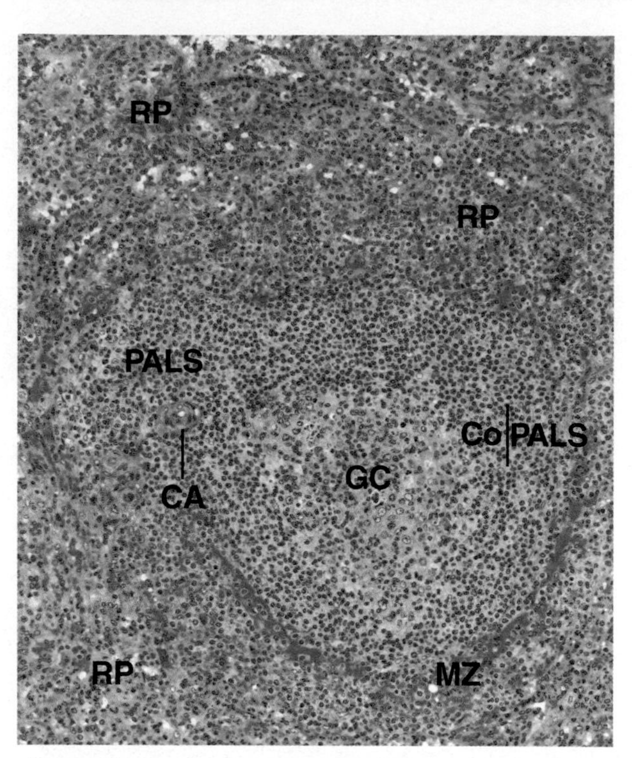

Fig. 12.22 This is a low-magnification photomicrograph of the white pulp and red pulp (RP) of the spleen. Note that the white pulp is composed of the periarterial lymphatic sheath (PALS) that surrounds a secondary lymphoid nodule whose corona (Co) and germinal center (GC) are clearly distinguishable. The PALS also displays its central artery (CA) and the entire white pulp is surrounded by the marginal zone (MZ). (×132)

bronchioles bifurcate. As in GALT, the epithelial cover over these lymphoid nodules changes from a pseudostratified ciliated columnar with goblet cells to **M cells**.

Afferent lymph vessels are absent, although lymph drainage has been demonstrated. The rich vascular supply of BALT indicates its possible systemic as well as localized role in the immune process. Most of the cells are B cells, although APCs and T cells are also present. Lymphocytes destined to enter BALT have homing receptors that are specific for the HEVs of this lymphoid tissue (see Chapter 15 for more information concerning immunity in the respiratory system).

Tonsils

The **tonsils** (palatine, pharyngeal, and lingual) collectively form the Waldeyer ring. They are incompletely encapsulated aggregates of lymphoid nodules, many with germinal centers, which guard the entrance to the oral pharynx. Because of their locations, the tonsils are interposed into the path of airborne and ingested antigens. They react to these antigens by forming lymphocytes and mounting an immune response. B and T lymphocytes are distributed differently in each tonsil, and their specific locations are signaled by **stromal cell–released CCLs** specific for those cells. Collectively, tonsils respond to bacterial and viral infections by increasing in size and by forming IgA antibodies against the invading pathogens.

Palatine Tonsils

The bilateral **palatine tonsils** are located at the boundary of the oral cavity and the oral pharynx, between the palatoglossal and the palatopharyngeal folds. The deep aspect of each palatine tonsil is isolated from the surrounding connective tissue by a dense, fibrous **capsule**. The superficial aspect of the tonsils is covered by a stratified squamous nonkeratinized epithelium that dips into the 10 to 12 deep **crypts** that invaginate the tonsillar parenchyma. The crypts frequently contain food debris, desquamated epithelial cells, dead leukocytes, bacteria, and other antigenic substances. The parenchyma of the tonsil is composed of numerous lymphoid nodules, many of which display germinal centers, indicative of B-cell formation (Fig. 12.29).

Pharyngeal Tonsil

The single **pharyngeal tonsil** is located in the roof of the nasal pharynx. It is similar to the palatine tonsil, but its incomplete capsule is thinner. Instead of crypts, the pharyngeal tonsil has shallow, longitudinal infoldings called **pleats**, whose bases receive the ducts of seromucous glands. Its superficial surface is covered by a pseudostratified ciliated columnar epithelium that is interspersed with patches of stratified squamous epithelium (Fig. 12.30).

The parenchyma of the pharyngeal tonsil is composed of lymphoid nodules, some of which have germinal centers. When this tonsil is inflamed, it is called the ***adenoid***.

Lingual Tonsil

The **lingual tonsil** is located on the dorsal surface of the posterior one-third of the tongue and is covered on its superficial aspect by a stratified squamous nonkeratinized epithelium. The deep aspect of the lingual tonsil has a flimsy capsule that separates it from the underlying connective tissue. The tonsil has numerous crypts whose bases receive the ducts of mucous minor salivary glands.

The parenchyma of the lingual tonsil is composed of lymphoid nodules, which frequently have germinal centers.

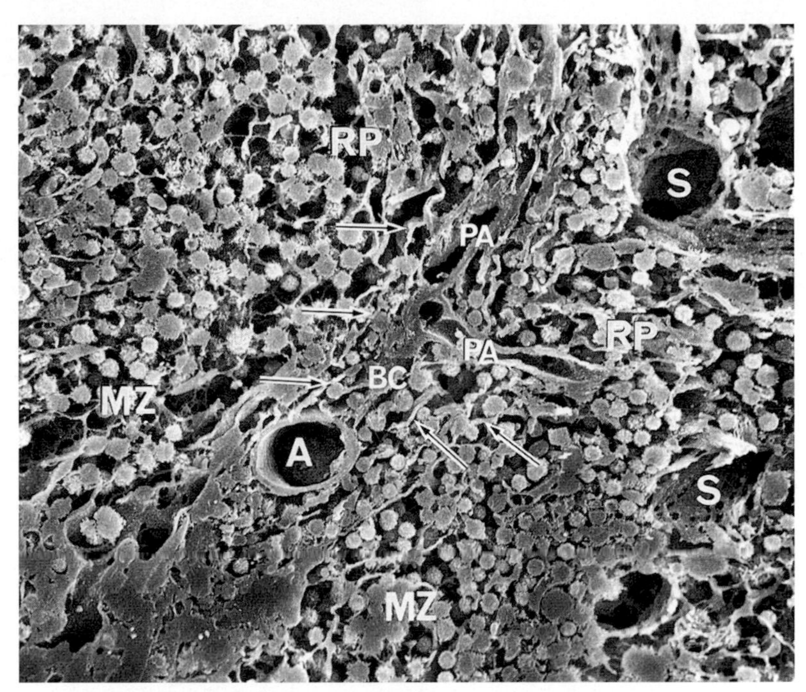

Fig. 12.23 Scanning electron micrograph of the marginal zone and adjoining red pulp of the spleen (×680). *Arrows* point to periarterial flat reticular cells. A, Central artery; BC, marginal zone bridging channel; MZ, marginal zone; PA, penicillar artery; RP, red pulp; S, venous sinus. (From Sasou S, Sugai T. Periarterial lymphoid sheath in the rat spleen: a light, transmission, and scanning electron microscopic study. *Anat Rec.* 1992;232:15-24. Reprinted with permission from Wiley-Liss, Inc., a subsidiary of John Wiley & Sons, Inc.)

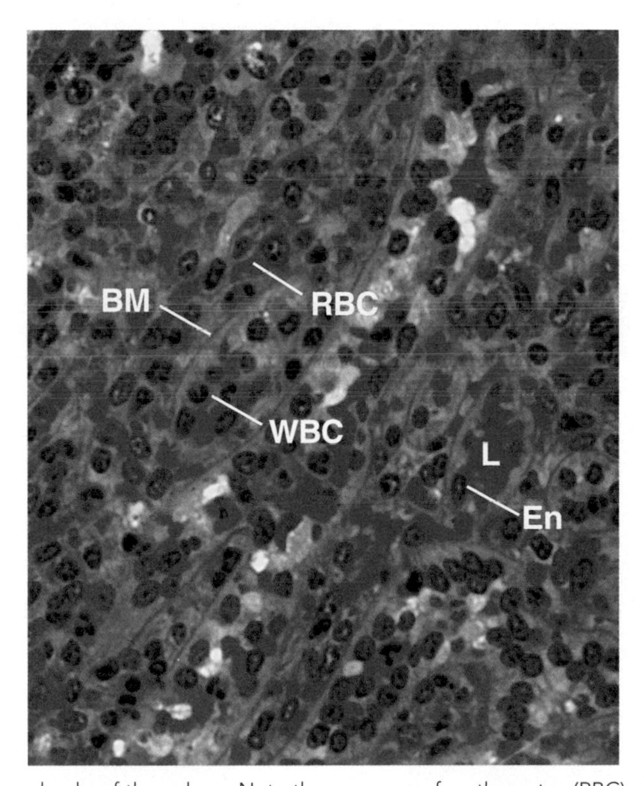

Fig. 12.24 A high magnification of the red pulp of the spleen. Note the presence of erythrocytes (RBC) and leukocytes (WBC) in the lumina (L) of the endothelial cell (En) lined sinusoids and the discontinuous basal lamina (BM) surrounding the endothelial cells. (×540)

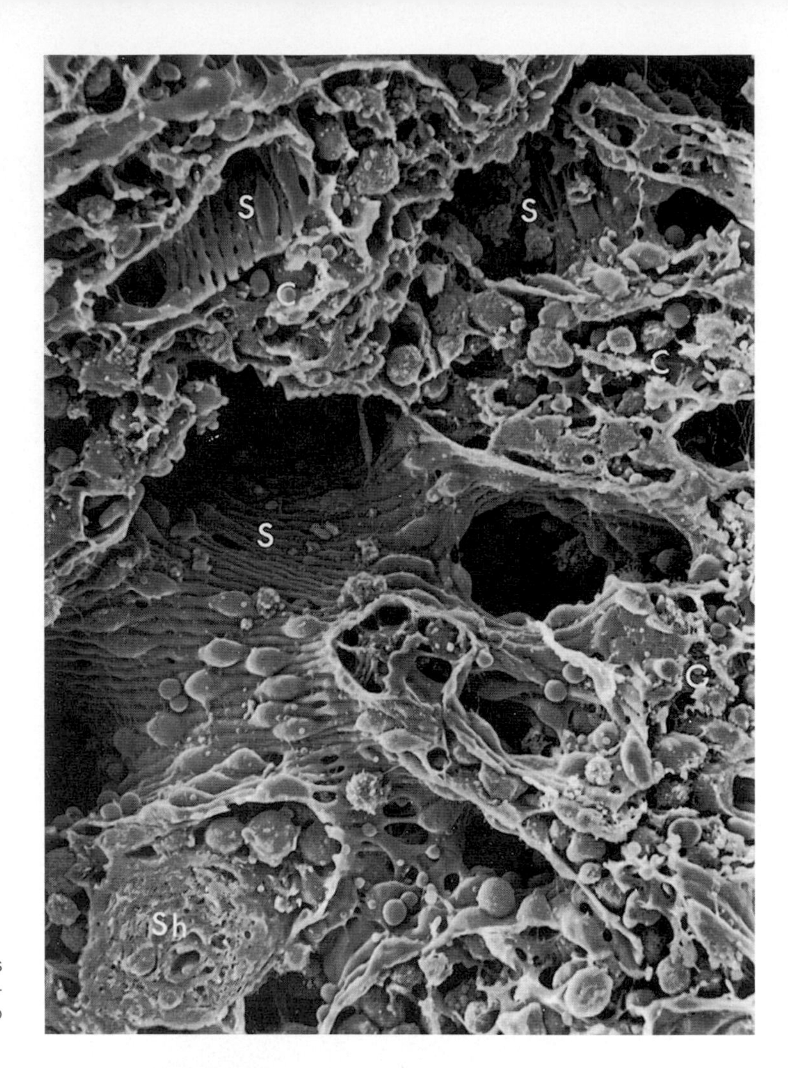

Fig. 12.25 Scanning electron micrograph of sinusoidal lining cells bounded by splenic cords (×500). C, Splenic cords; S, venous sinuses; Sh, sheathed arteriole. (From Leeson TS, Leeson CR, Paparo AA. *Text-Atlas of Histology*. Philadelphia: WB Saunders; 1988.)

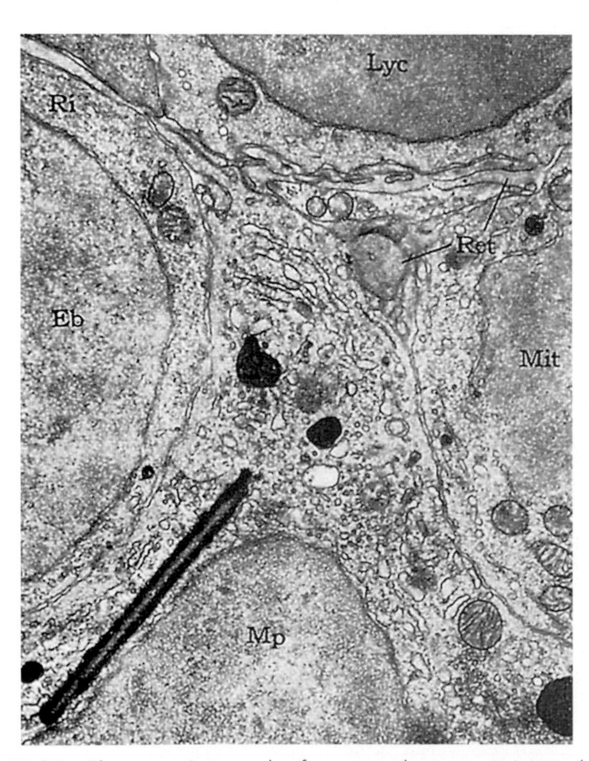

Fig. 12.26 Electron micrograph of a macrophage containing phagocytosed materials, including a crystalloid body. Mp, Macrophage; Mit, cell undergoing mitosis; Lyc, lymphocyte; Eb, erythroblast; Ret, reticular fibers in the interstitial spaces; Ri, ribosomes. (From Rhodin JAG. *An Atlas of Ultrastructure*. Philadelphia: WB Saunders; 1963.)

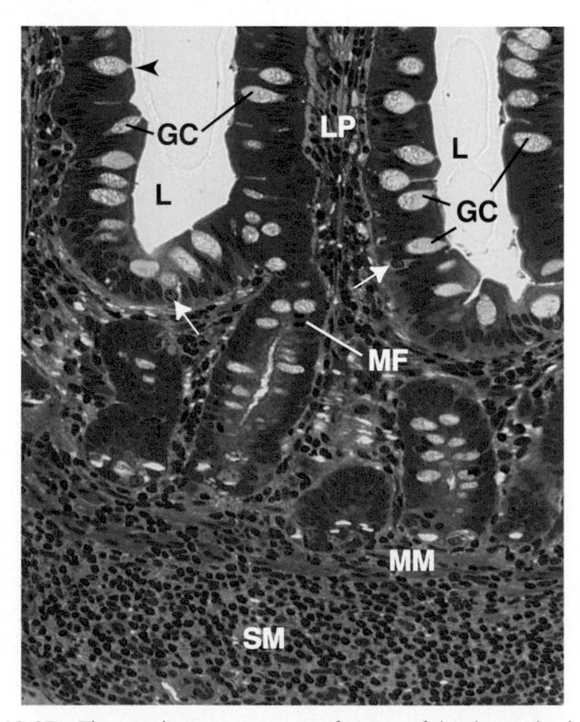

Fig. 12.27 This medium-power magnification of the ileum displays its lumen (L) lined by the epithelium housing goblet cells (GC), which release their mucinogen at the opening *(arrowhead)*. Mitotic figures (MF) are frequently noted in the epithelial lining of the crypts of Lieberkuhn. *Arrows* indicate the presence of DNES cells. Note that the muscularis mucosae (MM) separates the lamina propria (LP) from the submucosa (SM) overcrowded by large numbers of lymphoid cells, which constitute the gut-associated lymphoid tissue, a part of the diffuse lymphoid system, in the case of the ileum, known as Peyer patches. (×270)

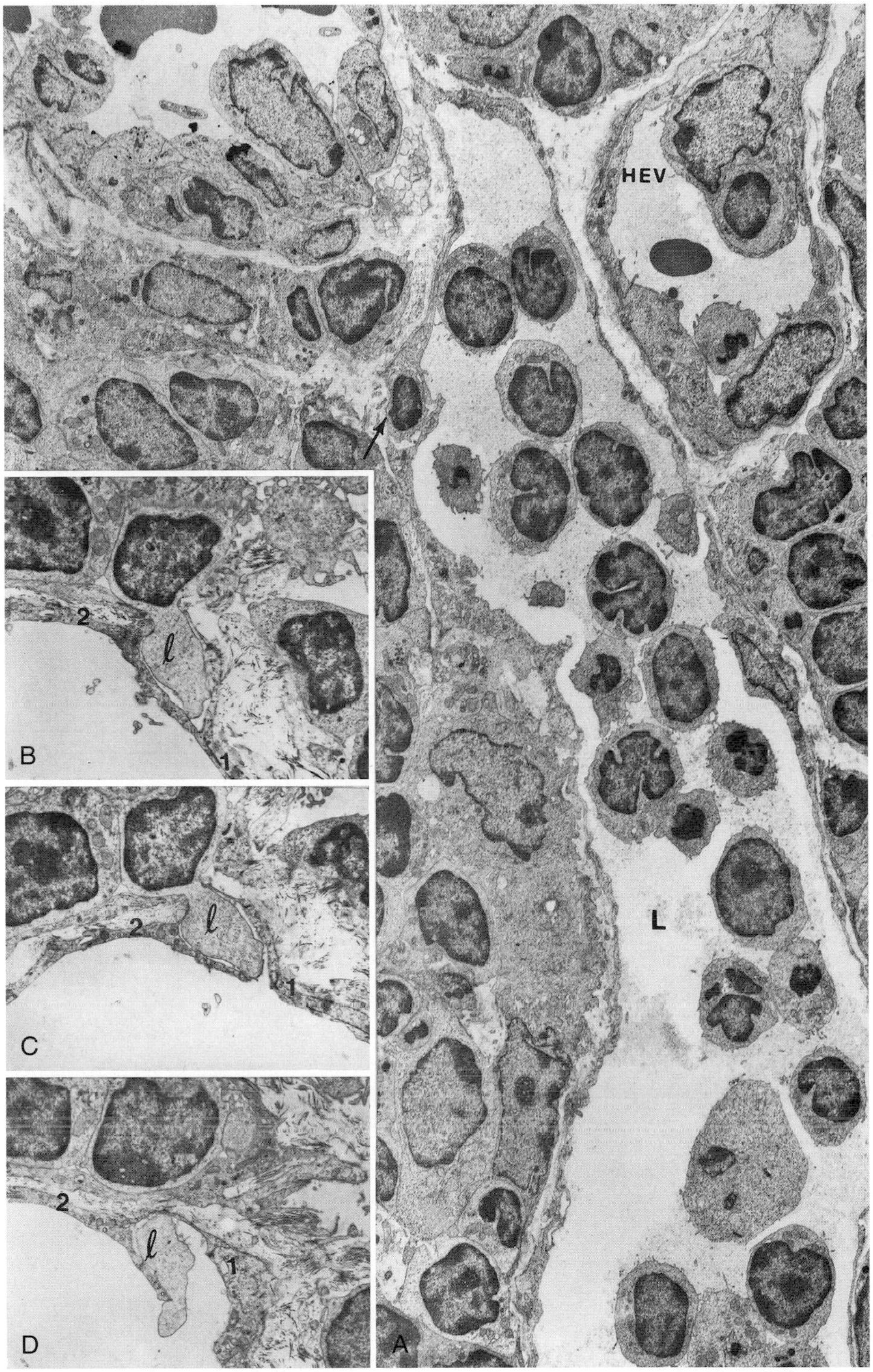

Fig. 12.28 (A) A transmission electron microscopy (TEM) micrograph of a rabbit's Peyer patches, showing absorbing peripheral lymphatic (ALPA) vessel (designated by the L) of the interfollicular area full of lymphocytes that has an intraendothelial channel that includes lymphocyte *(arrow)* in the endothelial wall (HEV, postcapillary high endothelium venula [×3000]). (B–D) TEM micrographs of ultrathin serial sections that document various stages of lymphocyte migration through an intraendothelial channel composed of one and two endothelial cells (×9000). (From Azzali G, Arcari MA. Ultrastructural and three-dimensional aspects of the lymphatic vessels of the absorbing peripheral lymphatic apparatus in Peyer patches of the rabbit. *Anat Rec.* 2000;258:76. Reprinted with permission from Wiley Liss, Inc., a subsidiary of John Wiley & Sons, Inc.)

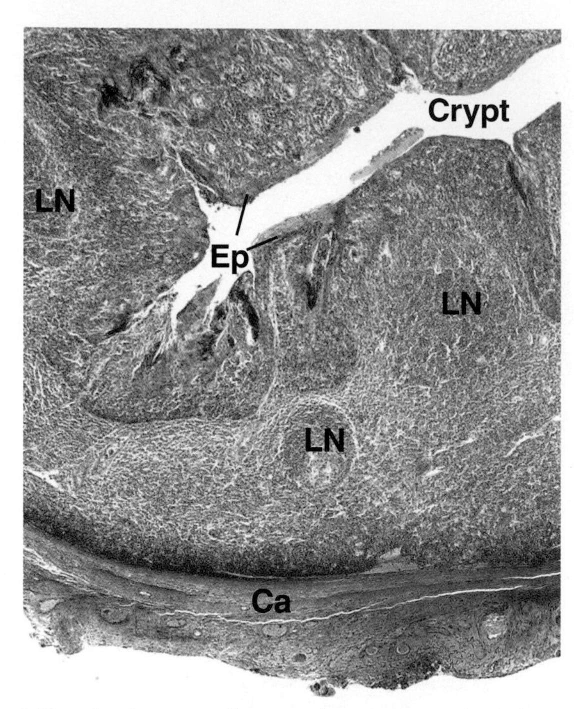

Fig. 12.29 This low-magnification photomicrograph of the palatine tonsil displays its deep, stratified squamous epithelial (Ep) lined crypt and the dense irregular collagenous connective tissue capsule (Ca). Observe the lymphoid nodules (LN) that form most of the substance of the palatine tonsil. (×14)

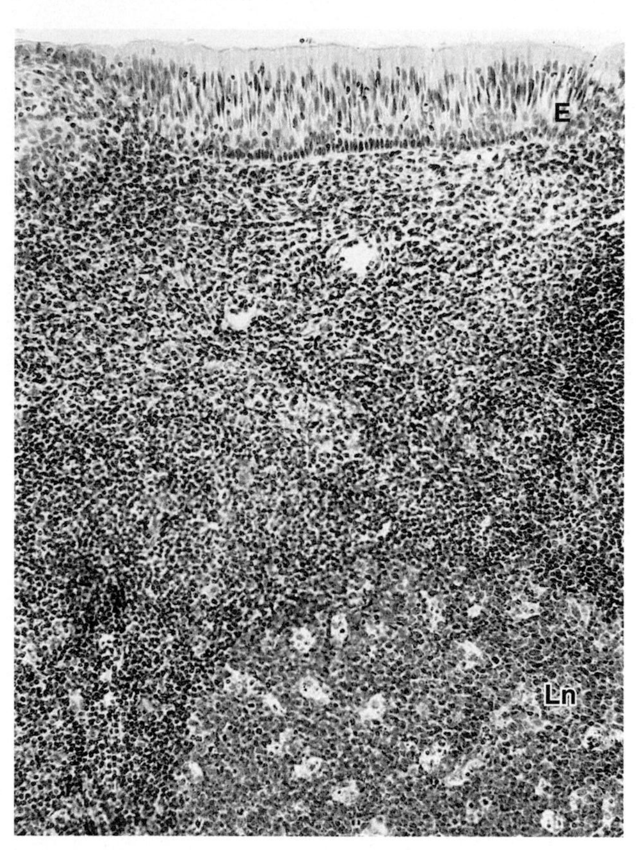

Fig. 12.30 Photomicrograph of a lymphoid nodule of the pharyngeal tonsil displaying its pseudostratified ciliated columnar epithelium (E) and a germinal center of the secondary nodule (Ln). (×132)

Pathological Considerations

See Figs. 12.31 through 12.33.

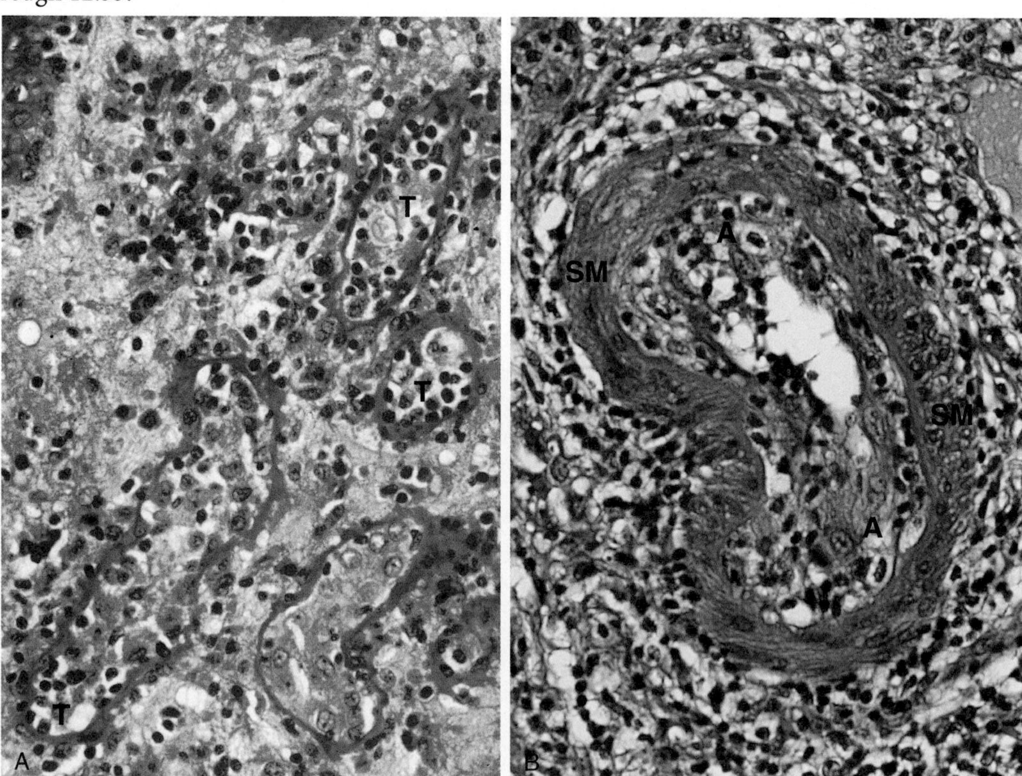

Fig. 12.31 These two photomicrographs display T cell–mediated rejection of a kidney transplant. (A) Banff type I T cell–mediated rejection is an acute rejection that is characterized by the presence of lymphocytes that infiltrate both the renal interstitium and the tubular epithelium. (B) Banff type II T cell–mediated rejection is characterized by the infiltration of the endothelium of the blood vessels, as well as by the enlargement and overpropagation of the endothelial cells. (Reprinted with permission from Young B, Stewart W, O'Dowd G. *Wheater's Basic Pathology: A Text, Atlas and Review of Histopathology.* 5th ed. Oxford: Churchill Livingstone/Elsevier Limited; 2011:190.)

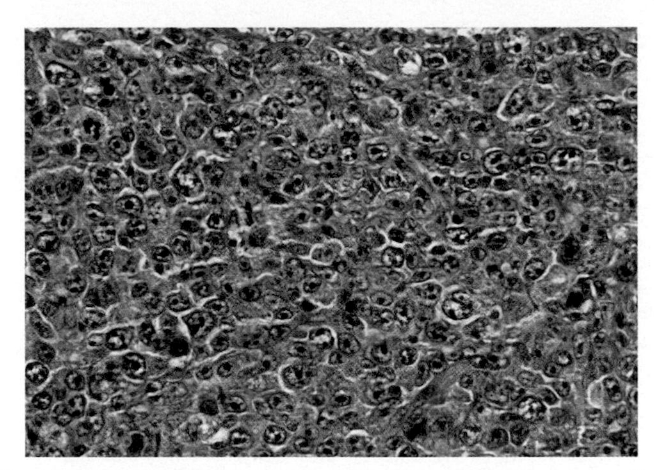

Fig. 12.32 Photomicrograph of a diffuse large B-cell lymphoma. The B cells are large and pleomorphic and are widely distributed throughout the tissue. (Reprinted with permission from Young B, Stewart W, O'Dowd G. *Wheater's Basic Pathology: A Text, Atlas and Review of Histopathology*. 5th ed. Oxford: Churchill Livingstone/Elsevier Limited; 2011:206.)

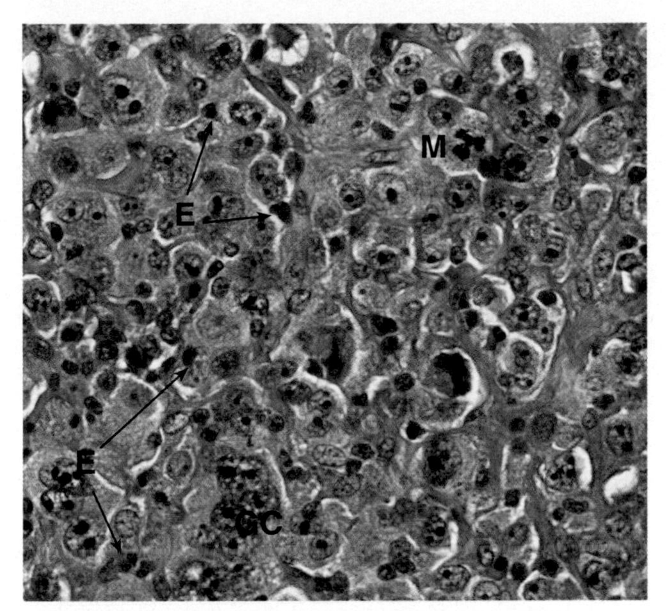

Fig. 12.33 Photomicrograph of an anaplastic large cell lymphoma, characterized by large, atypical cells whose nuclei are highly irregular in morphology. The presence of aberrant mitotic figures (M) and numerous eosinophils (E) is common. Occasionally, giant cells (GC) are also evident. (Reprinted with permission from Young B, Stewart W, O'Dowd G. *Wheater's Basic Pathology: A Text, Atlas and Review of Histopathology*. 5th ed. Oxford: Churchill Livingstone/Elsevier Limited; 2011:207.)

Histology Laboratory Instructions: Lymphoid (Immune) System

This section will not discuss the immune system. Instead, it will deal only with the lymphoid organs.

Thymus

The thymus is invested by a dense, irregular, collagenous connective tissue capsule that sends connective tissue septa into the substance of each lobe, partitioning the thymus into lobules. Each lobule is composed of a cortex and medulla. The cortex stains darker than the medulla, which sports one or more Hassall corpuscles (see Fig. 12.6, C, M, H; and Fig. 12.7, HC). A high magnification of the cortex displays a collagenous connective tissue septum separating neighboring cortices from each other. In order to provide an antigen-free environment, the capsule is lined by type I epithelial reticular cells. The cortex houses thymocytes, supported and tested by type II epithelial reticular cells (see Fig. 12.8, Se, *arrow*, *arrowhead*, ERC). The medulla is lighter in consistency than the cortex and its type VI epithelial reticular cells congregate to form Hassall corpuscles. The medulla also displays the presence of numerous lymphocytes (see Fig. 12.9, ERC, HC, L).

Lymph Node

At a very low magnification, much of the lymph node's morphology is evident. The dense, irregular, collagenous connective tissue capsule of the lymph node has afferent lymph vessels with valves that direct the lymph into the subcapsular sinus. The cortex of the lymph node is incompletely divided into compartments by collagenous connective tissue trabeculae derived from the capsule. Paratrabecular sinuses accept lymph from the subcapsular sinus and deliver the lymph into cortical sinusoids from which the lymph enters the medullary sinusoids to be drained by efferent lymph vessels, at the hilum, whose valves prevent backflow into the medullary sinusoids. The cortex houses primary and secondary lymphoid nodules, with germinal centers where B lymphocytes reside and, when necessary, proliferate to form more B cells, as well as plasma cells. Deep to the cortex, separating it from the medulla is the T cell–rich paracortex where high endothelial venules permit circulating T cells and B cells to enter the substance of the paracortex. The majority of the T cells remain in the paracortex and some, along with the B cells, migrate into the cortex. The medulla of the lymph node is richly endowed with veins and arterioles (see Fig. 12.11, Ca, LV, V, ScS, GC, Pc, BV, *arrows*). At a higher magnification of the cortical region, the valves of the afferent lymph vessel of the capsule is more evident, as is the adipose tissue that invests the capsules of most lymph nodes. The subcapsular sinus and its reticular cells are well defined, as are the paratrabecular sinuses. The corona and the germinal center of the secondary lymph nodules are well delineated (see Fig. 12.12, LVV, LV, AT, Ca, SCS, *arrows*, PTS, Co, GC).

A different view of the outer region of the lymph node displays the subcapsular sinus, the secondary lymphoid nodule with its corona and germinal center, and the deeper lying paracortex (see Fig. 12.13, S, C, G, P). A higher magnification of the paracortex displays the dense accumulation of T cells, as well as the HEVs. The medulla is easy to distinguish because of its scant cellular regions (see Fig. 12.14, *arrows*). A low magnification of the lymph node medulla displays its medullary sinusoids and the densely populated medullary cords. The trabeculae of dense, irregular, collagenous connective tissue conveys blood vessels into and out of the medulla (see Fig. 12.15, S, C, T). At a high magnification, the endothelial cells of the medullary sinusoids are clearly visible and the absence of erythrocytes is indicative that these sinusoids contain lymph rather than blood. Trabeculae convey blood vessels into and out of the lymph node. The medullary cords are composed of a network of reticular fibers in which reticular cells, plasma cells, macrophages, and lymphocytes are enmeshed (see Fig. 12.16, EC, Si, T, MC).

Continued

Histology Laboratory Instructions: Lymphoid (Immune) System—cont'd

Spleen

Viewing a section of a spleen stained with silver stain displays its capsule, as well as its reticular fiber architecture and how the cells are trapped in the meshwork of reticular fibers that form the lymphoid nodules of the white pulp (see Fig. 12.18, Ca, Ln). A very low magnification of a hematoxylin and eosin (H&E)–stained section of the spleen displays that its dense irregular collagenous connective tissue capsule is covered by a layer of simple squamous epithelium, known as the visceral peritoneum. Observe that the parenchyma of the spleen is composed of white pulp and red pulp. Connective tissue projections of the capsule, trabeculae, convey blood vessels into and out of the pulp (see Fig. 12.21, Ca, *arrowhead*, WP, RP, Tr). A low magnification of the white pulp displays the periarterial lymphatic sheath as it encloses a secondary lymphoid nodule with its corona and germinal center. The central artery of the PALS is well defined, as is the MZ that separates the white pulp from the red pulp (see Fig. 12.22, PALS, Co, GC, CA, MZ, RP). A high magnification of an H&E stained section of the red pulp displays that the lumen of the pulp sinusoids is lined by endothelial cells and that the sinusoids are filled with red and white blood cells. Observe that a discontinuous basal lamina covers the endothelial cells of the sinusoids (see Fig. 12.24, L, En, RBC, WBC, BM).

Mucosa-Associated Lymphoid Tissue

The ileum provides a very good example of MALT, in this case known as GALT. Observe that the lamina propria, located between the epithelial lining of the ileum and its muscularis mucosae, is richly endowed by lymphoid cells. The submucosa of the ileum also houses large groups of lymphoid elements, known as Peyer patches (see Fig. 12.27, LP, MM, SM).

Tonsils

Tonsils are incompletely encapsulated aggregates of primary and secondary lymphoid nodules. A very low magnification of a **palatine tonsil** displays its deep, stratified squamous epithelial-lined crypt and the dense, irregular, collagenous connective tissue capsule. Observe the lymphoid nodules that form most of the substance of the palatine tonsil (see Fig. 12.29, Ep, Ca, LN). A low magnification of a **pharyngeal tonsil** displays that its shallow pleats are lined by a pseudostratified ciliated columnar interspersed with a stratified squamous nonkeratinized epithelium. A secondary lymph nodule with its corona and germinal center are clearly evident (see Fig. 12.30, E, Ln).

13 Endocrine System

The **endocrine system** consists of **ductless glands**, distinct **clusters of cells** within certain organs of the body, and *individual* **endocrine cells** (known as the ***diffuse neuroendocrine system [DNES]***), situated in the epithelial lining of the respiratory system and in the digestive tract. (The latter are discussed in Chapters 15 and 17, respectively.) The **endocrine glands**, the subject of this chapter, are abundantly and richly vascularized so that their secretory product may be released into slender connective tissue spaces between cells and the capillary beds from which they enter the bloodstream. The endocrine glands include the **pituitary gland**, **thyroid gland**, **parathyroid glands**, **suprarenal glands**, and **pineal body**. Other endocrine glands, such as the *islets of Langerhans* in the pancreas, are discussed in the pertinent chapters.

The endocrine system and the autonomic nervous system (see Chapter 9) interact to modulate and coordinate the metabolic activities of the body, thereby helping to bring about homeostasis. Unlike the nervous system, which acts very rapidly, the endocrine system produces a slow and diffused effect via chemical substances called ***hormones***, which are released into the bloodstream of capillary beds to influence target cells at remote sites.

Hormones

Hormones are chemical messengers that are produced by endocrine glands and delivered by the bloodstream to target cells or organs on which they usually have regulatory effects.

The chemical nature of a hormone dictates its mechanism of action. Most hormones elicit several effects on their target cells (e.g., short- and long-term effects). A list of the hormones, their source, and functions is presented in Table 13.1.

Although there are various ways of categorizing hormones, one of the simplest classifications is to divide them into two types based on their water solubility (water soluble or lipid soluble) or into three types based on their chemical structure:

- Proteins and polypeptides—mostly water soluble (e.g., insulin, glucagon, follicle-stimulating hormone [FSH])
- Amino-acid derivatives—mostly water soluble (e.g., thyroxine, epinephrine)
- Steroid and fatty acid derivatives—mostly lipid soluble (e.g., progesterone, estradiol, testosterone)

When a hormone enters the bloodstream and arrives in the vicinity of its target cells, it first binds to specific receptors on (or in) the target cell. Receptors for certain hormones (mostly protein and peptide hormones, i.e., water-soluble hormones) are located on the plasmalemma (**cell-surface receptors**) of the target cell, whereas other receptors are located in the cytoplasm and bind only to hormones that have diffused through the plasmalemma (i.e., lipid-soluble hormones). The binding of a hormone to its receptor communicates a message to the target cell, initiating **signal transduction**, or translation of the signal into a biochemical reaction by the target cell.

HORMONES THAT TRANSLOCATE TO THE NUCLEUS

Steroid hormones pass through the cell membrane, where they bind to intracellular hormone receptors (Fig. 13.1). Thyroid hormones, for example, bind to membrane-bound iodothyronine transporters that, using an energy-requiring mechanism, transport the thyroid hormone into the cytoplasm, where it is transferred to an intracellular thyroid hormone receptor. The resulting *hormone–intracellular receptor complex* translocates to the nucleus, where it binds directly to deoxyribonucleic acid (DNA) close to a promoter site, stimulating gene transcription. However, at least some steroid hormones bind to receptors that are located in the target cell plasma membrane. Thus, the hormone's actions may be mediated directly without gene transcription or protein synthesis. Neither the hormone nor the receptor alone can initiate the target cell response.

HORMONES THAT BIND TO CELL-SURFACE RECEPTORS

Hormones that bind to cell-surface receptors located in the plasmalemma can use one of several different mechanisms to elicit a response in their target cells (Fig.13.1). In each instance, the hormone–receptor complex is believed to induce a protein kinase to phosphorylate certain regulatory proteins, generating a biological response to the hormone. For example, some hormone–receptor complexes stimulate adenylate cyclase to synthesize cyclic adenosine monophosphate (cAMP), which stimulates protein kinase A in the cytosol. In such an instance, cAMP acts as a **second messenger**. Several additional second messengers have been identified, including **cyclic guanosine 3′,5′ monophosphate**; **metabolites of phosphatidylinositol**; **calcium ions**; and, in neurons, **sodium ions**.

Certain hormone receptor complexes are associated with **guanosine triphosphate–binding proteins** (**G proteins**), which couple the receptor to the hormone-induced responses of the target cells. The receptors for epinephrine, thyroid-stimulating hormone (TSH), and serotonin, for example, use G proteins to activate a second messenger, which elicits a metabolic response. Other hormones, such as insulin and growth hormone, use **catalytic receptors** that activate protein kinases to phosphorylate target proteins.

TABLE 13.1 A Selected List of Hormones Produced by Endocrine Glands[a]

Hormone	Gland of Source	Major Function
Adrenocorticotropic hormone (ACTH)	Basophils of the anterior of the pituitary	Stimulates manufacture and release of hormones of the adrenal cortex.
Aldosterone (and deoxycorticosterone)	Cells of the zona glomerulosa of the suprarenal cortex	Stimulates the kidney to increase H^+ and K^+ secretion and Na^+ resorption.
Androgens (androstenedione)	Cells of the zona reticularis of the suprarenal cortex	Provides weak masculinizing characteristics.
Antidiuretic hormone (ADH; vasopressin)	Primarily the supraoptic nucleus of hypothalamus	Stimulates water resorption by the kidneys and smooth muscle contraction in arterioles.
Calcitonin	Thyroid parafollicular cells	Decreases serum calcium levels.
Corticotropin-releasing hormone (CRH)	Hypothalamus	Stimulates release of ACTH by basophils of the anterior pituitary.
Dopamine (prolactin-inhibiting factor [PIF])	Hypothalamus	Inhibits prolactin release.
Epinephrine	Chromaffin cells of the suprarenal medulla	Prepares body for stress ("flight, fight, freeze" response); releases glucose from the liver; increases heart rate and cardiac output.
Follicle-stimulating hormone (FSH)	Basophils of the anterior pituitary	Stimulates growth of ovarian follicles, estrogen secretion; stimulates spermatogenesis in testis.
Gonadotropin-releasing hormone (GnRH)	Hypothalamus	Stimulates release of LH and FSH by basophils of the anterior pituitary.
Glucocorticoids (cortisol and corticosterone)	Cells of the zona fasciculata of the suprarenal cortex	Suppresses immune reactions and inflammation; stimulates gluconeogenesis; decreases protein synthesis; releases fatty acids and glycerol.
Growth hormone (GH; somatotropin)	Acidophils of the anterior pituitary	Stimulates, via insulin-like growth factors, bone growth, hyperglycemia in muscles, and release of free fatty acids by fat cells.
Growth hormone–releasing hormone (GHRH)	Hypothalamus	Stimulates release of growth hormone by acidophils of the anterior pituitary.
Luteinizing hormone (LH)	Basophils of the anterior pituitary	Stimulates ovulation, estrogen and progesterone secretion, and corpus luteum formation; stimulates testosterone secretion by the testis.
Melanocyte-stimulating hormone (MSH)	Basophils of the anterior pituitary	Stimulates melanin synthesis by melanocytes.
Melatonin	Pinealocytes of the pineal body	May influence cyclic gonadal activity.
Norepinephrine	Chromaffin cells of the suprarenal medulla.	Causes vasoconstriction, thereby elevating blood pressure.
Oxytocin	Primarily, the paraventricular nucleus of the hypothalamus	Stimulates the milk ejection reflex and contraction of the smooth muscle of the uterus.
Parathyroid hormone (PTH)	Chief cells of the parathyroid gland	Increases calcium concentration in plasma.
Prolactin	Acidophils of the anterior pituitary	Promotes development of the mammary gland during pregnancy and stimulates milk secretion
Somatostatin (SRIF)	Hypothalamus	Inhibits growth hormone release.
Thyroid-stimulating hormone (TSH)	Basophils of the anterior pituitary	Stimulates thyroid hormone secretion.
Thyrotropin-releasing hormone (TRH)	Hypothalamus	Stimulates TSH and prolactin secretion.
Thyroxine (T_4) and Triiodothyronine (T_3)	Follicular cells of the thyroid	Increases cellular metabolism, growth rate, fatty acid synthesis; heart rate, respiration, and muscle activity. Decreases cholesterol, phospholipids, and triglycerides; body weight. Enhances development of the nervous system in the perinatal period.

[a]Hormones produced by other glands, such as the pancreas or diffuse neuroendocrine system cells, are discussed in the relevant chapters.

Clinical Correlations

Individuals with ***Laron syndrome****, an autosomal recessive condition, are short with truncated mandibles, overextending foreheads, flattened nasal bones, and excess fat in their abdominal region. Males frequently present with a small penis and adult females often possess normal-sized breasts that are too large for their body size. Individuals with Laron syndrome have mutated growth hormone receptors (GHRs) that are unable to bind growth hormone (GH). These patients have abnormally high GH blood levels but their level of insulin-like growth factor-1 (IGF-1) is very low. Patients with Laron syndrome can be treated with synthetic IGF-1 while still younger than 13 years of age. Interestingly, patients with this syndrome have been reported to have low incidence of cancer and type 2 diabetes mellitus.*

FEEDBACK MECHANISM AND INACTIVATION

Once a hormone activates its target cell, an inhibitory signal is generated and returned to the endocrine gland (**feedback mechanism**), either directly or indirectly, to halt hormone secretion. The feedback mechanism also operates in another way: when the hormone level is inadequate to elicit a sufficient metabolic response in the target, a positive feedback signal is released, travels to the endocrine gland, and initiates an increase in hormone secretion. Through the feedback mechanism, therefore, regulation of the endocrine glands maintains homeostasis.

Many of the hormones that circulate in the bloodstream are in oversupply. They are usually bound to plasma proteins, which make them biologically inactive, but they can be released from

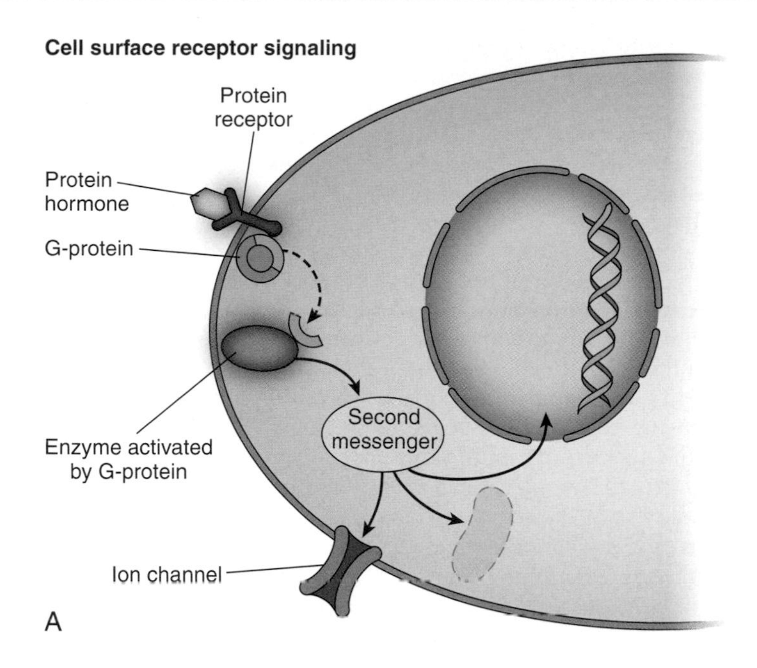

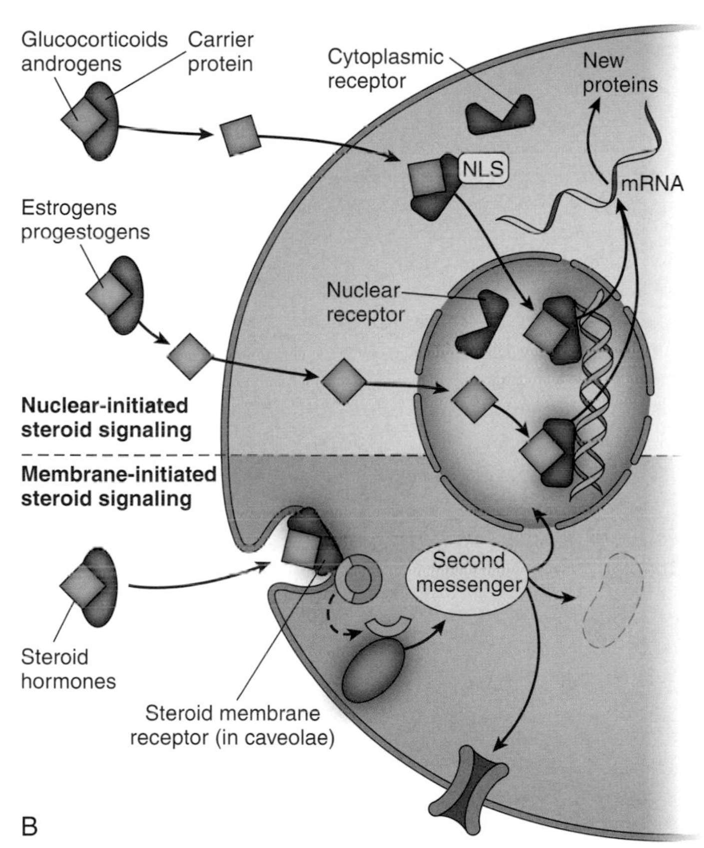

Fig. 13.1 (A) Hormones that bind to cell-surface receptors located in the plasmalemma are associated with G proteins, which couple the receptor to the hormone-induced responses of the target cells. The receptors for epinephrine, thyroid-stimulating hormone (TSH), and serotonin, for example, use G proteins to activate a second messenger, which elicits a metabolic response. Other hormones, such as insulin and growth hormone, use catalytic receptors that activate protein kinases to phosphorylate target proteins. (B) *Top:* Steroid hormones pass through the cell membrane, where they bind to intracellular hormone receptors. The resulting *hormone–intracellular receptor complex* translocates to the nucleus, where it binds directly to deoxyribonucleic acid (DNA) close to a promoter site, thereby stimulating gene transcription. (B) *Bottom:* However, at least some steroid hormones bind to receptors that are located in the target cell plasma membrane, activating a second messenger, thus the hormone's actions may be mediated directly without gene transcription or protein synthesis. Neither the hormone nor the receptor alone can initiate the target cell response. Modified from Hall, J.E. Guyton and Hall: *Guyton and Hall Textbook of Medical Physiology,* 12th ed. Figs. 74-5 and 74-6. Saunders/Elsevier, Philadelphia, 2011.

their bound state quickly, becoming active. Hormones become permanently inactivated in their target tissue; additionally, they may be degraded and destroyed in the liver and kidneys.

Pituitary Gland (Hypophysis)

The pituitary gland, composed of portions derived from oral ectoderm and neural ectoderm, produces hormones that regulate growth, metabolism, and reproduction.

The **pituitary gland**, or **hypophysis**, produces a number of hormones that are responsible for regulating growth, reproduction, and metabolism. This gland has two major parts that develop from two different embryological sources: (1) the **adenohypophysis** (**anterior pituitary**) develops from an evagination of the **oral ectoderm** (**Rathke pouch**) that lines the primitive oral cavity (stomadeum), and (2) the **neurohypophysis** (**posterior pituitary**) develops from neural ectoderm as a downgrowth of the developing diencephalon. Subsequently, the two parts are joined and encapsulated into a single gland. The evagination of the Rathke pouch occurs around the 4th to 5th week of embryogenesis. Once the pouch is established, the development of the neurohypophysis depends on various factors produced by cells of the Rathke pouch and by the diencephalon.

The pituitary gland lies below the hypothalamus of the brain, to which it is connected extending inferiorly from the diencephalon. It sits in the hypophyseal fossa, a bony depression in the sella turcica of the sphenoid bone that is lined by dura mater and covered over by a portion of the dura mater called the ***diaphragma sellae***. The gland measures approximately 1 cm × 1 to 1.5 cm; it is 0.5-cm thick and weighs about 0.6 g in men about 0.8 g in women who have never been pregnant, and approximately 1.2 g in pregnant women as well as in women who have given birth two or more times.

The pituitary is connected to the **hypothalamus** by neural pathways; it also has a rich vascular supply from vessels that supply the brain, attesting to the coordination of the two systems in maintaining a physiological balance. The neural pathways consist of the **hypothalamohypophyseal tract**, a group of axons whose somata reside in the **paraventricular** and **supraoptic nuclei** of the hypothalamus. The axons enter the pars nervosa of the pituitary gland and form dilatations that store and, when required, release the hormones produced in their somata.

- The **vascular supply** of the hypothalamus, via the **hypophyseal portal system**, drains into the capillary beds of the anterior pituitary (see later discussion) and carries releasing hormones produced in the **dorsal**, **paraventricular**, **medial paraventricular**, **arcuate**, **ventromedial**, and **periventricular nuclei** of the hypothalamus.
- A **retrograde blood flow** from the pituitary to the hypothalamus ensures a two-way communication between these interrelated systems.

In addition to controlling the pituitary, the hypothalamus also receives input from various areas of the central nervous system (i.e., information regarding plasma circulating levels of electrolytes and hormones) and controls the autonomic nervous system. Therefore, the hypothalamus is the brain center for the maintenance of homeostasis.

Within each subdivision of the hypophysis are various regions having specialized cells that release different hormones. The hypophysis is subdivided into two regions (Figs. 13.2 and 13.3): (1) the **adenohypophysis** (**anterior pituitary**), with its three component parts, the *pars distalis* (*pars anterior*), *pars intermedia*, and *pars tuberalis*; and (2) the **neurohypophysis** (**posterior pituitary**), with its three component parts, the *median eminence*, *infundibulum*, and *pars nervosa* (Figs. 13.4 and 13.5).

BLOOD SUPPLY AND CONTROL OF SECRETION

The hypophyseal portal system of veins delivers neurosecretory hormones from the primary capillary plexus of the median eminence to the secondary capillary plexus of the pars distalis.

Two pairs of arteries arising from the internal carotid artery (see Fig. 13.3) provide the blood supply to the pituitary gland. The **superior hypophyseal arteries** supply the pars tuberalis and infundibulum. They also form an extensive capillary network, the **primary capillary bed** (**plexus**), in the median eminence of the neurohypophysis. **Inferior hypophyseal arteries** primarily supply the posterior lobe, although they also send a few branches to the anterior lobe.

Hypophyseal portal veins drain the **primary capillary bed** (**plexus**) of the median eminence and deliver their blood into the **secondary capillary bed** (**plexus**), located in the pars distalis (see Fig. 13.3). The capillaries of both plexuses are **fenestrated**.

Axons of neurons that originate in various portions of the hypothalamus terminate around the primary capillary plexus of the median eminence. The endings of these axons differ from other axons of the body because, instead of delivering a signal to another cell, they liberate **hypothalamic secretory hormones** (either **releasing** or **inhibiting hormones** [**factors**]) directly into the connective tissue surrounding the primary capillary bed. These **hypothalamic secretory hormones** are taken by the blood of the hypophyseal portal system and delivered to the secondary capillary bed of the pars distalis, where these hormones leave the capillaries to regulate the secretion of various **anterior pituitary hormones**. Because of this arrangement of vascular flow, the releasing hormones do not have to enter the systemic circulation; therefore, they are not diluted by the larger blood volume and can act in a timely manner in the regulation of the release of the anterior pituitary hormones. The following are the main releasing and inhibitory hormones (factors):

- Thyroid-stimulating hormone–releasing hormone (thyrotropin-releasing hormone [TRH]) stimulates the release of thyroid-stimulating hormone (TSH).
- Corticotropin-releasing hormone (CRH) stimulates the release of adrenocorticotropin.
- Somatotropin-releasing hormone (SRH) stimulates the release of somatotropin (growth hormone).
- Luteinizing hormone–releasing hormone (LHRH) stimulates the release of luteinizing hormone (LH) and FSH.
- Prolactin-releasing hormone (PRH) stimulates the release of prolactin.
- Prolactin inhibitory factor (PIF) inhibits prolactin secretion.

The physiological effects of pituitary hormones are summarized in Table 13.2.

ADENOHYPOPHYSIS

The **adenohypophysis** (**pars anterior**) develops from the Rathke pouch and consists of three regions: pars distalis, pars intermedia, and pars tuberalis.

Pars Distalis

The parenchymal cells of the pars distalis consist of the chromophils and chromophobes.

A dense, irregular, collagenous fibrous capsule invests the **pars distalis** (anterior lobe). The parenchyma of the pars distalis, surrounded by reticular fibers, is composed of cords of cells, known as **chromophils** and **chromophobes**. Chromophils, the primary secretory cells of the pars distalis, have an affinity for dyes, whereas chromophobes have no affinity for dyes. Chromophils are further subdivided into **acidophils**, that stain with acid dyes and **basophils**, which stain with basic dyes. However, it should be noted that these latter designations refer to the affinity of the secretory granules within the cells to the dyes, not to the parenchymal cell cytoplasm. The release or the continued storage of the hormones housed in the secretory granules of

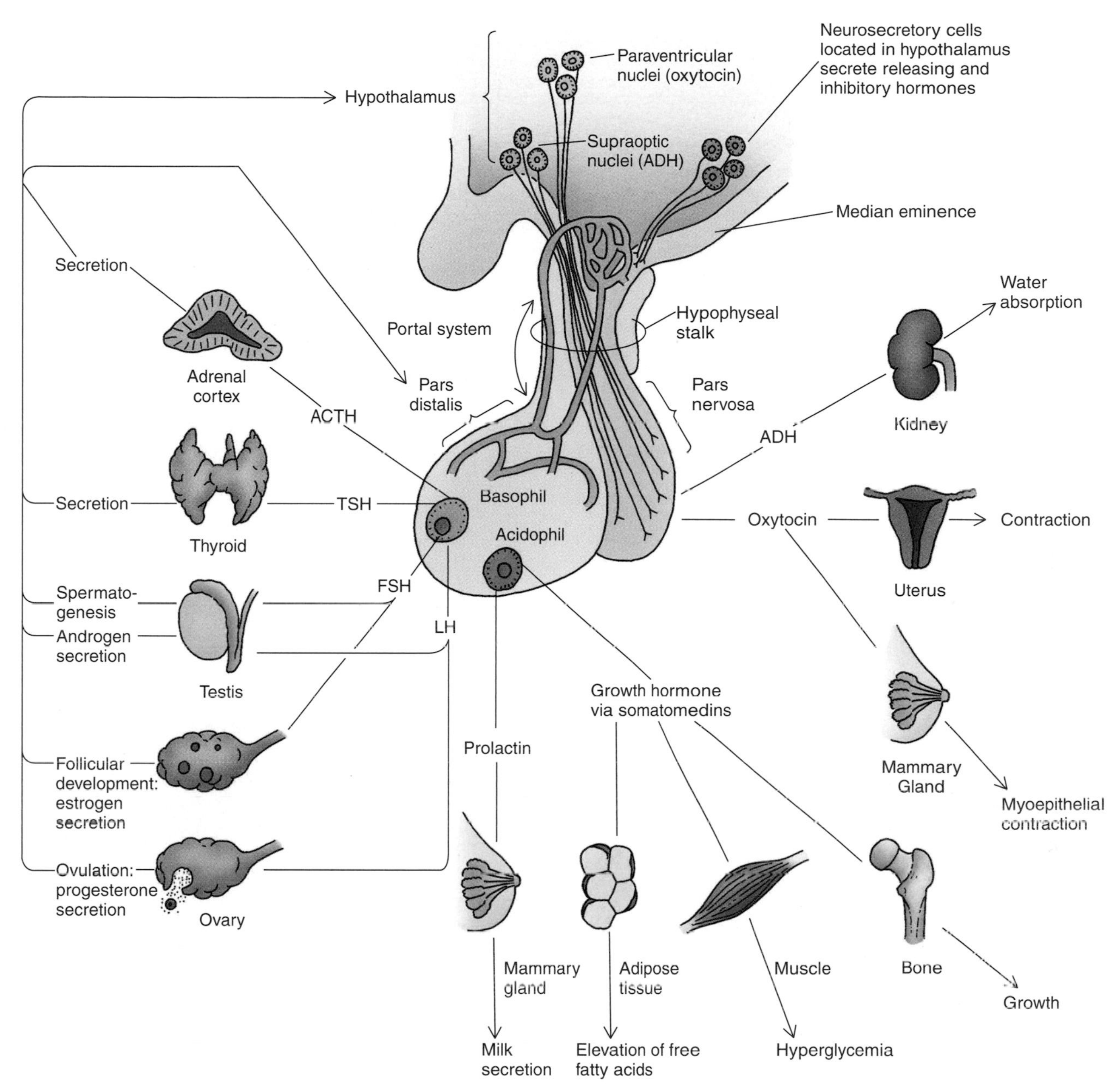

Fig. 13.2 Schematic diagram of the pituitary gland and its target organs. *ADH*, Antidiuretic hormone; *FSH*, follicle-stimulating hormone; *LH*, luteinizing hormone; *TSH*, thyroid-stimulating hormone.

the chromophils is controlled by the **releasing** (**stimulatory**) or **inhibitory hormones**, respectively. As indicated earlier, these stimulatory and inhibitory hormones are manufactured by neurons located in the hypothalamus and delivered by the hypophyseal portal system into the secondary capillary bed of the pars distalis. The endothelial lining of the secondary capillary bed is fenestrated, facilitating the diffusion of releasing/inhibiting factors to the parenchymal cells and providing entry sites for the secretions released by the parenchymal cells.

Chromophils

Secretory granules of chromophils have an affinity for histological dyes: those that stain orange-red with *acid* dyes and those that stain blue with *basic* dyes.

Acidophils

Acidophils, whose granules stain orange-red with eosin, are of two varieties: somatotrophs and mammotrophs.

The most abundant cells in the pars distalis are **acidophils**, whose granules are large enough to be seen by the light microscope and stain orange to red with eosin (Figs. 13.6 to 13.8). There are two types of acidophils, **somatotrophs** and **mammotrophs**.

Somatotrophs have a centrally placed nucleus, a moderate Golgi complex, small rod-shaped mitochondria, an abundant rough endoplasmic reticulum (RER), and numerous secretory granules 300 to 400 nm in diameter (Fig. 13.9). These cells

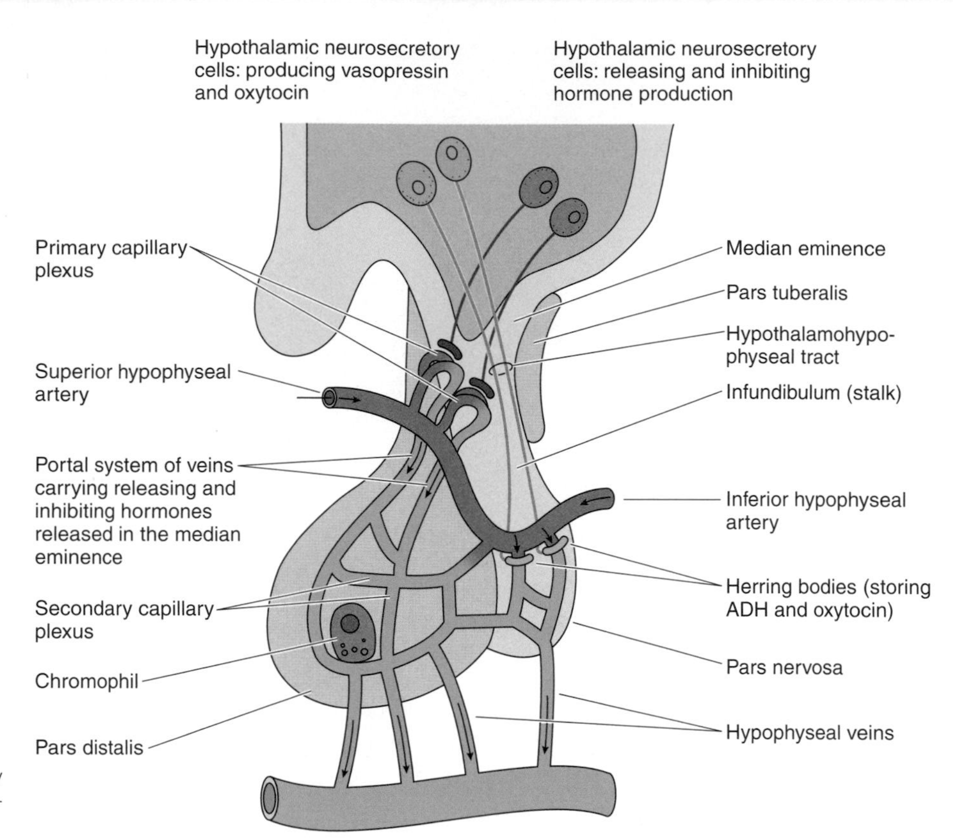

Fig. 13.3 Schematic diagram of the pituitary gland and its circulatory system. *ADH,* Antidiuretic hormone.

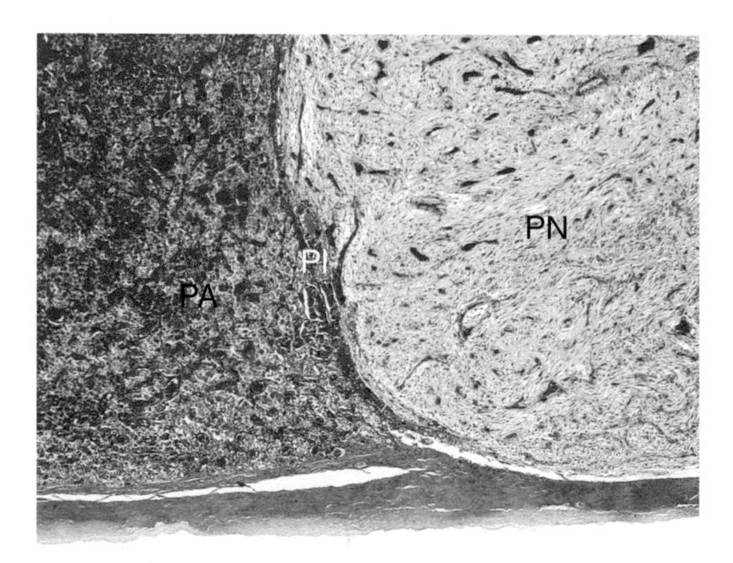

Fig. 13.4 This very-low-magnification photomicrograph presents the pars anterior (PA), pars intermedia (PI), and the pars nervosa (PN) of the pituitary gland. The collagenous connective tissue capsule (not labeled) is present at the bottom of the image. (×14)

secrete somatotropin (growth hormone), and are stimulated by somatotropin releasing hormone (SRH), also known as *growth hormone–releasing hormone*, and are inhibited by somatostatin. Somatotropin has a generalized effect of increasing cellular metabolic rates. This hormone also induces liver cells to produce insulin-like growth factor I and insulin-like growth factor II, which increase mitotic rates of epiphyseal plate chondrocytes, promoting the elongation of long bones and hence stimulating

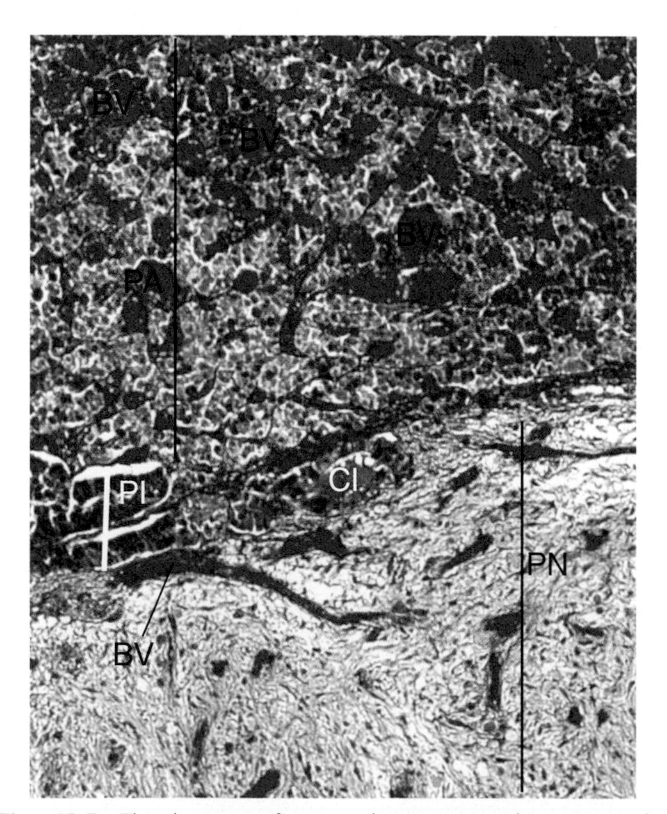

Fig. 13.5 This low-magnification photomicrograph presents the same area of the pituitary gland as Fig. 13.4 but at 90 degrees to it. Note the rich blood supply (BV) of the pars anterior (PA) and the pars nervosa (PN). A small island of colloid is evident in the pars intermedia (PI). (×132)

TABLE 13.2 **Physiological Effects of Pituitary Hormones**

Hormone	Releasing/Inhibiting	Function
PARS DISTALIS		
Somatotropin (growth hormone)	*Releasing:* SRH (GHRH) *Inhibiting:* Somatostatin	Generalized effect on most cells is to increase metabolic rates, stimulate liver cells to release insulin-like growth factors I and II, which increases proliferation of cartilage and assists in growth in long bones.
Prolactin	*Releasing:* PRH *Inhibiting:* PIF	Promotes development of mammary glands during pregnancy; stimulates milk production after parturition (prolactin secretion is stimulated by suckling).
Adrenocorticotropic hormone (ACTH; corticotropin)	*Releasing:* CRH	Stimulates synthesis and release of hormones (cortisol and corticosterone) from suprarenal cortex.
Follicle-stimulating hormone (FSH)	*Releasing:* GnRH and leptin *Inhibiting:* Inhibin (in males)	Stimulates secondary ovarian follicle growth and estrogen secretion; stimulates Sertoli cells in seminiferous tubules to produce androgen-binding protein.
Luteinizing hormone (LH) in women	*Releasing:* GnRH	Assists FSH in promoting ovulation, formation of the corpus luteum, and secretion of progesterone and estrogen, forming a negative feedback to the hypothalamus to inhibit LHRH in women.
Luteinizing hormone (LH) in men		Stimulates Leydig cells to secrete and release testosterone, which forms a negative feedback to the hypothalamus to inhibit LHRH in men.
Thyroid-stimulating hormone (TSH; thyrotropin)	*Releasing:* TRH *Inhibiting:* Negative feedback suppresses via CNS	Stimulates synthesis and release of thyroid hormone, which increases metabolic rate.
PARS NERVOSA		
Oxytocin		Stimulates smooth muscle contractions of the uterus during orgasm; causes contractions of pregnant uterus at parturition (stimulation of cervix sends signal to hypothalamus to secrete more oxytocin); suckling sends signals to hypothalamus, resulting in more oxytocin, causing contractions of myoepithelial cells of the mammary glands, assisting in milk ejection.
Vasopressin (antidiuretic hormone [ADH])		Conserves body water by increasing resorption of water by kidneys; thought to be regulated by osmotic pressure; causes contraction of smooth muscles in arteries, thus raising the blood pressure; may restore normal blood pressure after severe hemorrhage.

CNS, Central nervous system; *CRH,* corticotropin-releasing hormone; *FSH,* follicle-stimulating hormone; *GHRH,* growth hormone releasing hormone; *GnRH,* gonadotropin releasing hormone; *LHRH,* luteinizing hormone–releasing hormone; *PIF,* prolactin inhibitory factor; *PRH,* prolactin-releasing hormone; *SRH,* somatotropin-releasing hormone; *TRH,* thyrotropin-releasing hormone.

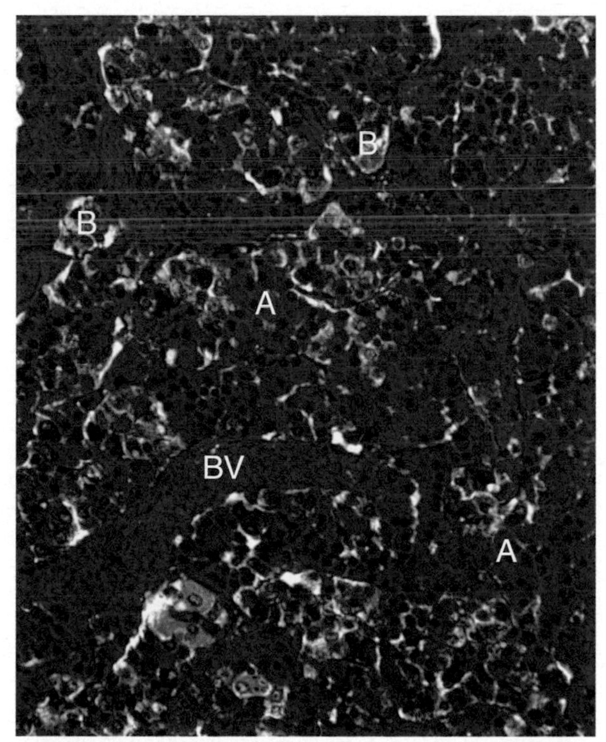

Fig. 13.6 This low-magnification photomicrograph of the pars anterior demonstrates the vascularity (BV) of this region and also displays the two types of chromophils: the orange-red acidophils (A) and the blue colored basophils (B). (×132)

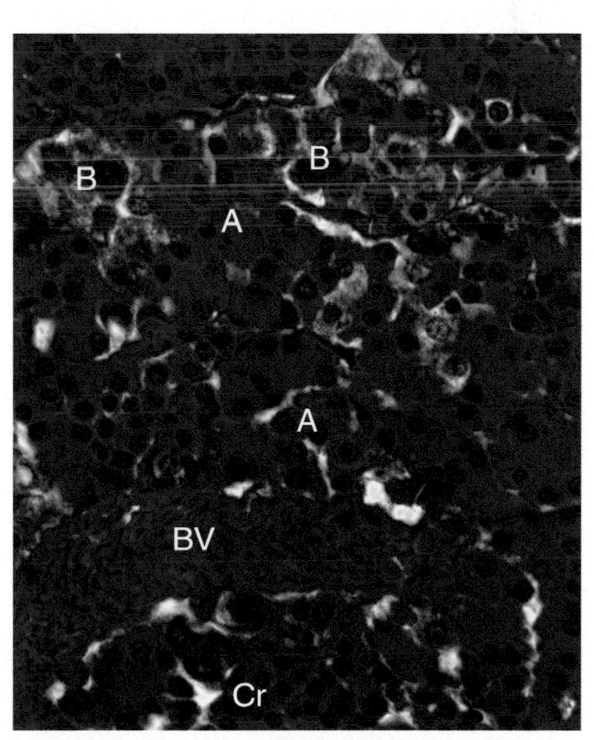

Fig. 13.7 This is a higher-magnification of Fig. 13.6 displaying the vascularity (BV) of the pars anterior and its chromophils, the acidophils (A) and the basophils (B), as well as the chromophobes (Cr).

growth. Approximately 50% of all chromophils are somatotrophs and reside mostly in the lateral aspect of the anterior pituitary.

Mammotrophs (lactotrophs), the other variety of acidophils, are arranged as individual cells rather than as clumps or clusters. These small, polygonal acidophils have the usual unremarkable organelle population. However, during lactation, the organelles enlarge and the Golgi complex may become as large as the nucleus. These cells can be distinguished by their large secretory granules, formed by the fusion of smaller granules that are released by the *trans*-Golgi network (see Fig. 13.9). These fused granules, which may be 600 nm in diameter, contain the hormone **prolactin**, which promotes mammary gland development during pregnancy as well as lactation after birth. Release of prolactin from mammotrophs is *stimulated* by the **prolactin-releasing hormone** (and to a certain limited extent by **thyrotropin-releasing hormone**, especially when nursing is taking place) and is *inhibited* by **dopamine**.

Clinical Correlations

Approximately 10% of all chromophils are mammotrophs in females who have never been pregnant and in males. However, in women who have had two or more pregnancies, mammotrophs may constitute as much as 30% of the chromophil population. Because the mammotroph population fluctuates, it is believed that there are stem cells present in the adenohypophysis that can differentiate into mammotrophs and probably into other acidophils and basophils. Some authors suggest that stem cells are members of the chromophobe cell population of the anterior pituitary, whereas others suggest that they are members of the folliculostellate cell population.

During pregnancy, circulating estrogen and progesterone inhibit secretion of prolactin. At birth, estrogen and progesterone levels are decreased; therefore, their inhibitory effect is lost. The number of mammotrophs also increases following birth. At the conclusion of nursing, the granules are degraded, and the excess mammotrophs regress.

Basophils

Basophils, the granules that stain blue with basic dyes, are of three varieties: corticotrophs, thyrotrophs, and gonadotrophs.

Basophils (see Figs. 13.6 to 13.8) granules stain blue with basic dyes. There are three types of basophils: **corticotrophs, thyrotrophs**, and **gonadotrophs**.

1. **Corticotrophs** are round to ovoid cells that constitute approximately 10% of the chromophils. They have an eccentric nucleus, relatively few organelles, and secretory granules that are approximately 250 to 400 nm in diameter. Corticotrophs synthesize **proopiomelanocortin (POMC)**, a large protein that is cleaved within the corticotrophs to produce **adrenocorticotropic hormone (ACTH)**, **melanocyte-stimulating hormone (MSH)**, **β-lipotropic hormone (β-LPH)**, and **β-endorphin.**
   - ACTH acts on melanocortin receptor type 2 in the suprarenal gland cortex, prompting the release of glucocorticoids by cells of the zona fasciculata (see later section on zona fasciculata).
   - MSH acts on melanocytes of the skin to produce melanin.
   - **β**-LPH induces lipolysis and the synthesis of steroids; it also prompts melanocytes to manufacture melanin pigments.
   - β-endorphins are natural analgesics that bind to opioid receptors.
2. **Thyrotrophs** constitute about 5% of the chromophil population and can be recognized by their small secretory granules (about 150 nm in diameter), which contain **TSH** (***thyrotropin***). Secretion is stimulated by **TRH** and inhibited by the presence of the thyroid hormones thyroxine (T_4) and triiodothyronine (T_3) in the blood. TSH functions in prompting the follicular cells of the thyroid gland to release thyroxine and triiodothyronine.
3. **Gonadotrophs** comprise approximately 10% of the chromophil population; they are round cells that have well-developed Golgi complexes and abundant RER and mitochondria. Their secretory granules vary in diameter from 300 to 400 nm. Gonadotrophs secrete **FSH** and **LH**; in males, some authors call LH ***interstitial cell–stimulating hormone (ICSH)***, because it stimulates steroid hormone production in interstitial cells of the testes. It remains unclear whether there are two subpopulations of gonadotrophs, one secreting FSH and the other LH, or whether both hormones are produced by one cell in different phases of the secretory cycle. Secretion is stimulated by **gonadotropin-releasing hormone (GnRH)** as well as by the hormone **leptin** and is inhibited by various hormones that are produced by the ovaries and testes.

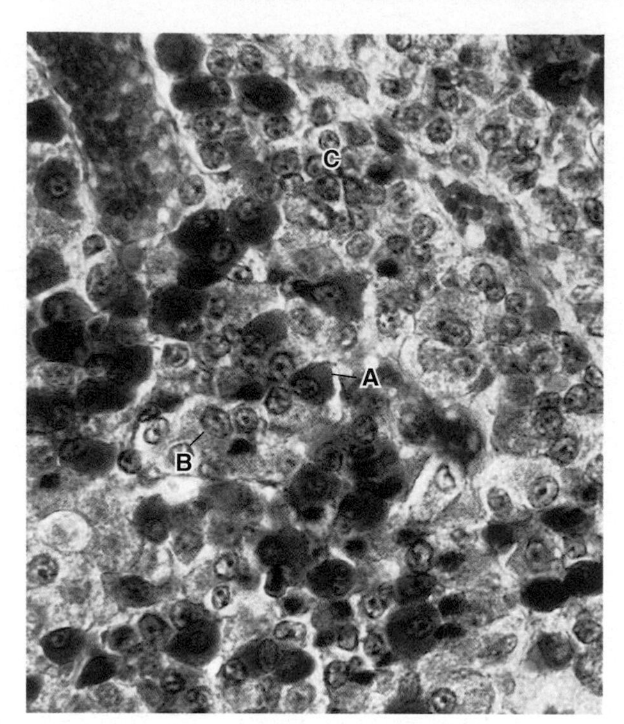

Fig. 13.8 Light micrograph of the pituitary gland displaying chromophobes (C), acidophils (A), and basophils (B). (×470)

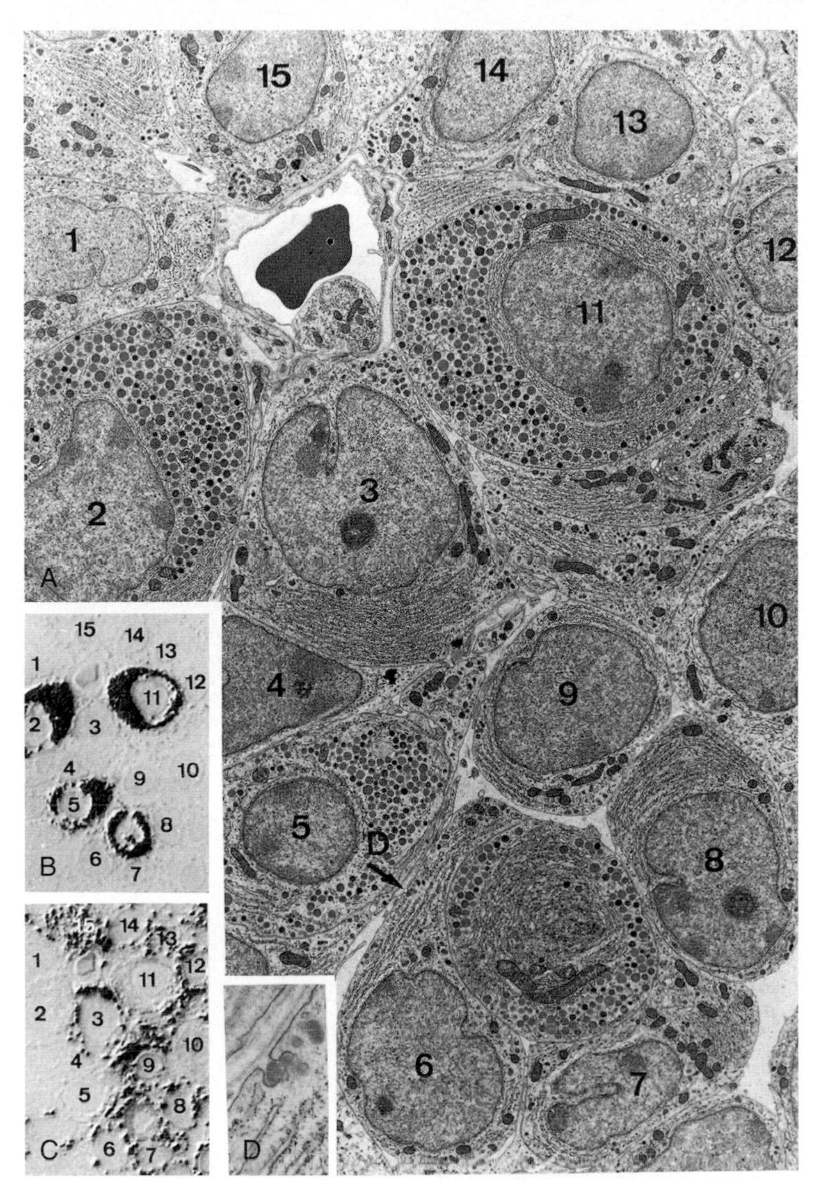

Fig. 13.9 Light and electron micrograph of mouse adenohypophysis (×4000). Observe the mammotropes (cells 3, 6–9, 12–15) and somatotropes (cells 2, 5, 11) and note the secretory granules of these cells. (From Yamaji A, Sasaki F, Iwama Y, Yamauchi S. Mammotropes and somatotropes in the adenohypophysis of androgenized female mice: morphological and immunohistochemical studies by light microscopy correlated with routine electron microscopy. *Anat Rec.* 1992;233:103-110. Reprinted with permission from Wiley-Liss, Inc., a subsidiary of John Wiley & Sons, Inc.)

Clinical Correlations

*Individuals with **Kallman syndrome** have very low levels of sex hormones. As a consequence, female patients present with lack of secondary sexual development (i.e., breasts and pubic hair are lacking, and menstruation does not begin). Males present with micropenis and delay in the beginning of puberty. This syndrome is caused by an **X-linked recessive disorder** that also presents with additional developmental disorders, such as atrophy of the optic nerve, cleft palate, color blindness, cryptorchidism, and deafness (among others). The mutation occurs in the gene in which the protein product (known as **anosmin-1**) facilitates during embryogenesis the migration of GnRH cells from their original location in the olfactory placodes into the developing hypothalamus.*

Chromophobes

Chromophobes have very little cytoplasm; therefore, they do not take up stain readily.

Chromophobes are clusters of small, weakly staining cells (see Figs. 13.7 and 13.8). These cells generally have much less cytoplasm than chromophils do and they may represent partially degranulated chromophils, although some retain a small amount of secretory granules. It is possible that some of the chromophobes are nonspecific stem cells that can replenish the chromophil population.

Folliculostellate Cells

Folliculostellate cells constitute a large population of nonendocrine cells in the pars distalis–occupying regions between chromophobes and chromophils. Although their function is not clear, they have long processes that form gap junctions with those of other folliculostellate cells and with chromophils. It has been suggested that these cells may have multiple functions, including the release of peptides that stimulate the chromophils to release their hormones; providing physical support for chromophils and chromophobes; phagocytosis; and, according to some, acting as stem cells to regenerate parenchymal cells of the anterior pituitary.

Pars Intermedia

The pars intermedia lies between the pars distalis and the pars nervosa and contains cysts that are remnants of the Rathke pouch.

The **pars intermedia** is characterized by many cuboidal cell-lined, colloid-containing cysts (Rathke cysts), which are remnants of the ectoderm of the Rathke pouch. It also houses cords of basophils along the networks of capillaries. These basophils synthesize the prohormone **POMC**, a large protein that, as indicated earlier, is cleaved within the basophils to produce **ACTH, β-LPH, MSH**, and **β-endorphin**.

Pars Tuberalis

The pars tuberalis surrounds the hypophyseal stalk and is composed of cuboidal to low-columnar basophilic cells.

The **pars tuberalis** surrounds the hypophyseal stalk but frequently is absent on its posterior aspect. Thin layers of pia arachnoid–like connective tissue separate the pars tuberalis from the infundibular stalk. The pars tuberalis is highly vascularized by arteries and the hypophyseal portal system, along which lie longitudinal cords of cuboidal to low-columnar epithelial cells. The cytoplasm of these basophilic cells contains small, dense granules; lipid droplets; interspersed colloid droplets; and glycogen. Although no specific hormones are known to be secreted by the pars tuberalis, some cells display secretory granules that may contain **FSH** and **LH**.

NEUROHYPOPHYSIS

The **posterior pituitary gland** (**neurohypophysis**) is divided into the median eminence, the infundibulum (continuation of the hypothalamus), and the pars nervosa (see Figs. 13.2 and 13.3).

Median Eminence

The **median eminence** is that region of the posterior pituitary gland that houses the **primary capillary bed** and where axons of various neurons that manufacture releasing and inhibitory hormones terminate to release their hormones indirectly into the primary capillary bed. The median eminence, along with the pars nervosa, pineal gland, and three other small regions of the brain (the subfornical organ, area postrema, and the vascular organ of the lamina terminalis), although belonging to the central nervous system, **lack the blood–brain barrier.** These structures are said to be **circumventricular organs** (**CVOs**). The first three are considered to be **secretory components** because they release hormones, and the last three are **sensory components** of the CVOs because they are sensory receptors that recognize alterations in temperature; osmotic pressure; hormone, peptide, and other biochemical levels of blood; and chemical composition of the cerebrospinal fluid. The CVOs are able to perform their functions because their lack of a blood–brain barrier permits substances present in the bloodstream to enter the extracellular spaces in the vicinity of the receptor cells and for hormones released by components of the CVOs to enter the capillary beds.

Hypothalamohypophyseal Tract

Axons of neurosecretory cells of supraoptic and paraventricular nuclei extend into the posterior pituitary as the hypothalamohypophyseal tract.

Unmyelinated axons, whose cell bodies reside in the supraoptic and paraventricular nuclei and project to the posterior pituitary to terminate in the vicinity of the capillaries, form the **hypothalamohypophyseal tract**, and constitute the bulk of the posterior pituitary gland. The soma of these cells synthesize **oxytocin** and **vasopressin** (**antidiuretic hormone** [**ADH**]), as well as adenosine triphosphate (ATP) and acetylcholine. Carrier proteins, **neurophysin I** and **neurophysin II**, also produced by the cells of these nuclei, bind to oxytocin and vasopressin, respectively, as they travel down the axons to the posterior pituitary, where they are released into the bloodstream from the axon terminals.

Pars Nervosa

The distal terminals of the axons of the **hypothalamohypophyseal tract** end in the **pars nervosa** and store the neurosecretions that are produced by their cell bodies in the hypothalamus (Fig. 13.10). As indicated earlier, cell bodies of neurons that secrete vasopressin are located chiefly in the supraoptic nucleus of the hypothalamus, whereas cell bodies of neurons that secrete oxytocin are located mostly in the paraventricular nucleus of the hypothalamus. Each of these peptide hormones travels down the axons of its respective neurons in association with a precursor protein known as a *neurophysin I* or *neurophysin II.* By the time they reach the pars nervosa of the hypophysis, the hormones have matured and cleaved from their precursors. Chrome-alum hematoxylin staining reveals blue-black distentions of the axons by light microscopy; these are called ***Herring***

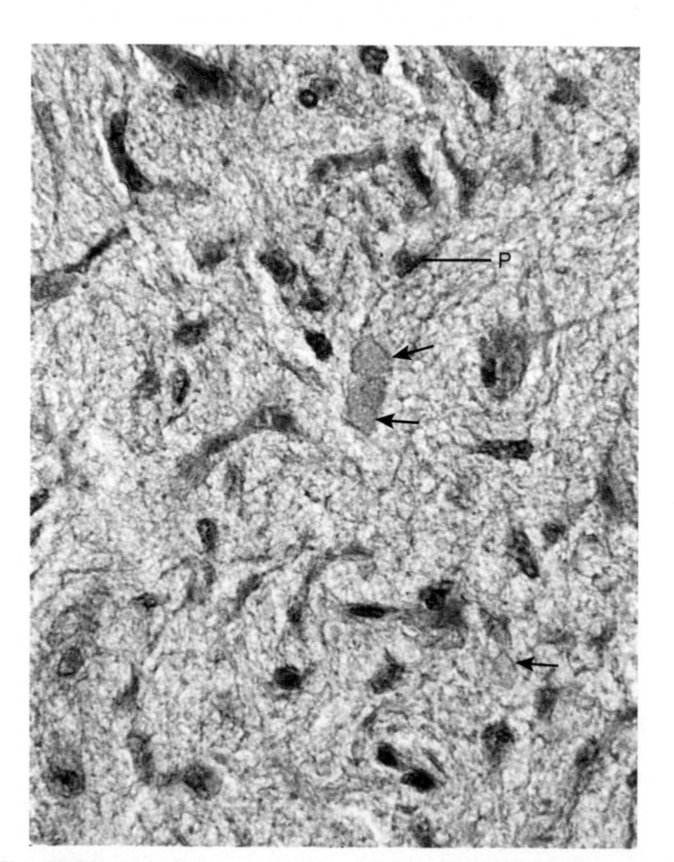

Fig. 13.10 Light micrograph of the pars nervosa of the pituitary gland displaying pituicytes (P) and Herring bodies *(arrows).* Herring bodies are the expanded terminals of the nerve fibers where the neurosecretory products vasopressin (antidiuretic hormone) and oxytocin are stored (×132).

bodies, which represent accumulations of neurosecretory granules (see Fig. 13.5) not only at the termini but also along the length of the axons. In response to nerve stimulation, the hormones are released from the Herring bodies into the perivascular space near the fenestrated capillaries of the capillary plexus.

The target for vasopressin (ADH) is the collecting ducts of the kidney, where it modulates plasma membrane permeability, which has the effect of lowering urine volume but increasing its concentration (see Chapter 19). The target for oxytocin is the myometrium of the uterus, where it is released in the late phases of pregnancy. During labor, oxytocin is believed to play a role in parturition by stimulating contraction of the smooth muscles of the uterus. Additionally, oxytocin functions in milk ejection from the mammary gland by stimulating contraction of the myoepithelial cells surrounding the glandular alveoli and the ducts of the mammary gland (see Chapter 20).

Pituicytes constitute about 25% of the volume of the pars nervosa. They are similar to neuroglial cells and help support the axons of the pars nervosa by ensheathing them as well as their dilatations. Pituicytes contain lipid droplets, lipochrome pigment, and intermediate filaments; they have numerous cytoplasmic processes that contact and form gap junctions with each other. Beyond supporting the neural elements in the pars nervosa, additional functions of pituicytes have not been elucidated. However, it is believed that they may contribute a trophic function to the normal operation of the neurosecretory axon terminals and neurohypophysis.

Clinical Correlations

1. ***Pituitary adenomas*** *are common tumors of the anterior pituitary gland. Their growth and enlargement may suppress hormonal production in other secretory cells of the pars distalis. When left unattended, these adenomas may erode surrounding bone and other neural tissues.*
2. ***Diabetes insipidus*** *may be caused by lesions in the hypothalamus or pars nervosa that reduce the production of ADH by neurosecretory cells whose axon terminals are located in the neurohypophysis. This condition has nothing to do with the hormone insulin but rather results in renal dysfunction, which leads to inadequate water resorption by the kidneys, with a consequential polyuria (high urinary output) and dehydration. Unlike in diabetes mellitus, in which the urine tastes sweet (mellitus = honey) due to its high sugar content, the urine in diabetes insipidus is tasteless (insipidus = insipid).*
3. ***Pituicytoma*** *is a very rare, slow-growing tumor originating from the pituicytes of the pars nervosa. Individuals with this benign tumor present with visual field disorders, hypopituitarism, as well as prolonged headaches and dizziness. The tumor usually appears in and above the sella turcica; the symptoms the patient exhibits depend on the compression effects of the lesion. The preferred treatment is surgical resection of the tumor because it results in minimal recurrence of the condition.*

Thyroid Gland

The thyroid gland, located in the anterior portion of the neck, secretes the hormones thyroxine, triiodothyronine, and calcitonin.

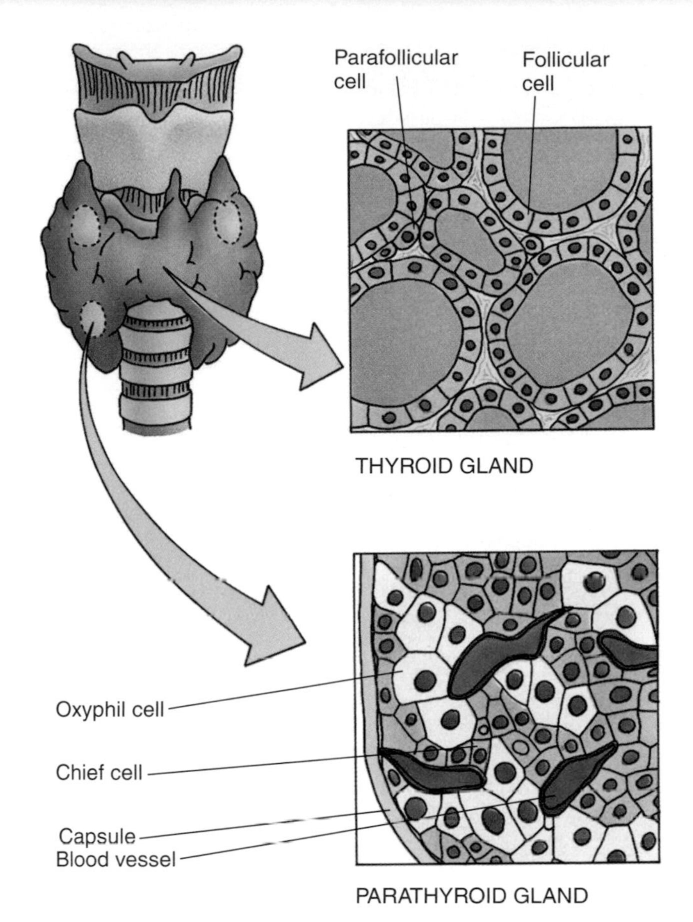

Fig. 13.11 Schematic diagram of the thyroid and parathyroid glands.

The **thyroid gland** is located just below the larynx, anterior to the junction of the thyroid and cricoid cartilages (Fig. 13.11). It is composed of a **right lobe** and **left lobe**, which are connected across the midline by an **isthmus**. In some individuals, the gland has an additional **pyramidal lobe** that ascends from the left side of the isthmus. This additional lobe is a vestige of the thyroglossal duct, indicative of the descent of the thyroid primordium through the forming tongue.

The thyroid gland is surrounded by a slender, dense, irregular collagenous connective tissue capsule, a derivative of the deep cervical fascia. Embedded within the capsule, on the posterior aspect of the gland, are the parathyroid glands. Connective tissue septa derived from the capsule invade the parenchyma and provide a conduit for blood vessels, lymphatic vessels, and nerve fibers. These connective tissue septa surround 20 to 40 follicles, forming a lobule that is served by a single arteriole, and each lobule acts independently from other lobules. Slender connective tissue elements, composed mostly of reticular fibers and housing a rich capillary plexus, arise from the connective tissue boundary of lobules to surround each follicle but are separated from the follicular and parafollicular cells by a thin **basal lamina**. Occasionally, follicular cells of neighboring follicles may come into contact with each other and disrupt the continuity of the basal lamina.

The thyroid gland produces the hormones **thyroxin** and **triiodothyronine** (**T_4** and **T_3**), which stimulate the rate of metabolism and **calcitonin** that functions in decreasing blood calcium levels and facilitates the storage of calcium in bones (Table 13.3).

TABLE 13.3 **Hormones and Functions of the Thyroid, Parathyroid, Adrenal, and Pineal Glands**

Hormone	Cell Source	Regulating Hormone	Function
THYROID GLAND			
Thyroxine (T_4) and triiodothyronine (T_3)	Follicular cells	Thyroid-stimulating hormone (TSH)	Facilitate nuclear transcription of genes responsible for protein synthesis; increase cellular metabolism and growth rates; facilitate mental processes; increase endocrine gland activity; stimulate carbohydrate and fat metabolism; decrease cholesterol, phospholipids, and triglycerides; increase fatty acids; decrease body weight; increase heart rate, respiration, muscle action.
Calcitonin (thyrocalcitonin)	Parafollicular cells	Feedback mechanism with parathyroid hormone	Lowers plasma calcium concentration by suppressing bone resorption.
PARATHYROID GLAND			
Parathyroid hormone (PTH)	Chief cells	Feedback mechanism with calcitonin	Increases calcium concentration in body fluids.
SUPRARENAL (ADRENAL) GLANDS			
Suprarenal Cortex			
Mineralocorticoids: aldosterone and deoxycorticosterone	Cells of the zona glomerulosa	Angiotensin II and adrenocorticotropic hormone (ACTH)	Control body fluid volume and electrolyte concentrations by acting on distal tubules of the kidney, causing excretion of potassium and resorption of sodium.
Glucocorticoids: cortisol and corticosterone	Cells of the zona fasciculata (spongiocytes)	ACTH	Regulate metabolism of carbohydrates, fats, and proteins; decrease protein synthesis, increasing amino acids in blood; stimulate gluconeogenesis by activating liver to convert amino acids to glucose; release fatty acid and glycerol; act as anti-inflammatory agents; reduce capillary permeability; suppress immune response.
Androgens: dehydroepiandrosterone and androstenedione	Cells of the zona reticularis	ACTH	Provides weak masculinizing characteristics.
Suprarenal Medulla			
Catecholamines: epinephrine and norepinephrine	Chromaffin cells	Preganglionic, sympathetic, and splanchnic nerves	*Epinephrine* Operates the "fight or flight or freeze" mechanism, preparing the body for severe fear or stress; increases cardiac heart rate and output, augmenting blood flow to the organs and release of glucose from the liver for energy. *Norepinephrine* Causes an elevation in blood pressure by vasoconstriction.
PINEAL GLAND			
Melatonin	Pinealocytes	Norepinephrine	May influence cyclic gonadal activity.

CELLULAR ORGANIZATION

The thyroid follicle is the structural and functional unit of the thyroid gland.

Unlike most of the endocrine glands, which store their secretory substances within the parenchymal cells, the thyroid gland stores its secretory substances in the lumina of **follicles** (Figs. 13.12 and 13.13). These cyst-like structures, ranging from 0.2 to 0.9 mm in diameter, have a simple cuboidal epithelium composed of **follicular cells** surrounding a central **colloid-filled** lumen and contacting the colloid, as well as larger **parafollicular cells** (**clear cells**; **C cells**) that are located at the periphery of the follicle and do not contact the colloid.

Follicular Cells (Principal Cells)

Follicular (principal) cells are squamous to low columnar in shape.

Follicular cells range from low cuboidal to low columnar in shape and are tallest when they are active. These cells have TSH receptors on their basal plasma membranes, a round to ovoid nucleus with two nucleoli, and basophilic cytoplasm. Frequently, their RER is distended and displays zones that are ribosome free. These cells also have numerous apically located lysosomes, rod-shaped mitochondria, a supranuclear Golgi complex, and numerous short microvilli that extend into the colloid (Fig. 13.14). Numerous small vesicles, dispersed throughout the cytoplasm, are believed to contain **thyroglobulin**, a large (660,000 D) secretory glycoprotein. *The presence of TSH is required both for the synthesis and release of thyroid hormones.*

SYNTHESIS OF THYROID HORMONES (T_3 AND T_4)

Thyroid hormone synthesis is regulated by iodide levels and by TSH binding to TSH receptors of follicular cells.

The synthesis of thyroid hormone is regulated by the iodide levels in the follicular cell, as well as by the binding of TSH to TSH receptors of the follicular cells. The occupation of TSH receptors triggers cAMP production, resulting in protein kinase A activity and synthesis of T_3 and T_4.

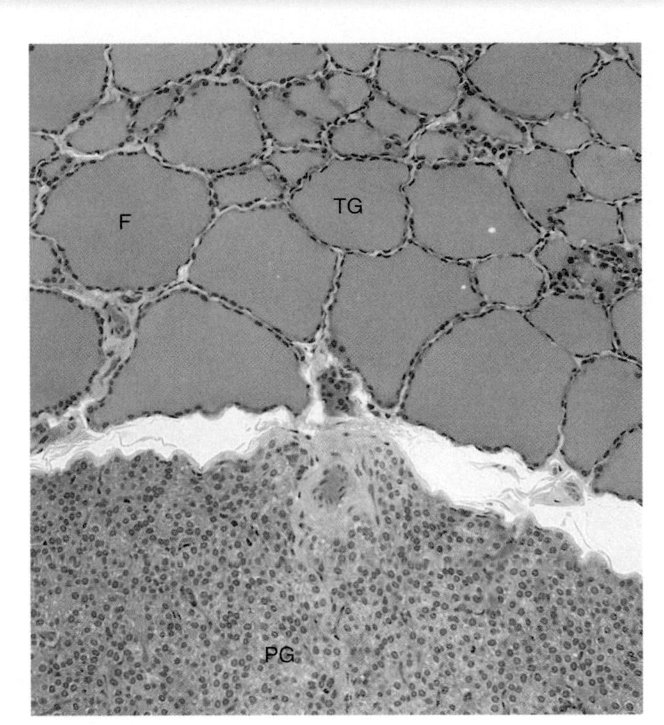

Fig. 13.12 Light micrograph of the thyroid and parathyroid glands. Observe the colloid-filled follicles (F) of the thyroid gland (TG) in the upper portion of the figure. The lower portion of this figure is the parathyroid gland (PG), as evidenced by the presence of chief and oxyphil cells. (×132)

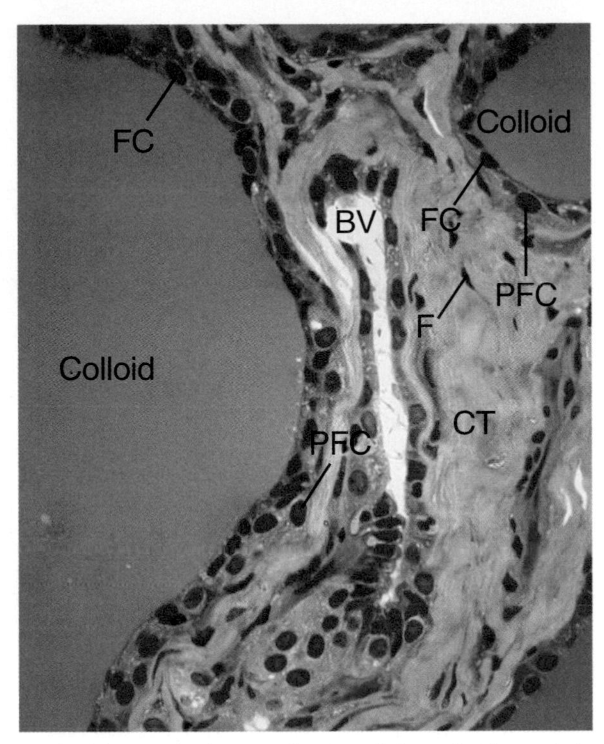

Fig. 13.13 This is a high magnification of the colloid-containing thyroid follicle and its surrounding connective tissue. Note the follicular cells (FC) that manufacture the colloid, as well as the thyroid hormones present in the colloid. Also, observe the larger, lighter staining parafollicular cells that manufacture the hormone calcitonin. The connective tissue of the thyroid gland displays the presence of blood vessels (BV) and fibroblasts (F). (×540)

Fig. 13.15 outlines the pathway for the synthesis and release of thyroid hormones. Thyroglobulin is synthesized in the RER and subsequently glycosylated in both the RER and the Golgi apparatus. The modified protein is packaged in the *trans*-Golgi network. The vesicles containing thyroglobulin are transported to the apical plasmalemma, where their contents are released into the colloid and stored in the lumen of the follicle.

Iodine is reduced to iodide (I^-) within the alimentary canal and is preferentially absorbed and conveyed by the bloodstream to the thyroid gland. Iodide is endocytosed via energy-requiring sodium/iodide symporters located in the basal plasmalemma of the follicular cells, so that the intracellular iodide concentration is 20- to 30-fold that of plasma. Once in the cytosol, iodide is transferred out of the follicular cell to the colloid-cell membrane interface via an iodide/chloride transporter, known as ***pendrin***. While the iodide is being transferred, noniodinated **thyroglobulin,** along with **thyroid peroxidase**, also leaves the follicular cell to enter the colloid. At the colloid–follicular cell interface, iodide is oxidized by the thyroid peroxidase, a process that requires the presence of hydrogen peroxide (H_2O_2). The activated iodide remains at the colloid–follicular cell interface. While there, it iodinates tyrosine residues of thyroglobulin, forming **monoiodinated tyrosine** (**MIT**) and **diiodinated tyrosine** (**DIT**). **Triiodinated** and **tetraiodinated tyrosines** are then formed by the coupling of an MIT and DIT or by the coupling of two DITs, respectively. Each thyroglobulin molecule has fewer than four T_4 molecules and fewer than 0.3 T_3 residues. The iodinated thyroglobulin is released from the follicular cell–colloid interface by the follicular cells and is stored in the colloid.

RELEASE OF THYROID HORMONES (T_3 AND T_4)

Thyroid-stimulating hormone stimulates follicular cells of the thyroid gland to release T_3 and T_4 into the bloodstream.

Binding of **TSH** to **TSH receptors** on the basal plasmalemma stimulates the low-cuboidal cells to become low-columnar cells (see Fig. 13.15). Additionally, they form filopodia at their apical cell membrane and endocytose aliquots of the colloid. Cytoplasmic vesicles containing colloid fuse with early (or late) endosomes. Within the endosomes, iodinated residues are cleaved from thyroglobulin by proteases and are transferred into the cytosol as free monoiodotyrosine, diiodotyrosine, T_3, and T_4.

Monoiodotyrosine and diiodotyrosine are stripped of their iodine by the enzyme **iodotyrosine dehalogenase**, and both the iodine and the amino acid tyrosine become part of their respective pools within the cytosol for later use.

T_3 and T_4 are released at the basal plasmalemma of the follicular cells, entering the connective tissue spaces of the thyroid for distribution by the bloodstream. Once in the bloodstream, both T_3 and T_4 bind to the carrier protein, **thyroxine-binding globulin**, to be transported to their target cells. It should be noted that both T_3 and T_4 can bind to other carrier proteins—**transerythrin**, **albumin**, and some **lipoproteins**. Transerythrin is responsible for ferrying T_3 and T_4 to the cerebrospinal fluid; albumin binds approximately 10% of the thyroid hormones, and lipoproteins bind approximately 5% of the thyroid hormones to transport them to their target cells. T_4 constitutes about 90% of the released hormone and, although it has a half-life of about 6 days, it is only 20% as effective as T_3, which has a half-life of only 1 day. Approximately one-third of T_4 enters the liver, heart, or kidney, where it is converted by the enzyme **5'-iodinase** to the more effective form of the hormone, T_3, also referred to as **reverse T_3 (rT_3)**.

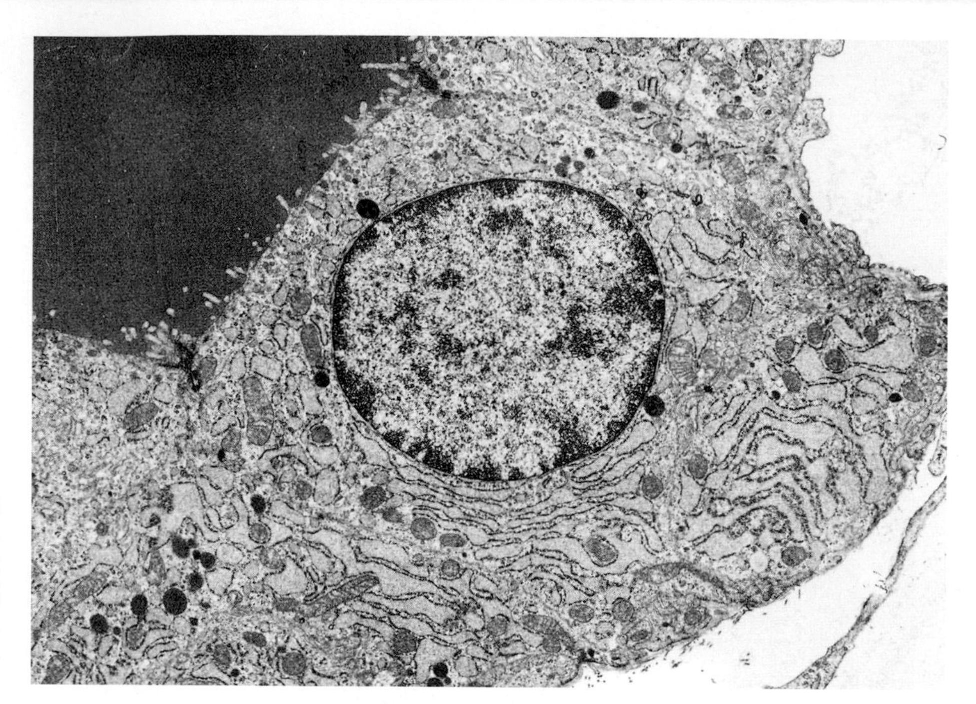

Fig. 13.14 Electron micrograph of a thyroid follicular cell bordering the colloid *(black area, upper left-hand corner)* (×10700). (From Mestdagh C, Many MC, Haalpern S, et al. Correlated autoradiographic and ion-microscopic study of the role of iodine in the formation of "cold" follicles in young and old mice. *Cell Tissue Res.* 1990;260:449-457.)

Clinical Correlations

1. ***Graves disease*** *is characterized by hyperplasia of the follicular cells, increasing the size of the thyroid gland two to three times above normal. Thyroid hormone production is also greatly increased, from 5 to 15 times normal (**hyperthyroidism**). Other symptoms include **exophthalmos**, or protrusion of the eyeballs. Although Graves disease may develop from several causes, the most common agent is the binding of autoimmune immunoglobulin G (IgG) antibodies to TSH receptors, which stimulates thyroid follicular cells.*
2. *Insufficient dietary intake of iodine causes the thyroid gland to enlarge, a condition called **simple goiter**. Goiter usually is not associated with hyperthyroidism or hypothyroidism. This condition can be treated with iodine in the diet.*
3. ***Hypothyroidism*** *is characterized by such conditions as fatigue, sleeping for up to 14 to 16 hours a day, muscular sluggishness, slowed heart rate, decreased cardiac output and blood volume, mental sluggishness, failure of body functions, constipation, and loss of hair growth. Patients with severe hypothyroidism may develop **myxedema**, which is characterized by bagginess under the eyes and a swollen face that is due to nonpitting edema of the skin and infiltration of excess glycosaminoglycans and proteoglycans into the extracellular matrix. **Cretinism** is an extreme form of hypothyroidism in fetal life through childhood that is characterized by failure of growth and mental retardation due to a congenitally missing thyroid gland.*
4. *The **external laryngeal** and **recurrent laryngeal nerves** supplying the laryngeal musculature are closely applied to the thyroid gland and must be isolated and protected during **thyroidectomy**. Damage to either of these two nerves results in hoarseness and, possibly, loss of speech.*

PHYSIOLOGICAL EFFECTS OF TRIIODOTHYRONINE AND THYROXINE

Once $\mathbf{T_3}$ and $\mathbf{T_4}$ enter the bloodstream, they bind to plasma-binding proteins. There, they are slowly released to the tissues to contact their target cells and pass through the cell membranes of these cells. Transport across the target cell membrane is effected by a number of transporter proteins, including **monocarboxylate transporter 8** (**MTC8**) in the body and **organic anion transporter polypeptide 1C1** (**OATP1C1**) in the brain. As they enter the target cell cytoplasm, they are bound to intracellular proteins and slowly used over a period of several days to weeks. Because only the free hormone has the ability to enter the cell and because T_3 is bound less avidly to transerythrin than is T_4, more T_3 gains entry into the cytoplasm than does T_4. Once in the target cell, both T_3 and T_4 bind to **nuclear thyroid hormone receptor proteins**, but T_3 binds with a much greater affinity than does T_4, which also accounts for the greater biological activity of T_3. The bound T_3 and T_4 enter the nucleus, where they stimulate transcription of many genes that encode various types of proteins (see Table 13.3), resulting in a generalized increase in cellular metabolism that may be as great as twice the resting rate. T_3 and T_4 also increase the growth rate in the young, facilitate mental processes, and stimulate endocrine gland activity.

Generally, thyroid hormones stimulate carbohydrate metabolism. They decrease synthesis of cholesterol, phospholipids, and triglycerides but increase synthesis of fatty acids and the uptake of various vitamins. Increased thyroid hormone production also decreases body weight and increases heart rate, metabolism, respiration, muscle function, and appetite. Excessive amounts of thyroid hormone cause muscle tremor, tiredness, impotence in men, and reduced or absence of menstrual bleeding in women.

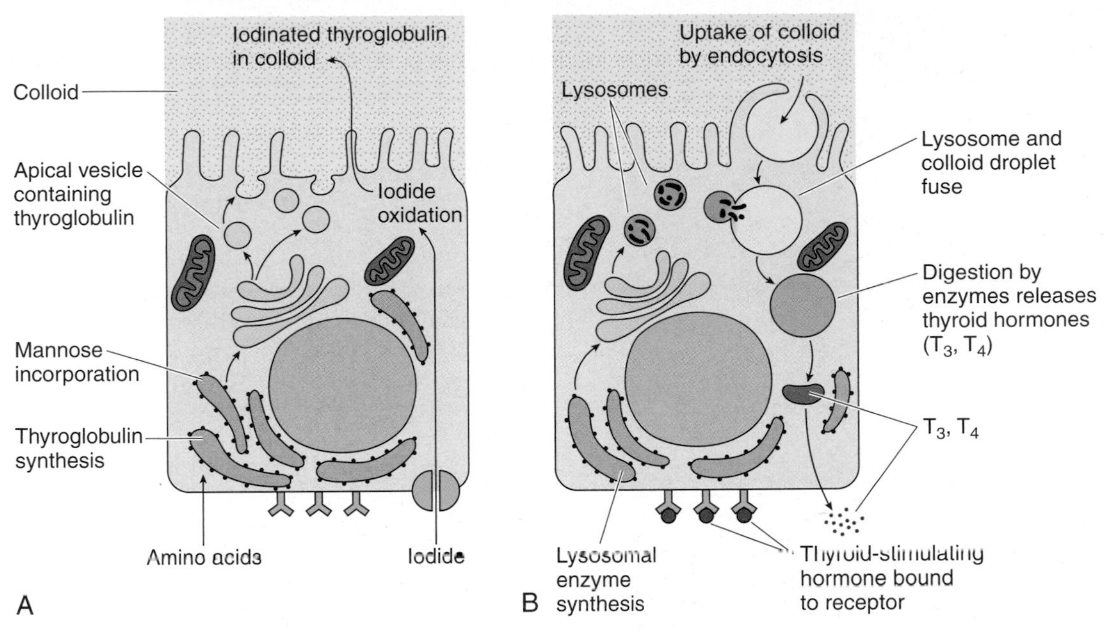

Fig. 13.15 Schematic diagram of the synthesis and iodination of thyroglobulin (A) and release of thyroid hormone (B).

Clinical Correlations

Individuals possessing a mutated form of the monocarboxylate transporter 8 (MTC8) have an X-linked hereditary condition known as the **Allen-Herndon-Dudley syndrome**. *This rare condition, affecting almost exclusively males, is distinguished by high T_3 serum levels and a number of developmentally caused neurological conditions, including severe intellectual disability, spastic movement, weak muscle tone, joint malformations, and speech impairment.*

Parafollicular Cells (Clear Cells, C Cells)

Parafollicular cells secrete calcitonin; they are found individually or may form small clusters of cells at the periphery of the follicle.

The pale-staining **parafollicular cells** (**clear cells; C cells**), considered to be part of the DNES, are derived from neural crest cells that migrate to the right and left 5th pharyngeal pouches and from there continue on to enter the developing thyroid gland. They lie singly or in clusters among the follicular cells, but they do not reach the lumen of the follicle (see Fig. 13.13). Although parafollicular cells are two to three times larger than follicular cells, they account for only about 0.1% of the follicular epithelium. Electron micrographs display a round to oval nucleus; moderate RER; elongated mitochondria; a well-developed Golgi complex; and small, dense secretory granules (0.1–0.4 µm in diameter) located in the basal cytoplasm. These secretory granules contain **calcitonin** (**thyrocalcitonin**), a peptide hormone that inhibits bone resorption by osteoclasts, thereby lowering calcium concentrations in blood. When the circulating level of calcium is high, release of calcitonin is stimulated (see Chapter 7).

Parathyroid Glands

The absence of parathyroid glands is incompatible with life because parathyroid hormone (PTH) regulates blood calcium levels.

The **parathyroid glands**, usually four in number, are located on the posterior surface on both poles (superior and inferior) of the right and left lobes of the thyroid gland. Each gland is enveloped in its own thin, collagenous connective tissue capsule (see Fig. 13.11).

Because of their embryological origin (the third and fourth pharyngeal pouches) and descent in the neck with the primordium of the thymus and thyroid tissues, the parathyroid glands may be located anywhere along that pathway; there may also be supernumerary parathyroid glands. Once they reach their final location, the glands grow slowly, reaching adult size at about 20 years of age. The glands function in producing **PTH** (**parathormone**), which acts on bone, kidneys, and intestines to increase blood calcium levels.

PARATHYROID CELLULAR ORGANIZATION

The parenchyma of the parathyroid glands consists of two cell types: chief cells and oxyphil cells.

Each parathyroid gland is a small, ovoid structure about 5 mm in length, 4 mm wide, and 2 mm in thickness and weighs about 25 to 50 mg. Extensions of the connective tissue capsule enter the gland as septa, accompanied by blood vessels, lymphatics, and nerves. The septa serve mainly to support the parenchyma, as well as a rich capillary network for the parenchymal cells that are arranged in cords or clusters. The connective tissue stroma in older adults often contains adipose cells that may occupy up to 60% of the gland. The parenchyma of the parathyroid glands is composed of two cell types: **chief cells** and **oxyphil cells** (Figs. 13.12 and 13.16).

Chief Cells

Chief cells synthesize parathyroid hormone (PTH).

The major functional parenchymal cells of the parathyroid glands are the slightly eosinophilic-staining **chief cells** (5–8 µm in diameter), which contain granules of lipofuscin

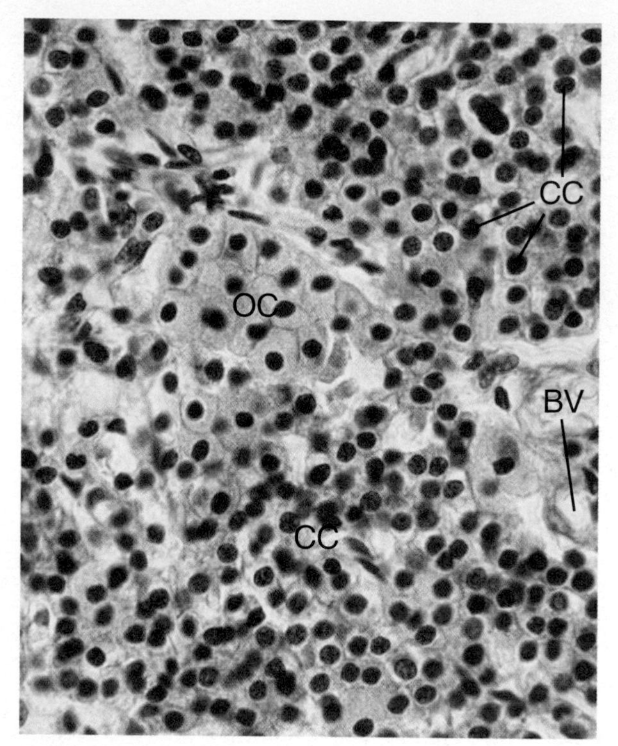

Fig. 13.16 High-magnification light micrograph of the parathyroid gland, displaying its rich vascular supply (BV) as well as its small, densely packed chief cells (CC) and its much larger and lighter-staining oxyphil cells (OC). (×540)

pigment that is scattered throughout the cytoplasm. Smaller, dense granules, 200 to 400 nm in diameter, arising from the Golgi complex and moving to the cell periphery, represent the secretory granules and contain **PTH**. Electron micrographs also reveal a juxtanuclear Golgi complex, elongated mitochondria, and abundant RER. Occasionally, desmosomes join adjacent chief cells to each other. A single primary cilium may extend into the extracellular space. Some chief cells have a smaller Golgi complex, scant secretory granules, and large amounts of glycogen; these cells are thought to be in an inactive phase.

Chief cells manufacture, store, and rapidly release PTH in response to alterations of blood calcium levels. If necessary, these cells can enter the cell cycle and increase their population. These properties of chief cells ensure that the parathyroid gland can respond to immediate, intermediate, and long-term adjustments to blood calcium level alterations and calcium homeostasis.

The precursor, **preproparathyroid hormone**, synthesized by chief cells on ribosomes of the RER, is rapidly cleaved as it is transported into the RER cisterna to form **proparathyroid hormone** and a polypeptide. On reaching the Golgi complex, proparathyroid hormone is cleaved again into PTH and another small polypeptide. The hormone is packaged into secretory granules at the *trans*-Golgi network and is released from the cell surface by exocytosis. The release of PTH is dependent on the cell membrane–bound calcium-sensing receptor, known as ***transmembrane calcium receptor*** (***CaSR***), which is associated with a G protein. If CaSR has calcium bound to it, indicating that the blood calcium level is adequate, CaSR compels the G protein to inhibit PTH release. However, if calcium is not bound to CaSR, indicating inadequate blood calcium levels, G protein becomes activated, and PTH is released by the chief cells (see Table 13.3).

Oxyphil Cells

Oxyphil cells are believed to be the inactive phase of chief cells.

The second cell type located in the parathyroid glands is the **oxyphil cell**. Its function is unknown, although some authors believe that oxyphil cells and a third cell, described as an **intermediate cell**, probably represent inactive phases of a single cell type, with chief cells being the actively secreting phase.

Oxyphil cells are less numerous, larger (6–10 μm in diameter), and more deeply stained with eosin than chief cells; they appear in groups and as isolated cells. They have more abundant mitochondria than do chief cells, but their Golgi apparatus is small and there is little RER. Glycogen is also located in the cytosol and is surrounded by mitochondria.

PHYSIOLOGICAL EFFECT OF PARATHYROID HORMONE

PTH helps maintain the proper extracellular fluid as well as the plasma concentration of calcium ions (8.5–10.5 mg/dL). This hormone acts on cells of the bones, kidneys, and, indirectly, the intestines, leading to an *increase* in serum **calcium ion concentration** and a *decrease* in **serum phosphate concentration** (see Table 13.3). When calcium ion concentration in body fluids falls below normal, the chief cells increase their production and release of PTH, quickly increasing their normal secretion rate as much as 10-fold. This rapid response is especially important because of the many functions of calcium in homeostasis, including its role in stabilizing ion gradients across the plasmalemmae of muscle and nerve cells and its role in the release of neurotransmitter at axon terminals.

The interplay of PTH and calcitonin represents a dual mechanism for regulating calcium levels in the blood: PTH acts to increase serum calcium levels, and calcitonin has the opposite effect.

In bone, PTH binds to receptors on osteoblasts, signaling the cells to increase their secretion of **osteoclast-stimulating factor**. This factor induces activation of osteoclasts, thereby increasing bone resorption and the ultimate release of calcium ions into the blood (see Chapter 7). In the kidneys, PTH (1) prevents loss of calcium in the urine by inducing the distal tubules to reabsorb it from the ultrafiltrate; (2) prompts the kidney proximal tubule cells to manufacture and release **calcitriol** (the physiologically active form of **vitamin D**); and (3) inhibits the proximal tubule cells from reabsorbing phosphate, thereby reducing serum phosphate concentration. In the gastrointestinal tract, PTH controls the rate of calcium uptake because vitamin D is necessary for intestinal uptake of calcium. Vitamin D functions to stimulate the intestinal mucosa to reabsorb calcium by inducing epithelial cells of the intestinal villus to form calcium-binding protein that becomes localized on the microvilli that facilitates the transport of calcium into the epithelial cells.

Clinical Correlations

1. *A condition called* **primary hyperparathyroidism***, which may be caused by a tumor in one of the parathyroid glands, is marked by high blood calcium levels, low blood phosphate levels, loss of bone mineral, and, sometimes, kidney stones.* ***Secondary hyperparathyroidism*** *may develop in patients with* **rickets***, because calcium cannot be absorbed from the intestines, owing to vitamin D deficiency; therefore, calcium ion concentrations in the blood are low.*
2. **Hypoparathyroidism** *results from deficiency in secretion of PTH, commonly caused by injury of the parathyroid glands or by their removal during thyroid gland surgery. This condition is marked by low blood calcium levels, retention of bone calcium, and increased phosphate resorption in the kidney. The main symptoms are numbness, tingling,* **carpopedal spasms** *(muscle cramps) in the hands and feet,* **muscle tetany** *(tremors) in the facial and laryngeal muscles, mental confusion, and memory loss. The only treatment for survival is large intravenous doses of calcium gluconate, vitamin D, and oral calcium.*
3. *Care must be taken during* **thyroidectomy** *to save the parathyroid glands and to maintain their blood supply because absence of the parathyroid glands is incompatible with life.*

Suprarenal (Adrenal) Glands

Suprarenal glands produce two different groups of hormones: steroids and catecholamines.

The **suprarenal (adrenal) glands** are located at the superior poles of the kidneys and are embedded in adipose tissue. The right and left suprarenal glands are not mirror images of each other; rather, the right suprarenal gland is pyramid shaped and sits directly on top of the right kidney, and the left suprarenal gland is more crescent shaped and lies along the medial border of the left kidney from the hilum to its superior pole.

Both glands are about 1 cm thick, 2 cm in width at the apex, and up to 5 cm at the base; each weighs 7 to 10 g. The parenchyma of the gland is divided into two histologically and functionally different regions: an outer yellowish portion, accounting for about 80% to 90% of the organ, called the ***suprarenal cortex***; and a small, dark, inner portion called the ***suprarenal medulla*** (Fig. 13.17). Although both regions have endocrine function, each develops from a different embryological origin and performs a different role. The **suprarenal cortex**, arising from mesoderm, produces a group of hormones called ***corticosteroids***, which are synthesized from **cholesterol**. Secretion of these hormones, including **cortisol** and **corticosterone**, is regulated by **ACTH**, a hormone secreted by the anterior pituitary gland. The **suprarenal medulla**, arising from the neural crest, is functionally related to and regulated by the sympathetic nervous system; it produces the hormones **epinephrine** and **norepinephrine** (see Table 13.3).

The suprarenal glands are retroperitoneal (located behind the peritoneum). They are surrounded by a connective tissue capsule that sends septa, accompanied by blood vessels and nerves, into the parenchyma of the gland. The capsule contains large amounts of adipose tissue.

BLOOD SUPPLY TO THE SUPRARENAL GLAND

Arteries from three separate sources provide the suprarenal glands with an abundant blood supply.

The suprarenal glands have one of the richest blood supplies in the body (Fig. 13.18) in that each gland is served by three separate arteries, the **superior**, **middle**, and **inferior suprarenal arteries**, each of which arises from a different source.

These arteries penetrate the capsule and form a **subcapsular plexus**. Arising from the plexus are **short cortical arteries**, which, in the cortical parenchyma, form a network of sinusoidal fenestrated capillaries (with diaphragms). The pore diameters of the fenestrated endothelial walls of the capillaries increase from 100 nm at the outer cortex to 250 nm in the deep cortex, where the sinusoidal capillaries become confluent with a venous plexus. Small venules arising from this area pass through the suprarenal medulla and drain into a suprarenal vein, emerging from the hilum. The right suprarenal vein joins the inferior vena cava, and the left suprarenal vein drains into the left renal vein.

Additional **long cortical arteries** pass unbranched through the cortex and into the medulla, where they form networks of capillaries. *Thus, the medulla receives a dual blood supply: (1) an arterial supply from the long cortical arteries and (2) numerous vessels from the cortical capillary beds.*

SUPRARENAL CORTEX

The suprarenal cortex is subdivided into three zones that produce three classes of steroid hormones.

The **suprarenal cortex** is subdivided histologically into three concentric zones named, from the capsule inward, the **zona glomerulosa**, **zona fasciculata**, and **zona reticularis** (Figs. 13.19 to 13.21; see Fig. 13.17), whose parenchymal cells secrete several **steroid hormones**. Each of the three identified zones of the suprarenal cortex is said to secrete specific hormones without storing them. The boundaries between these zones overlap; thus, it is better to remember the cortex as a secreting unit for the three classes of adrenocortical hormones (of course, the student's instructor may deem otherwise, in which case it is in the student's best interest to follow the instructor's point of view).

The three classes of adrenocortical hormones–**mineralocorticoids**, **glucocorticoids**, and **androgens**—are all synthesized from **cholesterol**, the major component of **low-density lipoprotein**. Cholesterol is taken up from the blood and stored esterified in lipid droplets within the cytoplasm of the cortical cells. When these cells are stimulated, cholesterol is freed and used in hormone synthesis in the **smooth endoplasmic reticulum (SER)** by enzymes that are located there and in the mitochondria. Cholesterol and the intermediate products of the hormone that is being synthesized are transferred between the SER and the mitochondria until the final hormone is produced. Therefore, the synthesis of these hormones is a function of the ability of cholesterol and the intermediate products to enter the mitochondria, a process regulated by **steroidogenic acute regulatory protein**.

Zona Glomerulosa

Parenchymal cells of the zona glomerulosa, when stimulated by angiotensin II and ACTH, synthesize and release the hormones aldosterone and deoxycorticosterone.

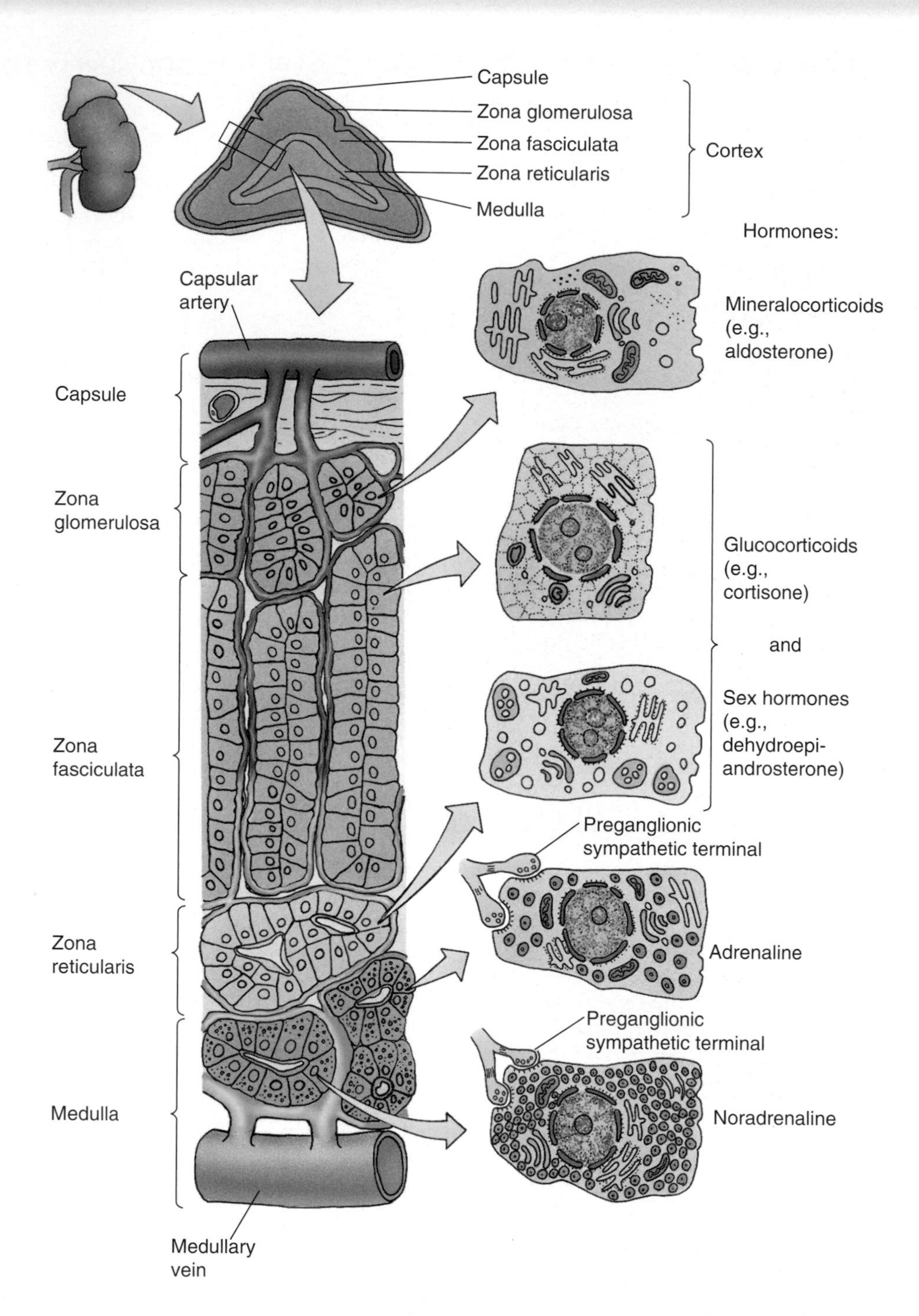

Fig. 13.17 Schematic diagram of the suprarenal gland and its cell types.

The outer concentric ring of parenchymal cells, located just beneath the suprarenal capsule, is the **zona glomerulosa**, which constitutes approximately 13% of the total adrenal volume (see Fig. 13.17). The small columnar cells composing this zone are arranged in cords and clusters. Their small, dark-staining nuclei contain one or two nucleoli, and their acidophilic cytoplasm contains an abundant and extensive SER, short **mitochondria** with **shelf-like cristae**, a well-developed Golgi complex, abundant RER, and free ribosomes. Some lipid droplets also are dispersed in the cytoplasm. Occasional desmosomes and small gap junctions join cells to each other, and some cells have short microvilli.

The parenchymal cells of the zona glomerulosa synthesize and secrete **mineralocorticoid hormones**, principally **aldosterone** and some **deoxycorticosterone**. Synthesis of these hormones is stimulated by **angiotensin II** and **ACTH**, both required for normal existence of glomerulosa cells. The mineralocorticoid hormones function in controlling fluid and electrolyte balance in the body by affecting the function of the renal tubules, specifically the distal convoluted tubules (see Chapter 19).

Progenitor cells located at the interface of the zona glomerulosa and zona fasciculata sustain the cell population of the adrenal cortex by entering the cell cycle and producing more adrenocortical parenchymal cells.

Zona Fasciculata

Parenchymal cells of the zona fasciculata (spongiocytes), when stimulated by ACTH, synthesize and release the hormones cortisol and corticosterone.

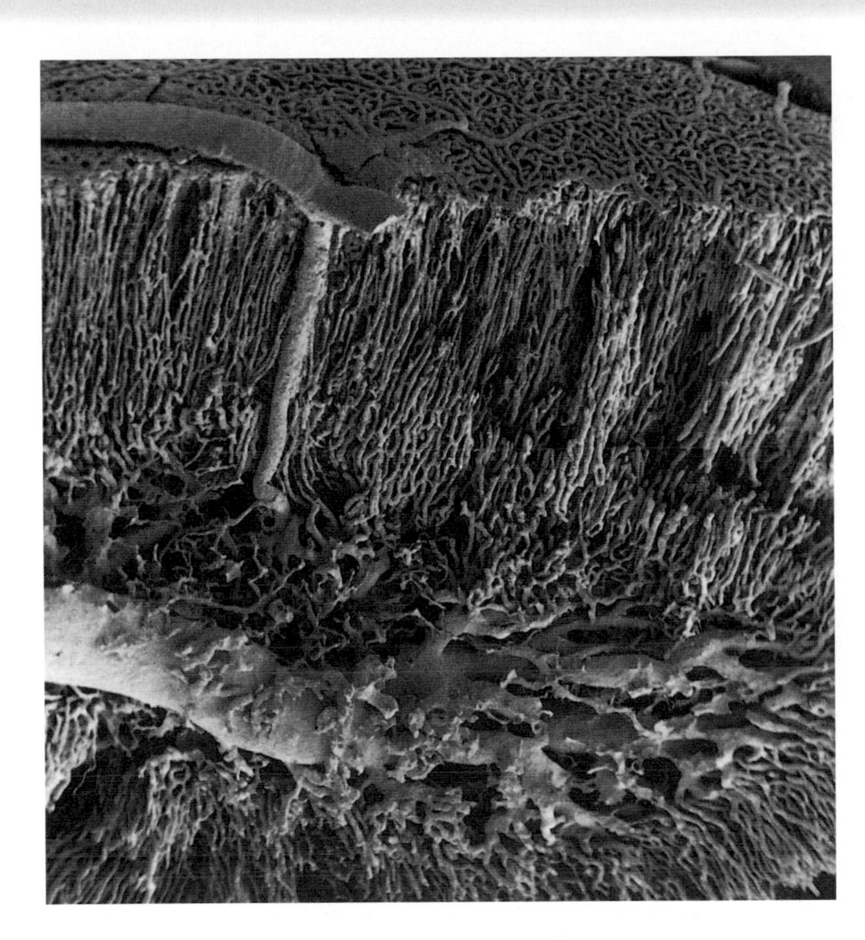

Fig. 13.18 Scanning electron micrograph of the rat adrenal gland demonstrating microcirculation in the cortex and medulla (×80). (From Kikuta A, Murakami T. Microcirculation of the rat adrenal gland: a scanning electron microscope study of vascular casts. *Am J Anat*. 1982;164:19-28. Reprinted with permission from Wiley-Liss, Inc., a subsidiary of John Wiley & Sons, Inc.)

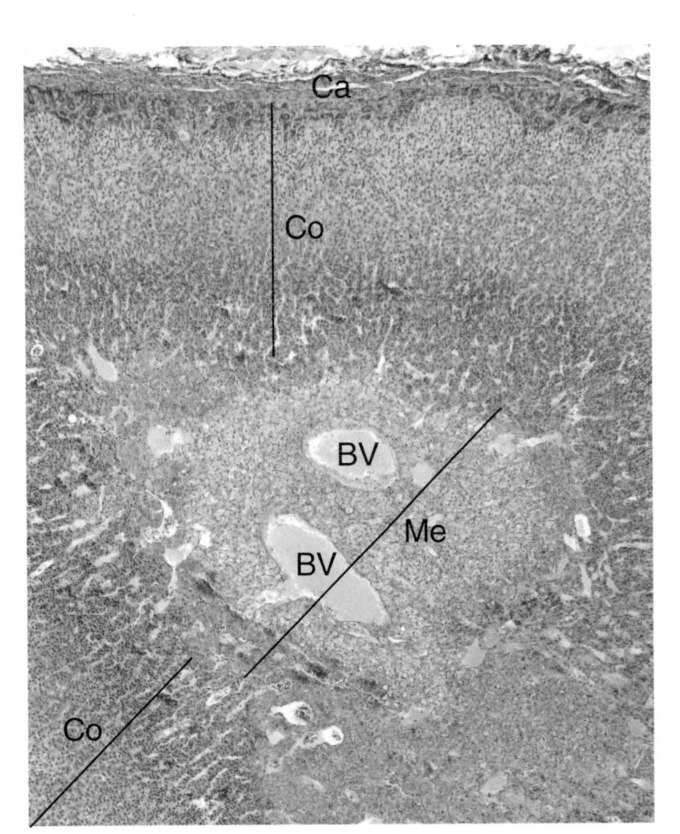

Fig. 13.19 Low magnification of the suprarenal gland displaying its dense irregular collagenous capsule (Ca), the cortex (Co) that envelopes the medulla (Me), and the blood vessels of the medulla (BV). (×56)

The intermediate concentric layer of cells in the suprarenal cortex is the **zona fasciculata**, the largest layer of the cortex, which accounts for up to 70% of the total volume of the gland. This zone houses sinusoidal capillaries that are arranged longitudinally between the columns of parenchymal cells. The polyhedral cells in this layer are larger than the cells of the zona glomerulosa and are arranged in radial columns, one to two layers thick, and stain lightly acidophilic. Because they have many lipid droplets in their cytoplasm, which are extracted during histological processing, these cells appear vacuolated and are called ***spongiocytes***. These cells have **spherical mitochondria** with **tubular** and **vesicular cristae**, extensive networks of SER, some RER, lysosomes, and granules of lipofuscin pigment.

When stimulated by ACTH, the cells of the zona fasciculata synthesize and secrete the **glucocorticoid hormones**, **cortisol** and **corticosterone**. Glucocorticoids function in the control of carbohydrate, fat, and protein metabolism.

Zona Reticularis

The cells of the zona reticularis, when stimulated by ACTH, synthesize and release dehydroepiandrosterone, androstenedione, and some glucocorticoids.

The innermost layer of the suprarenal cortex is the **zona reticularis**, constituting about 7% of gland volume. The darkly staining acidophilic cells in this layer are arranged in anastomosing cords. They are similar to the spongiocytes of the zona fasciculata but are smaller, with fewer lipid droplets. They frequently contain large amounts of lipofuscin pigment granules. Several cells near the suprarenal medulla are dark, with electron-dense

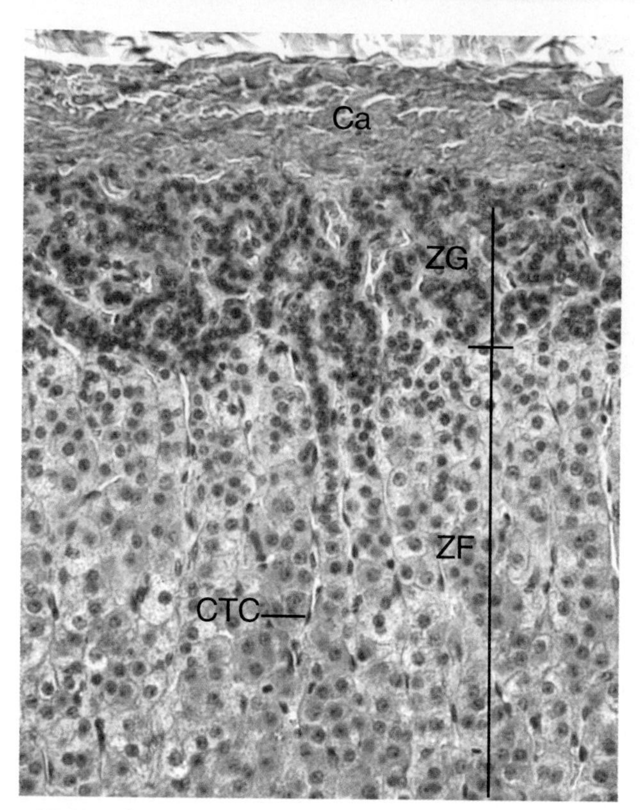

Fig. 13.20 This medium-power magnification of the suprarenal gland cortex displays its capsule (Ca) and zona glomerulosa (ZG), along with the outer portion of the zona fasciculata (ZF) with its slender amount of connective tissue and occasional connective tissue cell (CTC). (×270)

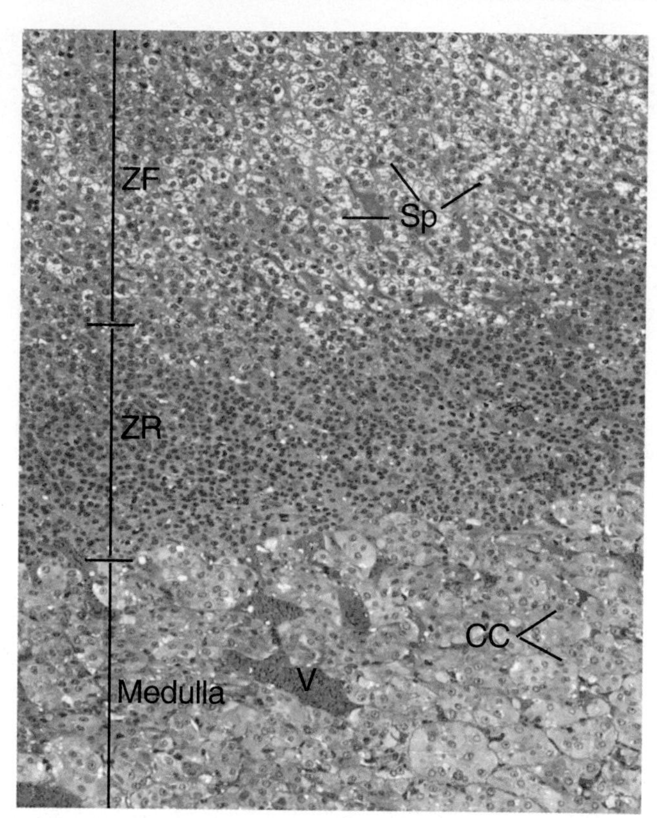

Fig. 13.21 This low-magnification photomicrograph displays the inner layers of the suprarenal cortex. Note that in the inner portion of the zona fasciculata (ZF), the parenchymal cells are referred to as spongiocytes (Sp) because of the empty spaces left after the histological preparation extracted the lipids. The innermost region of the cortex is occupied by the zona reticularis (ZR) that abuts the suprarenal medulla, whose chromaffin cells (CC) and sympathetic ganglion cells (not shown) are provided by a rich vascular supply (V). (×132)

cytoplasm and pyknotic nuclei, which suggests that this zone contains degenerating parenchymal cells.

Cells of the zona reticularis synthesize and secrete **androgens**, principally **dehydroepiandrosterone (DHEA)** and some **androstenedione**. Additionally, cells of the zona reticularis may synthesize and secrete small amounts of glucocorticoids. The secretion of these hormones is stimulated by ACTH. Both DHEA and androstenedione are weak, masculinizing hormones with negligible effects under normal conditions.

HISTOPHYSIOLOGY OF THE SUPRARENAL CORTEX

The three classes of steroid hormones that are secreted by the suprarenal cortex are (1) mineralocorticoids, (2) glucocorticoids, and (3) weak androgens. ACTH stimulates secretion of the suprarenal cortex hormones along with angiotensin II for the secretion of mineralocorticoids.

Mineralocorticoids

The **mineralocorticoids**, secreted by the zona glomerulosa, include **aldosterone** predominantly and some deoxycorticosterone. The targets of these hormones include the gastric mucosa, salivary glands, and sweat glands, where they stimulate absorption of sodium. However, the main target is the cells of the distal convoluted tubules of the kidney, where they function to stimulate the regulation of water balance and homeostasis of sodium and potassium by absorbing sodium and excreting potassium, a function regulated mostly by angiotensin II (see Chapter 19).

Glucocorticoids

Glucocorticoids, secreted by the zona fasciculata, include **hydrocortisone (cortisol)** and **corticosterone**. These steroid hormones have a wide range of functions that affect most tissues of the body and also control general metabolism. They exert an **anabolic** effect in the liver that promotes the uptake of fatty acids, amino acids, and carbohydrates for glucose synthesis and glycogen polymerization; in other tissues, however, the effect is **catabolic**. For example, in adipocytes, glucocorticoids stimulate **lipolysis**, and in muscle, these hormones stimulate **proteolysis**. Glucocorticoids, when circulating at above-normal levels, also influence anti-inflammatory responses by inhibiting macrophage and leukocyte infiltration at sites of inflammation. These hormones also suppress the immune response by inducing atrophy of the lymphatic system, thereby reducing the circulating lymphocyte population. Table 13.4 lists some of the deleterious effects of excess blood levels of glucocorticoids.

Clinical Correlations

*Glucocorticoids have an interesting relationship with the **circadian rhythm**. Individuals who sleep during the day have their highest cortisol levels in the evening and lowest in the morning, whereas those who sleep at night have the reverse condition, namely, the highest levels in the morning and lowest levels at night.*

TABLE 13.4 Deleterious Effects of Excess Blood Glucocorticoid Levels

Body/System/Organ/ Tissue/Activity	Effect
Brain	Psychosis and depression
Immune system	Suppression of immune system; anti-inflammatory response
Stature	Decrease in height
Endocrine system	Depressed levels of luteinizing hormone, follicle-stimulating hormone, growth hormone, and thyroid-stimulating hormone
Gastrointestinal tract	Formation of peptic ulcers
Adipose tissue	Induces fat deposition in the viscera.
Eye	Induces glaucoma.
Calcium metabolism	Decreases bone formation and bone mass.
Skin and muscle	Induces collagen proteolysis in skin; induces muscle atrophy.
Cardiovascular	Hypertension
Kidney	Induces salt and water preservation.
Carbohydrate metabolism	Increases gluconeogenesis in the liver; increases peripheral insulin resistance, thereby promoting diabetes.

The **negative feedback** mechanism for the glucocorticoids is partially controlled by their plasma concentration. When blood glucocorticoid levels are high, **CRH** cells of the hypothalamus are inhibited, which, in turn, inhibits **corticotrophs** of the pars distalis of the pituitary gland from releasing ACTH.

Weak Androgens

Androgens secreted by the zona reticularis include **dehydroepiandrosterone** and **androstenedione**, both weak, masculinizing sex hormones that are only a small fraction as effective as the androgens that are produced in the testes. Under normal conditions, the influence of these hormones is insignificant in males, but could have a masculinizing effect in females.

Clinical Correlations

1. *Addison disease is characterized by decreased secretion of the adrenocortical hormones as a result of destruction of the suprarenal cortex. This disease is most often caused by an autoimmune process; it also can develop as a sequela of tuberculosis or from some other infectious diseases. Death occurs if steroid treatment is not provided.*
2. *Cushing disease (hyperadrenocorticism) is caused by small tumors in the basophils of the anterior pituitary gland that lead to an increase in the output of ACTH. The excess ACTH causes enlargement of the suprarenal glands and hypertrophy of the suprarenal cortex, resulting in overproduction of cortisol. Patients are obese, predominantly in the face, neck, and trunk, and exhibit osteoporosis and muscle wasting. Men become impotent, and women have amenorrhea.*
3. *Primary adrenal carcinoma, a very rare disease, affects more than twice as many women than men. Usually, the cancer arises in individuals at least 40 years of age, and the cancerous cells are hormone producing: about 45% synthesize only glucocorticoids, 45% form both glucocorticoids and androgens, and 10% release androgens only. Only approximately 1% of the cancerous cells release aldosterone. Unfortunately, by the time the cancer is recognized, metastasis has occurred. Even with surgery and subsequent chemotherapy, the 5-year mortality rate is 80%.*

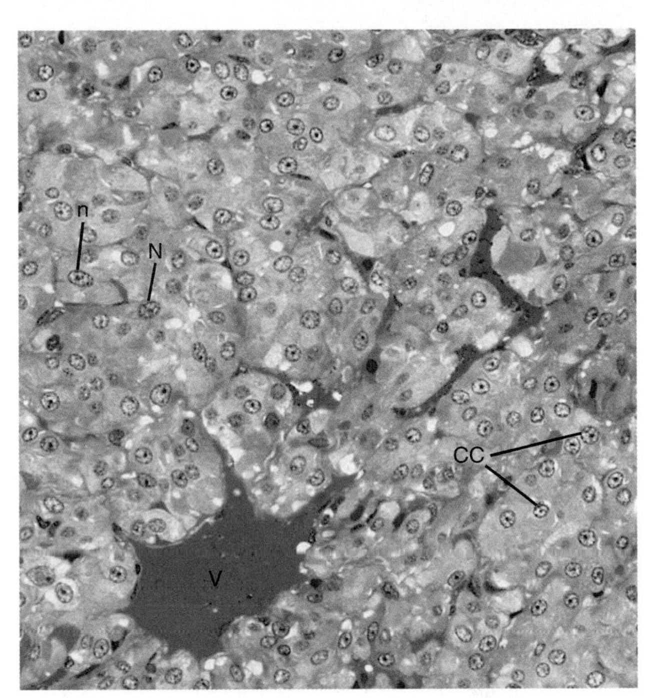

Fig. 13.22 Light micrograph of the medulla of the suprarenal gland. Note the chromaffin cells (CC) whose nucleus (N) houses a single nucleolus (n). Observe the rich arterial supply and venous drainage (V) of the suprarenal medulla (×270).

SUPRARENAL MEDULLA

Chromaffin cells of the suprarenal medulla are modified postganglionic neurons, without dendrites or axons, that have a secretory function.

The central portion of the suprarenal gland, the **suprarenal medulla**, is completely invested by the suprarenal cortex and forms only 10% of the volume of the suprarenal gland. The suprarenal medulla, which develops from ectodermal neural crest cells, comprises two populations of parenchymal cells: **chromaffin cells**, which produce the **catecholamines** (**epinephrine** and **norepinephrine**), and **sympathetic ganglion cells**, which are scattered throughout the connective tissue (see Table 13.3).

Chromaffin Cells

The suprarenal medulla functions as a modified sympathetic ganglion, housing postganglionic sympathetic cells, known as chromaffin cells, which lack dendrites and axons. The medulla also has a small number of sympathetic ganglion cells.

Chromaffin cells of the suprarenal medulla are large epithelioid cells arranged in clusters or short cords; they contain granules that stain intensely with chromaffin salts (see Figs. 13.19, 13.21, and 13.22). The reaction of the granules, which turn deep brown when exposed to chromaffin salts, indicates that the cells contain **catecholamines**, transmitters produced by postganglionic cells of the sympathetic nervous system. Thus, the suprarenal medulla functions as a modified sympathetic ganglion, housing postganglionic sympathetic cells that lack neurites (dendrites and axons). However, when grown in vitro, these cells sprout neurites; the addition of glucocorticoids to the culture medium inhibits neurite formation. The catecholamines synthesized by the chromaffin cells are the sympathetic transmitters **epinephrine (adrenaline)** and **norepinephrine (noradrenaline)**. Approximately 80% of the chromaffin cells produce epinephrine and 20% manufacture norepinephrine. These transmitters are secreted by the chromaffin cells in response to stimulation by **preganglionic sympathetic (cholinergic) splanchnic nerves** that synapse with these cells.

Chromaffin cells have a well-developed juxtanuclear Golgi complex, some RER, and numerous mitochondria. The identifying characteristic of the chromaffin cells is the 30,000 or so small, membrane-bound, dense granules in the cytoplasm; approximately 20% of these granules contain either epinephrine or norepinephrine (Fig. 13.23). The remaining granules are composed of **ATP**, **enkephalins**, and soluble proteins called **chromogranins**, which are believed to bind epinephrine and norepinephrine.

Clinical Correlations

*In some animals, but not in primates (or humans), two types of chromaffin cells have been identified via histochemical staining: those producing and storing **norepinephrine** and those producing and storing **epinephrine**. The granules of the norepinephrine-storing cells have an eccentric, electron-dense core within the limiting membrane of the granule, whereas the granules of chromaffin cells storing epinephrine are more homogeneous and less dense.*

HISTOPHYSIOLOGY OF THE SUPRARENAL MEDULLA

The secretory activity of the suprarenal medulla is controlled by the splanchnic nerves. Release of the aggregated **catecholamines** from **chromaffin cells** is induced by stimulation of the sympathetic ganglion cells in the suprarenal medulla. Release of **acetylcholine** from these preganglionic sympathetic nerve endings depolarizes the chromaffin cell membranes, leading to an influx of calcium ions. The rise in intracellular calcium then induces release of **epinephrine** or **norepinephrine** via exocytosis.

When the stimulus is derived from an emotional source, secretion of norepinephrine predominates; when the stimulus is physiological (e.g., pain), secretion of epinephrine predominates. Catecholamines released by the suprarenal medulla exhibit a more generalized overall effect than do the catecholamines released by sympathetic neurons. However, these effects are not uniform for all tissues. For example, they increase oxygen consumption, increase heat production, and mobilize fat for energy; in the cardiovascular system, they function in controlling the heart rate and the arterial smooth muscles, thus increasing blood pressure. Additionally, catecholamines regulate muscle contractions in some tissues (e.g., bladder sphincters); in other organs, they influence muscle relaxation (e.g., intestinal smooth muscle).

In severe fear or stress, increased epinephrine is released to prepare the body for "fight, flight, or freeze." The resulting plasma levels of epinephrine, up to 300 times the normal level, increase alertness, cardiac output, and heart rate, as well as increase the release of glucose from the liver.

Epinephrine is most effective in controlling cardiac output and heart rate and increasing blood flow through organs. Norepinephrine has little effect on these functions but brings about an elevation in blood pressure by vasoconstriction.

Norepinephrine is also produced in the brain and peripheral nerves, functioning as a neurotransmitter. However, norepinephrine produced in the suprarenal medulla has a short half-life because it is destroyed in the liver shortly after its release.

Clinical Correlations

*The most common tumor of the suprarenal medulla is **pheochromocytoma**, which may involve the chromaffin cells of one or both suprarenal glands. However, occasionally, the tumor resides in paraganglia located in various regions of the body, such as the posterior abdominal wall, heart, neck, and urinary bladder (in those cases, the condition is referred to as a paraganglioma). Pheochromocytoma is nonmalignant in 90% of the cases; if malignant, the tumor can metastasize to the liver, lungs, lymph nodes, and bones. Most commonly, the disease affects people between 20 and 50 years of age; the principal symptom is fluctuating or persistent high blood pressure that is resistant to being controlled. Other symptoms include tachycardia (rapid heartbeat), dyspnea (shortness of breath), pallor, headache, and profuse sweating. These symptoms may occur suddenly or may be triggered by strenuous exercise, nervous tension, and even certain foods containing large amounts of tyramine, such as chocolate, cheese, smoked meat, and fermented beverages. Diagnostic tests include urine and blood tests to look for elevated adrenaline and noradrenaline levels and imaging studies to search for tumors of the suprarenal glands (or sites of possible metastases). The key treatment protocol, subsequent to stabilization of the patient's blood pressure, is surgery to excise the suprarenal gland with the tumor. If both glands are involved, only the tumor is removed. If the tumor is malignant, then the surgical procedure is usually followed by chemotherapy and/or radiotherapy.*

Pineal Gland

The pineal gland, one of the circumventricular organs, is responsive to diurnal light and dark periods and is thought to influence gonadal activity.

The **pineal gland** (or **pineal body**), one of the circumventricular organs, is an endocrine gland whose secretions are influenced by the light and dark periods of the day. It is a cone-shaped, midline projection from the roof of the diencephalon, within a recess of the third ventricle extending into the stalk that is attached to it. It is 5 to 8 mm long and 3 to 5 mm wide; it weighs approximately 120 mg. The gland is covered by the pia mater, forming a capsule from which septa extend dividing the pineal gland into incomplete lobules. Blood vessels enter the gland via the connective tissue septa. The parenchymal cells of the gland are composed primarily of **pinealocytes** and **interstitial cells** (Figs. 13.24 and 13.25) The pineal gland produces **melatonin**, the hormone that controls the various circadian rhythms of the individual.

PINEALOCYTES

Pinealocytes are the parenchymal cells of the pineal gland that are responsible for secreting melatonin.

Pinealocytes constitute approximately 95% of the cell population of the pineal gland. These are slightly basophilic cells with one or two long processes whose terminal dilatations approximate capillaries and, occasionally, other parenchymal cells.

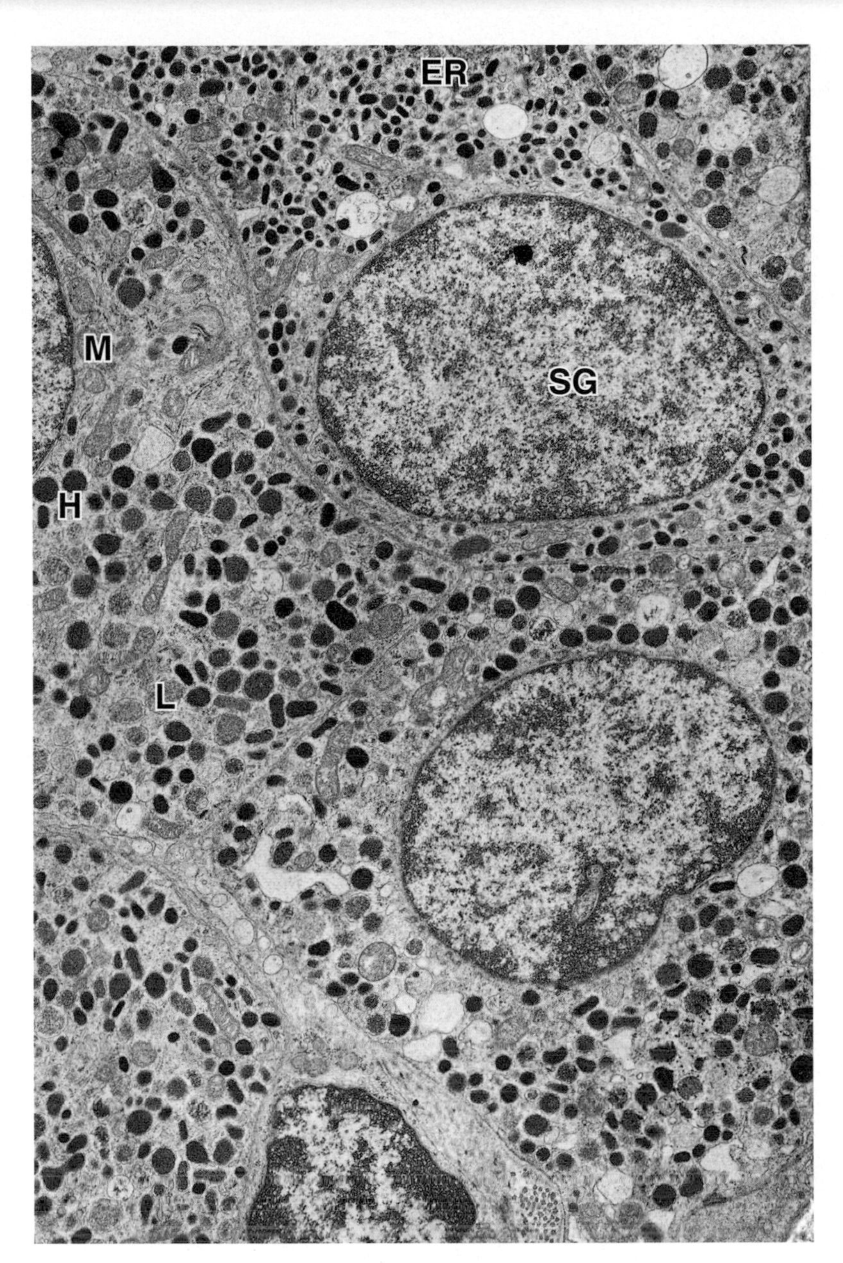

Fig. 13.23 Electron micrograph of baboon adrenal medulla (×14,000). The different osmiophilic densities of the vesicles may be a reflection of their maturational phases. ER, Endoplasmic reticulum; H, high-electron-density vesicle; L, low-electron-density vesicle; M, mitochondrion; SG, small granule cell. (From Al-Lami F, Carmichael SW. Microscopic anatomy of the baboon *[Papio hamadryas]* adrenal medulla. *J Anat.* 1991;178:213-221. Reprinted with permission from Cambridge University Press.)

Their spherical nuclei have a single prominent nucleolus. The cytoplasm contains SER and RER; a small Golgi apparatus; numerous mitochondria; and small secretory vesicles, some with electron-dense cores. Pinealocytes also contain a well-developed cytoskeleton composed of microtubules, microfilaments, and dense tubular structures invested by spherical vesicular elements. These unusual structures, known as ***synaptic ribbons*** (also observed in the retina and inner ear), increase in number during the dark period of the diurnal cycle, but the function of these synaptic ribbons is not understood.

The hormone **melatonin** is synthesized from tryptophan, through the serotonin pathway catalyzed by the rate-limiting enzyme **arylalkylamine *N*-acetyltransferase (AANAT)**, by pinealocytes and is released almost exclusively at night. Melatonin is not stored in pinealocytes but rather is released almost immediately after being synthesized. This hormone inhibits the release of growth hormone and gonadotropin by the hypophysis and hypothalamus, respectively. It should be noted that melatonin is not synthesized or released during daylight because the action of the enzyme AANAT is inhibited during the day.

Clinical Correlations

1. ***Melatonin** induces the feeling of sleepiness; therefore, some individuals use it as a supplement to combat sleep disorders, mood disorders, and depression, as well as to overcome the effects of jet lag.*
2. *It has been suggested that **melatonin** may act to protect the central nervous system by its ability to scavenge and eliminate free radicals that are produced during oxidative stress. Additional suggestions include that melatonin may alter human moods, causing depression during shortened daylight hours of winter months. It has been reported that exposure to bright artificial light may reduce the secretion of melatonin and may result in alleviation of depression.*
3. *There is some evidence that melatonin can reduce the incidence of heartburn because it facilitates a stronger contraction of the lower esophageal sphincter, thereby preventing the reflux of gastric content into the esophagus.*

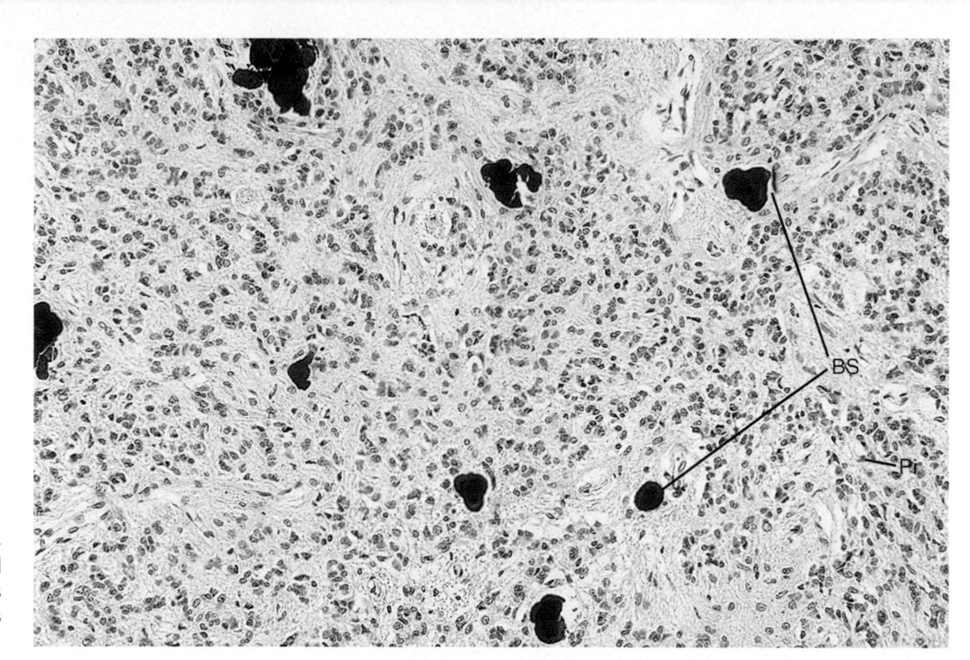

Fig. 13.24 Pineal gland. The large, dark-staining structures are brain sand (BS) scattered among the pinealocytes (Pi). Neuroglial cells are present but difficult to distinguish at this magnification. (×132)

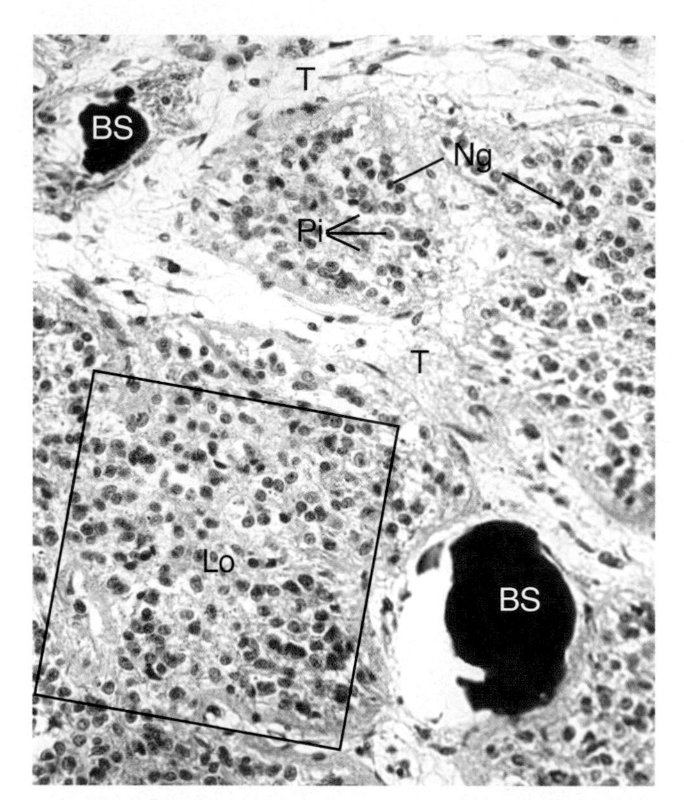

Fig. 13.25 A medium magnification of the pineal gland displays the connective tissue trabeculae (T) that subdivide the gland into lobules (Lo) and convey vascular and nerve supply to the pinealocytes (Pi). Note that the nuclei of the neuroglia (Ng) are smaller and darker than those of the pinealocytes. Observe the presence of brain sand (BS) in the substance of the gland. (×270)

INTERSTITIAL CELLS

Interstitial cells of the pineal gland are believed to be astrocyte-like neuroglia.

Interstitial cells, believed to be astrocyte-like neuroglia cells, are scattered throughout the pineal gland and are particularly abundant in the pineal stalk that leads to the diencephalon. These cells constitute approximately 5% of the cell population of the pineal gland. They have deeply staining, elongated nuclei and well-developed RER; some have deposits of glycogen. Their long cellular processes are rich in intermediate filaments, microtubules, and microfilaments.

CORPORA ARENACEA ("BRAIN SAND")

The pineal gland also contains concretions of calcium phosphates and carbonates, which are deposited in concentric rings around an organic matrix. These structures, called ***corpora arenacea*** (***"brain sand"***), appear in early childhood and increase in size throughout life. Although it is unclear how they are formed or function, they increase during short photoperiods and are reduced as the pineal gland is actively secreting.

HISTOPHYSIOLOGY OF THE PINEAL GLAND

It has been known for a long time that the pineal gland controls the various circadian cycles, but its location so far removed from access to daylight has intrigued researchers. It was recently discovered that approximately 5% of the **ganglion cells of the retina** of higher vertebrates, even those totally blind, react to light and *indirectly* relay this information to the pineal gland. The axons of these specialized ganglion cells join the retinohypothalamic tract to synapse with neurons located in the **suprachiasmatic nucleus (SCN)** of the hypothalamus. The neurons located in the SCN indirectly reach the preganglionic sympathetic neurons of the intermediolateral cell column. Axons of these preganglionic neurons synapse with postganglionic sympathetic neurons in the cervical chain ganglia whose postganglionic axons reach the pineal gland and induce the pinealocytes to manufacture and release melatonin.

Melatonin regulates not only the daily circadian rhythms but also controls the **reproductive axis**, probably by inhibiting FSH release by somehow acting on the release of GnRH from the hypothalamus. The role of melatonin in human reproduction is not understood, but in animals with seasonal reproductive strategies, melatonin inhibits the reproductive cycle until the length of the gestational period coincides with the most favorable time for the birth of the newborn animal.

Pathological Considerations

See Figs. 13.26 through 13.28.

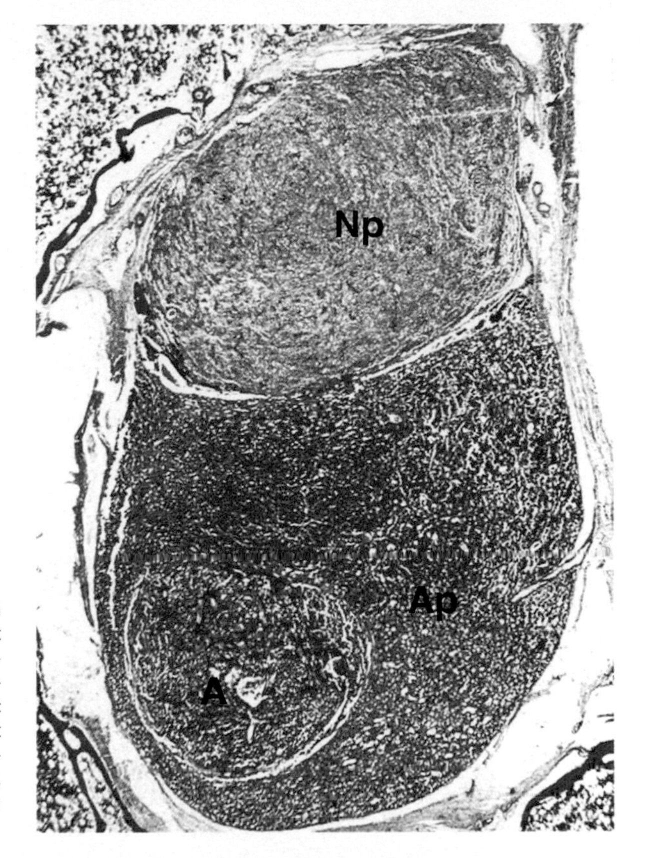

Fig. 13.26 This photomicrograph of the pituitary gland is from an individual with a benign tumor pituitary adenoma (A) present in the adenohypophysis (AP). The fact that the tumor is well defined and circumscribed by a connective tissue capsule indicates its nonmalignant nature. Unfortunately, the patient died shortly after the discovery of the tumor. The cells of the tumor produced so much adrenocorticotropic hormone that the patient developed a very aggressive form of Cushing disease that produced very strenuous metabolic and cardiac complications. (Reprinted with permission from Young B, Stewart W, O'Dowd G. *Wheater's Basic Pathology: A Text, Atlas and Review of Histopathology*. 5th ed. Oxford: Churchill Livingstone/Elsevier Limited; 2011:254.)

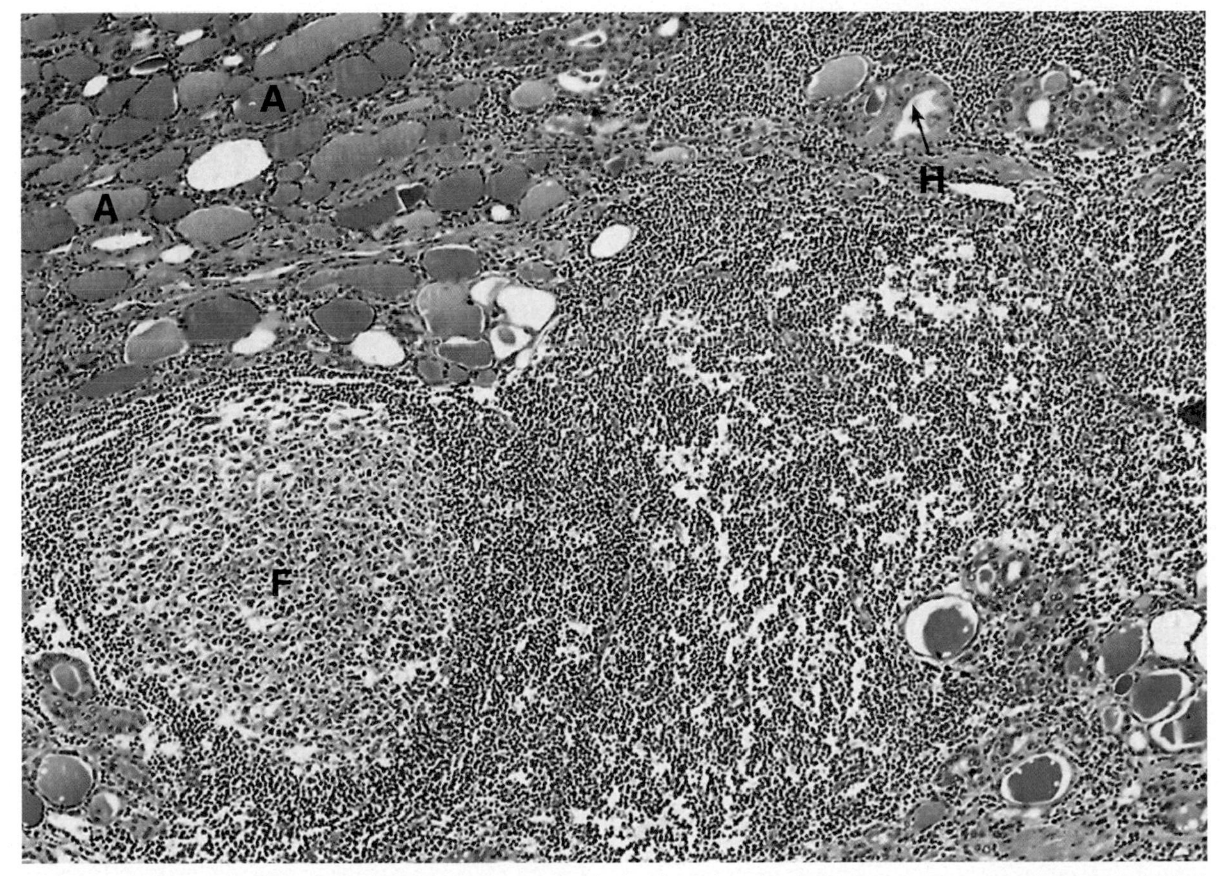

Fig. 13.27 This photomicrograph of the thyroid gland is from an individual with Hashimoto disease, an autoimmune disease in which the individual develops autoantibodies against one's own thyroid gland, destroying the thyroid follicles (A). The gland becomes infiltrated with lymphocytes, which even form lymphoid nodules (F). As the disease progresses, the follicular cells of the thyroid become transformed into Hurthle cells (H) that possess an eosinophilic granular cytoplasm but are not functional in the production of thyroid hormones. (Reprinted with permission from Young B, Stewart W, O'Dowd G. *Wheater's Basic Pathology: A Text, Atlas and Review of Histopathology*. 5th ed. Oxford: Churchill Livingstone/Elsevier Limited; 2011:256.)

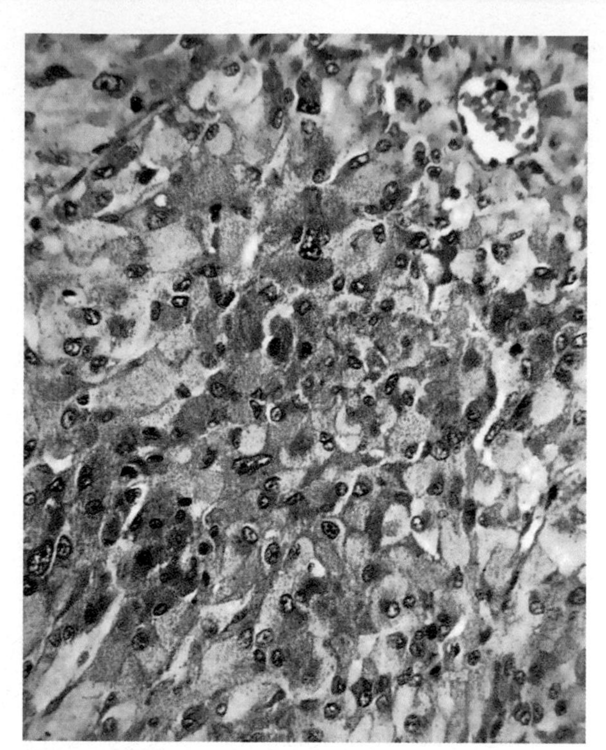

Fig. 13.28 This photomicrograph is from an individual presenting with pheochromocytoma, a tumor of the chromaffin cells of the suprarenal medulla. Although the tumor is benign, the patient may display symptoms that are caused by excess production of catecholamines, namely, heart palpitations, profuse sweating, and severe hypertensive disease that may lead to death. (Reprinted with permission from Young B, Stewart W, O'Dowd G. *Wheater's Basic Pathology: A Text, Atlas and Review of Histopathology*. 5th ed. Oxford: Churchill Livingstone/Elsevier Limited; 2011:263.)

Histology Laboratory Instructions: Endocrine System

Pituitary Gland

Before studying the histology of the pituitary gland, the student should review the regions of the pituitary gland that are usually examined in a histology laboratory: the adenohypophysis (anterior pituitary) and the neurohypophysis (posterior pituitary). The adenohypophysis has three regions: the pars anterior (pars distalis), pars intermedia, and pars tuberalis. The neurohypophysis also has three regions: the median eminence, infundibulum, and pars nervosa. Of these six regions, the student is usually expected to recognize the pars anterior and pars intermedia of the adenohypophysis and the pars nervosa of the neurohypophysis (of course, this is entirely dependent on the course director, whose opinion overrules this author's statement).

Viewing the pituitary gland at a very low magnification, the pars anterior is easy to recognize because of the vividly stained chromophils and the pars nervosa has a mostly uniform, grayish appearance. At the interface of the two is the very narrow pars intermedia that usually has colloid-filled cysts (Fig. 13.4, PA, PN, PI). At a low magnification of the three regions, the pars anterior displays a rich vascular supply, as does the pars nervosa, but the chromophils of the pars anterior provide a more vivid "landscape." The colloid-filled cysts of the pars intermedia make it relatively easy to identify (Fig. 13.5, PA, BV, PN, Cl, PI). Another low-magnification photomicrograph of the pars anterior demonstrates not only its numerous blood vessels but also the orange-red staining acidophils and the bluish staining basophils (Fig. 13.6, BV, A, B). A little higher magnification of the same region provides a better differentiation between the acidophils and basophils. Additionally, the chromophobes are also easy to see—their nuclei are clustered in a tight group because most of the hormones have been released by these cells; therefore, they have only a scant amount of cytoplasm. The vascular supply of the pars anterior is also evident (Fig. 13.7, A, B, Cr, BV). A high magnification of the pars anterior allows a clear differentiation between the acidophils and basophils. It also demonstrates how little cytoplasm remains in chromophobes (Fig. 13.8, A, B, C). Even a low-magnification photomicrograph permits an easy identification of the pars nervosa. Herring bodies are relatively easy to recognize, and most of the nuclei belong to the small pituicytes (Fig. 13.10, *arrows*, P).

Thyroid Gland

The thyroid gland is very easy to recognize even at a low magnification because of its large, colloid-filled follicles (whether seen under the student's microscope or with virtual microscopy). In some microscope slides, the thyroid and parathyroid glands are both present, and the contrast between the two also provides an excellent clue to recognizing the two glands (Fig. 13.12, TG, F, PG). At high magnifications, the follicular cell lining of the colloid can be recognized by their darker staining, smaller, oval nuclei in contrast to the parafollicular cell's larger, lighter staining oval nuclei. Note also that the follicular cells are in direct contact with the colloid, whereas the parafollicular cells are located farther from the colloid. The connective tissue of the thyroid gland displays the presence of blood vessels and fibroblasts (Fig. 13.13, FC, PFC, CT, BV, F).

Parathyroid Gland

The parathyroid gland is composed of small chief cells that bear a faint resemblance to lymphocytes that are crowded together. An additional cell type, the oxyphil cells, are larger than the chief cells and form small clusters of cells with a pale-pink cytoplasm; observe the slender connective tissue elements with their rich supply of blood vessels (Fig. 13.12, PG; Fig. 13.16 CC, OC, BV).

Suprarenal Gland (Adrenal Gland)

A very low magnification of the suprarenal gland displays its dense, irregular, collagenous connective tissue capsule, the three-layered cortex, and the centrally positioned medulla, with its large blood vessels. Observe that the cortex completely envelops the medulla, similar to the egg white surrounding the yolk of a hard-boiled egg (Fig. 13.19, Ca, Co, Me, BV). A medium magnification of the suprarenal cortex demonstrates the capsule, as well as two of the three layers of the cortex, the round-profiled zona glomerulosa and the column-like disposition of the cells of the zona fasciculata. The slender connective tissue elements between the columns of the zona fasciculata house connective tissue cells, as well as longitudinally disposed capillaries (Fig. 13.20, Ca, ZG, ZF, CTC). A low magnification of the inner region of the suprarenal cortex and adjoining medulla presents the spongiocytes of the zona fasciculata and the parenchymal cells of the zona reticularis. The vascular medulla is obvious due to its closely grouped, large chromaffin cells (Fig. 13.21, Sp, ZF, ZR, V, CC). Medium magnification of the suprarenal medulla demonstrates its rich vascular supply, as well as its closely packed chromaffin cells whose nuclei present a single, centrally placed nucleolus (Fig. 13.22, V, CC, N, n).

Pineal Gland

The pineal gland is easily recognizable if the image exhibits the dark, dense-appearing corpora arenacea ("brain sand") scattered among the light-staining pinealocytes (Fig. 13.24, BS). The pia mater that surrounds the pineal gland, forming its capsule, sends trabeculae into its substance, dividing it into lobules. In addition to its melatonin-producing pinealocytes, there are neuroglial cells whose smaller, darker nuclei make it easy to distinguish them from the pinealocytes. The presence of corpora arenacea provides an excellent clue to the recognition of the pineal gland (Fig. 13.25, T, Lo, Pi, Ng, BS).

14 Integument

The **integument** is composed of **skin** and its appendages: **sweat glands**, **sebaceous glands**, **hair**, and **nails**. It is the largest organ, constituting 16% of the body weight. The skin invests the entire body, becoming continuous with the mucous membranes of the digestive system at the lips and the anus, the respiratory system in the nose, and the urogenital systems where they surface. Additionally, the skin of the eyelids becomes continuous with the conjunctiva lining the anterior portion of the eye. Skin also lines the external auditory meatus and covers the external surface of the tympanic membrane. The mammary glands are also derivatives of the epidermis, but their histology is discussed in Chapter 20.

Skin

Skin, the largest organ of the body, is composed of an epidermis and the underlying dermis.

The skin performs many functions, such as **protection** against injury, bacterial invasion, and desiccation; **regulation of body temperature**; **reception** of continual sensations from the environment (e.g., touch, temperature, and pain); **excretion** from sebaceous glands, as well as from apocrine and eccrine sweat glands; and **absorption** of ultraviolet (UV) radiation from the sun, a requirement for vitamin D synthesis.

Skin is composed of an outer epidermis and a deeper connective tissue layer, known as the dermis (Fig. 14.1). The **epidermis** is an **ectodermally** derived stratified squamous keratinized epithelium, directly below which is the **dermis**, derived from **mesoderm** and composed of dense, irregular, collagenous connective tissue. The interface between the epidermis and dermis is formed by raised ridges of the dermis, the **dermal ridges** (**dermal papillae**), which interdigitate with invaginations of the epidermis, called **epidermal ridges**. Frequently, a dermal ridge is subdivided into two dermal ridges by a downgrowth of the epidermis, known as an **interpapillary peg**. Dermal and epidermal ridges are known, collectively, as the **rete apparatus**. Additional downgrowths of the epidermal derivatives (i.e., hair follicles, sweat glands, and sebaceous glands) that come to lie in the dermis also cause the interface to have an irregular contour.

The **hypodermis**, a loose connective tissue containing varying amounts of fat deep to the dermis, is not part of the skin. It is the **superficial fascia** of gross anatomical dissection; in those individuals who are overnourished or who live in cold climates, there is a large amount of fat deposited in this layer, which then is named **panniculus adiposus**.

Clinical Correlations

Skin displays different textures and thicknesses in different regions of the body. For example, skin of the eyelid is soft, fine, and thin and has fine hairs, whereas skin of the eyebrow is thicker and manifests coarse hair. Skin of the forehead produces oily secretions; the skin on the chin lacks oily secretions but develops much hair. The palms of the hands and soles of the feet are thick and do not produce hair but contain many sweat glands. In addition, finger and toe pad surfaces have well-defined, alternating ridges and grooves that form patterns of loops, curves, arches, and whorls called **dermatoglyphs** *(fingerprints), which develop in the fetus and remain unchanged throughout life. Dermatoglyphs are so individualized that they are used for identification purposes in forensic medicine and criminal investigations. Although fingerprints are determined genetically, perhaps by multiple genes, other grooves and flexure lines about the knees, elbows, and hands are, for the most part, related to habitual use and physical stresses in one's environment.*

EPIDERMIS

Epidermis, the surface layer of skin, is derived from ectoderm and is composed of stratified squamous keratinized epithelium.

The **epidermis** is 0.07 to 0.12 mm in thickness over most of the body but much thicker on the palms of the hands and soles of the feet (up to 0.8 mm and 1.4 mm in thickness, respectively). Thicker skin on the palms and soles is evident even in fetuses, but use, applied pressure, and friction result in continued increases in skin thickness in these areas over time.

The stratified squamous keratinized epithelium of skin is composed of four populations of cells: keratinocytes, melanocytes, Langerhans cells, and Merkel cells.

Keratinocytes of the Epidermis

Keratinocytes form the largest population of cells of skin and are arranged in five recognizable layers, due to the surfaceward migration of newly formed cells derived from mitotic activity of the keratinocytes in the basal layers of the epidermis. Mitosis occurs at night; as the new cells make their way to the surface, they differentiate, a process known as **cytomorphosis**, and begin to accumulate **keratin filaments** in their cytoplasm. Eventually, as they near the surface, the cells die and are sloughed off, a progression that takes approximately 30 days depending on the thickness of the epidermis.

Because of the continuous cytomorphosis of keratinocytes during their migration from the basal layer of the epidermis to its surface, five morphologically distinct zones of the epidermis can be identified. From the inner to the outer layer, these are the (1) **stratum basale (stratum germinativum)**, (2) **stratum spinosum**, (3) **stratum granulosum**, (4) **stratum lucidum**, and (5) **stratum corneum**.

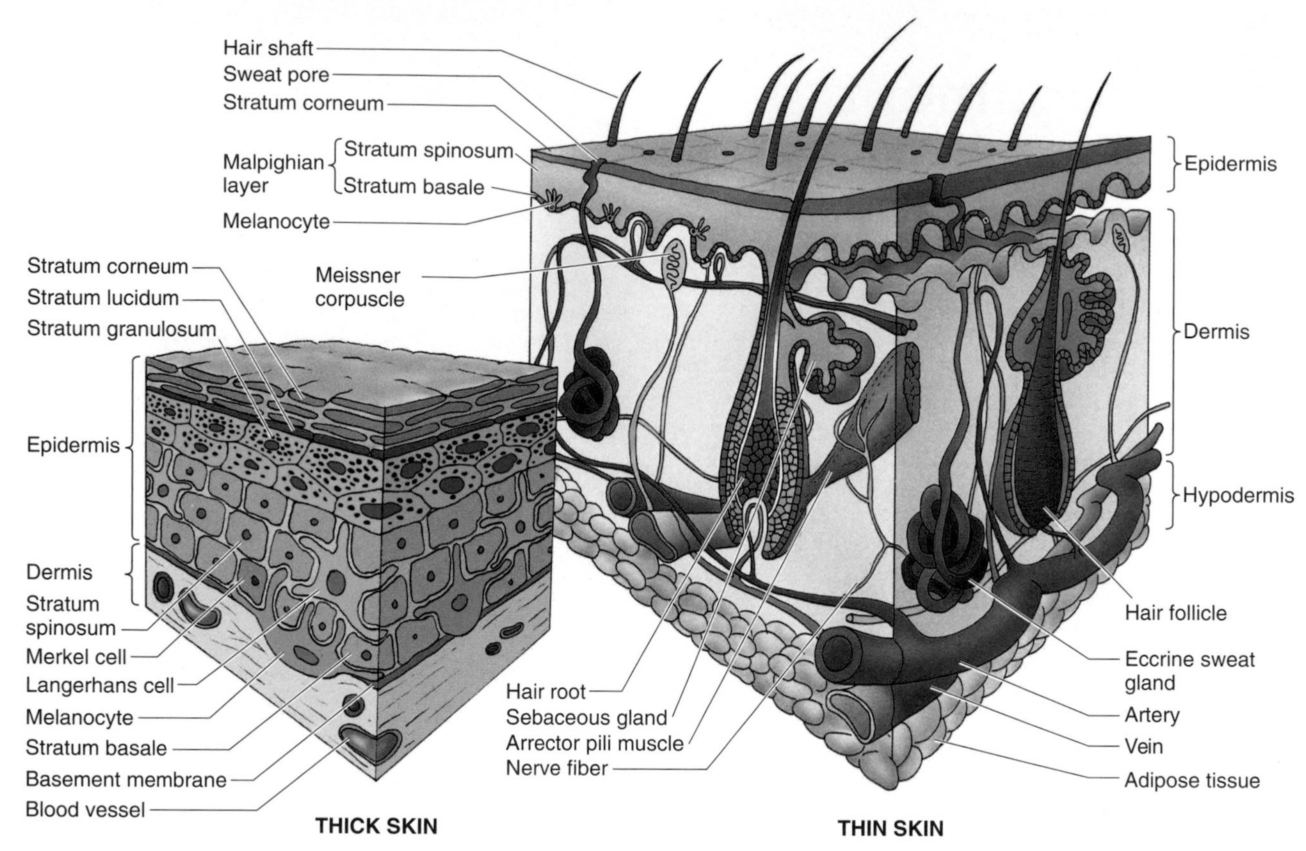

Fig. 14.1 Comparison of thick skin and thin skin.

Clinical Correlations

Keratinocytes synthesize and secrete signaling molecules, such as tumor necrosis factor, interleukins, colony-stimulating factors, and interferons, all of which contribute to the functioning of the immune system.

CLASSIFICATION OF SKIN

Skin is classified as thick skin or thin skin according to the thickness of the epidermis and, to a certain extent, thickness of the dermis.

Thick skin covers the palms and soles (Table 14.1). The epidermis of thick skin, which is 400 to 600 μm thick, is characterized by the presence of all five layers. Thick skin lacks hair follicles, arrector pili muscles, and sebaceous glands but does possess sweat glands (Fig. 14.2).

Thin skin covers most of the remainder of the body. The epidermis of thin skin, which ranges from 75 to 150 μm in thickness, has a thin stratum corneum, stratum spinosum, and stratum basale ; it lacks a definite stratum lucidum and stratum granulosum, although individual cells of these two layers are present in their proper locations. Thin skin has **hair follicles**, **arrector pili muscles**, **sebaceous glands**, and **sweat glands**.

EPIDERMIS

The epidermis of thick skin is composed of five layers, the deepest of which, the stratum basale, lies on the basement membrane that separated the epidermis from the dermis. The next four layers, moving toward the free surface, are the stratum spinosum, stratum granulosum, stratum lucidum, and the stratum corneum.

Stratum Basale

The stratum basale, the germinal layer that undergoes mitosis, forms interdigitations with the dermis and is separated from it by a basement membrane.

The **stratum basale** is the deepest layer of the epidermis, supported by a **basement membrane** separating it from the dermis. The stratum basale consists of a single layer of mitotically active, cuboidal to low columnar cells containing basophilic cytoplasm and a large nucleus (Fig. 14.3). Many desmosomes are located on their cell membranes attaching stratum basale cells to each other and to cells of the stratum spinosum. Basally located hemidesmosomes attach the cells to the basal lamina. Electron micrographs reveal a few mitochondria, a small Golgi complex, a few rough endoplasmic reticulum (RER) profiles, and abundant free ribosomes. Numerous bundles and single (10-nm) **intermediate filaments** (**tonofilaments**), composed of **keratin 5** and **keratin 14**, course through the plaques of the laterally placed desmosomes and end in plaques of hemidesmosomes.

Although **mitotic figures** would be expected to be common in the stratum basale because this layer is partially responsible for cell renewal in the epithelium, mitosis occurs mostly during the night and histological specimens are procured during the day. Thus, such figures are rarely seen in histological slides of skin. When new cells are formed via mitosis, the previous layer of cells is pushed toward the surface to join the next layer of the epidermis, the stratum spinosum. Melanocytes and Merkel cells are dispersed among the keratinocytes of the stratum basale.

TABLE 14.1 Strata and Histological Features of Thick Skin

Layer	Histological Features
Epidermis	Derived from ectoderm; composed of stratified squamous keratinized epithelium (keratinocytes).
Stratum corneum	Numerous layers of dead, flattened keratinized cells, keratinocytes, without nuclei or organelles (squames or horny cells) that will be sloughed off.
Stratum lucidum[a]	Lightly stained thin layer of keratinocytes without nuclei or organelles; cells contain densely packed keratin filaments and eleidin.
Stratum granulosum[a]	A layer three to five cell layers thick. These keratinocytes still retain nuclei; cells contain large, coarse keratohyalin granules as well as membrane-coating granules.
Stratum spinosum	Thickest layer of the epidermis, whose keratinocytes, known as prickle cells, interdigitate with one another by forming intercellular bridges and a large number of desmosomes; prickle cells have numerous tonofilaments and membrane-coating granules and are mitotically active; this layer also houses Langerhans cells.
Stratum basale (germinativum)	This single layer of cuboidal to low columnar, mitotically active cells is separated from the papillary layer of the dermis by a well-developed basement membrane; Merkel cells and melanocytes are also present in this layer.
Dermis	Derived from mesoderm; composed mostly of type I collagen and elastic fibers, the dermis is subdivided into two regions: the papillary layer and the reticular layer, a dense, irregular collagenous connective tissue.
Papillary layer	Interdigitates with the epidermis, forming the dermal papilla component of the rete apparatus; type III collagen and elastic fibers in loose arrangement and anchoring fibrils (type VII collagen); abundant capillary beds, connective tissue cells, and mechanoreceptors are located in this layer; occasionally, melanocytes are also present in the papillary layer.
Reticular layer	Deepest layer of skin; type I collagen, thick elastic fibers, and connective tissue cells; contains sweat glands and their ducts, hair follicles and arrector pili muscles, and sebaceous glands as well as mechanoreceptors (e.g., Pacinian corpuscles).

[a]Present in thick skin only. All layers are usually thinner in thin skin.

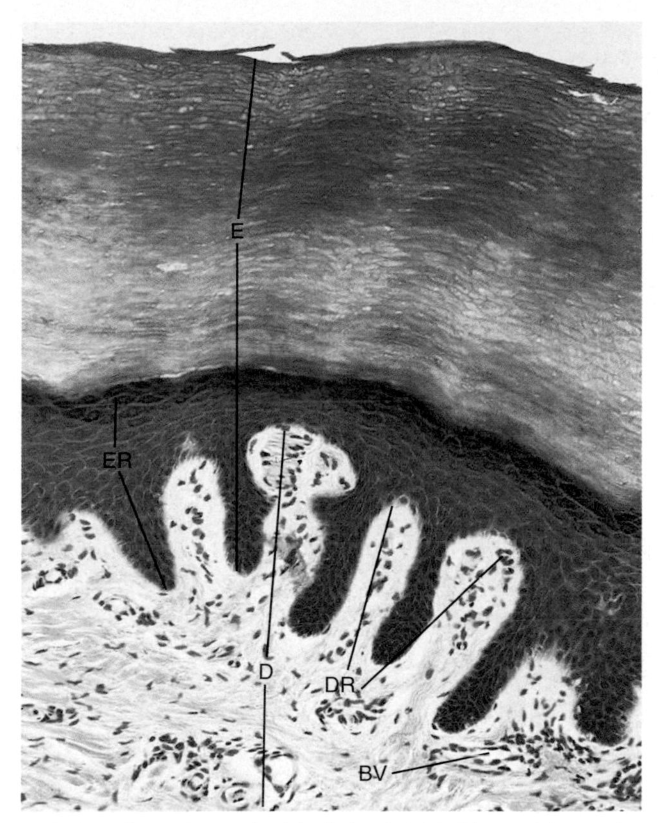

Fig. 14.2 Light micrograph of thick skin (×132). Observe the epidermis (E) and dermis (D) as well as the dermal ridges (DR) that are interdigitating with epidermal ridges (ER). Several blood vessels (BV) are present.

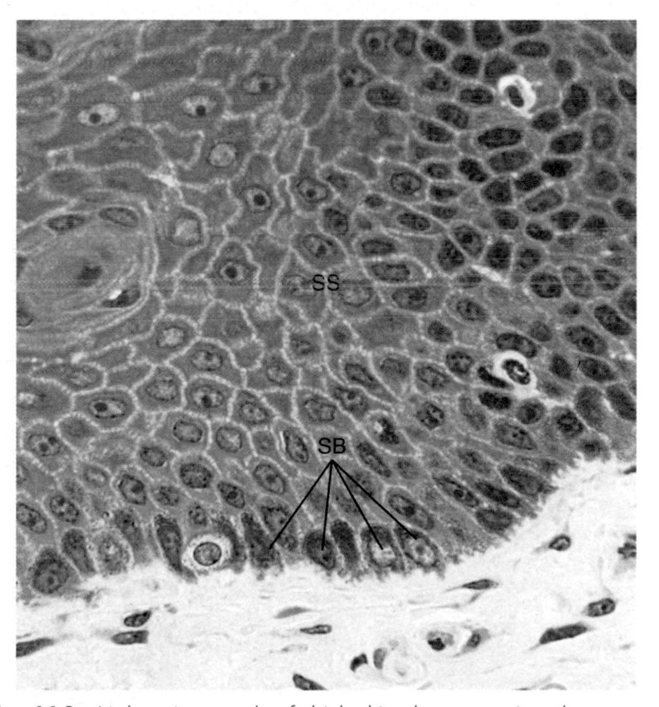

Fig. 14.3 Light micrograph of thick skin demonstrating the stratum basale (SB) and stratum spinosum (SS). (×540)

Stratum Spinosum

The stratum spinosum is composed of several layers of mitotically active polymorphous cells whose numerous processes give this layer a prickly appearance.

The thickest layer of the epidermis, the **stratum spinosum**, is composed of polyhedral to flattened cells. The basally located keratinocytes in the stratum spinosum also are mitotically active; the two strata together, frequently referred to as the ***Malpighian layer***, are responsible for the turnover of epidermal keratinocytes. Cellular proliferation in the Malpighian layer requires the presence of **epidermal growth factor (EGF)** and **interleukin-1 (IL-1)**, whereas **transforming growth factor (TGF)** inhibits mitotic activity. Keratinocytes of the stratum spinosum have the same organelle population as described for the stratum basale. However, the cells in the stratum spinosum are richer in thin bundles of intermediate (**keratin**) filaments (referred to as ***tonofilaments***) than are the cells of the stratum basale. Moreover, instead of keratins 5 and 14, these cells synthesize **keratin 1** and **keratin 10**. These tonofilament bundles radiate outward from the perinuclear region of the stratum spinosum cells toward the highly interdigitated cellular processes, known as **intercellular bridges**, which attach adjacent cells to each other by desmosomes, giving cells of the stratum spinosum a “prickle cell” appearance (see Fig. 14.3). As keratinocytes move toward the surface through the stratum spinosum, they continue to produce tonofilaments, which become enveloped by **keratohyalin**, a substance whose major constituents are **tricohyalin** and **filaggrin**. The combination of keratohyalin and tonofilaments creates groups of thickened bundles called **tonofibrils** (Fig. 14.4), causing the cytoplasm to become eosinophilic. Cells of the stratum spinosum also contain flattened secretory granules (0.1–0.4 μm in diameter) called **membrane-coating granules (lamellar bodies, Odland bodies)**. These vesicles house lipid substances—composed mostly of phospholipids, glycosphingolipids, and ceramides—arranged in a closely packed, lamellar configuration. Some of these granules release their contents into the extracellular space, forming a boundary that is impermeable to aqueous substances.

Stratum Granulosum

The stratum granulosum is composed of three to five layers of cells housing keratohyalin granules.

The **stratum granulosum** is composed of three to five layers of flattened keratinocytes; this is the most superficial layer of the epidermis whose cells still possess nuclei (see Fig. 14.2). The cytoplasm of these keratinocytes contains large, irregularly shaped, coarse, basophilic **keratohyalin granules**. Bundles of keratin filaments pass through these *non-membrane bound* granules.

Cells of the stratum granulosum also contain **membrane-coating granules**. The contents of these granules are released by exocytosis into the extracellular space, forming sheets of lipid-rich substance that acts as a **waterproof barrier**, achieving one of the functions of skin. This impermeable layer prevents cells lying superficial to this region from being bathed in the nutrient-filled aqueous extracellular fluid. Consequently, the cells enter the apoptosis pathway, their organelles self-destruct, and the cells are filled with **keratohyalin-embedded, keratin-based tonofibril complex**. The cytoplasmic aspect of their cell membrane becomes coated with a 10- to 12-nm thick reinforcing layer of dense material and the cells of the stratum granulosum make numerous **claudin-rich** tight junctions with each other.

Stratum Lucidum

Present only in thick skin, cells of the stratum lucidum are devoid of nuclei and organelles but contain eleidin.

The clear, homogeneous, lightly staining, thin layer of cells immediately superficial to the stratum granulosum is the **stratum lucidum**. This layer is present only in thick skin (i.e., palms of the hands and soles of the feet). Although the flattened cells of the stratum lucidum lack organelles and nuclei, they are filled with densely packed **keratohyalin-embedded, keratin-based tonofibril complex** known as ***eleidin***. The cytoplasmic aspect of the plasma membrane of these cells has a thickened appearance because of the deposition of a nonkeratin protein, known as ***involucrin***, which provides support for the cell membrane.

Stratum Corneum

The stratum corneum is composed of several layers of flattened, keratin-containing dead cells known as squames.

The most superficial layer of skin, the **stratum corneum**, is composed of as many as 20 layers of flattened, keratinized cells with a thickened plasmalemma (Figs. 14.2, 14.5–14.7). These cells also lack nuclei and organelles but are filled with **keratohyalin-embedded, keratin-based tonofibril complex**. Those cells farther away from the skin surface display desmosomes and tight junctions; assume the shape of highly flattened, 14-sided polygons; and are called ***squames*** or ***horny cells***. The cytoplasmic aspect of the plasmalemmae of these cells are lined by a thickened, dense material composed of three proteins that reinforce the cell membrane: **small proline-rich protein**, **involucrin**, and **loricrin**. This internally reinforced cell membrane is referred to as the ***cornified cell envelope***. The extracellular surface of the

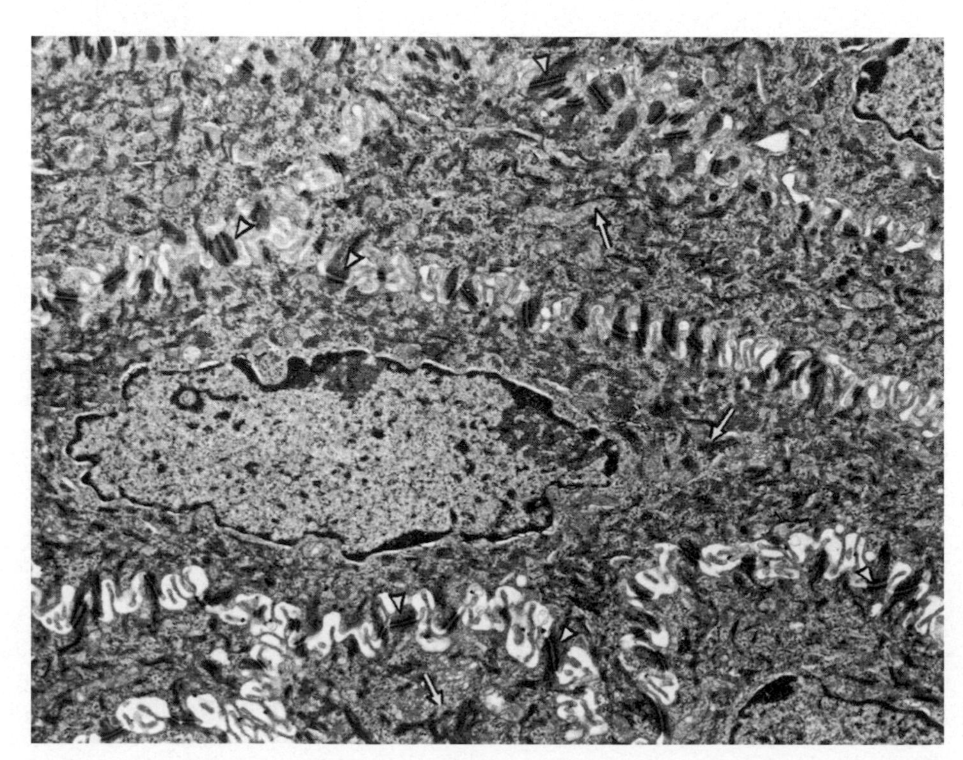

Fig. 14.4 Electron micrograph of the stratum spinosum (×6800). The tonofibrils *(arrows)* and the cytoplasmic processes are bridging the intercellular spaces. (From Leeson TS, Leeson CR, Paparo AA. *Text/Atlas of Histology*. Philadelphia: WB Saunders; 1988.)

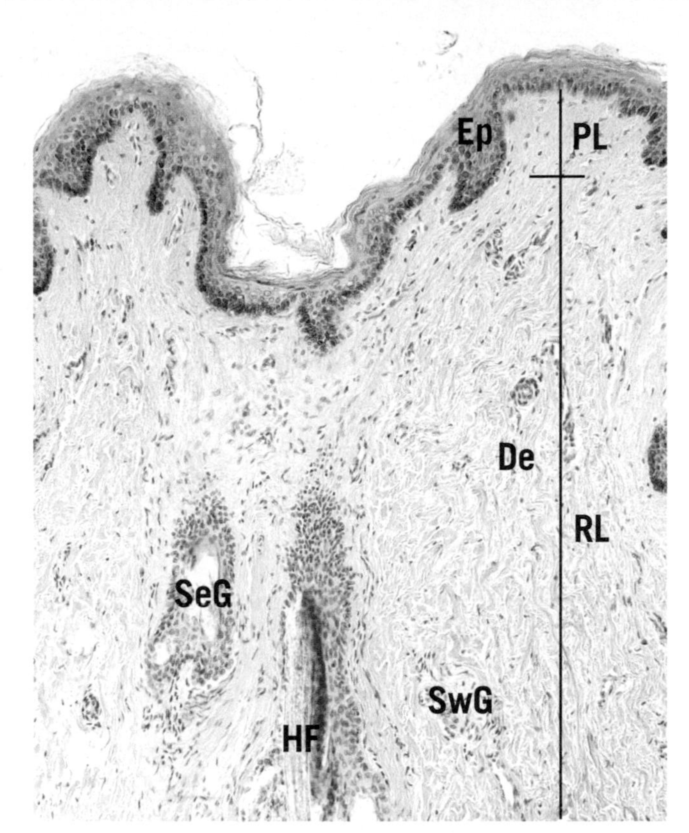

Fig. 14.5 This low-magnification light micrograph of thin skin displays the thin epidermis (Ep), papillary layer (PL) and reticular layer (RL) of the dermis, as well as a sweat gland (SwG) and a hair follicle (HF) with its associated sebaceous gland (SeG). (×132)

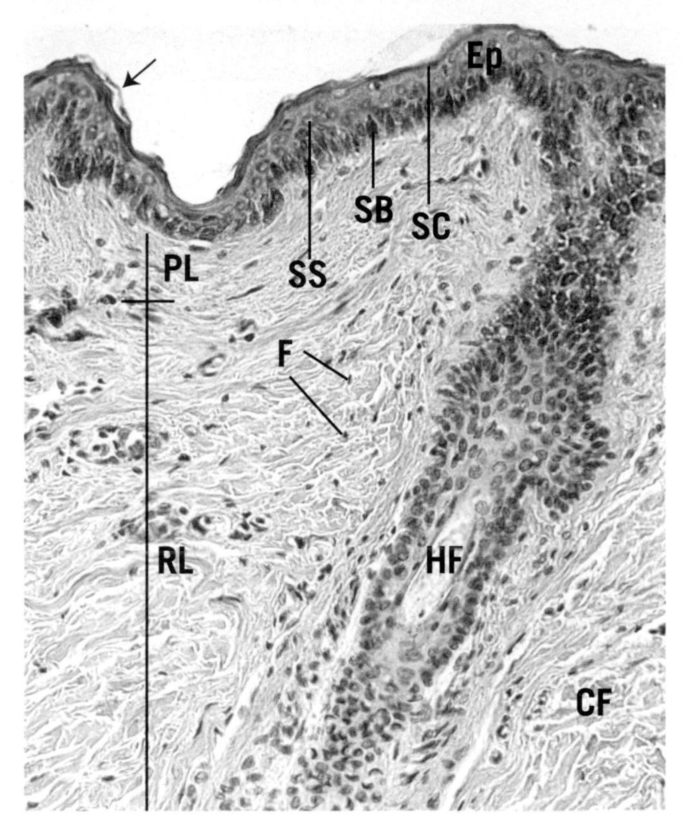

Fig. 14.6 This is a medium magnification of thin skin demonstrating that the stratum corneum (SC) of the epidermis (Ep) is sloughing off *(arrow)* and that both the stratum corneum and the stratum spinosum (SS) are much thinner than those of thick skin. Observe that the papillary layer (PL) of the dermis has a looser consistency than the reticular layer (RL), whose collagen fibers (CF) form thicker bundles and whose fibroblasts (F) have darker, denser nuclei. Note the presence of a hair follicle (HF). (×270)

stratum corneum cell membrane is embedded in the coat of **lipid material** that was released from the membrane-coating granules in the strata spinosum and the granulosum. The combination of the lipid coat and the cornified cell envelope together form a very strong impermeable barrier known as the ***compound cornified cell envelope***. The outermost squames lose their contact with each other and become **desquamated** (sloughed off). The pace at which the squames are desquamated from the stratum corneum equals the rate of new cell formation in the Malpighian layer; therefore, the epidermis retains its characteristic thickness.

Nonkeratinocytes in the Epidermis

Dispersed among the keratinocytes, the epidermis contains three other cell types: Langerhans cells, Merkel cells, and melanocytes (Table 14.2).

Langerhans Cells

Langerhans cells are antigen-presenting cells located among the cells of the stratum spinosum.

Although they are scattered throughout the epidermis, where they normally represent 2% to 4% of the epidermal cell population, **Langerhans cells**, sometimes called ***dendritic cells*** because of their numerous long processes, are located primarily in the stratum spinosum. These cells also may be found in the dermis, as well as in the stratified squamous epithelia of the oral cavity, esophagus, and vagina. However, they are most prevalent in the epidermis, where their numbers may reach 800 per square millimeter.

Langerhans cells display a dense nucleus, pale cytoplasm, and long slender processes that radiate out from the cell body

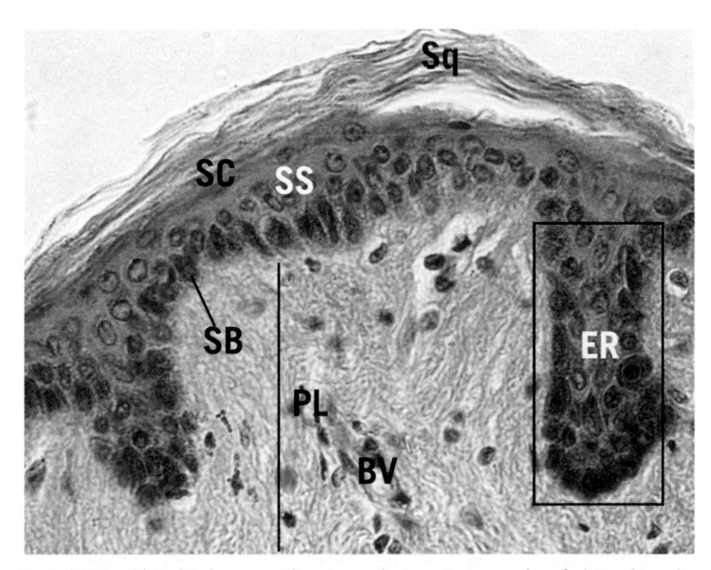

Fig. 14.7 This high-magnification photomicrograph of thin skin displays the three discernible layers of the epidermis— the stratum basale (SB), stratum spinosum (SS), and stratum corneum (SC)—whose surface layers are seen to be desquamating (Sq). The boxed area encloses an epithelial ridge (ER) that extends down to the interface of the papillary layer (PL) with the reticular layer (not shown). Observe the blood vessels (BV) of the papillary layer. (×540)

TABLE 14.2 Nonkeratinocyte Population of the Epidermis

Cell	Origin	Stratum Location	Function
Langerhans cell	Bone marrow	Spinosum	Antigen presentation to T cells
Merkel cell	Neural crest (epithelium?)	Basale	Mechanoreception and release of neuroendocrine substances
Melanocyte	Neural crest	Basale	Melanin synthesis

into the intercellular spaces between keratinocytes. Electron micrographs reveal the nucleus to be polymorphous; the electron-lucent cytoplasm houses sparse RER, few mitochondria, lysosomes, multivesicular bodies, and small vesicles but no intermediate filaments. Although the irregularly contoured nucleus and the absence of tonofilaments distinguish Langerhans cells from surrounding keratinocytes, the most unique feature of Langerhans cells is the membrane-bound **Birbeck granules** (**vermiform granules**), which in section resemble ping pong paddles (15–50 nm in length, 4 nm thick).

Langerhans cells originate from precursors in the bone marrow and are a part of the mononuclear phagocyte system. They very seldom divide; instead they are continually replaced by precursor cells that migrate into the epidermis and differentiate into Langerhans cells. These cells function in the immune response and have cell-surface Fc (antibody) and C3b (complement) receptors, as well as the proteins MHC I, MHC II, and CD1a. Birbeck granules of Langerhans cells contain **langerin**, an integral protein and lectin receptor, which assists the engulfing of antigens by Birbeck granules so that they can degrade them into their epitopes. Once the antigens are processed in the Birbeck granules, Langerhans cells migrate to lymph nodes in the vicinity, where they present epitopes of processed foreign antigens to T lymphocytes. Thus, Langerhans cells are **antigen-presenting cells** (**APCs**) that are responsible for triggering delayed-type hypersensitivity reactions.

Clinical Correlations

Individuals who suffer from an excess of Langerhans cells are said to have a condition known as **Langerhans cell histiocytosis (LCH)**, *also known as Hashimoto-Pritzker disease. Although some consider LCH to be a type of cancer, others consider it to be a granuloma, a type of inflammatory tumor consisting mostly of macrophages that surround foreign substances in order to isolate them from the body. In fact, 8 out of 10 patients diagnosed with LCH form granulomas in the long bones and/or the flat bones of the skull. As these granulomas increase in size they become responsible for fracturing the bones in which they reside. Additional sites where granulomas may form are the skin, where they form reddish blisters, and the pituitary gland, where they can cause endocrine malfunctions, such as diabetes insipidus or thyroid abnormalities. In 2 out of 10 patients, LCH may affect the lungs, causing respiratory problems; the bone marrow, resulting in reduced hemopoiesis with consequential anemia, leukopenia, and thrombocytopenia; the liver, causing jaundice, severe itching, and a feeling of exhaustion; as well as varied neurological conditions, such as memory loss, visual problems, loss of balance, and problems speaking. Although LCH is a disease of the very young, individuals of any age may be affected. Fortunately, the incidence of LCH is less than 2 per 100,000 individuals. Its cause is not understood completely, although almost 50% of the affected individuals present with a mutation in the BRAF gene. These individuals manufacture a defective form of* **signal transduction serine/threonine-protein kinase B-Raf**, *an intracellular messenger protein that controls cell division. Treatment depends on the location of the tumors and severity of the cases, but may include surgical excision, chemotherapy, radiation therapy, immunotherapy, drug therapy, and—in mild cases—observation and monitoring of the patient.*

Merkel Cells

Merkel cells, scattered among cells of the stratum basale, serve as mechanoreceptors.

Merkel cells originate from neural crest (but they may have an epithelial origin), are interspersed among the keratinocytes of the stratum basale of the epidermis, and are especially abundant in the fingertips, at the base of hair follicles, and in the oral mucosa. These cells are usually present as single cells oriented parallel to the basal lamina. However, they may extend their processes between keratinocytes, to which they are attached by desmosomes (Fig. 14.8). Merkel cell nuclei are deeply indented. Dense-cored granules are located in the perinuclear zone and in the processes; these granules are considered to be the distinguishing feature of Merkel cells.

Myelinated sensory nerves traverse the basal lamina to approximate the Merkel cells, thus forming **Merkel cell–neurite complexes**. These complexes may function as **mechanoreceptors**. These cells exhibit a synaptophysin-like immunoreactivity, indicating that Merkel cells may release neurocrine-like substances, suggesting that Merkel cells display diffuse neuroendocrine system-related activity.

Clinical Correlations

A recently discovered virus, Merkel cell polyoma virus, is responsible for at least 8 out of 10 cases of the aggressive skin cancer known as **Merkel cell carcinoma (MCC)**. *The cause of the other 20% of MCC is not known. These tumors are usually small nodules less than 2 cm in diameter or lumps that are at least 5 cm in diameter that exhibit rapid increase in size. Most of the patients are at least 50 years of age with fair skin, whose lesions are located in regions of the body that are exposed to the sun or to tanning beds in tanning salons. This aggressive carcinoma metastasizes readily to nearby lymph nodes but can also spread via blood vessels to bone, liver, lung, and the brain. The survival rate depends on how early the treatment begins; in stage Ia, the 5-year survival rate is 80%, but in stage IV it is only 20%. Fortunately, the incidence is rare, less than 1 person per 100,000. Treatment includes surgery, radiation therapy, chemotherapy, and a relatively new drug therapy that targets programmed cell death protein 1/programmed cell death protein-1 ligand pathway (PD-1/PD-L1 pathway).*

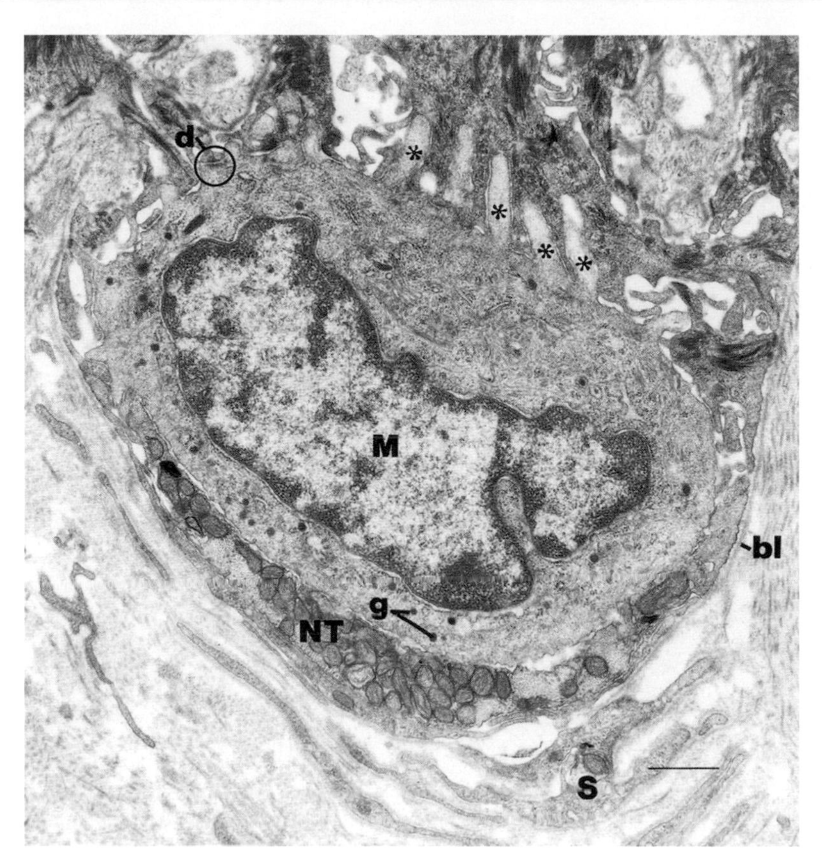

Fig. 14.8 Electron micrograph of a Merkel cell (M) and its nerve terminal (NT) from an adult rat (scale bar = 0.5 μm). Note the spine-like processes *(asterisks)* that project into the intercellular spaces of the stratum spinosum. Merkel cells form desmosomes (d) with cells of the stratum spinosum and share the basal lamina (bl) of cells of the stratum basale. (From English KB, Wang ZZ, Stayner N, et al. Serotonin-like immunoreactivity in Merkel cells and their afferent neurons in touch domes from hairy skin of rats. *Anat Rec.* 1991;232:112–120. Reprinted with permission from Wiley-Liss, Inc., a subsidiary of John Wiley & Sons, Inc.)

Melanocytes

Melanocytes, derived from neural crest cells, produce melanin pigment that imparts a brown coloration to skin.

Melanoblasts, derived from neural crest, migrate to the epidermis where they differentiate into **premelanocytes.** Premelanocytes continue their migration into the stratum basale, where they take up residence, although some melanoblasts may continue on to enter the superficial portions of the dermis to remain there (Fig. 14.9). Premelanocytes form hemidesmosomes with the basal lamina but do not form adhering junctions with the adjacent keratinocytes. **Stem cell factor**, permeating throughout the dermis and the extracellular spaces of the stratum basale and stratum spinosum, bind to **stem cell factor receptors** on the premelanocytes, inducing these cells to differentiate into **melanocytes**, cells that form processes known as ***dendrites***. These processes extend into the stratum spinosum and contact a number of keratinocytes. Each melanocyte and the keratinocytes that its processes contact is referred to as an ***epidermal melanin unit***.

Tyrosinase produced by the RER of the melanocyte is packaged by its Golgi apparatus into oval granules, known as ***melanosomes*** (although the melanosomes of red-haired individuals are spherical instead of oval). The amino acid tyrosine is preferentially transported into melanosomes. Under the influence of **melanocyte-stimulating hormone**, melanocytes express **microphthalmia-associated transcription factor.** This factor triggers the UV light–sensitive **tyrosinase** to convert **tyrosine** within the **melanosomes** into **melanin** through a series of reactions progressing through 3,4-dihydroxyphenylalanine (dopa, methyldopa) and dopaquinone.

Clinical Correlations

There are three types of melanin: brown eumelanin, black eumelanin, and pheomelanin. ***Brown melanin*** *and* ***black melanin*** *are both dark (it is customary to drop the "eu" from "eumelanin" and refer to it simply as "melanin"); as the individual ages, brown melanin is no longer produced. They are packaged in oval-shaped melanosomes and give skin a darker hue.* ***Pheomelanin*** *is yellow to red, present only in red-haired individuals, and is packaged in round melanosomes. Individuals with pheomelanin have the tendency to burn rather than tan when exposed to strong sunlight for an extended period of time.*

Ultraviolet light darkens the melanin and speeds tyrosinase synthesis, thus increasing melanin production. Also, pituitary adrenocorticotropic hormone (ACTH) influences pigmentation. In ***Addison disease***, *there is insufficient production of cortisol by the adrenal cortex; thus, excess ACTH is produced, which leads to hyperpigmentation.*

Albinism *is the absence of melanin production, resulting from a genetic defect in* ***tyrosinase synthesis***. *Melanosomes are present, but the melanocytes fail to produce tyrosinase.*

As the melanin content of melanosomes increases in quantity, the melanosome is said to be maturing. Once mature, they are conveyed along microtubules into the dendrites of the melanosomes and are released into the extracellular spaces of the stratum spinosum to be phagocytosed by keratinocytes of the stratum spinosum. Within the keratinocytes, the melanosomes are ferried to the nuclear region, where they accumulate between the nucleus and the cell membrane closest to the free surface of the epidermis. As the sun's UV radiation strikes the skin, the melanin in the melanosomes shields the keratinocyte's chromosomes from UV radiation–induced injury. Eventually, the melanosomes are attacked and degraded by lysosomes of the keratinocyte. This process occurs over a period of several days.

Melanocytes constitute approximately 3% of the epidermal cell population. The number of melanocytes per square millimeter varies in different regions of skin of an individual, ranging from 800 to 2300/mm^2. For example, there are significantly fewer melanocytes on the insides of the arms and thighs than on the face. The difference in skin pigmentation is related more to location of the melanin than to the total number of melanocytes in the skin, which is nearly the same for all races. For instance, there are more melanocytes in the skin on the dorsum than on the palmar surface of the hand; however, these numbers are very similar among the various races. The reason for the darker pigmentation is due not to the effective number of melanocytes but to an increase in their tyrosinase activity.

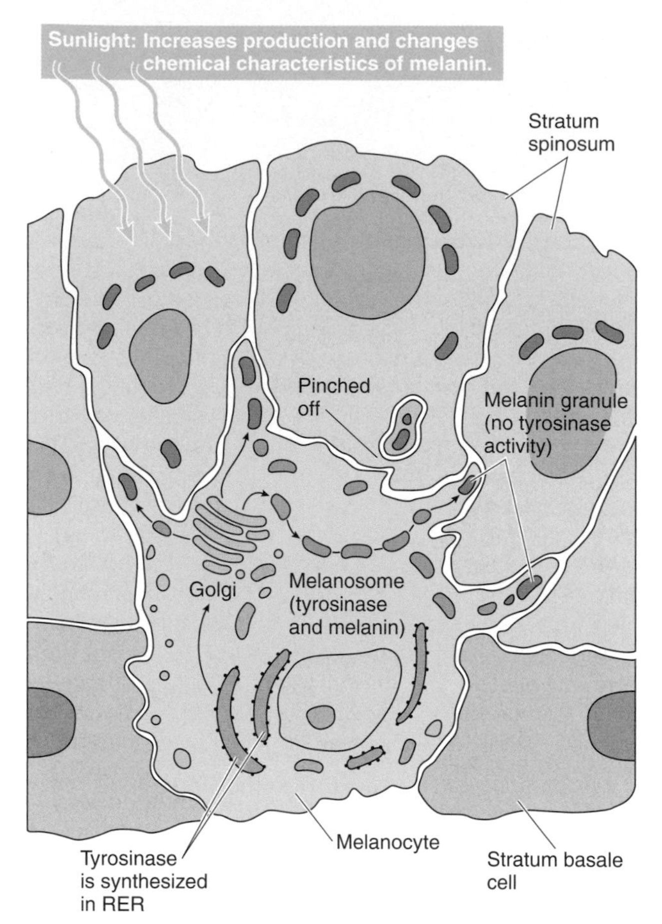

Fig. 14.9 Diagram of melanocytes and their function. *RER*, Rough endoplasmic reticulum.

Clinical Correlations

1. ***Ultraviolet (UV) rays*** *exist as three types. UVC is the shortest wave length and is absorbed by the ozone layer of the atmosphere. UVB, an intermediate wavelength, is the component in sunlight that is blocked by glass but still penetrates the epidermis and dermis, producing sunburn. UVA is the longest wavelength, is not blocked by glass, and is responsible for most of the damage to skin, including all forms of skin cancer. Until recently, it was believed that UVB was relatively safe, but it appears that it also causes damage to the superficial layers of skin, resulting in skin cancer.*
2. ***Xeroderma pigmentosum (XP)*** *is an uncommon autosomal-recessive genetic defect affecting 1 in 1 million individuals in the United States and Europe, but it is present with greater frequency in Morocco, the Middle East, and Japan. Individuals with XP are very sensitive to UV radiation and may get a severe sunburn after being exposed just a few minutes to sunlight. The condition expresses very early in childhood; affected children present with skin cancer, usually on the face and scalp, within the first decade of life. In some regions of the world, the average life span of patients with XP is less than 30 years. Approximately one-third of XP patients present not only with cloudy corneas and eye cancers but also with neurological conditions involving balance and movement disorders, seizures, and cognitive function disorders. There are a number of different forms of XP—fortunately, not all of them lead to neurological problems.*

DERMIS (CORIUM)

The dermis, the layer of skin immediately deep to the epidermis, is derived from mesoderm and is composed of a loose papillary layer and a deeper, denser reticular layer.

The region of the skin that is separated from the epidermis by the basement membrane is called the **dermis**. It is derived from the mesoderm and is divided into two layers: the superficial, loosely woven **papillary layer** and the deeper, much denser **reticular layer**. The reticular layer of the dermis is composed of dense, irregular, collagenous connective tissue, containing mostly **type I collagen fibers**, some **type III collagen fibers**, and broad bands of **elastic fibers**, all of which support the epidermis and bind the skin to the underlying **hypodermis** (superficial fascia). The dermis ranges in thickness from 0.6 mm in the eyelids to 3 mm or so on the palm of the hand and the sole of the foot. However, there is not a sharp line of demarcation at its interface with the underlying connective tissue of the superficial fascia. Normally, the dermis is thicker in men than in women and on the dorsal rather than on the ventral surfaces of the body.

Papillary Layer of the Dermis

The superficial layer of the dermis, the papillary layer, interdigitates directly with the epidermis but is separated from it by the basement membrane.

The superficial papillary layer of the dermis is uneven where it interdigitates with the epidermis, forming the dermal ridges (**dermal papillae**; see Fig. 14.2). It is composed of a loose connective tissue whose thin **type III collagen fibers** (reticular fibers) and slender **elastic fibers** are arranged in loose networks. **Anchoring fibrils**, composed of type VII collagen, extend from the basal lamina into the papillary layer, binding the epidermis to the dermis (see Chapter 4, Figs. 4.13 and 4.14). The papillary layer contains fibroblasts, macrophages, plasma cells, mast cells, and other cells common to connective tissue.

The papillary layer also possesses many capillary loops, which extend to the epidermis–dermis interface. These capillaries regulate body temperature and nourish the cells of the avascular epidermis. Located in some dermal papillae are oval- to pear-shaped encapsulated **Meissner corpuscles**, mechanoreceptors specialized to respond to slight deformations of the epidermis (Fig. 14.10). These receptors are most common in areas of the skin that are especially sensitive to tactile stimulation (e.g., lips, external genitalia, and nipples). Another encapsulated mechanoreceptor present in the papillary layer is the **Krause end bulb**. Although this receptor was once thought to respond to cold, its function is currently unclear. Additionally, unmyelinated pain fibers also course through the papillary layer to enter the epidermis, where they remain as free nerve endings that respond to pain sensations.

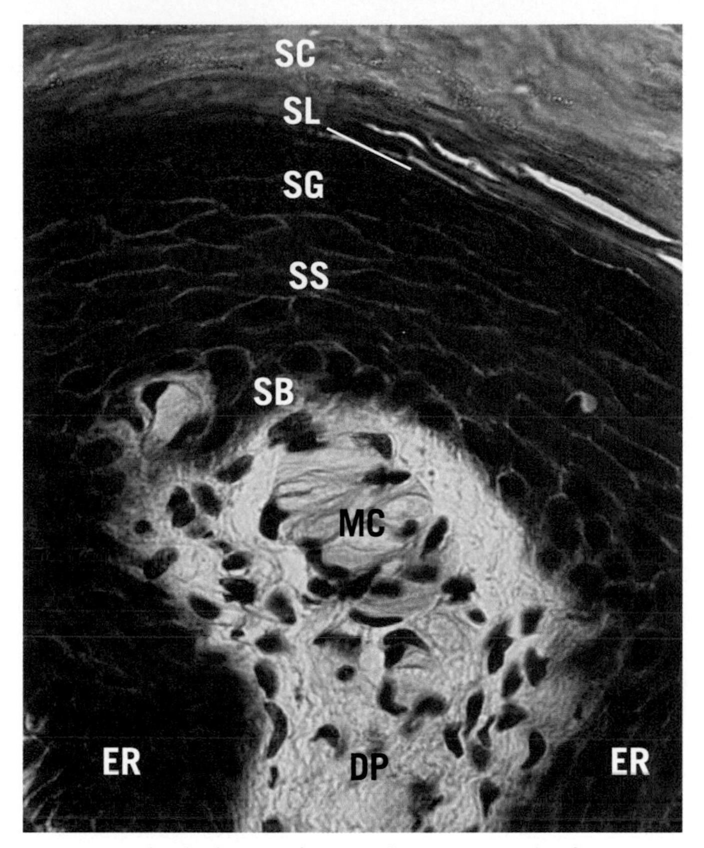

Fig. 14.10 This high-magnification photomicrograph of a Meissner corpuscle of a fingertip displays its oval structure and the prominent flattened nuclei of its modified Schwann cells. This encapsulated mechanoreceptor is located in the dermal papilla. Note the thick epidermis with its five layers: the stratum basale (SB), stratum spinosum (SS), stratum granulosum (SG), stratum lucidum (SL) and the stratum corneum (SC). Observe the epidermal ridges (ER) on either side of the dermal papilla. (×540)

Clinical Correlations

Itching (pruriception) is a somatic sensation that may be due to local causes, such as a tiny insect walking on one's arm or to generalized and systemic causes, such as a form of dermatitis or even to cancer and organ failure. The mechanism of an itch is better known in mice than in humans, but it is assumed that there may be a close correlation in the two species. It has been demonstrated in mice that itching sensation is conveyed by C fibers to the murine spinal cord, where secondary neurons reside that are capable of expressing gastrin-releasing peptide receptors (GRPR). Apparently, there are a number of GRPR types of neurons, which are activated by various types of G protein–coupled receptors that respond to a particular cause of the itching sensation. Moreover, there seems to be a relationship between pain and itching sensations because they share similar, but not identical, pathways; they both possess receptors in the skin, spinal cord, and brain.

Reticular Layer of the Dermis

The reticular layer of the dermis also contains epidermally derived structures, including sweat glands, hair follicles, and sebaceous glands.

The interface between the papillary layer and **reticular layer** of the dermis is indistinguishable because the two layers are continuous with each other. Characteristically, the reticular layer is composed of dense, irregular, collagenous connective tissue, displaying thick **type I collagen fibers** that appear to be closely packed into large bundles lying mostly parallel to the skin surface. In fact, it was recently demonstrated that previously unrecognized microscopic tissue spaces were discovered in dense, irregular, collagenous connective tissue. These fluid-filled **interstitial spaces**, bolstered by bundles of collagen fibers, appear to be lined by highly attenuated cells bearing CD34 molecules on their cell membranes. The fluid contained in these spaces is believed to be prelymphatic fluid that probably makes its way to lymph nodes. It is postulated that this tissue compartment has not been observed because the fluid is drained from the tissues during excision and the tissue collapses onto itself during routine histological preparation. In the living organism, these prelymphatic fluid–filled interstitial spaces act as "shock absorbers" that counter forces of compression (see Chapter 6). Networks of **thick elastic fibers** are intermingled with the collagen fibers, appearing especially abundant near sebaceous and sweat glands. Proteoglycans, rich in **dermatan sulfate**, are located in the interstices of the reticular layer of the dermis. Cells are sparser in this layer than in the papillary layer; they include fibroblasts, mast cells, lymphocytes, macrophages, and, frequently, fat cells in the deeper aspects of the reticular layer.

Sweat glands, **sebaceous glands**, and **hair follicles** are epidermal derivatives that invade the dermis and hypodermis during embryogenesis and remain there permanently (see Fig. 14.1). Groups of **smooth muscle cells** are located in the deeper regions of the reticular layer at particular sites, such as the skin of the penis and scrotum and the areola around the nipples; contractions of these muscle groups wrinkle the skin in these regions. Other smooth muscle fibers, called **arrector pili muscles**, are inserted into the hair follicles. When the individual is cold or is suddenly exposed to a cold environment, these muscle cells contract, elevating the hair and giving the skin the appearance of "goose bumps." Additionally, a particular group of striated muscles located in the face, parts of the anterior neck, and scalp (**muscles of facial expression**) originate in the superficial fascia and insert into the dermis.

At least three types of encapsulated mechanoreceptors are located in the deeper portions of the dermis: (1) **Pacinian corpuscles**, which respond to deep pressure and vibrations; (2) **Ruffini corpuscles**, which respond to tensile forces and torque, are most abundant in the dermis of the soles of the feet; and (3)

Krause end bulbs (**bulboid corpuscles**), whose function is not known but is assumed to be mechanoreception rather than cold receptors, as was previously believed.

HISTOPHYSIOLOGY OF SKIN

Keratinocytes manufacture 10-nm-wide intermediate filaments, known as **keratin**, the structural proteins located within their cytoplasm. Approximately 20 different species of keratin, classified as acidic or neutral basic, have been identified, four of which are present within the epidermis. Stratum basale cells synthesize two types of keratins that form finely woven bundles of filaments, whereas cells of the stratum spinosum synthesize the other two types, which tend to form coarser bundles of filaments. Cells of the stratum spinosum also produce and deposit the protein **involucrin** on the cytoplasmic aspect of their plasmalemma. Moreover, cells of the stratum spinosum also form the **membrane-coating granules**, which release their lipid-rich contents into the intercellular spaces, forming a permeability barrier.

The keratin-synthesizing machinery shuts down after keratinocytes enter the stratum granulosum. The cells in this layer produce **filaggrin**, a protein thought to help assemble keratin filaments into still coarser bundles. Once keratinocytes reach this stratum, they also become permeable to calcium ions, which assist in cross-linking involucrin with other proteins, thereby forming a tough layer beneath the plasmalemma. As keratinocytes move through the stratum granulosum into the stratum lucidum, enzymes released from lysosomes digest the organelles and the nucleus. When the cells finally enter the stratum corneum, they are nonliving, organelle-free, tough shells filled with bundles of keratin filaments.

GLANDS OF THE SKIN

The glands of the skin include eccrine sweat glands, apocrine sweat glands, sebaceous glands, and the mammary gland (a modified and highly specialized type of sweat gland). The mammary gland is described in Chapter 20.

Eccrine Sweat Glands

Eccrine sweat glands are abundant throughout the skin. They release their secretory product, sweat, via the merocrine method of secretion.

Eccrine sweat glands are about 0.4 mm in diameter and are located in the skin throughout most of the body. Numbering as many as 3 to 4 million, they are important organs of thermoregulation. Eccrine sweat glands develop as invaginations of the epithelium of the dermal ridge that grows down into the dermis, with its deep aspect becoming the glandular portion of the sweat gland. These glands, which begin to function soon after birth, excrete about 1 L of sweat per day but may form as much as 10 L of sweat a day under extreme conditions in highly active people engaged in vigorous exercise in hot weather. These glands are innervated by the sympathetic nervous system, but the nerve fibers innervating the secretory units are mostly **cholinergic**, that is, they release **acetylcholine**, and only some of the nerve fibers are adrenergic.

Eccrine sweat glands are simple coiled, tubular glands located deep in the dermis or in the underlying hypodermis (Figs. 14.11–14.14). Passing from the secretory portion of each gland is a slender, coiled duct that traverses the dermis and epidermis to open on the surface of the skin at a sweat pore. These

Clinical Correlations

Freckles are hyperpigmented spots located on sun-exposed areas of the skin, especially in fair-skinned individuals who sunburn easily. Freckles are usually exhibited by 3 years of age and are the result of increased melanin production and accumulation in the basal area of the epidermis without an increase in melanocytes. They tend to fade in the winter and darken with exposure to ultraviolet light.

Psoriasis is a disease characterized by patchy lesions caused by greater keratinocyte proliferation in the stratum basale and stratum spinosum and an accelerated cell cycle (turnover is increased as much as seven times), resulting in accumulations of keratinocytes and stratum corneum. The lesions are common on the scalp, elbows, and knees, but they may occur almost anywhere on the body. In some cases, the nails may also be involved. Psoriasis is an incurable but manageable chronic condition whose symptoms periodically escalate and then diminish with no apparent cause.

Warts are benign epidermal growths caused by infection of the keratinocytes with **papillomaviruses**. *The resulting epidermal hyperplasia thickens the epidermis with scaling. Deeper ingrowth of the dermis brings capillaries closer to the surface. Warts are common in children, young adults, and immunosuppressed patients.*

Basal cell carcinoma, the most common human malignancy, arises in the **stratum basale cells** *of the epidermis and usually is caused by exposure to ultraviolet radiation. Although basal cell carcinomas do not usually metastasize, they are destructive to local tissue. Of the several types of lesions that occur, the most common is the nodular variety, characterized by a papule or nodule with a central depressed "crater" that eventually ulcerates and crusts. These lesions are most common on the face, especially the nose. Surgery is the usual treatment, and up to 90% of patients recover with no additional sequela.*

Squamous cell carcinoma, *the second most common skin cancer, arises in the keratinocytes of the epidermis. It is locally invasive and may metastasize. It is characterized by a hyperkeratotic scaly plaque or nodule that often bleeds or ulcerates. It invades deeply, resulting in fixation to the underlying tissues. Several factors may cause this disease, including ultraviolet radiation, x-irradiation, soot, chemical carcinogens, and arsenic. The lesions are most common on the head and neck. Surgery is the usual treatment of choice.*

Malignant melanoma, *a skin cancer, is increasing in incidence, being most prevalent in fair-skinned individuals The malignant cells originate from transformed melanocytes and usually are associated with excessive exposure to the sun. Malignant melanoma is very invasive because the melanocytes penetrate the dermis and enter lymphatic vessels, as well as the bloodstream, to gain wide distribution throughout the body. Interestingly, even though the incidence of melanoma is much greater in whites than in individuals of African American and Hispanic descent, metastasis occurs in a much greater percentage of Hispanic (18%) and African American (26%) patients than in white (12%) patients. It is believed that the discrepancy is caused by the difference in the level of medical care in these populations.*

glands are merocrine in their method of releasing their secretory product. They are innervated by postganglionic fibers of the sympathetic nervous system.

Secretory Unit

The secretory portion of the gland is said to be a simple cuboidal to low columnar epithelium composed of dark cells and clear cells. Additionally, the secretory portion of eccrine sweat glands possesses myoepithelial cells. Some investigators consider the secretory portion to be pseudostratified; in this textbook, they are considered to be simple cuboidal.

Dark Cells (Mucoid Cells)

Dark cells line the lumen of the secretory unit and secrete a mucus-rich substance.

Dark cells resemble an inverted cone, with the broad end lining the lumen. The narrowed ends, which seldom reach the basal lamina, conform to fit between adjacent clear cells. Electron micrographs reveal some RER, numerous free ribosomes, elongated mitochondria, and a well-developed Golgi complex. Moderately dense glycoprotein-containing secretory granules are located in the apical cytoplasm of the dark cells, and the secretion released by these cells is **mucous** in nature.

Clear Cells

Clear cells do not possess secretory granules; they release a watery secretion.

Clear cells have a narrow apical area and a broader base that extends to the basal lamina. Unlike dark cells, clear cells do not contain secretory granules but do contain accumulations of **glycogen**; their organelles are similar to those of dark cells, except that they have little RER. The bases of the clear cells are tortuously infolded, similar to those of other cell types involved in transepithelial transport. Clear cells have limited access to the lumen of the gland because of the dark cells. Therefore, their **watery, electrolyte-rich secretion** enters **intercellular canaliculi** interposed between adjacent clear cells, where it mixes with the mucous secretion of the dark cells.

Myoepithelial Cells

Myoepithelial cells surrounding the secretory portion of the gland contain actin and myosin, imparting a contractile ability to these cells.

Myoepithelial cells surrounding the secretory portion of the eccrine sweat glands are enveloped by the basal lamina of the secretory cells. The cytoplasm of myoepithelial cells has **myosin filaments** as well as many deeply acidophil-staining **actin** filaments, which give the cell contractile capability. Contractions of the myoepithelial cells assist in expressing the fluid from the secretory portion of the gland.

Duct

The duct of eccrine sweat glands, composed of basal and luminal cells, is highly coiled and traverses the dermis and epidermis on its way to opening on the skin surface.

The **duct** of an eccrine sweat gland is continuous with the secretory unit at its base but narrows as it passes through the dermis on its way to the epidermal surface. The duct is composed of a stratified cuboidal epithelium made up of two layers (see Figs. 14.11–14.14). The **cells of the basal layer** have a large, heterochromatic nucleus and abundant mitochondria. The **cells of the luminal layer** have an irregularly shaped nucleus, little cytoplasm, only a few organelles, and a terminal web immediately deep to the apical plasma membrane.

The ducts follow a helical path through the dermis. As a duct reaches the epidermis, keratinocytes envelop the duct on its way to the sweat pore. The fluid secreted by the secretory portion of the gland is similar to blood plasma in regard to electrolyte balance, including potassium and sodium chloride, as well as ammonia and urea. However, most of the potassium, sodium, and chloride ions are reabsorbed by cells of the duct as the secretion travels through its lumen. Duct cells excrete ions, urea, lactic acid, and certain drugs into the lumen. Therefore, the sweat produced by the secretory unit is modified by the duct of the sweat gland so that the sweat released on the surface of the skin resembles a very dilute urine.

Apocrine Sweat Glands

Apocrine sweat glands are present only in the axilla, areola of the nipple, and anal region and may represent vestigial scent glands.

Apocrine sweat glands are present only in certain locations: the axilla (armpit), areola of the nipple, and anal region. Modified apocrine sweat glands constitute the **ceruminous (wax) glands** of the external auditory canal and the **glands of Moll** in the eyelids (see Chapter 22). Apocrine sweat glands are much larger than eccrine sweat glands; in fact, they may be as large as 3 mm in diameter. These glands are embedded in the deeper portions

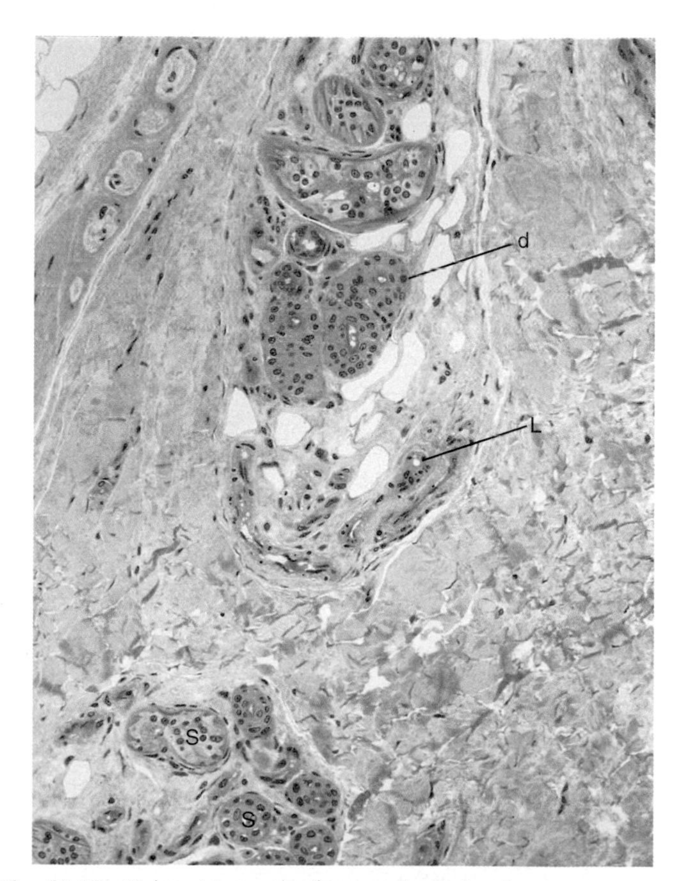

Fig. 14.11 Light micrograph of sweat gland showing secretory units (S) and ducts (d), some displaying a lumen (L). (×132)

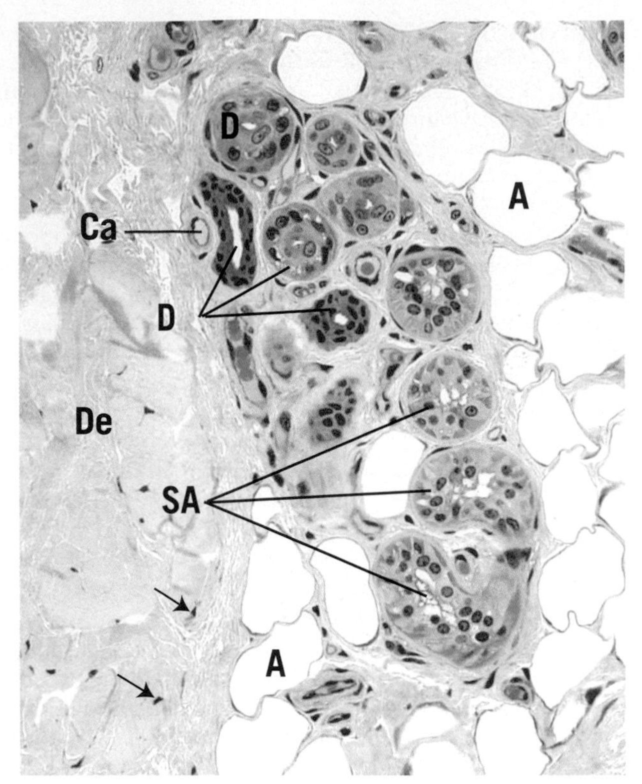

Fig. 14.12 This medium magnification of an eccrine sweat gland located in the dermis (De) of skin shows the simple cuboidal epithelium of the cross-sections of the secretory unit (SA) and the stratified cuboidal epithelium of the sweat gland duct (D). Observe the rich blood supply of the gland (Ca) and the adipocytes (A) flanking the gland. Nuclei of fibroblasts *(arrows)* scattered throughout the dermis are clearly evident. (×270)

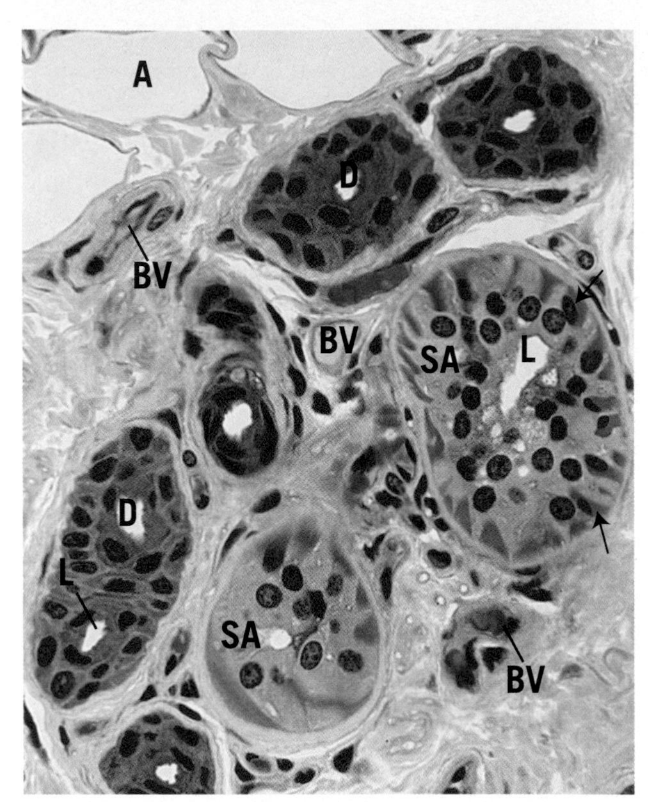

Fig. 14.13 This high-magnification photomicrograph of an eccrine sweat gland clearly demonstrates its rich vascular supply (BV) as well as the simple cuboidal epithelium constituting the secretory unit (SA) and the stratified cuboidal epithelium that forms the duct (D) of the gland. Observe the centrally located lumina (L) of the secretory unit and of the duct. Note the adipocytes (A) adjacent to the gland. (×540).

of the dermis and hypodermis. Unlike the ducts of eccrine sweat glands, which open onto the skin surface, the ducts of apocrine sweat glands open into canals of the hair follicles just superficial to the entry of the sebaceous gland ducts.

The secretory cells of apocrine glands are simple cuboidal to low columnar in profile. When the lumen of the gland is filled with secretory product, these cells may become squamous. The lumina of these glands are much larger than those of eccrine glands, and the secretory cells contain granules that are isolated from the apical membrane by the presence of a prominent terminal web. The viscous secretory product of apocrine glands is odorless upon secretion, but when metabolized by bacteria, it presents a distinctive odor. Myoepithelial cells surround the secretory portion of the apocrine sweat glands and assist in expressing the secretory product into the duct of the gland.

An apocrine sweat gland arises from the epithelium of the hair follicles as an epithelial bud that develops into a gland. Secretion by apocrine glands is under the influence of hormones and does not begin until puberty. Their innervation is provided by fibers of the postganglionic sympathetic nervous system. Because of the similarity of their location, their histology, and the fact that the odor is most likely due to the bacterial metabolism of 3-methyl-1-2 hexanoic acid (a volatile acid similar to pheromone signals), it is speculated that apocrine sweat glands evolved from glands that secrete sex attractants in lower animals. As an interesting note, apocrine sweat glands in women undergo cyclical changes that appear to be related to the menstrual cycle, so that the secretory cells and lumina enlarge before the premenstrual period and diminish during menstruation.

The name given to these special sweat glands, apocrine sweat glands, implies that the secretion contains a portion of the cytoplasm of the secreting cells. Although some researchers suggest that these cells release their secretion via the apocrine method, most investigators report that, despite their name, apocrine sweat glands release their secretory product via the merocrine mode of secretion.

Clinical Correlations

The ABCC11 ***gene*** *is responsible for the formation of a protein known as* ATP-binding cassette transporter subfamily C member 11. *This gene has two alleles, which differ from each other by the presence of a single nucleotide, in one case guanine and in the other case adenine, resulting in the coding for either glycine or arginine. The dominant inheritance is GG or GA, whereas the recessive genotype is AA. The* ***AA genotype*** *produces dry ear wax, an almost odorless sweat production by the apocrine sweat glands, and perhaps less susceptibility to breast cancer. There is a very specific demographic distribution of individuals with the AA allele: a large percentage of the Korean, Mongolian, western Japanese, and Chinese carry this allele. Consequently, they have dry earwax and practically odorless sweat from apocrine sweat glands. Other than the possible beneficial effect on breast cancer, there appears to be no known advantageous or deleterious effect of the presence of the AA allele in these populations.*

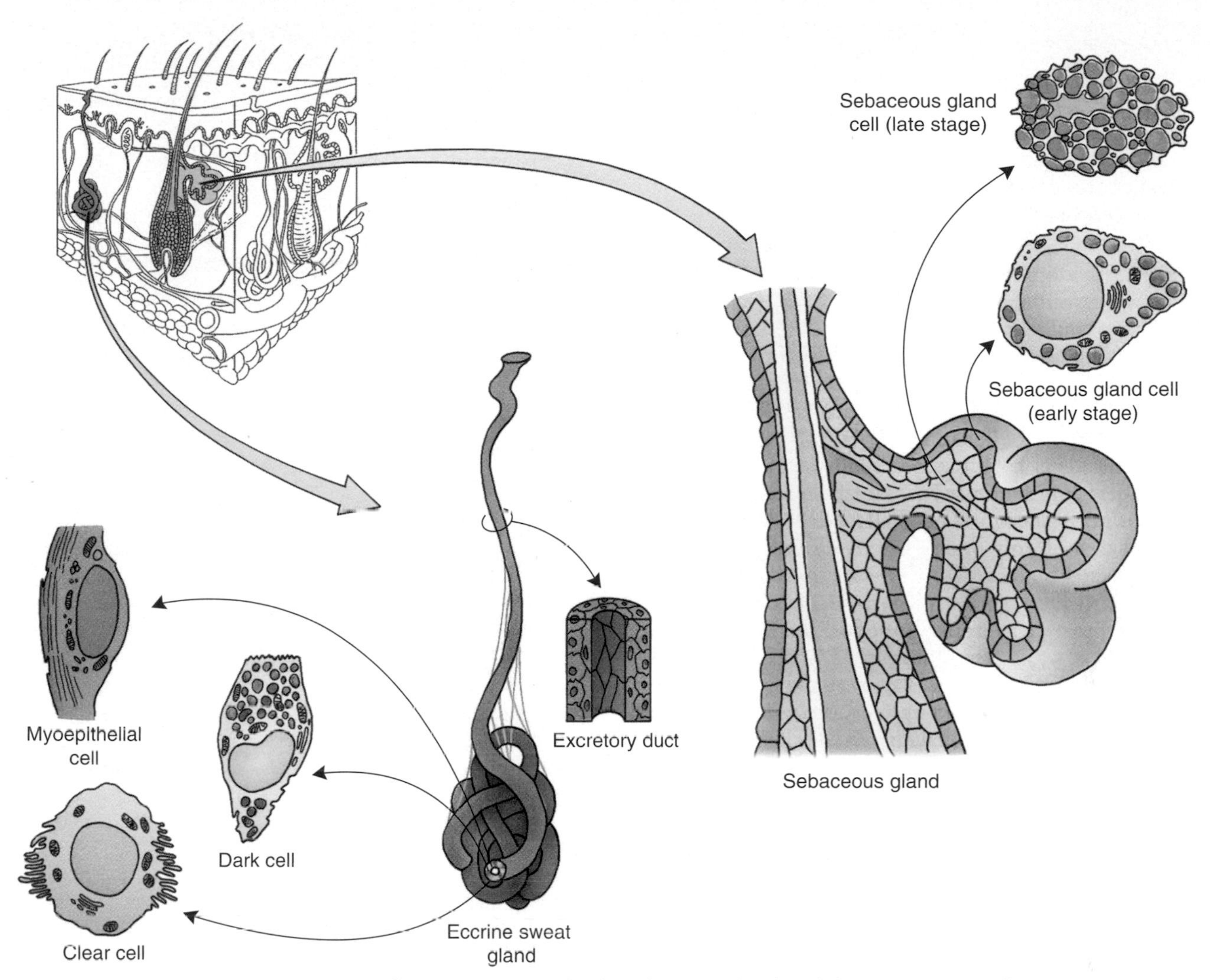

Fig. 14.14 Diagram of an eccrine sweat gland, a sebaceous gland, and their constituent cells.

Sebaceous Glands

Sebaceous glands secrete an oily substance known as sebum, which maintains the suppleness of the skin.

Except for the palms of the hands, soles of the feet, and sides of the feet inferior to the hairline, **sebaceous glands** are present throughout the body, embedded in the dermis and hypodermis. These glands are most abundant on the face, scalp, and forehead. The secretory product of the sebaceous glands, **sebum**, is a wax-like, oily mixture of cholesterol, triglycerides, and secretory cellular debris. Sebum is believed to facilitate the maintenance of proper skin texture and hair flexibility. Additionally, sebum has antimicrobial properties and assists in preventing watery fluids from entering or leaving skin.

Similar to apocrine sweat glands, sebaceous glands are appendages of hair follicles. The ducts of the sebaceous glands open into the upper third of the follicular canal, where they discharge their secretory product to coat the hair shaft and, eventually, coat the skin surface (see Fig. 14.14). The ducts of sebaceous glands in certain regions of the body lacking hair follicles (i.e., the lips, glans penis, areola of the nipples, labia minora, and mucous surface of the prepuce) open onto the surface of the skin to empty their secretions. These glands are under the influence of sex hormones and increase their activity greatly after puberty.

Sebaceous glands are lobular, with clusters of acini opening into single short ducts. Each acinus is composed of peripherally located small basal cells (resting on the basal lamina), which surround larger round cells that fill the remainder of the acinus (Figs. 14.15 and 14.16). The basal cells have a spherical nucleus, both smooth and RER, glycogen, and lipid droplets. These cells undergo cell division to form more basal cells and larger round cells. The larger cells have abundant smooth ER and cytoplasm filled with lipid droplets. The central region of the acinus is filled with cells in different stages of degeneration. These pale-staining cells display only strands of cytoplasm; deeply staining, pyknotic nuclei; ruptured plasmalemmae; and coalescing lipid droplets. Lipid synthesis continues for a short time followed by necrosis of the cells and the ultimate release of lipid and cellular debris, which form the secretory product (i.e., **holocrine secretion**). The secretory product is released into a duct lined with a stratified squamous epithelium that is continuous with the follicular canal at the hair follicle.

Clinical Correlations

Acne, the most common disease seen by dermatologists, is a chronic inflammatory disease involving the sebaceous glands and hair follicles. Obstructions resulting from impaction of sebum and keratinous debris within hair follicles is one cause of acne lesions. Anaerobic bacteria near these obstructions may contribute to development of acne, although the role of bacteria is not clear. However, the efficacy of antibiotic treatment for acne supports the idea of bacterial involvement in its pathogenesis. The disease is most severe in boys, with onset commonly from age 9 to 11 years, when increasing levels of sex hormones begin to stimulate the sebaceous glands. Acne usually subsides through the later teen years, but it may not resolve until the fourth decade of life. In some people, acne does not begin until adulthood.

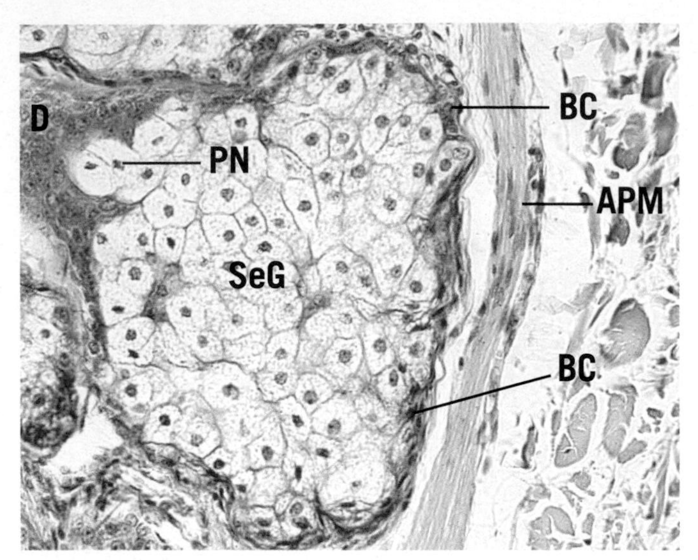

Fig. 14.16 Light micrograph of a medium magnification of a sebaceous gland (SeG) displaying the pyknotic nuclei (PN) of its dying cells that become the sebum emptied into the duct (D) of the sebaceous gland. The basal cells (BC) of the gland have a regenerative function in that they undergo mitotic activity to form new cells. An arrector pili (AP) muscle is present adjacent to the sebaceous gland (APM). (×270)

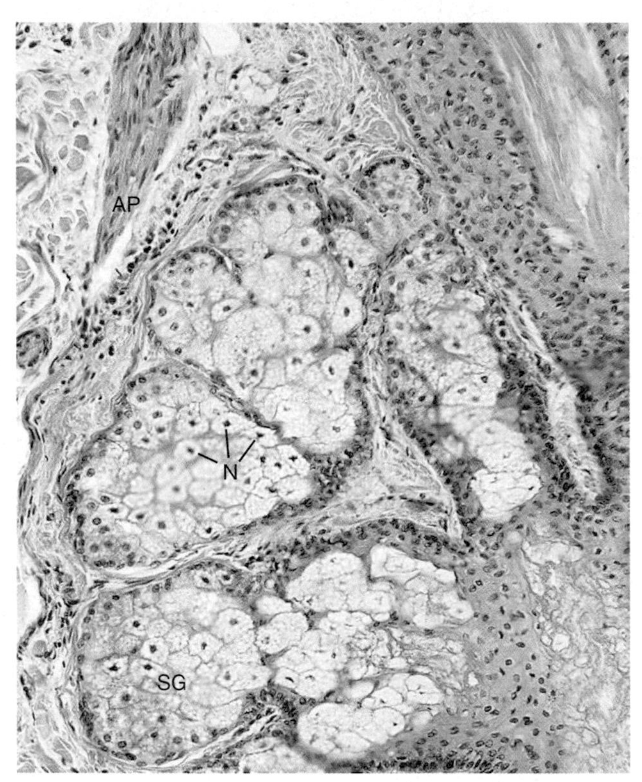

Fig. 14.15 Light micrograph of a human sebaceous gland (SG) whose cells are displaying nuclei (N) and the arrector pili muscle (AP). (×132)

HAIR

Hairs are filamentous, keratinized structures that project from the epidermal surface of the skin (see Fig. 14.1). Hair grows over most of the body except on the vermilion zone of the lips, palms and sides of the palms, soles and sides of the feet, dorsum of the distal phalanges of the fingers and toes, glans penis, glans clitoris, labia minora, and vestibular aspect of the labia majora.

Two types of hairs are present on the human body. Hairs that are soft, fine, short, and pale (e.g., those covering the eyelids) are called ***vellus hairs***; the hard, large, coarse, long, and dark hairs (e.g., those of the scalp and eyebrows) are called ***terminal hairs***. Additionally, very fine hair, called ***lanugo***, is present on fetuses.

The number of hairs on humans is essentially the same as on other primates, but most human hair is of the vellus type, whereas terminal hairs predominate on other primates. Human hair does not provide thermal insulation, as does the fur of animals. Instead, human hairs serve in tactile sensation, such that any stimulus that deforms a hair is translated down the shaft to sensory nerves that surround the hair follicle.

Hair growth is optimal from about 16 to 46 years of age; after age 50 years, hair growth begins to diminish. During pregnancy, hair growth is normal; after delivery, the cycle of hair growth subsides, and hair loss is temporarily increased.

Hair Follicles

Hair follicles develop from the epidermis and invade the dermis and hypodermis.

Hair follicles, the organs from which hairs develop, arise from invaginations of the epidermis that invade the dermis, hypodermis, or both. Hair follicles are surrounded by dense accumulations of fibrous connective tissue belonging to the dermis. A thickened basement membrane, the **glassy membrane**, separates the dermis from the epithelium of the hair follicle. The expanded terminus of the hair follicle, the **hair root**, is indented, and the concavity conforms to the shape of the **dermal papilla** occupying it. The hair root and the dermal papilla together are known as the ***hair bulb***. The dermal papilla contains a rich supply of capillaries that provide nutrients and oxygen for the cells of the hair follicle. Also, the dermal papilla acts as an inductive force controlling the physiological activities of the hair follicle (Figs. 14.17 and 14.18).

The bulk of the cells composing the hair root is called the ***matrix***. Proliferation of these matrix cells (**stem cells**) accounts for the growth of hair; thus, they are homologous to the stratum basale of the epidermis. These stem cells are present even in bald individuals, but the hair follicle cells produce prostaglandin D2, which, acting through the G protein-coupled receptors, prevents the stem cells from entering the cell cycle to form a new hair follicle. The outer layers of follicular epithelium form the **external root sheath**, which is composed of a single layer of cells at the hair bulb and several layers of cells near the surface of the skin (Figs. 14.19–14.21).

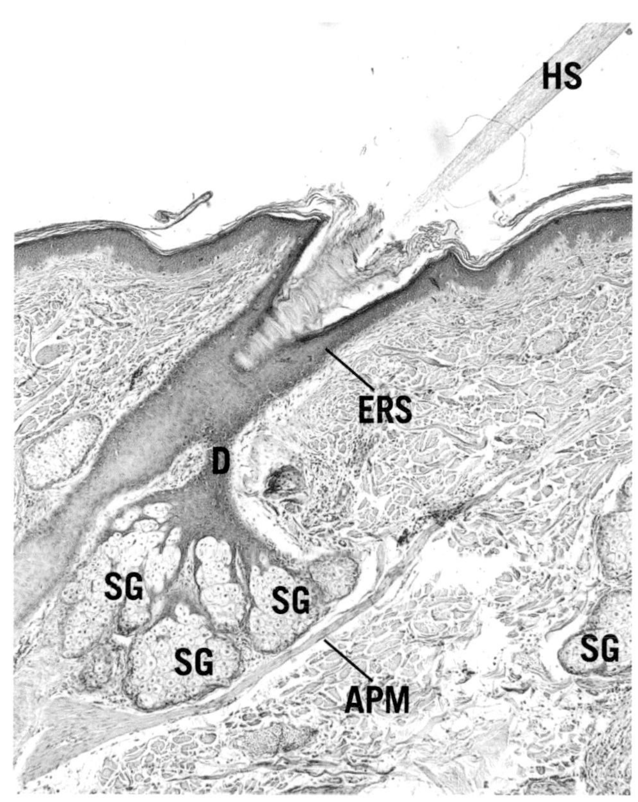

Fig. 14.17 This is a very-low-magnification photomicrograph of thin skin sporting a hair shaft (HS) as it arises from the hair follicle; its external root sheath (ERS) is labeled. Observe that the duct (D) of the sebaceous gland (SG) enters the hair follicle while still within the reticular layer of the dermis. An arrector pili muscle (APM) couches the gland and when the smooth muscle fibers contract, not only does it elevate the hair shaft but it also assists in expressing the sebum from the sebaceous gland. (×56)

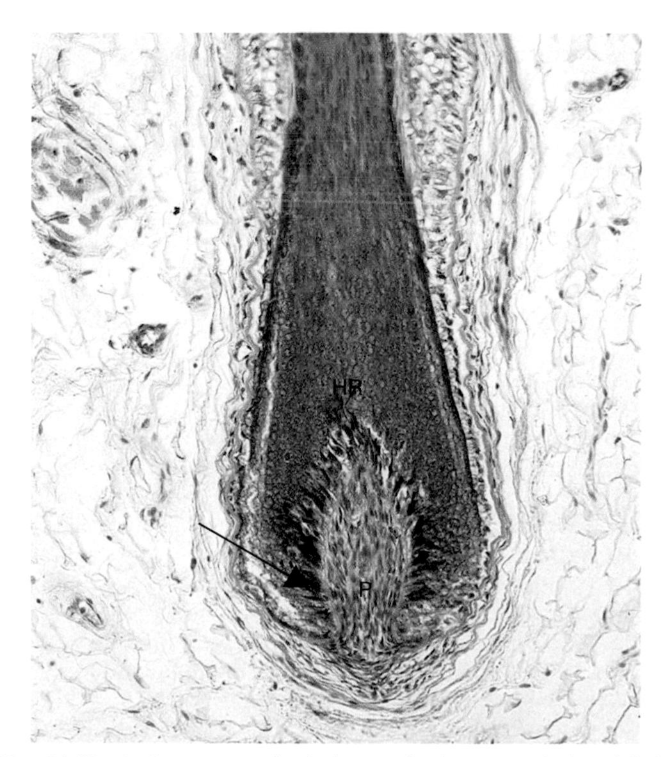

Fig. 14.18 Light micrograph of a longitudinal section of a hair follicle with its hair root (HR) and papilla (P). The dark structure at the tip of the arrow is pigment. (×122)

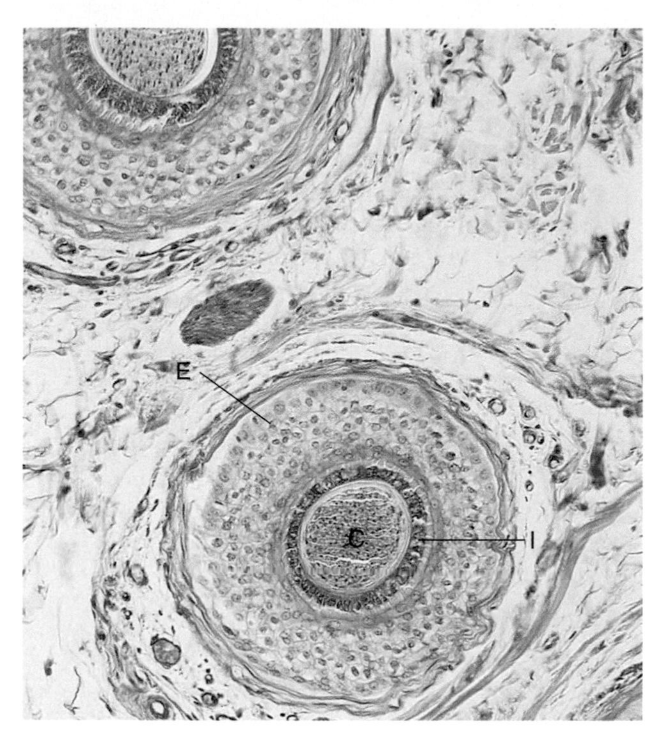

Fig. 14.19 Light micrograph of hair follicles in cross-section (×132). Observe the external root sheath (E), internal root sheath (I), and cortex (C).

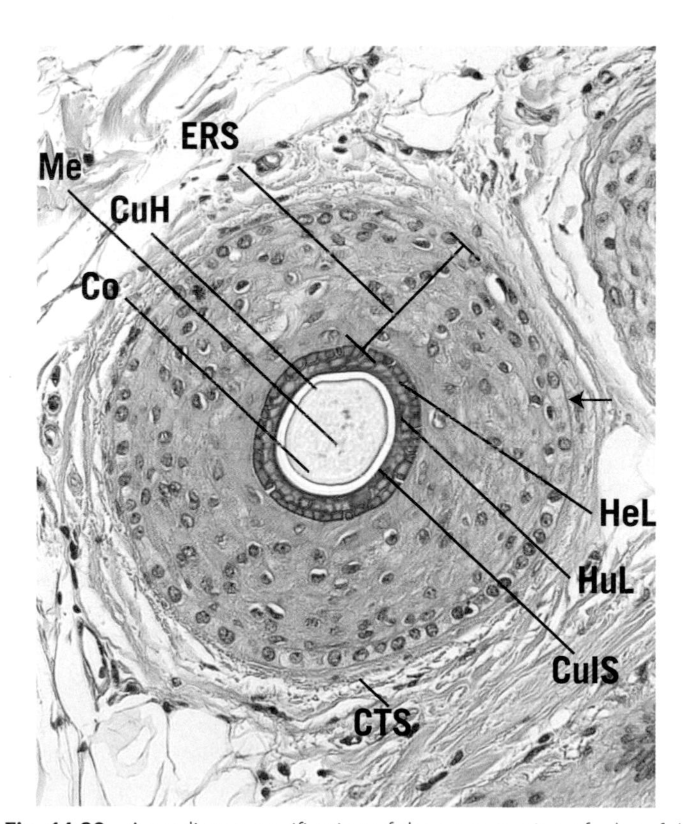

Fig. 14.20 A medium magnification of the cross-section of a hair follicle displays its various components. Note the outermost connective tissue sheath (CTS) that is separated from the epithelially derived components by the glassy membrane, a thickened basement membrane *(arrow)*. The bulk of the hair follicle at this level consists of the external root sheath (ERS) that extends from the basement membrane to the internal root sheath. The internal root sheath, composed of three layers—the Henle layer (HeL), Huxley layer (HuL), and cuticle of the internal root sheath (CuIS)—surrounds the cuticle of the hair (CuH), cortex (Co), and medulla (Me). (×270)

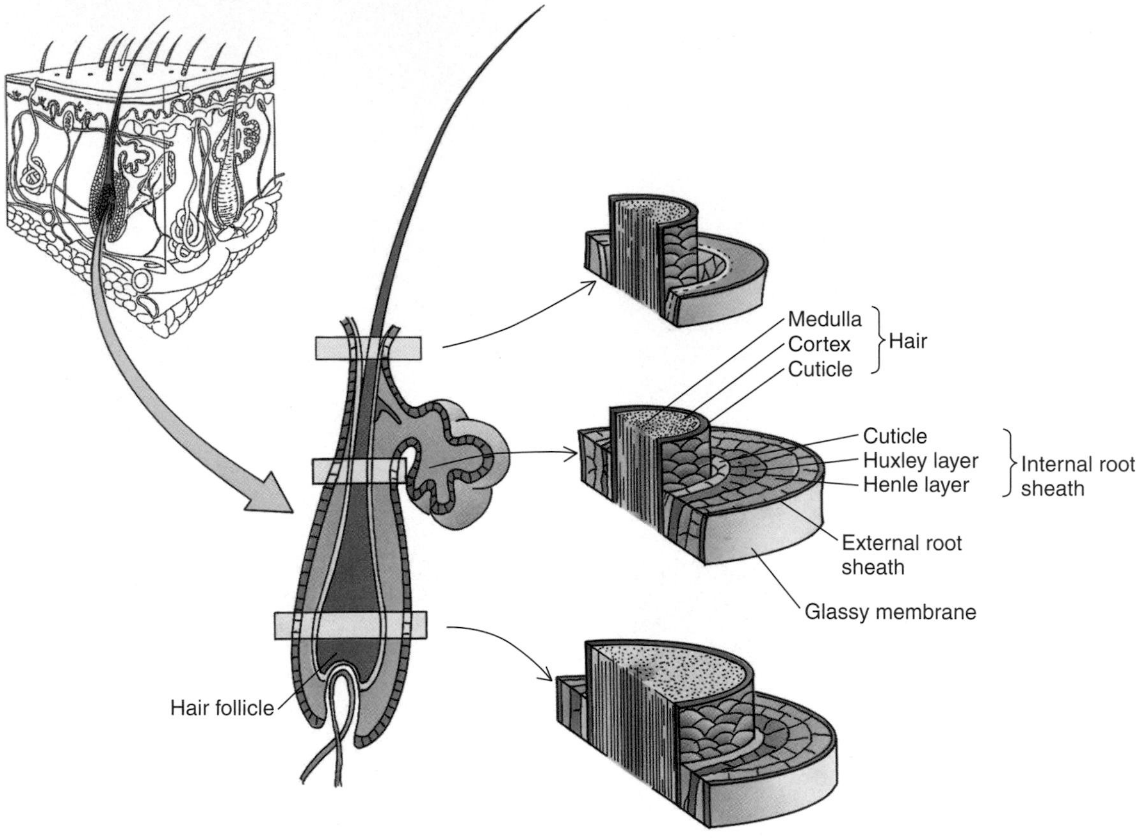

Fig. 14.21 Schematic diagram of the hair follicle.

The external root sheath surrounds several layers of epidermally derived cells, the **internal root sheath**, which consists of three components: (1) an outer single row of cuboidal cells, the **Henle layer**, which contacts the innermost layer of cells of the external root sheath; (2) one or two layers of flattened cells forming the **Huxley layer**; and (3) the **cuticle of the internal root sheath**, formed by overlapping scale-like cells whose free ends project toward the base of the hair follicle. The internal root sheath ends where the duct of the sebaceous gland attaches to the hair follicle (see Fig. 14.21).

The hair shaft is the long, slender filament that extends to and through the surface of the epidermis (Fig. 14.22). It consists of three regions: the **medulla**, **cortex**, and **cuticle of the hair**. As the cells of the matrix within the hair root proliferate and differentiate, they move toward the surface of the skin, eventually developing into the hair shaft (see Figs. 14.20 and 14.21). The cells in the center of the matrix are closest to the underlying dermal papilla and, thus, are most influenced by it. Cells lying increasingly peripheral to the matrix center are progressively less influenced by the dermal papilla. The distinctive layers of the follicle develop from different matrix cells. These matrix cells originate from a swelling of the external root sheath a little above the attachment of the arrector pili muscle known as the **follicular bulge**, which houses a group of slow-cycling **epidermal stem cells**. These stem cells migrate within the external root sheath toward the bulb of the hair follicle and join the cells of the hair matrix. Additional epidermal stem cells migrate toward the surface to enter the lobules of the sebaceous gland, where they replenish the population of basal cells. These epidermal stem cells have the ability to reprogram themselves and replace cells of the epidermis but only if the skin has experienced major trauma.

The distinctive layers of the follicle develop from different matrix cells, as follows:

- The *most central* matrix cells give rise to large vacuolated cells that form the core of the hair shaft (the **medulla**). This layer is present in thick hair only.
- Matrix cells *slightly peripheral* to the center become the **cortex** of the hair shaft.
- *More peripheral* matrix cells become the **cuticle** of the hair.
- The *most peripheral* matrix cells develop into the cells of the three components of the **internal root sheath**: the cuticle of the internal root sheath, Huxley layer, and Henle layer.

As the cells of the cortex are displaced toward the surface, they synthesize abundant **keratin filaments** and **trichohyalin granules** (resembling keratohyalin granules of the epidermis). These granules coalesce, forming an amorphous substance in which the keratin filaments are embedded. Scattered among the cells of the matrix nearest to the dermal papilla are large **melanocytes**, with long dendritic processes that transfer **melanosomes** to the cells of the cortex. The melanosomes remain in these cells, imparting to the hair a color based on the amount of melanin present. With age, the melanocytes gradually lose their ability to produce **tyrosinase**, which is essential for the production of melanin. Additionally, the production of the enzyme catalase is diminished, which increases hydrogen peroxide levels in these cells, bleaching the hair. Consequently, the reduction in the amount of these two enzymes results in the hair turning gray.

Clinical Correlations

As an individual ages, hair color becomes gray, silver, or white and is most noticeable in scalp hair. However, this change in color usually affects body and even pubic hair. There are some cases in which only the pubic hair turns white and may occur at a young age. If the hair becomes brittle and breaks easily, the condition, known as **tinea blanca (white piedra)**, *may be due to a fungal infection by* Piedria horti *and* Trichosporon ashaii *(and other* Trichosporon *species), which form soft nodules that coat the hair and turn it white. Individuals afflicted by this condition are young women who usually live in temperate climates throughout the world. The common cure is shaving the hair off or the use of antifungal creams, such as an ammoniated mercury ointment. If the problem persists, oral antifungal medication may be necessary to alleviate the condition.*

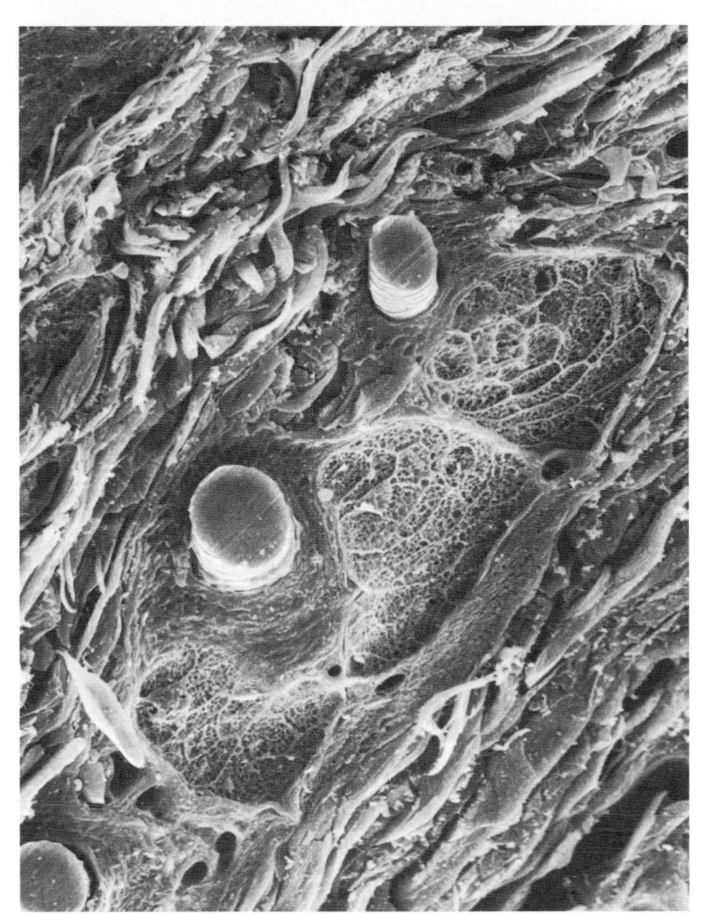

Fig. 14.22 Scanning electron micrograph of monkey scalp that shows three hair shafts and their sebaceous glands surrounded by the dense, irregular, collagenous connective tissue of the dermis (×235). (From Leeson TS, Leeson CR, Paparo AA. *Text/Atlas of Histology*. Philadelphia: WB Saunders; 1998.)

Arrector Pili Muscles

Arrector pili muscles are smooth muscle cells extending from the midshaft of the hair follicle to the papillary layer of the dermis.

Attached to the connective tissue sheath surrounding the hair follicles and to the papillary layer of the dermis are the **arrector pili muscles** (see Figs. 14.1, 14.16, and 14.17). These smooth muscles attach to the hair follicle above its middle at an oblique angle. Contractions of these muscles *depress* the skin over their attachment at the papillary layer of the dermis, *elevating* the hair shaft and the skin around the hair shaft, forming tiny "goose bumps" on the surface of the skin. These are easily observed when one is chilled or suddenly frightened.

Histophysiology of Hair

Although hair grows at an average rate of about 1 to 1.3 cm/month, the growth is not continuous. The hair growth cycle consists of three successive phases: (1) the growth period, the **anagen phase**; (2) a brief period of involution, the **catagen phase**; and (3) the final phase of rest, the **telogen phase**, in which the mature, aged hair is shed (falls out or is pulled out while comb ing or washing). Hairs shed in this fashion are called ***club hairs*** because they retain their club-shaped root. Soon afterward, a new hair is formed by the hair follicle and the hair growth cycle begins again.

The duration of the hair growth cycle varies in different areas of the body. For example, the life span of an axillary hair is roughly 4 months, whereas scalp hair may remain in the anagen phase for as long as 7 years and in the telogen phase for 4 months.

Hair follicles in certain regions of the body respond to male sex hormones. For this reason, men begin to develop more dark-pigmented terminal hairs about the chin, cheeks, and upper lip at puberty. Although women possess the same number of hair follicles in these regions, these hairs on women remain of the fine, pale, vellus type. In both sexes at puberty, however, heavily pigmented, coarse terminal hairs begin to grow in the axillary and pubic regions.

The keratinization processes in hair and skin, although generally similar, differ in some respects. The superficial cell layers of the epidermis of the skin form a **soft keratin**, consisting of keratin filaments embedded in trichohyalin and filaggrin; the keratinized cells are sloughed continuously. In contrast, not only does keratinization of hair form a **hard keratin**, consisting of keratin filaments embedded in trichohyalin, but not filaggrin, but the keratinizing cells are not shed. Instead, they accumulate, becoming compressed and hard.

The arrangement of cells composing the cuticle of the hair and cuticle of the internal root sheath interlocks the opposing free edges of these cells, making it difficult to pull the hair shaft out of its follicle (Fig. 14.23).

NAILS

Nails represent keratinized epithelial cells arranged in plates of hard keratin.

Nails, located on the distal phalanx of each finger and toe, are composed of plates of heavily compacted, highly keratinized epithelial cells that form the **nail plate**, lying on the epidermis, known as the ***nail bed*** (Figs. 14.24– 14.26). The nails develop from cells of the **nail matrix** that proliferate and become keratinized. The nail matrix, a region of the **nail root**, is located beneath the **proximal nail fold**. The stratum corneum of the proximal nail fold forms the **eponychium** (**cuticle**), which extends from the proximal end up on the nail for about 0.5 to 1 mm. Laterally, the skin turns under as **lateral nail folds**, forming the **lateral nail grooves**. The epidermis continues beneath

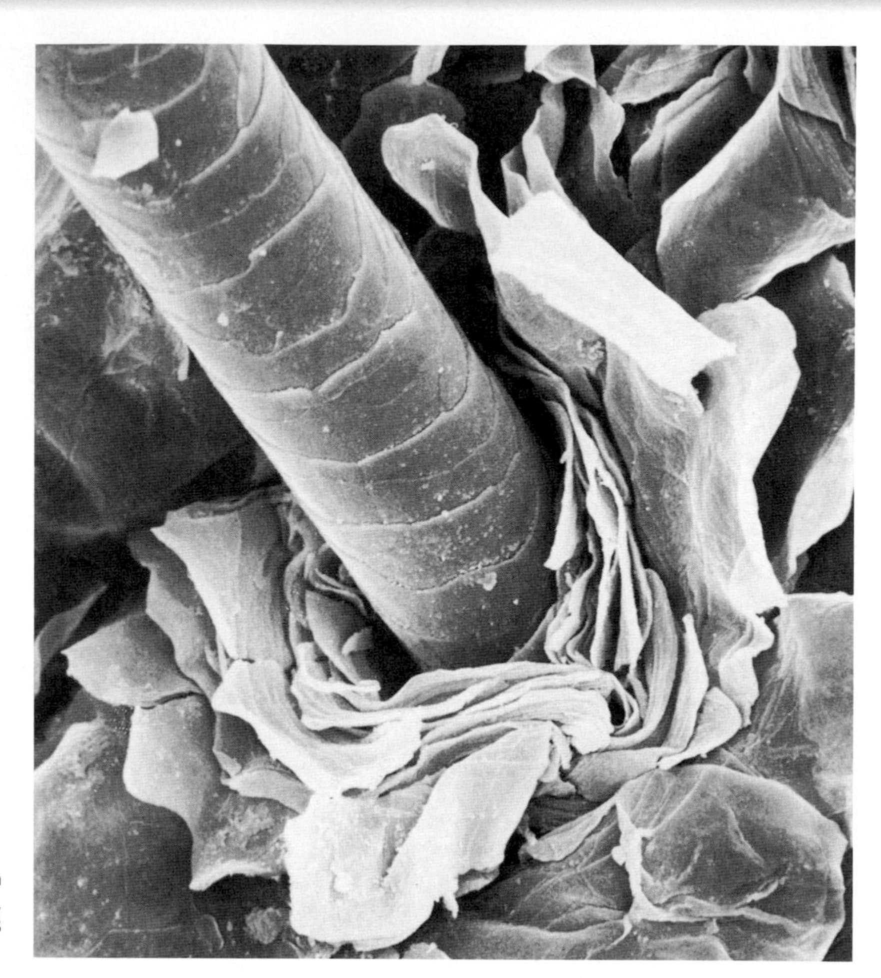

Fig. 14.23 Scanning electron micrograph of a hair from a monkey's scalp (×1115). (From Leeson TS, Leeson CR, Paparo AA. *Text/Atlas of Histology*. Philadelphia: WB Saunders; 1988.)

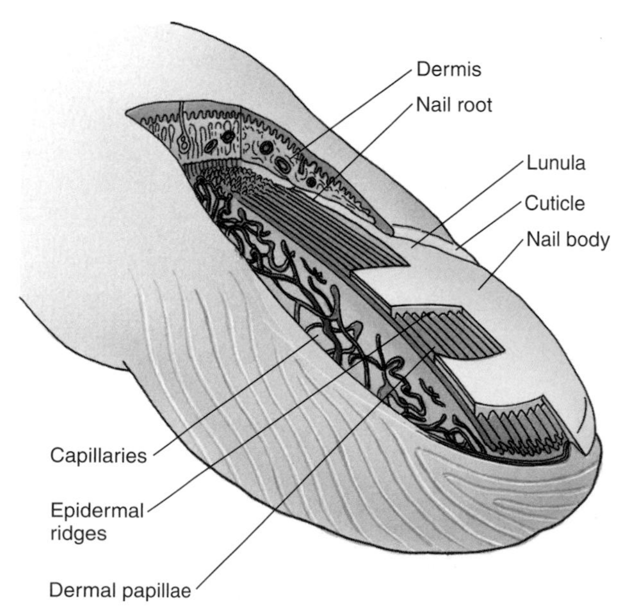

Fig. 14.24 Diagram of the structure of the thumbnail.

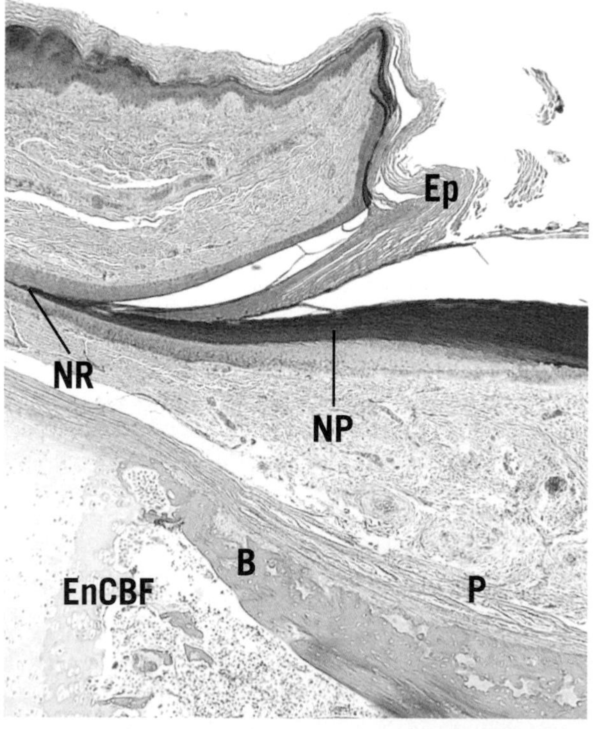

Fig. 14.25 This very-low-magnification photomicrograph of the nail root (NR), nail plate (NP), and eponychium (Ep) also displays the endochondral bone formation (EnCBF) of the distal phalanx with its subperiosteal bone collar (B) and its periosteum (P). The light-pink region just below the deep red of the nail plate is the nail bed. (×14)

the nail plate as the **nail bed**, and the nail plate occupies the position (and function) of the stratum corneum.

The **lunula**, the white crescent, is observed at the proximal end of the nail. The distal end of the nail plate is not attached to the nail bed, which becomes continuous with the skin of the finger (or toe) tip. Near this junction is an accumulation of stratum

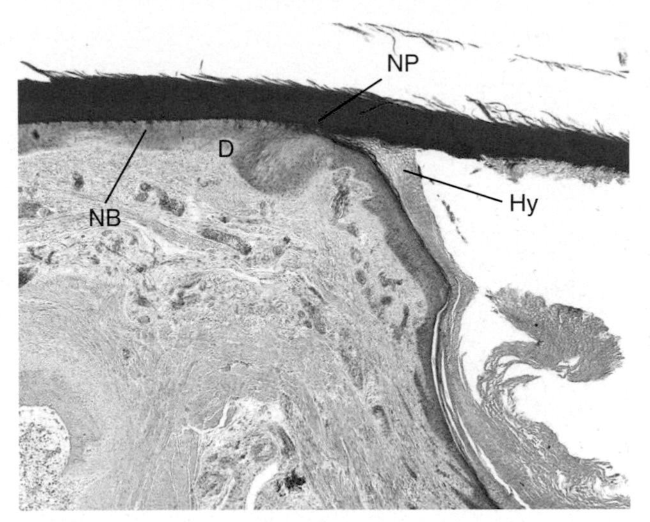

Fig. 14.26 Longitudinal section through a fingernail. Observe the dermis (D), hyponychium (Hy), nail bed (NB), and the nail plate (NP), whose continuation at and past the hyponychium is the nail. (×14)

corneum called the **hyponychium**. Fingernails grow continuously at the rate of about 0.5 mm/week; toenails grow somewhat slower. The translucency of the fingernails provides a quick indication of the health of an individual; pinkness indicates a well-oxygenated blood supply.

Pathological Considerations

See Figs. 14.27 through 14.30.

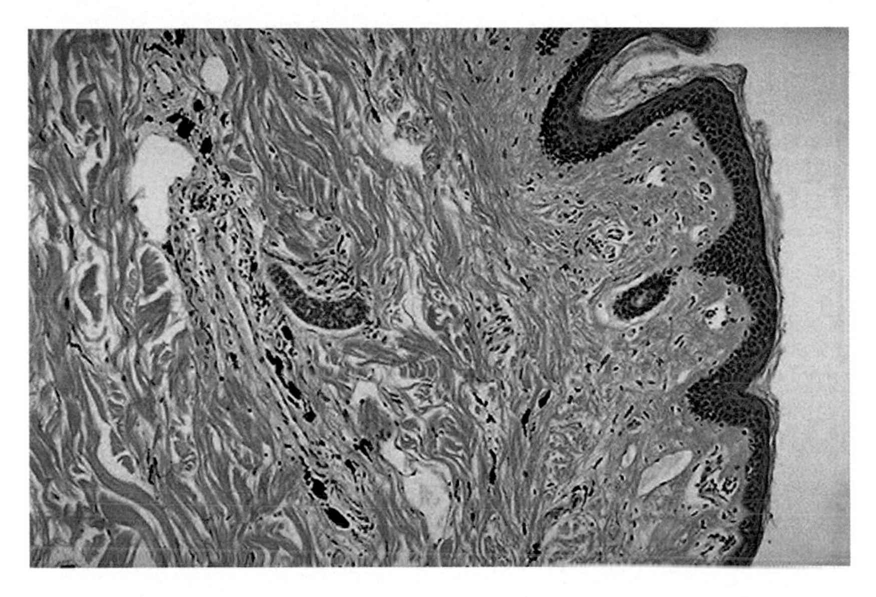

Fig. 14.27 Photomicrograph of a lateral surface of a hand with a tattoo. Note that there are tattoo pigments in the dermis. Because the pigment is deposited rather deep in the dermis, it is very difficult to remove it at a later date. Also, unless the tattooing conditions are very clean, infections may be introduced at the same time. (Reprinted with permission from Klatt EC. *Robbins and Cotran: Pathological Basis of Disease*. 2nd ed. Philadelphia: Elsevier; 2010:5.)

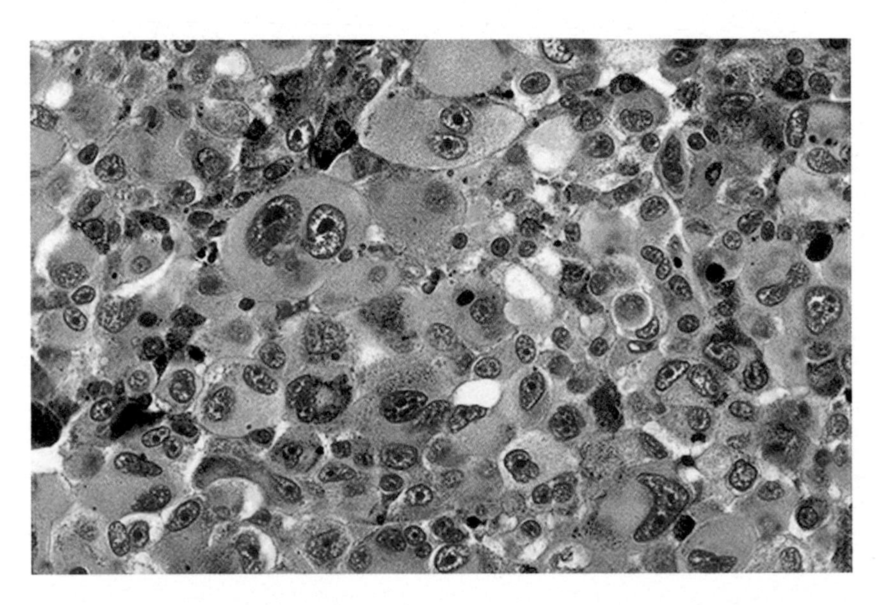

Fig. 14.28 Photomicrograph of a malignant melanoma. Note the large polygonal cells with pleomorphic nuclei and clearly evident nucleoli. The amount of pigment in melanoma cells is inconstant; this variability in pigment formation permits the differentiation of melanoma from a benign nevus. (Reprinted with permission from Klatt EC. *Robbins and Cotran: Pathological Basis of Disease*. 2nd ed. Philadelphia: Elsevier; 2010:406.)

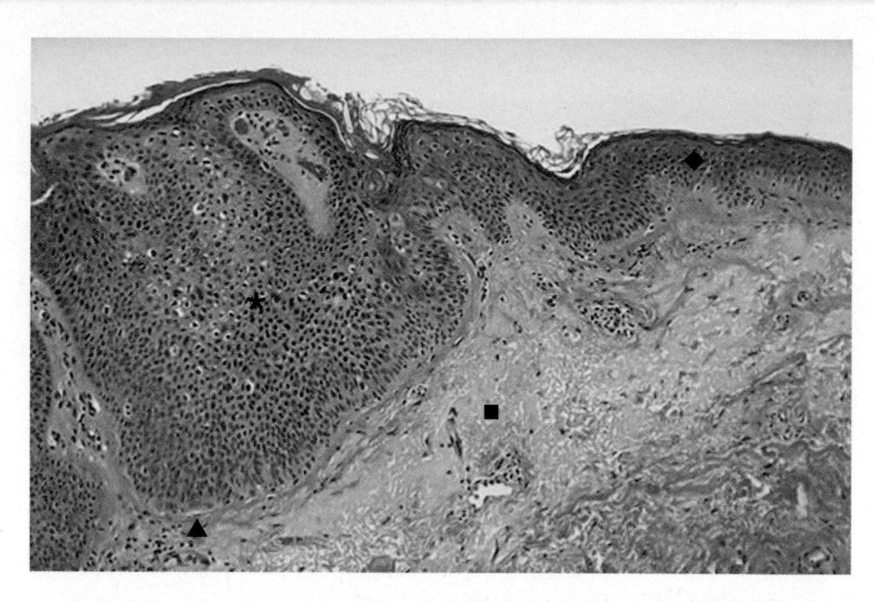

Fig. 14.29 Photomicrograph of a squamous cell carcinoma in situ. The reason for the term *in situ* is that the lesion did not pass through the basement membrane *(triangle)*. The right side of the photomicrograph presents healthy, normal skin *(diamond)*, whereas the cancerous epidermis is very thick *(asterisk)*. Observe the ultraviolet ray–damaged dermis, where the collagen fibers are pale, referred to as *solar elastosis*. (Reprinted with permission from Klatt EC. *Robbins and Cotran: Pathological Basis of Disease*. 2nd ed. Philadelphia: Elsevier; 2010:412.)

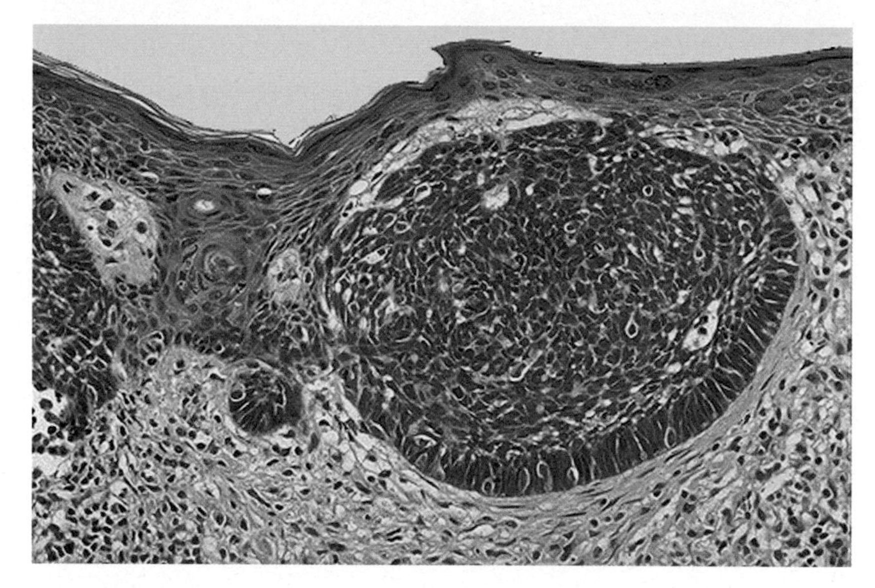

Fig. 14.30 Photomicrograph of a basal cell carcinoma. The dark-blue malignant cells are more or less elliptical, with very little cytoplasm. Most of the cells are similar to cells of the stratum basale of the normal epidermis. The tumor cells are compacted into islands or peninsulas that infiltrate the dermis and are surrounded by a fibrous stroma that displays variable degrees of inflammatory cells. Patients who have been chronically exposed to the sun and those who are immunosuppressed with xeroderma pigmentosum frequently develop basal cell carcinoma. (Reprinted with permission from Klatt EC. *Robbins and Cotran: Pathological Basis of Disease*. 2nd ed. Philadelphia: Elsevier; 2010:413.)

Histology Laboratory Instructions: Integument

Thick Skin

A low magnification of thick skin demonstrates that the epidermis and dermis interdigitate, forming epidermal ridges and dermal ridges, respectively. The thick layer of the stratum corneum shows that its superficial-most layer is in the process of sloughing off. The rich vascular supply of the dermis is clearly evident (see Fig. 14.2, E, D, ER, DR, BV). At high magnification, the single layer of cells of the stratum basale are noted to be separated from the dermis by a basement membrane. The stratum spinosum is composed of a thick layer of cells that form intercellular bridges with each other (see Fig. 14.3, SB, SS).

Thin Skin

Viewed at low magnification, the epidermis of thin skin is much thinner than that of thick skin and the interface between the epidermis and the papillary layer of the dermis is not nearly as convoluted as that of thick skin. The reticular layer of the dermis is considerably coarser than the papillary layer. Note the presence of hair follicles, sebaceous glands, and eccrine sweat glands in the reticular layer of the dermis (see Fig. 14.5, Ep, PL, De, RL, HF, SeG, SwG). At medium magnification, the three layers of the epidermis—the stratum basale, stratum spinosum, and stratum corneum, whose surface-most layer is sloughing off—are easily identified. The collagen fibers of the reticular layers are seen to be much coarser than those of the papillary layer and the nuclei of fibroblasts are darker and denser in the reticular layer. A hair follicle is sectioned longitudinally as it ascends in the dermis and meets the epidermis (see Fig. 14.6, Ep, SB, SS, SC, *arrow*, CF, RL, PL, F, HF). At high magnification, the three layers of the epidermis—the stratum basale, stratum spinosum, and the stratum corneum, with its desquamating surface-most layers—are well represented. The epithelial ridges interdigitate with the dermal ridges formed by the papillary layer of the dermis, with its rich blood supply (see Fig. 14.7, SB, SS, SC, Sq, boxed area, PL, BV).

Meissner Corpuscle

At high magnification, the skin of a fingertip displays the presence of a Meissner corpuscle, whose oval to pear shape is composed of three or four nerve terminals and their associated Schwann cells, all surrounded by connective tissue elements of the dermal ridge and flanked by epidermal ridges. The five layers of the epidermis of thick skin—the stratum basale, stratum spinosum, stratum granulosum, stratum lucidum, and the beginning layer of the stratum corneum—are well represented (see Fig. 14.10, MC, DP, ER, SB, SS, SG, SL, SC).

Eccrine Sweat Gland

Low magnification of an eccrine sweat gland demonstrates how tightly coiled sweat glands are. The secretory portion of the gland is composed of a simple cuboidal epithelium with its narrow lumen. The duct portion of the gland is composed of a stratified cuboidal epithelium consisting of two layers of cells. The duct portion stains darker than the secretory portion because its cells are shorter and have smaller, denser nuclei (see Fig. 14.11, S, d). At medium magnification, the differences between the duct and secretory portion of an eccrine sweat gland are very evident. The nuclei of fibroblasts of the dermis as well as the adipose tissue flanking the sweat gland are easy to see (see Fig. 14.12, D, SA, *arrows*, De, A). At high magnification, the rich vascularity of the eccrine sweat gland is very evident. The simple cuboidal epithelium composing the secretory portion as well as the stratified cuboidal epithelium of the duct portion are well demonstrated, as are the nuclei of the myoepithelial cells of the secretory component (see Fig. 14.13, BV, SA, D, *arrows*).

Sebaceous Gland

Lobules of a sebaceous gland open into a single duct that empties into the lumen of a hair follicle. The nuclei of the cells of the sebaceous gland are noted to vary from healthy to pyknotic, indicative of the status of the cell. Arrector pili muscles are able to squeeze the sebum into the duct by undergoing contraction (see Fig. 14.15, SG, N, AP). Medium magnification of a sebaceous gland lobule displays the basal cells that undergo mitosis to add to the number of sebum-forming cells. Nuclei of the new cells change from a normal, healthy appearance to pyknotic as the accumulation of sebum destroys the cell, which becomes the secretory product of this holocrine gland. Arrector pili muscles are always in close association with sebaceous glands, squeezing the sebum into the duct of the gland and, from there, into the lumen of the hair follicle (see Fig. 14.16, SeG, BC, pN, D, APM, D).

Hair

At very low magnification of thin skin, the hair shaft, external root sheath of the hair follicle, its associated sebaceous gland and duct, as well as the arrector pili muscle, are all evident (see Fig. 14.17, HS, ERS, SG, D, APM). At low magnification of the hair root, the dermal papilla and melanin pigment containing melanocytes are easily identified (see Fig. 14.18, HR, P, *arrow*). A low-magnification cross-section of a hair follicle from the scalp displays the thick external root sheath and narrow but more colorful internal root sheath, as well as the centrally positioned cortex (see Fig. 14.19, E, I, C). At medium magnification of a hair follicle in cross-section, all of the layers can be identified. The outermost connective tissue sheath is derived from the dermis and is separated from the external root sheath by a thickened basement membrane, known as the glassy membrane. The external root sheath varies in thickness, being only a single layer thick at the hair bulb to being several cell layers thick just below where the duct of the sebaceous gland attaches to the hair follicle. The external root sheath surrounds the internal root sheath, which is composed of three layers: the Henle layer, which contacts the external root sheath; the deeper Huxley layer; and the deepest cuticle of the internal root sheath. The central portion of the hair follicle is the hair shaft, composed of three layers: the cuticle of the hair, cortex, and medulla. The medulla is present only in thick hair (see Fig. 14.20, CTS, ERS, *arrow*, HeL, HuL, CuIS, CuH, Co, Me).

Nail

At very low magnification, the proximal portion of the nail presents the eponychium (cuticle) as well as the nail root and its outgrowth, the nail plate, which lies on an epidermal structure, known as the nail bed. Deep to that is the dermis of the finger, whose lower region merges with the periosteum of the distal phalanx. In a young individual, endochondral bone formation is lengthening the finger (see Fig. 14.25, Ep, NR, NP, P, B, EnCBF). A very low magnification photomicrograph of the distal portion of the nail presents the hyponychium, located at the region where the distal portion of the nail plate is no longer lying on the nail bed. At that point, the nail bed is continuous with the epidermis under the free edge of the nail plate and overlies the dermis (see Fig. 14.26, Hy, NB, D).

15 Respiratory System

The lungs and the airways leading to the external environment constitute the **respiratory system**, whose role is to provide oxygen (O_2) to and eliminate carbon dioxide (CO_2) from the cells of the body. The following four events, collectively known as **respiration**, have to occur in order to accomplish this task:

- Air has to move in and out of the lungs (**breathing** or **ventilation**)
- O_2 in the inspired air has to be exchanged for CO_2 in the blood (**external respiration**)
- O_2 and CO_2 have to be conveyed to and from the cells (**transport of gases**)
- CO_2 has to be exchanged for O_2 in the vicinity of the cells (**internal respiration**)

Only ventilation and external respiration occur within the confines of the respiratory system; the transport of gases is performed by the circulatory system, and internal respiration occurs in the cells throughout the body.

The respiratory system has two major components: the conducting portion and respiratory portion. The **conducting portion** conveys air from the external environment into the lungs. Therefore, it is located both within and external to the lungs. The **respiratory portion** functions in the actual exchange of oxygen for carbon dioxide (external respiration) and is located strictly within the lungs. Characteristic features of these two portions are listed in Table 15.1.

Conducting Portion of the Respiratory System

The conducting portion of the respiratory system conveys air to and from the respiratory portion of the respiratory system.

The **conducting portion** of the respiratory system, listed in order from the exterior to the inside of the lung, is composed of the nasal cavity, mouth, nasopharynx, pharynx, larynx, trachea, primary bronchi, secondary bronchi (lobar bronchi), tertiary bronchi (segmental bronchi), bronchioles, and terminal bronchioles. These structures not only transport but also filter, moisten, and warm the inspired air before it reaches the respiratory portion of the lungs.

A combination of bone, cartilage, and fibrous elements is responsible for keeping the conducting portion of the airways open. As the air progresses along the airway during inspiration, it encounters a branching system of tubules. Although the luminal diameter of each succeeding tubule continues to decrease, the total cross-sectional diameter of the various branches increases at each level of branching. As a result, the velocity of air flow for a given volume of inhaled air decreases as the air proceeds toward the respiratory portion.

NASAL CAVITY

The **nasal cavity** is divided into right and left halves by the cartilaginous and bony **nasal septum** (Figs. 15.1 and 15.2). Each half of the nasal cavity is bounded laterally by a bony wall and a cartilaginous **ala** (**wing**) of the nose; it communicates with the outside, anteriorly, via the **naris** (nostril) and with the nasopharynx by way of the **choana**. Projecting from the bony lateral wall are three thin, scroll-like bony shelves, situated one above the other: the superior, middle, and inferior **nasal conchae**.

Anterior Portion of the Nasal Cavity (Vestibule)

The anterior portion of the nasal cavity, in the vicinity of the nares, is dilated and is known as the ***vestibule***. This region is lined with thin skin and has **vibrissae**—short, stiff hairs that prevent larger dust particles from entering the nasal cavity. The dermis of the vestibule, housing numerous sebaceous and sweat glands, is anchored by an abundance of type I collagen fiber bundles to the perichondria of the hyaline cartilage segments that form the supporting skeleton of the ala.

Clinical Correlations

1. *Nasal bleeding usually occurs from the* **Kiesselbach area**, *the anteroinferior region of the nasal septum, which is the site of anastomosis of the arterial supply of the nasal mucosa. The bleeding may be arrested by applying pressure on the region or by packing the nasal cavity with cotton.*
2. *People who abuse drugs by intranasal inhalation frequently experience necrosis of the nasal and palatal tissues. Although the drugs of choice are most frequently cocaine, other narcotics, and prescription analgesics, there were several cases reported of combined opioid-acetaminophen inhalation-induced perforation of the nasopharynx, the posterior nasal septum, and of the palate.*

Posterior Aspect of the Nasal Cavity

Except for the vestibule and the olfactory region, the nasal cavity is lined by **respiratory epithelium** (**pseudostratified ciliated columnar epithelium**), which is well endowed with goblet cells in the more posterior regions of the nasal cavity. The subepithelial connective tissue (**lamina propria**) is richly vascularized, especially in the region of the conchae and the anterior aspect of the nasal septum, housing large arterial plexuses and venous sinuses. The lamina propria has many seromucous glands and abundant lymphoid elements, including occasional lymphoid nodules, mast cells, and plasma cells. Antibodies produced by plasma cells (immunoglobulins IgA, IgE, and IgG) protect the nasal mucosa against inhaled antigens, as well as against microbial invasion.

TABLE 15.1 **Characteristic Features of the Respiratory System**

Division	Region	Support	Glands	Epithelium	Cell Types	Additional Features
Extrapulmonary conducting	Nasal vestibule	Hyaline cartilage	Sebaceous and sweat glands	Stratified squamous keratinized	Epidermal	Vibrissae
	Nasal cavity: respiratory	Hyaline cartilage and bone	Seromucous glands	Respiratory	Basal, goblet, ciliated, brush, serous, and DNES	Erectile-like tissue
	Nasal cavity: olfactory	Bone	Bowman glands (serous)	Olfactory	Olfactory, sustentacular, and basal	Olfactory vesicle
Extrapulmonary conducting	Nasopharynx	Skeletal muscle	Seromucous glands	Respiratory	Basal, goblet, ciliated, brush, serous, and DNES	Pharyngeal tonsils and eustachian tubes
	Larynx	Hyaline and elastic cartilages	Mucous and seromucous glands	Respiratory and stratified squamous nonkeratinized	Basal, goblet, ciliated, brush, serous, and DNES	Epiglottis, vocal folds, and vestibular folds
	Trachea and primary bronchi	Hyaline cartilage and dense, irregular collagenous connective tissue	Mucous and seromucous glands	Respiratory	Basal, goblet, ciliated, brush, serous, and DNES	C-rings and trachealis muscle (smooth muscle) in adventitia
Intrapulmonary conducting	Secondary (intrapulmonary) bronchi	Hyaline cartilage and smooth muscle	Seromucous glands	Respiratory	Basal, goblet, ciliated, brush, serous, and DNES	Plates of hyaline cartilage and two ribbons of helically oriented smooth muscle
	(Primary) Bronchioles	Smooth muscle	No glands	Simple columnar to simple cuboidal	Ciliated cells and club cells (and occasional goblet cells in larger bronchioles)	Less than 1 mm in diameter; supply air to lobules; two ribbons of helically oriented smooth muscle
	Terminal bronchioles	Smooth muscle	No glands	Simple cuboidal	Some ciliated cells and many club cells (no goblet cells)	Less than 0.5 mm in diameter; supply air to lung acini; some smooth muscle
Respiratory	Respiratory bronchioles	Some smooth muscle and collagen fibers	No glands	Simple cuboidal and highly attenuated simple squamous	Some ciliated cuboidal cells, club cells, and types I and II pneumocytes	Alveoli in their walls; alveoli have smooth muscle sphincters in their opening
	Alveolar ducts	Type III collagen (reticular) fibers and smooth muscle sphincters of alveoli	No glands	Highly attenuated simple squamous	Type I and type II pneumocytes of alveoli	No walls of their own, only a linear sequence of alveoli
	Alveolar sacs	Type III collagen and elastic fibers	No glands	Highly attenuated simple squamous	Type I and type II pneumocytes	Clusters of alveoli
	Alveoli	Type III collagen and elastic fibers	No glands	Highly attenuated simple squamous	Type I and type II pneumocytes	200 μm in diameter; have alveolar macrophages

DNES, Diffuse neuroendocrine system.

Clinical Correlations

*There are approximately 50 species of bacteria that inhabit the human nasal passages. One of these species is present in 30% of humans—*Staphylococcus aureus*, whose methicillin-resistant strain (MRSA) causes severe, frequently lethal, infections. Interestingly, of the patients who had* Staphylococcus lugdunensis *in their nasal passages, less than 6% carried* S. aureus*, whereas more than 30% of patients without* S. lugdunensis *carried* S. aureus*. It appears that* S. lugdunensis *produces an antibiotic,* ***lugdunin****, that kills not only MRSA but also vancomycin-resistant* E. coli.

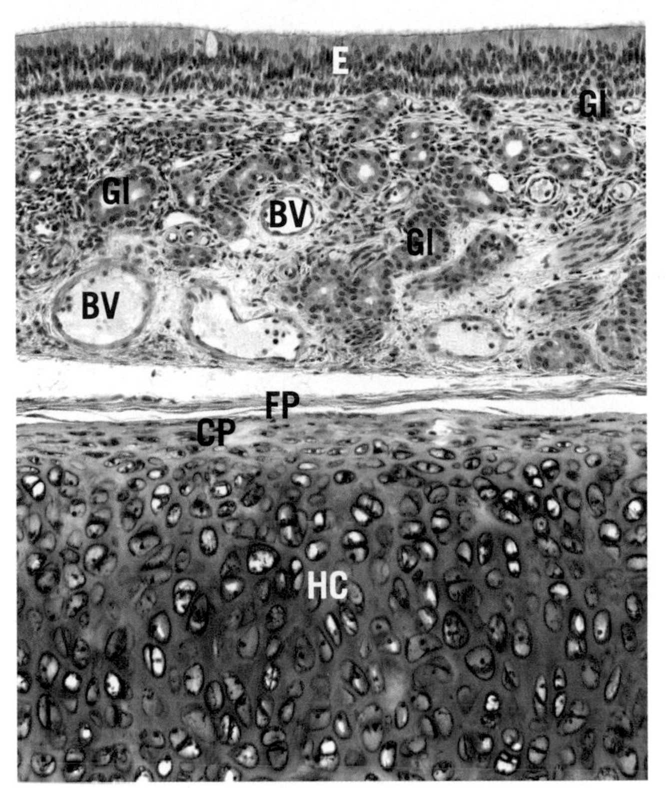

Fig. 15.1 This low-magnification photomicrograph is from the cartilaginous portion of the nasal septum. Observe the hyaline cartilage (HC) with its cellular (CP) and fibrous perichondria (FP). Observe the rich vascular supply (BV) and the seromucous glands (Gl) of the lamina propria whose ducts pierce the pseudostratified ciliated columnar epithelium that lines the nasal cavity. (×132)

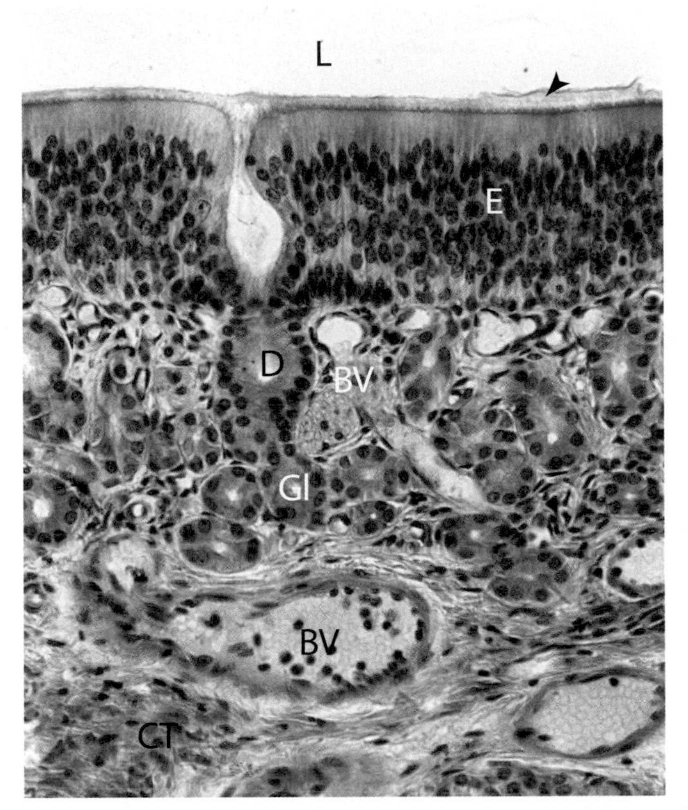

Fig. 15.2 This medium-magnification photomicrograph of the nasal septum highlights the vascularity (BV) of the lamina propria (CT). Observe that the duct (D) of a seromucous gland (Gl) pierces the pseudostratified ciliated columnar epithelium (E) that lines the nasal cavity (L). The cilia *(arrowhead)* of the columnar epithelial cells are well delineated. (×270)

Olfactory Region of the Nasal Cavity

The olfactory region comprises the olfactory epithelium and the underlying lamina propria that houses Bowman glands and a rich vascular plexus.

The roof of the nasal cavity, the superior aspect of the nasal septum, and the superior concha are covered by an olfactory epithelium 60 μm thick. The underlying lamina propria houses the serous fluid–secreting Bowman glands, a rich vascular plexus, and collections of axons that arise from the olfactory cells of the **olfactory epithelium**. The olfactory epithelium, which has a yellow color in the living person, is composed of three types of cells: olfactory, sustentacular, and basal (Fig. 15.3).

Olfactory Cells

Olfactory cells are bipolar neurons whose peripheral (distal) aspect is modified to form the olfactory vesicle and olfactory cilia, whereas its central aspect forms an axon that joins other axons to synapse in the olfactory bulb.

Olfactory cells are bipolar neurons whose apical aspect, the distal terminus of its slender dendrite, is modified to form a bulb, the **olfactory vesicle**, which projects above the surface of the sustentacular cells (Figs. 15.4 and 15.5). The nucleus of the olfactory cell is spherical and is slightly closer to the basal lamina than to the olfactory vesicle. Most of the organelles of the cell are located near the nucleus.

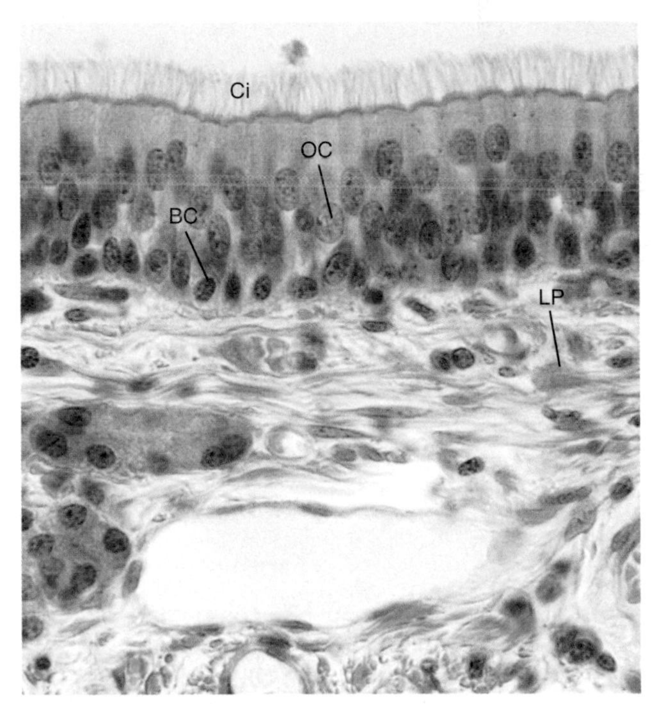

Fig. 15.3 Photomicrograph of the human olfactory mucosa. Observe that the olfactory cilia (Ci) are well represented and that the connective tissue displays the presence of Bowman glands (×540). BC, Basal cell; LP, lamina propria; OC, olfactory cell.

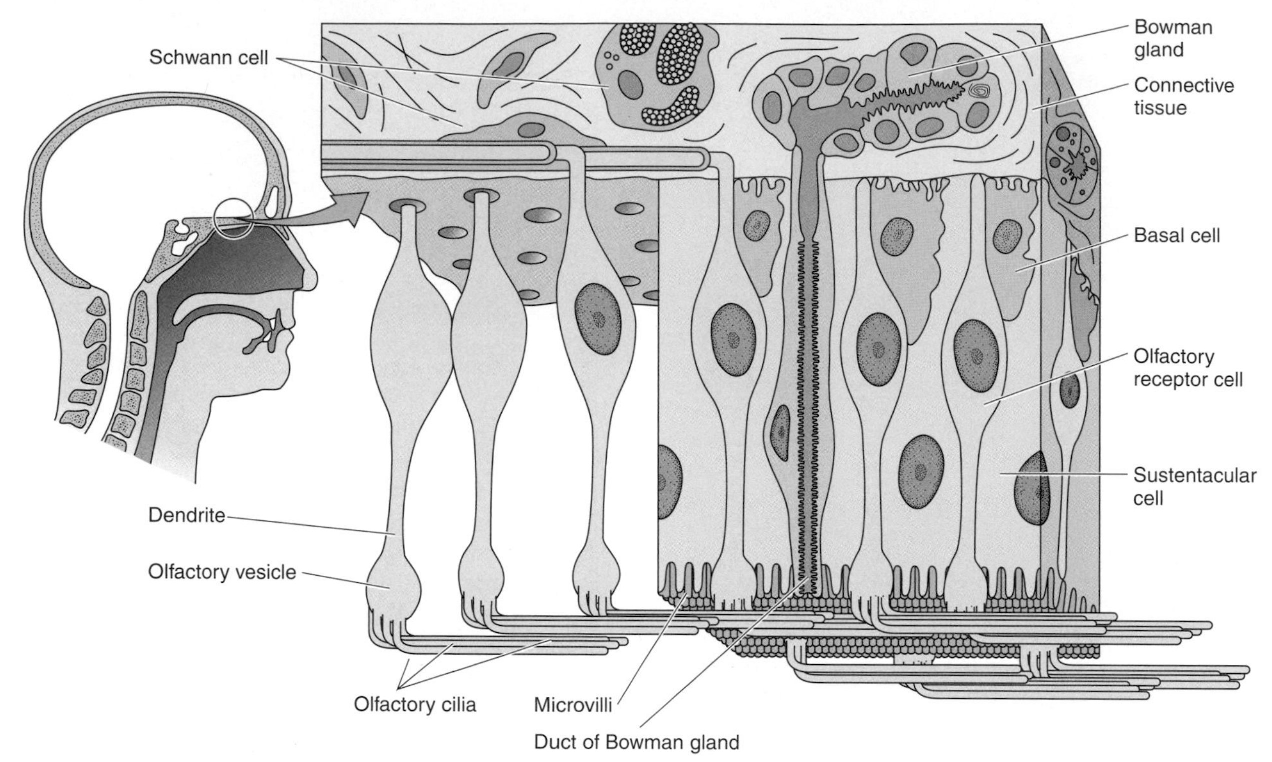

Fig. 15.4 Schematic diagram of the olfactory epithelium showing basal, olfactory, and sustentacular cells. Compare this diagram with the actual photomicrograph of the olfactory mucosa presented in Fig. 15.3.

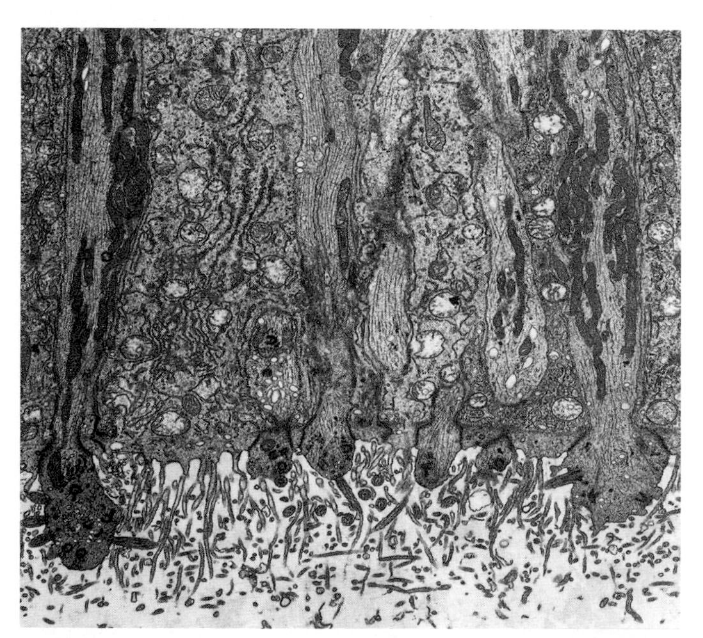

Fig. 15.5 Transmission electron micrograph of the apical region of the rat olfactory epithelium. Note the olfactory vesicles and cilia projecting from them. Compare this electron micrograph with Figs. 15.3 and 15.4 (×8260). (From Mendoza AS, Kühnel W. Postnatal changes in the ultrastructure of the rat olfactory epithelium: the supranuclear region of supporting cells. *Cell Tissue Res.* 1991;265:193-196. Copyright Springer-Verlag.)

Scanning electron micrographs demonstrate that six to eight long, nonmotile olfactory cilia extend from the olfactory vesicle and lie on the free surface of the epithelium. Transmission electron micrographs of these cilia display an unusual axoneme pattern that begins as a typical peripheral ring of nine **doublet** microtubules surrounding two central **singlets** (9 + 2 configuration) but without the characteristic dynein arms. The axoneme changes distally so that it is composed of nine **singlets** surrounding the two central singlets; near the end of the cilium, only the central singlets are present.

The basal region of the olfactory cell is its **axon**, which penetrates the basal lamina and joins similar axons to form bundles of nerve fibers. Each axon, although unmyelinated, has a sheath composed of Schwann cell–like olfactory ensheathing (glial) cells. The nerve fibers pass through foramina of the cribriform plate in the roof of the nasal cavity to synapse with secondary neurons in the olfactory bulb.

Clinical Correlations

Human herpes virus 6 (HHV-6) is responsible for a very common mild infection, known as ***roseola****, in infants and toddlers. In fact, most adults possess the HHV-6 that they acquired as an infant. During an HHV-6 infection, the virus can sometimes invade the nasal cavity and establish residence in the mucus. From there, the virus will follow the olfactory nerves through the cribriform plate and infect the olfactory bulb of the brain.*

Sustentacular and Basal Cells. **Sustentacular cells** are 50- to 60-μm-tall columnar cells whose apical aspects have a striated border composed of microvilli. Their oval nuclei are in the apical third of the cell, somewhat superficial to the location of the olfactory cell nuclei. The apical cytoplasm of these cells displays the presence of secretory granules housing a yellow pigment that provides the characteristic color of the olfactory mucosa. Electron micrographs of sustentacular cells demonstrate that they form junctional complexes with the olfactory vesicle regions of olfactory cells, as well as with other contiguous sustentacular cells. The morphology of sustentacular cells is not remarkable, although they do display a prominent terminal web of actin microfilaments. These cells are believed to provide physical support, nourishment, and electrical insulation for the olfactory cells.

Basal cells are of two types: horizontal and globose. Horizontal cells are flat and lie against the basement membrane, whereas globose cells are short, basophilic, pyramid-shaped cells; the apical aspects of the basal cells do not reach the epithelial free surface. Their nuclei are centrally located, but because these are short cells, the nuclei occupy the basal third of the epithelium. The globose type of basal cells has considerable proliferative capacity and can replace both sustentacular and olfactory cells. In a healthy person, the olfactory cells live for less than 3 months, and sustentacular cells have a life span of less than 1 year. The horizontal basal cells replicate to replace the globose basal cells.

Lamina Propria. The lamina propria of the olfactory mucosa is composed of a richly vascularized, loose to dense, irregular collagenous connective tissue that is firmly attached to the underlying periosteum. It houses numerous lymphoid elements, as well as the collection of axons of the olfactory cells, which form fascicles of unmyelinated nerve fibers. **Bowman glands** (**olfactory glands**), which produce a *serous* secretory product, are also present and are characteristic components of the olfactory mucosa. These glands release IgA, lactoferrin, lysozyme, and odorant-binding protein, a molecule that prevents the odorant from leaving the region of the olfactory epithelium, enhancing the individual's ability to detect odors.

Histophysiology of the Nasal Cavity

The nasal mucosa filters, warms, and humidifies the inhaled air and is also responsible for the perception of odors.

The moist nasal mucosa filters inhaled air. Particulate matter, such as dust, is trapped by the mucus produced by the goblet cells of the epithelium and the seromucous glands of the lamina propria. The serous fluid, produced by the seromucous glands, is situated between the mucus and the apical plasmalemmae of the respiratory epithelial cells. Because the cilia of the ciliated columnar cells do not reach the mucous layer, their movement is restricted to the serous fluid layer. Due to the ciliary motion within that watery fluid, the mucus is swept along (*hydroplaned*) at the interface of the two fluids. The particulate matter trapped in mucus is thus delivered, by ciliary action, to the pharynx to be swallowed or expectorated.

In addition to being filtered, the air is also warmed and humidified by being passed over the mucosa, which is kept warm and moist by its rich blood supply. Warming of the inspired air is facilitated by the presence of an extensive network of rows of arched vessels grouped in an anteroposterior arrangement. Capillary beds arising from these vessels lie just beneath the epithelium, and the flow of blood into this vascular network is directed from posterior to anterior, opposite to the flow of air; thus, heat is continuously being transferred to the inspired air by a countercurrent mechanism.

Antigens and allergens carried by the air are combated by lymphoid elements of the lamina propria. Secretory immunoglobulin (IgA), produced by plasma cells, is transported across the epithelium into the nasal cavity by ciliated columnar cells and by the acinar cells of the seromucous glands. IgE, which is also produced by plasma cells, binds to IgE receptors (FcεRI receptors) of mast cell and basophil plasmalemmae. Subsequent binding of a specific antigen or allergen to the bound IgE causes the mast cell (and basophil) to release various mediators of inflammation. These, in turn, act on the nasal mucosa, inducing the symptoms associated with colds and hay fever.

Clinical Correlations

1. *The nasal mucosa is protected from dehydration by alternating blood flow to the venous sinuses of the lamina propria overlying the conchae of the right and left nasal cavities. The erectile tissue–like region (**swell bodies**) of one side expands when its venous sinuses become engorged with blood, reducing the flow of air through that side. Seepage of plasma from the sinuses and seromucous secretions from the glands thus rehydrates the mucosa approximately every half hour.*
2. *Chemical irritants and particulate matter are removed from the nasal cavity by the **sneeze reflex**. The sudden explosive expulsion of air usually clears the nasal passage of the irritant.*

The olfactory epithelium is responsible for the perception of odors, which also makes a major contribution to the sense of taste discrimination. The plasmalemma of the olfactory cilia of a particular olfactory cell has numerous copies of one particular **odor receptor molecule**. Molecules of an odoriferous substance dissolved in the serous fluid bind to its specific receptor. When a threshold number of odor receptors is occupied, the olfactory cell becomes stimulated, an action potential is generated, and the information is transmitted via its axon to the olfactory bulb, a projection of the central nervous system, for processing. Axons of olfactory cells synapse with the dendrites of 1 of 30 mitral cells within small spherical regions of the olfactory bulb, known as ***glomeruli***. If a threshold level of impulses reaches a mitral cell, it becomes depolarized and relays the signal to the olfactory cortex for further processing.

Each glomerulus receives input (information) from approximately 2000 olfactory neurons, each specific for the same odoriferous substance. Similar to antigens, which may have several epitopes, each of which binds a specific antibody, odoriferous substances possess several small regions, each of which binds to a specific odor receptor molecule. Thus, a particular odoriferous substance may bind to several odor receptor molecules, activating a number of olfactory neurons and providing input to several glomeruli. To ensure that a single stimulus does not produce repeated responses, the continuous flow of serous fluid from **Bowman glands** provides a constant refreshing of the odorants impinging on the olfactory cilia.

Clinical Correlations

1. *Although there are only about 1000 glomeruli, each receiving information concerning a single odor receptor molecule, the human olfactory cortex has the ability to distinguish about 1 trillion different scents. It does so by recognizing information arising from a particular combination of glomeruli as a single scent. Thus, a particular glomerulus may be active in the recognition of several odors.*
2. *It appears that individuals who experience fear express that sense of fear as a specific scent in their sweat. Certain individuals have the ability to smell that fear and may react to it by also experiencing fear, suggesting that certain emotions, such as fear, may be transmitted from one person to another by the secretion and olfactory recognition of chemical signals.*

PARANASAL SINUSES

The ethmoid, sphenoid, frontal, and maxilla bones of the skull house large, mucoperiosteum-lined spaces, the **paranasal sinuses** (named after their location), which communicate with the nasal cavity. The mucosa of each sinus is composed of a vascular connective tissue lamina propria fused with the periosteum. The thin lamina propria resembles that of the nasal cavity in that it houses seromucous glands as well as lymphoid elements. The respiratory epithelial lining of the paranasal sinuses, similar to that of the nasal cavity, has numerous ciliated columnar cells whose cilia sweep the mucus layer toward the nasal cavity.

Clinical Correlations

The openings of the paranasal sinuses that communicate with the nasal cavity are quite small. Therefore, during a **sinus infection**, *when the mucosa becomes inflamed and swollen, the size of the opening is reduced even further and the fluid produced by the glands of the mucosa cannot drain into the nasal cavity. This causes an increased pressure within the sinus that places excess pressure on the periosteum of the bone, resulting in a "sinus headache."*

NASOPHARYNX

The pharynx begins at the choana and extends to the opening of the larynx. This continuous cavity is subdivided into three regions: (1) the superior **nasopharynx**, (2) middle **oral pharynx**, and (3) inferior **laryngeal pharynx**. The nasopharynx is lined by a respiratory epithelium, whereas the oral and laryngeal pharynges are lined by a stratified squamous epithelium. The lamina propria is composed of a loose to dense, irregular type of vascularized connective tissue housing seromucous glands and lymphoid elements. It is fused with the epimysium of the skeletal muscle components of the pharynx. The lamina propria of the posterior aspect of the nasopharynx houses the **pharyngeal tonsil**, an unencapsulated collection of lymphoid tissue described in Chapter 12.

Clinical Correlations

The lateral walls of the right and left nasopharynx display the openings of the **auditory tubes (eustachian tubes)**, *which connect the middle ear cavities of the respective side to the nasopharynx. Occasionally, the opening in the nasopharynx becomes plugged with mucus; when atmospheric pressure differences occur between the middle ear and the nasopharynx, as during the landing or take-off of an airplane or a fast-moving elevator in a skyscraper, the individual experiences an earache that can be alleviated by swallowing saliva or by blowing one's nose. This may dislodge the mucus that is plugging the opening of the auditory tube.*

LARYNX

The larynx, or voice box, is responsible for phonation and for preventing the entry of food and fluids into the respiratory system.

The **larynx**, situated between the pharynx and the trachea, is a rigid, short, cylindrical tube 4 cm in length and approximately 4 cm in diameter. It is responsible for phonation and prevents the entry of solids or liquids into the respiratory system during swallowing. The wall of the larynx is reinforced by several hyaline and elastic cartilages that are connected by ligaments; the movements of these cartilages are controlled by **intrinsic** and **extrinsic skeletal muscles**.

The thyroid and cricoid cartilages form the cylindrical support for the larynx, whereas the epiglottis provides a cover over the laryngeal **aditus (opening)**. During respiration, the epiglottis is in the vertical position, permitting the flow of air. During swallowing of food, fluids, or saliva, however, it becomes positioned horizontally, closing the laryngeal aditus. Yet, normally, even in the absence of an epiglottis, swallowed material bypasses the laryngeal opening. The arytenoid and corniculate cartilages are occasionally fused to each other, and most of the intrinsic muscles of the larynx move the two arytenoids with respect to each other and to the cricoid cartilage.

The lumen of the larynx is characterized by two pairs of shelf-like folds: the superiorly positioned vestibular folds and the inferiorly placed vocal folds (Fig. 15.6). The **vestibular folds** are immovable. Their lamina propria, composed of loose connective tissue, houses seromucous glands, adipose cells, and lymphoid elements. The free edge of each **vocal fold** is reinforced by dense, regular elastic connective tissue, called the ***vocal ligament***. The vocalis muscle, attached to the vocal ligament, assists the other intrinsic muscles of the larynx in altering the tension on the vocal folds. These muscles also regulate the width of the space between the vocal folds (the **rima glottidis**), permitting precisely regulated vibrations of their free edges by the exhaled air.

During silent respiration, the vocal folds are partially *abducted* (pulled apart); during forced inspiration, they are fully abducted. During phonation, however, the vocal folds are strongly *adducted*, forming a narrow interval between them.

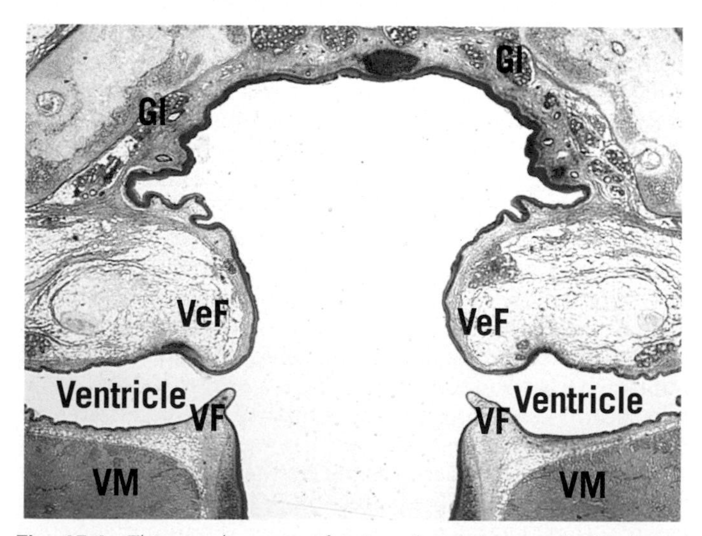

Fig. 15.6 This very-low-magnification photomicrograph of a frontal section of the larynx displays its three cavities: the centrally positioned ventricle, superiorly positioned vestibule, and the inferiorly located infraglottic cavity. The ventricular fold (VeF), also known as the false vocal fold, is the inferior boundary of the vestibule and the vocal fold (VF), housing the vocal cord, is the superior boundary of the infraglottic cavity. The vocalis muscle (VM) controls the tension placed on the vocal folds. The mucosa of the wall of the larynx houses seromucous glands. (×14)

The movement of air against the edges of the strongly adducted vocal folds produces and modulates sound (but not speech, which is formed by movements of the pharynx, soft palate, tongue, and lips). The longer and more relaxed the vocal folds, the deeper the **pitch** of the sound. Because the larynx of a post-pubescent male is larger than that of a female, men tend to have deeper voices than women.

The larynx is lined by **pseudostratified ciliated columnar epithelium**, except on the superior surfaces of the epiglottis and vocal folds, which are covered by stratified squamous nonkeratinized epithelium. The cilia of the larynx beat toward the pharynx, transporting mucus and trapped particulate matter toward the mouth to be expectorated or swallowed.

Clinical Correlations

1. *Laryngitis, inflammation of the laryngeal tissues, including the vocal folds, prevents the vocal folds from vibrating freely. Persons with laryngitis sound hoarse or can only whisper.*
2. *The presence of chemical irritants or particulate matter in the upper air passages, including the trachea or bronchi, elicits the* ***cough reflex****, producing an explosive rush of air that removes the irritant. The cough reflex begins with the inhalation of a large volume of air and the closure of the epiglottis and glottis (adduction of the vocal folds), followed by a powerful contraction of the muscles responsible for forced expiration (intercostal and abdominal muscles). The sudden opening of the glottis and epiglottis generates a rush of air whose velocity can exceed 100 miles per hour, removing the irritant with an enormous force.*
3. *Some patients who have been prescribed angiotensin-converting enzyme (ACE) inhibitors to control their blood pressure develop a dry cough, one of the side-effects of these medications. It is postulated that ACE inhibitors catabolize inflammatory peptides, such as bradykinin; the buildup of these agents starts the cough reflex.*

TRACHEA

The trachea has three layers: mucosa, submucosa, and adventitia. The hyaline cartilaginous support of the trachea is performed by a dozen or so C-shaped structures, known as C-rings, that are located in the adventitia.

The **trachea** is a tube, 12 cm long and 2 cm in diameter, that begins at the cricoid cartilage of the larynx and ends when it bifurcates to form the primary bronchi. The wall of the trachea is reinforced by 10 to 12 horseshoe-shaped hyaline cartilage rings (**C-rings**). The open ends of these rings face posteriorly and are connected to each other by smooth muscle: the trachealis muscle. Because of this arrangement of the C-rings, the trachea is rounded anteriorly but flattened posteriorly. The perichondrium of each C-ring is connected to the perichondria of other C-rings lying directly above and below it by fibroelastic connective tissue, which provides flexibility to the trachea and permits its elongation during inspiration. Contraction of the trachealis muscle decreases the diameter of the tracheal lumen, resulting in faster air flow, which assists in dislodging foreign material (or mucus or other irritants) from the larynx by coughing.

The trachea has three layers: mucosa, submucosa, and adventitia (Figs. 15.7 and 15.8).

Mucosa

The **mucosal lining** of the trachea is composed of **respiratory epithelium** (pseudostratified ciliated columnar epithelium), the subepithelial connective tissue (lamina propria), and a relatively thick bundle of elastic fibers separating the mucosa from the submucosa.

Respiratory Epithelium

The respiratory epithelium is a pseudostratified ciliated columnar epithelium composed of six cell types. Three of these—goblet cells, ciliated columnar cells, and basal cells—constitute 90% of the cell population.

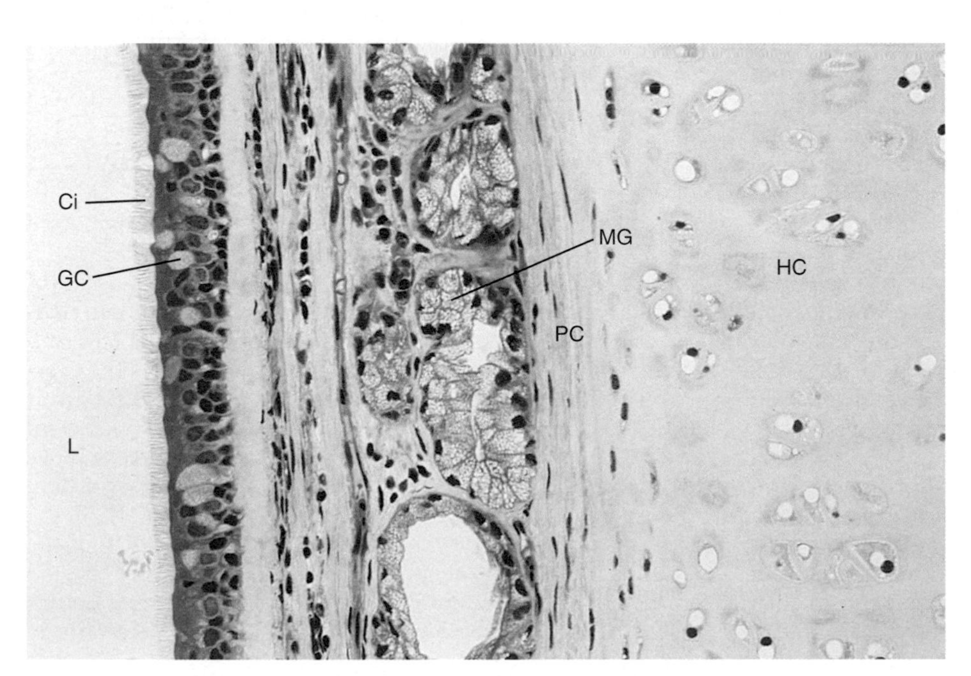

Fig. 15.7 Light photomicrograph of the trachea in a monkey. There are numerous cilia (Ci), as well as goblet cells (GC) in the epithelium. Also, observe the mucous glands (MG) in the subepithelial connective tissue, as well as the presence of the hyaline cartilage (HC) C-ring in the adventitia (×270). L, Lumen; PC, perichondrium.

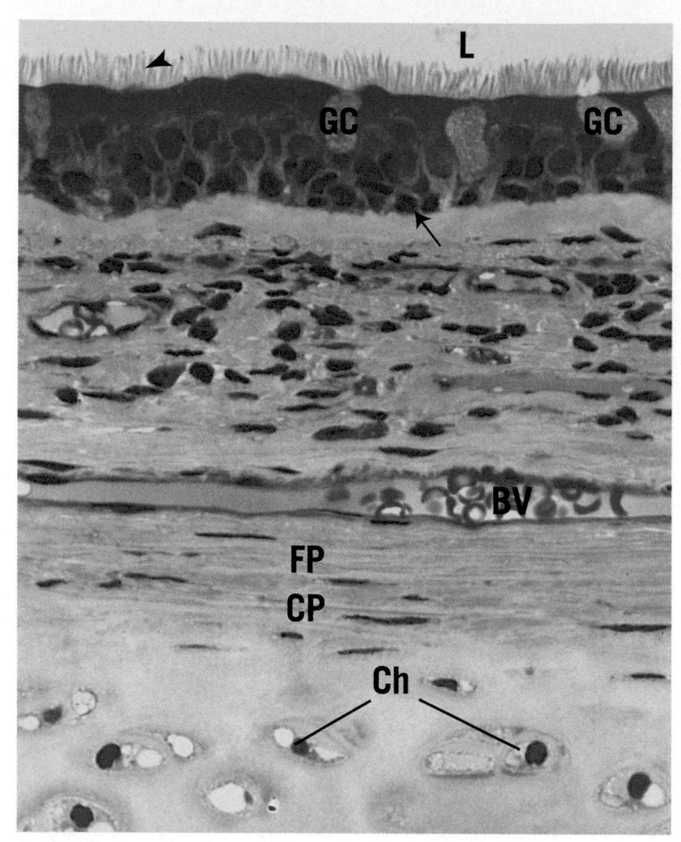

Fig. 15.8 This high-magnification photomicrograph of a monkey trachea displays the cilia *(arrowhead)* protruding into the lumen (L) of the trachea. Goblet cells (GC) and basal cells *(arrow)*, as well as the additional cell types of the respiratory epithelium all contact the basement membrane, located at the tip of the arrow denoting the basal cell. The subepithelial connective tissue is a combination of the lamina propria (which contacts the basement membrane) and the more deeply positioned submucosa. The blood vessel (BV) is located either in the submucosa or the adventitia. Observe the fibrous (FP) and cellular (CP) perichondrium of the hyaline cartilage whose chondrocytes (Ch) occupy lacunae in the cartilage matrix. (×540)

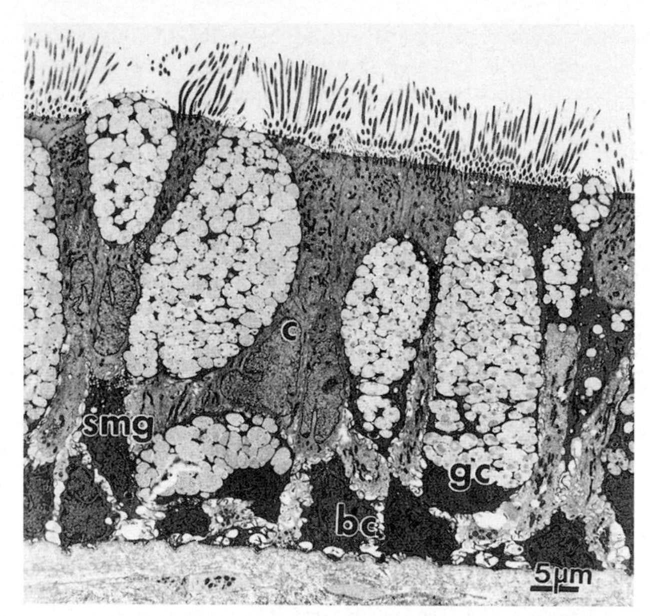

Fig. 15.9 Transmission electron micrograph of the monkey respiratory epithelium from the anterior nasal septum. Note the presence of goblet cells (gc), ciliated cells (c), basal cells (bc), and small granule mucous cells (smg). (From Harkema JR, Plopper CG, Hyde DM, et al. Nonolfactory surface epithelium of the nasal cavity of the bonnet monkey: a morphologic and morphometric study of the transitional and respiratory epithelium. *Am J Anat.* 1987;180:266-279. Reprinted with permission from Wiley-Liss, Inc., a subsidiary of John Wiley & Sons, Inc.)

The **respiratory epithelium**, a pseudostratified ciliated columnar epithelium, is separated from the lamina propria by a **thick basement membrane**. The epithelium is composed of five cell types: goblet cells, ciliated columnar cells, basal cells, brush cells, and cells of the diffuse neuroendocrine system (DNES). All of these cells come into contact with the basement membrane, but all do not reach the lumen (Fig. 15.9, Table 15.2).

Goblet cells constitute about 30% of the total cell population of the respiratory epithelium. They produce **mucinogen**, which becomes hydrated and is known as ***mucin*** when released into an aqueous environment. Once the mucin is mixed with other material in the watery environment, it is known as ***mucus***. Just as goblet cells elsewhere, goblet cells in the respiratory epithelium have a narrow, basally positioned **stem** and an expanded **theca** containing secretory granules. Electron micrography demonstrates that the nucleus and most organelles are located in the stem. This region displays a rich network of rough endoplasmic reticulum (RER), a well-developed Golgi complex, numerous mitochondria, and an abundance of ribosomes. The theca is filled with numerous mucinogen-containing secretory granules of varied diameters.

TABLE 15.2 Cells Composing the Respiratory Epithelium

Cells	% of cells	Function	Other Information
Goblet	30	Manufacture mucinogen	Theca houses secretory granules
Ciliated	30	Move mucus toward nasopharynx	Also have microvilli
Basal	30	Replace cells of the epithelium	Smallest cells
Brush	4-5	May have a chemosensory role	Associated with nerve endings
DNES*	4-5	Manufacture hormones	May have narrow cytoplasmic process that leads to the lumen

**DNES*, Diffuse neuroendocrine system.

The apical plasmalemma has a few short, blunt microvilli (see Fig. 15.9).

Ciliated columnar cells constitute approximately 30% of the total respiratory epithelial cell population. These tall, slender cells have a basally located nucleus and possess cilia and microvilli on their apical cell membrane (Fig. 15.10). The cytoplasm just below these structures is rich in mitochondria and has a Golgi complex. The remainder of the cytoplasm possesses some RER and a few ribosomes. The cilia of these cells move the mucus and its trapped particulate matter, via ciliary action, toward the nasopharynx for elimination.

Basal cells are short cells that compose about 30% of the total respiratory epithelial cell population. They are located on the basement membrane, but their apical surfaces do not reach the lumen (see Figs. 15.8 and 15.9). These relatively

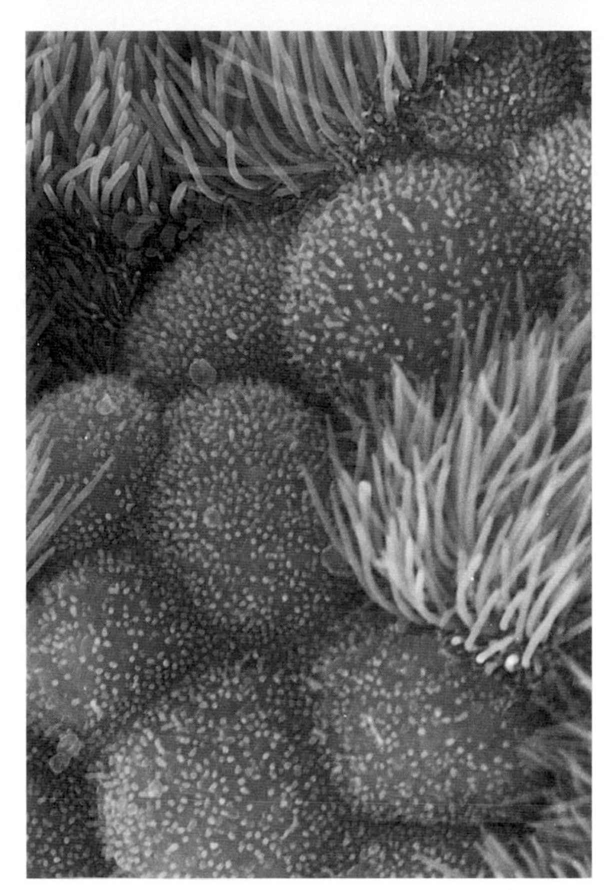

Fig. 15.10 Scanning electron micrograph of the human fetal trachea displaying ciliated and nonciliated cells (×5500). (From Montgomery PQ, Stafford ND, Stolinski C. Ultrastructure of the human fetal trachea: a morphologic study of the luminal and glandular epithelia at the mid-trimester. *J Anat.* 1990;173:43-59. Reprinted with permission from Cambridge University Press.)

undifferentiated cells are considered to be stem cells that proliferate to replace defunct goblet, ciliated columnar, and brush cells.

Brush cells (**small-granule mucous cells**) constitute about 4% to 5% of the total respiratory epithelial cell population. They are narrow, columnar cells with tall microvilli. Their function is unknown, but they have been associated with nerve endings. Thus, some investigators suggest that they may have a sensory role similar to gustatory cells (taste cells) of the tongue. Other investigators believe that brush cells are merely goblet cells that have released their mucinogen.

DNES cells, also known as ***small-granule cells*** or ***Kulchitsky cells***, constitute about 4% to 5% of the total cell population. Many of these cells possess long, slender processes that extend into the lumen. It is believed that they have the ability to monitor the oxygen and carbon dioxide levels in the lumen of the airway. These cells are closely associated with naked sensory nerve endings with which they make synaptic contact; together with these nerve fibers, they are referred to as ***pulmonary neuroepithelial bodies***. DNES cells contain numerous granules in their basal cytoplasm, which house pharmacological agents such as amines, polypeptides, acetylcholine, serotonin, and adenosine triphosphate. Under hypoxic conditions, these agents are released not only into the synaptic clefts but also into the connective tissue spaces of the lamina propria, where they act as paracrine hormones or may enter the vascular supply to act as hormones. Therefore, it has been suggested that these pulmonary neuroepithelial bodies can exert local effects to alleviate localized hypoxic conditions by regulating perfusion and ventilation in their vicinity or they may have generalized effects via the efferent nerve fibers that relay information about hypoxic conditions to the **respiratory regulators** located in the medulla oblongata.

Lamina Propria and Elastic Fibers

The **lamina propria** of the trachea is composed of a loose, fibroelastic connective tissue. It contains lymphoid elements (e.g., lymphoid nodules, lymphocytes, and neutrophils) as well as mucous and seromucous glands, whose ducts open onto the epithelial surface. A dense layer of elastic fibers, the **elastic lamina**, separates the lamina propria from the underlying submucosa (see Figs. 15.7 and 15.8).

Submucosa

The tracheal **submucosa** is composed of a dense, irregular fibroelastic connective tissue housing numerous **mucous** and **seromucous glands**. The short ducts of these glands pierce the elastic lamina and the lamina propria to open onto the epithelial surface. Lymphoid elements are also present in the submucosa. Moreover, this region has a rich blood and lymph supply, the smaller branches of which reach the lamina propria.

Adventitia

The adventitia of the trachea houses C-rings of hyaline cartilage.

The **adventitia** of the trachea is composed of a fibroelastic connective tissue (see Figs. 15.7 and 15.8). The most prominent features of the adventitia are the hyaline cartilage C-rings and the intervening fibrous connective tissue. The adventitia also is responsible for anchoring the trachea to the adjacent structures (i.e., the esophagus and connective tissues of the neck).

Clinical Correlations

The respiratory epithelium of people chronically exposed to irritants, such as cigarette smoke and coal dust, undergoes reversible alterations, known as metaplasia*, associated with an increase in the number of goblet cells relative to ciliated cells. The increased number of goblet cells produces a thicker layer of mucus to remove the irritants, but the reduced number of cilia retards the rate of mucus elimination, resulting in congestion. Moreover, the seromucous glands of the lamina propria and submucosa increase in size, forming a more copious secretion. A few months after elimination of the pollutants, the cell ratio returns to normal (1 : 1) and the seromucous glands revert to their previous size.*

BRONCHIAL TREE

The **bronchial tree** begins at the bifurcation of the trachea, as the **right** and left **primary bronchi**, which *arborize* (form branches that gradually decrease in size). The bronchial tree is composed of airways located outside of the lungs (the primary bronchi, extrapulmonary bronchi) and airways located inside of the lungs: the intrapulmonary bronchi (lobar [secondary] and segmental [tertiary] bronchi), bronchioles, terminal bronchioles, and respiratory bronchioles (Fig. 15.11). The bronchial tree divides 15 to 20 times before reaching the level of terminal bronchioles. As the airways progressively decrease in size, several trends are observed, including a *decrease* in all of the following: the amount of cartilage, numbers of glands and goblet cells, and height of epithelial cells. Also, there is an *increase* in smooth muscle and elastic tissue (but only with respect to the thickness of the wall).

Primary (Extrapulmonary) Bronchi

The structure of the **primary bronchi** is identical to that of the trachea, except that bronchi are smaller in diameter and their walls are thinner. Each primary bronchus—accompanied by the pulmonary arteries, veins, and lymph vessels—pierces the **root** (**hilum**) of the lung. The right bronchus is straighter than the left bronchus. The right bronchus trifurcates to lead to the three lobes of the right lung; the left bronchus bifurcates, sending branches to the two lobes of the left lung. These branches then enter the substance of the lungs as intrapulmonary bronchi.

Clinical Correlations

Parts of the conducting portion of the respiratory system manufacture mucinogen, which, when hydrated, becomes mucin. Once additional substances become mixed with mucin, it is known as **mucus** *and is conveyed into the oropharynx to be swallowed. Normal mucus is clear and has a thin, watery texture. If the individual becomes sick, especially with a cold or the flu, the mucus changes its color and texture because it accumulates various additional components, making it more difficult for the person to expel it into the oropharynx. It then is known as* **phlegm**, *which, once expectorated, is known as* **sputum**. *It should be stressed that phlegm does not originate in the nasal cavity; it is formed in the lower regions of the conducting portion of the respiratory system—the larger bronchioles, various bronchi, and trachea. An individual who is congested will have an opaque to white sputum that is somewhat thicker in consistency than normal mucus. As the patient's immune system begins to fight the infection, dead neutrophils and invasive microorganisms accumulate in the sputum, imparting a yellowish color to it. As the immune response accelerates and more dead leukocytes, microorganisms, and proteins populate the sputum, it then takes on a greenish color. With strenuous coughing, small capillaries break, releasing blood into the phlegm, which then becomes pink to red, depending on the amount of blood being released. However, if the blood that is present in the phlegm has coagulated, it turns light to dark brown. If the sputum is black, the patient may have a fungal infection, a situation that has to be investigated as soon as possible. If the patient is a coal miner or is exposed to very dusty work conditions, then the black sputum is explained by the presence of dark dust particles. Two important considerations are to be kept in mind: (1) the presence of a whitish, frothy sputum, which may be indicative of chronic obstructive pulmonary disease; and (2) an even more serious condition, when the sputum is pinkish and frothy and the patient is experiencing chest pain, shortness of breath, or profuse sweating. Patients who present with these symptoms may be suffering from left-sided heart failure and need medical intervention as soon as possible.*

Intrapulmonary (Secondary [Lobar] and Tertiary [Segmental]) Bronchi

Each secondary intrapulmonary bronchus serves a lobe of the lung; tertiary bronchi serve bronchopulmonary segments.

Each ***secondary*** (***lobar***) ***bronchus*** is the airway to a lobe of the lung. The left lung has two lobes and, thus, has two secondary bronchi. The right lung has three lobes and, thus, has three secondary bronchi. These airways are similar to primary bronchi, with the following exceptions. The C-rings are replaced by irregular plates of hyaline cartilage that completely surround the lumen of the secondary bronchus. Therefore, unlike the trachea, these airways do not have a flattened region but rather are completely round. The smooth muscle is located at the interface of the fibroelastic lamina propria and submucosa as two distinct smooth muscle layers spiraling in opposite directions. Elastic fibers, which radiate from the adventitia, connect to elastic fibers arising from the adventitia of other parts of the bronchial tree (Fig. 15.12).

As in the primary bronchi and trachea, seromucous glands and lymphoid elements are present in the lamina propria and submucosa of the secondary bronchi. Ducts of these glands deliver their secretory products onto the surface of the pseudostratified ciliated epithelial lining of the lumen.

As secondary bronchi enter the lobes of the lung, they subdivide into smaller branches, **tertiary** (**segmental**) **bronchi**. Each tertiary bronchus arborizes but leads to a discrete section of lung tissue, known as a ***bronchopulmonary segment***. Each lung has 10 bronchopulmonary segments that are completely separated from one another by connective tissue elements and are clinically important in surgical procedures involving the lungs. As the arborized branches of intrapulmonary bronchi decrease in diameter, they eventually lead to bronchioles. Lymphoid nodules are particularly evident where these airways branch to form increasingly smaller intrapulmonary bronchi. The smaller intrapulmonary bronchi have thinner walls, decreasing amounts of hyaline cartilage plates, and shorter epithelial-lining cells.

Clinical Correlations

Cystic fibrosis (CF), which currently affects approximately 30,000 patients in the United States alone, is a recessive hereditary disease caused by one of a number of mutations in the gene that codes for the protein known as **cystic fibrosis transmembrane conductance regulator (CFTR)**. *This protein is inserted into the parenchymal cell membranes of glands as a* **chloride channel** *and regulates the transport of Cl^- ions across the cell membrane. Although the disease affects most components of the digestive system and the conducting portion of the respiratory system, it is the effects on the bronchioles of the respiratory system that are the most problematic, causing bronchiolar infections and, eventually, the inability to breathe. The mechanism of the pathology involves problems with the transport of Cl^- ions out of the cell. Mucous glands of the bronchi and bronchioles release mucinogen into the lumen of their ducts. Normally, as Cl^- ions leave the secretory cells of the mucous acinus through the CFTR channel to enter the duct portion of the acinus, H_2O molecules also leave the cell, thereby hydrating and* *diluting the mucinogen, forming mucin that is sufficiently thin to flow through the ducts and away from the site of mucin production. However, in individuals with mutated CFTR, the Cl^- ions and water molecules are unable to leave the cell. The abnormally thick mucinogen that is released is unable to flow out of the duct and is trapped not only in the lumina of the acini but also in the ducts of the mucous glands. This rich, thick mucin becomes invaded by bacteria, usually* Pseudomonas aeruginosa, *which thrives in this nutrient-laden environment. Eventually, the blocked conducting system of the respiratory system becomes too inefficient and can no longer conduct enough air to the alveoli of the lungs and the individual dies. Before the advent of antibiotics, CF patients died at a very early age; currently, they can live to about 40 years of age. Almost every gland of the digestive system is affected by this disease, including the pancreas, but it is the respiratory effects of CF that are responsible for the death of the individual. Two recent clinical trials have demonstrated that a regimen of 3 drugs—tezakaftor, ivakaftor, and one of two currently unnamed experimental drugs—considerably improved the patients' lung functions with only mild side effects that included headache, cough, and an increased amount of mucus production. It is hoped that larger clinical trials of longer durations can maintain the improved lung function in these patients. Unfortunately, the improvement in breathing does not mean that the patients are cured, only that their condition is ameliorated.*

Bronchioles

Bronchioles possess no cartilage in their walls, are smaller than 1 mm in diameter, and have club cells (Clara cells) in their epithelial lining.

Each **bronchiole** (or **primary bronchiole**) supplies air to a pulmonary *lobule*. Bronchioles are considered the 10th to 15th generation of dichotomous branching of the bronchial tree. Their diameter commonly is described as less than 1 mm, although this number varies among authors from 5 mm to 0.3 mm. This disagreement concerning the diameter of bronchioles may lead to confusion in the descriptions of their structure (but should not be regarded as a purposeful attempt to complicate the life of the student).

The epithelial lining of bronchioles ranges from ciliated simple columnar with occasional goblet cells in larger bronchioles to simple cuboidal (many with cilia), with occasional club cells (previously known as *Clara cells*) and no goblet cells in smaller bronchioles.

Club cells (**Clara cells**) are columnar with dome-shaped apices that have short, blunt microvilli (Fig. 15.13). Their apical cytoplasm houses numerous secretory granules containing glycoproteins manufactured on their abundant RER. Club cells are believed to protect the bronchiolar epithelium by lining it with their secretory product, known as ***club cell secretory protein***. Additionally, these cells degrade toxins in the inhaled air via **cytochrome P-450 enzymes** in their smooth endoplasmic reticulum. Some investigators also suggest that club cells produce a **surfactant-like material** that reduces the surface tension of bronchioles and facilitates the maintenance of their patency. Moreover, club cells divide to regenerate the bronchiolar epithelium.

The lamina propria of bronchioles has no glands; it is surrounded by a loose meshwork of helically oriented smooth muscle layers (Figs. 15.14 and 15.15). The walls of bronchioles and their branches have no cartilage. Elastic fibers radiate from the fibroelastic connective tissue that surrounds the smooth muscle coats of bronchioles. These elastic fibers connect to elastic fibers ramifying from other branches of the bronchial tree. During inhalation, as the lung expands in volume, the elastic fibers exert tension on the bronchiolar walls; by pulling uniformly in all directions, the elastic fibers help maintain the patency of the bronchioles.

Clinical Correlations

1. *The smooth muscle layers of bronchioles are controlled by the parasympathetic nervous system. Normally, the smooth muscle coats contract at the end of expiration and relax during inspiration. In patients with* **asthma**, *the smooth muscle coat undergoes prolonged contraction during expiration; thus, they have difficulties in expelling air from their lungs. Steroids and β_2-agonists relax bronchiolar smooth muscle and are frequently used to relieve asthmatic attacks.*
2. *The risk of acquiring asthma by young children is decreased by consumption of milk and fruit as well as by a diet rich in eggs, vegetables, and cereals. However, consumption of fast foods and "junk food"—especially those rich in trans fats, saturated fats, carbohydrates, and sugar—increases the incidence of asthma in children.*
3. *It has been reported recently that bronchiolar smooth muscle cells possess taste receptors on their sarcolemmae that recognize bitter tastants. When exposed to bitter taste, these smooth muscle cells relax, permitting the bronchioles to open to 90% of their widest diameter. Current research is attempting to take advantage of this situation by developing inhalants that incorporate bitter tasting substances in their composition to assist asthmatic patients in relieving breathing problems without having to resort to steroids and β_2-agonists.*

Terminal Bronchioles

Terminal bronchioles form the smallest and most distal region of the conducting portion of the respiratory system.

Each bronchiole subdivides to form several smaller **terminal bronchioles**, which are less than 0.5 mm in diameter and constitute the terminus of the conducting portion of the respiratory system. The epithelium of terminal bronchioles is composed of club cells and cuboidal cells, some with cilia. The narrow lamina propria consists of fibroelastic connective tissue and is surrounded by one or two layers of smooth muscle cells. Elastic fibers radiate from the adventitia and, as with the bronchioles, bind to elastic fibers radiating from other members of the bronchial tree. Terminal bronchioles branch to give rise to respiratory bronchioles.

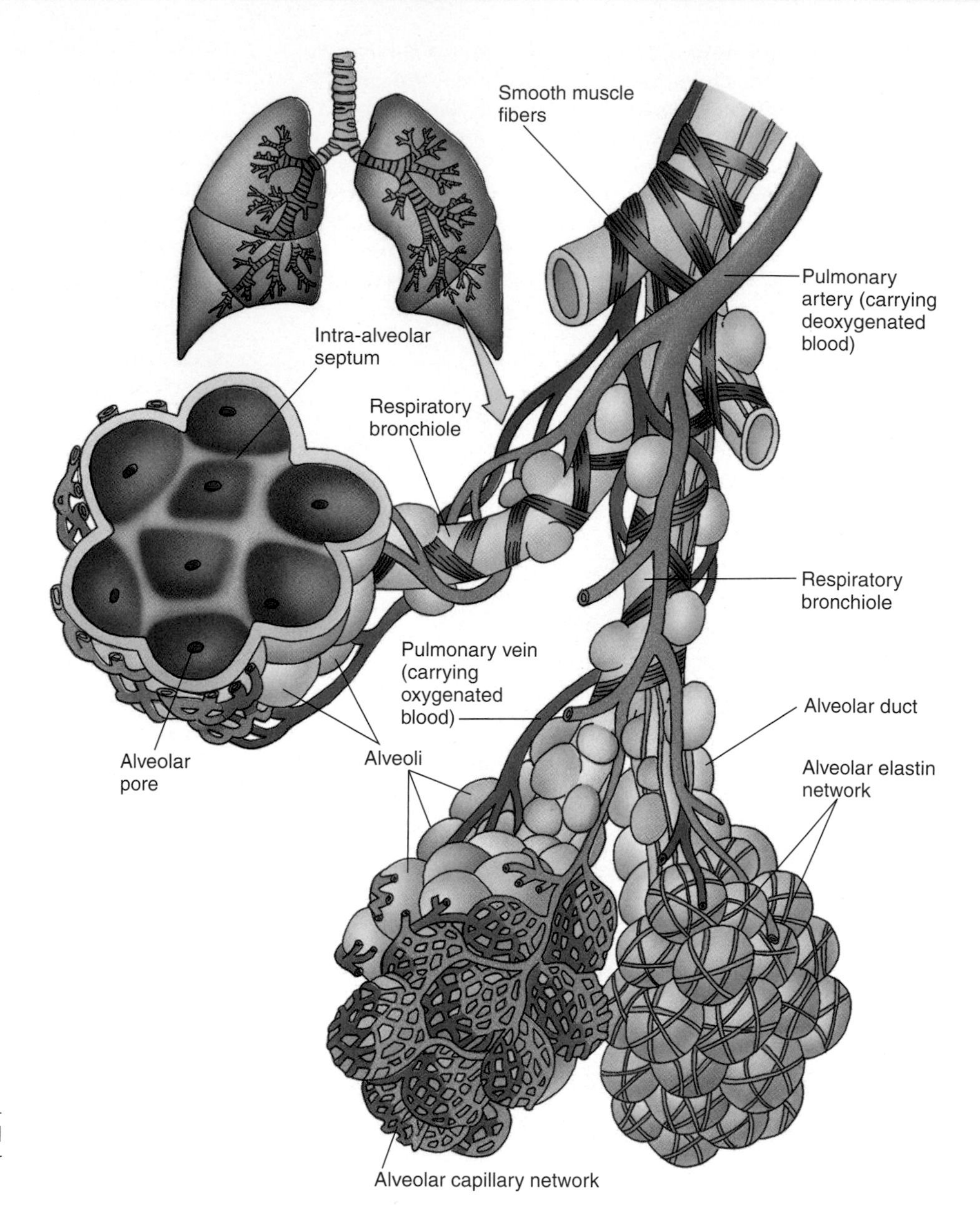

Fig. 15.11 Schematic diagram of the respiratory system, displaying bronchioles, terminal bronchioles, respiratory bronchioles, alveolar ducts, sacs, and alveoli.

Respiratory Portion of the Respiratory System

The respiratory portion of the respiratory system is composed of respiratory bronchioles, alveolar ducts, alveolar sacs, and alveoli.

RESPIRATORY BRONCHIOLES

Respiratory bronchioles are the first region of the respiratory system where exchange of gases can occur.

Respiratory bronchioles are similar in structure to terminal bronchioles in that their epithelium is a simple cuboidal epithelium rich in club cells and some ciliated cells. However, this epithelium is broken up by the presence of thin-walled, pouch-like structures known as **alveoli**, composed of an attenuated simple squamous epithelium, where gaseous exchange (O_2 for CO_2) can occur. As respiratory bronchioles branch, they become narrower in diameter and their population of alveoli increases. Subsequent to several branchings, each respiratory bronchiole terminates in an alveolar duct (Fig. 15.16).

ALVEOLAR DUCT, ATRIUM, AND ALVEOLAR SAC

Alveolar ducts, atria, and alveoli are supplied by a rich capillary network.

Alveolar ducts do not have walls of their own; they are merely a continuous sequence of alveoli (Figs. 15.17 and 15.18). An alveolar duct that arises from a respiratory bronchiole forms branches. Each of the resultant alveolar ducts usually ends as a blind outpouching composed of two or more small clusters of alveoli, in which each cluster is known as an alveolar sac. These alveolar sacs open into a common space, which some investigators call the *atrium*. The cells lining the alveolar ducts are of two types: type I and type II pneumocytes (described in later sections on pneumocytes).

Slender connective tissue elements between alveoli, the **interalveolar septa**, reinforce the alveolar duct, stabilizing it somewhat. Additionally, the opening of each alveolus to the alveolar duct is controlled by a single smooth muscle cell (viewed with the light microscope, this smooth muscle cell has a knob-like appearance), which forms a delicate sphincter regulating the diameter of the opening.

Fine elastic fibers ramify from the periphery of alveolar ducts and sacs to intermingle with elastic fibers radiating from other intrapulmonary elements. This network of elastic fibers not only maintains the patency of these delicate structures during inhalation but also protects them against damage during distention and is responsible for nonforced exhalation.

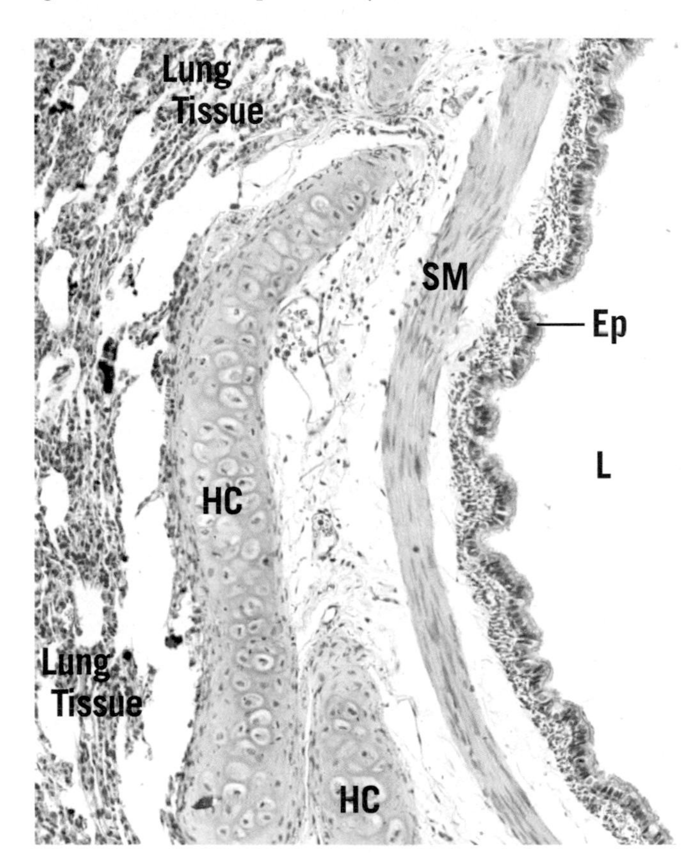

Fig. 15.12 Low-magnification photomicrograph of an intrapulmonary bronchus. Note that the lumen (L) is lined by a respiratory epithelium and that the interface of the lamina propria with the submucosa is occupied by spiraling smooth muscle bundles (SM) that control the diameter of the lumen. The submucosa houses plates of hyaline cartilage (HC) that completely surround the lumen of the intrapulmonary bronchus and the entire structure is embedded in lung tissue. (×132).

ALVEOLUS

Alveoli are small air sacs composed of highly attenuated type I pneumocytes and larger type II pneumocytes.

Each **alveolus** is a small outpunching, about 200 μm in diameter, of respiratory bronchioles, alveolar ducts, and alveolar sacs (Figs. 15.17–15.19). Alveoli form the primary structural and functional unit of the respiratory system because their thin walls permit the exchange of CO_2 for O_2 between the air in their lumina and blood in adjacent capillaries. Although

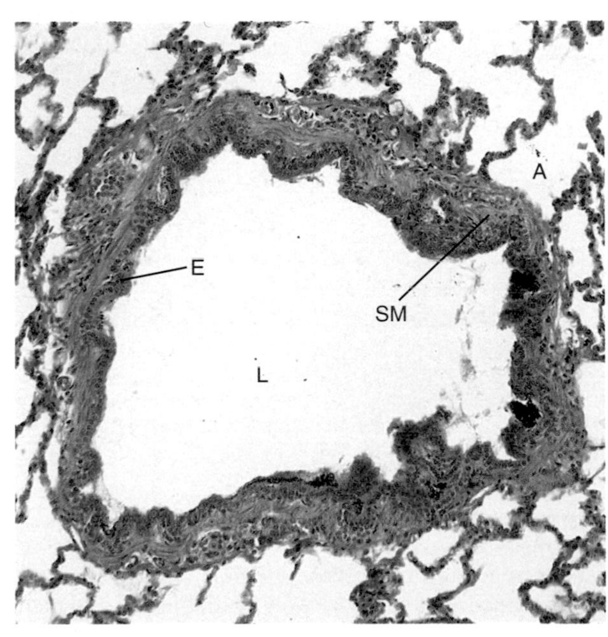

Fig. 15.14 Light photomicrograph of a larger-sized bronchiole. Note the presence of smooth muscle (SM) and the absence of cartilage in its wall. Observe that the entire structure is intrapulmonary and is surrounded by lung tissue. A, Alveolus; E, epithelium; L, lumen. (×117)

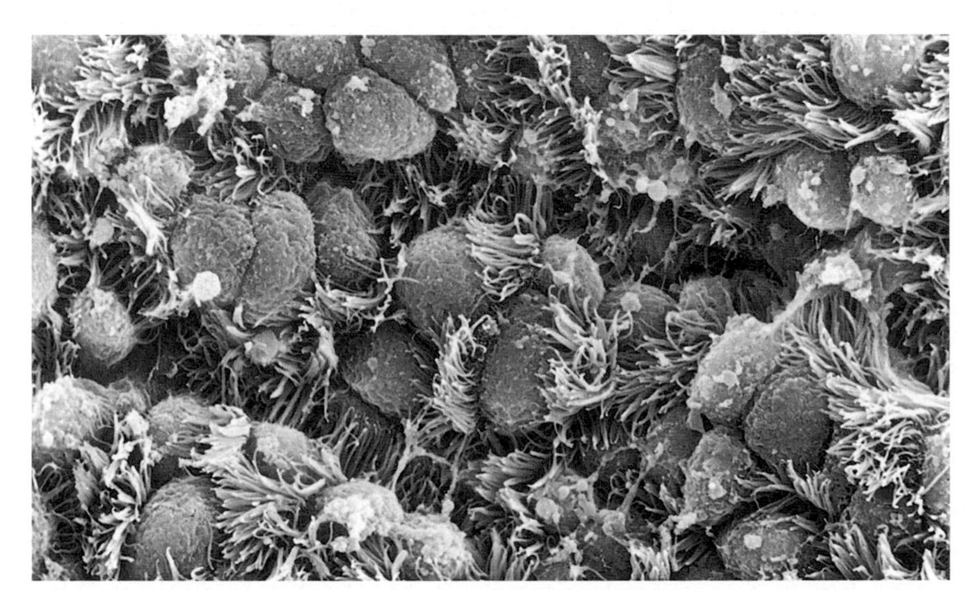

Fig. 15.13 Scanning electron micrograph of club cells and ciliated cuboidal cells of rat terminal bronchioles (×1817). (From Peao MND, Aguas AP, De Sa CM, Grande NR. Anatomy of Clara cell secretion: surface changes observed by scanning electron microscopy. *J Anat.* 1993;183:377-388. Reprinted with permission from Cambridge University Press.)

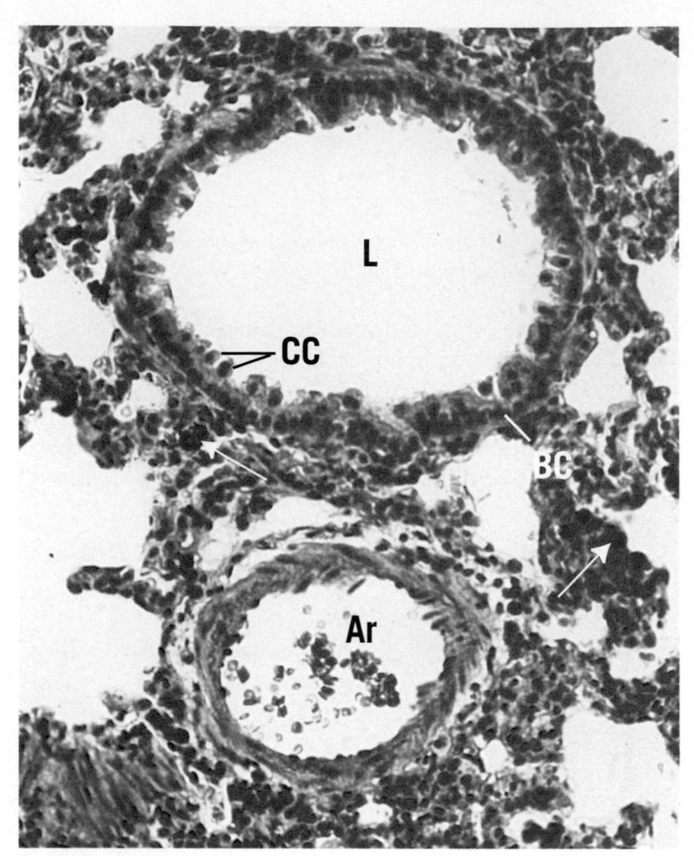

Fig. 15.15 This medium-magnification photomicrograph of a small bronchiole whose lumen (L) is lined by a simple cuboidal epithelium (BC) whose cuboidal cells are interspersed with club cells (CC). A small arteriole (Ar) accompanies the bronchiole and dark dust cells *(arrows)* are easily identified in the lung tissue. (×270)

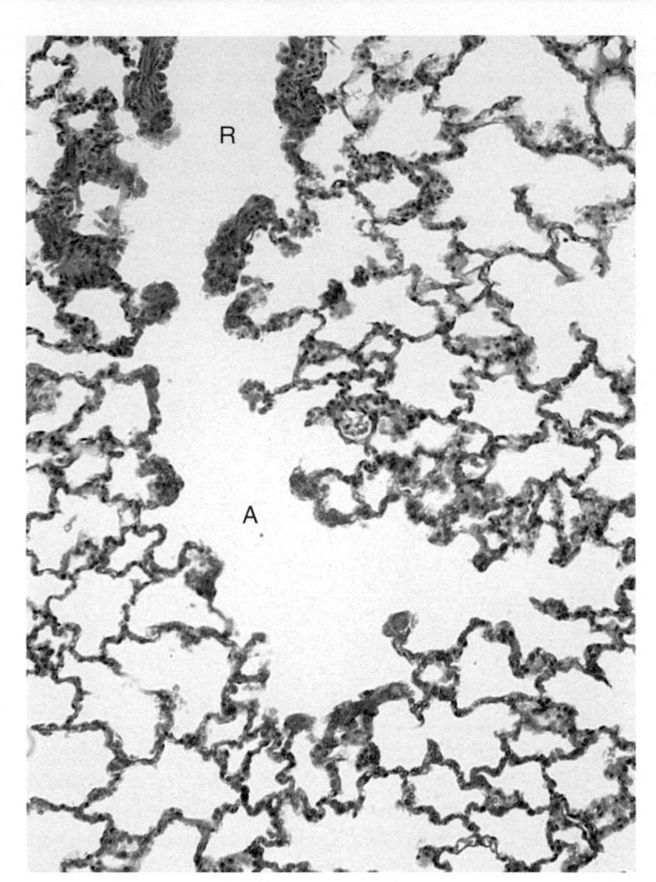

Fig. 15.16 Photomicrograph of a human respiratory bronchiole (R) giving rise to an alveolar duct (A). The respiratory bronchiole has a definite wall with alveoli interjected along its wall, whereas the alveolar duct has no wall of its own; instead, it is composed of alveoli.

each alveolus is a small structure, about 0.002 mm^3, their total number approximates 300 million, conferring on the lung its sponge-like consistency. It has been estimated that the total surface area of all alveoli available for gas exchange exceeds 140 m^2 (the approximate floor space of an average-sized two-bedroom apartment or the size of a singles tennis court).

Alveoli are separated by **interalveolar septa** of various widths containing diverse amounts of connective tissue elements (Fig. 15.20). In fact, because of their large number, alveoli are frequently pressed against each other and the connective tissue interstitium of the interalveolar septum is eliminated between them. In such areas of contact, the air spaces of the two alveoli may communicate with each other through an **alveolar pore (of Kohn)**, whose diameter varies from 8 to 60 μm (see Figs. 15.19 and 15.21).

These pores presumably function to equilibrate air pressure within pulmonary segments. In the region between adjacent alveoli, where the alveoli are not pressed against each other, the interalveolar septum is wider and occupied by an extensive capillary bed composed of **continuous capillaries** supplied by branches of the pulmonary artery and drained by tributaries of the pulmonary vein. The connective tissue of such an interalveolar septum is rich in elastic fibers and type III collagen (reticular) fibers.

Because alveoli and capillaries are composed of epithelial cells, they are invested by a prominent basal lamina. The openings of alveoli associated with alveolar sacs, unlike those of respiratory bronchioles and alveolar ducts, *are devoid of smooth muscle cells*. Instead, their orifices are circumscribed by elastic, and especially by reticular fibers. Walls of alveoli are composed mostly of two types of cells: type I pneumocytes and type II pneumocytes, although macrophages (dust cells) are also associated with the alveolar walls.

Type I Pneumocytes

Approximately 95% of the alveolar surface is composed of simple squamous epithelium, whose cells are known as **type I pneumocytes** (also called **type I alveolar cells** or **squamous alveolar cells**). Because the cells of this epithelium are highly attenuated, their cytoplasm may be as thin as 80 nm in width (Fig. 15.22). The region of the nucleus is—as expected—wider, and it houses much of the cell's organelle population, composed of a small number of mitochondria, a few profiles of RER, and a modest Golgi apparatus.

Type I pneumocytes form occluding junctions, preventing the seepage of extracellular fluid into the alveolar lumen. The adluminal aspect of these cells is covered by a well-developed basal lamina, which extends almost to the rim of the alveolar pores (of Kohn). The rim of each alveolar pore is formed by the fusion of the cell membranes of two closely apposed type I pneumocytes that belong to two discrete alveoli. The luminal aspect of type I pneumocytes is lined by surfactant, as detailed in the following discussion.

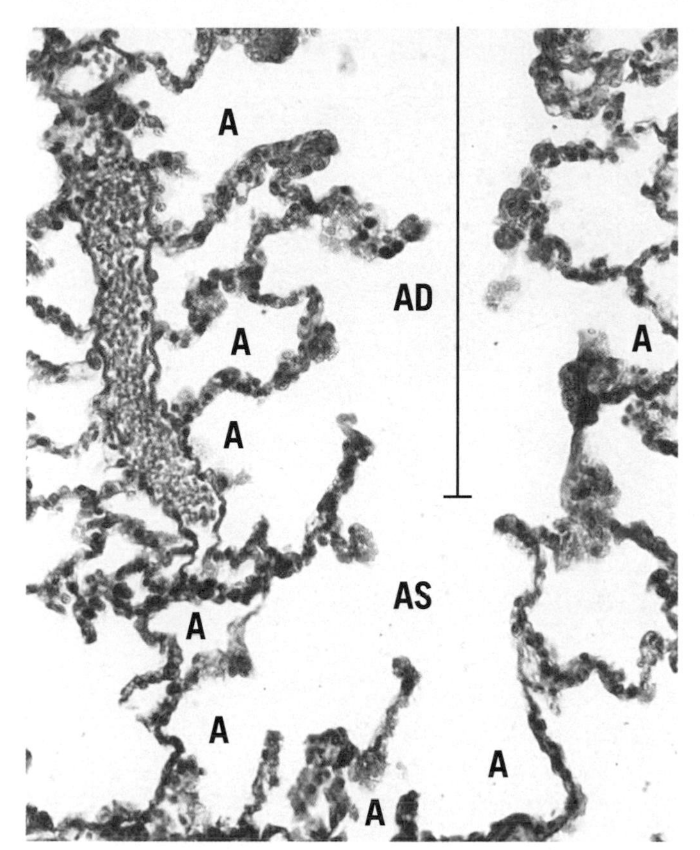

Fig. 15.17 Photomicrograph of alveoli (A) projecting off an alveolar duct (AD), which opens into an alveolar sac (AS) composed of several alveoli. (×270)

Type II Pneumocytes

Although **type II pneumocytes** (also known as **great alveolar cells**, **septal cells**, or **type II alveolar cells**) are more numerous than type I pneumocytes, they occupy only about 5% of the alveolar surface. These cuboidal-shaped cells are interspersed among type I pneumocytes and form occluding junctions with them. Their dome-shaped apical surface juts into the lumen of the alveolus (Fig. 15.23). Type II pneumocytes are usually located in regions where adjacent alveoli are separated by a septum (hence the name *septal cells*), and their adluminal surface is covered by basal lamina.

Electron micrographs of type II pneumocytes display short apical microvilli. They have a centrally placed nucleus, an abundance of RER profiles, a well-developed Golgi apparatus, and mitochondria. The most distinguishing feature of these cells is the presence of membrane-bound **lamellar bodies** that contain **pulmonary surfactant**, the secretory product of these cells.

Pulmonary surfactant, synthesized on the RER of type II pneumocytes, is composed primarily of two phospholipids—**dipalmitoyl phosphatidylcholine** and **phosphatidylglycerol**, **neutral lipid**, and **cholesterol**—and four unique proteins, **surfactant apoproteins SP-A, SP-B, SP-C**, and **SP-D**. The surfactant is modified in the Golgi apparatus and is then released from the *trans*-Golgi network into secretory vesicles, known as **composite bodies**, the immediate precursors of **lamellar bodies** (Fig. 15.24).

Clinical Correlations

At birth, an infant's lungs expand upon the first intake of breath and the presence of pulmonary surfactant permits the alveoli to remain patent. Premature infants (those born before 7 months of gestation) who have not as yet produced surfactant (or who have produced an inadequate supply of surfactant) have potentially fatal ***respiratory distress of the newborn****. These newborns are treated with a combination of synthetic surfactant and glucocorticoid therapy. The synthetic surfactant acts immediately to reduce surface tension, and glucocorticoids stimulate type II pneumocytes to produce surfactant.*

The surfactant is released by exocytosis into the lumen of the alveolus. Here, it forms a broad, lattice-like network, known as **tubular myelin**, which becomes a mononuclear film separated into lipid and protein portions. The lipid is inserted into a monomolecular phospholipid film forming an interface with air (the **superficial lipid phase**), and the protein enters an aqueous layer, the **lower aqueous phase**, between the pneumocytes and the phospholipid film. The surfactant not only decreases surface tension, preventing atelectasis (the collapse of the alveolus) but also resists (*but does not prevent*) fluid entry into the alveolar air space. It is continuously manufactured by type II pneumocytes plus also phagocytosed and recycled by type II pneumocytes and, less frequently, by alveolar macrophages (dust cells). The apoproteins SP-A and SP-D act as **opsonins**, which, by bonding to microorganisms, make them more attractive for phagocytosis by alveolar macrophages (dust cells). Additionally, SP-A controls the formation of surfactant by type II pneumocytes. SP-B and SP-C function in tandem to arrange the structure of surfactant so that it spreads along the alveolar surface at a rapid rate.

In addition to producing and phagocytosing surfactant, type II pneumocytes undergo mitosis to regenerate themselves as well as type I pneumocytes.

Alveolar Macrophages (Dust Cells)

Alveolar macrophages phagocytose particulate matter in the lumen of the alveolus, as well as in the interalveolar spaces.

Monocytes gain access to the pulmonary interstitium, become **alveolar macrophages** (**dust cells**), migrate between type I pneumocytes, and enter the lumen of the alveolus. These cells phagocytose particulate matter—such as dust, other inhaled particulate matter, and microorganisms—maintaining a sterile environment within the lungs. However, they are not nearly as avid phagocytes as are most other macrophages (see Figs. 15.21 and 15.25). Dust cells also assist type II pneumocytes in the uptake of surfactant. Interestingly, these cells are unusual in that, unlike macrophages in other regions of the body, they are programmed to be anti-inflammatory. Approximately 100 million macrophages migrate from the lungs to the bronchi each day and are transported from there, along with the mucus, by ciliary action to the pharynx to be eliminated by being swallowed or expectorated. Some alveolar macrophages, however, reenter the pulmonary interstitium and migrate into lymph vessels to exit the lungs.

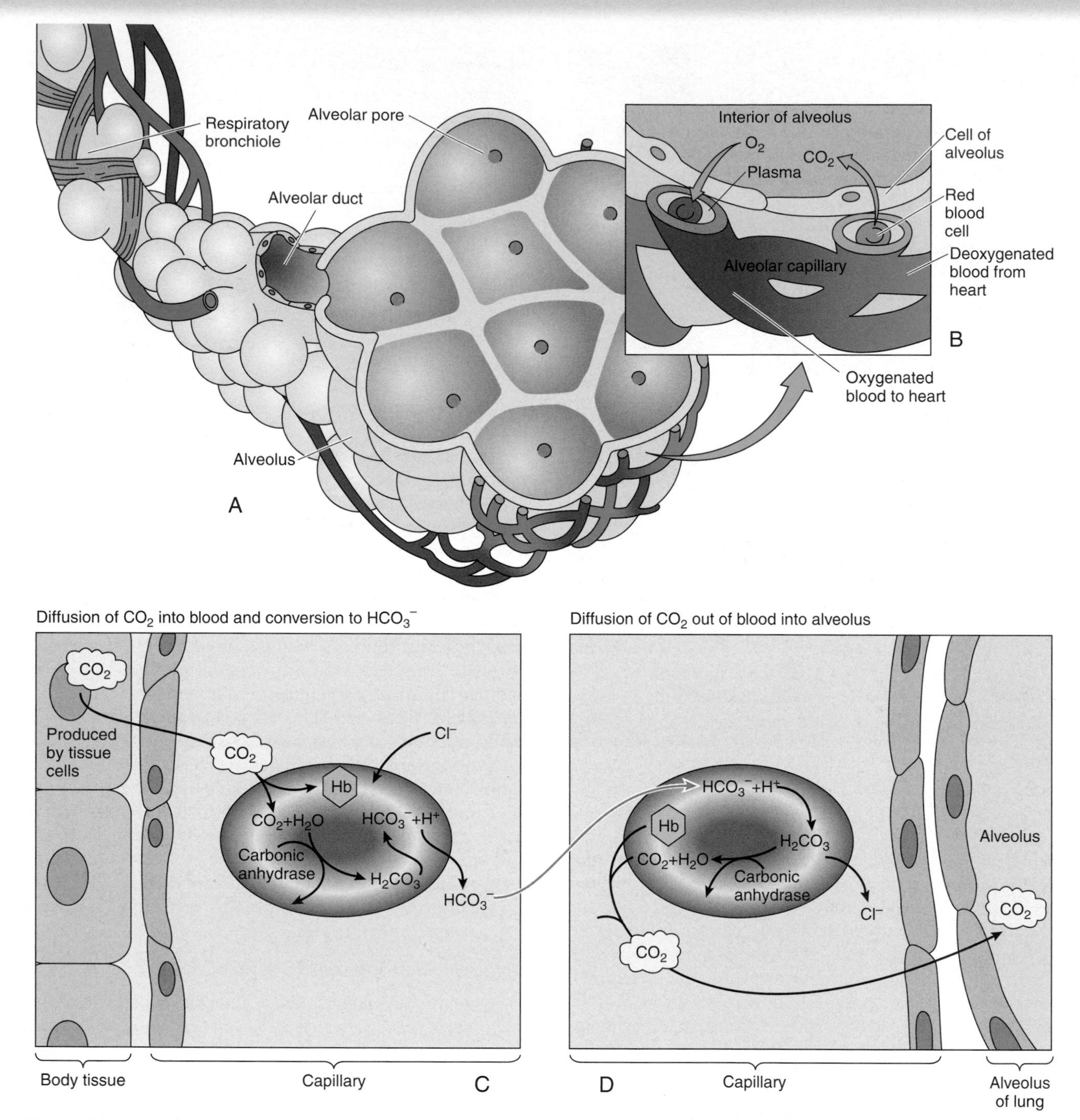

Fig. 15.18 Schematic diagram. (A) A respiratory bronchiole, alveolar sac, alveolar pore, and alveoli. (B) Interalveolar septum. (C) Carbon dioxide uptake from body tissues by erythrocytes and plasma. (D) Carbon dioxide release by erythrocytes and plasma in the lung. Compare (A) with Figs. 15.16 and 15.17 depicting a photomicrograph of the alveolar duct.

Clinical Correlations

1. *Alveolar macrophages of patients with pulmonary congestion and congestive heart failure contain phagocytosed, extravasated red blood cells. These macrophages are frequently called* **heart failure cells.**
2. **Emphysema** *is a disease usually associated with the sequelae of long-term exposure to cigarette smoke and/or other inhibitors of the protein α_1-antitrypsin. This protein safeguards the lungs against the destruction of elastic fibers by elastase synthesized by dust cells. In such patients, elasticity of the lung tissue is reduced, and large, fluid-filled sacs are present that decrease the gas-exchange capability of the respiratory portion of the respiratory system.*

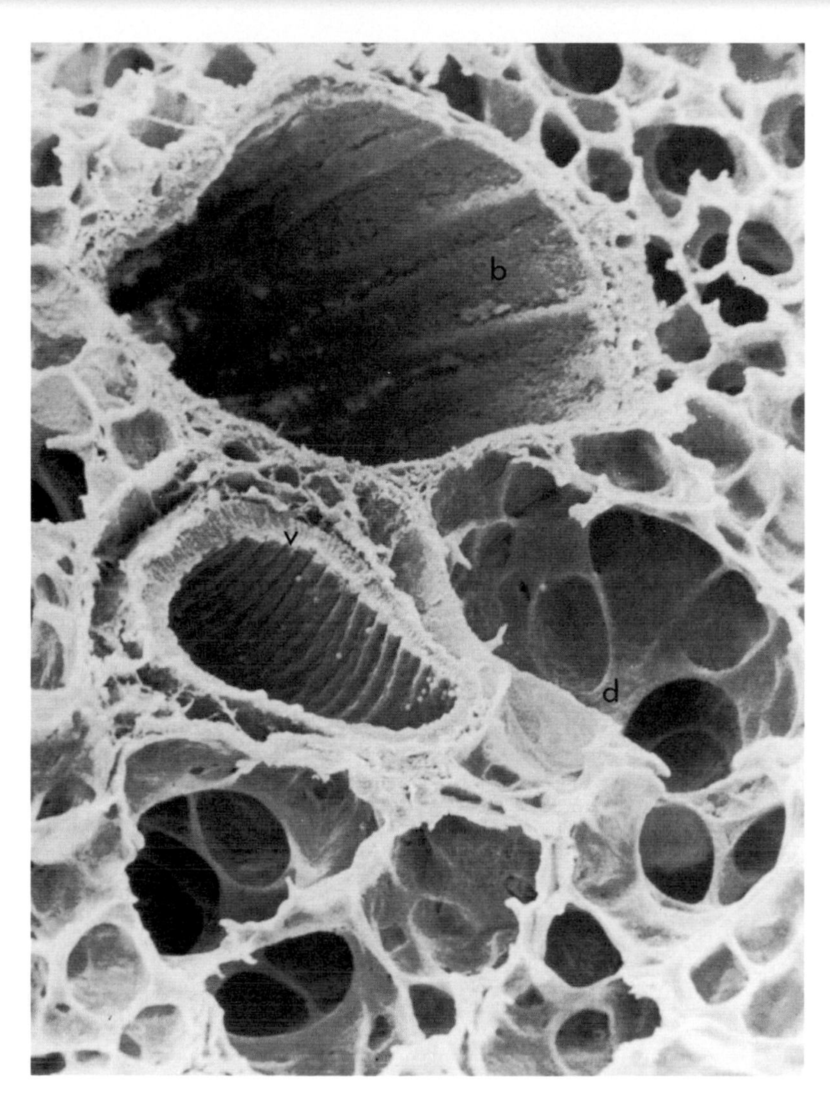

Fig. 15.19 Scanning electron micrograph of a rat lung displaying a bronchiole (b), a small artery (v), and alveoli (d), some of which present alveolar pores. (From Leeson TS, Leeson CR, Paparo AA. *Text/Atlas of Histology*. Philadelphia: WB Saunders; 1988.)

Interalveolar Septum

As indicated previously, the region between two adjacent alveoli is known as an ***interalveolar septum***, which is lined on both sides by alveolar epithelium (see Fig. 15.21). The interalveolar septum may be extremely narrow, housing nothing or only a **continuous capillary** and its basal lamina, or it may be somewhat wider, including connective tissue elements, such as type III collagen and elastic fibers, macrophages, fibroblasts (and myofibroblasts), mast cells, and lymphoid elements.

Blood–Gas Barrier

The blood–gas barrier is that region of the interalveolar septum that is traversed by O_2 and CO_2. These gases go from the lumen of the blood vessel to the lumen of the alveolus and vice versa.

The thinnest regions of the interalveolar septum where gases can be exchanged are called the ***blood–gas barriers*** (see Fig. 15.22). The narrowest blood–gas barrier, where the type I pneumocyte is in intimate contact with the endothelial lining of the capillary and the basal laminae of the two epithelia become fused, is the most efficient site for the exchange of O_2 (in the alveolar lumen) for CO_2 (in the blood). These regions are composed of the following three structures:

- Surfactant and type I pneumocytes
- Fused basal laminae of type I pneumocytes and endothelial cells of the capillary
- Endothelial cells of the continuous capillary

Exchange of Gases between the Tissues and Lungs

In the lungs, O_2 is exchanged for CO_2 carried by blood. In the tissues of the body, CO_2 is exchanged for O_2 carried by blood.

During inspiration, oxygen-containing air enters the alveolar spaces of the lung. Because the total surface area of all alveoli exceeds 140 m^2 and the total blood volume in all of the capillaries in the lungs at any one time is no more than 140 mL, the space available for diffusion of gases is enormous. Moreover, the diameter of the capillaries is small enough so that red blood cells may travel in a single file only, thus oxygen can reach each erythrocyte from all around, using all of the red blood cell surface area available for gas exchange. Oxygen diffuses through the blood–gas barrier to enter the lumina of the capillaries and binds to the **heme** portion of the erythrocyte hemoglobin, forming **oxyhemoglobin**. CO_2 leaves the blood, diffuses through the blood–gas barrier into the lumina of the alveolus, and exits the alveolar spaces as the CO_2-rich air is exhaled. The passage of O_2 and CO_2 across the blood–gas barrier is due to passive diffusion in response to the partial pressures of these gases within the blood and alveolar lumina (see also Chapter 10 in the section on hemoglobin). Carbon dioxide uptake from body tissues by erythrocytes and plasma and carbon dioxide release by erythrocytes and plasma in the lung are illustrated in Fig. 15.18.

Clinical Correlations

Hemoglobin also has two types of binding sites for ***nitric oxide (NO)****, a neurotransmitter substance that, when released by endothelial cells of blood vessels, causes relaxation of the vascular smooth muscle cells, with a resultant dilation of the blood vessels. Hemoglobin, S-nitrosylated (binding site 1) by NO manufactured by blood vessels of the lung, ferries bound NO to arterioles and metarterioles of the tissues, where NO is released and causes vasodilation. In this fashion, hemoglobin not only contributes to the modulation of blood pressure but also facilitates the more efficient exchange of O_2 for CO_2. Moreover, once O_2 leaves the heme portion of hemoglobin to oxygenate the tissues, NO takes its place on the iron atoms (binding site 2) and is transported into the lungs, where it is released into the alveoli to be exhaled along with CO_2.*

PLEURAL CAVITIES AND THE MECHANISM OF VENTILATION

Alteration of the volume of the pleural cavities by muscle action is responsible for the movement of gases into and out of the respiratory system.

The thoracic cage is separated into three regions: the left and right thoracic cavities and the centrally located mediastinum. Each thoracic cavity is lined by a serous membrane, the **pleura**, composed of simple squamous epithelium and subserous connective tissue. The pleura may be imagined as an inflated balloon; as the lung develops, it pushes against this serous membrane, as if a fist were pushing against the outer surface of a balloon. In this fashion, a portion of the pleura, the **visceral pleura**, covers and adheres to the lung; the remainder of the pleura, the **parietal pleura**, lines and adheres to the walls of the thoracic cavity.

The space between the visceral and parietal pleura (inside the balloon) is known as the ***pleural cavity***. This space contains a slight amount of serous fluid (produced by the serous membranes) that permits a nearly frictionless movement of the lungs during **ventilation** (breathing), which involves air moving into the lungs (inhalation) and out of the lungs (exhalation).

Inhalation is an energy-requiring process because it involves contraction of the diaphragm, intercostal, scalene, and other accessory respiratory muscles. As these muscles contract, the volume of the thoracic cage expands. Because the parietal pleura is firmly attached to the walls of the thoracic cage, the pleural cavities also increase in volume; consequently, the pressure within the pleural cavities decreases. The pressure differential between the atmospheric pressure outside of the body and the pressure within the pleural cavities drives air into the lungs. With the influx of air, the lungs expand, stretching the elastic fiber network of the pleural interstitium, and the visceral pleura is brought closer to the parietal pleura, reducing the volume of the pleural cavities and, thus, increasing the pressure inside of the pleural cavities.

For **exhalation** to occur, the respiratory (and accessory respiratory) muscles relax, decreasing the volume of the pleural cavities, with a consequent increase in pressure within the pleural cavities. Additionally, the stretched elastic fibers return to their resting length, driving air out of the lungs. Thus, normal expiration does not require energy. In forced expiration, the internal intercostal and abdominal muscles also contract further, decreasing the volume of the pleural cavity, forcing additional air to leave the lungs.

Clinical Correlations

In patients afflicted with ***poliomyelitis****, the muscles of respiration may become so weakened that the accessory muscles hypertrophy because they become responsible for the elevation of the thoracic cage. In other diseases, such as* ***myasthenia gravis*** *and* ***Guillain-Barré syndrome****, the weakness of the respiratory and accessory respiratory muscles may lead to respiratory failure and consequent death, even though the lungs function normally.*

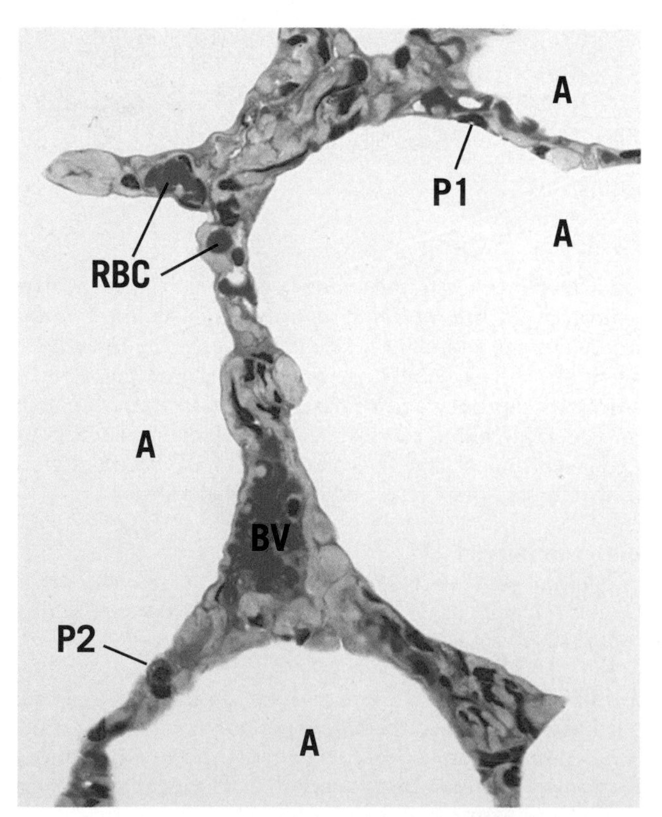

Fig. 15.20 Photomicrograph of several alveoli (A) composed of type 1 (P1) and type 2 pneumocytes (P2). The interalveolar septum is occupied by very small blood vessels (BV), continuous capillaries housing erythrocytes (RBC), and a slender amount of fibroelastic connective tissue. (×540)

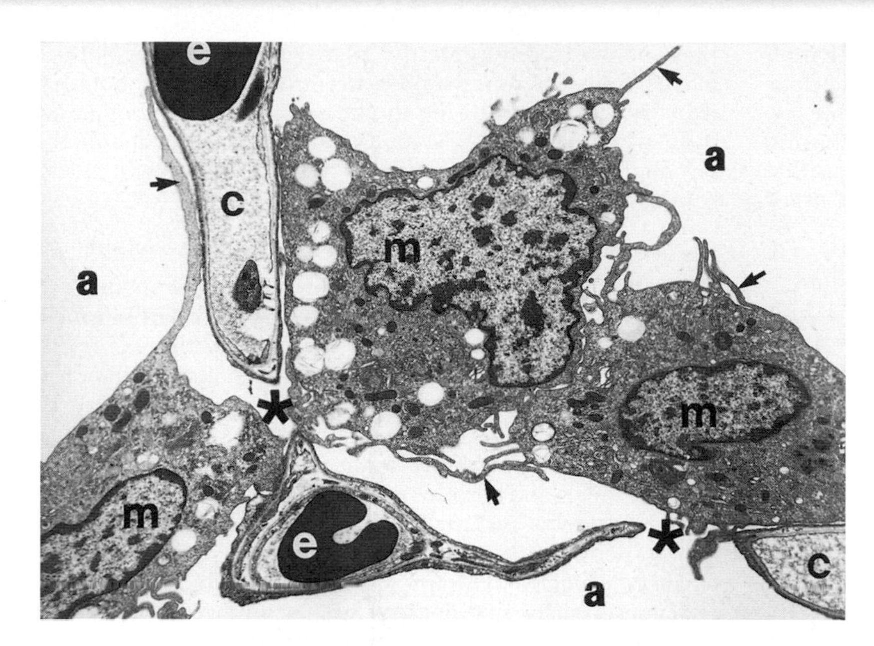

Fig. 15.21 Transmission electron micrograph of the interalveolar septum in a monkey. Note the presence of alveoli (a), erythrocytes (e) within capillaries (c), and alveolar macrophages (m). The filopodia *(arrows)* are evident. *Asterisks* indicate the presence of alveolar pores. (From Maina JN. Morphology and morphometry of the normal lung of the adult vervet monkey [*Cercopithecus aethiops*]. *Am J Anat.* 1988;183:258-267. Reprinted with permission from Wiley-Liss, Inc., a subsidiary of John Wiley & Sons, Inc.)

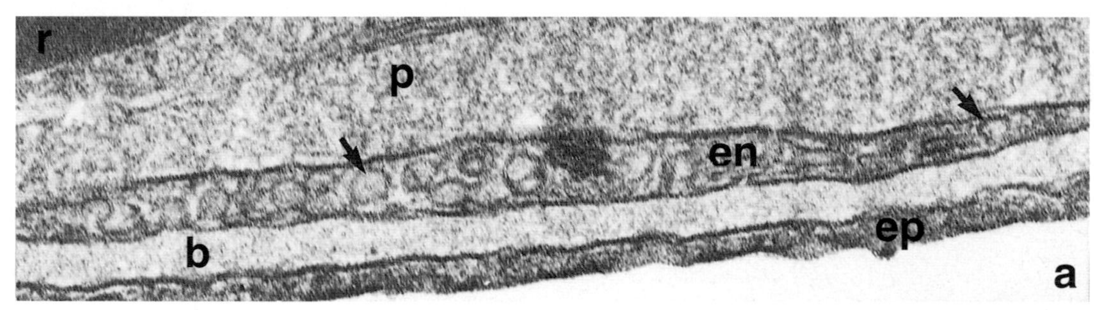

Fig. 15.22 Transmission electron micrograph of the blood–gas barrier (×71,250). Note the presence of the alveolus (a), attenuated type I pneumocytes (ep), fused basal laminae (b), attenuated endothelial cell of the capillary (en) with pinocytotic vesicles *(arrows)*, plasma (p), and erythrocyte (r) within the capillary lumen. (From Maina JN. Morphology and morphometry of the normal lung of the adult vervet monkey [*Cercopithecus aethiops*]. *Am J Anat.* 1988;183:258-267. Reprinted with permission from Wiley-Liss, Inc., a subsidiary of John Wiley & Sons, Inc.)

GROSS STRUCTURE OF THE LUNGS

The left lung has two lobes and the right lung has three lobes.

The left lung is subdivided into two lobes and the right lung is subdivided into three lobes. Each lung has a medial indentation, the **hilum**, where the primary bronchi, bronchiolar arteries, and pulmonary arteries enter and the bronchiolar veins, pulmonary veins, and lymph vessels leave the lung. This group of vessels and the airway that enter the hilum make up the **root** of the lung.

Each lobe is subdivided into several **bronchopulmonary segments** supplied by a tertiary intrapulmonary (segmental) bronchus. In turn, bronchopulmonary segments are subdivided into many **lobules**, each served by a bronchiole. Lobules are separated by connective tissue septa, in which lymph vessels and tributaries of pulmonary veins travel. Branches of bronchial and pulmonary arteries follow bronchioles in their passage through the center of the lobule.

Pulmonary Vascular and Lymphatic Supply

The pulmonary arteries supply deoxygenated blood to the lungs from the right side of the heart at a rate of 5 L per minute. Branches of these vessels follow the bronchial tubes into the lobules of the lung (see Fig. 15.11). When they reach the respiratory bronchioles, these vessels form an extensive pulmonary capillary network composed strictly of **continuous capillaries**. Because these capillaries are only 8 μm in diameter, erythrocytes, as indicated previously, follow each other in single file through them, reducing the space that gases have to traverse and maximally exposing the erythrocytes to oxygen.

The blood in the capillary bed becomes oxygenated and then drains into veins of increasing diameter. These tributaries of the pulmonary vein carry oxygenated blood and travel in the septa between lobules of the lung. Thus, the veins follow a path that is different from that of the arteries until they reach the apex of the lobule, where they accompany the bronchial tubes to the hilum of the lung to deliver oxygenated blood to the left side of the heart.

Bronchial arteries, which are branches of the thoracic aorta, bring nutrient-laden and oxygen-laden blood to the bronchial tree, interlobular septa, and pleura of the lungs. Many of the small branches anastomose with those of the pulmonary system. Others are drained by tributaries of the **bronchial veins**, which return the blood to the azygos system of veins.

The lung has a dual-lymph drainage, a superficial system of vessels in the visceral pleura and a deep network of vessels in the pulmonary interstitium, but these systems have numerous interconnections. The superficial system of lymph vessels forms several larger vessels, which drain into the hilar (bronchopulmonary) lymph nodes at the root of each lung. The deep network is organized into three groups following the pulmonary arteries, pulmonary veins, and bronchial tree down to the levels of the respiratory bronchioles. All of these networks drain into the hilar lymph nodes at the root of each lung. Efferent lymph vessels from these lymph nodes deliver their lymph to the thoracic duct or right lymphatic duct, which returns the lymph to the junction of the internal jugular and subclavian veins of the left and right sides, respectively.

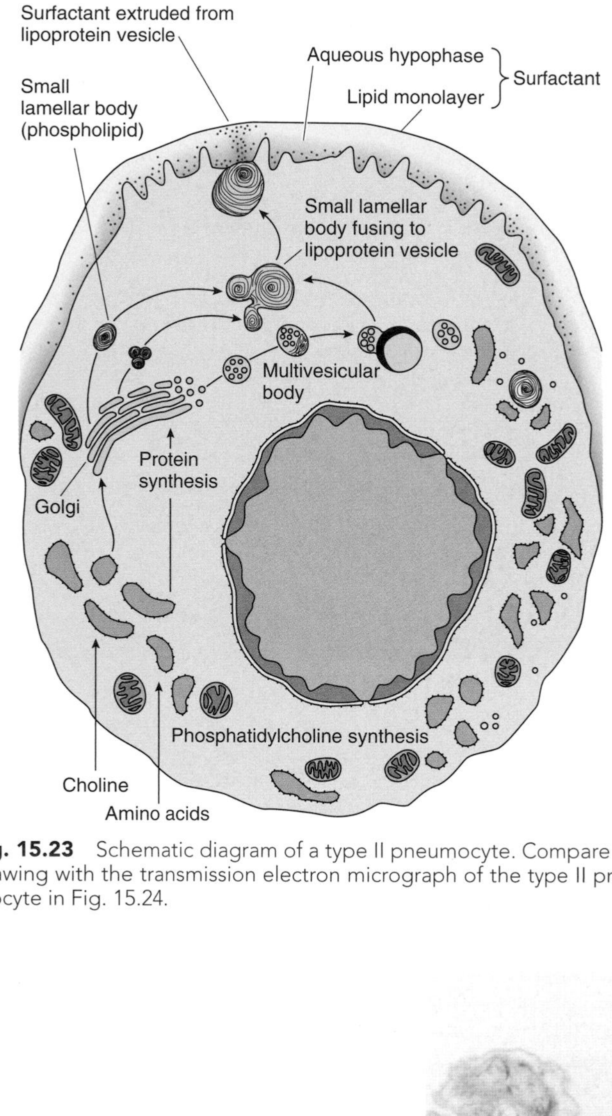

Fig. 15.23 Schematic diagram of a type II pneumocyte. Compare this drawing with the transmission electron micrograph of the type II pneumocyte in Fig. 15.24.

Mucosal Immune Defense of the Respiratory System

The respiratory system possesses its own regional immune system, **bronchus-associated lymphoid tissue (BALT)**, which creates a barrier to the invasion of various pathogens in its immediate milieu while maintaining an equilibrium between mounting a defense against invading pathogens and "ignoring" the presence of various commensal and symbiotic organisms. The barrier that is established by the respiratory system involves both the innate and adaptive immune systems. The components of these systems include the pharyngeal tonsil; bronchiolar lymph nodes and nodules; nasal/pharyngeal/tracheal/bronchial/bronchiolar epithelium and the **antimicrobial peptide**-containing mucus that lines its luminal surface; subepithelial lymphoid tissue and lymphoid cells (including dendritic cells); humoral antibodies (IgA, IgG, IgE); and the surfactant proteins SP-A and SP-D.

Although this particular aspect of the regional immune system is referred to as *bronchiolar*, it also includes the alveoli where **innate immune responses** are present but are finely modulated to ensure that inflammation, a process that would interfere with the exchange of gases, does not occur. Because there is no mucus production in the respiratory portion of the respiratory system, it is the presence of some of the surfactant proteins that act as components of the innate immune process. Some of these surfactant components bind to carbohydrate molecules, pathogen-associated molecular patterns that are expressed on many pathogen surfaces, opsonizing these pathogens, thus marking them for phagocytosis by macrophages (dust cells). Others, such as SP-A, prevent macrophage Toll-like receptors from activating dust cells, whereas SP-D diminishes the phagocytic activity of dust cells.

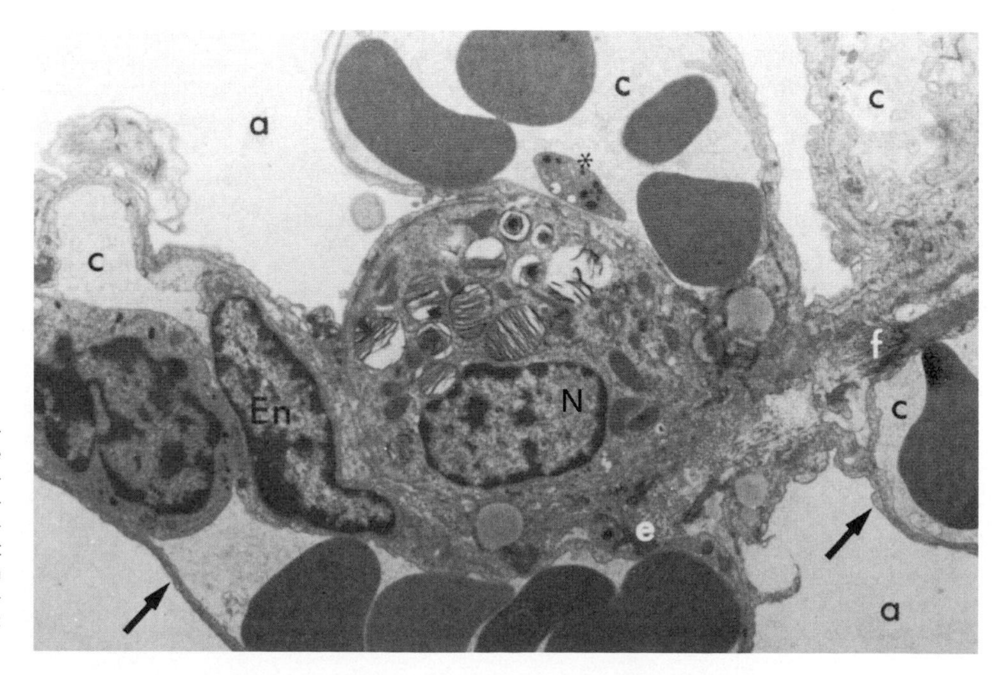

Fig. 15.24 Transmission electron micrograph of a type II pneumocyte. Observe the centrally placed nucleus (N) flanked by several lamellar bodies. a, Alveolus; c, capillaries; e, elastic fibers; En, nucleus of endothelial cell; f, collagen fibers. *Arrows* represent the blood–gas barrier; *asterisk* represents a platelet. (From Leeson TS, Leeson CR, Paparo AA. *Text/Atlas of Histology*. Philadelphia: WB Saunders; 1988.)

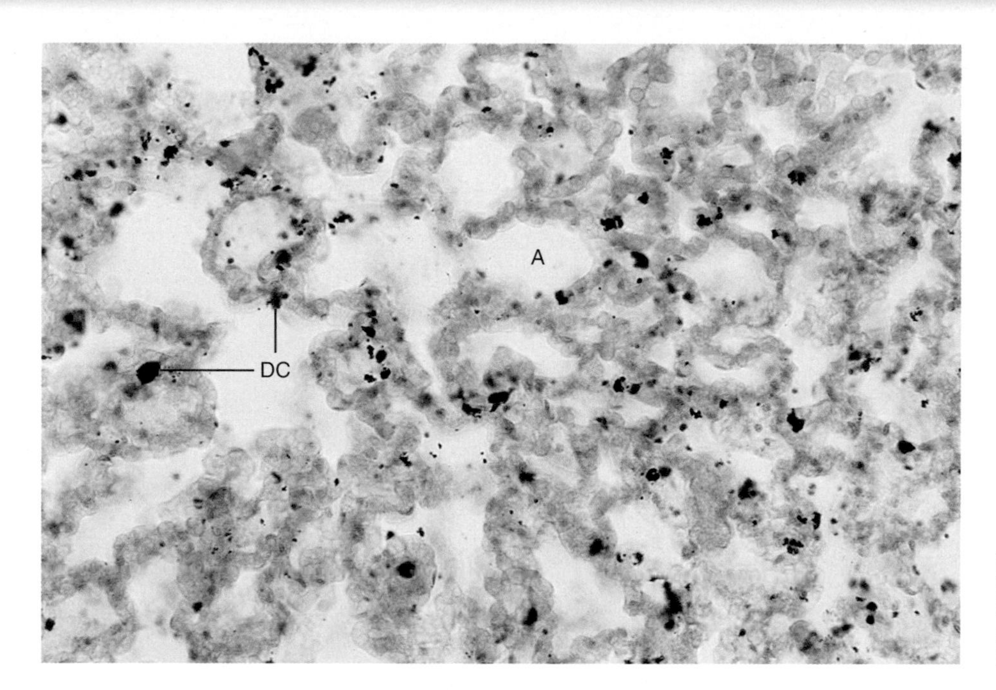

Fig. 15.25 Alveolar macrophages (dust cells) in the human lung. Dust cells (DC) appear as black spots on the image because they have phagocytosed dust particles that were present in the air spaces of the lung. A, Alveolus. (×270)

The **adaptive immunity** of the BALT depends on plasma cells and T cells. **Plasma cells** are recruited into the subepithelial connective tissue by chemokines released by the respiratory epithelium; the plasma cells secrete IgA, which passes through the epithelium into the lumina of the conducting portion of the respiratory system, where they bind to and inactivate antigens. Some IgE is also manufactured and released by plasma cells, but these remain in the connective tissue, where they bind to mast cells, eliciting inflammatory responses. T-cell responses are due to the activities of **dendritic cells** that protrude their processes into the lumina of the bronchiolar system of airways and sequester antigens. These dendritic cells then migrate to the pharyngeal tonsil, bronchiolar lymph nodes, and nodules and present their epitopes to T cells that reside in those structures to elicit a cell-mediated immune response.

Pulmonary Nerve Supply

The thoracic sympathetic chain ganglia provide sympathetic fibers and the vagus nerve supplies parasympathetic fibers to the smooth muscles of the bronchial tree. **Sympathetic fibers** (β-adrenergic) cause *relaxation* of bronchial smooth muscles and thus bronchodilation (while causing constriction of pulmonary blood vessels, known as a "paradoxical response"). **Parasympathetic fibers** are cholinergic; they elicit *contraction* of bronchial smooth muscles, causing bronchioconstriction. Nonadrenergic, noncholinergic fibers also travel with the vagus nerve, causing bronchodilation by releasing NO near bronchial smooth muscle, effecting their relaxation.

Occasionally, synapses have been noted to occur with type II pneumocytes, suggesting the possibility of some neural control over the production of pulmonary surfactant.

Clinical Correlations

*It has been demonstrated, at least in mice, that stretch sensing cation channels, formed by the multipass transmembrane protein **Piezo2**, are present in the nerve endings of pulmonary nerve fibers. These channels open when the lungs become stretched during inspiration and prevent them from becoming overinflated. People with mutations in the gene coding for Piezo2 display not only breathing disorders but also defects in their sensations of touch and proprioception.*

Pathological Considerations

See Figs. 15.26 through 15.29.

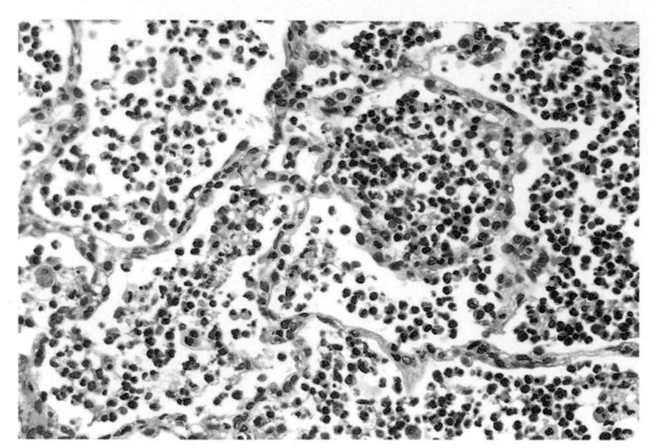

Fig. 15.26 Photomicrograph of the lung of an individual with acute bacterial pneumonia. Observe the congested capillaries of the interalveolar septa, as well as the large number of neutrophils occupying the alveolar air spaces. (Reprinted with permission from Kumar V, Abbas AK, Aster JC. *Robbins and Cotran Pathologic Basis of Disease*. 9th ed. Philadelphia: Elsevier; 2015:705.)

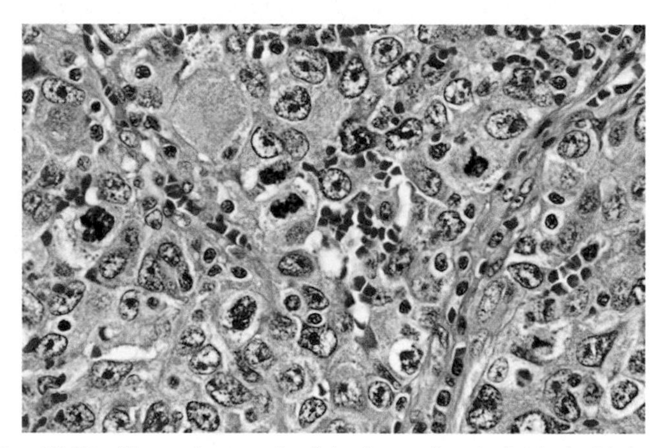

Fig. 15.27 Photomicrograph of the lung of an individual with large cell carcinoma. Observe the large, pleomorphic tumor cells and the absence of glandular differentiation. (Reprinted with permission from Kumar V, Abbas AK, Aster JC. *Robbins and Cotran Pathologic Basis of Disease*. 9th ed. Philadelphia: Elsevier; 2015:715.)

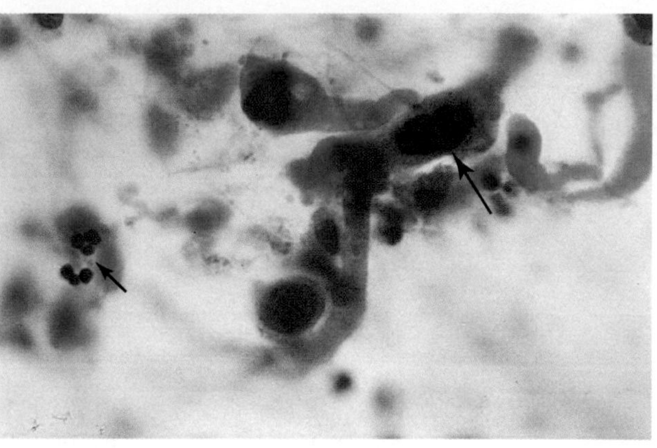

Fig. 15.28 Photomicrograph of sputum that is characteristic of an individual with cancer of the lung. Observe the characteristic large densely staining nucleus of keratinized squamous carcinoma cell *(large arrow)*. The size of the cancer cell is evident compared with the size of a normal neutrophil *(small arrow)*. (Reprinted with permission from Kumar V, Abbas AK, Aster JC. *Robbins and Cotran Pathologic Basis of Disease*. 9th ed. Philadelphia: Elsevier; 2015:717.)

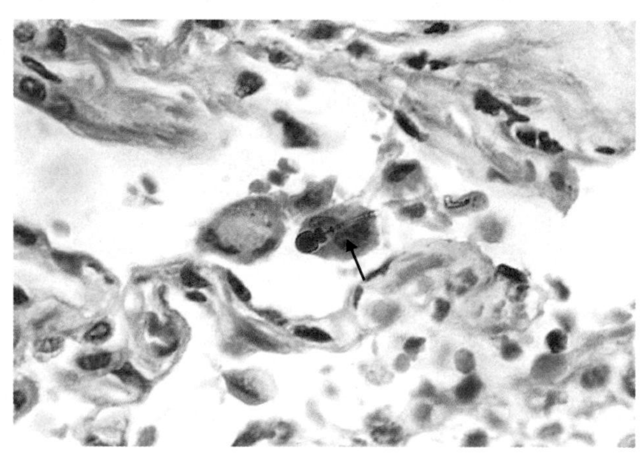

Fig. 15.29 Photomicrograph of the lung of an individual with asbestosis. Observe the asbestos body *(arrow)* characterized by the beaded appearance with knob-shaped ends. (Reprinted with permission from Kumar V, Abbas AK, Aster JC. *Robbins and Cotran Pathologic Basis of Disease*. 9th ed. Philadelphia: Elsevier; 2015:691.)

Histology Laboratory Instructions: Respiratory System

Nasal Cavity

A low-magnification photomicrograph of the cartilaginous portion of the nasal septum displays the hyaline cartilage skeleton with its cellular and fibrous perichondrium. The lamina propria is a highly vascular connective tissue housing seromucous glands. The pseudostratified ciliated columnar epithelium (E) covers the lamina propria (see Fig. 15.1, HC, CP, FP, BV, Gl, E). A higher magnification of a similar region of the nasal septum displays the cilia protruding into the nasal cavity. The ducts of the seromucous glands of the lamina propria pierce the pseudostratified ciliated columnar epithelium to deliver their secretory product into the nasal cavity. The connective tissue component of the lamina propria is richly endowed by blood vessels (see Fig. 15.2, *arrowhead*, L, D, Gl, E, CT, BV).

The olfactory region of the nasal cavity is lined by an olfactory epithelium whose olfactory cilia protrude into the nasal cavity. The basal cells and olfactory cells of the epithelium are easy to identify because their nuclei are located basally and at midlevel of the epithelium, respectively. The lamina propria has a rich vascular supply and is well endowed by Bowman glands (see Fig. 15.3, Ci, BC, OC, LP).

Larynx

At a very low magnification, the frontal section of the larynx displays some of its gross anatomy as well as its histological appearance. The three cavities of the larynx—the centrally positioned ventricle, superiorly positioned vestibule, and inferiorly located infraglottic cavity—are easily recognized. The ventricle is a deep recess between the superiorly positioned ventricular fold (also known as the false vocal fold) and the inferiorly positioned vocal fold that houses the vocal cord. The vocalis muscles that regulate the tension placed on the vocal cords are the medial fibers of the right and left thyroarytenoid muscles. The mucosa of the larynx houses seromucous glands (see Fig. 15.6, ventricle, VeF, VF, VM, Gl).

Trachea

A low magnification of the trachea displays the cilia of its pseudostratified columnar epithelium protruding into the lumen. The numerous goblet cells of the epithelium, along with the seromucous and mucous glands of the submucosa, produce a copious amount of mucinogen that becomes known as mucin upon hydration and mucus when additional substances become enmeshed in it. The C-rings of the trachea consist of hyaline cartilage with its perichondrium (see Fig. 15.7, Ci, L, GC, MG, HC, PC). At a high magnification, the cilia, goblet cells, and basal cells of the pseudostratified columnar epithelium are clearly evident. Observe that this particular section of the trachea has no glands and the lamina propria and submucosa are reduced in thickness. The location of the blood vessel cannot be clearly delineated; therefore, they may be in the submucosa or in the adventitia. The chondrocytes of the C-ring, as well as its cellular and fibrous perichondria, are located in the adventitia of the trachea (see Fig. 15.8, *arrowhead*, GC, *arrow*, BV, Ch, CP, FP).

Intrapulmonary (Secondary) Bronchus

At a low magnification, the various layers of the intrapulmonary bronchus are easy to identify. Its lumen is lined by a respiratory epithelium and the interface of the lamina propria and submucosa is occupied by spiraling smooth muscle bundles that replace the trachealis muscle located posteriorly, at the two ends of the C-rings. The hyaline cartilage of the intrapulmonary bronchus is composed of plates of hyaline cartilage that completely encircle this structure. Observe that it is embedded in lung tissue, which is the reason for its name, secondary bronchus (see Fig. 15.12, L, Ep, SM, HC, Lung tissue).

Bronchiole

A larger-sized bronchiole viewed at a low magnification displays that the epithelium lining its lumen contains no goblet cells, indicating that it is not a primary bronchiole. It has a thin layer of smooth muscle in its wall covered by a thin layer of connective tissue. The entire structure is surrounded by lung tissue whose alveoli are clearly evident (see Fig. 15.14, E, L, SM, A). A smaller-sized bronchiole viewed at medium magnification displays that its lumen is lined by a simple cuboidal epithelium composed of cuboidal cells and club cells. Observe that the bronchiole is accompanied by a small arteriole and that the lung tissue possesses numerous macrophages (dust cells) that engulf dark particulate matter (see Fig. 15.15, L, BC, CC, Ar, *white arrows*).

Respiratory Bronchiole, Alveolar Duct, Alveolar SAC, and Alveolus

A low magnification photomicrograph of a respiratory bronchiole displays occasional alveoli interrupting its wall. Each respiratory bronchiole terminates in a number of alveolar ducts, structures that do not have a wall. Instead, it has outpouchings of alveoli along its entire length. (see Fig. 15.16, R, A). At a higher magnification, an alveolar duct displays its outpocketings of alveoli along its length and demonstrates that the alveolar duct ends in one or more alveolar sacs that are composed of several alveoli (see Fig. 15.17, AD, A, AS, A). Alveoli are composed of type I and type II pneumocytes. Neighboring alveoli are separated by interalveolar septa of various thicknesses that house small blood vessels and capillaries, as well as alveolar macrophages (dust cells) and connective tissue elements (see Fig. 15.20, A, P1, P2, BV). Depending on the air quality, a lot of alveolar macrophages may display the presence of phagocytosed dust particles surrounding the alveoli (see Fig. 15.25, DC, A).

16

Digestive System: Oral Cavity

The digestive system—composed of the oral cavity, alimentary tract, and associated glands—functions in the ingestion, mastication, deglutition (swallowing), digestion, and absorption of food, as well as in the elimination of its indigestible remnants. Regions of the digestive system are modified and have specialized structures in order to be able to perform these varied tasks.

This and the following two chapters detail the histology and functions of the component parts of the digestive system. This chapter details the oral cavity and its contents; Chapter 17 describes the alimentary canal, including its intramural glands (esophagus, stomach, small and large intestines, rectum, and anus); and Chapter 18 discusses the glands of the digestive system that are external to the alimentary canal (major salivary glands, pancreas, and liver and gallbladder).

Oral Mucosa: Overview

The oral mucosa is composed of a wet, stratified squamous epithelium and an underlying dense, irregular, collagenous connective tissue. There are three categories of the oral mucosa: the lining mucosa, masticatory mucosa, and specialized mucosa.

The **oral mucosa** lines the oral cavity and is composed of a wet, **stratified squamous epithelium** (**keratinized**, **nonkeratinized**, or **parakeratinized**) and an underlying connective tissue. Those regions of the oral cavity that are exposed to considerable frictional and shearing forces (gingiva, dorsal surface of the tongue, and hard palate) are lined or covered by a **masticatory mucosa** composed of parakeratinized to completely keratinized stratified squamous epithelium with an underlying dense, irregular, collagenous connective tissue. The remainder of the oral cavity is lined or covered by a **lining mucosa**, composed of a nonkeratinized stratified squamous epithelium overlying a looser type of dense, irregular, collagenous connective tissue (Table 16.1). The regions of the oral mucosa that house taste buds in their epithelium (dorsal surface of the tongue and patches of the soft palate and pharynx) are said to be covered by **specialized mucosa**, that is, they are specialized to perceive taste.

Ducts of the three pairs of major salivary glands (parotid, submandibular, and sublingual) open into the oral cavity, delivering saliva to moisten the mouth. These major salivary glands (see Chapter 18) also manufacture and release the enzyme **salivary amylase** to break down carbohydrates; **lactoferrin** and **lysozymes**, antibacterial agents; and **secretory immunoglobulin (IgA)**. In addition, **minor salivary glands**, located in the connective tissue elements of the oral mucosa, add to the flow of saliva into the oral cavity. It is in the oral cavity that food is moistened with saliva, chewed, and formed, by the tongue, into spherical masses about 2 cm in diameter. These spherical masses, each known as a ***bolus***, are forced by the tongue into the oral pharynx to be swallowed.

The lips form the anterior boundary, and the palatoglossal folds form the posterior boundary of the oral cavity. The structures of interest in and about the oral cavity are the lips, teeth and their associated structures, palate, and the tongue.

Clinical Correlations

*Occasionally, bad breath (**halitosis**) occurs in almost everyone, especially when the individual's mouth is dry. However, in approximately a quarter of all adults, halitosis is a constant phenomenon. This chronic condition is caused mostly by anaerobic bacteria that reside in the crevices of the posterior aspect of the tongue and in the gingival sulcus (the shallow groove between the teeth and gums). These bacteria emit noxious gases—such as mercaptans, hydrogen sulfide, and methyl and dimethyl sulfides—and as they digest decomposing food remnants, they form malodorous compounds, such as indoles and skatoles. In most cases, gentle scraping of the tongue surface, meticulous dental hygiene, and the use of mouthwashes containing zinc and certain ions can alleviate the bad breath for a few hours. Unfortunately, as yet, there is no permanent solution to the problem of chronic bad breath. In fewer than 10% of individuals with chronic halitosis, other factors may be involved, such as deep cavities in the teeth, tonsillar crypts, sinuses, nasal cavity, and the stomach.*

LIP

The lip has three regions: the skin aspect, vermilion zone, and mucous (internal) aspect.

Entry into the oral cavity is guarded by the upper and lower **lips**. The core of the lips is composed of skeletal muscle fibers that are responsible for lip mobility. Each lip may be subdivided into three regions: the skin (external) aspect, vermilion zone, and mucous (internal, wet) aspect (Fig. 16.1).

The **skin aspect** (**external aspect**) of the lip is covered with thin skin and is associated with sweat glands, hair follicles, and sebaceous glands. This region is continuous with the **vermilion zone**, which is also covered by thin skin. However, the vermilion zone has neither sweat glands nor hair follicles, although occasional, nonfunctional sebaceous glands are present in its dermis. The interdigitation between the epidermis and dermis (**the rete apparatus**) is highly developed so that the capillary loops of the dermal papillae are close to the surface of the skin, imparting a pink color to the vermilion zone. The absence of functional glands in this region necessitates the occasional moistening of the vermilion zone by the tongue.

The **mucous aspect** (**internal aspect**) of the lip is always wet and is lined by stratified squamous nonkeratinized epithelium. The subepithelial connective tissue is of the dense, irregular

TABLE 16.1 Summary of the Histological Features of the Oral Mucosa

Mucosal Region	Type of Epithelium/Mucosa	Height of CT Papilla	Special Comments
Lip			
Skin aspect	Stratified squamous keratinized	Medium	Hair, sebaceous and sweat glands
Vermilion zone	Stratified squamous keratinized	High	Few sebaceous glands(?)
Mucosal aspect	Stratified squamous nonkeratinized	Medium	Mucous (mixed) minor salivary glands and Fordyce granules
Cheek			
Skin aspect	Stratified squamous keratinized	Medium	Hair, sebaceous and sweat glands
Mucosal aspect	Stratified squamous nonkeratinized	Medium	Mucous (mixed?) minor salivary glands and Fordyce granules
Gingiva			
Free and attached	Masticatory mucosa	High	Tightly bound to the periosteum
Sulcular	Lining mucosa	Low	Lines the gingival sulcus
Junctional epithelium	Stratified squamous nonkeratinized	None	Attached to tooth surface and to gingival CT by hemidesmosomes
Alveolar mucosa	Lining mucosa	Low	Some minor mucous salivary glands
Hard Palate (oral surface)	Masticatory mucosa	High	Adipose tissue in the CT
Anterior lateral	Masticatory mucosa	High	Minor mucous salivary glands in the CT
Posterior lateral	Masticatory mucosa	High	Tightly bound to periosteum
Raphe	Masticatory mucosa	High	Tightly bound to periosteum
Hard Palate (nasal surface)	Respiratory epithelium	NA	Mucous glands in the CT
Soft Palate (oral surface)	Lining mucosa	Low	Elastic lamina; minor mucous salivary glands
Uvula	Lining mucosa	Low	Minor mucous salivary glands in the CT
Soft Palate (nasal surface)	Respiratory epithelium	NA	Mucous glands in the CT
Uvula	Lining mucosa	Low	Mucous glands in the CT
Floor of the Mouth	Lining mucosa	Low	Minor mucous salivary glands in the CT
TONGUE			
Dorsal surface	Specialized mucosa embedded in masticatory mucosa	High	Taste buds; lingual papillae; serous, mucous, and mixed minor salivary glands
Ventral surface	Lining mucosa	Low	

CT, Connective tissue; NA, not applicable.
Modified with permission from Gartner LP. Oral Histology and Embryology, 3rd ed. Baltimore: Jen House Publishing; 2014 (Table 8.9).

collagenous type and houses numerous, mostly mucous, minor salivary glands.

The **core of the lip** is composed of dense, irregular, collagenous connective tissue that surrounds bundles of skeletal muscle, the orbicularis oris and other muscles of facial expression that control the movements of the upper and lower lips.

Clinical Correlations

Dormant herpes simplex virus type 1 (HSV type 1) inhabits the ganglia of the fifth cranial nerve (CN V, trigeminal ganglion). Occasionally, the virus migrates from the ganglion along the nerve fibers, infecting the oral cavity and the lips, forming small blisters that rupture. These blisters release a clear virus-rich fluid that makes this condition, known as ***herpetic stomatitis****, especially contagious. After the fluid is released, the blisters usually become ulcerated and exceptionally painful. Although herpetic stomatitis affects mostly children, when it affects adults, it becomes a more serious condition.*

TEETH

Each tooth, whether deciduous or permanent, has a crown, a cervix, and a root.

Humans have two sets of teeth: 20 **deciduous (milk) teeth**, which are replaced by 32 permanent (adult) teeth composed of 20 **succedaneous teeth** (i.e., teeth that succeed their deciduous forerunners) and 12 **molars** that did not have deciduous counterparts. Both the deciduous and permanent dentitions are evenly distributed between the maxillary and mandibular arches.

The various teeth have different morphological features, numbers of roots, and functions. They assist in seizing prey, cutting smaller pieces from large chunks, and macerating the chunks to form a bolus. Only the general structure of teeth is discussed here.

Each tooth is suspended in its bony socket, the **alveolus**, by a dense, irregular, collagenous connective tissue, the **periodontal ligament (PDL)**. The gingiva also supports the tooth, and its epithelium seals the oral cavity from the subepithelial connective tissue spaces (Fig. 16.2).

The portion of the tooth that is visible in the oral cavity is called the ***clinical crown***, and the region housed within the alveolus is known as the ***root***. The portion between the crown and the root is the **cervix**. The entire tooth is composed of three calcified substances, which enclose a soft, gelatinous connective tissue, the **pulp**, located in a continuous space subdivided into the pulp chamber and root canal. The root canal communicates with the **PDL** space via a small opening, the apical foramen, at the tip of each root. It is through this opening that blood and lymph vessels, as well as nerves, enter and leave the pulp (Figs. 16.3 and 16.4).

Enamel, Dentin, and Cementum

Enamel, dentin, and cementum are the mineralized components of the tooth.

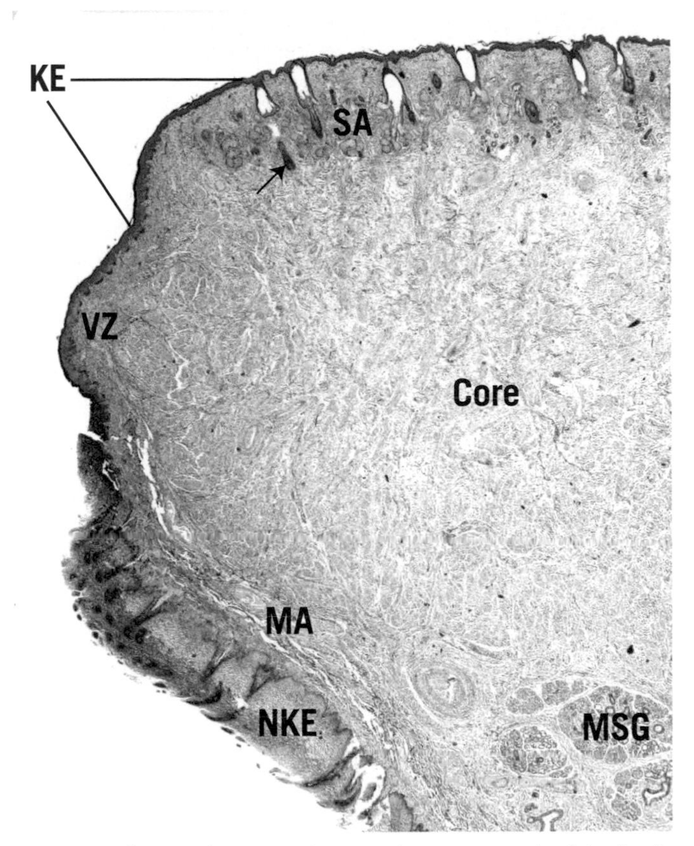

Fig. 16.1 This very-low-magnification photomicrograph of the lip displays its three regions and its core. Note that the skin aspect (SA) and the vermilion zone (VZ) are both covered by a stratified squamous keratinized epithelium (KE) and that the skin aspect sports hair follicles *(arrow)*. The mucous aspect (MA) is lined by a nonkeratinized stratified squamous epithelium (NKE) and has minor salivary glands (MSG) in its connective tissue. The core of the lip houses skeletal muscles surrounded by a dense, irregular, collagenous connective tissue. (×14)

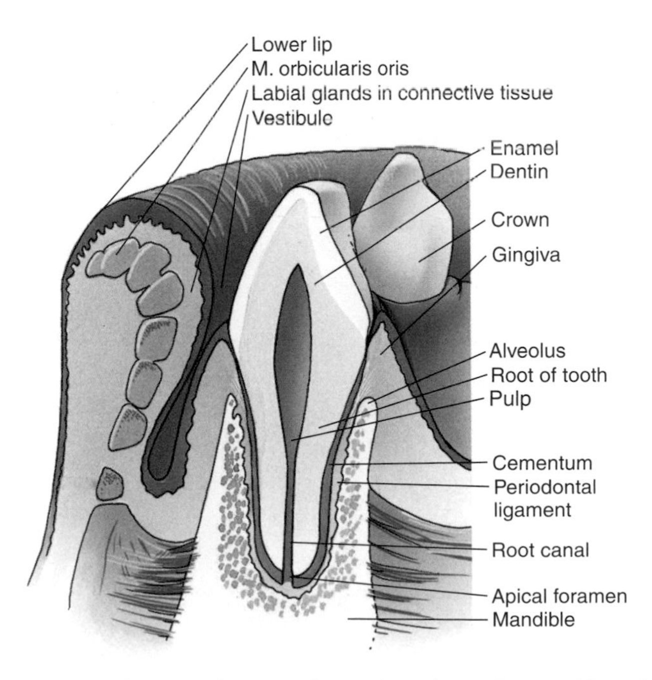

Fig. 16.2 Schematic diagram of a tooth in the oral cavity. Note the location of the vestibule between the lip and the labial aspect of the enamel of the tooth and gingiva, as well as the oral cavity on the buccal aspect of the teeth and gingiva.

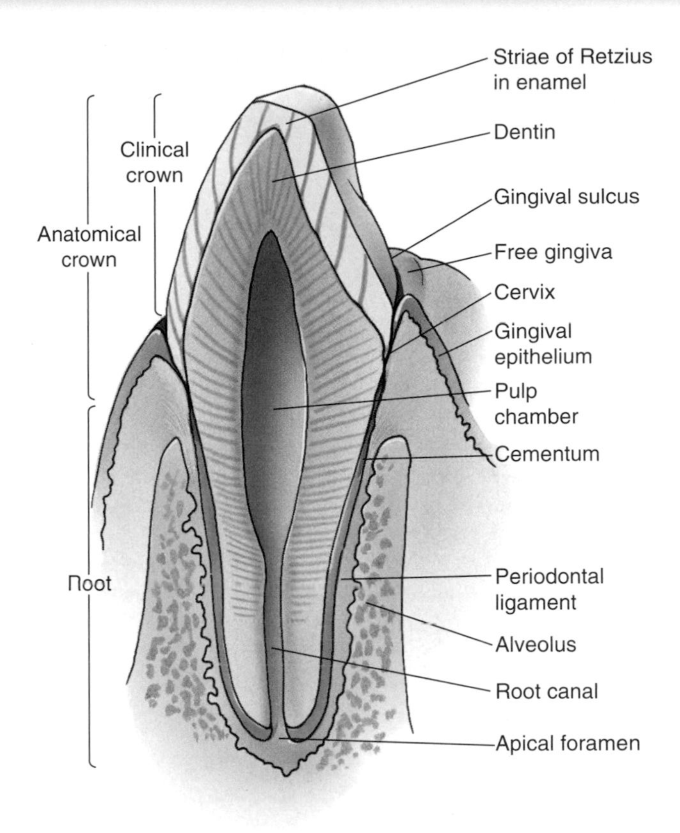

Fig. 16.3 Schematic diagram of a tooth and its surrounding structures. Note that the clinical crown is the portion of the crown that is visible in the oral cavity, and the anatomical crown extends from the cementoenamel junction to the occlusal surface of the tooth.

Enamel, dentin, and cementum are the mineralized structures of the tooth. Enamel covers dentin of the crown that surrounds the pulp chamber and cementum covers dentin of the root that surrounds the root canal. Thus, dentin is located both in the crown and the root and forms the bulk of the mineralized components of the tooth. Enamel and cementum meet each other at the cervix of the tooth.

Enamel

Enamel overlies dentin of the crown; it is composed of 96% calcium hydroxyapatite crystals and is the hardest substance in the body.

Enamel, the hardest substance in the body, consists of 96% calcium hydroxyapatite and 4% organic material and water. It is translucent; its coloration is due to the color of the underlying dentin. Enamel consists of large crystals. Each crystal is coated with a thin layer of keratin-like high-molecular-weight glycoproteins, tyrosine-rich **enamelins**, **amelogenins**, and **ameloblastin**.

Cells known as ***ameloblasts*** manufacture enamel daily in 4- to 8-μm segments known as ***rod segments*** that adhere to one another, forming cylindrical-like **enamel rods** (**enamel prisms**), which extend from the dentinoenamel junction (DEJ) to the enamel surface. The orientation of the crystals within rods varies so that the enamel rod has a cylindrical head to which a tail (interrod enamel), shaped like a rectangular solid, is attached. Because ameloblasts die before the tooth erupts into the oral cavity, enamel cannot be repaired by the body.

Clinical Correlations

Caries (cavities) usually result from the accumulation of microorganisms in and on slight defects of the enamel surface. As these bacteria metabolize nutrients in the saliva and on the tooth surface, they produce acids that begin to decalcify the enamel. As the bacteria proliferate in the cavity that they have "excavated," they and the toxins that they release enlarge the caries.

Fluoride increases the hardness of enamel, especially in young individuals, making the enamel more resistant to caries. The incidence of cavities has been greatly reduced by the addition of fluoride to the public water supply and toothpastes and by its topical application in the dental office. As the individual ages, the enamel crystals enlarge, and there is less space available for the exchange of hydroxyl ions for fluoride ions. Therefore, the use of fluoride treatments in adults is not nearly as effective as it is for young children.

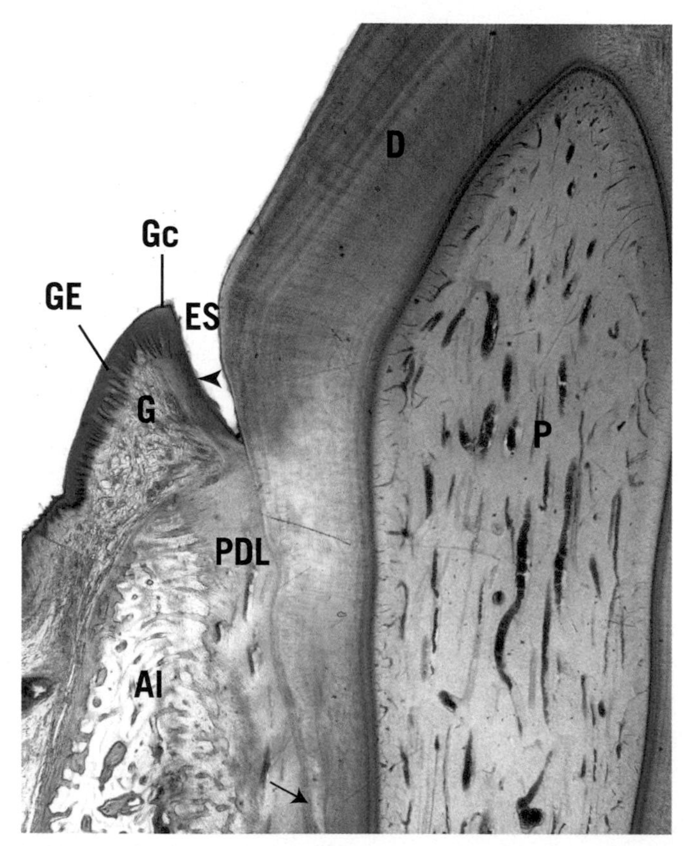

Fig. 16.4 This low-magnification photomicrograph of a decalcified incisor tooth and its surrounding structures displays its pulp (P), dentin (D), and cementum *(arrow)*. Note that the enamel is no longer present because it was removed during the decalcification process. The periodontal ligament (PDL) suspends the tooth in its socket by attaching to the cementum of the tooth and to the bony alveolus (Al). The gingiva (G) is attached to the enamel surface, represented by the enamel space (ES) where the enamel was before decalcification, by the nonkeratinized stratified squamous epithelial collar, known as the junctional epithelium *(arrowhead)*. The epithelium of the coronal-most aspect of the gingiva, the gingival crest (GC), is covered by a parakeratinized stratified squamous epithelium, as is the oral surface of the gingiva (GE). (×14)

Because enamel is elaborated in daily segments during its formation, the quality of the enamel produced varies with the health of the mother during prenatal stages. However, in enamel formed after birth, the quality of the enamel depends on the health of the individual. The **enamel rod** thus mirrors the metabolic state of the mother or the individual during the time of enamel formation, resulting in successive rod segment sequences of hypocalcified and normally calcified enamel. These alternating sequences, analogous to growth rings in a tree trunk, are evident histologically and are called ***striae of Retzius***.

The free surface of a newly erupted tooth is covered by a basal lamina–like substance, the **primary enamel cuticle**, manufactured by the same ameloblasts that elaborated enamel. This cuticle wears away shortly after the tooth's emergence into the oral cavity.

Dentin

Dentin forms the bulk of the tooth; it is composed of 70% calcium hydroxyapatite and is the second hardest substance in the body.

Dentin, the second hardest tissue in the body (Figs. 16.4 and 16.5), is somewhat elastic in nature, which acts to protect the brittle enamel covering it from becoming fractured. Dentin is yellow and composed of 65% to 70% calcium hydroxyapatite, 20% to 25% organic materials (specifically, **type I collagen**, proteoglycans, and glycoproteins), and 10% bound water.

Cells known as **odontoblasts** manufacture dentin and maintain their association with it for the life of the tooth. Odontoblasts are located at the periphery of the pulp; their cytoplasmic extensions, **odontoblastic processes**, occupy tunnel-like spaces within dentin. These extracellular fluid–filled spaces, known as **dentinal tubules**, extend from the pulp to the DEJ in the crown or dentinocemental junction in the root. Unlike ameloblasts,

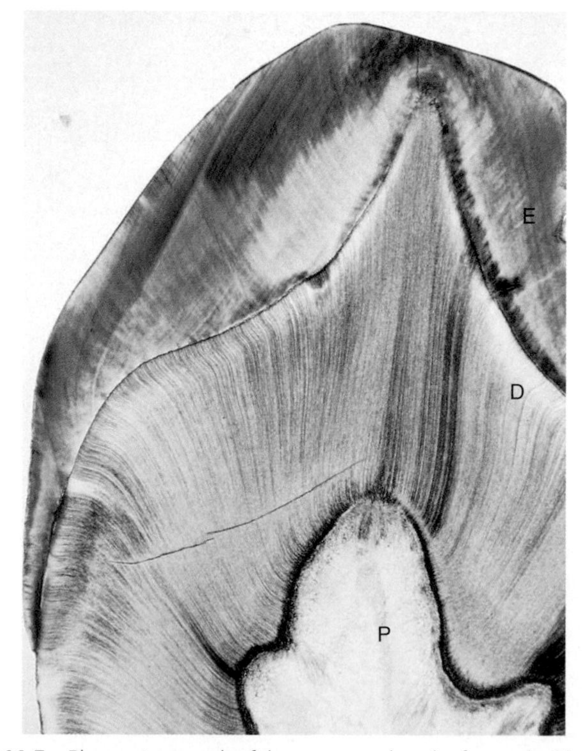

Fig. 16.5 Photomicrograph of the crown and neck of a tooth. Observe that this is a ground section (nondecalcified) and that the enamel (E) appears brown and the dentin (D) appears grayish in this preparation. The pulp (P) cavity occupies the center of the tooth. (×14)

odontoblasts remain functional for the life of the tooth. Therefore, dentin has the capability of self-repair; **reparative dentin** is elaborated on the surface of preexisting dentin within the pulp cavity, reducing the pulp cavity's size with age.

During dentinogenesis, odontoblasts manufacture about 4 to 8 μm of dentin every day. The quality of dentin, as of enamel, varies with the health of the mother prenatally or of the individual postnatally. Thus, along the length of the dentinal tubule, dentin displays alternating regions of normal calcification and hypocalcification. These are recognizable histologically as **lines of Owen** analogous to the striae of Retzius in enamel.

Clinical Correlations

Dentin sensitivity is mediated by sensory nerve fibers that are closely associated with odontoblasts, their processes, and the dentinal tubules. Disturbance of the tissue fluid within dentinal tubules is believed to depolarize the nerve fibers, sending a signal to the brain, where the signal is interpreted as pain.

Cementum

Cementum overlies dentin of the roots; it is composed of about 50% calcium hydroxyapatite and approximately 50% organic matrix and bound water. Therefore, it is approximately as hard as bone.

The third mineralized tissue of the tooth is cementum, a substance that is restricted to the root (Figs. 16.3, 16.4, 16.6, and 16.7). Cementum is composed of 45% to 50% calcium hydroxyapatite and 50% to 55% organic material and bound water. Most of the organic material is composed of types I, III, and XII collagen, with associated glycosaminoglycans, proteoglycans, and glycoproteins.

The apical region of cementum is similar to bone in that it houses cells called **cementocytes** within lenticular spaces, known as **lacunae**. Processes of cementocytes extend from lacunae within narrow **canaliculi** that extend toward the vascular PDL. Because of the presence of cementocytes, this type of cementum is called **cellular cementum**. The coronal region of cementum is very thin and has no cementocytes and is called **acellular cementum**. Both cellular cementum and acellular cementum have **cementoblasts**, cells that are responsible for the formation of cementum. These cells lie on a thin layer of uncalcified cementum, known as **cementum matrix**, that covers cementum and abuts the PDL. Cementoblasts continue to elaborate cementum for the life of the tooth.

Type I collagen fibers of the PDL, known as **Sharpey fibers**, are embedded in cementum and in the alveolus. In this fashion, the PDL suspends the tooth within its bony socket. **Odontoclasts (cementoclasts)** are large, multinucleated cells that resemble osteoclasts and are able to resorb both cementum and dentin. During exfoliation, the replacement of deciduous teeth by their succedaneous counterparts, odontoclasts resorb cementum (and dentin) of the root.

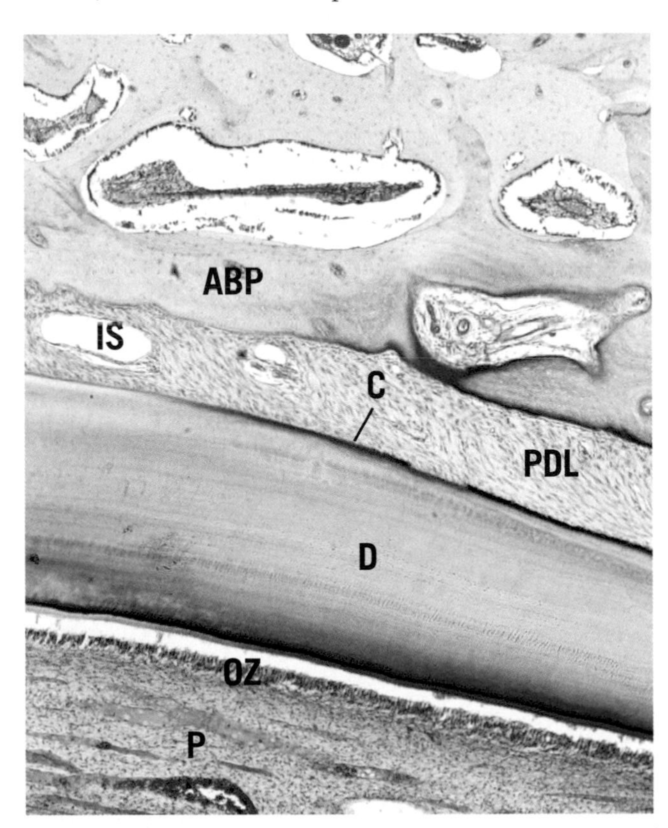

Fig. 16.6 Very-low-magnification photomicrograph of the root of a decalcified tooth in its socket, displaying the alveolus, its spongiosa, and alveolar bone proper (ABP); the periodontal ligament (PDL) with its interstitial spaces (IS) that usually house blood vessels and nerve fibers; the very thin layer of cementum (C) attached to the dentin (D), and the pulp (P), with its odontoblastic zone (OZ). Note that the apical foramen is to the right and the crown of the tooth is to the left. (×56)

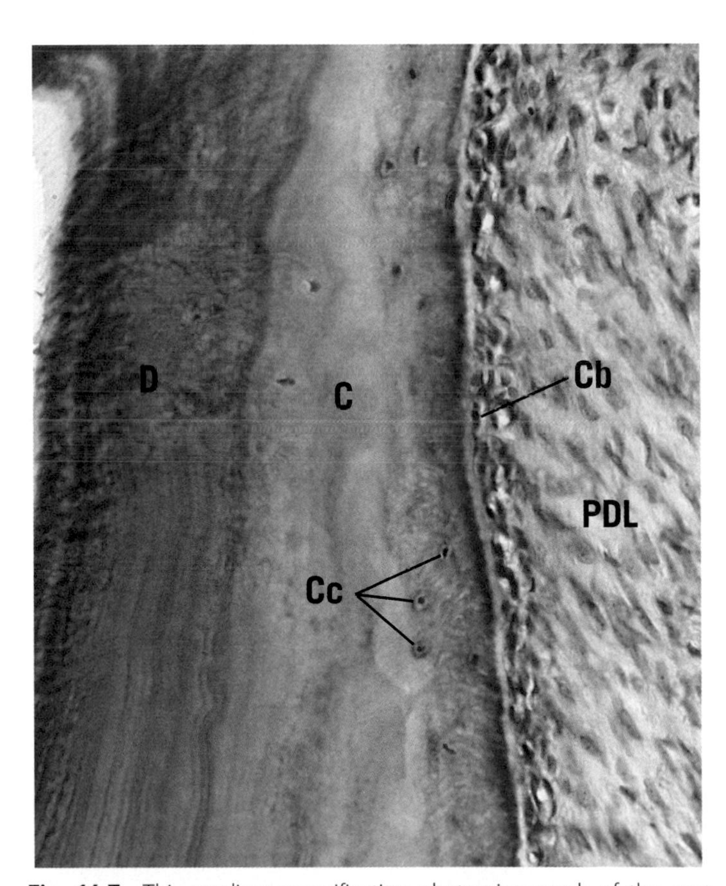

Fig. 16.7 This medium-magnification photomicrograph of the root of a decalcified incisor tooth near its apical foramen displays the thick region of cellular cementum (C) with its cementocytes (Cc) in their lacunae. Note that to the left of the cementum is dentin (D) of the root and to the right of the cementum is the periodontal ligament (PDL). Cementoblasts (Cb), the cells that manufacture cementum, are lined up against the uncalcified cementum matrix that separates the cementoblasts from the calcified cementum. Note that the crown of the root is above. (×270)

Clinical Correlations

1. *Cementum does not resorb as readily as does bone, a property that orthodontists use to their advantage in moving improperly positioned teeth. By placing the correct force on a tooth, the orthodontist reshapes the bony socket, causing the tooth to be moved into its proper position.*
2. *Cementum is continuously being elaborated, especially in the apical region of the root. This process compensates for the continuous eruption process of the tooth, which occurs in response to the abrasion of the occlusal surface due to the mechanical action of chewing. In order to maintain opposing teeth of the upper and lower arches in occlusion, the teeth must continuously erupt, albeit at a very slow rate. As the teeth move in an occlusal direction, the constant width of the periodontal ligament must also be maintained. All of these requirements are accomplished by the addition of cementum onto the root surface, especially in the region of the apex of the root. Due to the apposition of cementum, the diameter of the apical foramen becomes constricted, and, occasionally, even its location may be altered with age.*

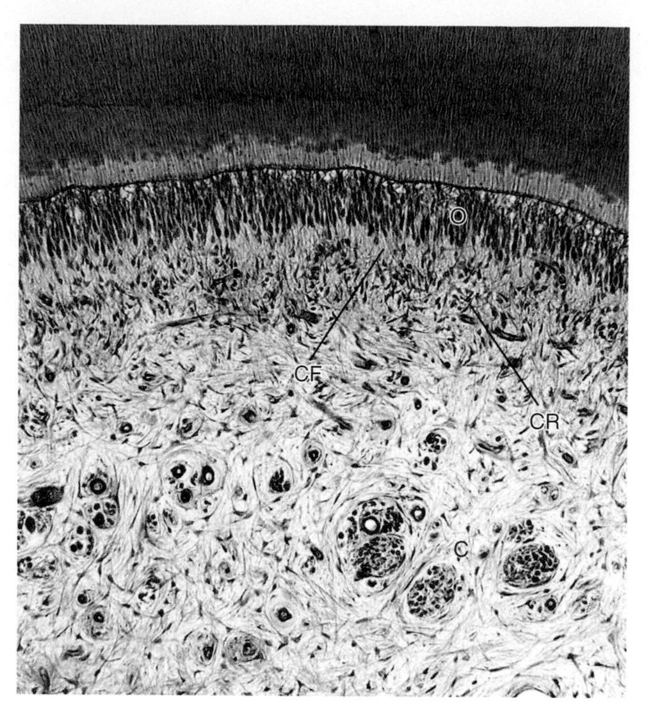

Fig. 16.8 Photomicrograph of the pulp of a tooth. Note the three layers—the odontoblastic zone (O), cell-poor (cell-free) zone (CF), and cell-rich zone—and the core of the pulp (C). (×132)

Pulp

Pulp, a richly vascularized and innervated loose connective tissue, is surrounded by dentin and communicates with the periodontal ligament via the apical foramen.

The **pulp** of the tooth, located in the pulp cavity, is a proteoglycans and glycosaminoglycans-rich loose, gelatinous connective tissue with some lymphatic elements and a very rich vascular and nerve supply. The pulp has two *anatomical* regions that are continuous with each other: the **coronal pulp**, located in the pulp chamber of the crown, and **radicular pulp**, located in the root canals of the roots. Blood vessels, lymph vessels, and nerve fibers exit and enter the pulp from the periodontal ligament via a small opening, the **apical foramen**, at the tip of each root. Therefore, teeth with multiple roots have an apical foramen at the tip of each root.

It is customary to subdivide the pulp histologically into three concentric zones around a central **core of the pulp**: the **odontoblastic zone** is composed of a single layer of **odontoblasts** whose processes, referred to as the **odontoblastic process**, extend into the adjacent dentinal tubules of dentin; the **cell-free zone** forms the layer deep to the odontoblastic zone, and as its name implies, is mostly devoid of cells; and the **cell-rich zone**, consisting of fibroblasts and mesenchymal cells, is the deepest zone of the pulp, adjacent to the **pulp core** (Figs. 16.8 and 16.9).

The core of the pulp resembles most other loose connective tissues but lacks adipose cells. Another notable difference is that the pulp core is highly vascularized and, occasionally, coronal pulp houses calcified elements called **pulp stones** (**denticles**).

The nerve fibers of the pulp are of two types: (1) **sympathetic** (vasomotor) fibers control the luminal diameters of blood vessels, and (2) **sensory** fibers are responsible for the transmission of pain sensation. Most of these **pain fibers** are thin myelinated fibers that form **Raschkow plexus**, just deep to the cell-rich zone and are believed to be Aδ fibers that conduct sharp pain. Additionally, some nonmyelinated C fibers also enter the

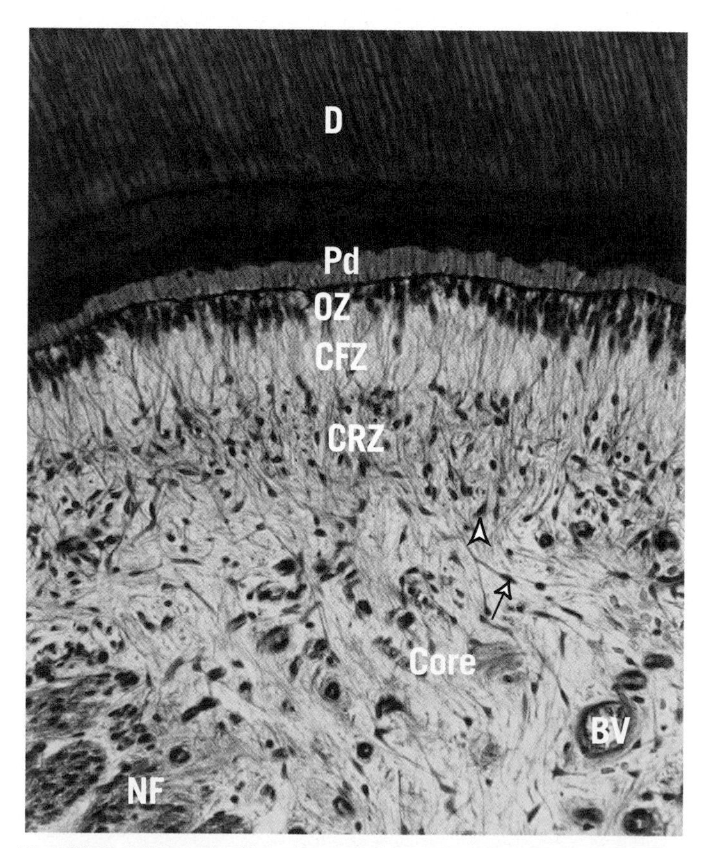

Fig. 16.9 The nerve fibers (NF) and blood vessels (BV) of the pulp core are easy to recognize. The three zones of the pulp—the cell-rich zone (CRZ), cell-free zone (CFZ), and odontoblastic zone (OZ)—are well defined in this photomicrograph of a decalcified tooth. Note that the odontoblasts abut the predentin (Pd), which protects them from the dentin (D) that is calcified in the living tooth. The *arrow* indicates a fibroblast, whereas the *arrowhead* points to mesenchymal cells. (×270).

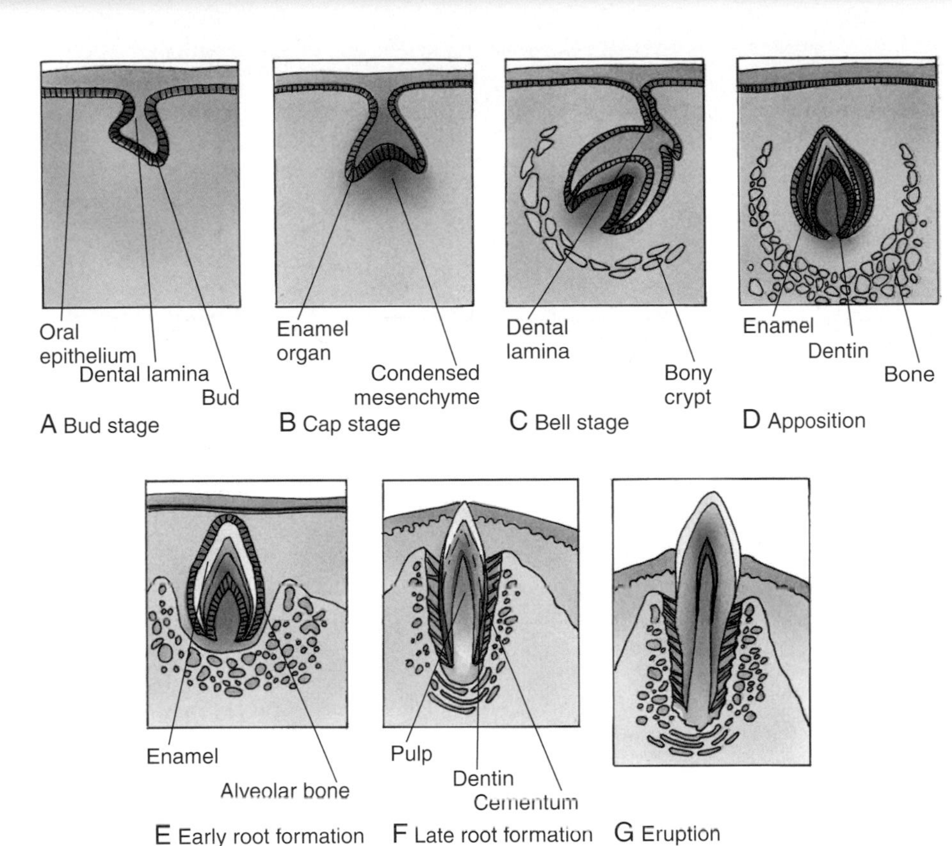

Fig. 16.10 Schematic diagram of odontogenesis.

Raschkow plexus and are responsible for the conveyance of dull pain. As nerve fibers continue through this plexus, the Aδ fibers lose their myelin sheath, pass through the cell-free zone, and penetrate the space between odontoblasts to enter the dentinal tubule. Some nerve fibers synapse on the odontoblasts or their processes instead of entering the dentinal tubules. Others enter the dentinal tubule where they may or may not synapse with the odontoblastic process.

Clinical Correlations

Hemorrhage of the pulp is evident clinically as dark discoloration of the tooth. Because the pulp may recover, hemorrhage should not be the sole indicator for extirpation of the pulp. If the pulp is determined to be diseased, then endodontic procedures should be performed. Otherwise, it may become necrotic and the infection may spread to the adjacent periapical tissues of the periodontal ligament via the apical foramen (or accessory foramina).

Odontogenesis

Odontogenesis begins with the appearance of the dental lamina.

The first sign of **odontogenesis** (tooth development) occurs between the sixth and seventh weeks of gestation, when the ectodermally derived **oral epithelium** of the maxillary and mandibular arches undergoes mitotic activity (Fig. 16.10), forming a horseshoe-shaped band of epithelial cells known as the **dental lamina**. The connective tissue surrounding the dental lamina is known as an **ectomesenchyme** because it is derived from **neural crest** material. The dental lamina and the ectomesenchyme are separated from each other by a well-defined **basement membrane**.

TABLE 16.2 Signaling Molecules and Gene Products During Odontogenesis

Tissue	Signaling Molecules	Gene Products
Oral epithelium	Fibroblast growth factor 8 Transforming growth factor-β	Wnt sonic hedgehog
Ectomesenchyme	Activin βA Bone morphogenic protein 4	MSX-1 and MSX-2 or DLX-1 and DLX-2

The process of tooth development is dependent on **epithelial-mesenchymal interaction**, accomplished by the synchronized release of a number of signaling molecules and gene products by the oral epithelium and the ectomesenchyme (Table 16.2).

Bud Stage

Shortly after the appearance of the dental lamina, mitotic activity increases in ten regions of the inferior aspect of this epithelial band of the maxillary and mandibular arches. This activity is responsible for the formation of 10 discrete epithelial structures known as ***buds***, initiating the **bud stage** of tooth development on both arches (Fig. 16.11).

These buds presage the 10 deciduous teeth of both the maxillary and mandibular arches and are separated from the ectomesenchyme by a basement membrane. At the inferior tip of each bud, ectomesenchymal cells congregate to form the presumptive **dental papilla**. Further development, although similar for each bud, is asynchronous, corresponding to the order of emergence into the oral cavity of the various teeth of the child.

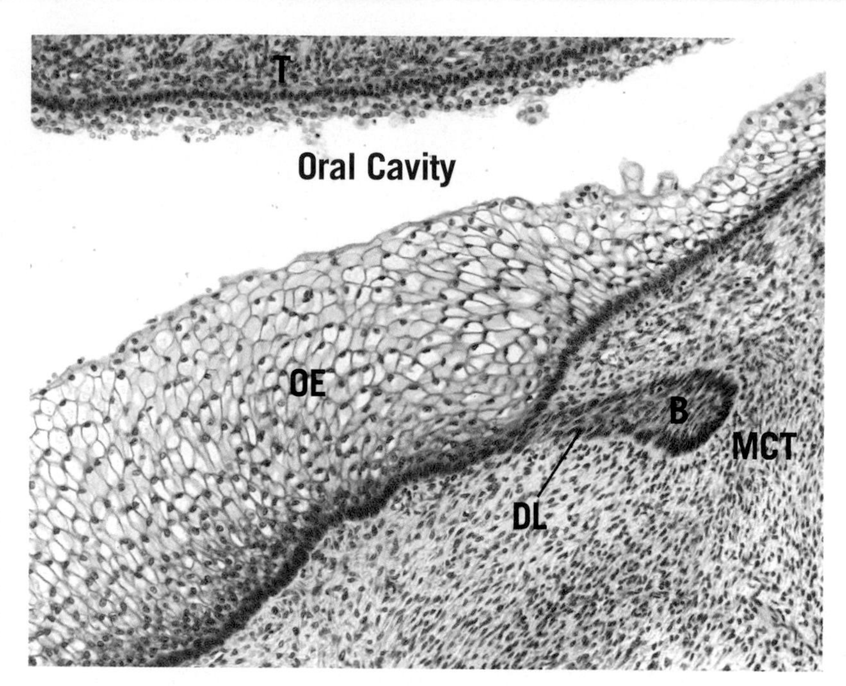

Fig. 16.11 This photomicrograph of the bud stage of tooth development displays the tongue (T) lying in the oral cavity above the oral epithelium (OE) of the mandibular arch. Observe the dental lamina (DL) and the attached bud (B) surrounded by the ectomesenchymal connective tissue (MCT), whose cells are just beginning to congregate around the forming bud. (×132)

Cap Stage

The cap stage of tooth development is recognized by the three-layered enamel organ, composed of the outer enamel epithelium, stellate reticulum, and inner enamel epithelium.

As cells of the bud proliferate, the bud increases in size and changes its morphology to become a three-layered structure, known as the **cap**, initiating the **cap stage** of tooth development. The outer layer, the convex *simple squamous* **outer enamel epithelium (OEE)**, and the inner layer, the concave *simple squamous* **inner enamel epithelium (IEE)** remain continuous with each other at a rim-like region, known as the **cervical loop**. They sandwich between them the third layer, known as the **stellate reticulum (SR)**, whose cells have numerous processes that are in contact with one another. These three epithelially derived layers form the **enamel organ** and are separated from the surrounding ectomesenchyme by a basement membrane. The concavity of the cap is occupied by a congregation of ectomesenchymal cells, the **dental papilla**, which becomes vascularized and innervated during the cap stage of tooth development, and occupies the concavity of the inner enamel epithelium. The dental papilla and the enamel organ together are known as the **tooth germ**. Viewed in three dimensions, the enamel organ resembles an insulated cup in which the handle is the dental lamina that is connected to the oral epithelium; the outer surface of the cup is the OEE; the inner surface is the IEE; and the rim of the cup, where the inner and outer surface meet, is the cervical loop. The insulation located between the inner and outer surfaces is the SR, and the cup is filled with the dental papilla; the glaze on the cup is the basement membrane.

The process of morphodifferentiation is responsible for the establishment of the template of the presumptive tooth; that is, the enamel organ assumes the shape of an incisor (incisiform), canine (caniniform), or a molar (molariform). This event is controlled by the **primary enamel knot**, a dense clump of cells located between the SR and the IEE within the substance of the enamel organ. It appears that the ectomesenchymal cells of the dental papilla induce the cells of the enamel knot to begin to express signaling molecules, transforming the enamel knot into one of the principal signaling centers of tooth morphogenesis.

Cells of the primary enamel knot synthesize **bone morphogenic proteins 2 and 4 (BMP-2** and **BMP-4)**, **sonic hedgehog**, and **fibroblast growth factor-4 (FGF-4)**, and proteins encoded by the ***Wnt* genes** in a particular sequential relationship that result in cusp formation in the developing tooth. To be able to establish this time-specific relationship, the ectomesenchymal cells of the dental papilla release **epidermal growth factor (EGF)** and **FGF-4**. Without EGF and FGF-4, the primary enamel knot cells are driven into apoptosis and cusps will not develop, which is exactly what happens in incisiform and caniniform tooth germs. Therefore, cusp formation is the responsibility of the primary enamel knot. As the cusps are being formed, cells from the primary enamel knot migrate to the regions of cusp formation and thereby seed the formation of the **secondary enamel knots** that preside over the development of the future cusps. Once the primary and secondary enamel knots have performed their functions, the ectomesenchymal cells cease their release of EGF and FGF-4, and the presence of BMP-4 drives the cells of the primary and secondary enamel knots into apoptosis.

The dental papilla, whose most peripheral layer of cells is separated from the IEE by the basement membrane, is responsible for the formation of the pulp and dentin of the tooth. Ectomesenchymal cells surrounding the tooth germ form a vascularized membranous capsule, the **dental sac (dental follicle)**, which gives rise to the cementum, PDL, and alveolus. Cells of the IEE differentiate into preameloblasts, which mature into ameloblasts to form enamel. Therefore, except for enamel, the tooth and its associated structures are derived from cells of neural crest origin.

During the cap stage of tooth development, a solid cord of epithelial cells, the **succedaneous lamina**, derived from the dental lamina, grows deep into the ectomesenchyme. The cells at the tip of the succedaneous lamina proliferate to form a bud, the precursor of the **succedaneous tooth** that eventually replaces the **deciduous tooth** being developed. Because there are only 20 deciduous teeth, only 20 succedaneous teeth are formed. The remaining 12 permanent teeth are known as ***accessional***

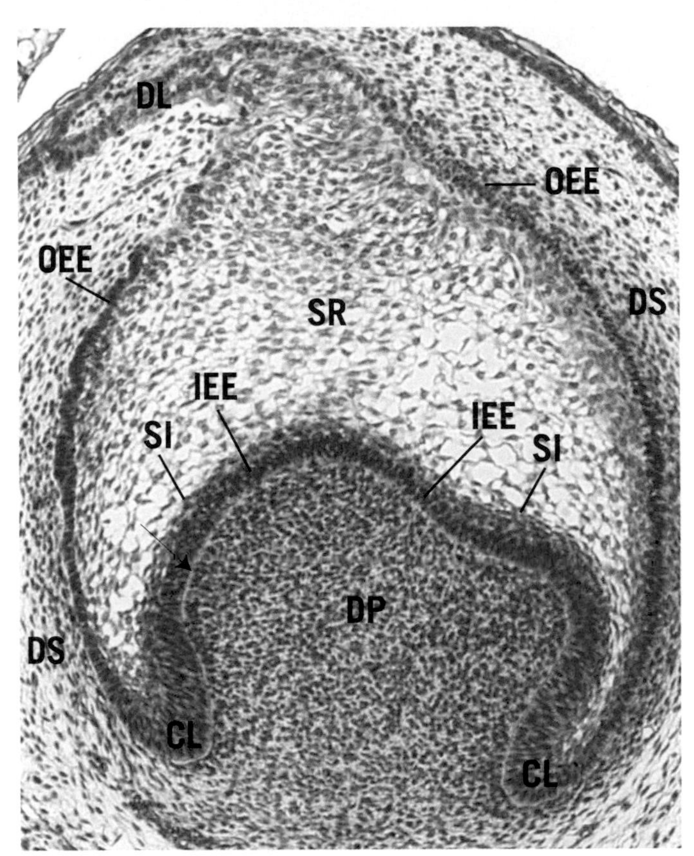

Fig. 16.12 This photomicrograph of the bell stage of tooth development displays the dental lamina (DL) to which the bell is attached. The four layers of the enamel organ—the outer enamel epithelium (OEE), inner enamel epithelium (IEE), stellate reticulum (SR), and stratum intermedium (SI), which is adjacent to and follows the contour of the inner enamel epithelium—are well represented. The OEE and the IEE join at the cervical loop (CL) and the entire enamel organ is separated from the ectomesenchymal components of the tooth germ by the basement membrane *(arrow)*. The dental papilla (DP) occupies the concavity formed by the IEE, and the dental sac (DS) surrounds the tooth germ. (×132)

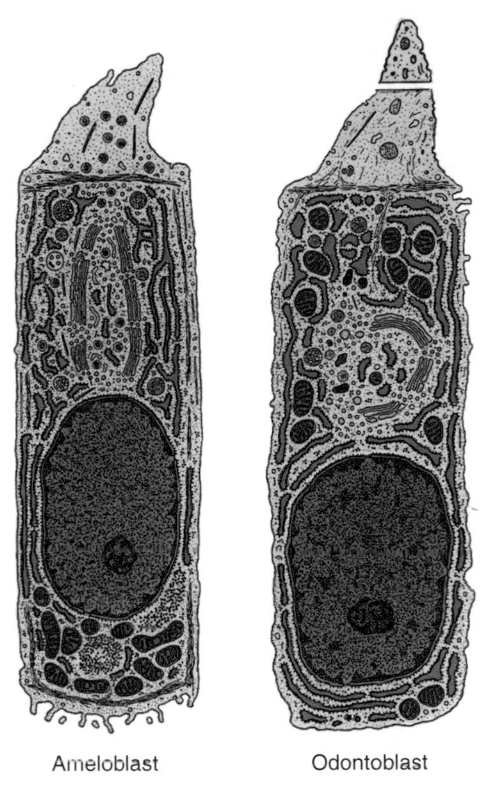

Fig. 16.13 Diagram of an electron micrograph of an ameloblast and odontoblast. Note that the odontoblastic process is very long, and a large section of it has been cut out—white space. (From Lentz TL. *Cell Fine Structure: An Atlas of Drawings of Whole-Cell Structure.* Philadelphia: WB Saunders; 1971.)

teeth (three permanent molars in each quadrant) because they do not replace existing deciduous dentition. Instead, they arise from the posterior extensions of the maxillary and mandibular dental laminae. The formation of the posteriorly directed extension of the original dental laminae begins in the fifth month of gestation.

Bell Stage and Appositional Stage

The bell stage is recognized by the four-layered enamel organ, composed of the outer enamel epithelium, stellate reticulum, stratum intermedium, and inner enamel epithelium.

Proliferation of the cells of the tooth germ increases its size, and the accumulation of fluid within the enamel organ increases its plump appearance. In addition, its concavity deepens and another layer of cells develops between the IEE and SR of the enamel organ. This new layer of cells is the **stratum intermedium**; its appearance characterizes the **bell stage** of tooth development (Fig. 16.12). Because of changes in the morphology of the enamel organ and changes in the shape of certain cells of the tooth germ, this stage of odontogenesis is also called the **stage of morphodifferentiation and histodifferentiation**.

As most of the fluid within the enamel organ is resorbed, much of the OEE collapses over the stratum intermedium, bringing the vascularized dental sac close to that new layer. The proximity of blood vessels apparently causes the stratum intermedium to induce the simple squamous cells of the IEE to differentiate into preameloblasts that will mature into enamel-producing columnar cells known as **ameloblasts** (Fig. 16.13). In response to the histodifferentiation of the inner enamel epithelial cells, the most peripheral cells of the dental papilla (those in contact with the basal lamina) also differentiate to become preodontoblasts that will mature into dentin-producing columnar cells known as **odontoblasts** (see Figs. 16.13 and 16.14).

Shortly after the odontoblasts begin to elaborate dentin matrix (a noncalcified material) into the basal lamina, the ameloblasts also begin to manufacture enamel matrix (also a noncalcified material). The dentin and enamel matrices adjoin, and the junction between them is the **dentinoenamel junction (DEJ**; see Fig. 16.5). The tooth germ is now said to be in the **appositional stage** of tooth development (Figs. 16.15 and 16.16). The process of dentin and enamel formation depends on the presence of various signaling molecules, such as FGF-8, bone morphogenetic protein-2, transforming growth factor-β, and insulin-like growth factors I and II.

During the formation of dentin, as the odontoblasts move away from the DEJ, the distal tip of their process remains at that junction, and the process continues to elongate. This cytoplasmic extension, known as the **odontoblastic process**, is surrounded by dentin. The space occupied by the odontoblastic process is the dentinal tubule.

As the ameloblasts secrete enamel matrix, their apical region becomes constricted by the matrix, forming the **Tomes process**. The ameloblasts then move away from the newly elaborated enamel, and the constricted region expands to its previous size. The cyclic nature of the Tomes process formation continues until enamel formation ceases. As dentin matrix becomes calcified to form **dentin**, the process of calcification spreads into the enamel matrix, which also calcifies and becomes known as **enamel**.

Root Formation

Root formation begins after the completion of the crown and is organized by the Hertwig epithelial root sheath.

When all of the enamel has been manufactured, the tooth germ enters the next stage of odontogenesis, known as **root formation**. The outer and inner enamel epithelia of the cervical loop elongate forms a two-layered (OEE and IEE) sleeve-like structure known as the **Hertwig epithelial root sheath (HERS)**, which encompasses ectomesenchymal cells located deep to the developing crown, forming an elongation of the dental papilla.

The absence of the stratum intermedium prevents the cells of the IEE from differentiating into ameloblasts; thus, enamel is not formed on the developing root surface. However, the most peripheral cells of the root dental papilla differentiate into preodontoblasts, which release **nuclear factor Ic**, a transcription factor that triggers the initiation of dentin formation and the

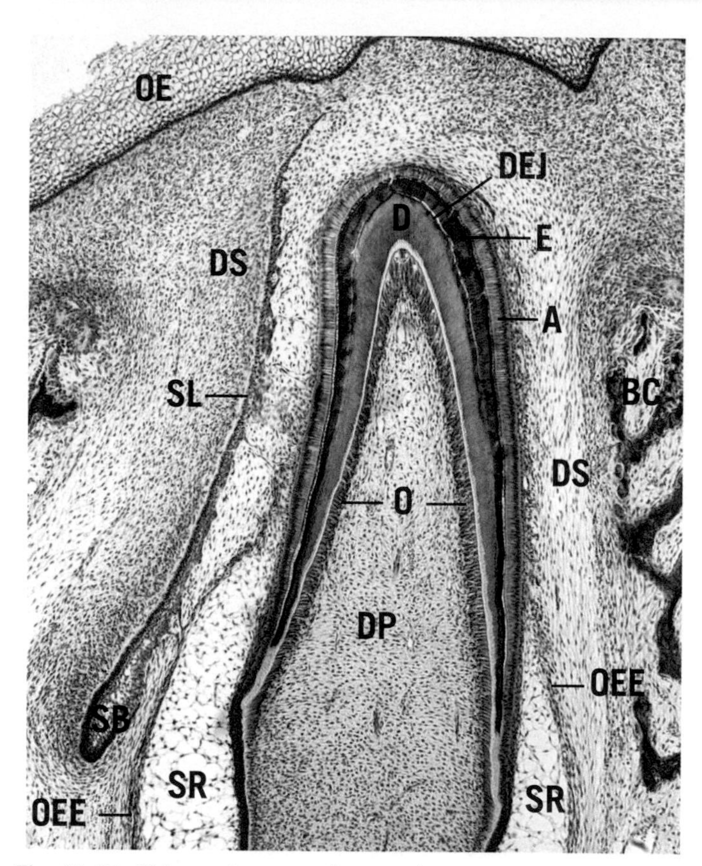

Fig. 16.15 This very-low-magnification photomicrograph displays the oral epithelium (OE) and the succedaneous lamina (SL) with the succedaneous bud (SB) that is forming while the deciduous tooth is in its early appositional stage of tooth development. Observe that the outer enamel epithelium (OEE) and stellate reticulum (SR) are clearly represented in the radicular half of the forming crown of this deciduous incisor. The odontoblasts (O) of the dental papilla (DP) are actively forming dentin (D), whereas the ameloblasts (A) of the enamel organ are manufacturing enamel matrix (E) and the dentinoenamel junction (DEJ) has already been established. The tooth germ is surrounded by the dental sac (DS), which is enclosed by the bony capsule (BC). (×56)

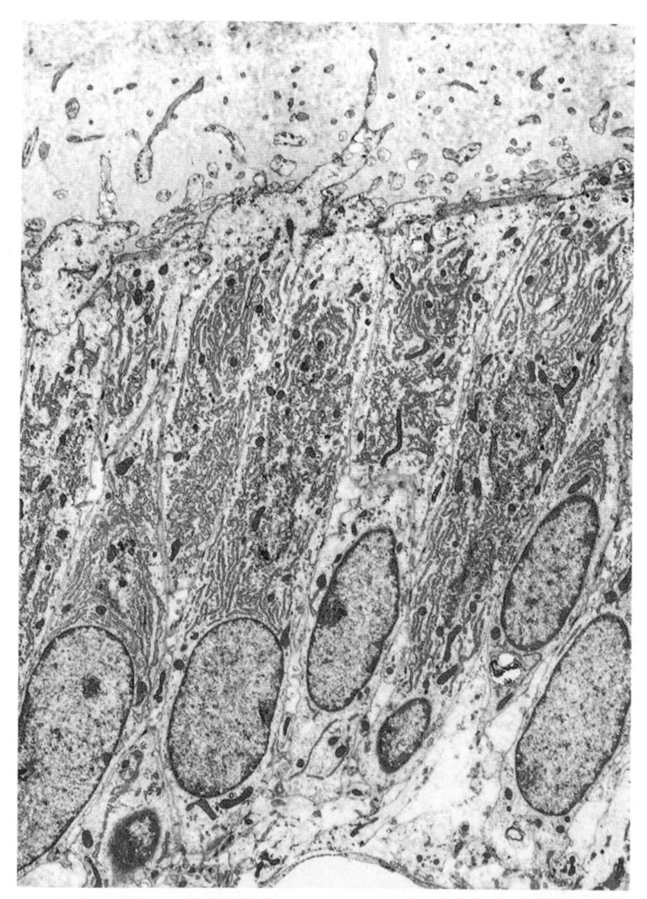

Fig. 16.14 Electron micrograph of rat incisor odontoblasts (×3416). (From Ohshima H, Yoshida S. The relationship between odontoblasts and pulp capillaries in the process of enamel-related cementum-related dentin formation in rat incisors. *Cell Tissue Res.* 1992;268:51–63.)

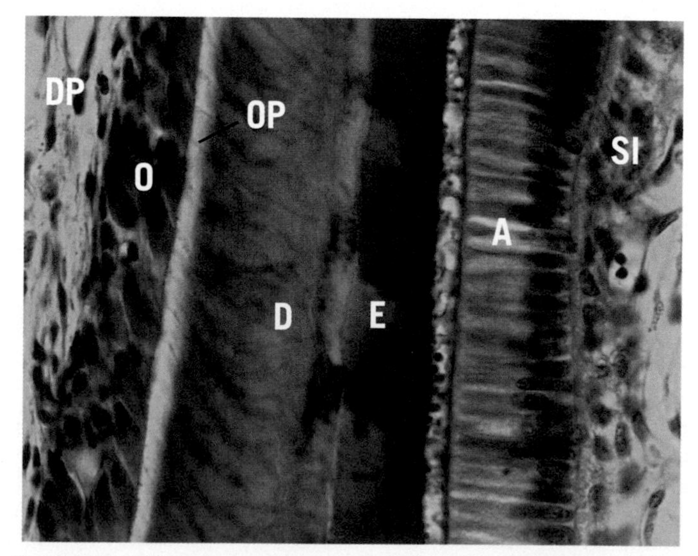

Fig. 16.16 This high-magnification photomicrograph of the appositional stage of tooth development of Fig. 16.15 displays the dental papilla (DP) and its odontoblasts (O), whose odontoblastic processes (OP) may be observed to enter and occupy the dentinal tubule of the forming dentin (D). Enamel (E) is formed by the tall columnar ameloblasts (A) whose basal surfaces are adjoined by cells of the stratum intermedium (SI). (×540)

differentiation of these cells into odontoblasts, the cells that continue to elaborate root dentin. As the HERS elongates, the root continues to be manufactured, and the region of HERS closer to the cervical loop begins to disintegrate, forming perforations in this sleeve-like structure. As an increasing amount of spaces develop in the HERS, the structure begins to lose continuity and forms clusters of epithelial cells known as **rest cells of Malassez** that are surrounded by a basement membrane. Ectomesenchymal cells from the **dental sac** migrate through the openings in the HERS, approximate the newly formed dentin, and differentiate into **cementoblasts**. These newly differentiated cells manufacture cementum matrix, which subsequently calcifies and is referred to as ***cementum***. It has been suggested by some authors that, in addition to the ectomesenchymal cells, cementoblasts may also form from cells of the HERS.

The elongation of the root is a consequence of the lengthening of the HERS. As the root becomes longer, the crown approaches and eventually erupts into the oral cavity. However, the lengthening of the root is not responsible for tooth eruption; instead, the two processes merely happen to occur simultaneously.

Clinical Correlations

For a very long time, epithelial rest cells of Malassez (ERM), remnants of Hertwig epithelial root sheath, have been considered to be cell islands that remained present in the periodontal ligament but had no functions. Research in the past few years has suggested that ERM may function in maintaining the homeostasis of the periodontal ligament (PDL) by ensuring that the PDL space is not decreased, thereby preventing the possibility of ankylosis of the tooth to the bony alveolus. Additionally, the cells of ERM may possess stem cell–like properties and can become cementoblasts for the repair of cementum and fibroblasts for the repair of the PDL.

Structures Associated with Teeth

The structures associated with teeth are the PDLs, alveolus, and gingiva.

Periodontal Ligament

The periodontal ligament is a dense, irregular, collagenous connective tissue whose principal fiber groups, composed of type I collagen, suspend the tooth in its alveolus.

The **PDL**, a richly vascularized connective tissue, occupies the PDL space, which is defined as the region between the cementum of the root of the tooth and the bony alveolus, a space that is less than 0.5 mm wide in a healthy mouth (Figs. 16.17 and 16.7). Although the PDL is classified as dense, irregular, collagenous connective tissue, it has **principal fiber groups**, composed mostly of **type I collagen fibers**, that are arranged in specific, predetermined patterns designed to absorb and counteract masticatory forces. The ends of the principal fiber groups are embedded in the alveolus and cementum as **Sharpey fibers**, which assist the PDL in suspending the tooth in its socket.

As in any dense, irregular, collagenous connective tissue, the most populous cells of the PDL are **fibroblasts**, which not only manufacture the collagen and amorphous intercellular components of the PDL, but also **resorb** collagen fibers, thus are responsible for the *high turnover of collagen* in the PDL. In addition, mast cells, macrophages, plasma cells, and leukocytes are also present in the PDL.

Nerves of the PDL include (1) **autonomic fibers**, which regulate the luminal diameter of the arterioles; (2) **pain fibers**, which mediate pain sensation; and (3) **proprioceptive fibers**, which are responsible for the perception of spatial orientation.

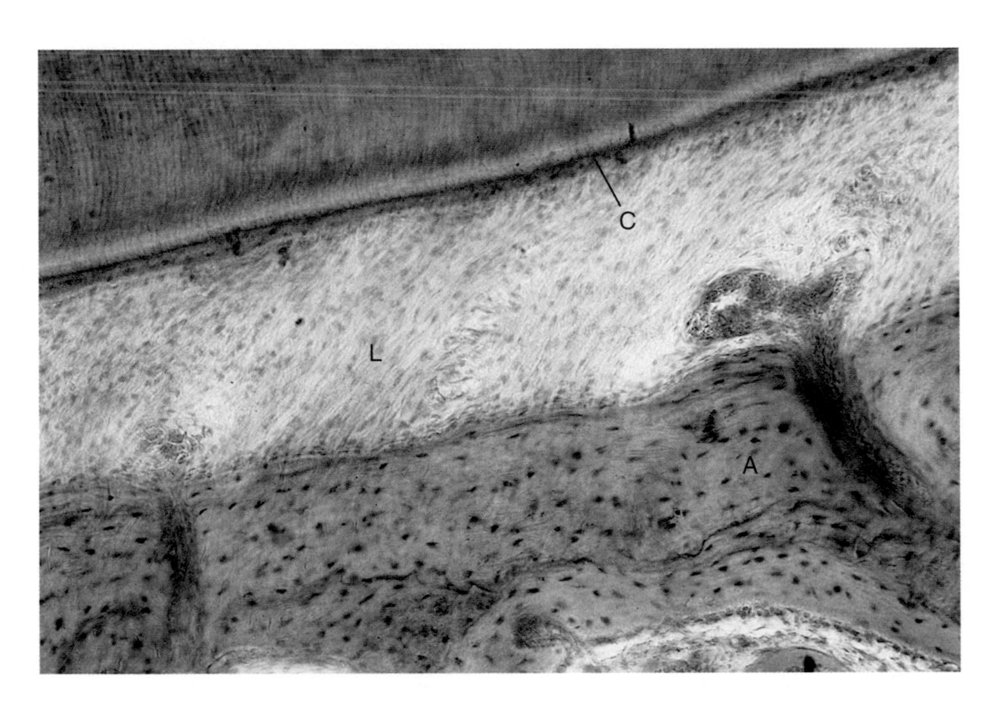

Fig. 16.17 The periodontal ligament (L) is a dense, irregular, collagenous connective tissue located between the cementum (C) of the root and the bony alveolus (A). (×132)

Clinical Correlations

1. *Proprioceptive fibers in the periodontal ligament are responsible for the **jaw-jerk reflex**, an involuntary opening of the jaw when one unexpectedly bites down on something hard. This reflex causes relaxation of the muscles of mastication and contraction of muscles responsible for opening the jaw, protecting the teeth from fracture.*
2. ***Periodontitis** is an inflammatory disease of the periodontal ligament that has been shown to have more serious consequences than just the health of the individual's dentition. It has been demonstrated that patients who are on dialysis and received periodontal treatment had approximately 30% fewer incidence of pneumonia and infection that required hospitalization. Additionally, patients on dialysis who had periodontitis had a 10% higher mortality rate over a 10-year period than dialysis patients without periodontitis.*

Alveolus

The alveolus is the bony socket in which the tooth is suspended by fibers of the PDL.

The alveolar process, a bony continuation of the mandible and maxilla, is divided into compartments, each known as an **alveolus**, that houses the root or, in the case of multirooted teeth, roots of a tooth. Adjacent alveoli are separated by a bony interalveolar septum. The alveolus has three regions: (1) the **cortical plates**, located labially and lingually, are composed of thick compact bone; (2) the **spongiosa**, located between the cortical plates, is composed of cancellous bone; and (3) the **alveolar bone proper**, a thin layer of compact bone surrounded by the spongiosa, whose shape mirrors that of the root suspended in it (see Figs. 16.2–16.4).

Nutrient arteries, traveling in **nutrient canals** within the spongiosa, supply the bony alveolus. The alveolar bone proper, supported by the cortical plate and spongiosa, has numerous perforations through which branches of the nutrient artery, named **perforating arteries**, pass from the spongiosa into the PDL, contributing to its vascularization.

Gingiva (Gums)

The gingiva is attached to the enamel surface by a thin, wedge-shaped, stratified squamous nonkeratinized epithelium, known as the junctional epithelium.

Because the **gingiva** is exposed to strenuous frictional forces, its stratified squamous epithelium is either fully keratinized (**orthokeratinized**) or partially keratinized (parakeratinized; see Figs. 16.2–16.4). Deep to the epithelium is a dense, irregular, collagenous connective tissue whose type I collagen fibers form principal fiber groups that resemble those of the PDL.

As the epithelium of the gingiva approaches the tooth, it forms a hairpin turn, proceeds apically (toward the root tip) for approximately 1 mm in a healthy mouth, and then attaches to the enamel surface by the formation of hemidesmosomes. The 1-mm-deep space between the gingiva and the tooth is the **gingival sulcus**. It is lined by a stratified squamous nonkeratinized epithelium, known as the **sulcular epithelium**.

The region of the gingival epithelium that attaches to the enamel surface is known as the ***junctional epithelium***, which forms a collar around the neck of the tooth. The junctional epithelium forms a robust barrier between the bacteria-laden oral cavity and the sterile environment of the gingival connective tissue. The principal fiber groups of the gingiva assist in the adherence of the junctional epithelium to the tooth surface, maintaining the integrity of the epithelial barrier. This barrier is about 1 mm long, and is only about 35 to 50 cells wide coronally and 5 to 7 cells wide apically.

Palate

The palate—composed of the hard palate, soft palate, and uvula—separates the oral cavity from the nasal cavity.

The oral and nasal cavities are separated by the **hard palate** and **soft palate**. The hard palate, positioned anteriorly, is immovable and receives its name from the bony plate contained within it. In contrast, the soft palate is movable, and its core is occupied by skeletal muscle that is responsible for its movements.

The **masticatory mucosa** on the oral aspect of the **hard palate** is composed of a wet, stratified squamous keratinized (or parakeratinized) epithelium and a dense, irregular, collagenous connective tissue (Fig. 16.18). The connective tissue of the anterior lateral region of the hard palate displays clusters of adipose tissue, whereas its posterior lateral aspect exhibits acini of mucous minor salivary glands. This connective tissue is fused with and indistinguishable from the periosteum of the hard palate. Therefore, the palatal epithelium and underlying connective tissue together are referred to as the **mucoperiosteum**. The nasal aspect of the hard palate is covered by respiratory epithelium, with occasional patches of stratified squamous nonkeratinized epithelium.

The oral surface of the **soft palate** is covered by a **lining mucosa**, composed of a wet stratified squamous nonkeratinized epithelium and a subjacent dense, irregular, collagenous connective tissue housing mucous minor salivary glands that are continuous with glands of the hard palate. The

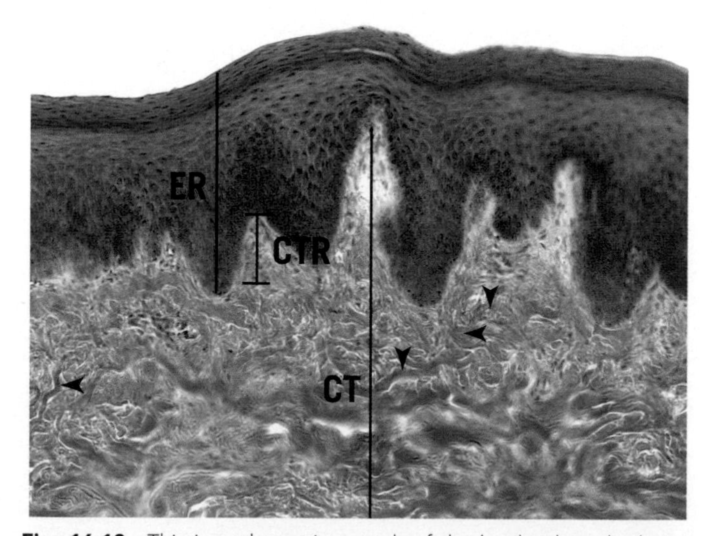

Fig. 16.18 This is a photomicrograph of the hard palate displaying its masticatory mucosa, composed of a parakeratinized stratified squamous epithelium and the dense, irregular, collagenous connective tissue (CT). Observe that the epithelial ridges (ER) are highly developed and that they interdigitate with the connective tissue ridges (CTR). The *arrowheads* demonstrate the irregular arrangement of the collagen fiber bundles. (×132)

epithelium of its nasal aspect, similar to that of the hard palate, is of the pseudostratified ciliated columnar type. The core of the soft palate is composed of skeletal muscle bundles that control its movements. The most posterior extension of the soft palate is the **uvula**, whose histological appearance is similar to that of the soft palate, but its epithelium is composed of a stratified squamous nonkeratinized epithelium all around the uvula. The connective tissue of the uvula is also a dense irregular collagenous type possessing mucous minor salivary glands, and its core is composed of skeletal muscle that is responsible for its movements.

Clinical Correlations

Wound healing in the oral cavity occurs approximately three times as fast as wound healing on the upper arm. When circular wounds were created in the oral cavity and on the anterior aspect of the upper arm of volunteers, the oral wounds healed at a rate of 0.3 mm per day whereas the wounds on the arm healed at a rate of 0.1 mm per day. It appears that the products of regulator genes SOX2, PAX9, PITX1, and PITX2 were responsible for shortening the time required to heal the wounds in the oral cavity. Additionally, they were responsible for inhibiting the inflammation that normally accompanies wound healing of skin. Thus, wounds in the oral cavity heal without the formation of scars.

Tongue

The tongue has three regions: the anterior two-thirds, the posterior one-third, and a root.

The **tongue** is the largest structure in the oral cavity. Its extreme mobility is due to the large intertwined mass of skeletal muscle fibers that compose its bulk (Fig. 16.19). The muscle fibers may be classified into two groups: those that originate outside of the tongue and insert into the tongue, known as the **extrinsic muscles**, and those that originate within and insert into the tongue, the **intrinsic muscles**. The extrinsic muscles are responsible for moving the tongue in and out of the mouth as well as from side to side and up and down, whereas the intrinsic muscles alter the shape of the tongue. The intrinsic muscles are arranged in four groups: superior longitudinal, inferior longitudinal, vertical, and transverse.

Interspersed among the intrinsic muscles of the tongue are the minor salivary glands:

- Anterior lingual glands (Blandin-Nuhn glands) near the tip of the tongue
- Posterior mucous glands in the core of the posterior one-third of the tongue
- Glands of von Ebner, located in the posterior aspect of the anterior one-third of the tongue and whose ducts deliver their serous saliva into the epithelially lined groove of circumvallate papillae and the furrows of the foliate papillae

The tongue has a dorsal surface, a ventral surface, and two lateral surfaces. The dorsal surface is observed to have

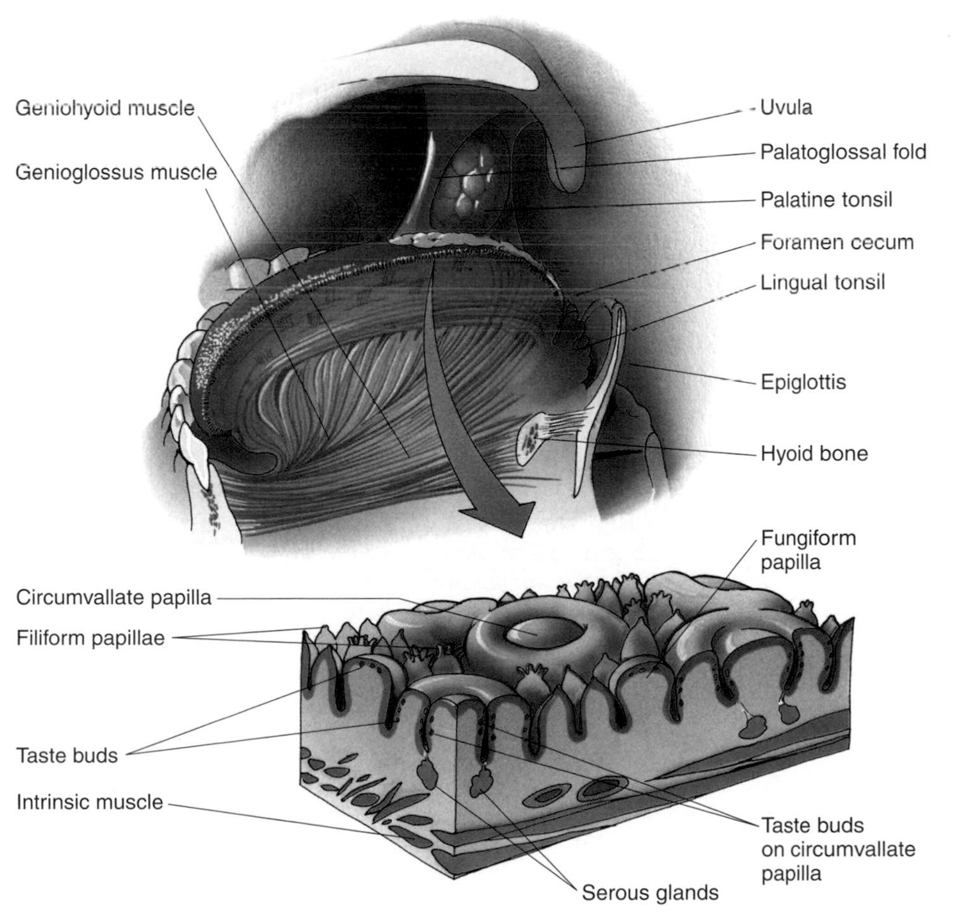

Fig. 16.19 Schematic diagram of the tongue and its lingual papillae.

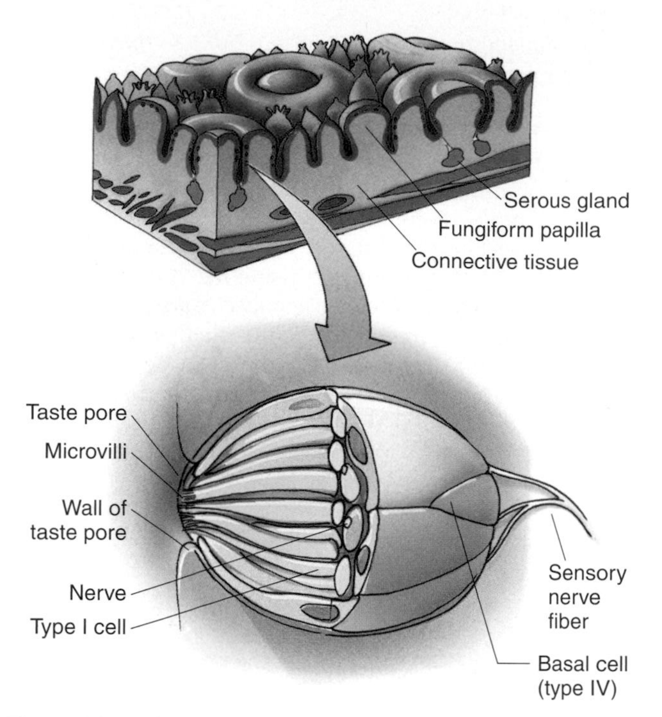

Fig. 16.20 Schematic diagram of lingual papillae and a taste bud.

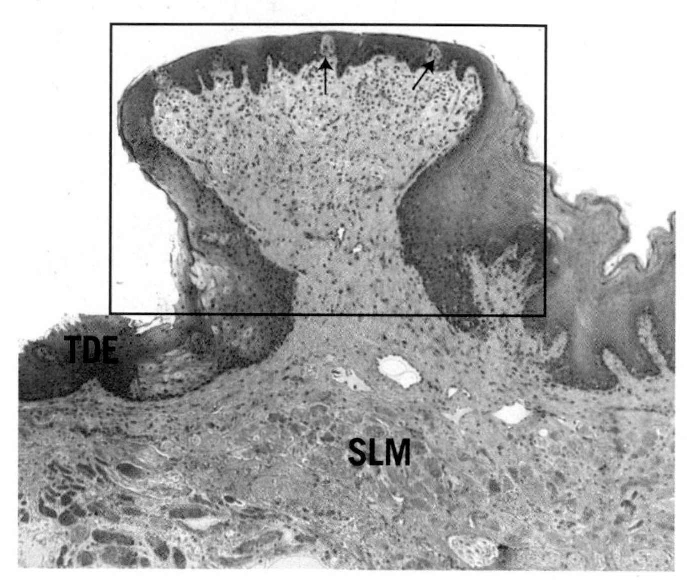

Fig. 16.21 This is a very-low-magnification photomicrograph of a fungiform papilla (inside the rectangle) demonstrating that it is above the tongue's dorsal epithelium (TDE). The *arrows* indicate taste buds on the dorsal surface of the fungiform papilla. The skeletal muscle fibers of the superior longitudinal muscle are cut in cross-section. (×56)

two unequal regions, the larger **anterior two-thirds** and the smaller **posterior one-third**. The two regions are separated by a shallow, V-shaped groove, the **sulcus terminalis**, whose apex points posteriorly and contains a deep concavity, the **foramen cecum**.

The dorsal surface of the posterior one-third of the tongue is uneven because of the presence of the **lingual tonsils** (see Chapter 12). The most posterior portion of the tongue is known as the ***root of the tongue***.

Lingual papillae, most of which project above the surface, cover the anterior two-thirds of the tongue's dorsal surface.

Lingual Papillae

There are four types of lingual papillae: filiform, fungiform, foliate, and circumvallate.

On the basis of their structure and function, the lingual papillae are of four types: filiform, fungiform, foliate, and circumvallate (see Figs. 16.19 and 16.20). They are all located anterior to the sulcus terminalis on the dorsal or lateral aspect of the tongue.

The numerous **filiform papillae** are slender structures that impart a velvety appearance to the dorsal surface (see Figs. 16.19 and 16.20). These papillae are covered by stratified squamous keratinized epithelium and help scrape food off a surface. The high degree of keratinization is especially apparent in the sandpaper-like quality of a cat's tongue. Filiform papillae do not have taste buds.

Each fungiform papilla resembles a mushroom whose slender stalk connects a broad cap to the tongue surface (see Figs. 16.19–16.21). The epithelial covering of these papillae is stratified squamous nonkeratinized; thus, the blood coursing through the subepithelial capillary loops is evident as red dots distributed randomly among the filiform papillae on the dorsum of the tongue. Fungiform papillae have taste buds on the dorsal aspect of their cap.

Foliate papillae are located along the posterolateral aspect of the tongue and appear as vertical furrows, reminiscent of pages of a book. Foliate papillae have functional taste buds in the neonate, but these taste buds degenerate by the second or third year of life. Slender ducts of serous minor salivary **glands of von Ebner**, located in the core of the tongue, empty into the base of the furrows.

Circumvallate papillae are 8 to 12 in number, arranged in a V-shaped configuration just anterior to the sulcus terminalis. These papillae are submerged into the surface of the tongue so that they are surrounded by an epithelially lined groove whose base is pierced by slender ducts of glands of von Ebner (Figs. 16.22 and 16.23). The epithelial covering of the circumvallate papillae (but not the dorsum) have numerous taste buds.

Taste Buds. Approximately 2000 to 8000 **taste buds**, intraepithelial sensory organs that function in the perception of taste, are located on the surface of the tongue and the posterior aspect of the oral cavity. Each taste bud, distinctly paler than the epithelium surrounding it, is an oval structure, 70 to 80 μm long and 30 to 40 μm wide, composed of 60 to 80 spindle-shaped cells (see Figs. 16.20, 16.22, and 16.23). The narrow end of the taste bud, located at the free surface of the epithelium, projects into an opening, the **taste pore**, formed by the stratified squamous epithelial cells that overlie the taste bud (see Figs. 16.23 and 16.24).

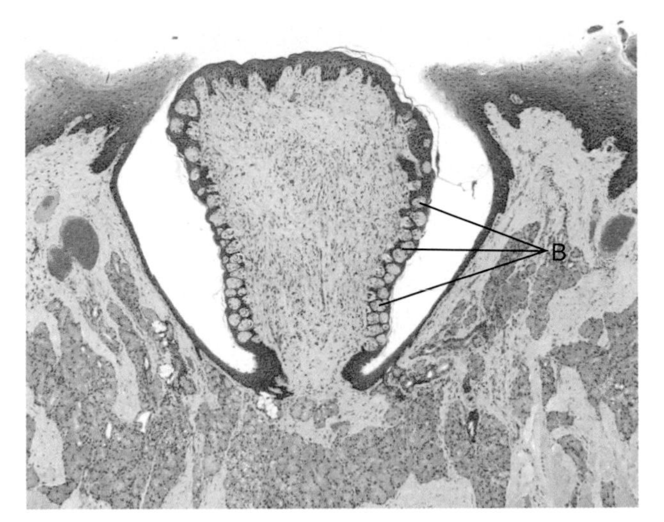

Fig. 16.22 Low-power photomicrograph of a monkey circumvallate papilla. (×58)

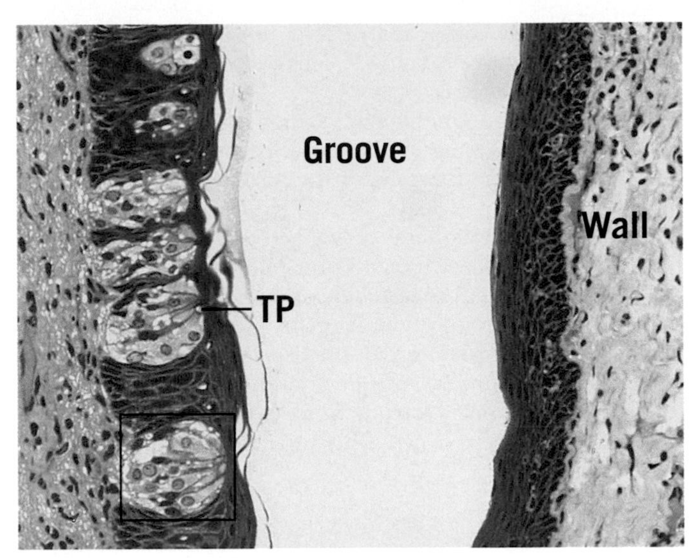

Fig. 16.23 The epithelial covering of the circumvallate papilla has numerous taste buds (square box). Each taste bud has a taste pore (TP) through which microvilli of gustatory cells protrude into the saliva-laden groove located between the circumvallate papilla and the wall of the moat-like groove. (×270)

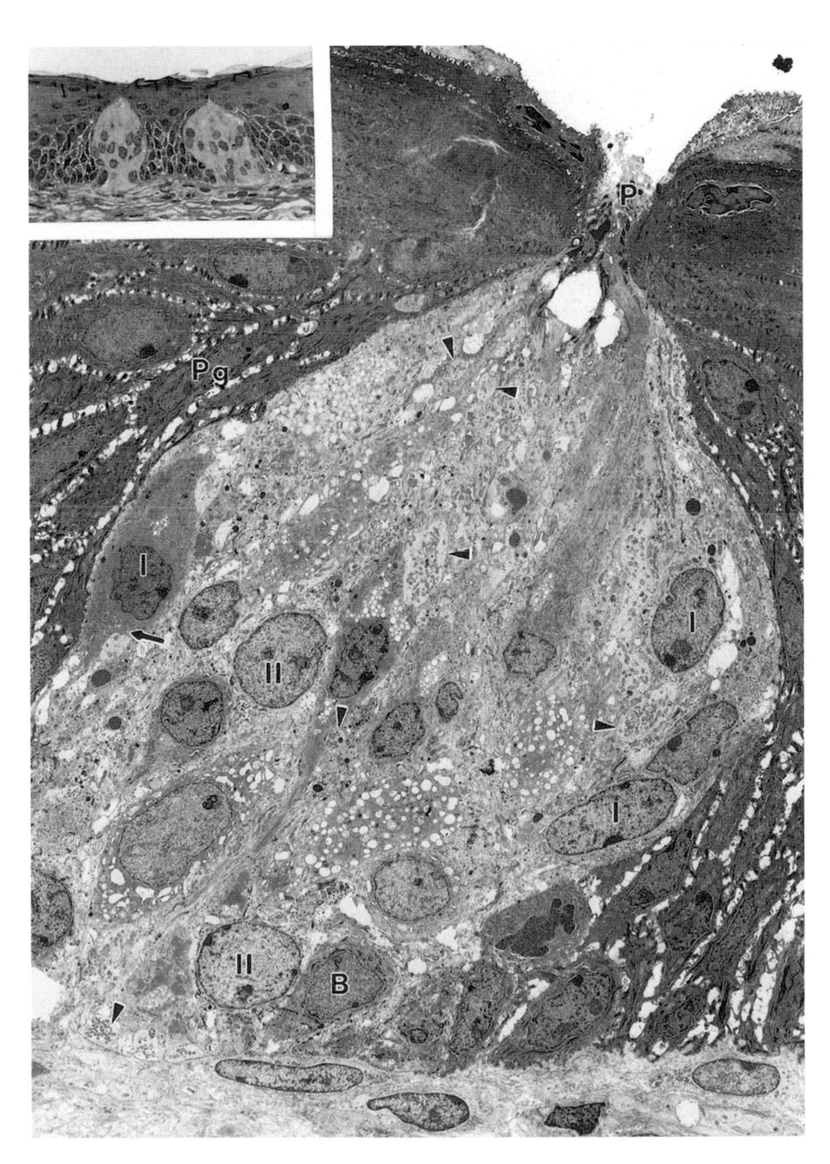

Fig. 16.24 Low-power electron micrograph of a taste bud from a lamb epiglottis (×2353). B, Basal cell; I, type I cell; II, type II cell; P, taste pore; Pg, perigemmal cell. *Arrowheads* represent nerve fibers; *arrow* represents synapse-like structure between a type I cell and a nerve fiber. (From Sweazy RD, Edwards CA, Kapp BM. Fine structure of taste buds located on the lamb epiglottis. *Anat Rec.* 1994;238:517–527. Reprinted with permission from Wiley-Liss, Inc., a subsidiary of John Wiley & Sons, Inc.)

A taste bud is composed of four types of cells: dark cells (type I cells); light cells (type II cells); intermediate cells (type III cells); and basal cells.

The relationship among the various cell types is not clear, although researchers agree that basal cells function as reserve cells and regenerate the cells of the taste bud, which have an average life span of 10 days. Most investigators believe in the following progression: basal cells give rise to dark cells, which mature into light cells, which become intermediate cells and die.

Nerve fibers enter the taste bud and form synaptic junctions with type I, type II, and type III cells, indicating that all three cell types probably function in the discernment of taste and are known as *neuroepithelial cells*. Each of these cell types has long, slender microvilli that protrude from the taste pore. In the past, these microvilli were noted with light microscopes and were called *taste hairs*.

Clinical Correlations

Some investigators suggest the following about the different types of cells: type I cells constitute about half of the cells of a taste bud and function as glia cells; type II cells, which constitute about one-third of the cells of a taste bud and communicate with nearby afferent nerve fibers (without forming synapses), are responsible for reacting to taste sensations; type III cells, which constitute less than 20% of taste bud cells, also react to taste sensations and relay them via synaptic contact with afferent sensory nerve fibers. These investigators suggest that type I cells remove neurotransmitters from the extracellular spaces of the taste bud and also monitor and modify the extracellular potassium ion levels. Type II cells are of different types depending on their ability to detect sweet and umami or bitter and umami. There may be two groups of type III cells that can detect either salt or sour tastes.

Tastants, chemicals from food dissolved in saliva, interact either with ion channels or with receptors located on the microvilli of the taste cells. The binding causes electrical alterations in the resting potentials of these cells, resulting in depolarization of the cell and initiating an action potential that is transmitted to the brain, where the signals are interpreted as specific taste sensations. There are five primary taste sensations: salty, sweet, sour, bitter, and umami (a savory taste sensed via glutamate receptors). It is believed that, although every taste bud can discern each of the five sensations, each taste bud specializes in two of the four tastes. The reaction to these taste modalities is due to the presence of specific ion channels (for salty and sour tastes) and G protein–linked membrane receptors (for bitter, sweet, and umami tastes) in the plasmalemma of the cells of the taste bud. Recently, another receptor was localized on taste buds, CD36, a fatty acid transporter, that has the ability to detect fat. Individuals possessing these receptors prefer foods that are fatty.

It is now known that three of the five taste sensations—bitter, sweet, and umami—depend on the presence of **G protein–linked membrane receptors** in the membranes of the microvilli protrudes through the taste pores. The taste receptors for sweet and umami are coded for by three genes: ***T1R1***, ***T1R2***, and ***T1R3***. Each receptor is coded for by **two** of these three genes. The receptors for bitter are coded for by at least 43 different genes, known as ***T2R#***; the best known of these is **T2R38**, whose protein product recognizes a large number of different tastants that register as bitter. The receptors for sour and salt depend on the presence of hydrogen and sodium ion channels, respectively; the sour taste also depends on the expression of the ***PKD2L1*** **gene** (codes for **polycystic kidney disease 2-like 1 protein**). Lipid taste depends on the presence of a cluster of differentiation molecule (**CD36**) on the cell membrane of the microvilli protruding from the taste pore (Table 16.3).

These five (six, including lipid) taste sensations are only part of what one considers to be the taste of food. The flavor perception also involves olfaction, temperature, and the consistency of the food being consumed. The process of complex taste perception is due more to the olfactory apparatus than to the taste buds, as evidenced by the decreased taste ability of people with nasal congestion from colds. Interestingly, visual cues also play a part in taste—when wine connoisseurs were asked to critique a white wine that, unknown to them, was dyed red, they used terminology specific to red wines to describe its characteristics.

TABLE 16.3 Properties of Taste Buds

Taste Sensation	Receptor or Protein Expressed	G Protein or Ion Channel
Bitter	T2R38	G protein–linked
Sweet	T1R2–T1R3	G protein–linked
Umami	T1R1–T1R3	G protein–linked (glutamate receptors)
Sour	PKD2L1	Hydrogen ion channels
Salt	?	Sodium ion channels
Fat	CD36	

CD36, Cluster of differentiation-36 receptor; *PKD2L1*, polycystic kidney disease 2-like 1 protein; *T2R, T1R*, taste receptor gene product.

Clinical Correlations

Recent investigations using mice placed on a high-fat diet demonstrated that, as the mice gained weight, they lost up to one-quarter of their taste buds 8 weeks into the experiment when compared with mice on a normal diet that did not gain weight. The taste buds of the experimental mice degenerated at a faster rate and their cells were replenished at a slower rate than those of control mice. Taste buds of obese mice had a higher level of tumor necrosis factor alpha (TNF-α); this cytokine has a deleterious effect on taste buds.

Pathological Considerations

See Figs. 16.25 and 16.26.

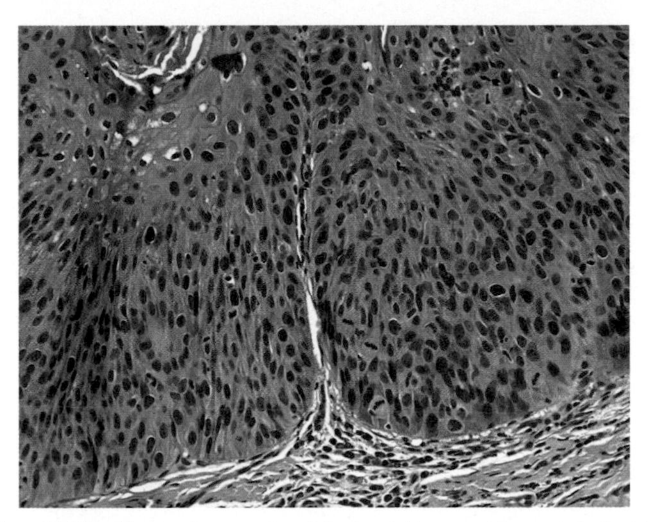

Fig. 16.25 Photomicrograph of leukoplakia, a white patch that is premalignant in less than 25% of the cases and cannot be removed by gentle scraping, in the oral cavity. Note that the epithelium presents a severe dysplasia, with a large population of immature epithelial cells and a higher than normal incidence of mitotic activity. (Reprinted with permission from Kumar V, Abbas AK, Aster JC. *Robbins and Cotran Pathologic Basis of Disease.* 9th ed. Philadelphia: Elsevier; 2015:732.)

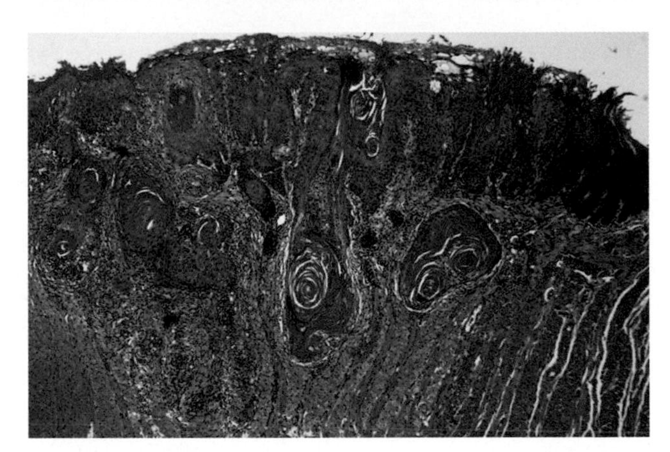

Fig. 16.26 Photomicrograph of squamous cell carcinoma in the oral cavity. Observe the islands of keratinocytes that have invaded the subepithelial connective tissue and skeletal muscle. (Reprinted with permission from Kumar V, Abbas AK, Aster JC. *Robbins and Cotran Pathologic Basis of Disease.* 9th ed. Philadelphia: Elsevier; 2015:733.)

Histology Laboratory Instructions: Digestive System—Oral Cavity

Lip

In a very-low-magnification photomicrograph of the lip, stratified squamous keratinized epithelium is seen to be present on the skin aspect and the vermilion zone. The mucous aspect is lined by a stratified squamous nonkeratinized epithelium. Hair follicles are present on the skin aspect and mucous (to mixed) minor salivary glands are located in the connective tissue of the mucous aspect of the lip. The core of the lip has skeletal muscles surrounded by a dense, irregular, collagenous connective tissue (see Fig. 16.1, KE, SA, VZ, NKE, *arrow*, MSG).

Tooth

Viewing a decalcified incisor tooth in situ at a very low magnification displays the coronal and radicular pulp of the tooth, surrounded by coronal and radicular dentin. Because enamel is 96% calcified material, decalcification removes all of it, leaving behind the enamel space. Cementum covers radicular dentin, and the space between cementum and the alveolus, known as the periodontal ligament space, is occupied by the periodontal ligament. The gingival crest separates the sulcular epithelium from the epithelium of the attached gingiva. The gingiva adheres to the enamel surface by a narrow band of nonkeratinized stratified squamous epithelium, known as the junctional epithelium, an apical continuation of the sulcular epithelium (see Fig. 16.4, P, D, ES, *arrow*, AL, PDL, Gc, GE, *arrowhead*). A ground section of an undecalcified tooth displays enamel covering dentin, which surrounds the pulp cavity (see Fig. 16.5, E, D, P). A very-low-magnification decalcified section of the coronal aspect of the root of a tooth displays the odontoblastic zone of the pulp and its surrounding dentin. A thin layer of acellular cementum covers the dentin, and collagen fibers from the periodontal ligament extend from the cementum to the alveolar bone proper of the alveolus. The interstitial spaces of the periodontal ligament are occupied by blood vessels and nerve fibers surrounded by indefinite tissue (see Fig. 16.6, OZ, P, D, C, PDL, ABP, IS). The fiber bundles of the periodontal ligament are composed mostly of type I collagen; they extend from the bony alveolus to the cementum of the root (see Fig. 16.17, L, A, C). A medium-power magnification of the decalcified root near the apical foramen presents the cementocytes in the lacunae of a thick layer of cellular cementum covering the dentin. Cementoblasts, located in the periodontal ligament space, lie against the thin layer of cementoid (uncalcified cementum) that covers the cementum surface. Observe that collagen fibers of the periodontal ligament are embedded in the cementum (see Fig. 16.7, Cc, C, D, Cb, PDL). At low magnification, the pulp of the decalcified tooth displays its core. The three zones of the pulp are also clearly identifiable: the cell-rich zone adjoining the core, the cell-free zone, and the odontoblastic zone (see Fig. 16.8, CR, CF, O). At medium magnification, the core of the pulp of the decalcified tooth displays mesenchymal cells, as well as blood vessels and nerve fibers and various connective tissue cells, such as fibroblasts. The cell-rich zone of the pulp, adjacent to the core, is well represented, as are the two other zones—the cell-free zone and odontoblastic zone. Observe that the odontoblasts adjoin the uncalcified predentin, which separates them from the calcified dentin (see Fig. 16.9, *arrowhead*, BV, NF, *arrow*, CRZ, CFZ, OZ, Pd, D).

Odontogenesis

The dental lamina, derived from the oral epithelium, provides cells that form a cluster of cells at the inferior aspect of the dental lamina. This cell cluster, known as the bud, indicates the bud stage of tooth development. Mesenchymal connective tissue, derived from neural crest material, begins to congregate at the inferior aspect of the bud. The location of the tongue and oral cavity indicate that this bud is in the mandibular arch (see Fig. 16.11, DL, OE, B, MCT, T). Cells of the bud proliferate, forming the cap and then the bell stage of tooth development. The enamel organ of the bell stage, still attached to the dental lamina, is composed of four layers: the outer enamel epithelium, stellate reticulum, stratum intermedium, and inner enamel epithelium. The dental papilla fills the concavity formed by the inner enamel epithelium and is separated from the dental sac at its inferior aspect by the cervical loop. The arrow indicates the basement membrane that isolates the epithelially derived components from the ectomesenchymally derived components of the bell (see Fig. 16.12, DL, OEE, SR, SI, IEE, DP, CL, *arrow*). A very-low-magnification photomicrograph of an undecalcified deciduous incisor tooth germ in the appositional stage of tooth development shows the very long succedaneous lamina whose inferior aspect sports the developing succedaneous bud.

Histology Laboratory Instructions: Digestive System—Oral Cavity—cont'd

The deciduous tooth germ still has its outer enamel epithelium and stellate reticulum. The dental papilla and the dental sac are well developed and the odontoblasts of the crown are actively producing dentin. The ameloblasts are manufacturing enamel in the crown and the dentinoenamel junction is very evident. The entire tooth germ is partially enveloped in a bony capsule (see Fig. 16.15, SL, SB, OEE, SR, DP, DS, O, A, E, DEJ, BC). A high magnification of the appositional stage the dental papilla and its odontoblasts, each with its odontoblastic process, are easily distinguishable. The dentin and enamel meet at the dentinoenamel junction. The tall columnar ameloblasts and the adjacent layer of stratum intermedium are clearly evident (see Fig. 16.16, DP, O, OP, D, E, A, SI).

Hard Palate

The stratified squamous parakeratinized epithelium of the hard palate forms epithelial ridges that interdigitate with the connective tissue ridges of the subepithelial dense, irregular, collagenous connective tissue. Observe that the bundles of collagen fibers are oriented in an almost haphazard fashion (see Fig. 16.18, ER, CTR, CT, *arrowheads*).

Tongue

The very-low-magnification photomicrograph of a fungiform papilla demonstrates that it projects above the dorsal surface of the tongue, which is covered by a stratified squamous keratinized epithelium. However, the dorsal surface of the fungiform papilla is covered by a stratified squamous nonkeratinized epithelium that houses a few taste buds. The core of the tongue possesses intrinsic and extrinsic skeletal muscles. One of the intrinsic muscles, the superior longitudinal muscle, is evident in this section (see Fig. 16.21, boxed area, TDE, *arrows*, SLM). The circumvallate papilla is located mostly below the dorsal surface of the tongue and is surrounded by a moat-like groove, as is evident in this very-low-magnification photomicrograph. The stratified squamous nonkeratinized covering, but not the dorsal surface, of the circumvallate papilla has taste buds (see Fig. 16.22, B). At a medium magnification of a circumvallate papilla, the taste buds are clearly evident, as is the taste pore. The groove separates the circumvallate papilla from the wall of the groove, which is lined by a stratified squamous nonkeratinized epithelium (see Fig. 16.23, boxed area, TP, groove, wall).

17 Digestive System: Alimentary Canal

The **alimentary canal**, the tubular portion of the digestive tract, extends from the oral cavity to the anus. Aliquots of food that was swallowed at the level of the oral cavity enters the alimentary canal to be churned, liquefied, and digested so that its nutritional elements and water can be absorbed and its indigestible components eliminated. The approximately 9-m-long alimentary canal is subdivided into several morphologically recognizable regions: the esophagus, stomach, small intestine (duodenum, jejunum, and ileum), and large intestine (cecum, colon, rectum, anal canal, and appendix). The time that is spent by the ingested food in the various regions of the alimentary canal depends on many factors, including its chemical composition. However, a "standard" meal spends 5 seconds in the esophagus, 3 to 5 hours in the stomach, 6 to 12 hours in the small intestine, and 30 to 40 hours in the large intestine.

The alimentary canal has a general plan that will now be presented. Once the conceptual design of the alimentary canal is understood, variations on that common theme are easier to assimilate.

General Plan of the Alimentary Canal

The alimentary canal is composed of the following concentric layers: mucosa, submucosa, muscularis externa, and serosa (adventitia).

The alimentary canal is composed of several histological layers, which are schematically illustrated in Fig. 17.1. These layers are innervated by the enteric nervous system and modulated by parasympathetic and sympathetic nerves; they are also served by sensory fibers.

HISTOLOGICAL LAYERS

The histology of the alimentary canal displays four layers: **mucosa**, **submucosa**, **muscularis externa**, and **serosa** (or **adventitia**). Although these layers are similar along the entire length of the digestive tract, they display regional modifications and specializations.

Mucosa

The lumen of the alimentary canal is lined by the mucosa, composed of an **epithelium**; a subepithelial loose connective tissue known as the **lamina propria**, a richly vascularized connective tissue that houses glands as well as lymph vessels and occasional lymphoid nodules; and the **muscularis mucosae**, always composed of smooth muscle that usually has two layers—an inner circular layer and an outer longitudinal layer.

Submucosa

The mucosa is surrounded by a dense, irregular, fibroelastic connective tissue layer, the **submucosa** (see Fig. 17.1), which houses glands in only two regions of the alimentary canal—the esophagus and duodenum. The submucosa also contains blood and lymph vessels, as well as a component of the **enteric nervous system** known as the **Meissner submucosal plexus** (**Meissner plexus**). This plexus, which also houses postganglionic parasympathetic nerve cell bodies, controls the motility of the mucosa (and, to a limited extent, the motility of the submucosa) and the secretory activities of its glands.

Muscularis Externa

The muscularis externa is usually composed of inner circular and outer longitudinal smooth muscle layers.

A thick muscular layer, the **muscularis externa**, surrounds the submucosa and is responsible for **peristaltic activity**: the movement of the contents of the lumen along the alimentary tract. The muscularis externa, composed of smooth muscle (except in the esophagus), is usually disposed in two layers: the inner circular layer and outer longitudinal. Certain modified smooth muscle cells, the **interstitial cells of Cajal**, undergo rhythmic contractions. Therefore, they are considered to be the pacemakers for the contraction of the muscularis externa. A second component of the enteric nervous system, known as the **Auerbach myenteric plexus** (**Auerbach plexus**), is situated between these two muscle layers. It regulates the activity of the muscularis externa (and, to a limited extent, the activity of the mucosa). The Auerbach plexus also houses postganglionic parasympathetic nerve cell bodies.

The inner circular and the outer longitudinal layers are arranged in a helical configuration. The pitch of the helices differs, however: the inner circular layer displays a tight helix, whereas the outer longitudinal layer presents a loose helix.

Serosa or Adventitia

The muscularis externa is enveloped by a thin connective tissue layer that may or may not be surrounded by the simple squamous epithelium of the visceral peritoneum. If the region of the alimentary canal is intraperitoneal, it is invested by peritoneum, and the simple squamous epithelial covering is known as the **serosa**. If the organ is retroperitoneal, it adheres to the connective tissue of the body wall by its dense irregular connective tissue component and is known as the **adventitia**.

INNERVATION OF THE DIGESTIVE TRACT

The enteric nervous system, innervating the alimentary canal, is modulated by sympathetic and parasympathetic nervous systems.

The alimentary canal is innervated by two nervous components: an intrinsic element, the **enteric nervous system**, and the extrinsic constituents, the **sympathetic** and **parasympathetic nervous systems**. The enteric nervous system is completely self-sufficient; however, its functions are usually modified by the sympathetic and parasympathetic components. In fact, severing the sympathetic and parasympathetic connections to the entire gut does not interfere with the functions of the alimentary canal.

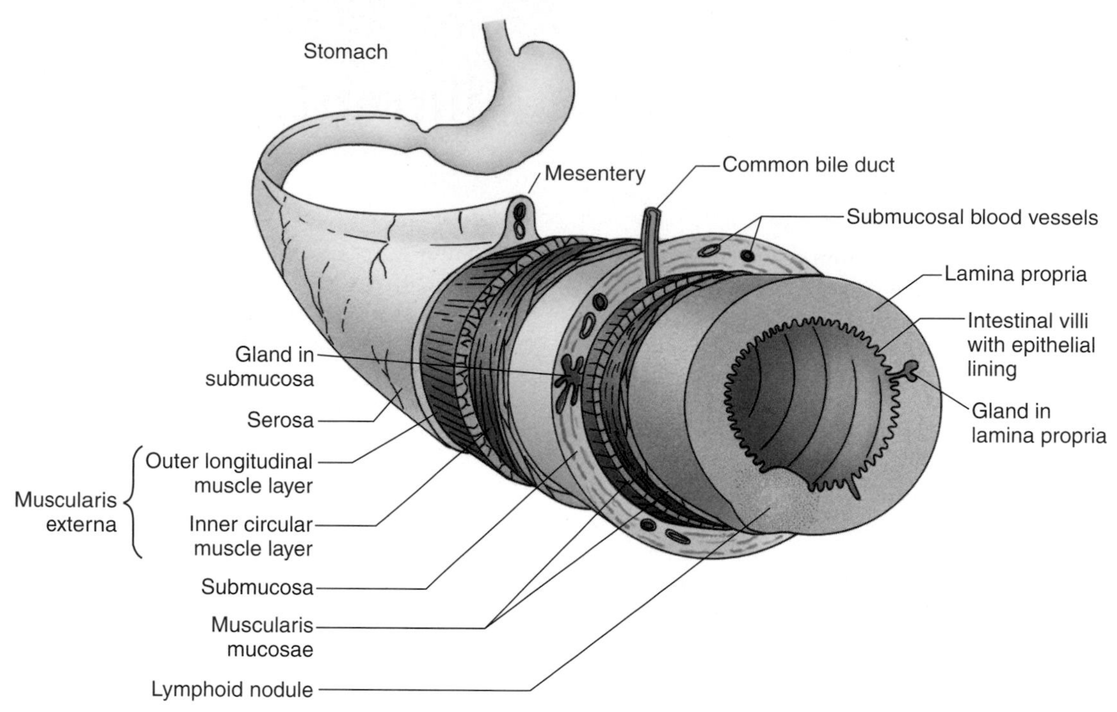

Fig. 17.1 Schematic diagram of the alimentary tract displaying its various layers and the generalized contents of each layer.

Enteric Nervous System

The enteric nervous system is a self-contained nervous system composed of numerous repeating ganglia known as the Meissner submucosal plexus and Auerbach myenteric plexus.

The **enteric nervous system**, considered to be the third component of the autonomic nervous system, extends the entire length of the alimentary canal from the esophagus to the anus and is dedicated to controlling the secretory and motile functions of the alimentary canal. The 500 million or so neurons of the enteric nervous system are distributed in a large number of small clusters of nerve cell bodies and associated nerve fibers in the **Auerbach myenteric plexus** and **Meissner submucosal plexus**. The number of neurons associated with the enteric nervous system exceeds by a factor of 5 the total number of neurons contained within the spinal cord, suggesting that the enteric nervous system is an exceptionally important entity.

Generally speaking, the peristaltic motility of the digestive tract is under the direction of the myenteric plexus, whereas its secretory function and mucosal movement, as well as the regulation of localized blood flow, are governed by the submucosal plexus. Moreover, the myenteric plexus is concerned not only with local conditions but also with conditions along much of the digestive tract, whereas the submucosal plexus is attentive primarily to local conditions in the vicinity of the particular cluster of nerve cells in question. As with all generalizations, there are exceptions to these rules. Therefore, it must be appreciated that there is a great deal of interaction between the two sets of plexuses, and the possibility of cross-controls has been suggested.

Sensory components located in the wall of the alimentary canal convey information concerning the luminal contents, muscular status, and secretory status of the gut to the plexuses in the vicinity of the information, as well as to plexuses at considerable distances from the location of the information source. In fact, some of the information is transmitted to sensory ganglia, as well as to the central nervous system (CNS), by nerve fibers that accompany fibers of the sympathetic and parasympathetic nerve supplies of the digestive tract.

Parasympathetic and Sympathetic Supply to the Gut

Parasympathetic innervation stimulates peristalsis, inhibits sphincter muscles, and triggers secretory activity. Sympathetic nerves inhibit peristalsis and activate sphincter muscles.

Much of the digestive tract receives its **parasympathetic nerve supply** from the vagus nerve (cranial nerve [CN] X). However, the descending colon and rectum are innervated by the **sacral spinal nerves** (**spinal outflow**). Most of the fibers of the vagus nerve are sensory and deliver information from receptors in the mucosa and muscle layers of the alimentary canal to the CNS. Frequently, responses to the information are then conveyed by the efferent vagal fibers from the CNS to the digestive tract. The parasympathetic fibers synapse with postganglionic parasympathetic nerve cell bodies, as well as with nerve cell bodies of the enteric nervous system in both plexuses. The parasympathetic innervation is responsible for inducing secretions from the glands of the digestive tract and for smooth muscle contraction.

The **sympathetic innervation**, controlling blood flow to the alimentary canal, is derived from the splanchnic nerves. As a generalization, it may be stated that parasympathetic innervation stimulates peristalsis, inhibits sphincter muscles, and triggers secretory activity; whereas sympathetic innervation inhibits peristalsis and activates sphincter muscles.

The remainder of this chapter discusses the various regions of the alimentary canal, highlighting how they differ from the general plan.

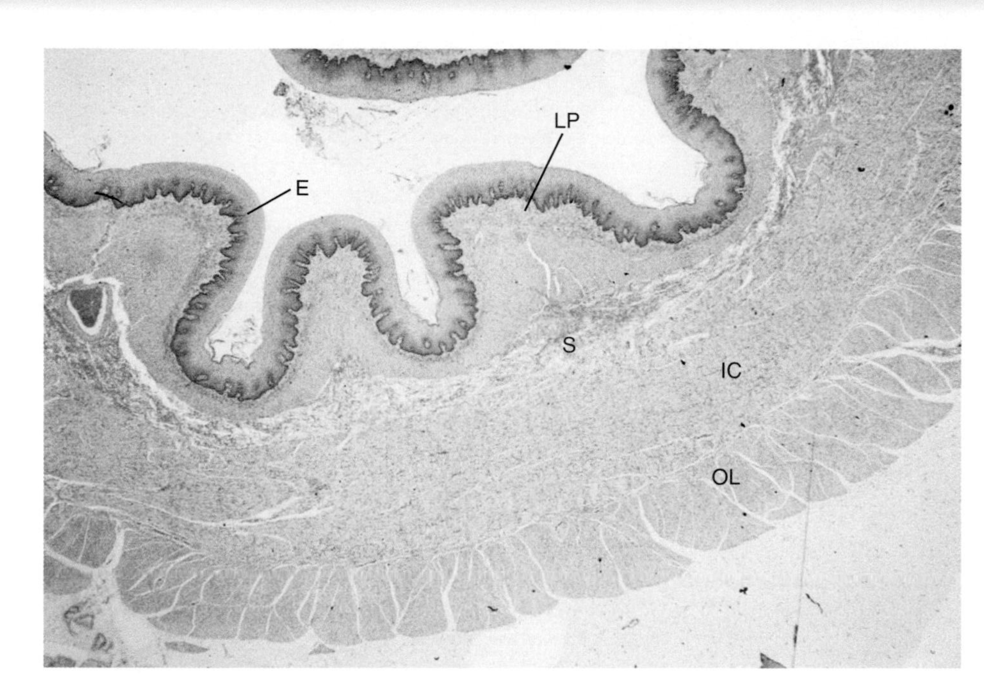

Fig. 17.2 Esophagus. Note that its lumen is lined by a relatively thick, stratified squamous epithelium (E) that forms a well-developed rete apparatus with the underlying lamina propria (LP). The submucosa (S) is surrounded by a thick muscularis externa composed of an inner circular (IC) and outer longitudinal (OL) muscle layer (×17).

Esophagus

The **mucosa** of the approximately 25-cm-long **esophagus**, a muscular tube connecting the oral pharynx to the stomach, presents numerous longitudinal folds that cause the lumen to appear to be obstructed. However, when the bolus travels down the esophagus to the stomach, the folds disappear, the esophagus becomes distended, and the lumen becomes patent.

ESOPHAGEAL HISTOLOGY

Mucosa

> *The esophageal mucosa is composed of a stratified squamous epithelium, fibroelastic lamina propria, and a smooth muscle layer that is composed only of the longitudinally disposed muscularis mucosae.*

The mucosa of the esophagus is composed of three layers: the epithelium, lamina propria, and muscularis mucosae (Figs. 17.2 and 17.3).

The 0.5-mm-thick **stratified squamous nonkeratinized epithelium** lining the lumen of the esophagus interdigitates with the lamina propria, forming a well-developed rete apparatus. The epithelium is regenerated at a much slower rate than that of the remainder of the gastrointestinal (GI) tract; the newly formed cell in the basal layer of the epithelium reaches the free surface in about 3 weeks after formation. Interspersed within the keratinocytes of the epithelium are **antigen-presenting cells**, known as **Langerhans cells**, which phagocytose and degrade antigens into small polypeptides, known as **epitopes** (Langerhans cells are discussed in Chapter 14, Integument).

The **lamina propria** houses **esophageal cardiac glands** located in only two regions of the esophagus, one cluster near the pharynx and the other near its juncture with the stomach. It also houses occasional lymphoid nodules, members of the **gut-associated lymphoid system** (**GALT**). The **muscularis mucosae** is unusual in that it consists of only a *single layer* of longitudinally oriented smooth muscle fibers that become thicker in the vicinity of the stomach.

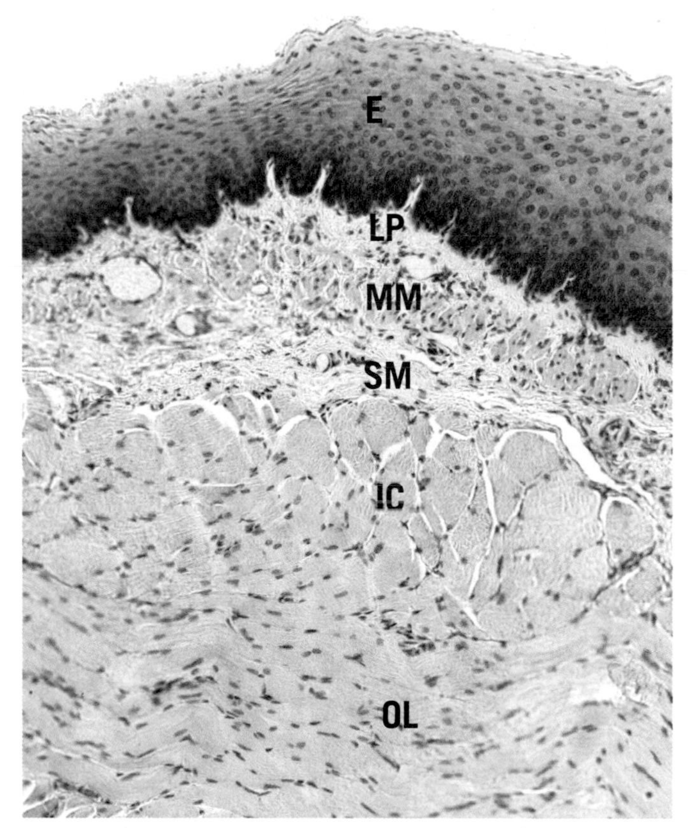

Fig. 17.3 This low-magnification photomicrograph of the esophagus displays its stratified squamous nonkeratinized epithelium (E), its narrow lamina propria (LP) and the muscularis mucosae (MM) as well as submucosa (SM). Note that the inner circular (IC) and outer longitudinal (OL) muscle layers of the muscularis externa are composed of skeletal muscle fibers, indicating that this section was taken from the upper third of the esophagus. (×132)

The **esophageal cardiac glands** produce a mucous secretion that coats the lining of the esophagus, lubricating it to protect the epithelium and to make it easier to convey the bolus into the stomach.

Submucosa

The submucosa of the esophagus houses mucous glands known as the esophageal glands proper.

A dense, fibroelastic connective tissue forms the **submucosa** of the esophagus, which houses the **esophageal glands proper**. The esophagus and the duodenum are the only two regions of the alimentary canal with glands in the submucosa.

Electron micrographs of these tubuloacinar glands indicate that their secretory units are composed of mucous cells and serous cells. **Mucous cells** have basally located, flattened nuclei and apical accumulations of mucinogen-filled secretory granules. **Serous cells** possess round, centrally placed nuclei and numerous cytoplasmic secretory granules that house the proenzyme **pepsinogen** and the antibacterial agent **lysozyme**. The ducts of these glands deliver their secretions into the lumen of the esophagus.

The **submucosal plexus** is in its customary location within the submucosa, in the vicinity of the inner circular layer of the muscularis externa.

Muscularis Externa and Adventitia

The muscularis externa of the esophagus is composed of both skeletal and smooth muscle cells.

The **muscularis externa** of the esophagus is arranged in the customary two layers, inner circular and outer longitudinal. However, these muscle layers are unusual in that they are composed of both skeletal and smooth muscle fibers. The muscularis externa of the upper third of the esophagus has mostly skeletal muscle and is served by the vagus nerve (CN X), the middle third has both skeletal and smooth muscle, and the lowest third has only smooth muscle fibers that are served by nerve fibers of the enteric nervous system. The **Auerbach plexus** occupies its usual position between the inner circular and outer longitudinal smooth muscle layers of the muscularis externa.

The esophagus is covered by an **adventitia** until it pierces the diaphragm, after which it is covered by a **serosa**.

HISTOPHYSIOLOGY OF THE ESOPHAGUS

A bolus entering the esophagus is conveyed, via peristaltic action of the muscularis externa, into the stomach at a rate of about 50 mm/sec. The esophagus possesses physiological sphincters at two levels, the *upper esophageal sphincter (pharyngoesophageal sphincter)*, which is designed to prevent reflux into the pharynx from the esophagus; and the two *lower esophageal sphincters (gastroesophageal sphincters)*, composed of the **internal sphincter** (composed of smooth muscle) and **external sphincter** (composed of skeletal muscle from the diaphragm). These two lower esophageal sphincters normally prevent reflux into the esophagus from the stomach. The internal gastroesophageal sphincter is located at the region where the esophagus pierces the diaphragm and joins the stomach. The muscle fibers of this sphincter are always in tonus except when a bolus is about to pass into the stomach or if the individual is vomiting. The external esophageal sphincter encircles the esophagus to close its lumen during inspiration and during elevation of the intraabdominal pressure (as during defecation).

Clinical Correlations

1. *As the esophagus passes through the diaphragm, it is reinforced by fibers of that muscular structure. In some people, development is abnormal, causing a gap in the diaphragm around the wall of the esophagus that permits herniation of the stomach into the thoracic cage. This condition, known as* **hiatal hernia***, weakens the gastroesophageal sphincter, allowing reflux of the stomach contents into the esophagus.*
2. *Weakened or malfunctioning gastroesophageal sphincters permit the return of stomach content into the esophagus, a condition known as* **gastroesophageal reflux disease (GERD)***. Because the acidic content of the stomach enters the lumen of the esophagus, it usually creates a burning feeling (heartburn) in the midsternum area of the chest, occasionally accompanied by regurgitation. GERD affects approximately 15% to 20% of the population in the "developed" world. In most cases, GERD can be treated by alteration of the patient's lifestyle, such as weight loss; restrained exercise; elevating of the head at night; and elimination of acidic foods, spicy foods, fatty foods, coffee, alcohol, and other foods that the patient notices aggravate the condition. If lifestyle changes do not control the condition then medications, such as* **proton pump inhibitors (PPIs)***, and even surgery may be required. It has been reported that patients taking PPIs have a greater incidence of vitamin B_{12} deficiency than those who are not taking those drugs. Additionally, individuals taking PPIs have a 33% greater risk for chronic kidney disease or end-stage renal disease than patients treated with another type of medication against GERD, namely, Histamine-2 receptor antagonists.*
3. **Barrett syndrome** *is believed to be a premalignant condition initially caused by GERD. Part of the stratified squamous nonkeratinized epithelium of the esophagus, usually in the lowest region, is replaced by a simple columnar epithelium that resembles the lining of the stomach. Endoscopically, this metaplastic area is reddish in color; in order to be classified as Barrett syndrome, at least 3 cm of the esophagus must be involved. If there are numerous red patches in the lower esophagus, esophageal resection may be necessary.*

Stomach

The stomach is responsible for the formation and processing of the ingested food into a thick, acidic fluid known as chyme.

The **stomach** is a sac-like structure that, in the resting state in the average adult, has a volume of only 50 mL. When completely distended, however, it can hold as much as 1500 mL of food and gastric juices. Yet, as the stomach expands, its intraluminal pressure remains relatively constant because of ghrelin and the vagovagal reflex. The hormone **ghrelin**, released by the diffuse neuroendocrine system (DNES) cells, not only induces the sensation of hunger but also modulates receptive relaxation of the smooth muscle fibers of the muscularis externa. In the **vagovagal reflex**, the vagus nerve, by providing feedback information to the muscularis externa of the stomach, maintains the muscle in a relaxed condition. The vagus nerve also prompts three additional effects: (1) the stimulation of **hydrochloric acid (HCl)** production by parietal cells; (2) release of histamine by enterochromaffin-like (ECL) cells; and (3) inhibition of delta cells, whose function is to hinder the release of gastrin by G cells (see later section on HCl production).

Anatomically, the stomach has a concave lesser curvature and a convex greater curvature. Gross observations disclose that the stomach has four regions:

- **Cardia**: a narrow region at the gastroesophageal junction, 2 to 3 cm wide
- **Fundus**: a dome-shaped region to the left of the esophagus, frequently filled with gas
- **Body** (**corpus**): the largest portion, responsible for the formation of chyme
- **Pylorus** (**pyloric antrum**): a funnel-shaped, constricted portion equipped with a thick **pyloric sphincter** that controls the intermittent release of chyme into the duodenum

GASTRIC HISTOLOGY

Histologically, the stomach is said to have three regions: cardiac, fundic, and pyloric regions. Because the fundus and body are identical, the two together are referred to as the **fundic region**. All three regions display **rugae**, longitudinal folds of the mucosa and submucosa (but transverse in the pyloric antrum), which disappear in the distended stomach. Rugae permit expansion of the stomach as it fills with food and gastric juices. Additionally, the epithelial lining of the stomach invaginates into the mucosa, forming **gastric pits** (**foveolae**), which are shallowest in the cardiac region and deepest in the pyloric region. Gastric pits increase the surface area of the gastric lining. Five to seven **gastric glands** of the lamina propria empty into the bottom of each gastric pit.

The ensuing discussion of the stomach details the fundic region because the microscopic anatomy of each of the remaining regions is a variation of the fundic region. Fig. 17.4 schematically depicts the major histological elements of the fundic region.

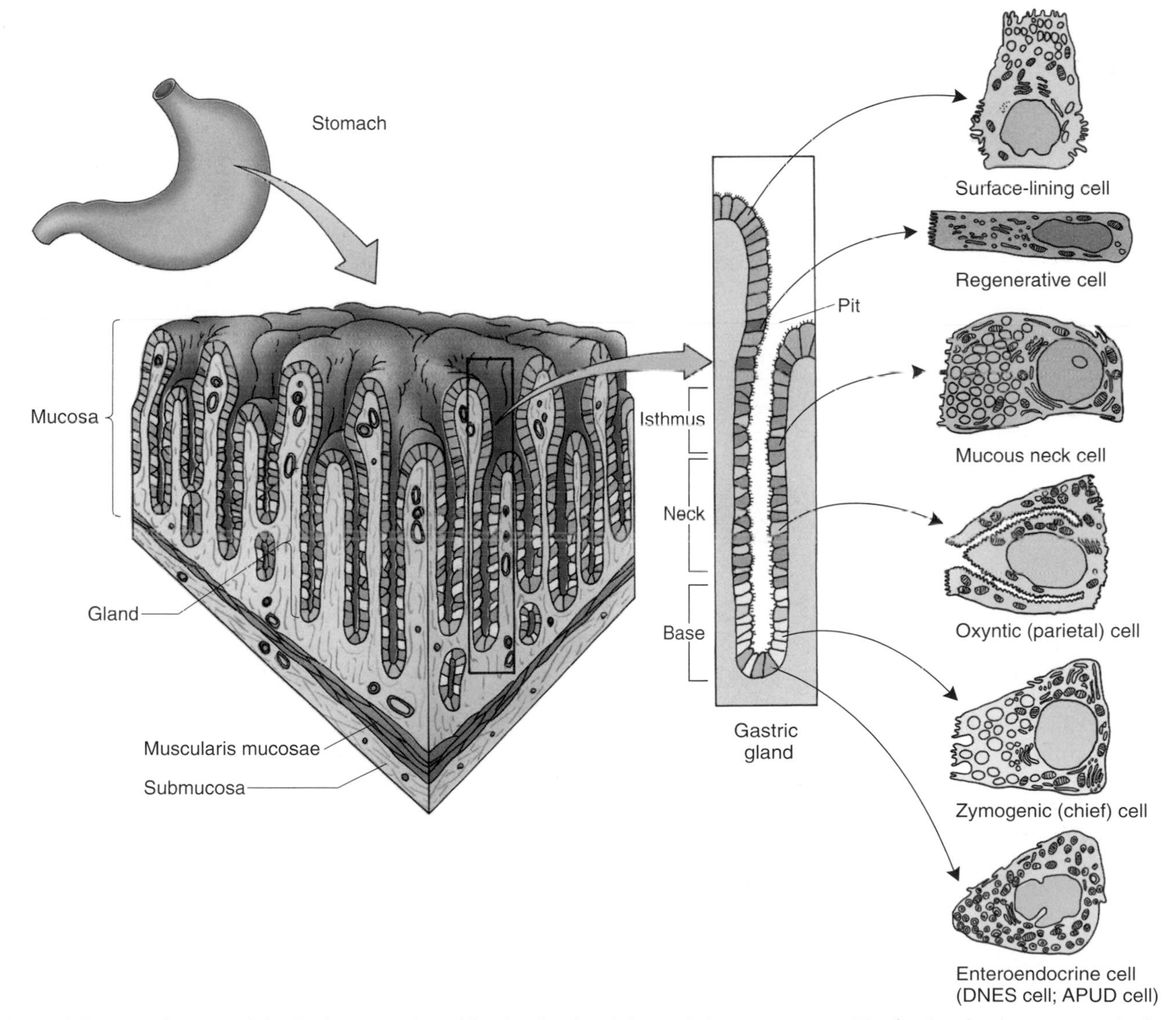

Fig. 17.4 Schematic diagram of the fundic stomach and fundic gland and their cellular composition. The fundic glands open into the bottom of the gastric pits. Each gland is subdivided into an isthmus, neck, and base. APUD, Amine precursor uptake and decarboxylation; DNES, diffuse neuroendocrine system.

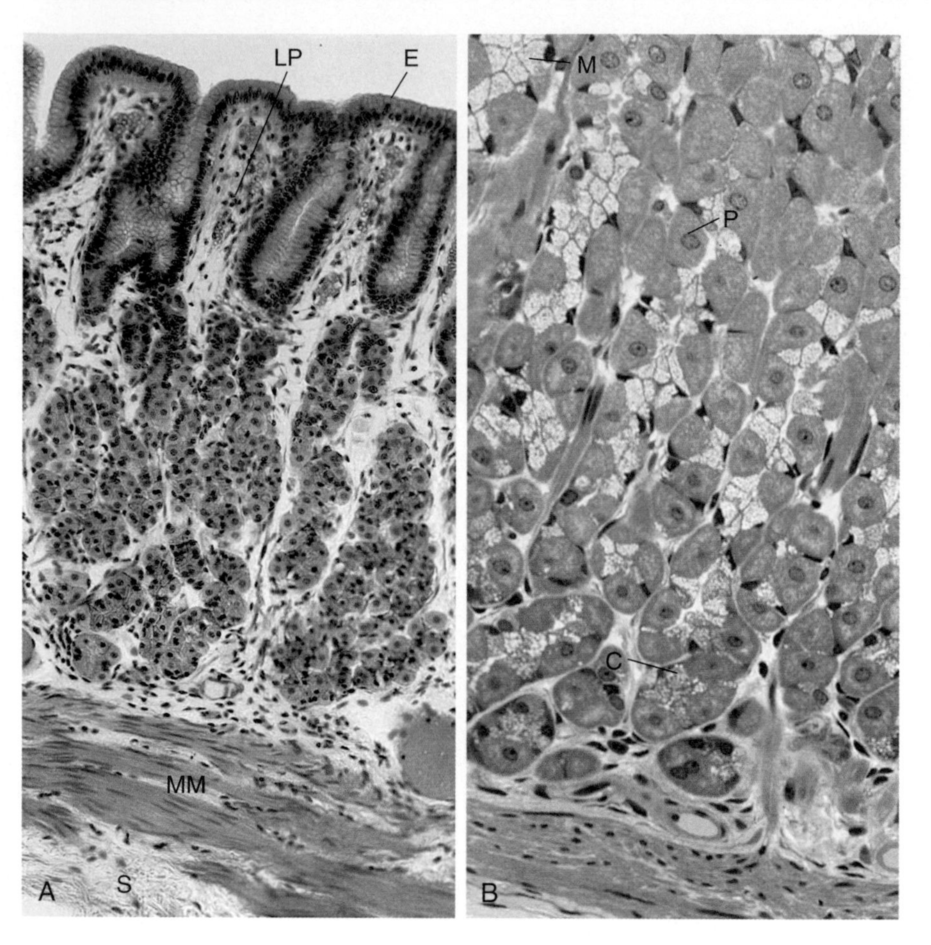

Fig. 17.5 (A) Photomicrograph of the mucosa of the fundic stomach. The mucosa is composed of the simple columnar epithelium (E), the connective tissue lamina propria (LP), and the muscularis mucosae (MM). A little section of the submucosa (S) is evident at the bottom left-hand corner of the photomicrograph (×132). (B) Photomicrograph of fundic glands. Note that the glands are very tightly packed, and much of the connective tissue is compressed into thin wafers occupied by capillaries (×270). C, Chief cell; M, mucous neck cell; P, parietal cell.

Fundic Mucosa

The **mucosa** of the fundic stomach is composed of the usual three components: (1) an epithelium lining the lumen; (2) an underlying connective tissue, the lamina propria; and (3) the smooth muscle layers forming the muscularis mucosae.

Epithelium

The epithelial lining of the stomach secretes visible mucus that adheres to and protects the stomach lining.

The lumen of the fundic stomach is lined by a simple columnar epithelium composed of surface-lining cells, regenerative cells, and a few gustatory cells (taste cells). **Surface lining cells** manufacture a thick gel-like mucus layer, known as **visible mucus** (Fig. 17.5), which adheres to the lining of the stomach and protects it from autodigestion. Moreover, bicarbonate ions that are trapped in this mucus layer assist in maintaining a relatively neutral pH at its interface with the cell membranes of the surface-lining cells despite the low (acidic) pH of the luminal contents. Surface-lining cells continue into the gastric pits, contributing to the formation of their epithelial lining. **Regenerative cells** are also present in the base of these pits, but because they are more numerous in the neck of the gastric glands, they are discussed along with the glands. A small number of **taste cells** that recognize sweet, bitter, and umami taste sensations are also present in the fundic epithelium (see the later section on the small intestine and Chapter 16, the section on taste buds).

The apical surfaces of surface-lining cells possess glycocalyx-covered, short, stubby microvilli and their apical cytoplasm displays the presence of secretory granules containing the precursor of the visible mucus (Fig. 17.6). These cells form intricate zonulae occludentes and zonulae adherentes with those of neighboring cells and their basal cytoplasm is occupied by their nuclei, mitochondria, and their protein synthesis and packaging apparatus.

Lamina Propria

The highly vascularized **lamina propria** is populated by fibroblasts, plasma cells, lymphocytes, mast cells, and additional components of the **GALT**, as well as occasional smooth muscle cells. However, much of the lamina propria is occupied by the approximately 15 million closely packed gastric glands, known as ***fundic* (*oxyntic*) *glands*** in the fundic region (see Figs. 17.5 and 17.7).

Fundic Glands. **Fundic glands** are composed of six cell types: surface-lining cells, parietal (oxyntic) cells, regenerative (stem) cells, mucous neck cells, chief (zymogenic) cells, and DNES cells. Each gland extends from the base of the gastric pit to the muscularis mucosae and is subdivided into three regions: (1) the isthmus, (2) neck, and (3) base, of which the base is the longest (see Fig. 17.4). The distribution of these cells within the three regions of the gland is presented in Table 17.1.

The **surface-lining cells** in the isthmus region were described previously. The structure and function of the other five cell types are discussed in the following sections.

Mucous Neck Cells

Mucous neck cells produce soluble mucus that is mixed with and lubricates the chyme, reducing friction as it moves along the digestive tract.

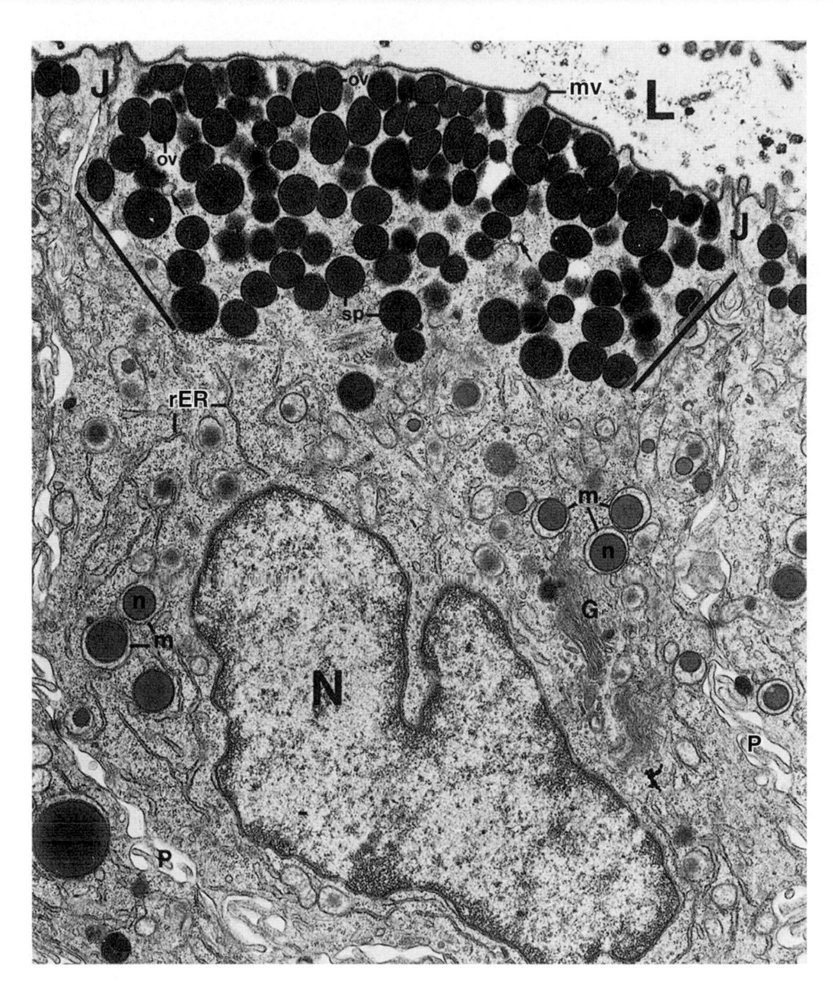

Fig. 17.6 Electron micrograph of a surface-lining cell from the body of a mouse stomach (×11,632). G, Golgi apparatus; J, junctional complex; L, lumen; m, mitochondria exhibiting large spherical densities known as *nodules* (n); mv, microvillus; N, nucleus; ov, oval secretory granules; P, intercellular projections; rER, rough endoplasmic reticulum; sp, spherical granules. (From Karam SF, Leblond CP. Identifying and counting epithelial cell types in the "corpus" of the mouse stomach. *Anat Rec.* 1992;232:231–246. Reprinted with permission from Wiley-Liss, Inc., a subsidiary of John Wiley & Sons, Inc.)

The columnar-shaped **mucous neck cells** have short microvilli, basally located nuclei and mitochondria, a well-developed Golgi apparatus and rough endoplasmic reticulum (RER; Fig. 17.8). Their apical cytoplasm is filled with secretory granules containing **soluble mucus** (not the visible mucus synthesized by surface-lining cells), which functions to lubricate the lining of the stomach, thereby reducing frictional forces as the gastric contents is being churned. The lateral membranes of mucous neck cells form zonulae occludentes and zonulae adherentes with the adjacent cells.

Regenerative (Stem) Cells

A relatively few thin **regenerative cells** are interspersed among the mucous neck cells of fundic glands (see Fig. 17.4). These cells are organelle poor but have a rich supply of ribosomes; their nuclei are basally situated, have little heterochromatin, and display a large nucleolus. The lateral cell membranes of these cells also form zonulae occludentes and zonulae adherentes with those of adjacent cells.

Regenerative cells proliferate to replace all of the specialized cells lining the fundic glands, gastric pits, and luminal surface. Newly formed cells migrate to their new locations, either deep into the gland or up into the gastric pit and gastric lining. Surface-lining cells, DNES cells, and mucous neck cells are replaced every 5 to 7 days; thus, regenerative cells have a high proliferative rate.

Parietal (Oxyntic) Cells

Parietal cells manufacture hydrochloric acid and gastric intrinsic factor; both products are released into the lumen of the stomach.

Large, round to pyramid-shaped **parietal cells** are located mainly in the upper half of the fundic glands and only occasionally in the base (see Figs. 17.4, 17.5, and 17.7). They are about 20 to 25 μm in diameter and are situated at the periphery of the gland. These cells manufacture **HCl** and **gastric intrinsic factor**.

Clinical Correlations

Gastric intrinsic factor, a glycoprotein secreted into the lumen of the stomach, is necessary for vitamin B_{12} absorption from the ileum. Absence of this factor results in deficiency of vitamin B_{12}, with the consequent development of ***pernicious anemia****. Because the liver stores high quantities of vitamin B_{12}, a deficiency of this vitamin may take several months to develop after production of gastric intrinsic factor ceases.*

Parietal cells have round, basally located nuclei, and their cytoplasm is eosinophilic. Their most remarkable characteristic is the invaginations of their apical plasmalemma to form deep **intracellular canaliculi** lined by microvilli (Figs. 17.9 and 17.10). The cytoplasm bordering intracellular canaliculi is richly endowed by round and tubular vesicles, the **tubulovesicular system**. Parietal cells are rich in mitochondria, whose combined volume constitutes almost half that of the cytoplasm. Only a scant amount of RER and Golgi are present.

The abundance of vesicles of the tubulovesicular system and the number of microvilli are indirectly related to each other and vary with the HCl secretory activity of the cell. During active

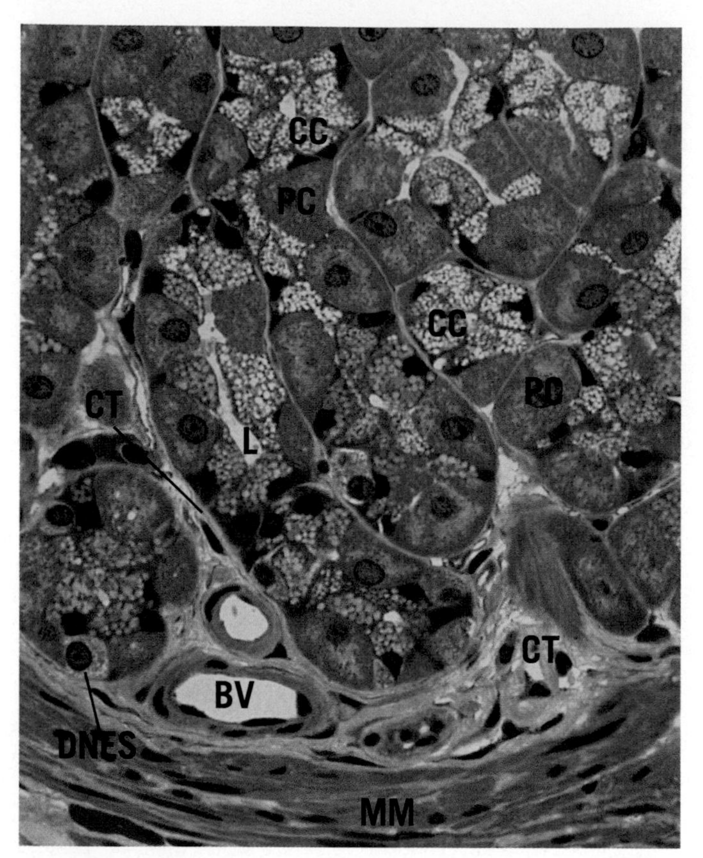

Fig. 17.7 This high-magnification photomicrograph of the fundic region of the stomach displays chief cells (CC), parietal cells (PC), (DNES cells (DNES), the narrow lumina (L) of the fundic glands, the sparse amount of connective tissue (CT), blood vessels (BV), and the muscularis mucosae (MM). (×540).

HCl production, the tubulovesicular system decreases and the number of microvilli increases, indicating that the membrane being stored as tubules and vesicles is probably used for microvillar assembly, increasing the surface area of the cell by a factor of 4 or 5 in preparation for HCl production.

The process of microvillus formation requires energy and involves polymerization of soluble forms of actin and myosin into filaments, which then interact to transport membranes from the tubulovesicular system to those of the intracellular canaliculi. The stored membranes have a high content of **H^+, K^+-ATPase** (a protein that pumps protons from the cytoplasm into the intracellular canaliculus).

Chief (Zymogenic) Cells

Chief cells manufacture the enzymes pepsinogen, rennin, and gastric lipase and release them into the lumen of the stomach.

Most of the cells in the base of fundic glands are **chief cells** whose blunt, glycocalyx-covered microvilli project from the apical aspect of the cell into the lumen of the gland (see Figs. 17.4, 17.5, and 17.7). These columnar cells have a basophilic cytoplasm, basally located nuclei, occasional lysosomes, and are richly endowed with RER, Golgi apparatus, and apically situated secretory granules that house the proenzymes **pepsinogen**, **rennin**, and **gastric lipase** (Fig. 17.11). Exocytosis of pepsinogen from chief cells is induced by neural stimulation by the vagus nerve and by the binding of the hormone **secretin** to receptors in the basal plasma membrane.

Chief cells also manufacture the hormone **leptin**, which acts on the arcuate nucleus of the hypothalamus to inhibit the sensation of hunger. Thus, it is antagonistic to the hormone ghrelin.

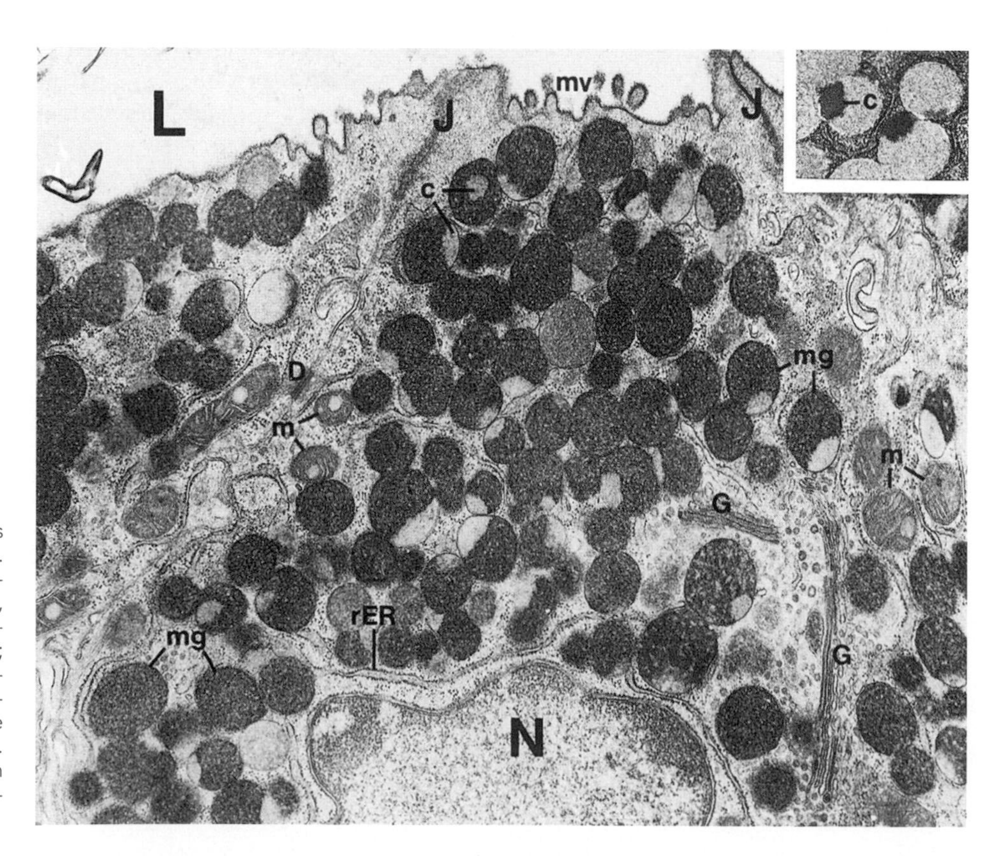

Fig. 17.8 Electron micrograph of a mucous neck cell from the body of a mouse stomach. *Inset*: Secretory granule. c, Dense-cored granule; D, desmosome; G, Golgi apparatus; J, junctional complex; L, lumen; m, mitochondria; mg, mucous granules; mv, microvillus; N, nucleus; rER, rough endoplasmic reticulum. (From Karam SF, Leblond CP. Identifying and counting epithelial cell types in the "corpus" of the mouse stomach. *Anat Rec.* 1992;232:231–246. Reprinted with permission from Wiley-Liss, Inc., a subsidiary of John Wiley & Sons, Inc.)

TABLE 17.1 Distribution of Cell Types in Fundic Glands

Region	Cell Types
Isthmus	Surface-lining cells and few DNES cells
Neck	Mucous neck cells, regenerative cells, parietal cells, and few DNES cells
Base	Chief cells, occasional parietal cells, and few DNES cells

DNES, Diffuse neuroendocrine system.

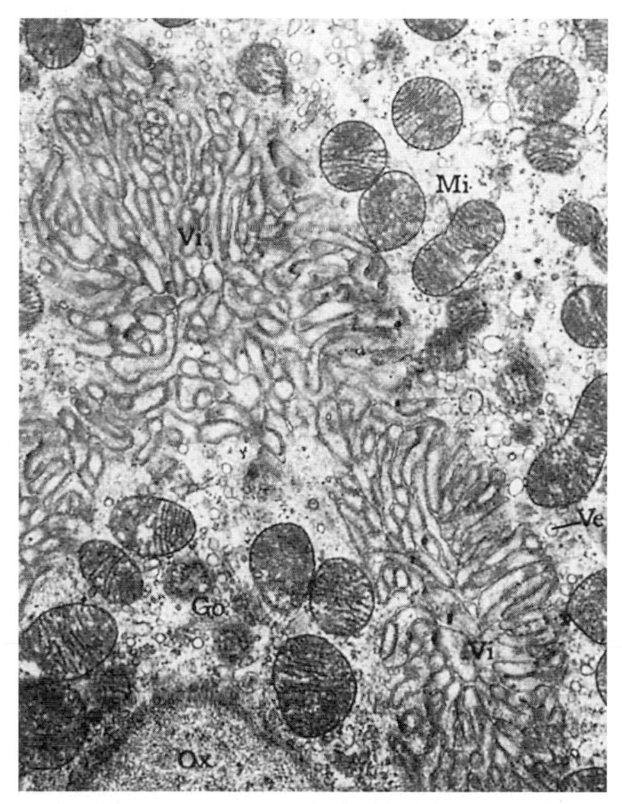

Fig. 17.9 Electron micrograph of a parietal cell from the body of a mouse stomach (×14,000). Go, Golgi apparatus; Mi, mitochondria; Ox, nucleus of oxyphil cell; Ve, tubulovesicular apparatus; Vi, microvilli. (From Rhodin JAG. *An Atlas of Ultrastructure*. Philadelphia: WB Saunders; 1963.)

Diffuse Neuroendocrine System Cells (Enteroendocrine Cells; APUD Cells)

DNES cells may be open or closed; they manufacture endocrine, paracrine, and neurocrine hormones.

There are two types of DNES cells, **open type** and **closed type**. The open-type DNES cells reach the lumen via long, thin apical processes with microvilli, which may serve to monitor the contents of the gastric lumen. The closed-type DNES cells do not possess such processes; therefore, they have no access to the gastric lumen. The cytoplasm of DNES cells has a well-developed RER and Golgi apparatus and numerous mitochondria. Additionally, small secretory granules are evident, disposed **basally** in most cells (Fig. 17.12). All DNES cells release the contents of their granules basally into the lamina propria. The hormones that these cells release either travel short distances in the interstitial tissue to act on target cells in the immediate vicinity of the signaling cell (paracrine effect) or enter the circulation and travel a distance to reach their target cell (endocrine effect). Furthermore, the substance released may be identical with neurosecretions. Because of these three possibilities, some researchers have used the

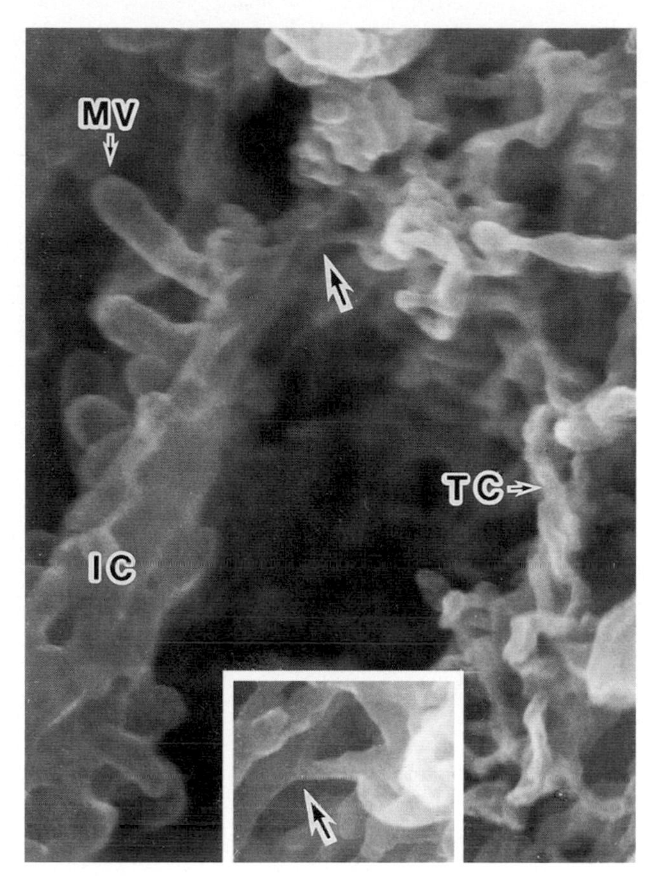

Fig. 17.10 Scanning electron microscopy of the fractured surface of a resting parietal cell. The cytoplasmic matrix is removed by the aldehyde-osmium-DMSO-osmium method (or A-ODO method), exposing the cytoplasmic membranes. The tubulovesicular network (TC) is connected to the intracellular canaliculus (IC) lined with microvilli (MV, *arrow*) (×50,000). *Inset*: A higher magnification of the area indicated by the *arrow* in panel (×100,000). (From Ogata T, Yamasaki Y. Scanning EM of the resting gastric parietal cells reveals a network of cytoplasmic tubules and cisternae connected to the intracellular canaliculus. *Anat Rec*. 2000;258:15–24. Reprinted with permission from Wiley-Liss, Inc., a subsidiary of John Wiley & Sons, Inc.)

terms ***endocrine***, ***paracrine***, and ***neurocrine*** to differentiate among the three variations of the secreted substances.

Some DNES cells are individually designated according to the substance that they produce. Generally, a single type of DNES cell secretes only one hormone, although occasional cell types may secrete two different hormones. There are at least 13 different DNES cell types, only some of which are located in the mucosa of the stomach. Table 17.2 lists most of the better-known cells; their locations, granule size, and the substance being secreted; and the action of the released substances. Cells of the DNES have been localized not only in the digestive tract but also in the respiratory system and endocrine pancreas. Additionally, some of the secretory products synthesized and released by these DNES cells are identical with neurosecretions localized in the CNS. The significance of their diverse location and the substances that they produce is only incompletely understood.

MUSCULARIS MUCOSAE OF THE STOMACH

The smooth muscle cells that compose the **muscularis mucosae** are arranged in three layers. The inner circular and outer longitudinal layers are well defined. An occasional third layer,

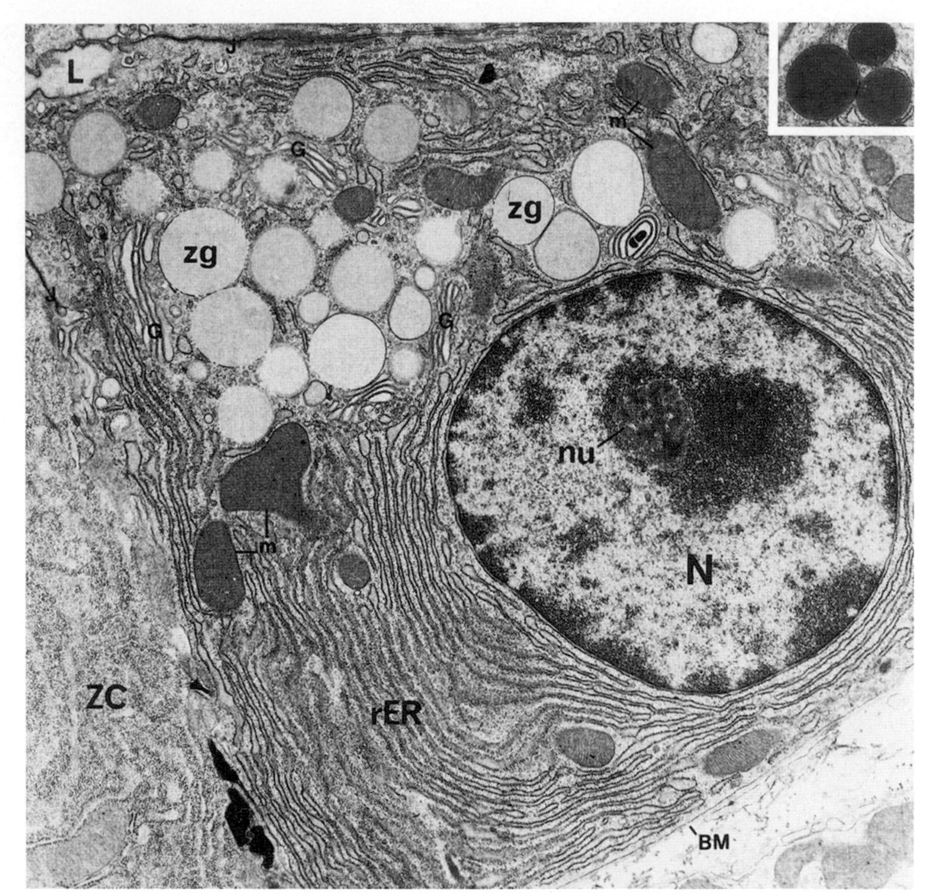

Fig. 17.11 Electron micrograph of a chief cell from the fundus of a mouse stomach (×11,837). BM, Basement membrane; G, Golgi apparatus; L, lumen; m, mitochondria; N, nucleus; nu, nucleolus; rER, rough endoplasmic reticulum; ZC, zymogenic (chief) cell; zg, zymogen granules. (From Karam SF, Leblond CP. Identifying and counting epithelial cell types in the "corpus" of the mouse stomach. *Anat Rec*. 1992;232:231–246. Reprinted with permission from Wiley-Liss, Inc., a subsidiary of John Wiley & Sons, Inc.)

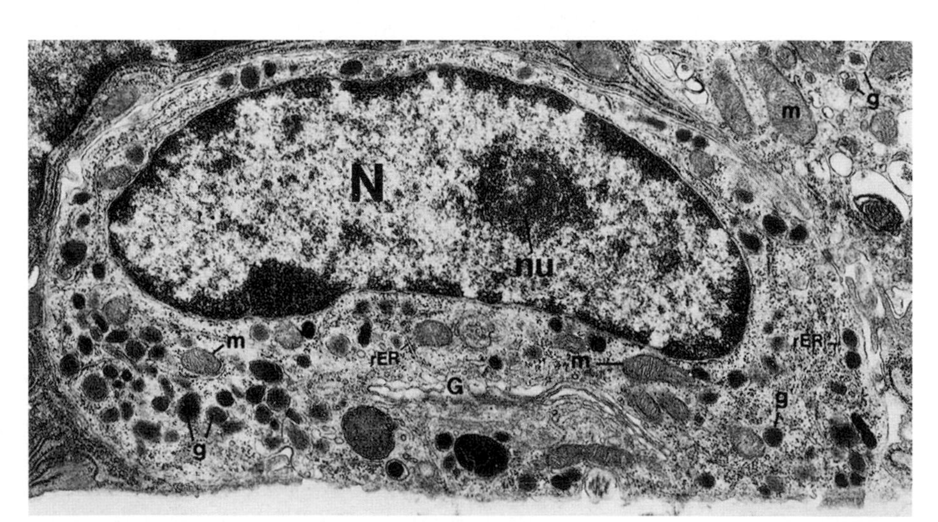

Fig. 17.12 Electron micrograph of a diffuse neuroendocrine system cell from the body of a mouse stomach. g, Secretory granules; G, Golgi apparatus; N, nucleus; nu, nucleolus; m, mitochondria; rER, rough endoplasmic reticulum. (From Karam SF, Leblond CP. Identifying and counting epithelial cell types in the "corpus" of the mouse stomach. *Anat Rec*. 1992;232:231–246. Reprinted with permission from Wiley-Liss, Inc., a subsidiary of John Wiley & Sons, Inc.)

Clinical Correlations

Diffuse neuroendocrine system (DNES) *cells are located throughout the respiratory system, digestive tract, and pancreas. These cells manufacture various hormones and have been known by various names, such as* ***argentaffine cells*** *and* ***argyrophilic cells****, because they are stained with silver salts;* ***enterochromaffin cells*** *because they are stained with chromium salts;* ***APUD cells*** *because some of them undergo* ***amine precursor uptake and decarboxylation****; and* ***enteroendocrine cells*** *because they are located in the epithelium of the digestive tract and manufacture and release hormones. With the exception of APUD cells that are derived from neural crest cells, DNES cells are derived from regenerative cells of the epithelium of the alimentary canal.*

TABLE 17.2 Diffuse Neuroendocrine System Cells and Hormones of the Gastrointestinal Tract

Cell	Location	Hormone Produced	Granule Size (nm)	Hormonal Action
A	Stomach and small intestine	Glucagon (enteroglucagon)	250	Stimulates glycogenolysis by hepatocytes, elevating blood glucose levels.
D	Stomach, small and large intestines	Somatostatin	350	Inhibits release of hormones by DNES cells in its vicinity.
EC	Stomach, small and large intestines	Serotonin; Substance P	300	Increases peristaltic movement.
ECL	Stomach	Histamine	450	Stimulates HCl secretion.
G	Stomach and small intestine	Gastrin	300	Stimulates HCl secretion, gastric motility (especially contraction of the pyloric region and relaxation of pyloric sphincter to regulate stomach emptying), and proliferation of regenerative cells in the body of the stomach.
GL	Stomach, small and large intestines	Glicentin	400	Stimulates hepatocyte glycogenolysis, elevating blood glucose levels.
Gr (P/D1 cell)	Stomach and small intestine as well as in Gr cells of the islands of Langerhans in the pancreas (secreted mostly by adipocytes)	Ghrelin *and also* Leptin	?	Ghrelin induces the sensation of hunger and modulates receptive relaxation of the smooth muscle fibers of the muscularis externa. Leptin inhibits hunger sensation.
I	Small intestine	Cholecystokinin	250	Stimulates the release of pancreatic enzymes and contraction of the gallbladder; also reduces food intake and counteracts the effects of gastrin.
K	Small intestine	Gastric inhibitory peptide (GIP)	350	Inhibits HCl secretion.
L	Small and large intestines	PYY	?	Reduces appetite, decreases gastric motility; boosts function of the colon.
		GLP-1		Stimulates insulin and inhibits glucagon secretion; reduces appetite.
		GLP-2		Encourages mitotic activity in the crypts of Lieberkühn.
		OXM		Reduces appetite and increases energy use.
Mo	Small intestine	Motilin		Increases intestinal peristalsis
N	Small intestine	Neurotensin	300	Increases blood flow to ileum and decreases peristaltic action of small and large intestines.
PP (F)	Stomach and large intestine (mostly by the islets of Langerhans)	Pancreatic polypeptide	180	Reduces appetite.
S	Small intestine	Secretin	200	Stimulates release of bicarbonate-rich fluid from pancreas.
VIP	Stomach, small and large intestines	Vasoactive intestinal peptide		Increases peristaltic action of small and large intestines and stimulates elimination of water and ions by the GI tract

DNES, Diffuse neuroendocrine system; EC, enterochromaffin cell; ECL, enterochromaffin-like cell; G, gastrin-producing cell; GI, gastrointestinal; GL, glicentin-producing cell; GLP-1, glucagon-like peptide; Gr, ghrelin-producing cells; HCl, hydrochloric acid; MO, motilin-producing cell; N, neurotensin-producing cell; OXM, oxyntomodulin; PP, pancreatic polypeptide–producing cell; PYY, peptide YY; VIP, vasoactive intestinal peptide–producing cell.

whose fibers are disposed circularly (**outermost circular**), is not always evident.

Differences in the Mucosa of the Cardiac and Pyloric Regions

The mucosa of the **cardiac region** of the stomach differs from that of the fundic region in that the gastric pits are shallower and the base of its glands is highly coiled. The cell population of these cardiac glands is composed mostly of surface-lining cells, some mucous neck cells, a few DNES cells and parietal cells, and *no chief cells* (Figs. 17.13 and 17.14).

The glands of the **pyloric region** contain the same cell types as those in the cardiac region, but the predominant cell type in the pylorus is the mucous neck cell. In addition to producing soluble mucus, these cells secrete **lysozyme**, a bactericidal enzyme. Pyloric glands are highly convoluted and tend to branch. Additionally, the gastric pits of the pyloric region are deeper than in the cardiac and fundic regions, extending approximately halfway down into the lamina propria (Fig. 17.15; Table 17.3).

Submucosa of the Stomach

The dense, irregular, collagenous connective tissue of the gastric **submucosa** has a rich vascular and lymphatic network that supplies and drains the vessels of the lamina propria. The cell population of the submucosa resembles that of any connective tissue proper. The **Meissner submucosal**

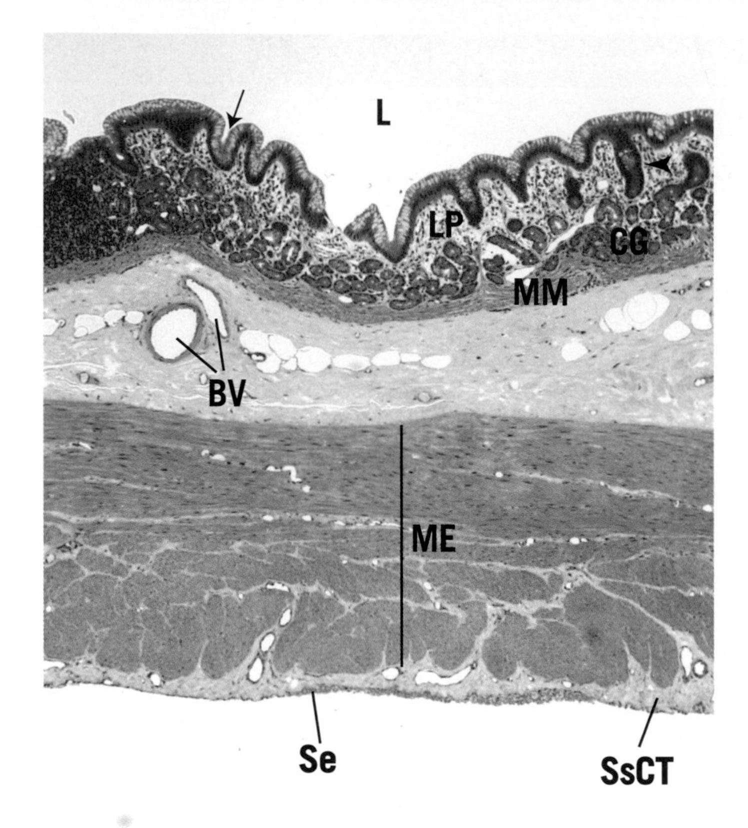

Fig. 17.13 This very-low-magnification photomicrograph displays the gastric pit *(arrow)* opening into the lumen (L) of the cardiac stomach. The lamina propria (LP) and its cardiac glands (CG), and the muscularis mucosae (MM) are clearly evident. The blood vessels (BV) of the submucosa (SM) and of the muscularis externa (ME) are easily identifiable. Note the presence of the serosa (S) and the subserous connective tissue (SsCT). (×56)

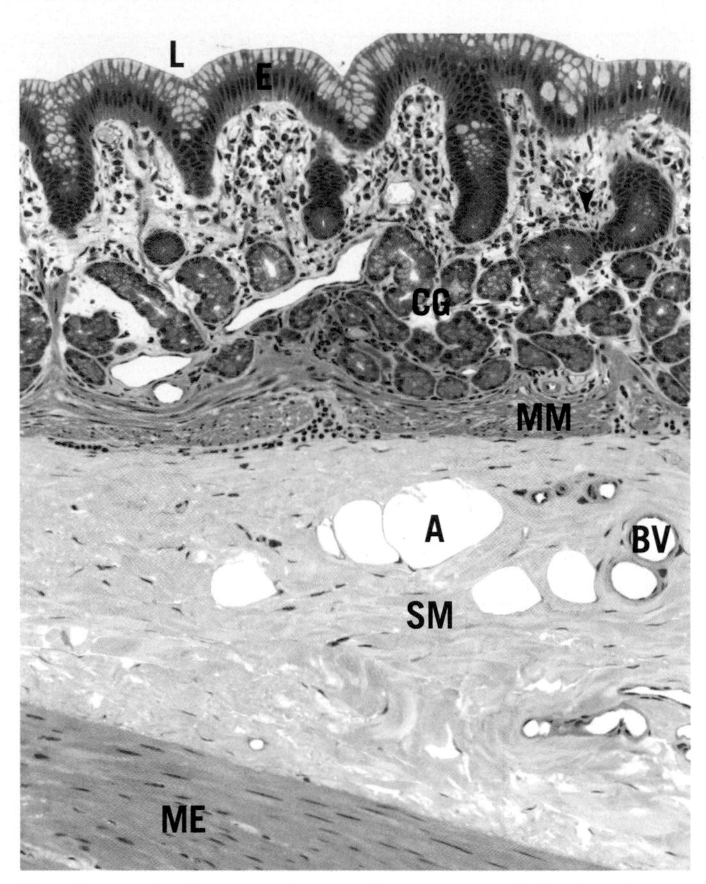

Fig. 17.14 This low-magnification photomicrograph displays the epithelial lining (E) of the lumen (L) of the cardiac stomach. The connective tissue cells *(arrowhead)* of the lamina propria, its cardiac glands (CG), and the muscularis mucosae (MM) are clearly evident. The blood vessels (BV) and adipose cells (A) of the submucosa (SM) are easily recognized. Observe a small section of the muscularis externa (ME) at the bottom left. (×132)

plexus is in its accustomed location, within the submucosa in the vicinity of the muscularis externa.

Clinical Correlations

Infrequently, one of the arteries that serves the lesser curvature of the stomach, instead of arborizing as it enters the submucosa into capillaries 0.1 to 0.5 mm in diameter, remains as an arteriole between 1 and 5 mm in diameter. The pulsatility of this aberrant arteriole may slowly erode the submucosa and the vessel approaches the epithelial lining of the gastric mucosa. This developmental defect may have a very serious complication, known as the **Dieulafoy lesion**, *characterized by erosion of the arterial wall and bleeding into the lamina propria, eventually bleeding into the lumen of the stomach. The presenting symptoms are* **hematemesis** *(vomiting of blood) and* **melena** *(black feces). If the condition is not diagnosed early and if the offending arteriole is large enough, the patient may die from sudden blood loss.*

Muscularis Externa of the Stomach

The muscularis externa of the stomach is composed of three layers of smooth muscle: the innermost oblique layer, middle circular layer, and outer longitudinal layer.

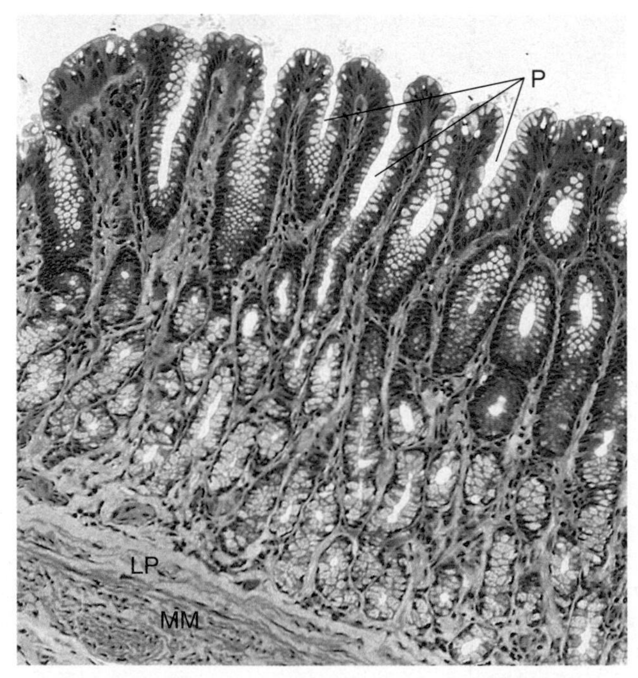

Fig. 17.15 Photomicrograph of the pyloric stomach. The gastric pits are much deeper here than in the cardiac or fundic regions of the stomach (×132). P, Gastric pits; LP, lamina propria; MM, muscularis mucosae.

TABLE 17.3 **Histology of the Alimentary Canal**

Organ	Epithelium	Cell Type of Epithelium	Lamina Propria	Cells of Glands	Muscularis Mucosae	Submucosa	Muscularis Externa	Serosa or Adventitia
Esophagus	Stratified squamous nonkeratinized		Esophageal cardiac glands	Mucus secreting	Longitudinal layer only	Esophageal glands proper	Inner circular and outer longitudinal	Adventitia (except serosa in abdominal cavity)
Cardiac stomach	Simple columnar	Surface-lining cells (no goblet cells)	Cardiac glands; shallow gastric pits	Surface-lining mucous neck cells, regenerative cells, DNES cells, parietal cells	Inner circular, outer longitudinal and, in places, outermost circular	No glands	Inner oblique, middle circular, outermost longitudinal	Serosa
Fundic stomach	Simple columnar	Surface-lining cells (no goblet cells)	Fundic glands	Surface-lining cells, mucous neck cells, parietal cells, regenerative cells, chief cells, DNES cells	Inner circular, outer longitudinal and, in places, outermost circular	No glands	Inner oblique, middle circular, outermost longitudinal	Serosa
Pyloric stomach	Simple columnar	Surface-lining cells (no goblet cells)	Pyloric glands; deep gastric pits	Mucous neck cells, surface-lining cells, parietal cells, regenerative cells, DNES cells	Inner circular, outer longitudinal and, in places, outermost circular	No glands	Inner oblique, middle circular (well developed to form pyloric sphincter), outermost longitudinal	Serosa
Duodenum	Simple columnar (goblet cells)	Surface absorptive cells, goblet cells, DNES cells, occasional M cells	Crypts of Lieberkühn	Surface absorptive cells, goblet cells, regenerative cells, DNES cells, Paneth cells	Inner circular, outer longitudinal	Brunner glands	Inner circular, outer longitudinal	Serosa and adventitia
Jejunum	Simple columnar (goblet cells)	Surface absorptive cells, goblet cells, DNES cells, occasional M cells	Crypts of Lieberkühn	Surface absorptive cells, goblet cells, regenerative cells, DNES cells, Paneth cells	Inner circular, outer longitudinal	No glands	Inner circular, outer longitudinal	Serosa
Ileum	Simple columnar (goblet cells)	Surface absorptive cells, goblet cells, DNES cells, occasional M cells	Crypts of Lieberkühn; Peyer patches	Surface absorptive cells, goblet cells, regenerative cells, DNES cells, Paneth cells	Inner circular, outer longitudinal	No glands (Peyer patches may extend into this layer)	Inner circular, outer longitudinal	Serosa
Colon[a]	Simple columnar (goblet cells)	Surface absorptive cells, goblet cells, DNES cells	Crypts of Lieberkühn	Surface absorptive cells, goblet cells, regenerative cells, DNES cells	Inner circular, outer longitudinal	No glands	Inner circular, outer longitudinal modified to form taeniae coli	Serosa and adventitia
Rectum	Simple columnar (goblet cells)	Surface absorptive cells, goblet cells, DNES cells	Shallow crypts of Lieberkühn	Surface absorptive cells, goblet cells, regenerative cells, DNES cells, Paneth cells	Inner circular, outer longitudinal	No glands	Inner circular, outer longitudinal	Adventitia
Anal canal	Simple cuboidal; stratified squamous nonkeratinized; stratified squamous keratinized		Rectal columns; circumanal glands; at *anus:* hair follicles and sebaceous glands		Inner circular, outer longitudinal	No glands; internal and external hemorrhoidal plexuses	Inner circular (forms internal and sphincter), outer longitudinal (becomes fibroelastic sheet)	Adventitia
Appendix	Simple columnar (goblet cells)	Surface absorptive cells, goblet cells, DNES cells, occasional M cells	Shallow crypts of Lieberkühn; lymphoid nodules	Surface absorptive cells, goblet cells, regenerative cells, DNES cells, Paneth cells	Inner circular, outer longitudinal	No glands; *occasional* lymphoid nodules; possible fatty infiltration	Inner circular, outer longitudinal	Serosa

[a]Includes cecum.
DNES, Diffuse neuroendocrine system.

The **muscularis externa** of the stomach is arranged in three layers, an ill-defined **innermost oblique layer;** a well-developed **middle circular layer**, which is especially pronounced in the pyloric region, where it forms the **pyloric sphincter**; and the **outer longitudinal muscle layer**, which is most evident in the cardiac region and the body of the stomach but is poorly developed in the pylorus. Located between the middle circular and outer longitudinal layers of smooth muscle is the **Auerbach myenteric plexus.**

Serosa of the Stomach. A **serosa**, composed of a thin, loose, subserous connective tissue covered by a smooth, wet, simple squamous epithelium, invests the entire outer surface of the stomach. This external covering provides an almost friction-free environment during the stomach's churning movements.

Clinical Correlations

Three familiar organisms—Pseudomonas, Legionella, and Cryptosporidium—which can withstand the lethal effects of disinfectants commonly used to disinfect pools, hot tubs, and water features in water parks, have been shown to cause most of the water-related infections in the United States. Approximately one-third of the 27,000 illnesses that were caused by these three organisms between 2000 and 2014 occurred in hotel swimming pools and hot tubs, approximately 25% occurred in public pools, and another 25% occurred in clubs and water parks. The remaining 20% or so were probably caused by private swimming pools. The best way of limiting exposure, of course, is not to get in the water; however, people who get in the water should make sure not to swallow any pool water.

HISTOPHYSIOLOGY OF THE STOMACH

The lining and glands of the stomach produce and release secretions into the lumen of the stomach; these secretions are composed of water, hydrochloric acid, gastric intrinsic factor, pepsinogen, rennin, gastric lipase, visible mucus, and soluble mucus.

Once the bolus passes from the esophagus through the gastroesophageal junction into the stomach, it is churned into a viscous fluid known as **chyme**. Intermittently, the stomach releases small aliquots of its contents through the **pyloric valve** into the duodenum. The stomach liquefies the food, continuing its digestion via the production of **HCl** and the enzymes **pepsin**, **rennin**, and **gastric lipase** and via production of paracrine hormones.

Approximately 2 to 3 L of gastric juices are produced by the glands of the stomach on a daily basis. These gastric juices are very acidic (pH of 2.0) and are composed of (1) **water** (derived from the extracellular fluid in the interstitial connective tissue and delivered into the lumen of the stomach by parietal cells); (2) the enzymes **pepsinogen**, **rennin**, and **gastric lipase** (manufactured by chief cells); (3) **HCl** and **gastric intrinsic factor**, manufactured by parietal cells, where the HCl causes the gastric juice to be very acidic (which facilitates the conversion of the inactive pepsinogen to its active form of **pepsin**); (4) a glycoprotein, **visible mucus** (manufactured by surface-lining cells), which forms a coat of mucus that lines and protects the epithelium of the stomach from the acidic chyme and serves as a favorable, mostly neutral pH environment for the bacterium *Helicobacter pylori*; and (5) **soluble mucus** that becomes part of the gastric content (produced by mucous neck cells). Little absorption of food products occurs in the stomach, although some substances, such as alcohol, can be absorbed by the gastric mucosa.

The three muscle layers of the muscularis externa interact in such a fashion that during their contraction, the contents of the stomach are churned and the ingested food is liquefied to form **chyme**, a viscous fluid with the consistency of split pea soup. Independent contraction of the muscularis mucosae exposes the chyme to the entire surface area of the gastric mucosa.

Emptying of Gastric Contents

Owing to interaction between neurons of the myenteric and submucosal plexuses, as well as owing to the effect of the hormone **ghrelin**, a relatively constant intraluminal pressure is maintained irrespective of the degree of distention of the stomach. In an empty stomach, the pylorus is always open; however, during peristalsis, the pyloric sphincter is closed. Coordinated contraction of the muscularis externa and momentary relaxation of the pyloric sphincter permit emptying of the stomach by intermittently delivering small aliquots of the chyme into the duodenum. The rate at which the stomach releases its chyme into the duodenum is a function of the acidity, caloric and fat content, and osmolality of the chyme. The production of the peristaltic waves occurs in a rhythmic fashion and is generated by the gastric pacemaker at a rate of about three per minute. Receptors in the duodenum, in response to the arrival of the chyme, cause a sudden closure of the pyloric sphincter and contraction of the muscularis externa of the pyloric antrum, driving the chyme back into the body of the stomach to continue the thorough mixing of the chyme with the stomach's digestive enzymes.

The factors that facilitate emptying of the stomach are the degree of its distention and the action of **gastrin**, a hormone that stimulates contraction of the muscularis externa of the pyloric region and relaxation of the pyloric sphincter. Factors that inhibit gastric emptying include distention of the duodenum; overabundance of fat, proteins, or carbohydrates in the chyme; and increased osmolarity and excessive acidity of the chyme delivered into the duodenum. These factors activate a neural feedback mechanism by stimulating release of cholecystokinin, which counteracts gastrin, and by the release of gastric inhibitory peptide, which also inhibits gastric contractions.

Clinical Correlations

Patients who feel full after eating only a little amount of food and who experience frequent bloating, nausea, vomiting, and pain in the region of the stomach may have difficulties in emptying the contents of their stomach. If this problem is not caused by blockage of the pyloric orifice or obstruction in the small intestine, then it is possible that the patient is suffering from **gastroparesis***. In many cases, the cause of this condition is idiopathic (unknown), although individuals who have had type I diabetes for five years or more are predisposed to suffer from gastroparesis. Moreover, injury to CN X (vagus nerve), Parkinson disease, hyperglycemia, viral infection, autoimmune disorders, and certain prescription drugs—such as opioids, psychotropic medications, and chemotherapeutic agents—have also been indicated as possible causative factors. Treatment modalities have to address the known underlying conditions, drug side effects, and, in case of an idiopathic cause, the careful administration of drugs that induce emptying of the stomach.*

Gastric Hydrochloric Acid Production

The three phases in the production of hydrochloric acid are cephalic, gastric, and intestinal.

Hydrochloric acid activates the proenzyme **pepsinogen** to become the active proteolytic enzyme **pepsin**, thereby assisting in the breakdown of food material in the stomach. Because pepsin requires a low pH for its acidity, the presence of HCl also provides the necessary acidic conditions of **pH 2** or less.

There are three phases of hydrochloric acid production:

- **Cephalic.** Secretion caused by psychological factors (e.g., the thought, smell, or sight of food, as well as stress) initiates parasympathetic impulses via the vagus nerve, resulting in the release of the neurotransmitter **acetylcholine.**
- **Gastric.** Secretion of the paracrine hormones **gastrin** (by G cells) and **histamine** (by ECL cells) and acetylcholine (from the vagus nerve) due to the presence of certain food substances in the stomach, as well as to the stretching of the stomach wall.
- **Intestinal.** Secretion due to the presence of food in the small intestine is elicited by the endocrine hormone **gastrin**, released by G cells of the small intestine.

Mechanism of Gastric Hydrochloric Acid Production

HCl production is initiated when gastrin, histamine, and acetylcholine bind to the basal plasma membrane of parietal cells.

Parietal cells have receptors for gastrin, histamine-2, and acetylcholine on their basal plasmalemma. Binding of these signaling molecules to the appropriate receptors causes the cells to manufacture and release HCl into the intracellular canaliculus. The process occurs as follows (Fig. 17.16):

1. The enzyme **carbonic anhydrase** facilitates the production of carbonic acid (H_2CO_3) from water (H_2O) and carbon dioxide (CO_2), which then dissociates into hydrogen ions (H^+) and bicarbonate (HCO_3^-) within the cytoplasm of the parietal cell.
2. A **H^+, K^+-ATPase**, using adenosine triphosphate (ATP) as an energy source, pumps intracellular H^+ ions out of the cell into the intracellular canaliculi and transfers extracellular potassium ions (K^+) into the cell.
3. Carrier proteins, using ATP as an energy source, pump K^+ and chloride ion (Cl^-) out of the cell and into the intracellular canaliculi. Thus, **Cl^-** and **H^+** ions enter the lumen of the intracellular canaliculi separately, to combine into HCl there.
4. K^+ is actively transported into the cell at the basal plasmalemma, as well as at the microvilli jutting into the intracellular canaliculi, increasing the intracellular level of K^+. The high intracellular K^+ concentration forces K^+ to leave the cell via ion channels located in the basal plasmalemma and in the plasma membrane of the microvilli. Thus, K^+ is constantly recirculated in and out of the parietal cell.
5. Water, derived from the extracellular fluid, enters the parietal cell and then leaves the cytoplasm to enter the intracellular canaliculus as a consequence of the osmotic forces generated by the movement of ions just described. Because the intracellular canaliculus is continuous with the lumen of the stomach, HCl, manufactured by the parietal cells, enters the gastric lumen.

Clinical Correlations

*The lining of the stomach is protected from the acidic pH by the buffering activity of the HCO_3^- present in the layer of mucus manufactured by the surface-lining cells and, to a certain limited extent, by mucous neck cells. Additionally, the zonulae occludentes of the epithelial cells prevent the influx of HCl into the lamina propria, protecting the mucosa from damage. Moreover, evidence suggests that **prostaglandins**, released by DNES cells, protect the cells lining the gastric lumen and also increase local circulation, especially if the integrity of the epithelial barrier is compromised. This increased blood flow removes the accidentally escaped H^+ ions from the lamina propria.*

Inhibition of Hydrochloric Acid Release

The hormones **somatostatin** (produced by D cells), **prostaglandin** (PGE_2), and **gastric inhibitory peptide (GIP**, produced by K cells) inhibit gastric HCl production. Somatostatin acts on G cells and ECL cells, inhibiting their release of gastrin and histamine, respectively. Prostaglandins and GIP act directly on parietal cells and inhibit their ability to produce HCl.

Additionally, **urogastrone** (**epidermal growth factor**), produced by Brunner glands of the duodenum, acts directly on parietal cells to inhibit HCl production.

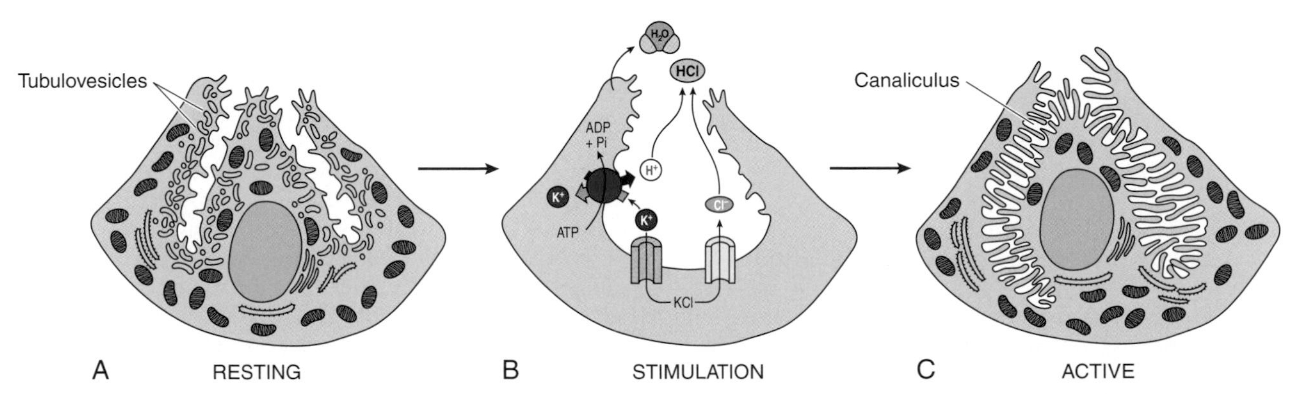

Fig. 17.16 Schematic diagram of a parietal cell. Note the well-developed tubulovesicular apparatus in the resting cell (A) and the mechanism of hydrochloric acid release (B). (C) Numerous microvilli in the active cell.

Clinical Correlations

1. *Possibly the most common cause of* **ulcers** *in the United States is the prevalent use of the nonsteroidal anti-inflammatory drugs (NSAIDs)* **ibuprofen** *and* **aspirin.** *Both of these drugs inhibit the manufacture of prostaglandins, precluding their protective effects on the stomach lining.*
2. *The bacterium* **Helicobacter pylori**, *which is localized in the mucus layer protecting the gastric epithelium, has also been implicated as a possible factor in ulcer formation.*
3. *Almost 12% of cancer-related fatalities are due to* **gastric carcinoma**, *one of the most common gastrointestinal (GI) malignancies. Although the cancer may be localized to any region of the stomach, usually the region of the lesser curvature and the pyloric antrum are the sites that are most generally involved.*
4. *Many individuals who had type 2 diabetes and, owing to obesity or other conditions, underwent gastric bypass surgery, experienced a quick reduction in their blood glucose levels. Currently, there is no explanation for this unexpected result, although it has been suggested that hormones released by the DNES cells of the GI tract may play an important role in this outcome.*

Small Intestine

The small intestine has three regions: the duodenum, jejunum, and ileum.

The **small intestine** at 7 m in length is the longest region of the alimentary tract. It is divided into three regions: the duodenum, jejunum, and ileum. It not only continues the digestion of food material that began in the oral cavity and stomach but also absorbs the end products of the digestive process. To perform its digestive functions, the duodenum receives enzymes and an alkaline buffer from the pancreas and bile from the liver. Additionally, epithelial cells and glands of the duodenal mucosa contribute buffers and enzymes to facilitate digestion.

COMMON HISTOLOGICAL FEATURES

Because the three regions of the small intestine are similar histologically, the common features are described first. Following this discussion, variations from this plan are depicted for each segment (see Table 17.3). Then, the functional aspects are considered.

Modifications of the Luminal Surface

The surface area of the intestinal lumen is enlarged by the formation of plicae circulares, villi, microvilli, and to a certain extent, crypts of Lieberkühn.

The luminal surface of the small intestine is modified to increase its surface area. Three types of modifications have been noted:

- **Plicae circulares (valves of Kerckring)**, transverse folds of the submucosa and mucosa that form semicircular to helical elevations, some as large as 8 mm in height and 5 cm in length. Unlike rugae of the stomach, these are permanent fixtures of the duodenum and jejunum and end in the proximal half of the ileum. They not only increase the surface area by a factor of 2 to 3 but also function to decrease the velocity of the movement of chyme along the alimentary canal.
- **Villi** are epithelially covered, finger-like or oak leaf–like protrusions of a loose connective tissue rich in lymphoid cells, known as the **lamina propria.** The core of each villus contains capillary loops, a blindly ending lymphatic channel (**lacteal**), and a few smooth muscle fibers. Villi are permanent structures ranging in number from 10 to 40 per mm^2 (Figs. 17.17–17.20). Their numbers are greater in the duodenum than in the jejunum or the ileum, and their height decreases from 1.5 mm in the duodenum to about 0.5 mm in the ileum. These delicate structures confer a velvety appearance to the lining of the living organ. Villi increase the surface area of the small intestine by a factor of 10.
- **Microvilli**, modifications of the apical plasmalemma of the epithelial cells covering the intestinal villi, increase the surface area of the small intestine by a factor of 20.

Thus, these three types of intestinal surface modifications increase the total surface area available for absorption of nutrients by a factor of 400 to 600.

Invaginations of the epithelium into the lamina propria between the villi form intestinal glands, **crypts of Lieberkühn**, which also augment the surface area of the small intestine.

Intestinal Mucosa

The mucosa of the small intestine is composed of the usual three layers: a simple columnar epithelium, the lamina propria, and the muscularis mucosae.

Epithelium

The simple columnar epithelium covering the villi and the surface of the intervillar spaces is composed of surface absorptive cells, goblet cells, DNES cells, M cells (microfold cells), and occasional tuft cells.

Surface Absorptive Cells

Surface absorptive cells are tall columnar cells that function in terminal digestion and absorption of water and nutrients.

The most numerous cells of the epithelium, the **surface absorptive cells**, are tall cells, about 25 μm in length, with basally located oval nuclei and an apically located **striated border** (see Figs. 17.19 and 17.21). The principal functions of these cells are terminal digestion and absorption of nutrients and water. Additionally, these cells re-esterify fatty acids into triglycerides, form chylomicrons, and transport them, as well as the bulk of the absorbed nutrients, into the lamina propria for distribution to the rest of the body (see later discussion).

Using electron microscopy, the striated border of surface absorptive cells is resolved into as many as 3000 **microvilli**, each approximately 1 μm long, whose tips are covered with a thick **glycocalyx** layer. The glycocalyx coat not only protects the microvilli from autodigestion, but its enzymatic components also function in terminal digestion of dipeptides and disaccharides into their monomers. The actin core of the microvilli is anchored into the actin and intermediate filaments of the cell web. The cytoplasm of surface absorptive cells is rich in organelles, especially endosomes, smooth endoplasmic reticulum, RER, and Golgi apparatus.

The lateral cell membranes of these cells form zonulae occludentes, zonulae adherentes, desmosomes, and gap junctions with

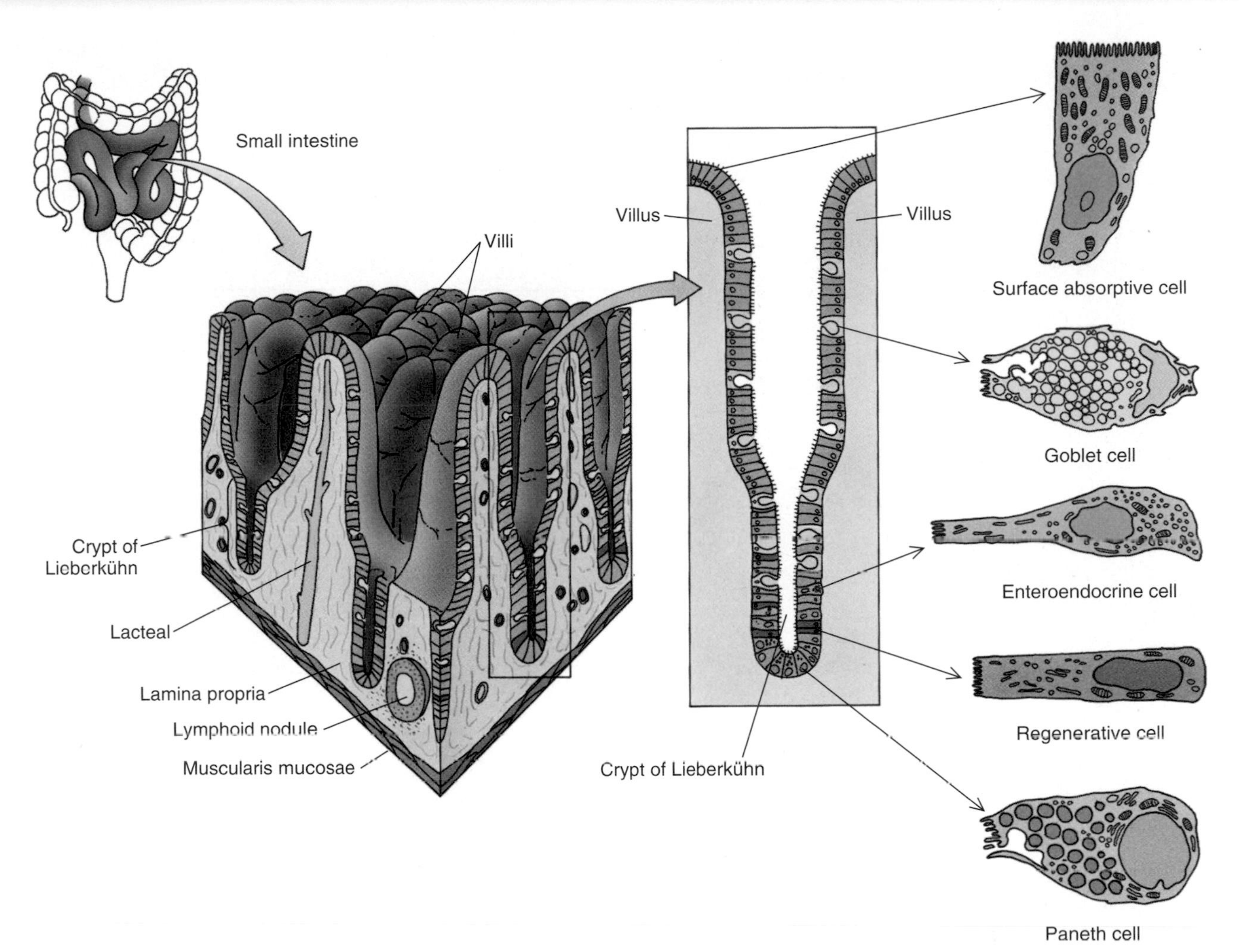

Fig. 17.17 Schematic diagram of the mucosa, villi, crypts of Lieberkühn, and component cells of the small intestine. Note that the crypts of Lieberkühn open into the intervillar spaces; a solitary lymphoid nodule is shown in the lamina propria.

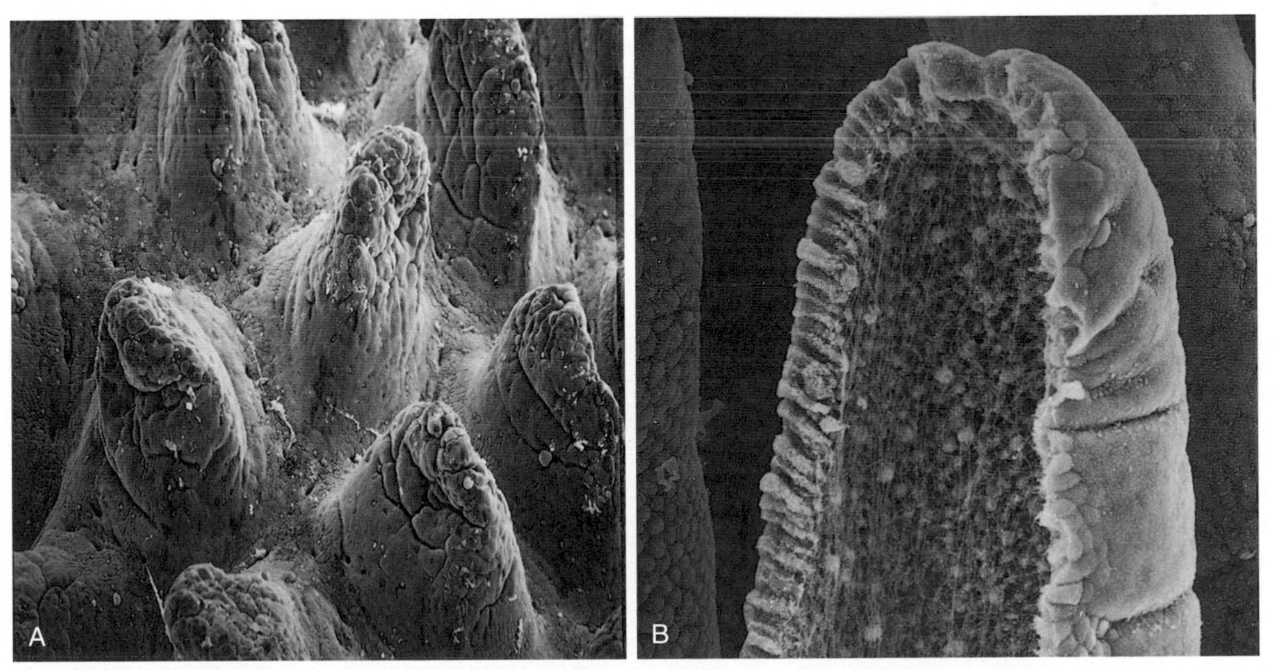

Fig. 17.18 Scanning electron micrographs of villi from the mouse ileum. (A) Observe the villi and the openings of the crypts of Lieberkühn in the intervillar spaces (×160). (B) Note that the villus is fractured, revealing its core of connective tissue and migrating cells (×500). (From Magney JE, Erlandsen SL, Bjerknes ML, Cheng H. Scanning electron microscopy of isolated epithelium of the murine gastrointestinal tract: morphology of the basal surface and evidence for paracrine-like cells. *Am J Anat.* 1986;177:43–53. Reprinted with permission from Wiley-Liss, Inc., a subsidiary of John Wiley & Sons, Inc.)

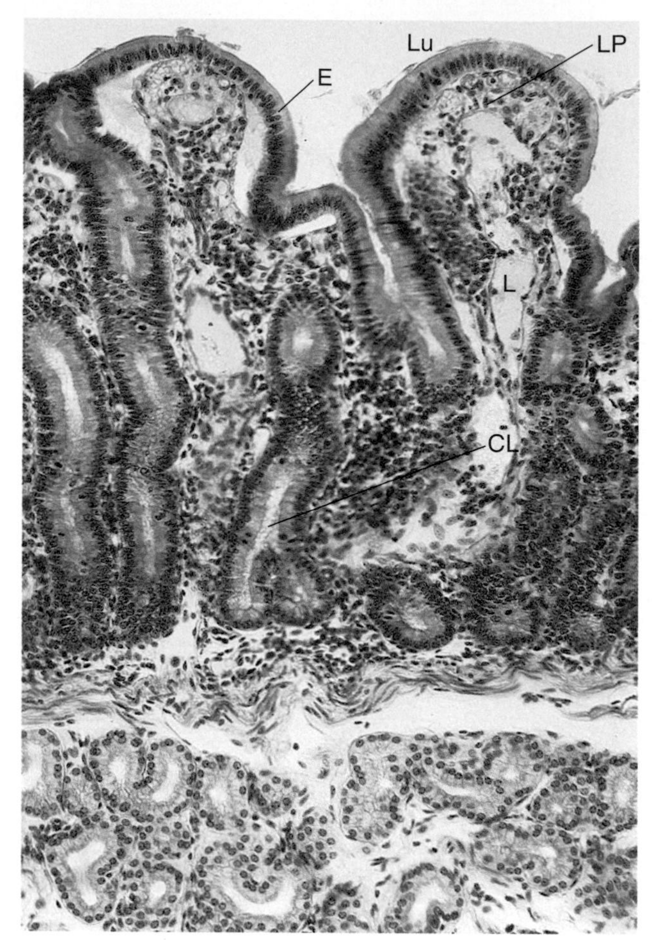

Fig. 17.19 Photomicrograph of the duodenal mucosa, displaying the simple columnar epithelium (E), the cellular lamina propria (LP) with its lacteal (L) and the muscularis mucosae. The submucosa houses Brunner glands, a clear indication that this is a section of the duodenum (×132). L, Lacteals of villus.

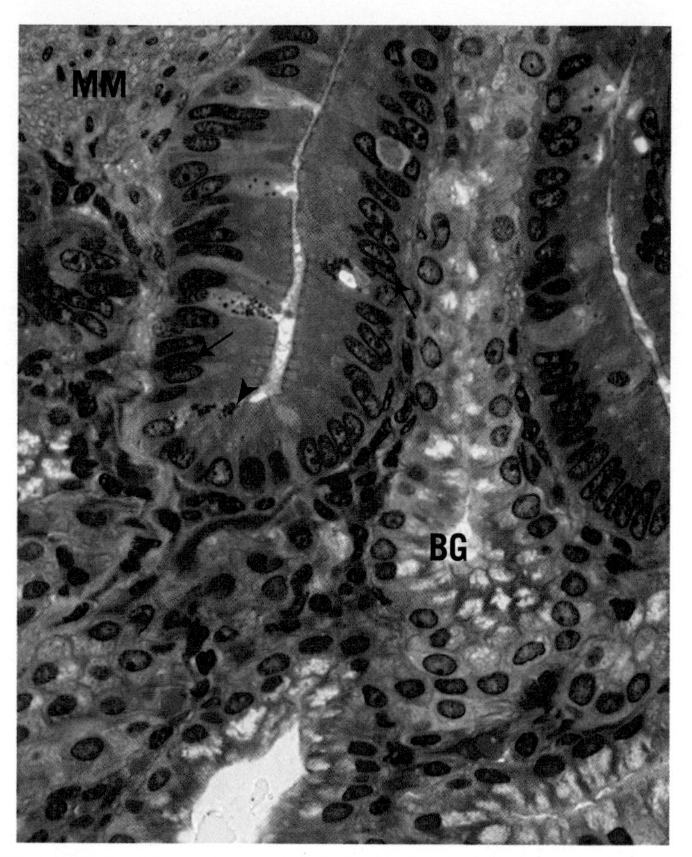

Fig. 17.20 This medium magnification of the duodenum displays the muscularis mucosae (MM), Brunner glands (BG), and, between them, the base of a crypt of Lieberkuhn. Observe that the arrows point to narrow regenerative and intermediate cells and the arrowhead depicts the large eosinophilic granules of Paneth cells, all three cell types components of the crypts of Lieberkühn. (×270)

adjacent cells. The tight junctions prevent the passage of material via the paracellular route to or from the lumen of the gut.

Goblet Cells. **Goblet cells** are unicellular glands (see Figs. 17.17 and 17.19; see also Chapter 5) that manufacture **mucinogen**, whose hydrated form **mucin** is a component of **mucus**, a protective layer lining the lumen. The number of goblet cells increases from the duodenum, being most numerous in the ileum.

DNES Cells. Approximately 1% of the cells covering the villi and intervillar surface of the small intestine are composed of DNES cells, both open and closed types, that produce paracrine and endocrine hormones (see Table 17.2). A small percentage of the open form of the DNES cells expresses the taste receptor protein products of the genes *T2R38*, *T1R1*, *T1R2*, and *T1R3*, acting as "taste cells" in the small intestine recognizing bitter, sweet, and umami tastes. When sweet components of the intestinal contents are detected, these DNES cells signal the β cells of the islets of Langerhans to release the hormone insulin into the bloodstream.

M Cells (Microfold Cells)

M cells phagocytose and transport antigens from the lumen to the lamina propria.

The simple columnar epithelial lining of the small intestine is replaced by squamous-like **M cells** in regions where lymphoid nodules abut the epithelium. These M cells—which are believed to belong to the mononuclear phagocyte system of cells—sample, phagocytose, and transport antigens present in the intestinal lumen.

Tuft cells (brush cells). **Tuft cells** (also referred to as **brush cells**) have been discovered in the epithelia of the respiratory tract, stomach, small intestine, and large intestine. They are pear-like tall cells whose apical extent possesses a tuft of microvilli that protrude into the lumen. An interesting characteristic of tuft cells of the alimentary canal is the presence of α-gustducin, indicative of their ability to react to certain taste sensations. Tuft cells can recognize and react to the presence of helminths, large parasitic worms, in the alimentary canal. These cells release interleukin 25 (IL-25) into the lamina propria, activating **type 2 innate lymphoid cells (ILC2s)** to proliferate and to release **IL-13**, a cytokine that prompts regenerative cells to differentiate into more tuft cells and to activate **T helper cells (T_H2 cells)**. Both ILC2s and T_H2 cells function in regulating an immune response against parasitic invaders.

Lamina Propria

The loose connective tissue of the **lamina propria** forms the core of the villi, which, similar to trees of a forest, rise above the luminal surface of the small intestine. The remainder of the lamina propria, extending down to the muscularis mucosae, is compressed into thin sheets of highly vascularized connective tissue by the numerous tubular intestinal glands, the **crypts of Lieberkühn**. Moreover, the lamina propria is well endowed

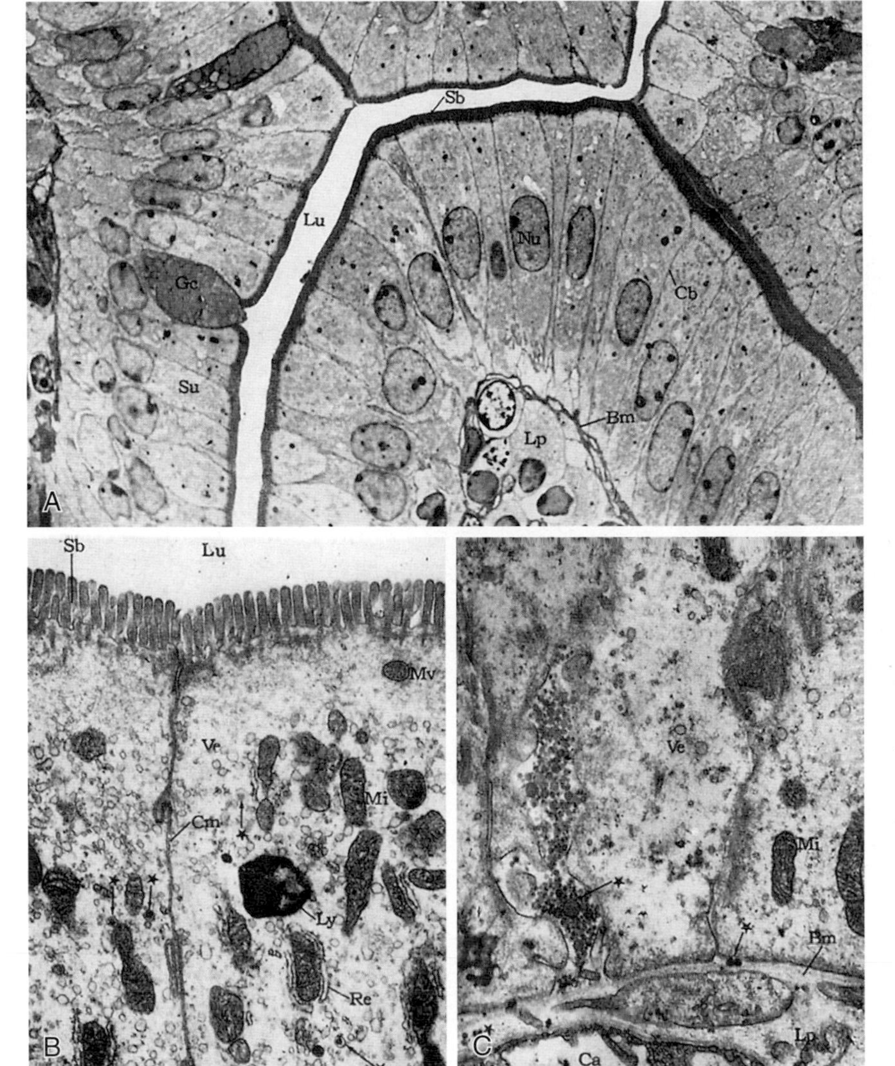

Fig. 17.21 Surface absorptive cells from a villus of the mouse jejunum. (A) Low-magnification electron micrograph displaying two goblet cells (Gc) and numerous surface absorptive cells (Su) (×1744). Note the striated border (Sb) facing the lumen (Lu). Nuclei (Nu) and cell boundaries (Cb) are clearly evident. Observe also that the epithelium is separated from the lamina propria by a well-defined basement membrane (Bm). (B) A higher-magnification electron micrograph of two adjoining surface absorptive cells (×10,500). The striated border (Sb) is clearly composed of numerous microvilli that project into the lumen (Lu). The adjoining cell membranes (Cm) are close to each other. Ly, Lysosomes; Mi, mitochondria; Re, rough endoplasmic reticulum; Ve, vesicles; *asterisk* indicates membrane-bound lipid droplets. (C) Electron micrograph of the basal aspect of the surface absorptive cells (×11,200). Bm, Basement membrane; Lp, lamina propria; Mi, mitochondria; Ve, Vesicles; *asterisk* indicates chylomicrons. (From Rhodin JAG. *An Atlas of Ultrastructure*. Philadelphia: WB Saunders; 1963.)

with lymphoid cells and contains occasional lymphoid nodules, which help protect the intestinal lining from invasion by microorganisms (see Figs. 17.18–17.20). These lymphoid cells and lymphoid nodules belong to the GALT.

Crypts of Lieberkühn

Crypts of Lieberkühn increase the surface area of the intestinal lining. They are composed of DNES cells, surface absorptive-like columnar cells, goblet cells, regenerative cells, M cells, intermediate cells, and Paneth cells.

Crypts of Lieberkühn are simple tubular (or branched tubular) glands (see Fig. 17.17) that open into the intervillar spaces as perforations of the epithelial lining. Scanning electron micrographs indicate that the base of each villus is surrounded by the openings of several crypts (see Fig. 17.18). These tubular glands are composed of surface absorptive-like columnar cells, goblet cells, DNES cells, M cells, regenerative cells, intermediate cells, and Paneth cells.

Surface absorptive-like columnar cells and goblet cells occupy the upper half of the gland. The goblet cells have a short life span; it is believed that after they disgorge their mucinogen, they die and are desquamated. The basal half of the gland has no surface absorptive–like columnar cells and only a few goblet cells; instead, most of the cells are intermediate and regenerative cells. The crypt epithelium also houses DNES cells, some M cells, and Paneth cells. Only regenerative cells, intermediate cells, and Paneth cells are described here; the others were discussed earlier.

Regenerative Cells

The **regenerative cells** of the small intestine are stem cells that undergo extensive proliferation to repopulate the epithelium of the crypts, mucosal surface, and villi. These narrow cells appear to be wedged into limited spaces among the newly formed cells (see Figs. 17.20 and 17.22). Their rate of cell division is high, with a relatively short cell cycle of 24 hours. It has been suggested that 5 to 7 days after the appearance of a new cell, that cell has progressed to the tip of the villus and has been exfoliated. Electron micrographs of these undifferentiated cells display few organelles but many free ribosomes. Their single, basally located, oval nuclei are electron-lucent, indicating the presence of a large amount of euchromatin.

Intermediate cells

The intermediate cells constitute the largest cell population of the lining of the crypts of Lieberkühn; they resemble and are the progeny of regenerative cells. Although their function is to replace

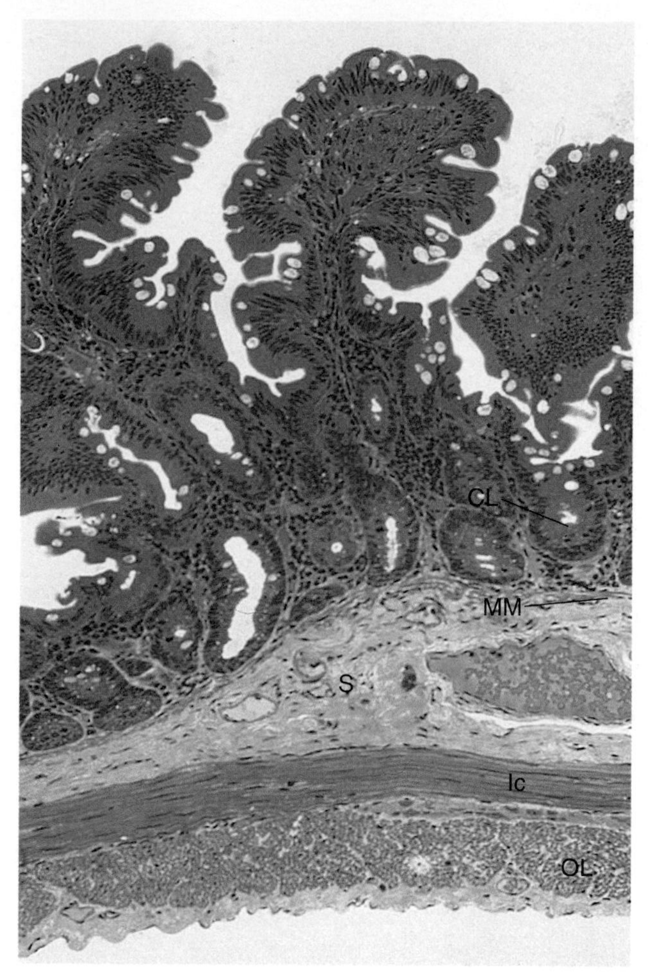

Fig. 17.22 Photomicrograph of the mucosa of a monkey jejunum. Observe the well-developed villi, and note that there are no Peyer patches in the lamina propria or any Brunner glands in the submucosa; therefore, this must be a section of the jejunum (×132). CL, Crypts of Lieberkühn; Ic, inner circular muscle layer of the muscularis externa; MM, muscularis mucosae; OL, outer longitudinal layer of the muscularis externa; S, submucosa.

defunct cells of the epithelial lining of the intestinal lumen, they have not as yet shown a preference to a particular cell line.

Paneth Cells

Paneth cells produce the antibacterial agent lysozyme.

Paneth cells are clearly distinguishable because of the presence of large, eosinophilic, apical secretory granules (see Fig. 17.20). These pyramid-shaped cells occupy the bottom of the crypts of Lieberkühn and manufacture the antibacterial agent **lysozyme**, defensive proteins (**defensins**), and **tumor necrosis factor-α**. Unlike the other cells of the intestinal epithelium, Paneth cells have a comparatively long life span of approximately 20 days and secrete lysozyme continuously. Electron micrographs of these cells display a well-developed Golgi apparatus, a large complement of RER, numerous mitochondria, and large apical secretory granules housing a homogeneous secretory product (Fig. 17.23).

Muscularis Mucosae

The **muscularis mucosae** of the small intestine are composed of an inner circular layer and an outer longitudinal layer of smooth muscle cells. Muscle fibers from the inner circular layer enter the villus and extend through its core to the tip of the connective tissue, as far as the basement membrane. During digestion, these muscle fibers rhythmically contract, shortening the villus several times a minute.

Submucosa

The **submucosa** of the small intestine is composed of dense, irregular fibroelastic connective tissue with a rich lymphatic, neural, and vascular supply. The intrinsic innervation of the submucosa is from the **submucosal (Meissner) plexus**. The submucosa of the **duodenum** is unusual because it houses glands known as ***Brunner glands*** (***duodenal glands***).

Brunner Glands

Brunner glands produce a mucous, bicarbonate-rich fluid, as well as urogastrone (human epidermal growth factor).

Brunner glands are branched, tubuloalveolar glands whose secretory portions resemble mucous acini and whose ducts penetrate the muscularis mucosae, pierce the base of the crypts of Lieberkühn (or occasionally into the intervillar spaces) to deliver their secretory product into the lumen of the duodenum (see Figs. 17.19 and 17.20). Electron micrographs of the acinar cells display a well-developed RER and Golgi apparatus, numerous mitochondria, and flattened to round nuclei.

Brunner glands secrete a mucous, alkaline fluid in response to parasympathetic stimulation. This fluid helps neutralize the acidic chyme that enters the duodenum from the pyloric stomach. The glands also manufacture the polypeptide hormone **urogastrone** (also known as ***human epidermal growth factor***), which inhibits production of HCl (by directly inhibiting parietal cells) and amplifies the rate of mitotic activity of the regenerative and intermediate cells.

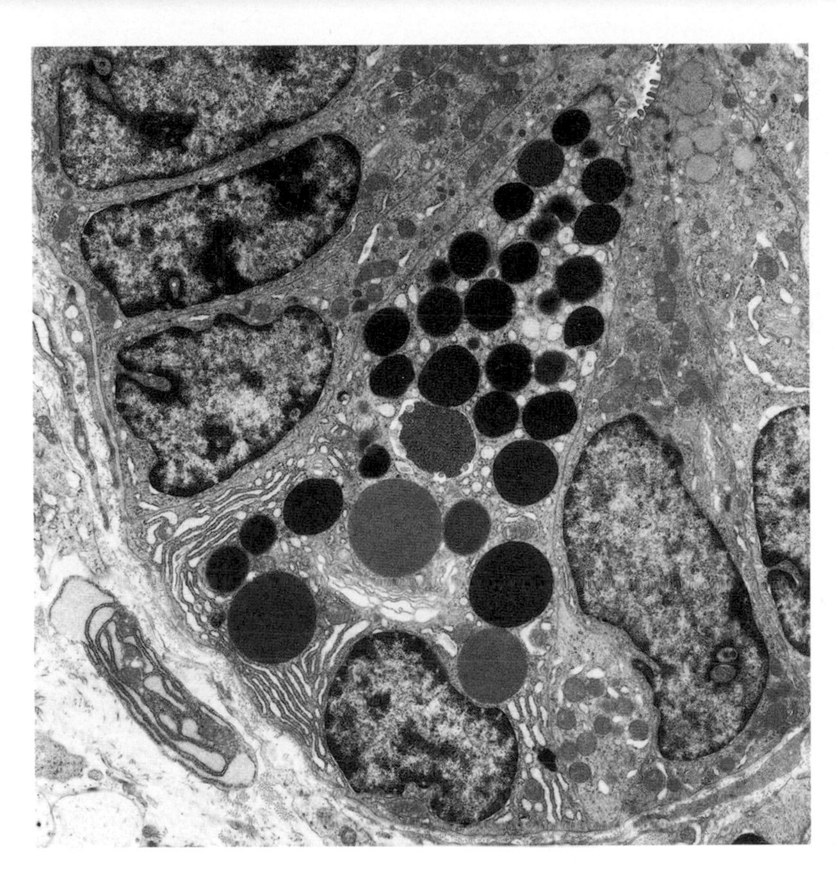

Fig. 17.23 Electron micrograph of a Paneth cell from the rabbit ileum (×5900). Note the large, round granules in the cytoplasm of the Paneth cell. (From Satoh Y, Yamano M, Matsuda M, Ono K. Ultrastructure of Paneth cell in the intestine of various mammals. *J Electron Microsc Tech.* 1990;16:69–80. Reprinted with permission from Wiley-Liss, Inc., a subsidiary of John Wiley & Sons, Inc.)

Muscularis Externa and Serosa/Adventitia

The **muscularis externa** of the small intestine is composed of an inner circular layer and an outer longitudinal smooth muscle layer. The **Auerbach myenteric plexus**, located between the two muscle layers, is the intrinsic neural supply of the external muscle coat. The muscularis externa is responsible for the peristaltic activity of the small intestine.

Except for the second and third parts of the duodenum, which have **adventitia**, the entire small intestine is invested by a **serosa**.

Lymphatic and Vascular Supply of the Small Intestine

Lymph drainage in the small intestine begins as blindly ending lymphatic vessels known as lacteals.

The small intestine has a well-developed lymphatic and vascular supply. Blindly ending lymph capillaries called **lacteals** (see Fig. 17.19), which are located in the cores of villi, deliver their contents into the **submucosal lymphatic plexus**. From here, lymph passes through a series of lymph nodes to be delivered to the thoracic duct, the largest lymph vessel in the body. The thoracic duct empties its content into the circulatory system at the junction of the left internal jugular and subclavian veins.

Capillary loops adjacent to the lacteals are drained by blood vessels that are tributaries of the **submucosal vascular plexus**. Blood from here is delivered to the hepatic portal vein to enter the liver for processing.

REGIONAL DIFFERENCES

The **duodenum** is the shortest segment of the small intestine, only 25 cm in length. It receives bile from the liver and digestive juices from the pancreas via the common bile duct and pancreatic duct, respectively. These ducts open into the lumen of the duodenum at the **duodenal papilla (of Vater)**. The duodenum differs from the jejunum and ileum in that its villi are broader, taller, and more numerous per unit area. It has fewer goblet cells per unit area than the other segments, and there are **Brunner glands** in its submucosa (see Figs. 17.19 and 17.20).

The villi of the **jejunum** are narrower, shorter, and sparser than those of the duodenum. The number of goblet cells per unit area is greater in the jejunum than in the duodenum (see Figs. 17.22 and 17.24).

The villi of the **ileum** are the sparsest, shortest, and narrowest of the three regions of the small intestine. The lamina propria of the ileum houses permanent clusters of lymphoid nodules, known as ***Peyer patches***. These structures are located in the wall of the ileum that is opposite the attachment of the mesentery. In the region of Peyer patches, the villi are reduced in height and may even be absent (Figs. 17.25 and 17.26).

Clinical Correlations

Meckel diverticulum is a very common congenital anomaly occurring in about 2% of the white population. The diverticulum, a remnant of the vitelline duct—an embryonic connection between the midgut and yolk sac—is a short, wide-mouthed extension of the distal aspect of the ileum about 100 cm from the cecum. Most Meckel diverticula are asymptomatic, but some can have bleeding and intestinal obstruction. The obstruction is usually caused by intussusception, which is prolapse of the ileum into the diverticulum.

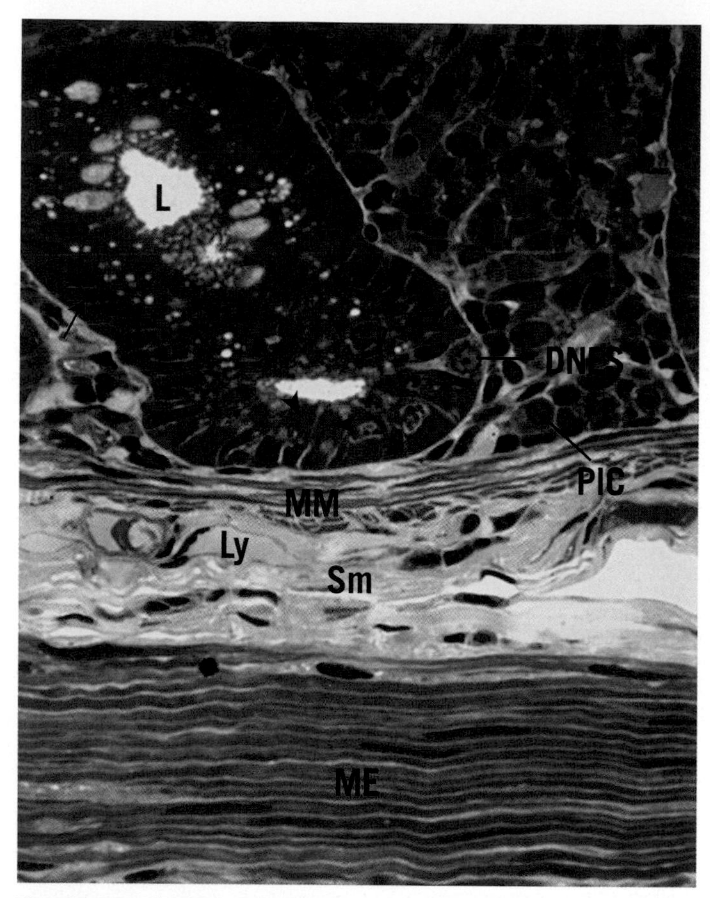

Fig. 17.24 This high-magnification photomicrograph of the lower half of the crypt of Lieberkühn of the jejunum displays three of the cell types of the crypt: regenerative/intermediate cells *(arrow)*, the DNES cell (DNES), and Paneth cells *(arrowhead)*. The lamina propria has numerous lymphoid cells, such as plasma cell (PlC). The muscularis mucosae is well defined, as is the lymph vessel (Ly) in the submucosa (Sm). The inner circular layer of the muscularis externa (ME) is easily distinguished. Lumen of the crypt of Lieberkühn (L). (×540)

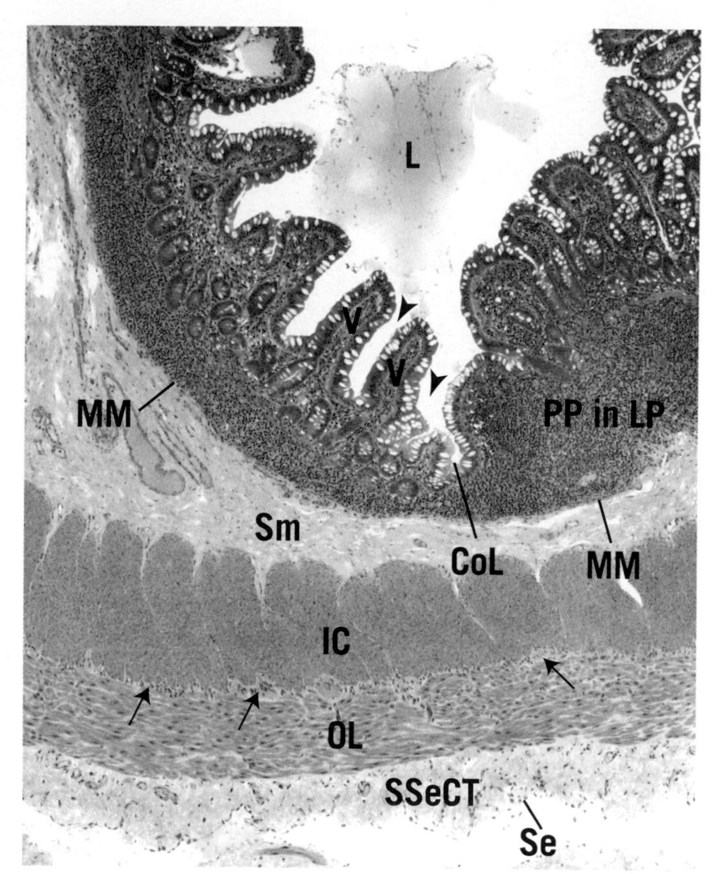

Fig. 17.25 This very-low-magnification photomicrograph displays the short villi (V) jutting into the lumen (L) of the ileum and the crypts of Lieberkühn (CoL) opening into the intervillar space. Observe the dense accumulation of lymphoid elements, Peyer patches (PP), in the lamina propria (LP). Note that the submucosa (Sm) is separated from the mucosa by the muscularis mucosae (MM). The inner circular (IC) and outer longitudinal (OL) layers of the muscularis externa display the presence of the Auerbach myenteric plexus *(arrows)* between them. The ileum as well as the jejunum and much of the duodenum are covered by a serosa (Se). Note the subserous connective tissue (SSeCT) between the serosa and the outer longitudinal layer of the muscularis externa. (×56)

HISTOPHYSIOLOGY OF THE SMALL INTESTINE

In addition to its roles in digestion and absorption, the small intestine exhibits immunological and secretory activities. These activities are considered first, followed by the discussion of digestion and absorption in the small intestine.

Immunological Activity of the Lamina Propria

Immunoglobulin A produced by plasma cells in the lamina propria is recirculated through the liver and gallbladder.

Plasma cells, lymphocytes, mast cells, extravasated leukocytes, and fibroblasts constitute a large population of cells in the lamina propria of the small intestine. Additionally, solitary lymphoid nodules are frequently present in the lamina propria adjacent to the epithelial lining of the mucosa and the ileum has permanent clusters of lymphoid nodules; these groups of lymphoid nodules are referred to as ***Peyer patches***.

The columnar epithelial cells lining the small intestine are replaced by **M cells**, where a lymphoid nodule contacts the epithelium. M cells phagocytose luminal antigens, viruses, and bacteria (Figs. 17.27 and 17.28). The endocytosed materials enter the endosomal system of M cells, where they are packaged (*without being processed*) in clathrin-coated vesicles, conveyed to the basal aspect of the cell, and exocytosed into the lamina propria. Antigen-presenting cells and dendritic cells of the lymphoid nodule present in the immediate vicinity of M cells endocytose the transferred material, process them, and present the epitopes to lymphocytes, activating them to initiate an immune response.

Once activated, the lymphocytes migrate to mesenteric lymph nodes, where they form secondary lymphoid nodules with germinal centers, regions where B cells proliferate. The newly formed B cells leave the secondary lymphoid nodules differentiating into **plasma cells** that produce monomeric **immunoglobulin A (IgA)**. Still within the cytoplasm of the plasma cell, two monomeric IgAs are complexed together by **J protein**, also synthesized by the plasma cell, to form **IgA dimers**, which they then release into the lamina propria. The IgA dimers attach to **polymeric immunoglobulin receptor molecules (pIgR)** of surface absorptive cell that endocytose the IgA–pIgR complex and transport it to early endosomes. Within the early endosome, the pIgR molecule is modified to become

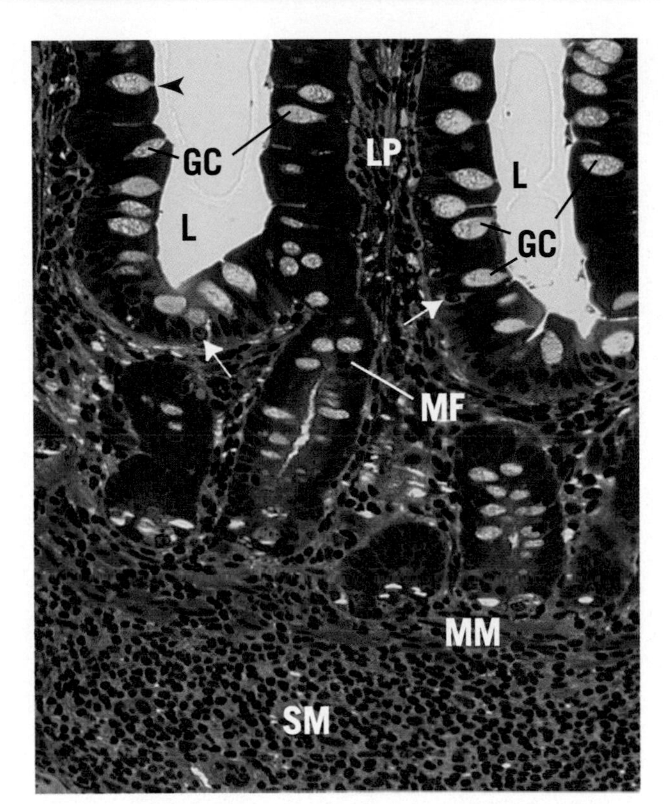

Fig. 17.26 This is a medium magnification of the ileum displaying the lower portions of the villi. Note the numerous goblet cells (GC) and their apically located openings *(arrowhead)* that disgorge their mucinogen into the intervillar spaces (L). Observe also the DNES cells *(white arrows)* and the mitotic figure (MF) as the regenerative cells give rise to intermediate cells. The lamina propria (LP) is inundated with lymphoid elements that press through the muscularis mucosae (MM) to enter and infiltrate the submucosa (SM). (×270)

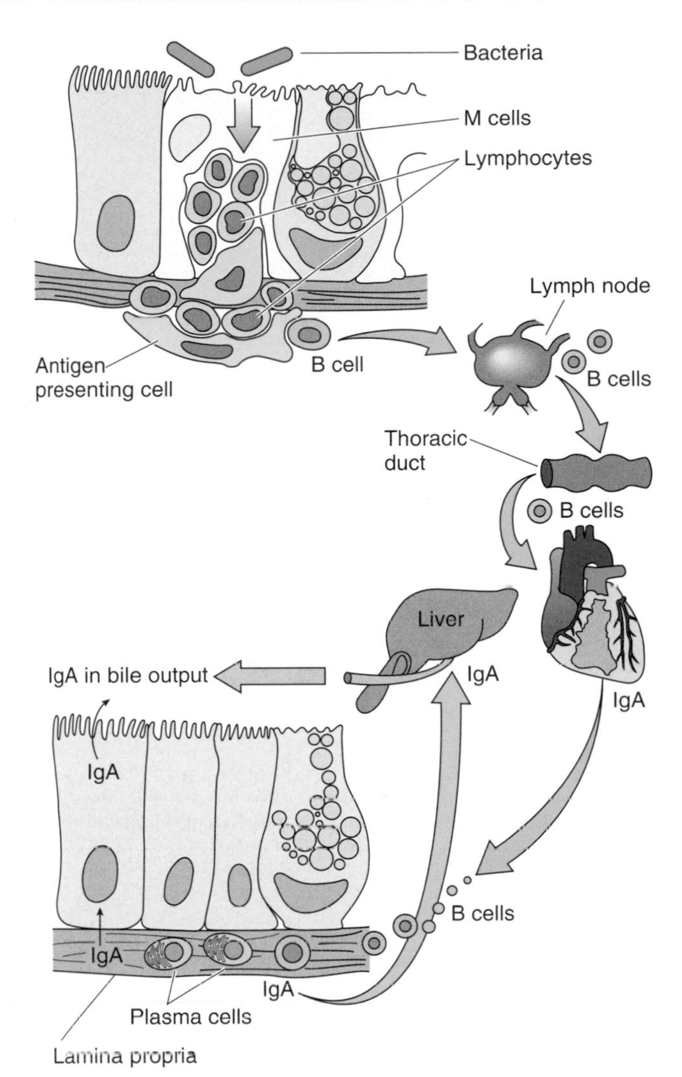

Fig. 17.27 Schematic diagram of an M cell and its immunological relationship to the alimentary canal. Observe that immunoglobulin A (IgA) is produced by plasma cells in the lamina propria. From there, some of it enters the lumen of the duodenum directly via the surface absorptive cells, whereas most of the IgA enters the hepatic portal system. Hepatocytes of the liver complex it with secretory protein and deliver it into the gallbladder, where it is stored with bile. As bile is released into the duodenum, it will be rich in IgA. Therefore, most of the IgA enters the lumen of the duodenum via the bile.

the *secretory component* of the IgA dimer, now referred to as **secretory IgA** (**sIgA**), and is released via **transcytosis** into the intestinal lumen, where it combats antigens, viruses, and pathogenic bacteria. A large portion of the sIgA is reabsorbed by the surface absorptive cells to be released into the lamina propria and enter blood vessels that convey it to the **liver**. Hepatocytes endocytose the sIgA, and it becomes a component of bile that is transported into the gallbladder to be released as bile as needed into the duodenum, a route known as the **enterohepatic circulation**, to defend the body against pathogenic onslaught. Thus, much of the luminal IgA enters the intestine through the common bile duct as a constituent of bile.

Secretory Activity of the Small Intestine

Intramural glands of the small intestine secrete mucus and a watery fluid in response to neural and hormonal stimulation. Neural stimulation, originating in the submucosal plexus, is the principal trigger, but the hormones **secretin** and **cholecystokinin** also play a part in regulating the secretory activities of Brunner glands in the duodenum, as well as of the crypts of Lieberkühn, which collectively produce almost 2 L of slightly alkaline fluid per day.

The DNES cells of the small intestine produce numerous hormones that affect movement of the small intestine and help regulate gastric HCl secretion and the release of pancreatic secretions (see Table 17.2).

Clinical Correlations

The rate of fluid secretion into the small intestine is greatly increased in response to **cholera toxin***. The amount of fluid lost as diarrhea may amount to as much as 10 L/day and, if not replaced, may lead to circulatory shock and death within a few hours. The fluid loss is accompanied by electrolyte imbalance, a contributory factor in the lethal effect of cholera.*

Contractions of the Small Intestine

The small intestine participates in two types of contraction: mixing and propulsive.

Contractions of the small intestine may be subdivided into two interrelated phases:

- **Mixing contractions** are more localized and sequentially redistribute the chyme to expose it to the digestive juices.

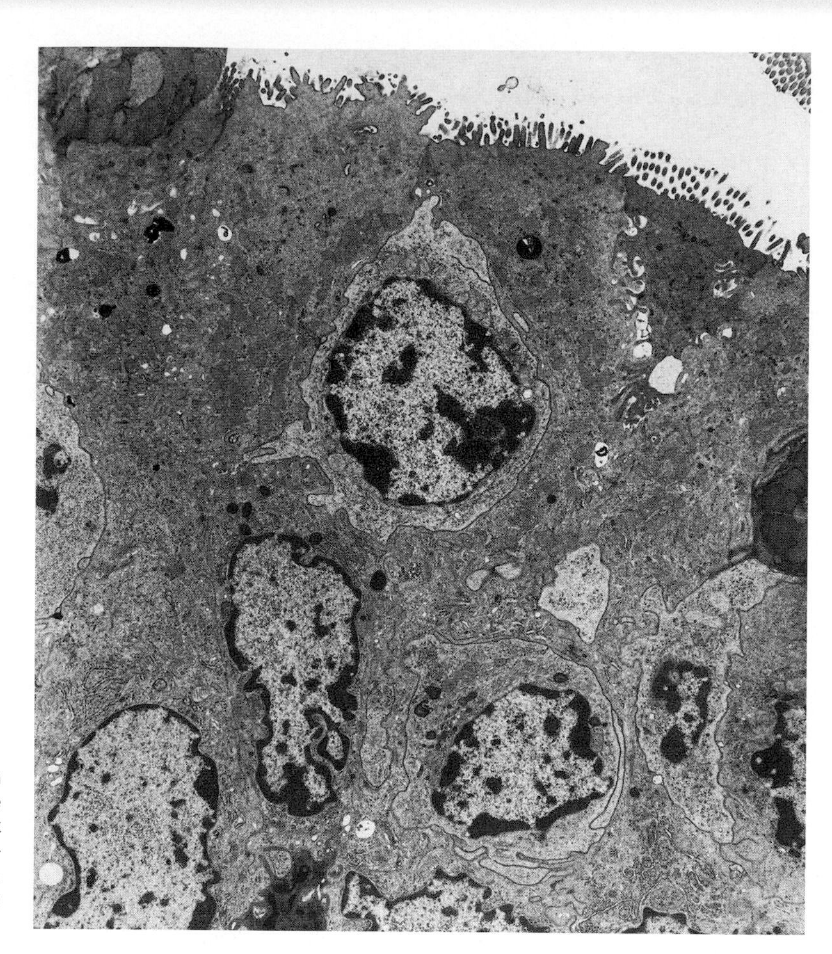

Fig. 17.28 Electron micrograph of M cells of the mouse colon (×6665). Observe the electron-dense M cells surrounding the electron-lucent lymphocytes. (From Owen RL, Piazza AJ, Ermak TH. Ultrastructural and cytoarchitectural features of lymphoreticular organs in the colon and rectum of adult BALB/c mice. *Am J Anat.* 1991;190:10_18. Reprinted with permission from Wiley-Liss, Inc., a subsidiary of John Wiley & Sons, Inc.)

- **Propulsive contractions** occur as **peristaltic waves** that facilitate the movement of the chyme along the small intestine. Because the chyme moves at an average of 1 to 2 cm/min, it spends 6 to 12 hours in the small intestine. The rate of peristalsis is controlled by neural impulses and hormonal factors. In response to gastric distention, a **gastroenteric reflex** mediated by the **myenteric plexus** provides the neural impetus for peristalsis in the small intestine (Fig 17.29). The hormones **cholecystokinin**, **gastrin**, **motilin**, **substance P**, and **serotonin** *increase* intestinal motility, whereas **secretin** and **glucagon** *decrease* motility.

Clinical Correlations

The exposure of the intestinal mucosa to profound irritation by foreign substances such as parasites, viruses, bacteria, or toxins results in a condition known as ***gastroenteritis****. With this condition, a large volume of watery fluid is released by the intestinal lining, causing the muscularis externa to undergo intense, swift contractions of long duration known as* ***peristaltic rush****. These strong contractions propel the highly diluted gastric and intestinal contents into the colon within minutes for elimination of a very watery stool. Gastroenteritis is usually caused by ingestion of food or water contaminated by fecal matter, may last two or three days and, as a result of the loss of a profound volume of water in the stool, known as* ***diarrhea****, may cause dehydration. Fecal culture can determine whether the cause is due to infection or one of the noninfectious causes of diarrhea, such as certain drugs, irritable bowel syndrome, celiac disease, and Crohn disease, among others.*

Digestion

Digestion of the chyme that enters the duodenum from the pyloric stomach is intensified due to the presence of enzymes contributed by the exocrine pancreas. Proteins and carbohydrates that were broken down in the lumen of the duodenum into dipeptides and disaccharides undergo final digestion at the microvilli of the surface absorptive cells, where **dipeptidases** and **disaccharidases**, adherent to the glycocalyx, release individual amino acids and monosaccharides (mostly **glucose**, **fructose**, and **galactose**). These monomers are transported into the surface absorptive cells by specific carrier proteins; however, dipeptides and tripeptides are also endocytosed by the surface absorptive cells. Lipids are **emulsified** by bile salts into small fat globules that are split into monoglycerides and fatty acids by pancreatic lipase. Bile salts segregate monoglycerides and free fatty acids into **micelles**, 2 nm in diameter, which diffuse into the surface absorptive cells through their plasmalemma.

Absorption

Each day, surface absorptive cells of the small intestine absorb approximately 6 to 7 L of water, 30 to 35 g of sodium, 0.5 kg of carbohydrates and proteins, and 1 kg of fat. **Water**, **amino acids**, **dipeptides and tripeptides**, **ions**, and **monosaccharides** enter the surface absorptive cells at their apices and are released into the lamina propria at their basolateral membrane. The processes of absorption and release of nutrients use specific carrier molecules, ion channels, and aquaporins both at the luminally located entry points and the basolaterally located exit points. Once in the lamina propria, these nutrients

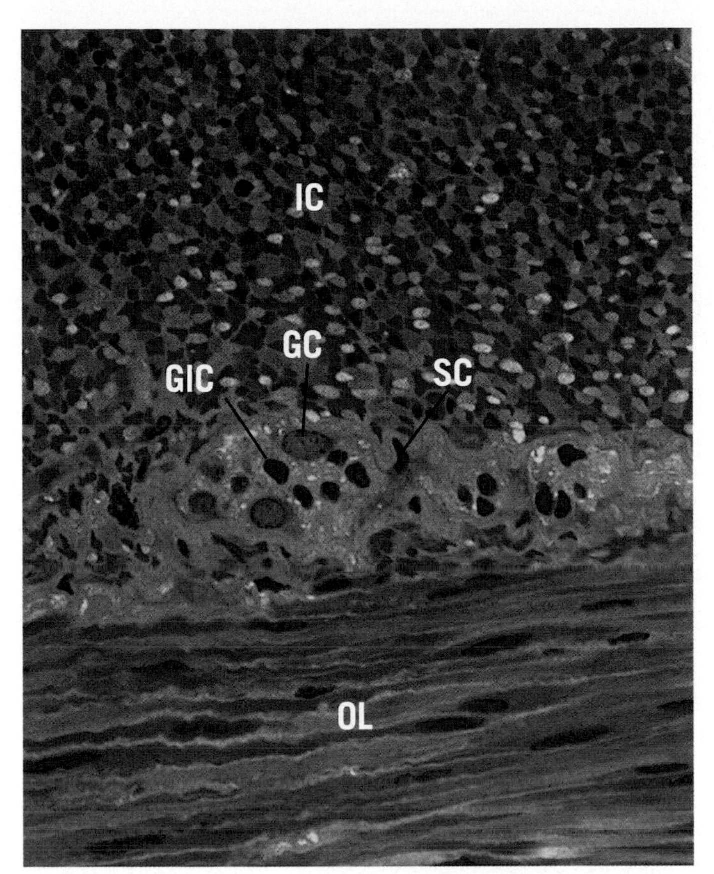

Fig. 17.29 This high-magnification photomicrograph presents the Auerbach myenteric plexus, located between the inner circular (IC) and outer longitudinal (OL) layers of the muscularis externa. Observe the nucleus of a Schwann cell (SC) surrounding the nerve fiber that modifies the activity of the neurons (GC) of the enteric nervous system. There are many enteric glial cells (GC) that act similar to neuroglia of the central nervous system. (×540)

enter the capillary beds of the villi and are transported to the liver for processing.

Long-chain fatty acids and **monoglycerides** enter the smooth endoplasmic reticulum of the surface absorptive cells, where they are **reesterified** to triglycerides that are transferred to the Golgi apparatus. Here, they are combined with a β-lipoprotein coat, manufactured on the RER, and form large lipoprotein droplets, known as **chylomicrons.** These chylomicrons, after being packaged and released from the Golgi apparatus, are transported to the basolateral cell membrane to be released into the lamina propria (Fig. 17.30). The chylomicrons enter blindly ending lymphatic vessels, known as lacteals, where this lipid-rich substance becomes known as ***chyle***. Rhythmic contractions of the smooth muscle cells located in the cores of the villi, derived from the muscularis mucosae, cause shortening of each villus and, acting as a syringe, inject the chyle from the lacteal into the **submucosal plexus of lymph vessels**. These lymph vessels drain into ever larger lymph vessels and eventually into the largest lymph vessel of the body, known as the *thoracic duct*, which delivers its chyle-rich lymph into the systemic circulation and is conveyed to the liver. Therefore, unlike the products of carbohydrate and protein digestion, long-chain fatty acids do not go *directly* to the liver but enter the systemic circulation and, only then, *indirectly* make their way to the liver to be processed.

Short-chain fatty acids (< 12 carbons in length) do not enter the smooth endoplasmic reticulum for reesterification. These free fatty acids, which are short enough to be somewhat water soluble, progress to the basolateral membrane of the surface absorptive cell, diffuse into the lamina propria, and enter the capillary loops to be delivered *directly* to the **liver** for processing.

Clinical Correlations

Malabsorption in the small intestine may occur even though the pancreas delivers its normal complement of enzymes. The various diseases that result in malabsorption are called ***sprue****. An interesting form of sprue,* ***gluten enteropathy (nontropical sprue)****, is caused by* ***gluten****, a substance present in rye and wheat, which, perhaps as a result of an allergic response to gluten, destroys the microvilli and even villi of susceptible individuals. In patients with this disorder, the destruction of microvilli and villi causes a reduction in the surface area available for absorption of nutrients. Treatment involves elimination of gluten-containing grains from the diet.*

Large Intestine

The large intestine is subdivided into the cecum, colon, rectum, and anus; the appendix is a small, blind outpouching of the cecum.

The approximately 1.5-m-long **large intestine** has several named regions: the cecum, colon (ascending, transverse, descending, and sigmoid), rectum, and anus (see Table 17.3). It absorbs most of the water and ions from the chyme that it receives from the small intestine, as well as much of the gases present in its luminal content. Additionally, it compacts the chyme into feces for elimination. The cecum and colon are indistinguishable histologically and are discussed as a single entity, called the **colon**. The **appendix**, a blind outpocketing of the cecum, is described separately.

COLON

The **colon** accounts for almost the entire length of the large intestine. It receives chyme from the ileum at the **ileocecal valve**, an anatomical and physiological sphincter that prevents reflux of the cecal content into the ileum.

Histology of the Colon

The colon has no villi, but its lamina propria is richly endowed with **crypts of Lieberkühn** that are similar in composition to those of the small intestine, except that there are no Paneth cells in the colon (Figs. 17.31–17.35). The number of goblet cells of its simple columnar epithelium increases from the cecum to the sigmoid colon, but throughout most of the colon, the surface absorptive cells are the most numerous cell type. **DNES** cells, including L cells that secrete the appetite-reducing hormone **peptide YY (PYY)**, are also present, although they are few in number. Rapid mitotic activity of the regenerative cells replaces the epithelial lining of the crypts and of the mucosal surface every 6 to 7 days.

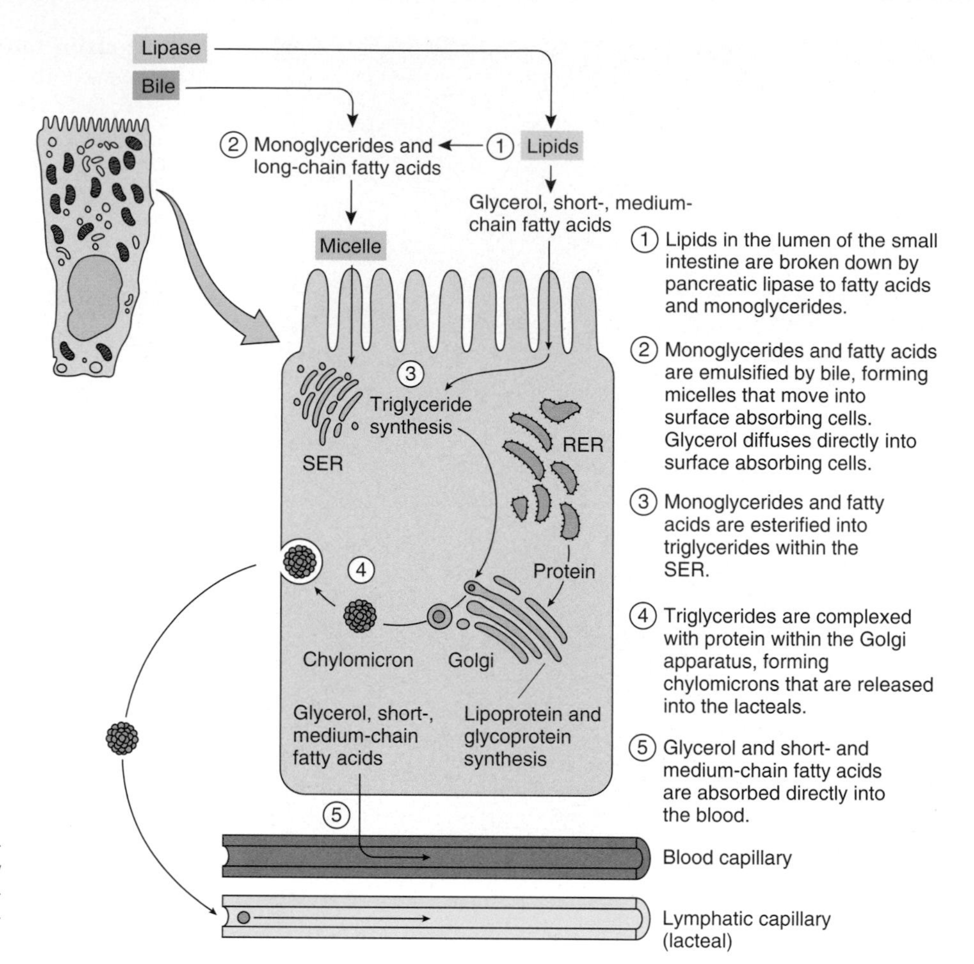

Fig. 17.30 Schematic diagram of fat absorption, fat processing, and chylomicron release by surface absorptive cells. RER, Rough endoplasmic reticulum; SER, smooth endoplasmic reticulum.

There are two types of **fibroblast** in the lamina propria: one is the normal fibroblast of any connective tissue that is scattered throughout the lamina propria and the other is located at the bases of the crypts of Lieberkühn, pericryptal fibroblasts, which migrate along the length of the crypts at the same rate as the epithelial cells. When they reach the vicinity of the opening of the crypts, these fibroblasts differentiate into macrophage-like cells and function as if they were monocyte-derived macrophages. The lamina propria is also richly endowed with components of **GALT:** lymphoid cells and lymphoid nodules. However, there is only a scant amount of lymph drainage in the colon, which accounts for the limited incidence of metastasis of colon cancers.

The **muscularis mucosae** and **submucosa** of the colon resemble those of the small intestine. The **muscularis externa** is unusual in that the outer longitudinal layer is not of continuous thickness along the surface; rather, most of it is gathered into three narrow ribbons of muscle fascicles, known as ***taeniae coli***. The constant tonus maintained by the taeniae coli puckers the large intestine into sacculations, called ***haustra coli***. The **serosa** displays numerous fat-filled pouches, called ***appendices epiploicae***.

Histophysiology of the Colon

The colon functions in absorption of water, electrolytes, and gases as well as in the compaction and elimination of feces.

The colon absorbs almost 1.5 L of water and electrolytes on a daily basis and compacts and eliminates approximately 100 mL feces per day.

Feces are composed of water (75%), dead bacteria (7%), roughage (7%), fat (5%), inorganic substances (5%), and undigested protein, dead cells, and bile pigment (1%). The odor of feces varies with the individual and is a function of the diet and bacterial flora, which produce varied amounts of **indole, hydrogen sulfide**, and **mercaptans**. The color of feces is due to **urobilin** and **stercobilin**, both the by-products of bilirubin. Bacterial by-products include riboflavin, thiamin, vitamin B_{12}, and vitamin K.

Bacterial action in the colon produces gases, released as **flatus**, composed of CO_2, methane, and H_2, which then is mixed with the nitrogen and oxygen from swallowed air. The gas is combustible and, very infrequently, it may explode when electrical cauterization is used during sigmoidoscopy or colonoscopy. The large intestine holds 7 to 10 L of gases each day, of which only 0.5 to 1.0 L is expelled as flatus; the remainder is absorbed through the lining of the colon.

The colon also produces mucus and HCO_3^-. Mucus not only protects the mucosa of the colon but also facilitates the compaction of feces because it is the mucus that permits adherence of the solid wastes into a compact mass. HCO_3^- adheres to the mucus and acts as a buffer, protecting the mucosa from the acid by-products of bacterial metabolism within the feces.

Clinical Correlations

1. *Intense irritation of the colonic mucosa, as in* **enteritis**, *results in the secretion of large quantities of mucus, water, and electrolytes. Voiding of copious quantities of liquid stool, known as* **diarrhea**, *protects the body by diluting and eliminating the irritant. Long-term diarrhea and loss of a large amount of fluid and electrolytes without a regimen of replacement therapy may result in circulatory shock and even death.*
2. **Pseudomembranous colitis**, *an inflammatory disease of the bowel, may result from mercury poisoning, intestinal ischemia, and bronchopneumonia, but most frequently it is due to prolonged antibiotic therapy. Patients most at risk are those who are weak, immunocompromised, and/or elderly. As the intestinal flora is disrupted due to the antibiotic therapy,* Clostridium difficile *assumes a major role in the genesis of this disease, whose clinical manifestations include fluid accumulation in the small intestine as well as epithelial shedding and the formation of a thick, viscous membrane composed of fibrin, mucus, neutrophils, and mononuclear cells. The symptoms include a low-grade fever (38°C–40°C [100.4°F–104°F]), copious watery diarrhea, severe abdominal cramps, and abdominal tenderness. Mortality is relatively high (10%–15% of affected individuals) if the condition is not treated in a timely manner by restoring electrolyte balance and maintaining adequate fluid volume by fluid replacement therapy, as much as 10 to 15 L per 24 to 36 hours.*
3. *Individuals with recurrent abdominal pain, usually beginning between 15 and 30 years of age and who have diarrhea or very loose stool occurring several times a day, may have* **Crohn disease.** *Accompanying the pain and diarrhea, especially in 15- to 20-year-olds, growth retardation is common (30% of cases). In fact, this is one of the contributing indications to the diagnosis of Crohn disease in youth. The underlying causes of this condition are not understood, but they involve inflammation of the gastrointestinal tract and an immune response, not to the individual's own tissues but to antigens of the patient's bacterial flora. The disease has a genetic component, at least in approximately 50% of the patients with this condition. The prevalent locations that are affected by Crohn disease are the ileum and colon. Unfortunately, there is no cure for the disease, but the patient may be kept in remission by smoking cessation, decreased meat and dairy intake, an increase in vegetable-based proteins, and the consumption of smaller meals several times a day. Moderate daily exercise and an adequate amount of sleep and rest have also proved beneficial to patients with this condition.*

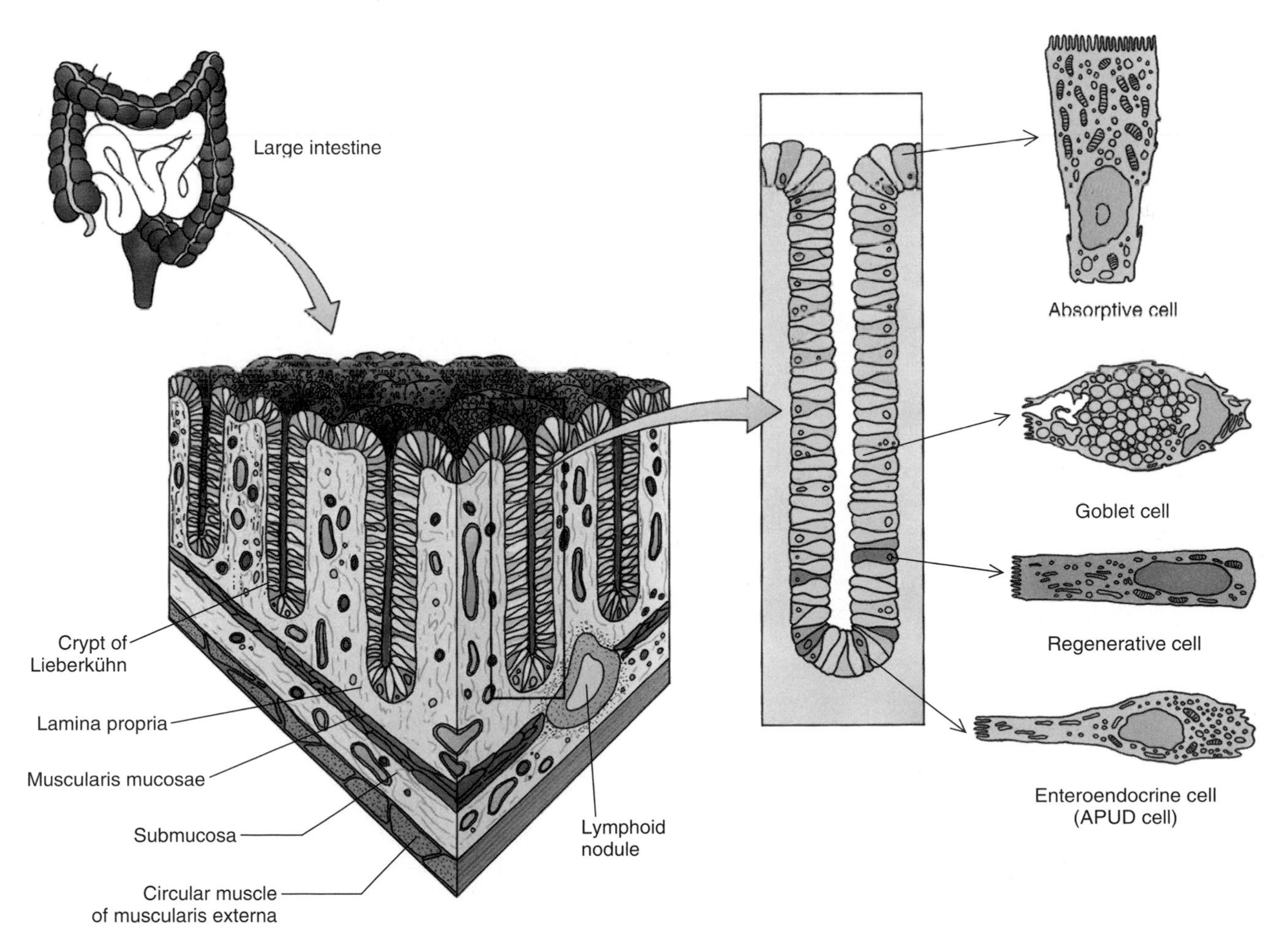

Fig. 17.31 Schematic diagram of the colon, crypts of Lieberkühn, and associated cells. APUD, Amine precursor uptake and decarboxylation.

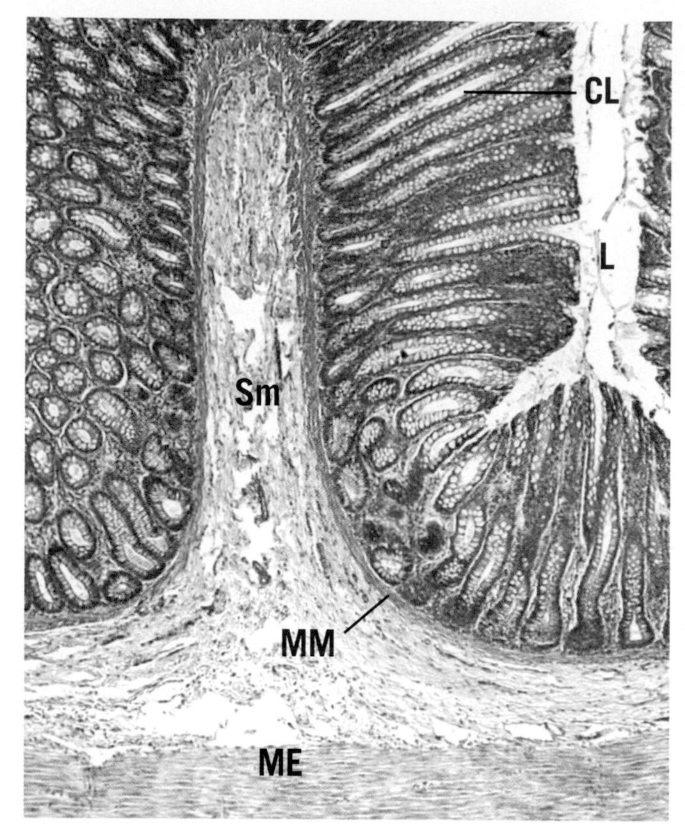

Fig. 17.32 This very-low-magnification photomicrograph of the colon displays the half moon–shaped folds of the submucosa (Sm) caused by the contraction of the narrow bands of the taeniae coli. The lumen (L) of the colon is lined by a simple columnar epithelium composed mostly of surface absorptive cells and goblet cells that continue into the crypts of Lieberkühn (CL). Note that there is only a scant amount of connective tissue separating the crypts of Lieberkühn. The lamina propria is separated from the submucosa by the muscularis mucosae (MM) and the inner circular layer of the muscularis externa (ME) borders the submucosa. (×56)

Clinical Correlations

1. *It is interesting to note that human breast milk contains nutrients, such as some oligosaccharides, that neonates are unable to digest. Instead, it is now believed that these oligosaccharides are actually prebiotics that are designed to sustain the intestinal flora of the newborn.*
2. *Recent reports have demonstrated that artificial sweeteners have a deleterious effect on the intestinal microbial flora, altering it to present an unhealthy state. These changes to the flora disposed the individuals to obesity, as well as to glucose intolerance, a condition that is considered to be a precursor of type 2 diabetes.*
3. *Recent studies have indicated that the microorganism* Akkermansia muciniphila *in the colons of mice and monkeys ameliorated insulin resistance in these animals, reducing their chances of acquiring type 2 diabetes. Although this microorganism constitutes less than 5% of the microbiota, they are essential for colon health because they manufacture the short-chain fatty acid butyrate, the primary nutrient used by the epithelial cells of the large intestine. As the mice and monkeys aged, the population of* A. muciniphila *declined and the levels of butyric acid were depressed. With this decrease of the short-chain fatty acid, the health of the colon decreased, its wall became thinner, leaky, inflamed, initiated an immune response, and brought on insulin resistance. Additionally, the population of other butyrate-producing members of the microbiota also declined. When the aged animals were given butyrate, the* A. muciniphila *population increased, as did the population of the other butyrate-producing members of the microbiota, the inflammation and immune response were halted, and the insulin resistance of the older animals reverted back to the levels present in younger animals. Current research is examining whether the population of* A. muciniphila *in older humans mirrors those found in mice and monkeys.*

Microbiota of the Colon

The human body is composed of approximately 1 trillion human cells, a number dwarfed by the estimated 10 trillion microbes that inhabit the surface of the skin as well as the lining of the respiratory, genitourinary, and GI tracts. Of course, these numbers are conjectures; more research is required to improve the reality of the estimates. Irrespective of the actual numbers, this population of microorganisms is known as the **microbiota**. The collective genome of the microbiota is known as the **microbiome**. The bulk of the microbiota that inhabit the large intestine are commensal organisms. It has been shown that the physiological condition of this intestinal flora directly affects the health of the individual in whom it resides. Because fetuses develop under sterile conditions, it is only during its passage through the birth canal that the baby acquires a microbial flora from the maternal vagina; thus, the baby's flora mirrors that of the mother. It is believed that some of the fecal microbes are swallowed and, later on, during breastfeeding, the baby's intestinal flora becomes expanded. It is only after the maternal milk is supplemented and later supplanted by the baby's diet that the intestinal flora resembles that of the adult members of the nuclear family. It was believed that the adult microbial flora may be classified into three enterotypes according to the predominant organisms that reside in the intestine. However, recent reports suggest that instead of enterotypes, there are gradients of organisms that predominate, which may be categorized as groups that coexist in the gut lumen. There are two phyla that may be described as the predominant residents in the intestinal lumina of some populations of humans but not in others. Therefore, in some individuals *Prevotella* is in the majority whereas, in others, *Bacteriodes* is in the majority. Both of these populations of people of any age group are considered to be healthy. However, in older, frail, unhealthy individuals, the predominant flora consisted of various species of the genera *Oscillobacter* and *Alistipes*, suggesting such a flora to be indicative of an unhealthy condition. It has also been demonstrated that diet plays a major role in the composition of the intestinal flora and that this flora can be altered within a few days of dietary changes. Indeed, a predominantly Western-type diet has been shown to alter the intestinal flora, which has been suggested to have serious health consequences, leading to conditions such as type 2 diabetes and obesity.

Regulation of Appetite

It may appear strange to discuss the regulation of appetite following the description of the colon, but the entire GI tract appears to have roles in this sensation. Therefore, it is advisable to understand the structure and function of almost every region of the intestinal tract before treating appetite control.

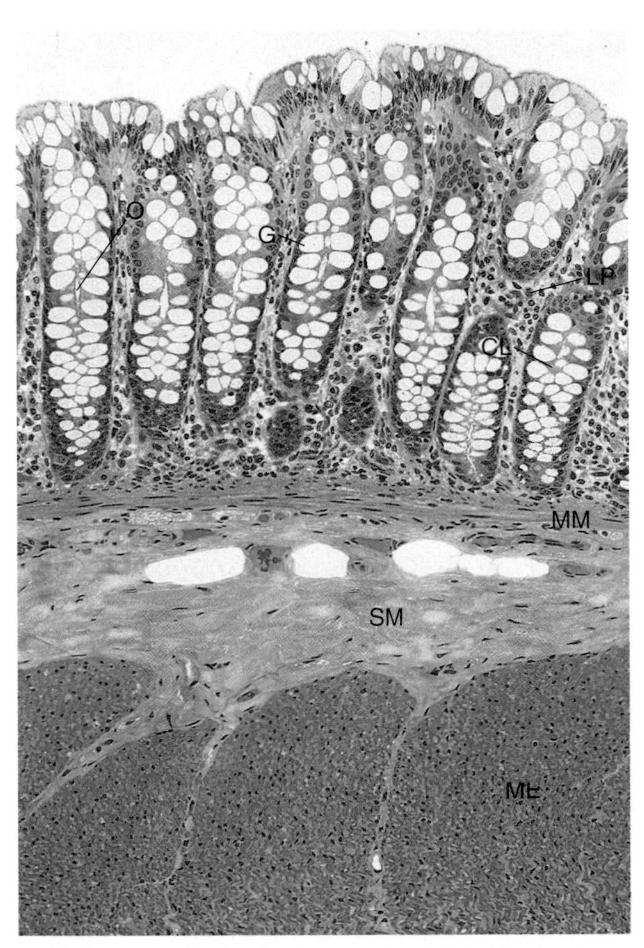

Fig. 17.33 Photomicrograph of the monkey colon. Observe that it appears as if most of the cells of the epithelial lining are goblet cells. However, in fact, the surface absorptive cells constitute the largest population of this epithelium (×132). G, Goblet cells; CL, crypts of Lieberkühn; LP, lamina propria; ME, muscularis externa; MM, muscularis mucosae; O, open lumen of crypts of Lieberkühn; SM, submucosa.

The control of appetite is a multifactorial process that has psychological, physical, microbial, physiological, neuronal, and hormonal components.

- The **psychological component** involves the smell, sight, and thoughts of food. However, these may be superseded by the physical and physiological components.
- The **physical components** involve an empty stomach or duodenum that induces a feeling of hunger, whereas a full stomach or duodenum induces a feeling of satiety and a lack of desire for food intake.
- The physical components are actually controlled by **physiological factors**, such as blood nutrient levels. Therefore, the following section concentrates on the physiological aspect of appetite regulation, which involves neuronal and hormonal factors.
- Although the **microbial component** is not understood, it has been demonstrated that the microbiota residing in the lumen of an individual's colon has a direct influence on an individual's amount of body fat accompanied by a decrease in the blood concentration of hormones, PYY and glucagon-like peptide-1 (GLP-1), that are known to reduce food intake. Manipulation of the microbiota, specifically by the administration of probiotics and prebiotics, shifts the microbiota, reducing the individual's body fat by altering the release of the appropriate DNES-manufactured hormones.

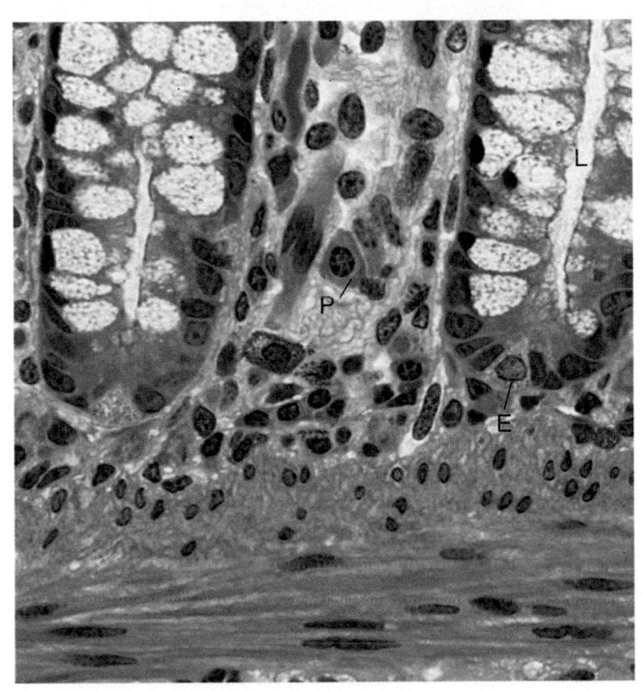

Fig. 17.34 Photomicrograph of the crypts of Lieberkühn of the monkey colon. Observe that the base of the crypt displays DNES cells whose granules are basally oriented (×270). E, Diffuse neuroendocrine system (DNES) cell; L, lumen of crypt; P, plasma cell.

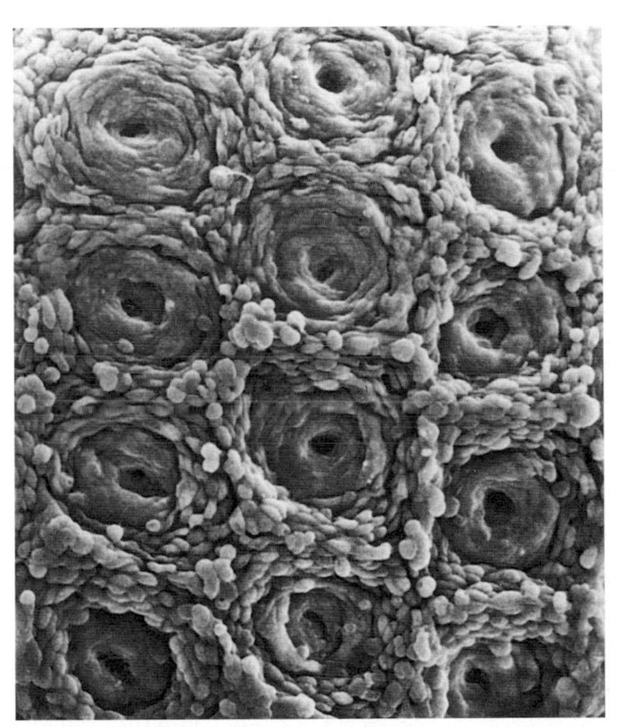

Fig. 17.35 Scanning electron micrograph of a monkey colon (×516). Observe the opening of the crypts. (From Specian RD, Neutra MR. The surface topography of the colonic crypt in rabbit and monkey. *Am J Anat.* 1981;160:461–472. Reprinted with permission from Wiley-Liss, Inc., a subsidiary of John Wiley & Sons, Inc.)

Neuronal Factors of Appetite Control

It has been demonstrated in mice that neurons located in the bed nucleus of the stria terminalis (BNST) project to nuclei of the lateral hypothalamus (the feeding center), whose signals initiate feeding behavior. Conversely, if the BNST neurons stop signaling the nuclei of the lateral hypothalamus, the feeding behavior stops, and the animals stop eating. Unfortunately, at this point, it is not known how the BNST neurons are activated or silenced.

The control of appetite has both positive signals and negative feedback signals. The latter is under the control of the vagus nerve (CN X), which senses the amount of food in the small intestine and the length of time that the ingested food spends in the various regions of the alimentary canal. The sensory fibers of the vagus provide information to the dorsal vagal complex to provide a sensation of satiety and inhibit further intake of food.

Hormonal Factors of Appetite Control

Most of the hormones that control the appetite are manufactured by the DNES cells of the GI tract. These hormones control not only food intake but also many regulate the expenditure of energy, as well as additional functions of the digestive tract. See Table 17.2 for the list of hormones produced by the DNES cells of the GI tract and their functions, including their effects on appetite.

Insulin, produced by the beta cells of the islets of Langerhans in the pancreas, function in the control of blood glucose level (see Chapter 18) but also reduce appetite. The hormone leptin, produced by adipocytes (and, to a limited extent, by P/D1 cells [Gr cells] of the stomach and small intestine), inhibits hunger sensation, thereby reducing food intake.

RECTUM AND ANAL CANAL

Histologically, the **rectum** resembles the colon, but the crypts of Lieberkühn are deeper and number fewer per unit area (see Table 17.3).

The **anal canal**, the constricted continuation of the rectum, is about 3 to 4 cm long. Its crypts of Lieberkühn are short and few and are present only in the proximal half of the canal. The mucosa also displays longitudinal folds, the **anal columns** (**rectal columns of Morgagni**). These meet one another to form pouch-like outpocketings, the **anal valves** with intervening **anal sinuses**. The anal valves assist the anus in supporting the column of feces.

Anal Mucosa

The **epithelium** of the anal mucosa is *simple cuboidal* from the rectum to the **pectinate line** (at the level of the anal valves), *stratified squamous nonkeratinized* from the pectinate line to the external anal orifice, and *stratified squamous keratinized* (epidermis) at the anus. The **lamina propria**, a fibroelastic connective tissue, houses **anal glands** at the rectoanal junction and **circumanal glands** at the distal end of the anal canal. Hair follicles and sebaceous glands are also present at the anus. The **muscularis mucosae** is composed of an inner circular layer and an outer longitudinal layer of smooth muscle. These muscular layers do not extend beyond the pectinate line.

Anal Submucosa and Muscularis Externa

The **submucosa** of the anal canal is composed of fibroelastic connective tissue. It houses two venous plexuses, the **internal hemorrhoidal plexus**, situated above the pectinate line, and the **external hemorrhoidal plexus**, located at the junction of the anal canal with its external orifice, the **anus**.

Clinical Correlations

1. *An increase in the size of the vessels of the submucosal venous plexuses of the anal canal results in the formation of* ***hemorrhoids****, a condition common in pregnancy and in people older than 50 years. This condition may manifest as painful defecation, appearance of fresh blood with defecation, and anal itching.*
2. *As a* ***rectal examination*** *is performed by insertion of the index finger through the external anal orifice, the external anal sphincter tightens around the finger. Continued penetration results in activation of the internal anal sphincter, which also tightens around the finger. In males, structures that may be palpated through the anal canal include the bulb of the penis, the prostate, enlarged seminal vesicles, the inferior aspect of the distended bladder, and enlarged iliac lymph nodes; in females, palpable structures include the cervix of the uterus and, in pathological conditions, the ovaries and broad ligament.*

The **muscularis externa** consists of an inner circular and outer longitudinal smooth muscle layer. The inner circular layer becomes thickened as it encircles the region of the pectinate line to form the **internal anal sphincter muscle**. The smooth muscle cells of the outer longitudinal layer continue as a fibroelastic sheet surrounding the internal anal sphincter.

Skeletal muscles of the floor of the pelvis form an **external anal sphincter muscle** that surrounds the fibroelastic sheet and internal anal sphincter. The external sphincter is under voluntary control, exhibits a constant tonus, and is the muscle that prevents spontaneous defecation.

APPENDIX

The histological appearance of the appendix resembles that of the colon, except it is much smaller in diameter, has a richer supply of lymphoid elements, and contains many more DNES cells in its crypts of Lieberkühn.

The **vermiform appendix** is a 5- to 6-cm-long diverticulum of the cecum with a stellate-shaped lumen that usually is occupied by debris. The mucosa of the appendix is composed of a simple columnar epithelium, consisting of surface absorptive cells, occasional goblet cells, and M cells where lymphoid nodules adjoin the epithelium (see Table 17.3). The lamina propria is a loose connective tissue with numerous lymphoid nodules and shallow crypts of Lieberkühn. The cells composing these crypts are surface absorptive cells, goblet cells, regenerative cells, intermediate cells, numerous DNES cells, and infrequent Paneth cells. The muscularis mucosae, submucosa, and muscularis externa do not deviate from the general plan of the alimentary canal, although lymphoid nodules and occasional fatty infiltration are present in the submucosa, especially in older individuals. The appendix is completely invested by a serosa (Figs. 17.36 and 17.37).

Function of the Appendix

Until recently, it has been suggested that the appendix is a vestigial organ with no known functions, but recent studies have suggested otherwise. It is now believed that the lumen of this

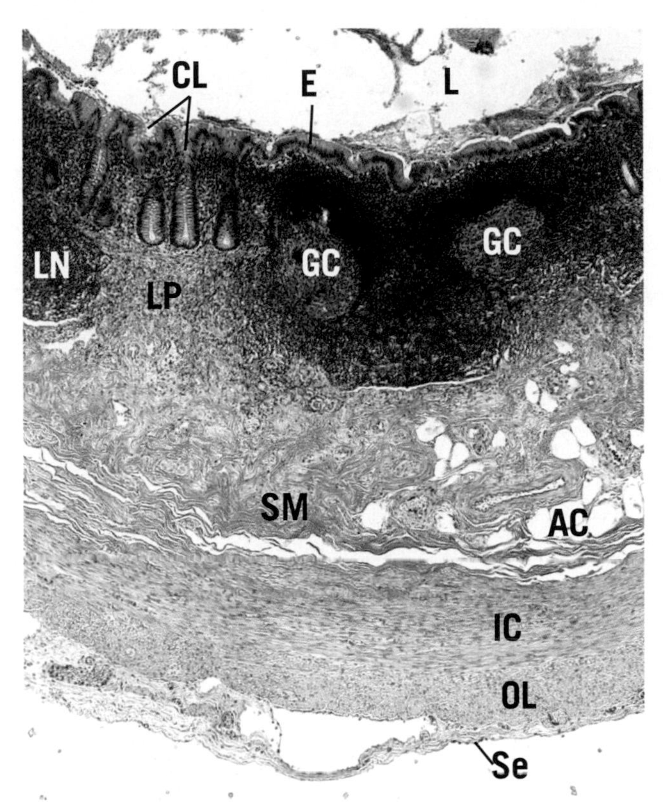

Fig. 17.36 This very-low-magnification photomicrograph of the appendix demonstrates the entire thickness of its wall. Note that the lumen (L) is lined by a simple columnar epithelium and that the lamina propria (LP) has shallow crypts of Lieberkühn (CL) as well as lymphoid nodules (LN), some with germinal centers (GC). Observe that the submucosa (SM) is composed of a dense, irregular, collagenous connective tissue with a few adipocytes (AC). The inner circular (IC) and outer longitudinal (OL) layers of the muscularis externa are well represented, as is the serosa (Se). (×56)

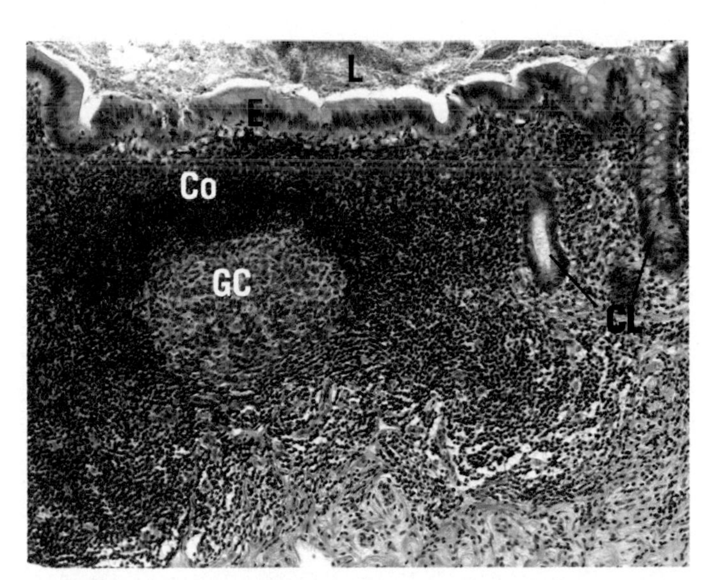

Fig. 17.37 This low-magnification photomicrograph of the appendix displays the debris in its lumen (L) and the simple columnar epithelium (E) lining the lumen. Note the crypts of Lieberkühn (CL) as well as the corona (Co) and germinal center (GC) of the lymphoid nodule and the numerous lymphoid elements in the lamina propria. (×132)

slender structure houses a bacterial biofilm of colonies that represent the normal intestinal flora and, in the case of pathogenic invasion that annihilates much of the individual's intestinal bacteria, colonies sequestered in the appendix may have the capability of restoring the person's normal flora, thus repairing the biological damage.

Clinical Correlations

The incidence of inflammation of the appendix, ***appendicitis****, is greater in teenagers and young adults than in older people; it also occurs more frequently in males than in females. Appendicitis usually is caused by obstruction of the lumen, which results in inflammation accompanied by swelling and an unremitting, severe pain in the lower right quadrant of the abdomen. Additional clinical signs are nausea and vomiting, fever (usually below 102°F), tense abdomen, and an elevated leukocyte count. If the condition is not treated within 1 to 2 days, the appendix may rupture, leading to the onset of peritonitis, which may result in death if untreated. However, recent investigations from Finland demonstrated that if computed tomography scans show that the appendix is not in a critical stage of possible rupturing, then a regimen of antibiotics may be a good alternative for surgery. Five hundred people were selected for the experiment; 250 were given an antibiotic regimen and 250 had surgery. One hundred patients on the antibiotic regimen had to have surgery in the first five years, indicating that 60% of the patients were able to avoid surgery without any complications. Currently, there are several clinical studies in the United States that are evaluating antibiotic administration versus surgery.*

Pathological Considerations

See Figs. 17.38 through 17.41.

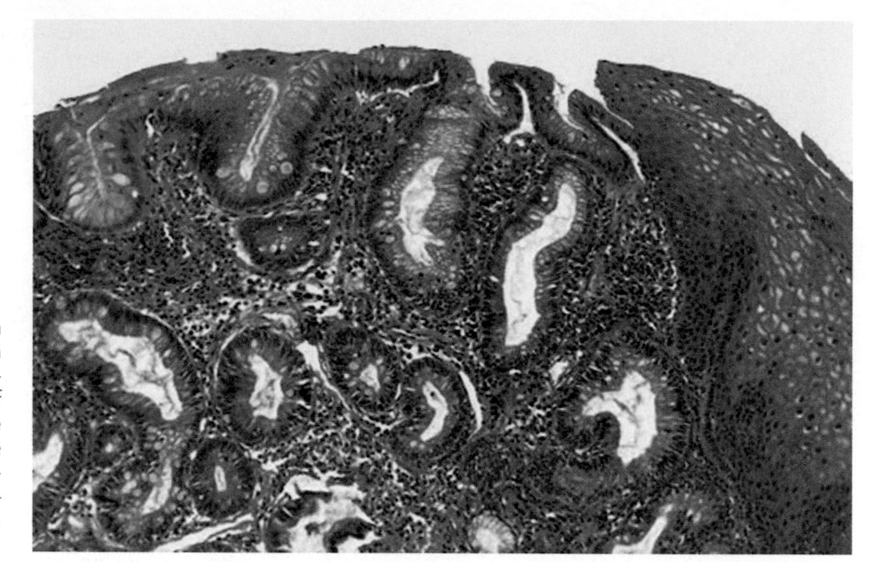

Fig. 17.38 Photomicrograph of Barrett esophagus, a condition caused by long-term gastroesophageal reflux in which the esophageal epithelium changes from the normal stratified squamous epithelium (on the right side of the image) to an abnormal columnar epithelium (left side of the image). The epithelium in this patient displays the presence of goblet cells, reminding one of intestinal epithelium. (Reprinted with permission from Klatt EC. *Robbins and Cotran: Pathological Basis of Disease*. 2nd ed. Philadelphia: Elsevier; 2010:173.)

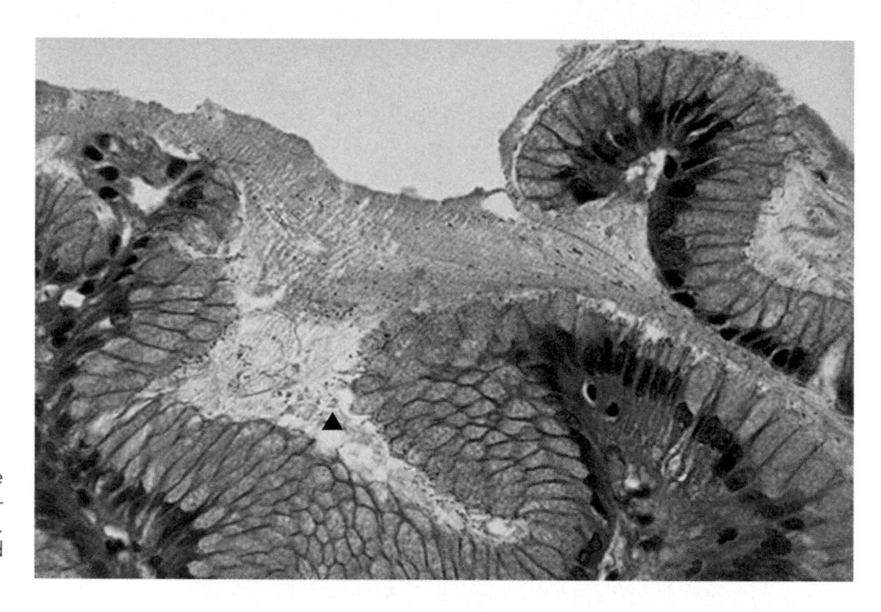

Fig. 17.39 Photomicrograph of a stomach whose visible mucous houses small, spiral Gram-negative rods, *Helicobacter pylori*. (Reprinted with permission from Klatt EC. *Robbins and Cotran: Pathological Basis of Disease*. 2nd ed. Philadelphia: Elsevier; 2010:179.)

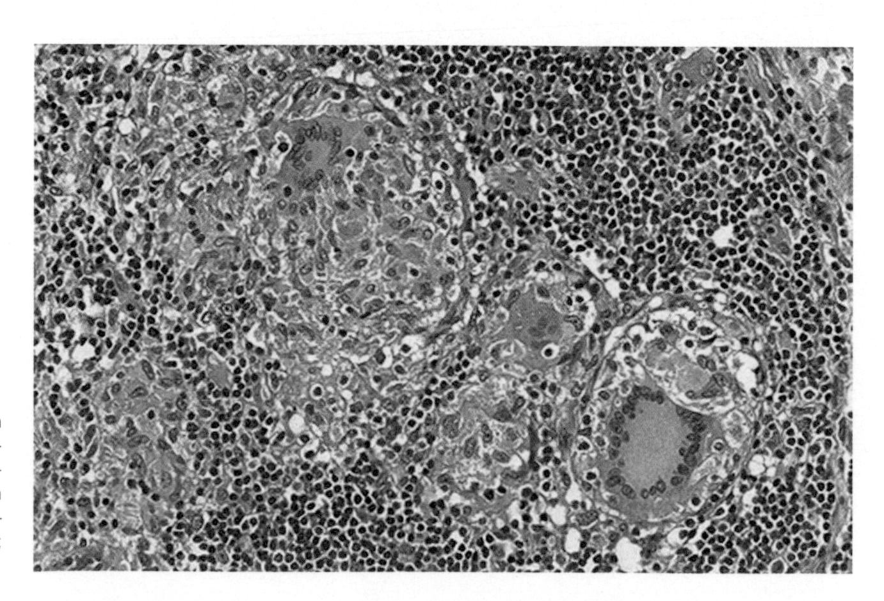

Fig. 17.40 Photomicrograph of a patient afflicted with Crohn disease. Note that the inflammation has granulomatous characteristics with the presence of many lymphocytes as well as giant and epithelioid cells. (Reprinted with permission from Klatt EC. *Robbins and Cotran: Pathological Basis of Disease*. 2nd ed. Philadelphia: Elsevier; 2010:192.)

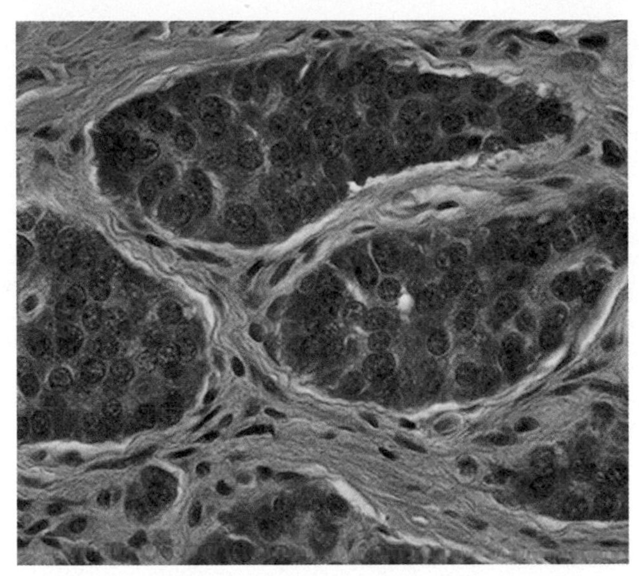

Fig. 17.41 Photomicrograph of a patient afflicted with carcinoid tumor of the small intestine. Note that the tumor is composed of clusters of endocrine-resembling small, round cells with round nuclei. (Reprinted with permission from Klatt EC. *Robbins and Cotran: Pathological Basis of Disease.* 2nd ed. Philadelphia: Elsevier; 2010:208.)

Histology Laboratory Instructions: Digestive System—Alimentary CanaL

Esophagus

A very-low-magnification photomicrograph of the esophagus demonstrates how its thick, stratified squamous epithelium forms a well-developed rete apparatus with its lamina propria. The submucosa is interposed between the muscularis externa and the inner circular layer of the muscularis externa. The outer longitudinal layer is easily distinguished (see Fig. 17.2, E, LP, S, IC, OL). A low-magnification photomicrograph taken from the upper third of the esophagus also displays the well-developed rete apparatus formed by the stratified squamous epithelium and underlying lamina propria. The lamina propria, muscularis mucosae, and submucosa are readily distinguishable. Observe that the muscularis mucosae is composed of only a longitudinal layer of smooth muscle cells. At this level, the submucosa is very narrow; the inner circular and outer longitudinal layers of the muscularis externa are easily recognized (see Fig. 17.3, E, LP, MM, SM, IC, OL).

Stomach

A low-magnification photomicrograph displays that the simple columnar epithelium lining the fundic stomach dips down into the lamina propria to form gastric pits and the bottom of each gastric pit receives a number of fundic glands that extend to the muscularis mucosae that contact the submucosa (see Fig. 17.5A, E, LP, MM, S). At medium magnification, at least three cell types can be recognized as components of the fundic glands: mucous neck cells, parietal cells, and chief cells (see Fig. 17.5B, M, P, C). At high magnification, the cells composing the deeper aspect of the fundic glands (neck and base) are clearly represented: chief cells, parietal cells, and DNES cells. The lumen of the fundic glands as well as the connective tissue elements, blood vessels, and the muscularis mucosae are also easy to identify (see Fig. 17.7, CC, PC, DNES, L, CT, BV, MM).

A very-low-magnification photomicrograph of the cardiac stomach displays the very shallow gastric pits opening up into the lumen. The lamina propria has cardiac glands that extend from the gastric pits to the muscularis mucosae. The submucosa has larger blood vessels and contacts the muscularis externa. Note also the serosa and the subserosal connective tissue between the serosa and the muscularis externa (see Fig. 17.13, *arrow*, L, LP, CG, MM, SM, BV, ME, Se, SsCT). At a low magnification, the surface-lining cells lining the lumen of the cardiac stomach are well displayed. The lamina propria is occupied by cardiac glands and numerous connective tissue cells. The muscularis mucosae contact the submucosa, which has occasional adipose cells and is richly endowed with blood vessels. The submucosa is surrounded by the muscularis externa (see Fig. 17.14, E, CG, *arrowhead*, MM, SM, A, BV, ME).

A low magnification of the pyloric stomach displays the gastric pits that extend deep into the lamina propria. The pyloric glands of the lamina propria extend down to the muscularis mucosae (see Fig. 17.15, P, LP, MM).

Small Intestine

Duodenum

The simple columnar epithelium lining the lumen of the duodenum dips into the crypts of Lieberkühn, which extend to the muscularis mucosae. Observe in this low-magnification photomicrograph that the lamina propria of the villi house large, blindly ending lymphatic vessels, known as lacteals. Observe Brunner glands in the submucosa (see Fig. 17.19, E, Lu, CL, LP, L). This medium-magnification photomicrograph of the duodenum presents the base of the crypts of Lieberkühn with Paneth cells and regenerative (or intermediate) cells. Brunner glands open into the base of the crypts of Lieberkühn and, occasionally, into the intervillar spaces (see Fig. 17.20, *arrowhead*, *arrows*, BG).

Jejunum

A low-magnification photomicrograph of the jejunum displays the well-developed villi and the crypts of Lieberkühn reaching the muscularis mucosae. Observe the absence of Brunner glands in the submucosa, as well as the lack of Peyer patches in the lamina propria. The inner circular and outer longitudinal layers of the muscularis externa are well differentiated, as is the Auerbach myenteric plexus between the two smooth muscle layers. Note the subserosal connective tissue and the serosa covering the muscularis externa (see Fig. 17.22, CL, MM, S, Ic, OL). At a high magnification, the lumen of the crypts of Lieberkühn are well demonstrated, as are their Paneth cells, regenerative or intermediate cells, as well as the DNES cells. A plasma cell of the lamina propria is also identified. Observe the muscularis mucosae bordering the submucosa in which blood vessels and lymph vessels abound. The inner circular layer of the muscularis externa is also identified (see Fig. 17.24, L, *arrowheads*, *arrow*, DNES, PlC, MM, Sm, Ly, ME).

Continued

 Histology Laboratory Instructions: Digestive System—Alimentary CanaL—cont'd

Ileum

At a very low magnification, the entire wall of the ileum—from the lumen to the serosa—and subserosal connective tissue are evident. Observe the short villi and the crypts of Lieberkühn as they empty into the intervillar spaces. The lamina propria has a great deal of lymphoid infiltration, including aggregates of lymphoid nodules known as Peyer patches that, frequently but not in this specimen, extend into the submucosa. The muscularis mucosae is clearly visible, as are elements of the Auerbach myenteric plexus, located between the inner circular and outer longitudinal smooth muscle layers of the muscularis externa (see Fig. 17.25, L, Se, SSeCT, V, CoL, PPinLP, Sm, MM, *arrows*, IC, OL). At a medium magnification of the lower portion of the villi of the ileum, the goblet cell components of the villar epithelium are very obvious, as is their disgorging of their mucinogen into the intervillar spaces. DNES cells are also evident, as is a mitotic figure of a crypt of Lieberkühn regenerative cell. Observe that the lamina propria is separated from the submucosa by the muscularis mucosae. In this specimen, Peyer patches extend from the lamina propria into the submucosa (see Fig. 17.26, GC, *arrowhead*, *white arrows*, MF, MM, SM). A high magnification photomicrograph of the Auerbach myenteric plexus, located between the inner circular and outer longitudinal smooth muscle layers of the muscularis externa, displays its ganglion cells and associated enteric glial cells. Additionally, observe the myelin sheath of the Schwann cell that surrounds the axon of a neuron that modifies the activity of the enteric nervous system neurons (see Fig. 17.29, IC, OL, GC, GlC, SC).

Large Intestine

Colon

Looking at a very low magnification of the colon, the first thing to note is that there are no villi protruding into the lumen, but crypts of Lieberkühn are present and their simple columnar epithelial lining displays numerous goblet cells. The submucosa, located between the muscularis mucosae and the muscularis externa, is thrown into half moon–shaped folds (see Fig. 17.32, L, CL, Sm, MM, ME). A low-magnification photomicrograph of the colon displays the presence of surface absorptive cells and goblet cells lining the lumina of the crypts of Lieberkühn, as well as the lining of the colon's lumen. Careful observation demonstrates the absence of Paneth cells at the bottom of the crypts of Lieberkühn, which contacts the muscularis mucosae. The submucosa and the inner circular layer of the muscularis externa are easily recognized (see Fig. 17.33, G, O, CL, MM, SM, ME). Medium magnification of the lower portions of the crypts of Lieberkühn displays goblet cells, surface absorptive cells, regenerative cells/intermediate cells, and DNES cells. The lamina propria is rich in lymphoid cells, especially plasma cells (see Fig. 17.34, E, P).

Appendix

A very-low-magnification photomicrograph of the appendix demonstrates that its lumen, frequently occupied by debris, is lined by a simple columnar epithelium that dips into the shallow crypts of Lieberkühn. The lamina propria is highly infiltrated by lymphoid elements, including numerous primary and secondary (displaying germinal centers) lymphoid nodules. The submucosa has a sparse amount of adipose cells. The muscularis externa, surrounded by a serosa, has an inner circular and outer longitudinal smooth muscle layer (see Fig. 17.36, L, E, CL, LP, LN, GC, SM, A C, Se, IC, OL). A low-magnification photomicrograph of the appendix displays its lumen, lined by a simple columnar epithelium. Crypts of Lieberkühn are sparsely distributed and the lamina propria and submucosa are occupied by a large secondary lymphoid nodule whose corona and germinal center are well differentiated. Much of the field is densely populated by lymphoid cells (see Fig. 17.37, L, CL, Co, GC).

18 Digestive System: Glands

The major salivary glands associated with the oral cavity, pancreas, and liver are considered to be the **extramural glands** of the digestive system. Each of these glands has numerous functions aiding the digestive process; their secretory products are delivered to the lumen of the alimentary tract by a system of ducts.

Major Salivary Glands

There are three pairs of major salivary glands: parotid, sublingual, and submandibular.

The paired parotid, sublingual, and submandibular glands, constituting the major salivary glands, are branched (**compound**) **tubuloacinar glands** whose dense, irregular, collagenous connective tissue capsule provides connective tissue septa that subdivide the glands into lobes and lobules. The vascular and neural components of the glands reach the secretory units via their connective tissue elements. Individual acini are also invested by thin connective tissue elements. Each of the major salivary glands has a secretory and duct portion (Fig. 18.1), where the secretory portion manufactures and releases saliva, known as **primary saliva**, into the system of ducts whose cells are impermeable to water. Cells of the striated ducts use active and passive transports to remove sodium and chloride ions from and add bicarbonate and potassium ions to the primary saliva. In effect, the isotonic primary saliva loses electrolytes, thereby making it hypotonic. This more dilute saliva is known as **secondary saliva** and is delivered into the oral cavity. The flow rate of saliva is in an indirect relationship to its tonicity; the faster the saliva flows along the striated duct, the less time the ductal cells have to alter salivary composition, and the closer the tonicity of the secondary saliva is to that of the primary saliva. The only exception to this is the concentration of bicarbonate ion, whose secretion is stimulated in concert with stimulation of primary saliva secretion.

SECRETORY PORTION

The secretory portion of salivary glands is composed of serous and/or mucous secretory cells arranged in acini or tubules that are couched by myoepithelial cells.

The **secretory portion**, arranged in tubules and acini, is composed of serous cells, mucous cells, and myoepithelial cells.

Serous Cells

Serous cells (Fig. 18.2) resemble truncated pyramids with a single, round, basally located nucleus, a well-developed rough endoplasmic reticulum (RER) and Golgi complex, and numerous basal mitochondria. These cells also possess an abundance of apically situated secretory granules rich in **salivary amylase** (**ptyalin**), an enzyme that initiates the digestion of complex carbohydrates into sugars, which they secrete along with **secretory component** (of the secretory immunoglobulin A [IgA] molecule), **lactoferrin**, **lysozyme**, and **thiocyanate** (the last three control the microbial levels of the oral cavity). The lateral plasmalemma, basal to the tight junctions, forms many processes that interdigitate and form tight junctions with those of neighboring cells.

The basal aspect of the serous cells possesses **IgA dimer receptor molecules** that bind IgA dimers manufactured by plasma cells located in the connective tissue. The bound **IgA dimer–IgA dimer receptor molecule complex** becomes internalized into the serous cell and is transferred into early endosomes, where a portion of the receptor molecule is cleaved. The remainder of the receptor molecule, known as the ***secretory component***, remains attached to the IgA dimer, which becomes known as ***secretory IgA (sIgA)***. The sIgA is released into the saliva, where the secretory component protects it from enzymatic digestion while the immunoglobulin is still capable of combating antigens.

Mucous Cells

Mucous cells are similar in shape to the serous cells. Their nuclei are also basally located but are flattened instead of being

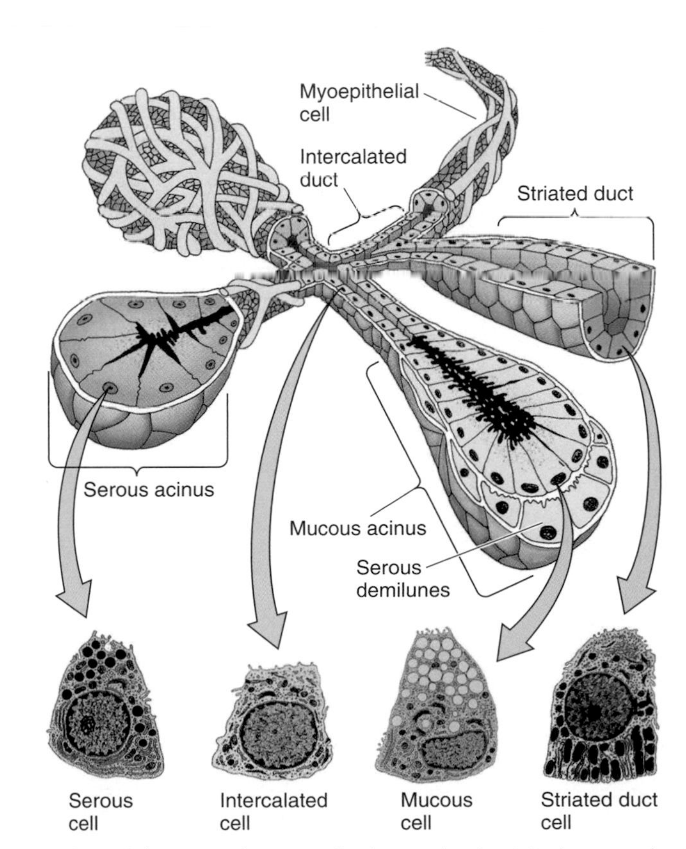

Fig. 18.1 Schematic diagram of salivary gland acini, ducts, and cell types.

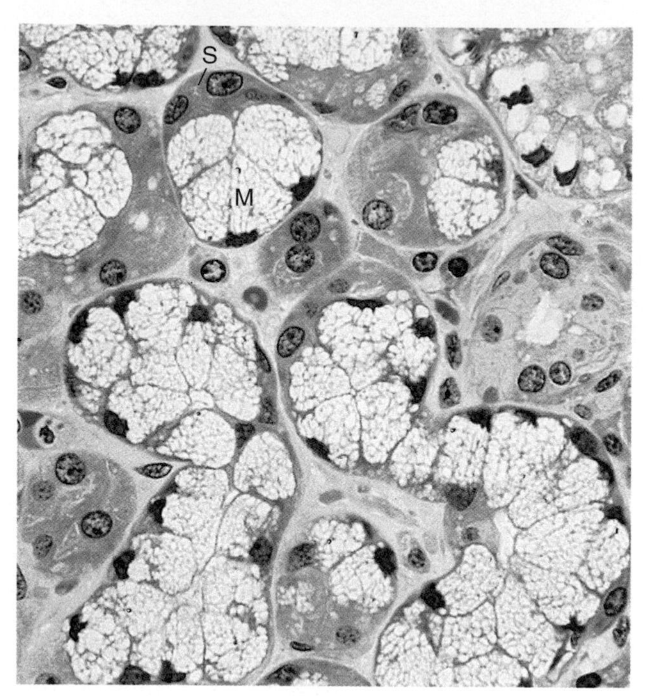

Fig. 18.2 Photomicrograph of the monkey sublingual gland displaying mucous acini (M) with serous demilunes (S). Note that serous demilunes may be fixation artifacts. (×540)

round (see Fig. 18.2). The organelle population of these cells differs from that of the serous cells in that mucous secretory cells have fewer mitochondria, a less extensive RER, and a considerably greater Golgi apparatus, indicative of the greater carbohydrate component of their secretory product (Fig. 18.3). The apical region of the cytoplasm is occupied by abundant secretory granules housing **mucinogen**, which, when released into the ducts of the gland, becomes hydrated and is known as ***mucin***, a slippery, viscous substance. When mucin contacts and is intermixed with substances present in the oral cavity, it becomes known as ***mucus***. The intercellular canaliculi and processes of the basal cell membranes are much less extensive than those of serous cells.

Myoepithelial Cells

Myoepithelial cells (**basket cells**) share the basal laminae of the acinar cells. They have a cell body and several long processes that envelop the secretory acinus and intercalated ducts (see Fig. 18.1). The cell body houses a small complement of organelles in addition to the nucleus and makes hemidesmosomal attachments with the basal lamina. The cytoplasmic processes, which form desmosomal contacts with the acinar and duct cells, are rich in actin and myosin; in electron micrographs, these processes resemble smooth muscle cells. As the processes of myoepithelial cells contract, they compress the acinus, facilitating release of the secretory product into the duct of the gland.

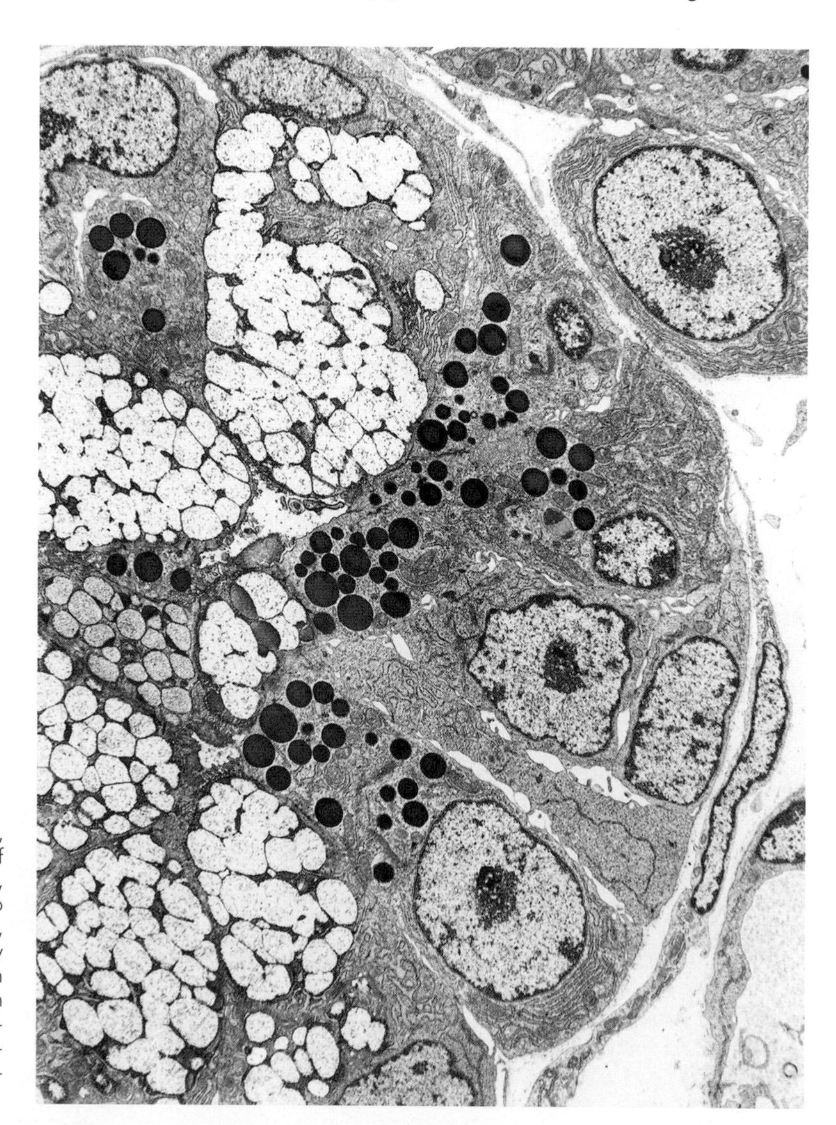

Fig. 18.3 Electron micrograph of the rat sublingual gland, displaying serous and mucous granules in the cytoplasm of their acinar cells. Note that the nuclei of serous cells are round, whereas the nuclei of mucous cells are flattened. Observe also that the serous secretory products are present as round, dense, dark structures, and the mucous secretory products are mostly dissolved and appear light in color and spongy (×5400). (From Redman RS, Ball WD. Cytodifferentiation of secretory cells in the sublingual glands of the prenatal rat: a histological, histochemical, and ultrastructural study. *Am J Anat.* 1978;153:367-390. Reprinted with permission from Wiley-Liss, Inc., a subsidiary of John Wiley & Sons, Inc.)

DUCT PORTION

The ducts of major salivary glands are highly branched and range from very small intercalated ducts to very large principal (terminal) ducts.

The ducts of major salivary glands are highly branched structures. The smallest branches of the system of ducts are the **intercalated ducts**, to which the secretory acini (and tubules) are attached. These small ducts are composed of a single layer of low cuboidal cells and possess some myoepithelial cells. Several intercalated ducts merge to form **striated ducts**, composed of a single layer of cuboidal to low columnar cells (see Fig. 18.1). Accentuated infoldings of the basolateral cell membranes subdivide the basal aspect of the cytoplasm into longitudinal compartments that are occupied by elongated mitochondria.

Striated ducts join together, forming **intralobular ducts** of increasing caliber, which are surrounded by more abundant connective tissue elements. Ducts arising from lobules unite to form **interlobular ducts**, which, in turn, form **intralobar** and **interlobar ducts**. The **terminal** (**principal**) **duct** of the gland delivers saliva into the oral cavity.

SALIVON

The acinus, intercalated duct, and striated duct together, according to some authors, constitute the **salivon**, the functional unit of a salivary gland.

HISTOPHYSIOLOGY OF THE SALIVARY GLANDS

Secretory cells of acini produce primary saliva that is modified by striated ducts to form secondary saliva.

The major salivary glands produce approximately 700 to 1100 mL of saliva per day. Minor salivary glands are located in the mucosa and submucosa of the oral cavity, but they contribute only 3 to 5 mL to the total daily salivary output. In order to be able to provide such a large salivary output, the major salivary glands have an extraordinarily rich vascular supply. In fact, it has been estimated that the basal rate of blood flow to salivary glands is 20 times greater than the flow of blood to skeletal muscle. During maximal secretion, the blood flow is correspondingly increased.

Saliva has numerous functions, including lubricating and cleansing of the oral cavity, antibacterial activity, participating in taste sensation by dissolving food material, initial digestion via the action of salivary amylase (ptyalin) and salivary lipase, aiding swallowing by moistening the food and permitting the formation of bolus, and participating in the clotting process and wound healing because of the clotting factors and epidermal growth factor present in saliva.

Acinar cells and duct cells also synthesize the secretory component required to transfer IgA from the connective tissue into the lumen of the secretory acinus or duct (see section on ducts). **Secretory IgA** complexes with antigens in the saliva, mitigating their deleterious effects. Saliva also contains lactoferrin, lysozyme, and thiocyanate ions. **Lactoferrin** binds iron, an element essential for bacterial metabolism; **lysozyme** breaks down bacterial capsules, permitting the entry of **thiocyanate ions**, a bactericidal agent, into the bacteria.

The cells of the salivary gland striated ducts secrete the enzyme **kallikrein** into the connective tissue. Kallikrein enters the bloodstream, where it converts kininogens, a family of plasma proteins, into **bradykinin**, a vasodilator that dilates blood vessels and enhances blood flow to the region.

ROLE OF AUTONOMIC NERVE SUPPLY IN SALIVARY SECRETION

The major salivary glands do not secrete continuously. Secretory activity is stimulated via **parasympathetic** and **sympathetic innervation**. Innervation may be intraepithelial (i.e., formation of a synaptic contact between the end-foot and acinar cell) or subepithelial. In subepithelial innervation, the end-feet of axons do not make synaptic contact with the acinar cells. Instead, they release their acetylcholine in the vicinity of the secretory cell at a distance of approximately 100 to 200 nm from its basal plasmalemma. The cell, thus activated, stimulates neighboring cells via **gap junctions** to release their serous secretory product into the lumen of the acinus.

Parasympathetic innervation is the major initiator of salivation and is responsible for the formation of serous saliva. Acetylcholine, released by the postganglionic parasympathetic nerve fibers, binds to muscarinic cholinergic receptors, with consequent release of inositol triphosphate, prompting the liberation of calcium ions, a second messenger, into the cytosol, which facilitates the secretion of serous saliva from the acinar cells.

Initially, **sympathetic innervation** reduces blood flow to the salivons, but that reduction is reversed in short order. Norepinephrine, released by the postganglionic sympathetic fibers, binds to β-adrenergic receptors, resulting in the formation of **cyclic adenosine monophosphate** (**cAMP, cyclic AMP**). This secondary messenger activates a cascade of kinases that result in the secretion of the mucous and enzymatic components of saliva by the acinar cells. The mucous element is responsible for the adhesion of food particles to one another in the bolus, as well as for the creation of a slippery surface, facilitating swallowing.

Salivary output is enhanced by the taste and smell of food, as well as by the process of chewing. Inhibitors of salivation include fatigue, fear, and dehydration; moreover, salivary flow is greatly reduced while the individual is asleep.

Properties of Individual Salivary Glands

PAROTID GLAND

Although physically the largest of the salivary glands, the two parotid glands produce only about 30% of the total salivary output; the saliva that they produce is serous.

The largest of the salivary glands, the two **parotid glands**, each weigh about 20 to 30 g but produce only approximately 30% of the total salivary output. Although the parotid gland is said to produce a purely **serous secretion** (Figs. 18.4 and 18.5), the secretory product does have a small amount of mucous component. Electron micrographs of the apical regions of serous cells display numerous secretory granules filled with an electron-dense product that has an even more electron-dense core of unknown composition.

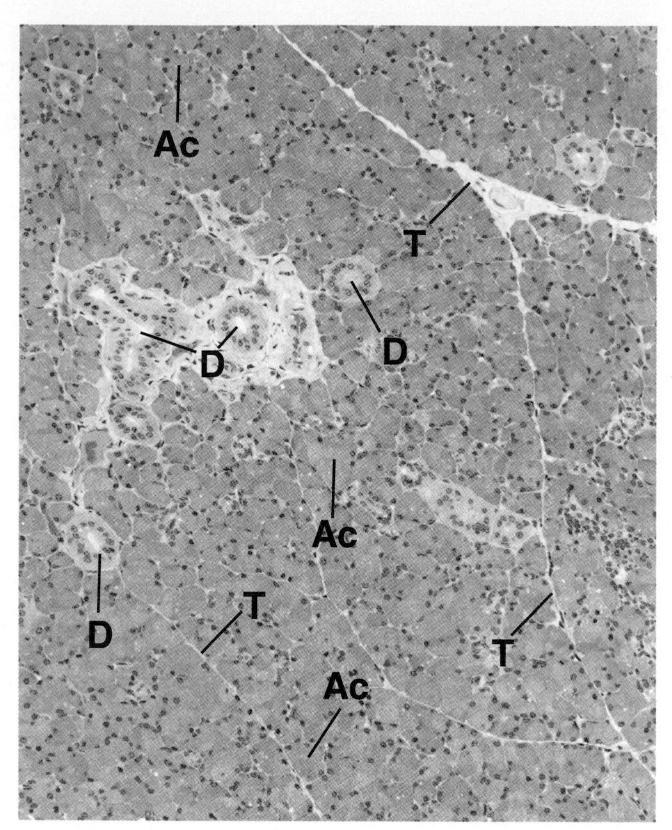

Fig. 18.4 This low-magnification photomicrograph of the parotid gland lobe displays how the septa (T) subdivide the gland into lobules. Note that the acini (Ac) are composed of serous cells with round nuclei. The numerous ducts deliver the saliva into the oral cavity. (×132)

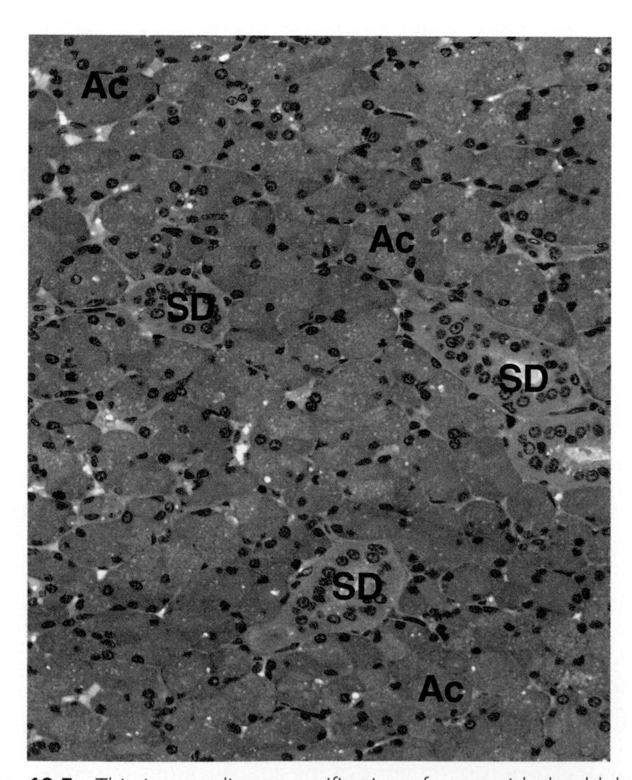

Fig. 18.5 This is a medium magnification of a parotid gland lobule displaying that the cells of the acini (Ac) possess basally located round nuclei. The striated ducts (SD) are characterized by round nuclei located near the center of the cells composing the duct and by the scant amount of connective tissue surrounding them. (×270)

The saliva produced by the parotid gland has high levels of the enzyme **salivary amylase** (**ptyalin**), responsible for digestion of most of the starch in food, and secretory IgA, which inactivates antigens located in the oral cavity.

The connective tissue capsule of the parotid gland is well developed and forms numerous septa, which subdivide the gland into lobes and lobules. By the fifth decade of life, the gland becomes invaded by adipose tissue, which spreads from the connective tissue into the glandular parenchyma.

SUBLINGUAL GLAND

The paired sublingual glands are very small, are composed mostly of mucous acini with serous demilunes, and produce mixed saliva.

The smallest of the three pairs of major salivary glands, the **sublingual glands**, is almond shaped and each weighs only 2 to 3 g, producing only about 5% of the total salivary output. Each gland is composed of mucous tubular secretory units, many of which are capped by a small cluster of serous cells, known as ***serous demilunes*** (Figs. 18.2, 18.6, and 18.7). Although routine light microscopy demonstrates the presence of serous demilunes, if the tissue is flash frozen, serous demilunes are absent, indicating that they may be fixation artifacts and are merely small clusters of serous cells that deliver their secretion into a lumen in common with the mucous tubular secretory units. Under normal fixation at room temperature, the mucinogen of the mucous cells become swollen, and they enlarge the cells containing

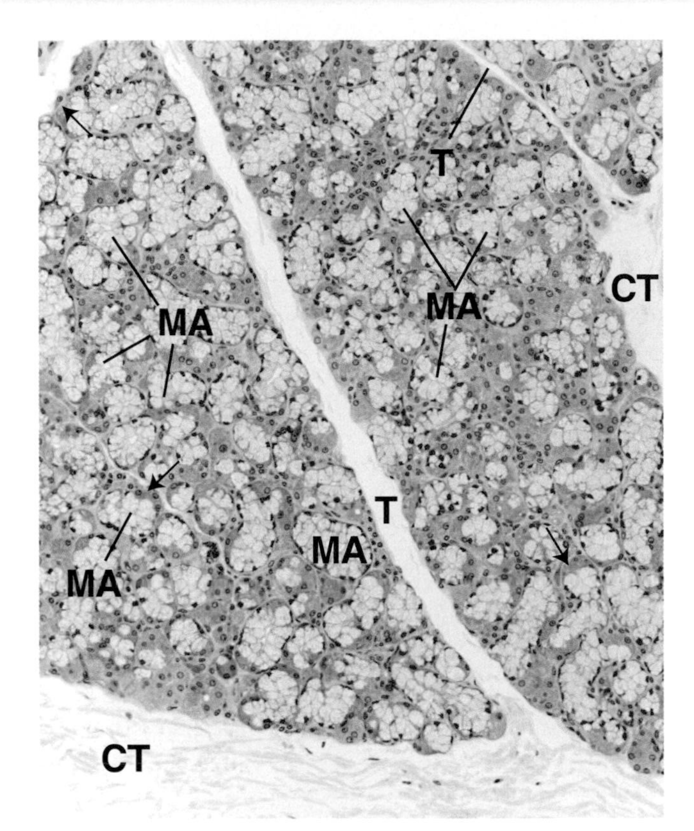

Fig. 18.6 This low-magnification photomicrograph of the sublingual gland displays connective tissue (CT) organized into septae (T) of various thicknesses that subdivide the gland into lobes and lobules. Observe the preponderance of mucous acini (MA) with their serous demilunes *(arrows)*. (×132).

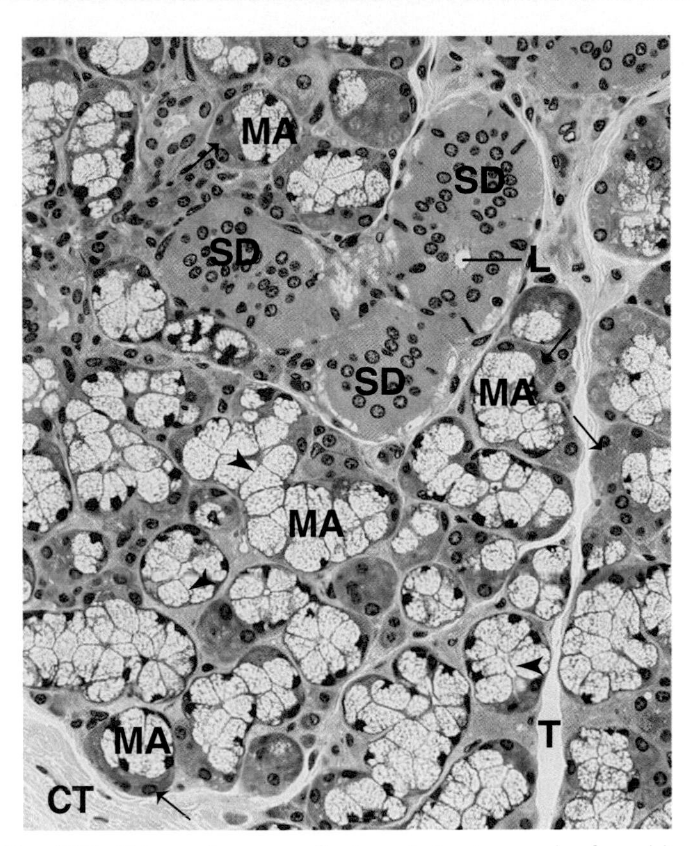

Fig. 18.7 This medium-magnification photomicrograph of a sublingual gland displays sections of one of the more striated ducts (SD) with a central lumen (L). Observe that the nuclei are more or less centrally placed within the cells composing the duct. The mucous acini (MA) are composed of several cells whose cell membranes are indicated by *arrowheads* and are filled with secretory vesicles whose contents have been extracted during the slide preparation. Note that the nuclei of the mucinogen-producing cells are basally located and present a flattened morphology. The serous demilunes *(arrows)* are composed of serous cells with round, centrally located nuclei. Connective tissue septa (T) subdivide the gland into lobes and lobules. (×270)

them to such an extent that they squeeze most of the serous cells away from the lumen of the acinus; thus, the serous cells form a cap between the swollen mucous cells and the basement membrane. If the tissue is flash frozen, the mucinogen does not swell and the serous cells remain in their normal position, adjacent to the mucous cells. These serous cells have been shown to secrete lysozyme. The sublingual gland produces a mixed, but mostly mucous, saliva. The intercellular canaliculi are well developed between the mucous cells of the secretory units. Electron micrographs of the cells of the serous demilunes display apical accumulations of secretory vesicles. However, unlike the cells of the parotid and submandibular glands, these vesicles do not have an electron-dense core (see Fig. 18.3).

The sublingual gland has a slender connective tissue capsule, and its duct system does not form a terminal duct. Instead, several ducts open into the floor of the mouth and into the duct of the submandibular gland. Because of the organization of the ducts, some authors consider the sublingual gland to be composed of several smaller glandular subunits.

SUBMANDIBULAR GLAND

The paired submandibular glands produce 60% of the total salivary output. Although these glands manufacture a mixed saliva, the saliva that they produce is mostly serous.

The pair of **submandibular glands**, although only 12 to 15 g in weight each, produces approximately 60% of the total salivary output. About 90% of the acini produce serous saliva, whereas the remainder of the acini manufactures a mucous saliva. Electron micrographs of the apical aspects of the serous cells display electron-dense secretory products, with a denser core, within membrane-bound secretory granules. The number of serous demilunes is limited. The striated ducts of the submandibular gland are much longer than those of the parotid or sublingual glands; therefore, histological sections of this gland display many cross-sectional profiles of these ducts, a characteristic feature of the submandibular gland (Figs. 18.8–18.10).

The connective tissue capsule of the submandibular gland is extensive and forms abundant septa, which subdivide the gland into lobes and lobules. Fatty infiltration of the connective tissue elements into the parenchyma is evident by midlife.

Clinical Correlations

1. *Benign pleomorphic adenoma, a noncancerous salivary gland tumor, usually affects the parotid and submandibular glands. Surgical removal of the parotid gland must be performed with care because of the presence of the facial nerve plexus within the substance of the gland. Because the facial nerve supplies motor innervation to*

Continued

Clinical Correlations—cont'd

the muscles of facial expression, damage to its branches during parotidectomy may cause temporary or even permanent paralysis of the muscles served by the damaged fibers.

2. *The parotid gland (and occasionally other major salivary glands) is also affected by viral infections, causing* **mumps**, *a painful disease in children that may result in sterility when it affects adults.*
3. *About 25% of the cancers involving the parotid gland are considered to be* **acinic cell carcinoma**, *a slow-growing malignancy that can recur after surgical removal. Occasionally, the carcinoma metastasizes to other organs.*

Pancreas

The pancreas is both an exocrine gland that produces digestive juices and an endocrine gland that manufactures hormones.

The **pancreas**, about 25 cm long, 5 cm wide, and 1 to 2 cm thick, weighing approximately 150 g, is situated on the posterior body wall, deep to the peritoneum. It has four regions: uncinate process, head, body, and tail. Its flimsy connective tissue capsule forms septa, which subdivide the gland into lobules and conveys its vascular and nerve supply, as well as its system of ducts. The pancreas produces exocrine and endocrine secretions. Scattered among its exocrine **secretory acini** are the endocrine components of the pancreas, known as **islets of Langerhans** (Figs. 18.11 and 18.12).

EXOCRINE PANCREAS

The exocrine pancreas is a compound tubuloacinar gland that produces daily about 1200 mL of a bicarbonate-rich fluid containing digestive proenzymes. Forty to 50 acinar cells form a round to oval **acinus** whose lumen is occupied by three or four **centroacinar cells**, the beginning of the duct system of the pancreas. The presence of **centroacinar cells** in the center of the acinus is a distinguishing characteristic of the exocrine portion of this gland.

Secretory and Duct Portions

The acinar cells of the pancreas have receptors for the hormone ***cholecystokinin (CCK)*** *and the neurotransmitter* ***acetylcholine****, whereas the centroacinar cells and intercalated ducts have receptors for secretin and for acetylcholine.*

Each **acinar cell** is shaped like a truncated pyramid, with its base positioned on the basal lamina separating the acinar cells from the connective tissue compartment. The round nucleus of the cell is basally located and surrounded by basophilic cytoplasm. The apex of the cell, facing the lumen of the acinus, is filled with proenzyme-containing **secretory granules** (**zymogen granules**), whose number diminishes after a meal (Fig. 18.13 and 18.14).

Electron micrographs of acinar cells display an abundance of basally located RER, a rich supply of polysomes, and numerous mitochondria exhibiting matrix granules. The Golgi apparatus is well developed but fluctuates in size, being smaller when the zymogen granules are numerous and larger after the granules release their contents. The zymogen granules may release their contents individually, or several secretory vesicles may fuse, forming a channel to the lumen of the acinus from the apical cytoplasm.

The basal cell membranes of acinar cells have receptors for the hormone **CCK**, released by diffuse neuroendocrine system (DNES) cells of the small intestine, and for the neurotransmitter **acetylcholine**, released by postganglionic parasympathetic nerve fibers.

The **duct system** of the pancreas begins within the center of the acinus with the terminus of the **intercalated ducts**, composed of pale, low cuboidal **centroacinar cells** (see Figs. 18.11 and 18.13). Centroacinar cells and intercalated ducts both have receptors on their basal plasmalemma for

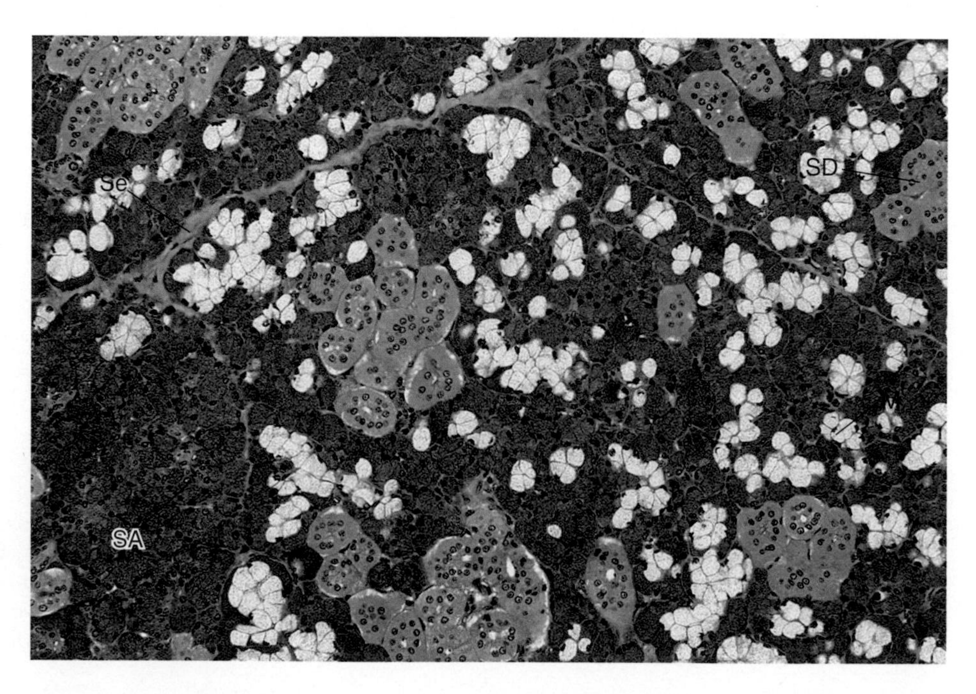

Fig. 18.8 The submandibular gland is characterized by the numerous cross-sectional profiles of striated ducts. Note that the ducts appear pale pink, and many display a very small but clear lumen. The mucous secretory product has a frothy-looking appearance. Se, Septum; SA, serous acinus; SD, serous demilune; M, mucous cell of the acinus. (×132)

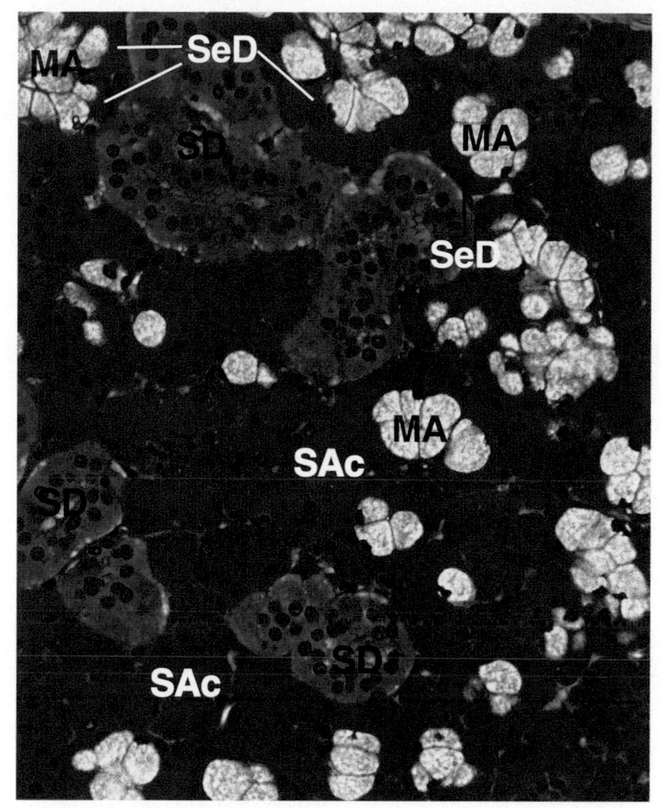

Fig. 18.9 The submandibular gland produces mainly serous saliva. Accordingly, most of its acini are serous (SAc) with some mucous tubules (MA) capped with serous demilunes (SeD). One of the most characteristic features of the submandibular gland is the presence of a large number of striated duct (SD) profiles. (×270)

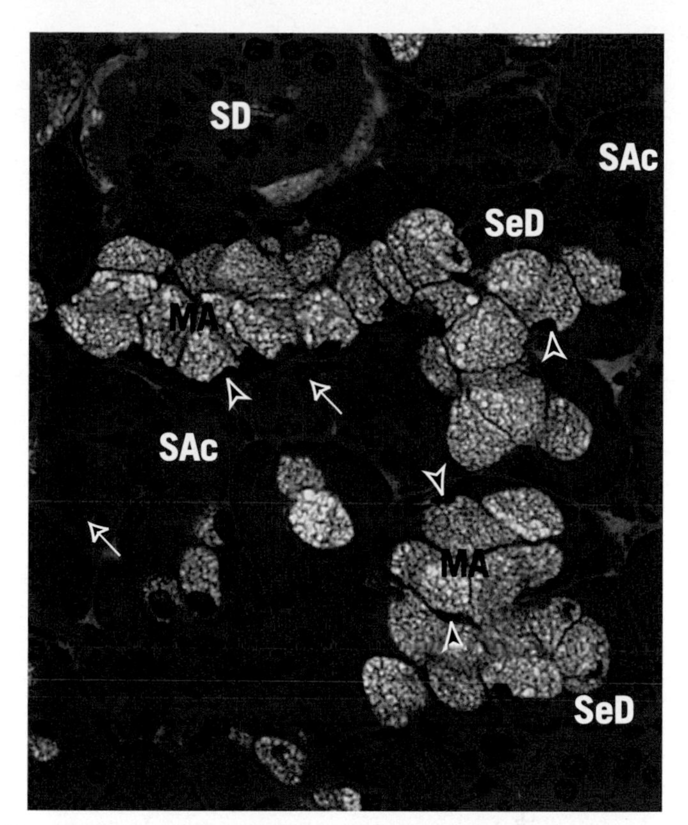

Fig. 18.10 This high-magnification photomicrograph of the submandibular gland demonstrates the flattened nuclei of the mucous cells *(arrowheads)* in contrast with the round nuclei of the serous cells *(arrows)*. Observe the numerous serous acini (SAc), as well as the serous demilunes (SeD) capping the mucous acini (MA). (×270)

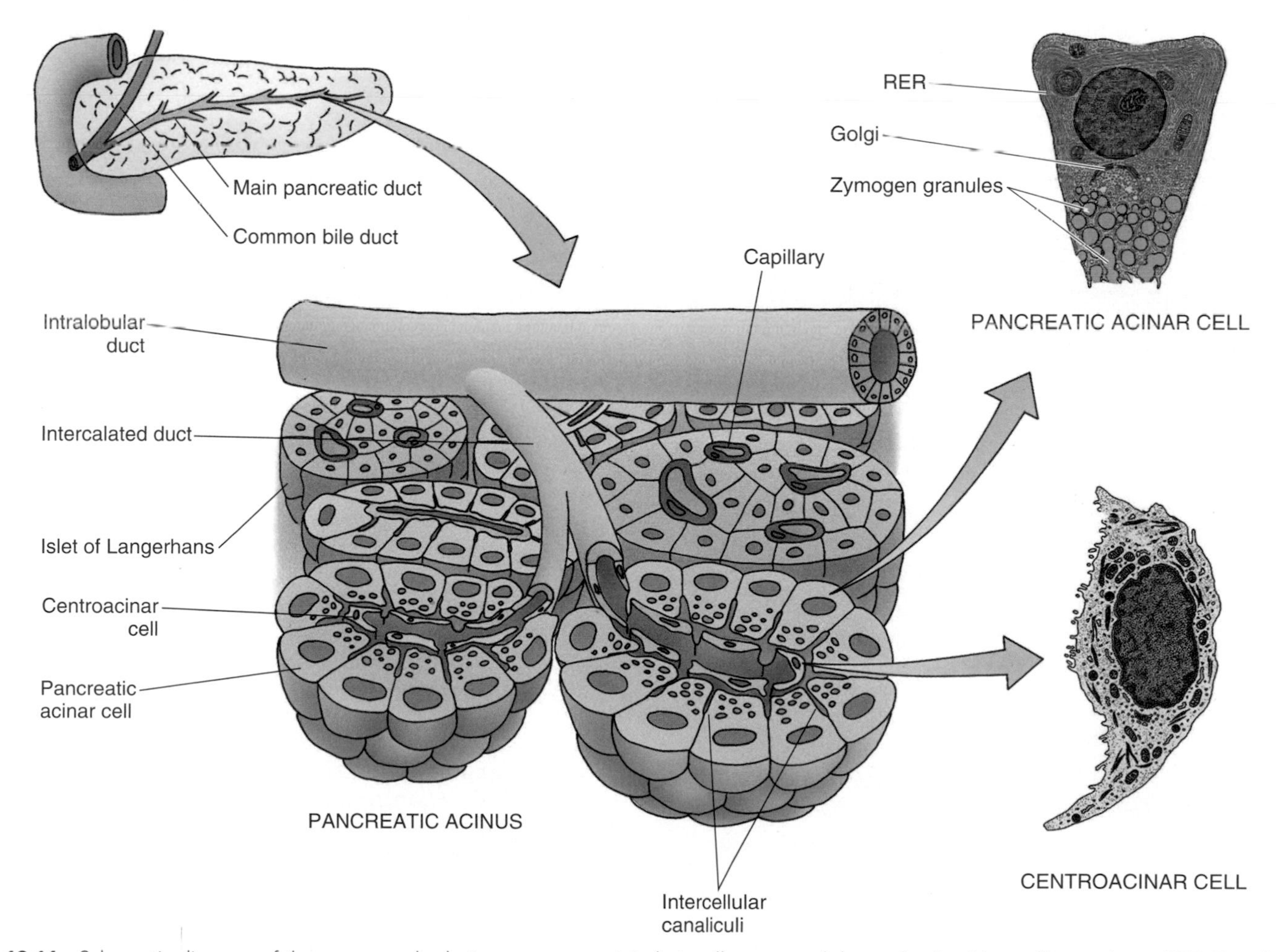

Fig. 18.11 Schematic diagram of the pancreas displaying secretory acini, their cell types, and the endocrine islets of Langerhans. RER, Rough endoplasmic reticulum.

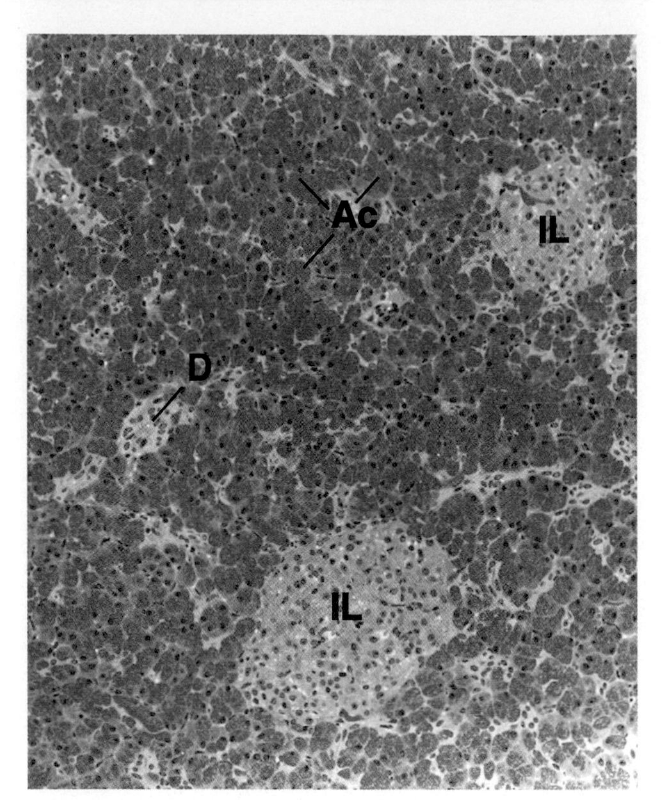

Fig. 18.12 This low-magnification photomicrograph displays the exocrine portion of the pancreas, the secretory acini (Ac), some of the duct system (D), the endocrine portion, and the islets of Langerhans (IL). (×132)

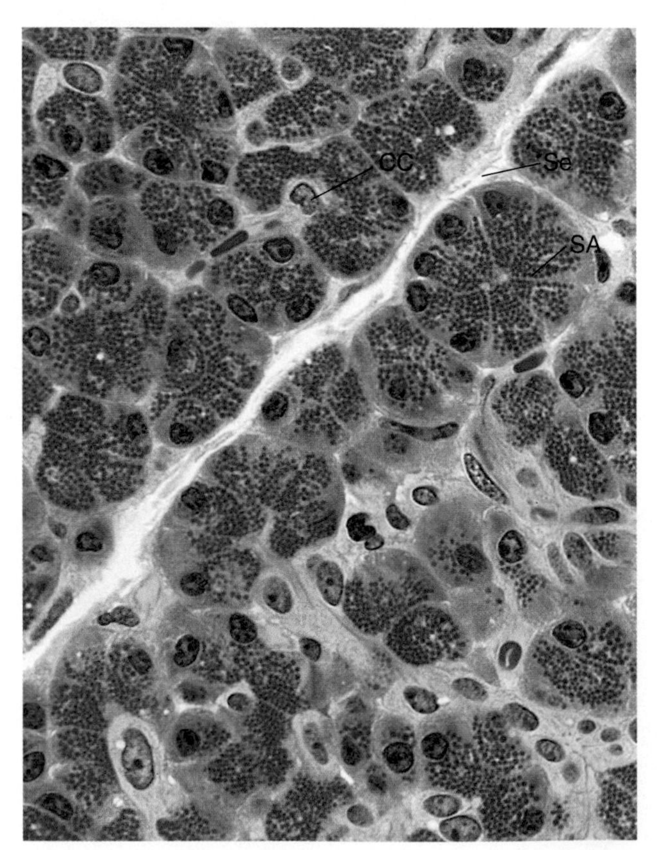

Fig. 18.13 Photomicrograph of the monkey exocrine pancreas. Observe that the acini in section appear to be round structures, and much of the acinar cells have many secretory granules, known as *zymogen granules*. CC, Centroacinar cell; Se, septum; SA, serous acinus. (×540)

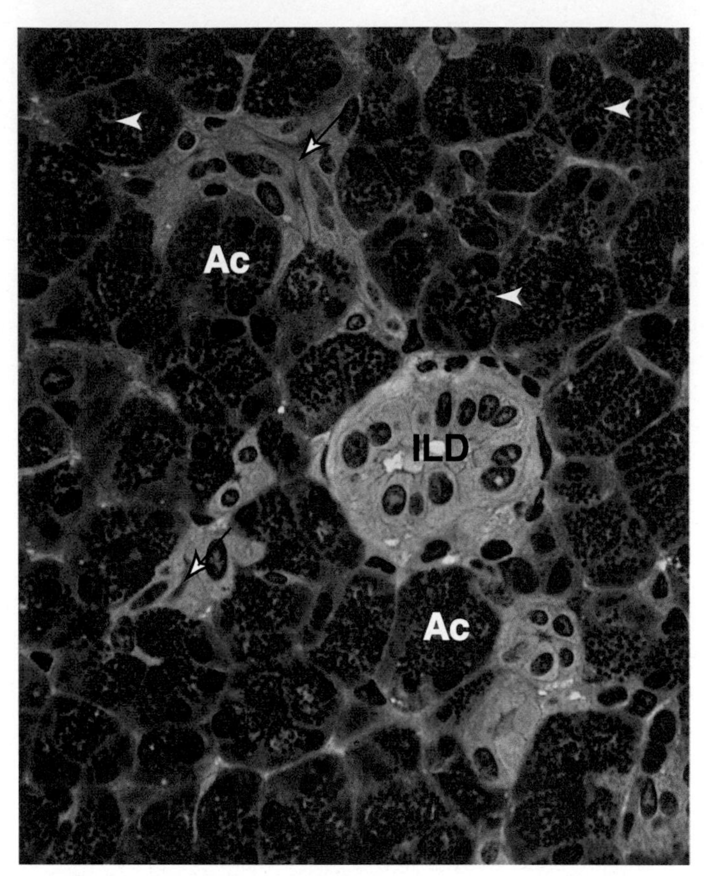

Fig. 18.14 Observe that at high magnification the intercalated ducts *(arrows)*, which deliver their contents into the interlobular ducts (ILD), are occasionally evident. Observe that the cells of the acini (Ac) are packed with secretory granules *(arrowheads)*. (×540)

the hormone **secretin**, released by DNES cells of the small intestine, and **acetylcholine**, released by postganglionic parasympathetic fibers. Intercalated ducts join to form larger **intralobular ducts**, several of which converge to form **interlobular ducts**. These ducts are surrounded by a considerable amount of connective tissue and deliver their contents into the **main pancreatic duct**, which joins the **common bile duct** before opening in the duodenum at the **papilla of Vater**.

Histophysiology of the Exocrine Pancreas

The acinar cells manufacture and release digestive enzymes, whereas the centroacinar cells and intercalated duct cells release a bicarbonate-rich buffer solution.

The acinar cells of the exocrine pancreas manufacture, store, and release a large number of enzymes: pancreatic amylase; pancreatic lipase; pancreatic cholesterol esterase; ribonuclease (RNase); deoxyribonuclease (DNase); elastase; and the proenzymes trypsinogen, chymotrypsinogen, and procarboxypolypeptidase (Table 18.1). The cells also manufacture **trypsin inhibitor**, a protein that protects the cell from accidental intracellular activation of trypsin, as well as its activation in the pancreatic duct.

Release of the pancreatic enzymes is effected by the hormone **CCK** manufactured by DNES cells of the small intestine (especially of the duodenum), as well as by **acetylcholine** released by the postganglionic parasympathetic nerve fibers. Both CCK and acetylcholine have to bind to their respective receptors located in

TABLE 18.1 Digestive Enzymes and Proenzymes Secreted by the Exocrine Pancreas

Enzyme/Proenzyme	Function
ENZYMES	
Pancreatic amylase	Breaks down starches, carbohydrates (although it cannot hydrolyze cellulose or chitin), and glycogen into disaccharides
Pancreatic lipase	Breaks down fats into fatty acids and monoglycerides
Pancreatic cholesterol esterase	Breaks down cholesterol esters into cholesterol and fatty acids
DNase and RNase	Break down DNA and RNA, respectively
Elastase	Breaks down the major component of elastic fibers, namely, elastin
PROENZYMES	
Trypsinogen	Converted into trypsin: breaks down proteins into short peptides
Chymotrypsinogen	Converted into chymotrypsin: breaks down proteins into short peptides
Procarboxypolypeptidase	Converted into carboxypolypeptidase: breaks down small peptides to form dipeptides and amino acids

the basal plasmalemmae of the pancreatic acinar cells before the enzymes and proenzymes can be released from the acinar cells.

The centroacinar cells and intercalated ducts manufacture a serous, bicarbonate-rich alkaline fluid, which neutralizes and buffers the acid chyme that enters the duodenum from the pyloric stomach. This fluid is enzyme poor, and its release is effected by the hormone **secretin**, produced by enteroendocrine cells of the small intestine in conjunction with **acetylcholine**, released by the postganglionic parasympathetic nerve fibers. Both secretin and acetylcholine have to bind to their respective receptors located in the basal plasmalemmae of the duct cells before the bicarbonate-rich fluid can be released from the duct cells. Thus, the enzyme-rich and enzyme-poor secretions are regulated separately, and the two secretions may be released at different times or concomitantly.

The mechanism of sodium bicarbonate secretion is facilitated by the enzyme **carbonic anhydrase**, which catalyzes the formation of carbonic acid (H_2CO_3) from water (H_2O) and carbon dioxide (CO_2). In the aquatic medium of the cytosol, H_2CO_3 dissociates to form H^+ and HCO_3^-; the HCO_3^- is *actively* transported into the lumen of the duct, and the hydrogen (H^+) ion is *actively* transported into the connective tissue elements in exchange for sodium ions (Na^+). The Na^+ passively enters the lumen, where it joins the HCO_3^- to form sodium bicarbonate. The movement of sodium and bicarbonate ions from the cell into the lumen of the duct establishes an osmotic gradient that is followed (*passively*) by the movement of water from the connective tissue into the duct cell and then into the lumen of the duct. This results in the creation of a buffer solution of sodium bicarbonate that is conveyed by the pancreatic duct into the duodenum to buffer the highly acidic chyme that enters the duodenum from the pyloric stomach.

Clinical Correlations

Occasionally, the pancreatic digestive enzymes become active within the cytoplasm of the acinar cells, resulting in ***acute pancreatitis****, which is often fatal. The histological changes involve inflammatory reaction, necrosis of the blood vessels, proteolysis of the pancreatic parenchyma, and enzymatic destruction of adipose cells, not only within the pancreas but also in the surrounding region of the abdominal cavity.*

Pancreatic cancer *is the fifth leading cause of mortality from all cancers, killing about 25,000 people in the United States per year. Fewer than 50% of patients survive more than 1 year, and fewer than 5% survive 5 years. Men are more susceptible to this disease than women. Cigarette smokers have a 70% greater risk for development of pancreatic cancers than nonsmokers.*

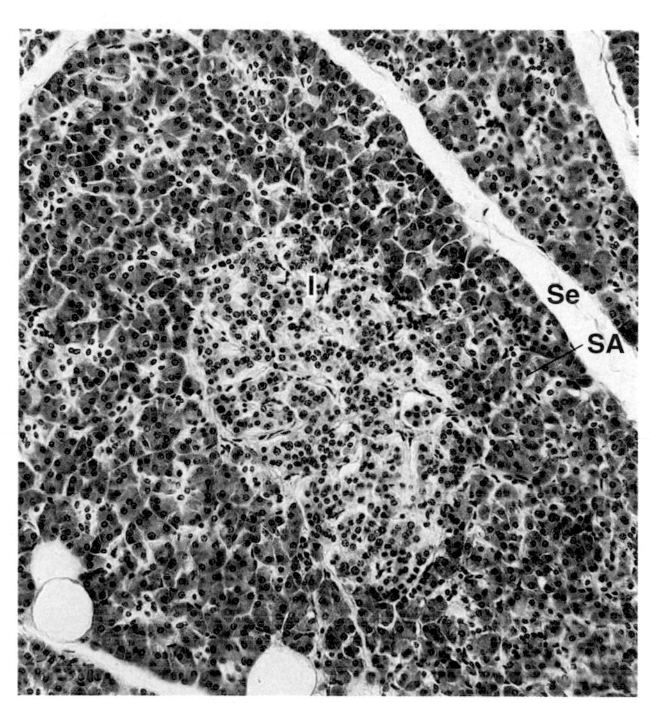

Fig. 18.15 Photomicrograph of the human pancreas displaying secretory acini and an islet of Langerhans (I). The histological difference between the exocrine and endocrine pancreas is very evident in this photomicrograph because the islet is much larger than individual acini and is much lighter in color. Se, Septum; SA, serous acinus. (×132)

ENDOCRINE PANCREAS

The endocrine pancreas is composed of spherical aggregates of cells, known as islets of Langerhans, that are scattered among the acini.

Each **islet of Langerhans** is a richly vascularized spherical conglomeration of approximately 3000 cells. The approximately 1 to 2 million islets distributed throughout the human pancreas constitute the endocrine pancreas. A somewhat greater number of islets are present in the tail than in the remaining regions. Each islet is about 300 μm in diameter and is surrounded by reticular fibers, which also enter the substance of the islet to encircle the network of capillaries that pervade it (Figs. 18.12 and 18.15).

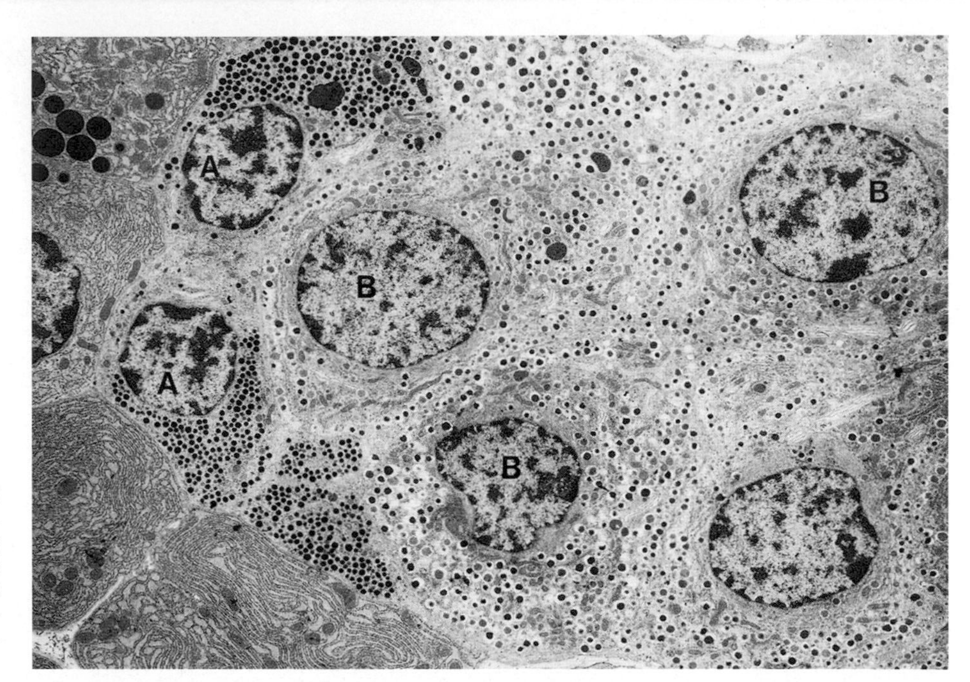

Fig. 18.16 Electron micrograph of α cells (A) and β cells (B) of the rabbit islet of Langerhans. Note that the granules of α cells are much more numerous, more tightly packed, smaller, and denser than those of β cells (×5040). (From Jorns A, Grube D. The endocrine pancreas of glucagon-immunized and somatostatin-immunized rabbits. *Cell Tissue Res.* 1991;265:261–273.)

TABLE 18.2 Cells and Hormones of the Islets of Langerhans

Cell	% of Total	Location	Fine Structure of Granules	Hormone and Molecular Weight	Function
β Cell	70	Scattered throughout islet (but concentrated in center)	300 nm in diameter; dense core granule surrounded by a wide electron-lucent halo	Insulin, 6000 Da Amylin, ~3200 Da	Decreases blood glucose levels Inhibits gastric emptying and glucagon release from α cells
α Cell	20	Islet periphery	250 nm in diameter; dense core granule with a narrow electron-lucent halo	Glucagon, 3500 Da	Increases blood glucose levels
δ Cell D	5	Scattered throughout islet	350 nm in diameter; electron-lucent homogeneous granule	Somatostatin, 1640 Da	*Paracrine:* inhibits hormone release from endocrine pancreas and enzymes from exocrine pancreas *Endocrine:* reduces contractions of alimentary tract and gallbladder smooth muscles
D_1				Vasoactive intestinal peptide, 3800 Da	Induces glycogenolysis; regulates smooth muscle tonus and motility of gut; controls ion and water secretion by intestinal epithelial cells
G cell	1	Scattered throughout islet	300 nm in diameter	Gastrin, 2000 Da	Stimulates production of hydrochloric acid by parietal cells of stomach
PP cell (F cell)	1	Scattered throughout islet	180 nm in diameter	Pancreatic polypeptide, 4200 Da	Inhibits exocrine secretions of pancreas
ε Cell (Epsilon cell)	1	Scattered throughout islet	?	Ghrelin	Induces the sensation of hunger and modulates receptive relaxation of the smooth muscle fibers of the muscularis externa of the gastrointestinal tract

Cells Composing the Islets of Langerhans

Each islet of Langerhans is composed of 5 types of parenchymal cells: beta (β) cells, alpha (α) cells, delta (δ) cells (D and D_1 cells), PP cells, and G cells. These cells cannot be differentiated by routine histological examination, but immunocytochemical procedures allow them to be recognized. Electron micrographs also display the features that distinguish the various cells, especially the size and electron density of their granules. Otherwise, the cells do not exhibit any unusual morphological features but rather resemble cells that specialize in protein synthesis. The characteristic features, locations, and hormones synthesized by these cells are presented in Table 18.2.

TABLE 18.3 Control of Insulin Release by Beta Cells

Induction of Insulin Release	Inhibition of Insulin Release
Elevated blood glucose levels	Decreased blood glucose levels
Elevated levels of free fatty acids in the blood	Leptin
Elevated levels of amino acids in the blood	Somatostatin
Cortisol and growth hormone	Fasting
Obesity	
Insulin resistance	
Gastric inhibitory peptide, secretin, CCK, and gastrin from intestinal DNES cells	

CCK, Cholecystokinin; *DNES*, diffuse neuroendocrine system.

Histophysiology of the Endocrine Pancreas

The cells of the islets of Langerhans produce insulin, glucagon, somatostatin, vasoactive intestinal peptide, gastrin, pancreatic polypeptide, ghrelin, and amylin.

The two hormones produced in the greatest amounts by the endocrine pancreas—insulin and glucagon—act to decrease and increase blood glucose levels, respectively (Table 18.3***).***

Insulin production begins with synthesis of a single polypeptide chain, **preproinsulin**, on the RER of **β cells**. Within the RER cisternae, this initial product is converted to **proinsulin** by enzymatic cleavage of a polypeptide fragment. Within the *trans*-Golgi network, proinsulin is packaged into clathrin-coated vesicles and a segment of the proinsulin molecule near its center is removed by self-excision. This process forms insulin, which is released into the intercellular space in response to increased blood glucose levels, as occurs after consumption of a carbohydrate-rich meal (see Table 18.3).

The released insulin binds to cell-surface insulin receptors on many cells, especially skeletal muscle, liver, and adipose cells. The plasma membranes of these cells also have glucose transport proteins, **glucose transporter protein-4** (**GLUT-4**), which are activated to take up glucose, thus decreasing blood glucose levels. Subplasmalemmal vesicles, rich in GLUT-4, are added to the cell membrane during insulin stimulation and returned to their intracellular position when insulin levels are reduced.

Glucagon, a peptide hormone produced by **α cells**, is released in response to low blood glucose levels, as well as by the consumption of a meal low in carbohydrates and high in proteins. As in insulin production, a prohormone is produced first, and it undergoes proteolytic cleavage to yield the active hormone. Glucagon acts mainly on hepatocytes, causing these cells to activate a cascade of enzymes that eventually leads to the activation of **glycogenolytic enzymes**. It does that by activating the hepatocyte cell membrane-bound enzyme **adenylyl cyclase** that, in turn, responds by the formation of the second messenger, **cAMP**. It is the cAMP that activates a **protein kinase regulator protein** that results in the formation of the enzyme **glycogen phosphorylase**, which liberates **glucose-1-phosphate** (**G-1-P**) molecules from glycogen. The newly formed G-1-P is dephosphorylated, forming glucose, and is released into the bloodstream, increasing blood glucose levels. Once the intracellular glycogen depot in liver cells is depleted, glucagon activates **hormone-sensitive lipase** and **adipose triglyceride lipase** in fat cells. These enzymes break down the stored fats into fatty acids that leave the adipocytes, entering blood vessels, from where they are endocytosed by hepatocytes. Within the liver cells, hepatic enzymes responsible for **gluconeogenesis** (the synthesis of glucose from noncarbohydrate sources) are activated by glucagon, and glucose is manufactured to reestablish the intracellular glycogen depot.

Hormones produced by cells of the islets of Langerhans in lesser quantities include somatostatin, vasoactive intestinal peptide, gastrin, pancreatic polypeptide, ghrelin, and amylin (see Table 18.3).

Somatostatin, manufactured by one of the two types of **δ cells**, **D cells**, has both paracrine and endocrine effects. The hormone's paracrine effects are to inhibit the release of endocrine hormones by nearby α cells and β cells. Its endocrine effects are on smooth muscle cells of the alimentary tract and gallbladder, reducing the motility of these organs. Somatostatin is released in response to the increased levels of blood glucose, amino acids, or chylomicrons that occur after a meal. Somatostatin also hinders the release of enzymes synthesized by the acinar cells of the pancreas and reduces hydrochloric acid (HCl) production by parietal cells of the stomach.

Vasoactive intestinal peptide (**VIP**) is produced by the second type of δ cells, known as ***D1 cells***. This hormone induces glycogenolysis and hyperglycemia and regulates intestinal motility and the tone of smooth muscle cells of the wall of the gut. VIP also controls the secretion of ions and water by intestinal epithelial cells.

Gastrin, released by **G cells**, stimulates gastric release of HCl (by parietal cells), gastric motility and emptying, and the rate of cell division in gastric regenerative cells.

Pancreatic polypeptide, produced by **PP cells**, inhibits the exocrine secretions of the pancreas and the release of bile from the gallbladder. It also stimulates the release of enzymes by the gastric chief cells while depressing the release of HCl by parietal cells of the stomach.

Ghrelin, produced by **ε (epsilon) cells**, induces the sensation of hunger and modulates receptive relaxation of the smooth muscle fibers of the muscularis externa of the gastrointestinal tract.

Amylin, a hormone produced by **β cells** and released along with insulin, inhibits emptying of the stomach. It has been suggested that amylin also inhibits glucagon release.

Blood Supply of the Pancreas

The arterial blood supply to the pancreas is unusual in that the supply to the exocrine portion and to the endocrine portion of the gland are completely separate. However, the venous drainage is designed so that venous blood from the islets of Langerhans drains directly into the exocrine pancreas so that the acinar cells have direct access to blood into which the endocrine cells of the islets of Langerhans have delivered their hormones. Therefore, hormones such as **somatostatin** released by **δ cells** of the islets of Langerhans can control the secretory function of the acinar cells.

Clinical Correlations

1. ***Diabetes mellitus*** *is a hyperglycemic metabolic disorder that results from (1) lack of insulin production by β cells of the islets of Langerhans or (2) defective insulin receptors on the target cells. There are two major forms of diabetes mellitus:* ***type 1*** *and* ***type 2*** *(Table 18.4). The incidence of type 2 diabetes is about five to six times that of type 1. If uncontrolled, both types of diabetes may have debilitating sequelae, including circulatory disorders, renal failure, blindness, gangrene, stroke, and myocardial infarcts. The most significant laboratory result indicative of diabetes is elevated blood glucose levels after an overnight fast.*

Type 1 diabetes *(insulin-dependent diabetes; juvenile-onset diabetes) usually affects persons younger than 20 years of age. It is characterized by the three cardinal signs of* ***polydipsia*** *(constant thirst),* ***polyphagia*** *(undiminished hunger), and* ***polyuria*** *(excessive urination). It has been demonstrated in genetically susceptible mice that too much* ***zonulin****—a haptoglobin-2 precursor produced by epithelial cells of the small intestine that temporarily opens tight junctions of the intestinal surface absorptive cells—is formed, permitting macromolecules of the intestinal lumen to use the paracellular route to enter the lamina propria. Once there, the immune reaction forms antibodies against them, some of which can attack* ***β cells*** *of the* ***islets of Langerhans****, resulting in type 1 diabetes and other autoimmune diseases, such as celiac disease.*

Type 2 diabetes *(non–insulin-dependent diabetes) is the most common and usually affects obese persons older than 40 years of age. The cause is not the lack of insulin production—as in type 1 diabetes—but rather the inability of insulin to bind to insulin receptors on cells such as hepatocytes, smooth muscle cells, and adipocytes, which prevent these cells from adding GLUT-4 transporters to their plasmalemma that would otherwise transport glucose into these cells. Recent studies of aged mice and rhesus monkeys with type 2 diabetes have disclosed that there is a diminished level of the intestinal bacteria* Akkermansia muciniphila. *This organism catalyzes dietary fibers into butyrate and acetate, fatty acids that trigger certain cells to carry out specific tasks. The low levels of intestinal* A. muciniphila *results in the onset of inflammation, leading to insulin resistance. When these elderly animals were treated with the antibiotic enrofloxacin or with butyrate, they reestablished their normal levels of intestinal* A. muciniphila. *Hepatocytes, smooth muscle cells, and adipocytes were once again able to respond to insulin, thus reversing their type 2 diabetes.*

2. ***Verner-Morrison syndrome (pancreatic cholera)*** *is characterized by explosive, watery diarrhea that results in hypokalemia (reduced potassium levels) and hypochlorhydria (reduced chloride levels). It is caused by the excessive manufacture and release of vasoactive intestinal peptide due to the adenoma of the D_1 cells that produce this hormone. Frequently, tumors of D_1 cells are malignant.*

TABLE 18.4 Comparison of Type 1 and Type 2 Diabetes Mellitus

Type	Common Synonyms	Clinical Characteristics	Patient Weight	Hereditary Component	Islets of Langerhans
Type 1 (insulin-dependent)	Juvenile-onset diabetes; juvenile diabetes; idiopathic diabetes	Abrupt onset of symptoms; age younger than 20 years; decreased blood insulin level; ketoacidosis is common; antibodies present against β cells; possible autoimmune disease; reacts to insulin; polyphagia, polydipsia, polyuria	Normal (or weight loss despite increase in food intake)	About 50% concordance in identical twins; environmental factors important in the development of the disease	Decrease in the size and number of β cells; islets are atrophied and fibrotic
Type 2 (non–insulin-dependent)	Adult-onset diabetes; ketosis-resistant diabetes	Onset after 40 years of age; mild decrease in blood insulin levels; ketoacidosis is rare; no antibodies against β cells; impaired insulin release; insulin-resistant; decrease in number of insulin receptors; impaired postreceptor signaling	80% of the affected individuals are obese	About 90%–100% concordance in identical twins	Some decrease in number of β cells; amylin present in the tissue surrounding β cells

Liver

The **liver**, located in the upper right-hand quadrant of the abdominal cavity just inferior to the diaphragm and weighing approximately 1500 g, is the largest gland in the body. It is subdivided into four lobes: right, left, quadrate, and caudate. The first two constitute its bulk (Fig. 18.17A).

Similar to the pancreas, the liver has both endocrine and exocrine functions. Unlike the pancreas, however, the same cell, the **hepatocyte**, is responsible for the formation of the liver's exocrine secretion, **bile**, as well as its numerous endocrine products. In addition, hepatocytes convert noxious substances into nontoxic materials that are excreted in bile.

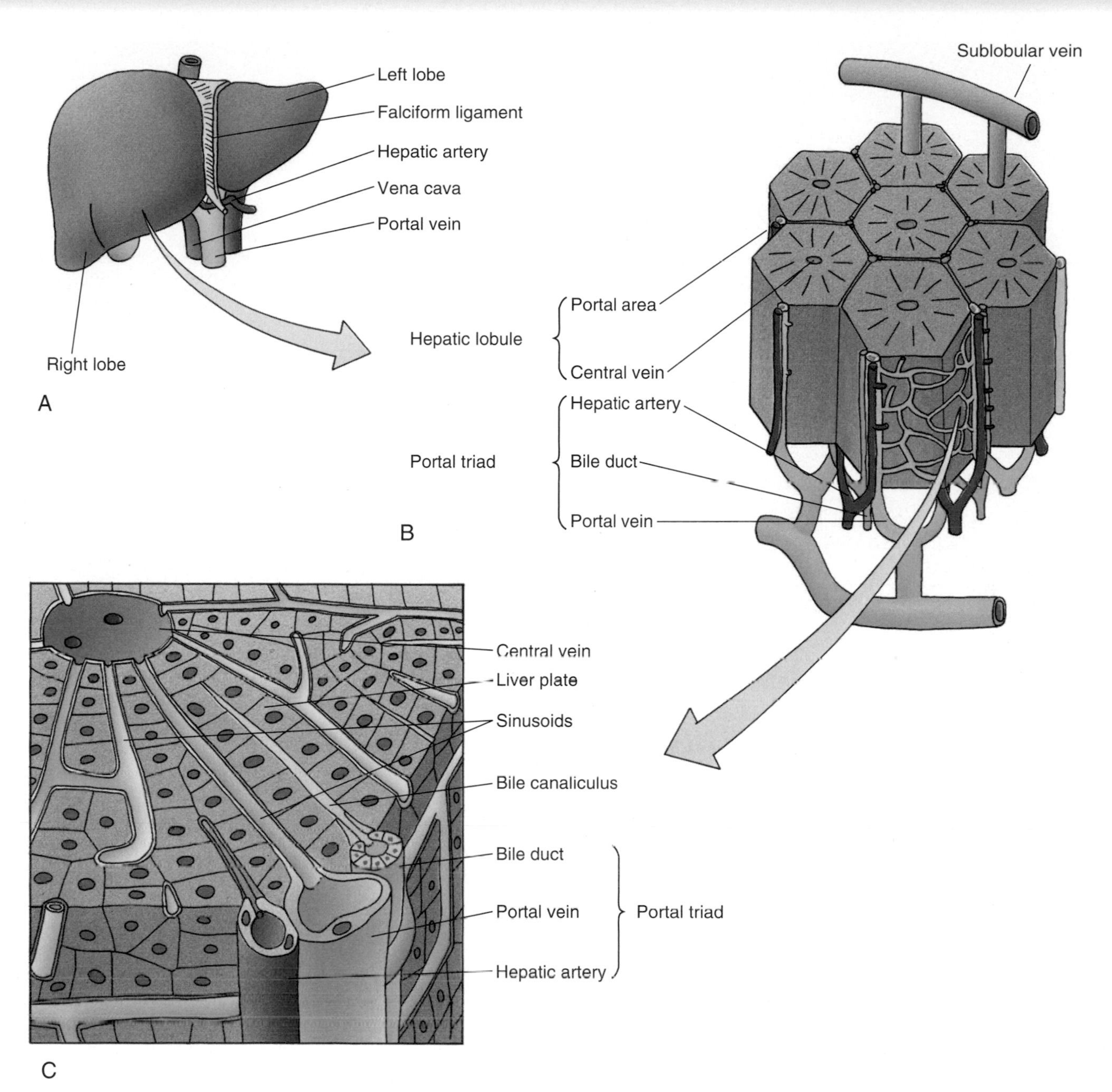

Fig. 18.17 Schematic diagram of the liver. (A) Gross anatomy of the liver. (B) Liver lobules displaying the portal areas and the central vein. (C) Portion of the liver lobule displaying the portal area, liver plates, sinusoids, and bile canaliculi.

GENERAL HEPATIC STRUCTURE AND VASCULAR SUPPLY

The inferior, concave aspect of the liver houses the porta hepatis, through which the portal vein and hepatic artery bring blood into the liver and through which the bile ducts drain bile from the liver.

The liver is almost completely enveloped by peritoneum, a simple squamous epithelium, deep to which is a dense, irregular, collagenous connective tissue **capsule**, known as the **Glisson capsule**. This capsule is loosely attached over the entire surface of the liver except at the hilum-like indentation, the **porta hepatis**, where connective tissue septa derived from the capsule enter the liver, forming a conduit for blood and lymph vessels and bile ducts. The substance of the liver is unusual in that its connective tissue elements are sparse; thus, the bulk of the liver is composed of its uniform parenchymal cells, the **hepatocytes**.

The liver has a dual blood supply, receiving oxygenated blood from the **left** and **right hepatic arteries** and hemoglobin-rich venous blood from the spleen, as well as nutrient-rich venous blood from the digestive tract via the **portal vein**. Thus, 25% of the blood supply comes from the arteries and 75% is derived from the veins. The hepatic arteries and the portal vein enter the liver at the porta hepatis, bringing blood into the liver. Blood leaves the liver at the posterior aspect of the organ through the **hepatic veins**, which deliver their contents into the inferior vena cava. Bile also leaves the liver at the porta hepatis by way of the right and left hepatic ducts, to be delivered to the **gallbladder** for concentration and storage.

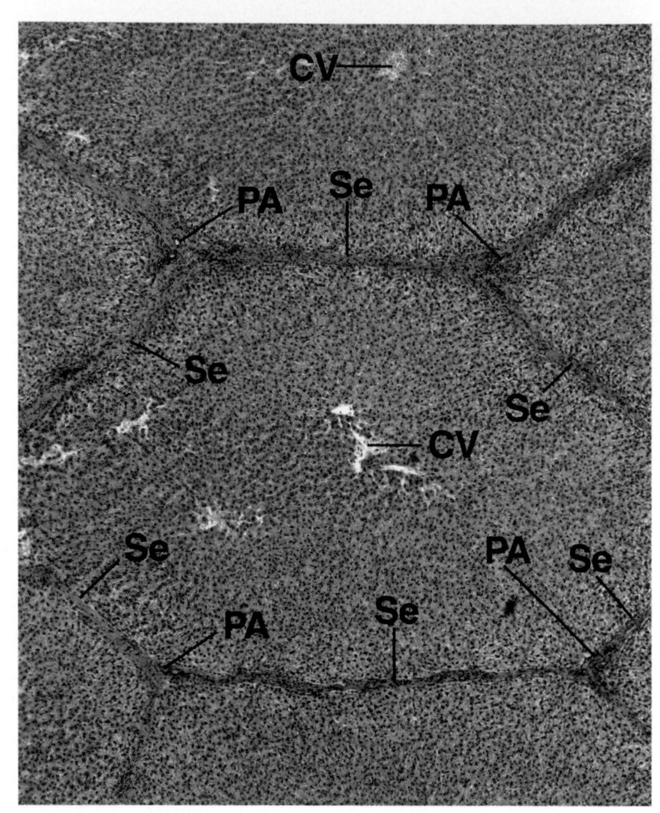

Fig. 18.18 This very-low-magnification photomicrograph of a pig liver displays the hexagonal liver lobule, classical lobule, circumscribed by connective tissue septa (Se). Observe that in regions where three classical lobules contact each other, the septa are wider and are known as portal areas (PA). The center of the classical lobule is occupied by the central vein (CV). (×56)

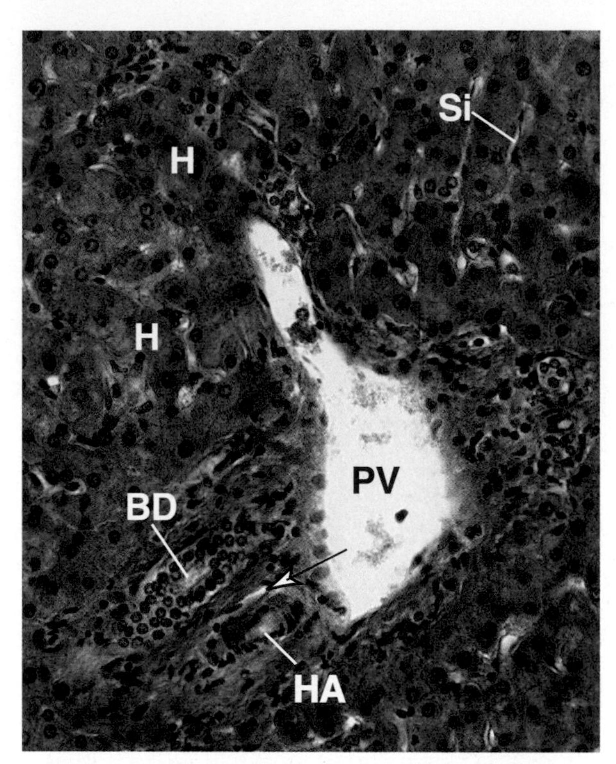

Fig. 18.19 This is a medium magnification of the portal area displaying the portal vein (HV), hepatic artery (HA), lymph vessel (LV), and the bile duct (BD). The bile duct is distinguished by its simple cuboidal epithelium. Observe the large hepatocytes (H) and sinusoids (Si) between plates of hepatocytes. (×270)

Because the liver occupies a central position in metabolism, all nutrients (except for chylomicrons) absorbed in the alimentary canal are transported directly to the liver via the portal vein. In addition, iron-rich blood from the spleen is routed, by way of the portal vein, directly to the liver for processing. Much of the nutritive material delivered to the liver is converted by the **hepatocytes** into storage products, such as glycogen, to be released as glucose when required by the body.

Hepatocytes are arranged in hexagon-shaped lobules (**classical lobules**) about 2 mm in length and 700 μm in diameter. These lobules are clearly demarcated by slender connective tissue elements (known as *portal tracts*) in animals such as the pig and camel (Fig. 18.18). However, because of the scarcity of connective tissue and the closely packed arrangement of the lobules in humans, the boundaries of the classical lobules can only be approximated.

Where three classical lobules are in contact with each other, the connective tissue elements are increased. These regions are known as ***portal areas*** (***portal triads, portal canals***). In addition to lymph vessels, portal areas house the following three structures, each of which follows the longitudinal axis of each lobule (see Figs. 18.17–18.19):

- Slender branches of the hepatic artery
- Relatively large limbs of the portal vein
- Interlobular bile ducts (recognized by their simple cuboidal epithelium)

The portal areas are isolated from the liver parenchyma by the **limiting plate**, a sleeve of modified hepatocytes. A narrow space, the **space of Moll**, separates the limiting plate from the connective tissue of the portal area.

Although one would expect six portal areas around each classical lobule, usually only *three* more or less equally distributed portal areas are present at a random section. Along the length of each slender branch of the hepatic artery within the portal area, fine branches, known as ***distributing arterioles***, arise. Similar to outstretched arms, they reach toward their counterparts in the neighboring portal areas. Smaller vessels, known as ***inlet arterioles***, branch from the distributing arterioles (or from the parent vessel). In addition, the interlobular bile ducts are vascularized by a **peribiliary capillary plexus**. Venules belonging to the portal vein are also two sizes: the larger **distributing veins** and the smaller **inlet venules**.

The longitudinal axis of each classical lobule is occupied by the **central vein**, the initial branch of the **hepatic vein. Hepatocytes** radiate, similar to spokes of a wheel, from the central vein, forming anastomosing, fenestrated plates of liver cells, separated from each other by large vascular spaces known as ***hepatic sinusoids*** (Figs. 18.17C, 18.20, and 18.21). **Inlet arterioles**, **inlet venules**, and branches from the **peribiliary capillary plexus** pierce the limiting plate (of modified hepatocytes) to join the hepatic sinusoids (see Fig. 18.20) As blood enters the sinusoids, its flow slows considerably, and it slowly percolates into the central vein.

Because there is only one central vein in each classical lobule, it receives blood from every sinusoid of that lobule, and its diameter increases as it progresses through the lobule. As the central vein leaves the lobule, it terminates in the **sublobular vein**. Numerous central veins deliver their blood into a single sublobular vein; sublobular veins join each other to form **collecting veins**, which, in turn, form the right and left hepatic veins.

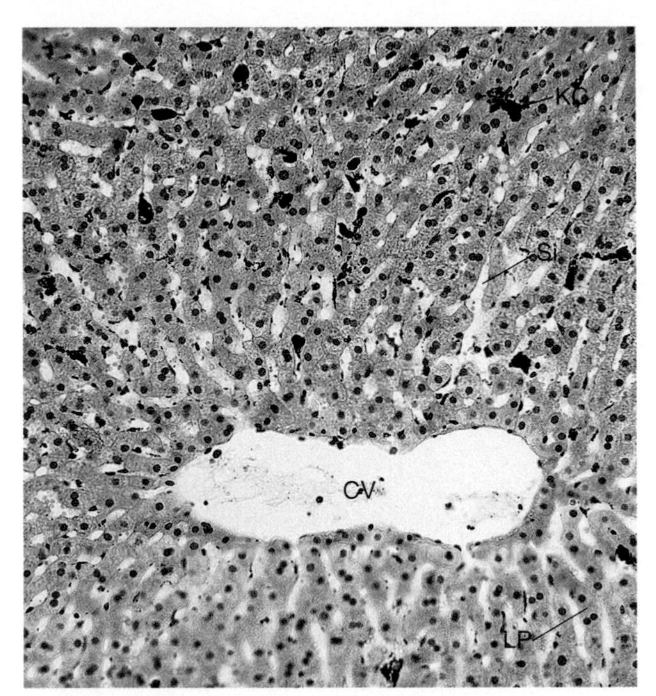

Fig. 18.20 Photomicrograph of a dog liver displaying the central vein (CV), liver plates (LP), and sinusoids (Si). This animal was injected with India ink that was phagocytosed by Kupffer cells (KC), which, consequently, appear as black spots. (×132)

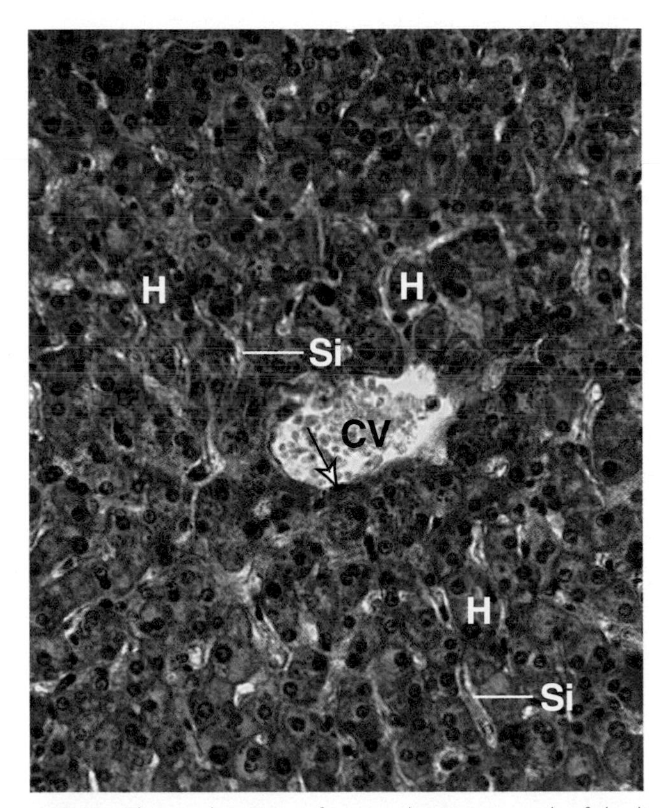

Fig. 18.21 This medium-magnification photomicrograph of the liver displays the central vein (CV) lined by endothelial cells *(arrow)*. Observe that the plates of hepatocytes (H) border sinusoids (Si). (×270)

Lymph Flow in the Liver

Lymph formed in the liver flows to the **space of Moll** and enters slender tributaries of the lymph vessel located in the portal area (see Fig. 18.19). These lymph vessels merge to form increasingly

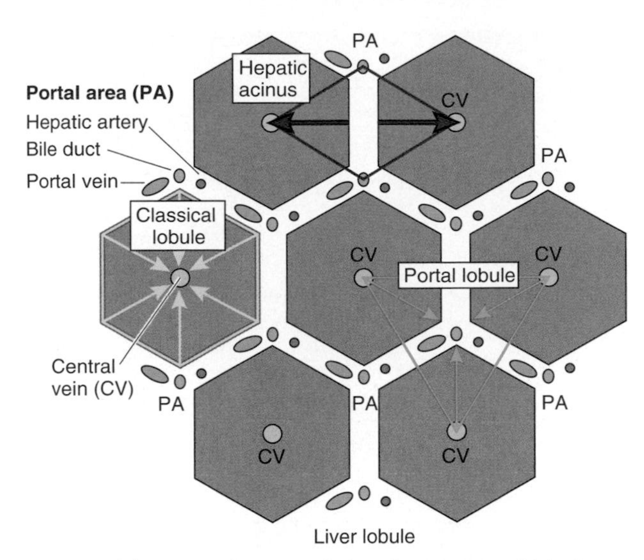

Fig. 18.22 Schematic diagram of the three types of lobules in the liver: classic, portal, and liver acinus.

larger structures, creating a small number of large vessels that deliver their lymph into the thoracic duct to be transported into the vascular system at the junction of the left internal jugular and left subclavian veins. Lymph from the liver constitutes almost 50% of all of the lymph formed in the entire body. Because the walls of the liver sinusoids are quite leaky, lymph formed in the liver has a much higher concentration of proteins than lymph formed almost anywhere else in the body.

Three Concepts of Liver Lobules

The three types of liver lobules are the classical lobule, portal lobule, and the hepatic acinus (acinus of Rappaport).

There are three basic conceptualizations of the liver lobule (Fig. 18.22). The **classical liver lobule** was the first to be defined histologically because the connective tissue arrangement in the pig liver afforded an obvious rationale (see Fig. 18.18) that could be easily transferred to the histology of the human liver. A view of the classical lobule demonstrates that blood flows from the periphery of the lobule to the *center of the lobule* into the central vein. Bile, manufactured by liver cells, enters into small intercellular spaces, **bile canaliculi**, located between hepatocytes and flows to the *periphery of the lobule* to the interlobular bile ducts of the portal areas (Fig. 18.23).

The concept of an exocrine secretion flowing to the periphery of a lobule was not consistent with the situation in the acini of most glands, where the secretion enters a central lumen of the acinus. Therefore, histologists suggested that all hepatocytes that deliver their bile to a particular bile duct constitute a lobule, called the ***portal lobule***. In histological sections, the portal lobule is defined as the triangular region whose center is the portal area and whose periphery is bounded by imaginary straight lines connecting the three surrounding central veins that form the three apices of the triangle where the bile flows into the centrally located portal area. Transferring the two-dimensional image to three dimensions, the lobule would resemble a pyramid with the bile flows into the center of the pyramid.

A third conceptualization of hepatic lobules is based on blood flow from the distributing arteriole and, consequently, on the order in which hepatocytes degenerate subsequent to toxic or hypoxic insults. This ovoid- to diamond-shaped lobule is

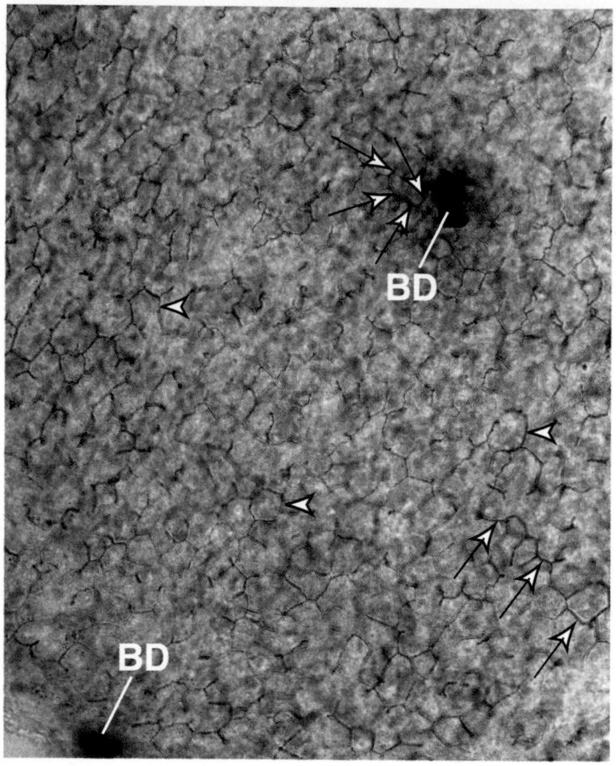

Fig. 18.23 This medium-magnification photomicrograph was prepared to demonstrate the bile canaliculi *(arrowheads)* located between adjacent hepatocytes. Observe that the bile canaliculi form a continuous channel *(arrows)* that will lead the bile to the bile duct. (×270)

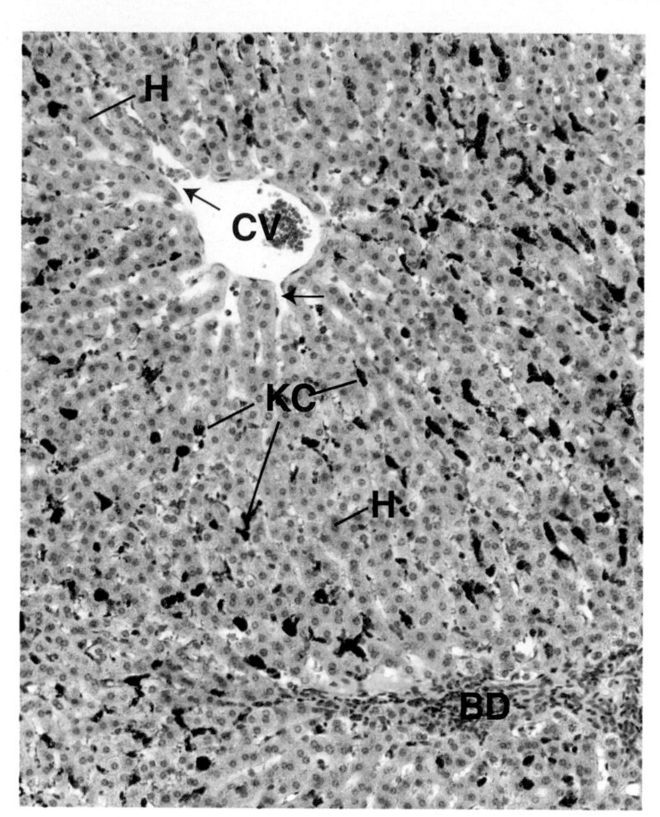

Fig. 18.24 This low-magnification photomicrograph of a liver injected with India ink demonstrates the presence of numerous resident macrophages, known as Kupffer cells (KC), located among the sinusoidal lining cells. Observe that this image includes both the portal area (BD) and the central vein (CV). Note that the sinusoids, located between plates of hepatocytes (H), open into the central vein *(arrows)*. (×132)

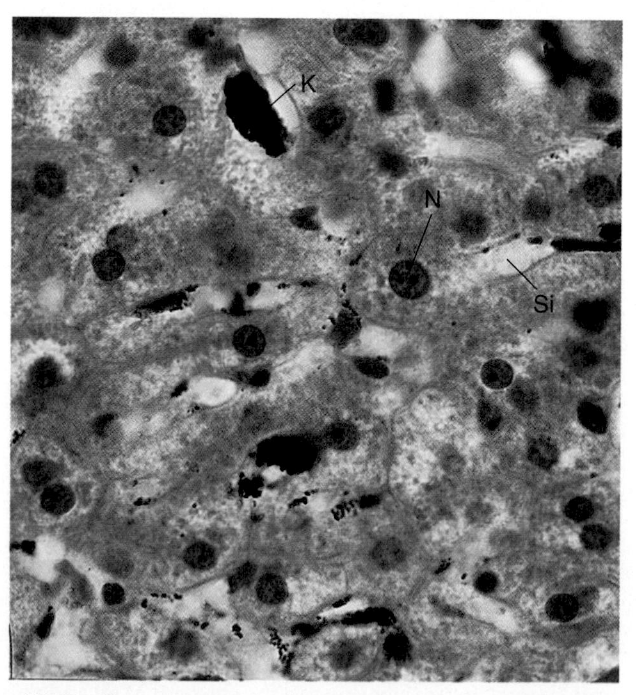

Fig. 18.25 Photomicrograph of a canine liver demonstrating plates of hepatocytes, sinusoids (Si), and India ink–containing Kupffer cells (K). N, Nucleus. (×540)

known as the ***hepatic acinus*** (***acinus of Rappaport***). It is viewed, in two dimensions, as three poorly defined, concentric regions of hepatic parenchyma surrounding a distributing artery in the center. The outermost layer, **zone 3**, extends as far as the central vein and is the most oxygen-poor of the three zones. The remaining region is equally divided into two zones (1 and 2). **Zone 1** is the richest in oxygen and **zone 2** has characteristics in between the other two zones. In three dimensions, the hepatic acinus would resemble a solid parallelogram.

Hepatic Sinusoids and Hepatocyte Plates

Plates of liver cells delineate vascular spaces between them that are lined by sinusoidal lining cells; the vascular spaces are known as hepatic sinusoids.

Anastomosing **plates of hepatocytes**, no more than two cells thick prior to the age of 7 years and one cell thick after that age, radiate from the central vein toward the periphery of the classical lobule (see Fig. 18.17C). The spaces between the plates of hepatocytes are occupied by hepatic sinusoids. The blood flowing in these wide vessels is prevented from coming in contact with the hepatocytes by the presence of an endothelial lining composed of **sinusoidal lining cells**. Often, the cells of this endothelial lining do not make contact with each other, leaving gaps of up to 0.5 μm between them. The sinusoidal lining cells also have fenestrae that are present in clusters, known as ***sieve plates***. Thus, particulate matter less than 0.5 μm in diameter may leave the lumen of the sinusoid with relative ease.

Resident macrophages, known as *Kupffer cells*, are intermingled with the sinusoidal lining cells of the sinusoids (Figs. 18.24 and 18.25). Frequently, phagosomes of Kupffer cells contain

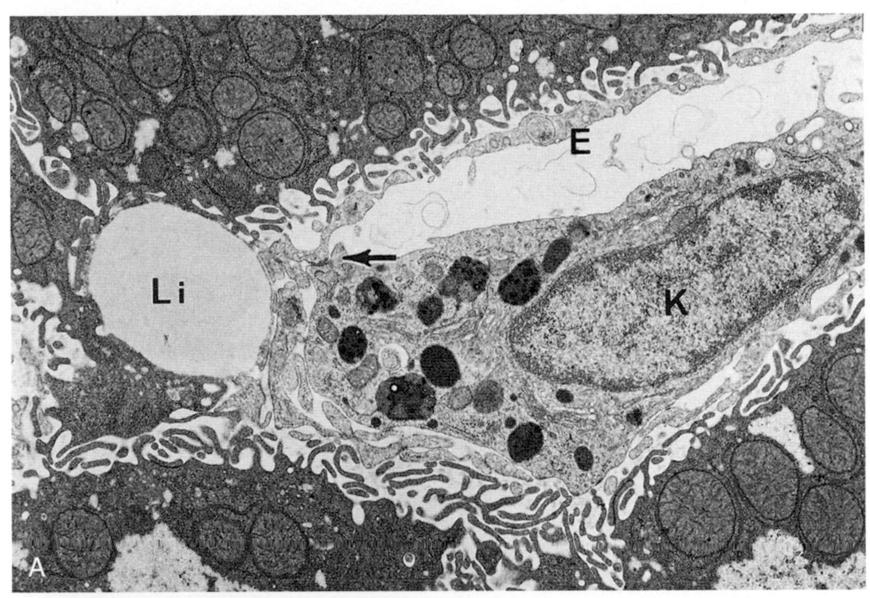

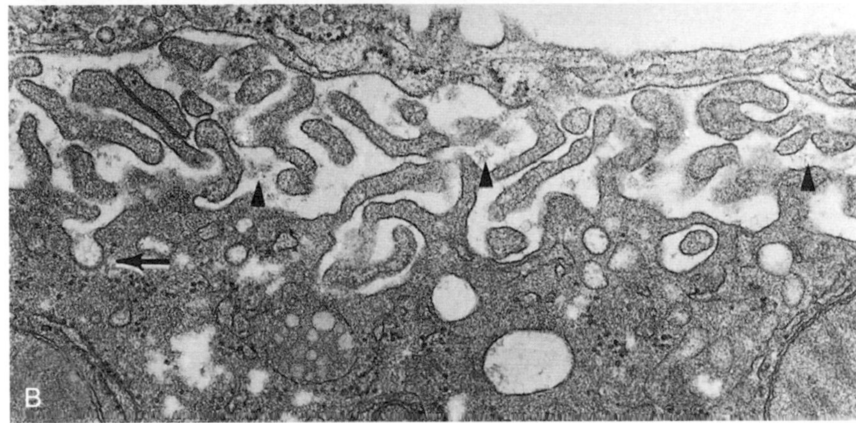

Fig. 18.26 Electron micrograph of the shrew liver. (A) Observe the sinusoid, with its sinusoidal lining cell (E), Kupffer cell (K), and a small region of a lipid droplet (Li)–containing Ito cell (×8885). (B) A higher magnification of the hepatocyte displays its numerous microvilli *(arrowheads)* protruding into the space of Disse (×29,670). The *arrow* indicates the process of pinocytosis. (From Matsumoto E, Hirosawa K. Some observations on the structure of *Suncus* liver with special reference to the vitamin A–storing cell. *Am J Anat.* 1983;167:193-204. Reprinted with permission from Wiley-Liss, Inc., a subsidiary of John Wiley & Sons, Inc.)

endocytosed particulate matter and cellular debris, especially defunct erythrocytes that are being destroyed by these cells. Electron micrographs of Kupffer cells display numerous filopodia-like projections, mitochondria, some RER, a small Golgi apparatus, and an abundance of lysosomes and late endosomes (Fig. 18.26). Because these cells do not make intercellular junctions with the neighboring cells, it has been suggested that they may be migratory scavengers.

Perisinusoidal Space of Disse

The narrow space between a plate of hepatocytes and sinusoidal lining cells is known as the perisinusoidal space of Disse.

The sinusoidal lining cells are separated from the hepatocytes by a narrow **space of Disse** (**perisinusoidal space**); plasma escaping from the sinusoids has free access to this space (Figs. 18.26 and 18.27). Microvilli of the hepatocytes occupy much of the space of Disse; the extensive surface area of the microvilli facilitates exchange of materials between the plasma escaping from the bloodstream and the hepatocytes. ***Hepatocytes do not come into contact with the bloodstream; instead, the space of Disse acts as an intermediate compartment between them.***

Although the perisinusoidal space of Disse contains type III collagen fibers (reticular fibers) that support the sinusoids, as well as a limited amount of type I and type IV collagen fibers, a basal lamina is absent. Occasionally, nonmyelinated nerve fibers and stellate **perisinusoidal stellate cells** (also known as ***Ito cells*** and ***fat storing cells***) have been noted in this space (see Fig. 18.26). Perisinusoidal stellate cells store vitamin A; manufacture and release type III collagen into the space of Disse; secrete growth factors required by the liver for generating new hepatocytes; and, by differentiating into myofibroblasts, form fibrous connective tissue to replace damaged hepatocytes. They do that in response to the presence of **tumor growth factor β** released by hepatocytes of a compromised liver. In addition, **pit cells**, which display short pseudopodia and cytoplasmic granules, have been noted in the perisinusoidal space of mice and rats. These cells, believed to be **natural killer cells (NK cells)**, are also assumed to be in the human liver.

Clinical Correlations

1. *Chronic inflammation of the liver—caused by factors such as long-term alcoholism, portal hypertension, hepatitis B, and hepatitis C—causes hepatocytes to begin to die at a higher than normal rate. Also, perisinusoidal cells (Ito cells) are induced to differentiate into myofibroblasts and form collagen, eventually resulting in fibrosis and, later, cirrhosis of the liver. Fortunately, these*

Continued

Clinical Correlations—cont'd

conditions can be reversed if treated in time. Frequently, however, the patient will experience liver failure; in the absence of a liver transplant, the patient will die.

2. *Although many physicians consider* **fatty liver disease** *to be due to excessive alcohol consumption, this disease is more often present due to other factors, giving rise to the term* **non-alcoholic fatty liver disease.** *This condition, in many cases, leads to cirrhosis. Individuals with* **metabolic syndrome** *are most commonly diagnosed with nonalcoholic fatty liver disease. These individuals do not consume much alcohol, but they are obese and diagnosed with type 2 diabetes, high blood pressure, and hyperlipidemia (especially cholesterol and triglycerides). Due to the high levels of obesity in the United States, an increasing number of individuals will have nonalcoholic* **steatohepatitis,** *a serious form of nonalcoholic fatty liver disease, which will require more liver transplants than all other forms of liver disease combined. Individuals who have been diagnosed with nonalcoholic fatty liver disease are highly susceptible to liver cancer. If the disease is permitted to progress and the patient cannot get a liver transplant in time, the patient will die. However, if diagnosed early enough, the condition can be reversed by lifestyle changes, including weight reduction and control of hypertension, blood glucose levels, triglycerides, and cholesterol. The patients have to be monitored at least twice a year for liver cancer, as well as for hepatitis A, B, and C. Additionally, patients have to be screened for the possible development of esophageal and gastric varices to prevent the possibility of death due to bleeding as a result of portal hypertension caused by cirrhosis-induced vascular obstruction within the liver.*

Hepatic Ducts

The hepatic duct system is composed of cholangioles, canals of Hering, and bile ducts leading to increasinlgy larger bile ducts that finally culminate in the right and left hepatic ducts.

Bile canaliculi anastomose, forming labyrinthine tunnels among the hepatocytes. As these bile canaliculi reach the periphery of the classic lobules, they merge with **canals of Hering**, slender conduits that are formed by hepatocytes in combination with low cuboidal (or ovoid) cells known as ***cholangiocytes***. Bile from the canals of Hering flow into **bile ducts** (composed of cholangiocytes) located in the portal areas of the classical lobules. These bile ducts merge to form increasingly larger conduits, which eventually unite to form the **right hepatic duct** and the **left hepatic duct**. The extrahepatic system of bile ducts is described later. The **ovoid cells** of the canals of Hering are capable of proliferation. The progeny of these oval cells may give rise to cuboidal cells of the bile duct system, as well as to hepatocytes.

The cuboidal epithelial cells of the canals of Hering and of the bile ducts secrete a bicarbonate-rich fluid similar to that produced by the duct system of the pancreas. The formation and release of this alkaline buffer are controlled by the hormone **secretin**, produced by DNES cells of the duodenum. This fluid acts, with fluid from the pancreas, to neutralize the acidic chyme that enters the duodenum.

Hepatocytes

Hepatocytes are polygonal-shaped cells, possessing 5 to 12 sides, approximately 20 to 30 μm in diameter, that are closely packed together to form anastomosing plates of liver cells, one cell in thickness, with a life span of approximately 150 days. These cells exhibit variations in their structural, histochemical, and biochemical properties, depending on their location within liver lobules.

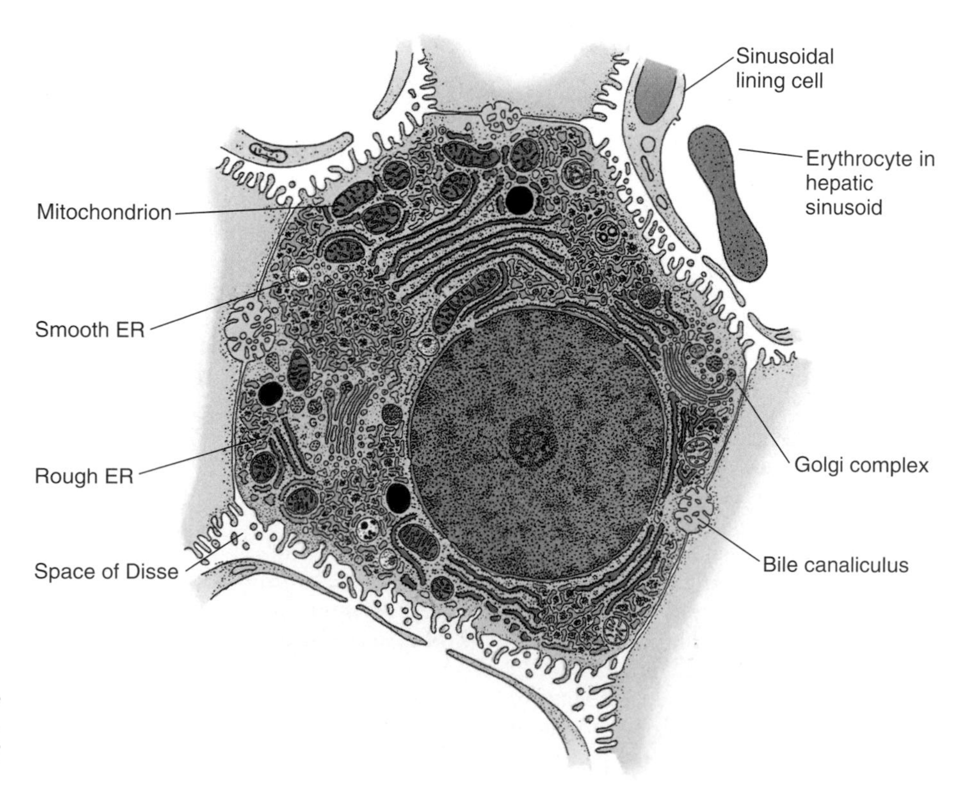

Fig. 18.27 Schematic diagram of a hepatocyte indicating its sinusoidal and lateral domains. ER, Endoplasmic reticulum. (From Lentz TL. Cell Fine Structure: An Atlas of Drawings of Whole-Cell Structure. Philadelphia: WB Saunders; 1971.)

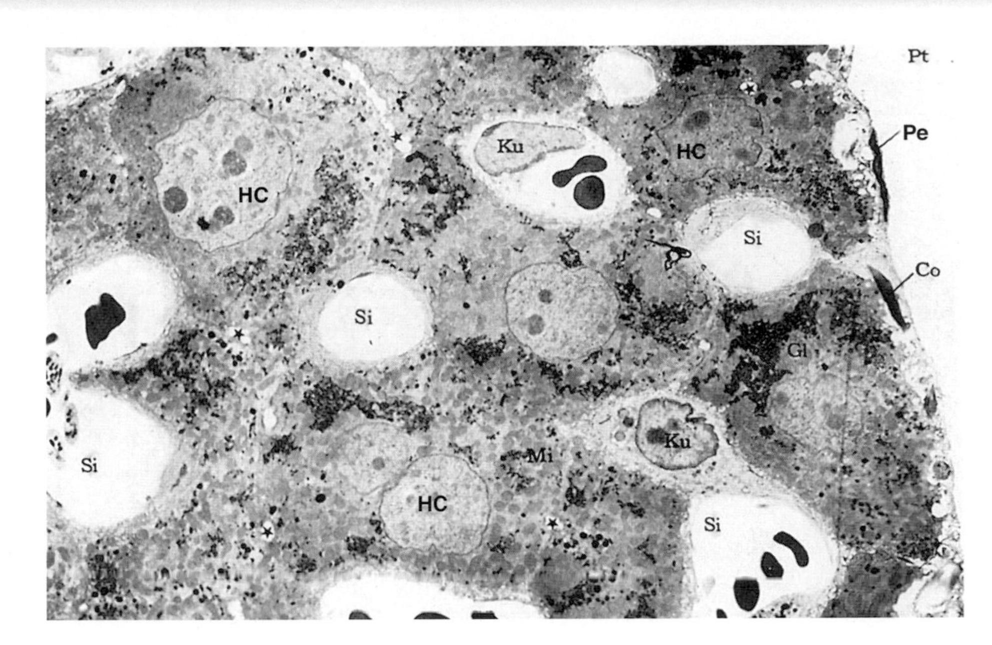

Fig. 18.28 Low-magnification electron micrograph of a mouse liver (×2535). The liver is covered over most of its surface by peritoneum (Pe), which overlies the collagenous capsule (Co) of the liver. Observe the sinusoids (Si), Kupffer cells (Ku), and glycogen deposits (Gl) in the hepatocyte (HC) cytoplasm. Bile canaliculi are denoted by *asterisks*. Mi, Mitochondria; PT, peritoneal cavity. (From Rhodin JAG. *An Atlas of Ultrastructure*. Philadelphia: WB Saunders; 1963.)

Domains of Hepatocyte Plasmalemma

The plasma membranes of hepatocytes are said to have two domains, lateral and sinusoidal.

Hepatocytes are arranged in such a manner that each cell not only comes in contact with other hepatocytes, their **lateral domains**, but they also have sides that face the space of Disse, their **sinusoidal domains**.

Lateral Domains

The lateral domains are responsible for the formation of bile canaliculi.

The **lateral domain** of hepatocytes contacts adjacent hepatocytes and forms elaborate, labyrinthine intercellular spaces, 1 to 2 μm in diameter, known as *bile canaliculi*, channels that conduct bile between hepatocytes to the periphery of the classical lobules (see Figs. 18.17, 18.23, and 18.27). Short, blunt microvilli project from the hepatocyte into the bile canaliculi, increasing the surface areas through which bile can be secreted. The actin cores of these microvilli mingle with the thickened network of actin and intermediate filaments that reinforce the region of the hepatocyte plasmalemma participating in the formation of bile canaliculi. Liver cells participating in the formation of bile canaliculi form fasciae occludentes to prevent leakage of bile into the remaining extracellular space. The cell membranes that form the walls of bile canaliculi display high levels of **Na^+-K^+ ATPase** activity and the enzyme **adenylate cyclase**, which most probably provide the energy to release bile into the bile canaliculi. The lateral domains also have isolated gap junctions whereby hepatocytes are able to communicate with each other.

Sinusoidal Domains

The sinusoidal domains form microvilli that protrude into the perisinusoidal space of Disse.

The **sinusoidal domains** of hepatocyte plasma membranes also have microvilli, which project into the space of Disse (see Figs. 18.26 and 18.27). It has been calculated that these microvilli increase the surface area of the sinusoidal domain by a factor of 6, facilitating the exchange of material between the hepatocyte and the plasma in the perisinusoidal space (space of Disse). This cell membrane is rich in mannose-6-phosphate receptors, Na^+-K^+ ATPase, and adenylate cyclase because it is here that the endocrine secretions of the hepatocyte are released and enter the sinusoidal blood and material carried by the bloodstream is transported into the hepatocyte cytoplasm.

Hepatocyte Organelles and Inclusions

Hepatocytes are large, organelle-rich cells that manufacture the exocrine secretion bile as well as a large number of endocrine secretions; in addition, these cells can perform a large array of metabolic functions.

Hepatocytes constitute only 60% of the total cell number, but they account for about 75% of the weight of the liver. These cells manufacture **primary bile**, which is modified by the epithelial cells lining the bile ducts and gallbladder—becoming known as **secondary bile**, called simply ***bile***. Approximately 75% of the hepatocytes have a single nucleus; the remainder have two nuclei. The nuclei vary in size, the smallest (50% of the nuclei) being diploid and the larger ones being polyploid, with the largest nuclei reaching 64 N.

Hepatocytes actively synthesize proteins for their own use as well as for export. Thus, they have an abundance of organelles, such as free ribosomes, RER, and Golgi apparatus (Figs. 18.28 and 18.29). Each cell houses numerous sets of Golgi apparatuses, located preferentially in the vicinity of bile canaliculi.

Hepatocytes have a very high energy requirement, as evidenced by the more than 2000 mitochondria that each cell possesses. Cells near the central vein (zone 3 of the liver acinus) have nearly twice as many, but considerably smaller, mitochondria as hepatocytes in the periportal area (zone 1 of the liver acinus). Liver cells also have a rich complement of endosomes, lysosomes, and peroxisomes.

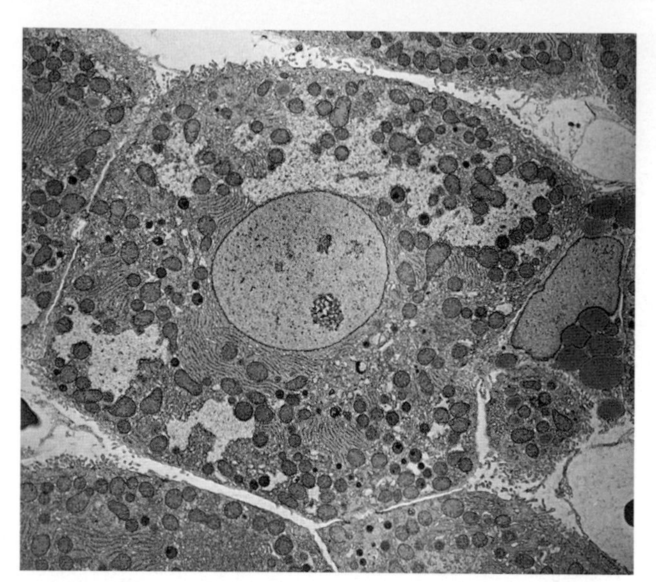

Fig. 18.29 Electron micrograph of a rat hepatocyte (×2500). (From Tandler B, Krahenbuhl S, Brass EP. Unusual mitochondria in the hepatocytes of rats treated with a vitamin B12 analogue. *Anat Rec.* 1991;231:1-6. Reprinted with permission from Wiley-Liss, Inc., a subsidiary of John Wiley & Sons, Inc.)

The complement of smooth endoplasmic reticulum (SER) of hepatocytes varies not only by region but also with function. Cells in zone 3 of the liver acinus have a much richer endowment of SER than those in the periportal area. Moreover, the presence of certain drugs and toxins in the blood induces an increase in the SER content of liver cells because detoxification occurs within the cisternae of this organelle.

Clinical Correlations

1. *Persons who have consumed* ***hepatotoxic substances****, such as alcohol, display an increased number of lipid deposits in their zone 3 hepatocytes. In addition, persons who are taking barbiturates display an increase in the SER content of zone 3 liver cells. Because this zone has the lowest oxygen levels of the three zones, this is the region of the liver acinus that is most susceptible to necrosis in the case of severe liver injury.*
2. ***Wilson disease*** *is a hereditary condition in which the liver does not eliminate copper by transferring it into bile. Instead, copper accumulates in the eyes, where it appears as green to gold rings in the cornea; in the brain, where it interferes with normal brain function, causing tremors, aphasia, and, occasionally, psychosis; and in the liver, where it causes cirrhosis. If left untreated, the disease is fatal. The disease can be treated by use of a chelating agent, such as penicillamine, which binds with copper and facilitates its elimination from the body.*

Hepatocytes contain varying amounts of inclusions in the form of lipid droplets and glycogen (Fig. 18.30). The lipid droplets are mostly **very-low-density lipoprotein** and are especially prominent after the consumption of a fatty meal.

Glycogen deposits are present as accumulations of electron-dense granules 20 to 30 nm in size, known as ***β particles***, in the vicinity of SER. The distribution of glycogen varies with hepatocyte location. Liver cells in the vicinity of the portal area (zone 1 of liver acinus) display large clumps of β particles surrounded by SER, whereas pericentral hepatocytes (zone 3 of liver acinus) exhibit diffuse glycogen deposits (Fig. 18.30). The number of these particles varies with the dietary state of the individual. They are abundant subsequent to feeding and fewer after fasting.

HISTOPHYSIOLOGY OF THE LIVER

The liver has both exocrine and endocrine roles, as well as the protective function of detoxification of toxins and elimination of defunct erythrocytes.

The liver has as many as 100 different functions, most of which are performed by the hepatocytes. Each hepatocyte produces not only the exocrine secretion bile but also various endocrine secretions. They metabolize the end products of absorption from the alimentary canal, store them as inclusion products, and release them in response to hormonal and neural signals. Liver cells also detoxify drugs and toxins (protecting the body from their deleterious effects) and transfer secretory IgA from the space of Disse into bile. In addition, Kupffer cells phagocytose blood-borne foreign particulate matter, as well as defunct erythrocytes, and perisinusoidal stellate cells (Ito cells) store vitamin A.

Bile Manufacture

Bile, a fluid manufactured by the liver, is composed of water, bile salts, phospholipids, cholesterol, bile pigments, and IgA.

The liver produces approximately 600 to 1200 mL of bile per day. This fluid, which is mostly water, contains **bile salts** (**sodium and potassium salts of conjugated bile acids**), **bilirubin glucuronide** (**bile pigment**), phospholipids, lecithin, cholesterol, plasma electrolytes (especially sodium, bicarbonate, and excess calcium), and IgA. Bile emulsifies fats in the lumen of the small intestine, assisting the surface absorptive cells of the small intestine in absorbing lipids. It eliminates approximately 80% of the cholesterol synthesized by the liver and excretes waste products such as bilirubin, the end result of hemoglobin destruction.

Bile salts constitute almost half of the organic components of bile. Most of the bile salts are resorbed from the lumen of the small intestine, enter the liver via the portal vein, are endocytosed by hepatocytes, and are transported into the bile canaliculi for subsequent re-release back into the duodenum (**enterohepatic recirculation of bile salts**). The remaining 10% of bile salts are manufactured de novo in the SER of hepatocytes by the conjugation of cholic acid, a metabolic by-product of

Clinical Correlations

Because ***bile salts*** *are amphipathic molecules, their hydrophilic regions are dissolved in aqueous media, and their hydrophobic (lipophilic) regions surround lipid droplets. In the lumen of the duodenum, therefore, bile salts emulsify fats and facilitate their digestion. Absence of bile salts prevents fat digestion and absorption, resulting in* ***fatty stool****.*

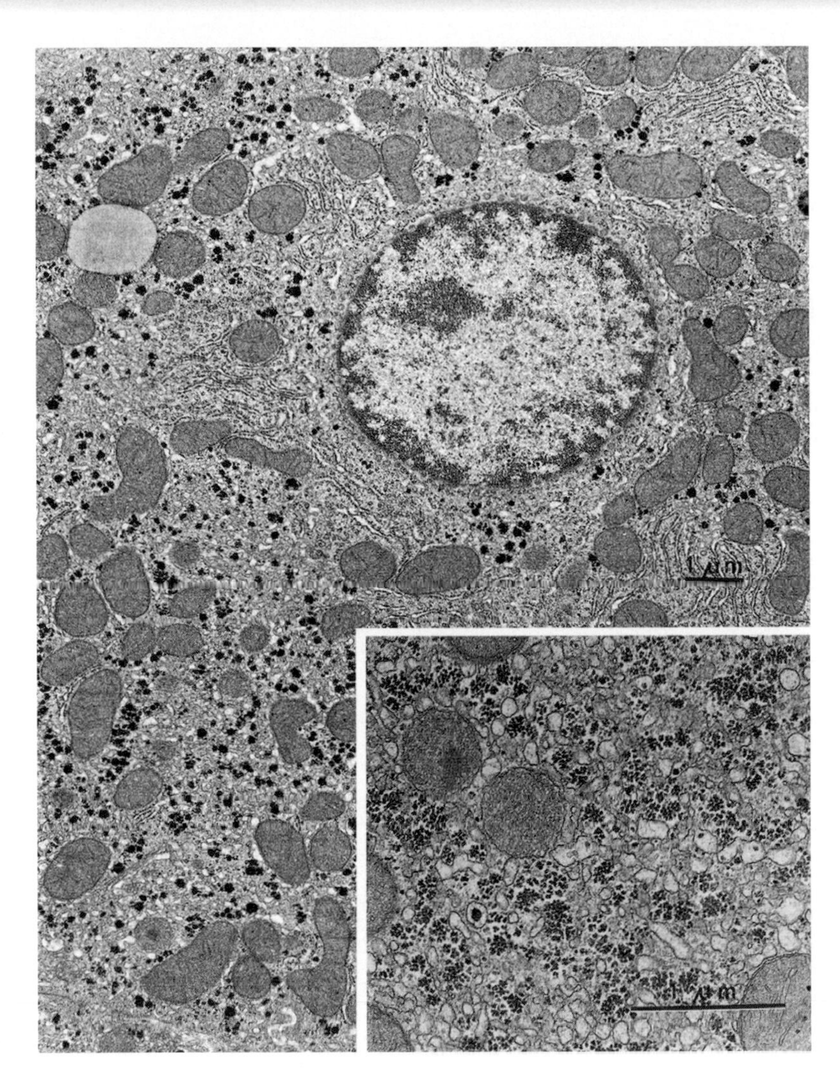

Fig. 18.30 Electron micrograph of glycogen and lipid deposits in the pericentral hepatocyte of a rat. Inset shows the presence of glycogen particles at a higher magnification. (From Cardell RR, Cardell EL. Heterogeneity of glycogen distribution in hepatocytes. *J Electron Microsc Tech.* 1987;14:126-139. Reprinted with permission from Wiley-Liss, Inc., a subsidiary of John Wiley & Sons, Inc.)

cholesterol, to either taurine (taurocholic acid) or glycine (glycocholic acid).

Bilirubin, a water-insoluble, yellowish green pigment, is the *toxic degradation product* of hemoglobin. As defunct erythrocytes are destroyed by macrophages in the spleen and by Kupffer cells in the liver, bilirubin is released into the bloodstream and is bound to plasma albumin. In this form, known as ***free bilirubin***, it is endocytosed by hepatocytes. The enzyme **glucuronyltransferase**, located in the SER of the hepatocyte, catalyzes the conjugation of bilirubin with glucuronide to form the water-soluble, nontoxic **bilirubin glucuronide** (**conjugated bilirubin**). Some of the bilirubin glucuronide is released into the bloodstream, but most of it is excreted into the bile canaliculi for delivery into the alimentary canal for subsequent elimination with the feces (Fig. 18.31).

Lipid Metabolism

Hepatocytes remove chylomicrons from the space of Disse and degrade them into fatty acids and glycerol.

Chylomicrons released by surface absorbing cells of the small intestine enter the lymphatic system and reach the liver through branches of the hepatic artery. Within hepatocytes, they are degraded into **fatty acids** and **glycerol**. The fatty acids are subsequently desaturated and are used to synthesize phospholipids and cholesterol or are degraded into **acetyl coenzyme A**. Two molecules of acetyl coenzyme A are combined to form the **ketone body** called **acetoacetic acid**, most of which is converted into β-hydroxybutyric acid and some into acetone, two other ketone bodies. Phospholipids, cholesterol, and ketone bodies are stored in hepatocytes until their release into the space of Disse. In addition, the liver manufactures **very-low-density lipoproteins**, which are also released into the space of Disse as droplets 30 to 100 nm in diameter. If the need arises, hepatocytes can synthesize fats from carbohydrates and proteins. The newly manufactured fats are released as lipoproteins to be ferried by the bloodstream to adipose cells, where they are stored as triglycerides.

Clinical Correlations

1. *The yellowish discoloration of the skin that is the hallmark of* ***jaundice*** *results from excessively high levels of the yellowish green–colored substances, free or conjugated bilirubin, in the bloodstream. The two primary types of jaundice have different causes. A decrease in bilirubin conjugation—because of either hepatocyte malfunction*

Continued

Clinical Correlations—cont'd

*(as in hepatitis) or, more commonly, obstruction of the bile ducts—causes **obstructive jaundice.** Increased hemolysis of erythrocytes, producing so much free bilirubin that hepatocytes, even though unimpaired, cannot eliminate bilirubin rapidly enough, causes **hemolytic jaundice.***

2. ***Ketosis** occurs when the concentration of ketone bodies in the blood becomes too high (as in persons with diabetes or starvation). It is recognizable by the typical acetone breath of affected persons. If untreated, ketosis results in decreased blood pH (**acidosis**), possibly leading to death. The smell of "nail polish remover" (acetone) on the breath of a patient is an indicator that the physician should suspect that the patient has diabetes, and the proper diagnostic tests should be performed.*
3. *Excessive blood ammonia levels, indicative of impaired liver function or drastic reduction in blood flow to the liver, may lead to **hepatic coma**, a condition that is incompatible with life.*

Carbohydrate and Protein Metabolism

Additional responsibilities of the liver include maintenance of normal blood glucose levels, deamination of amino acids, and synthesis of many blood proteins.

The liver maintains normal levels of glucose in the blood by transporting glucose from the blood into the hepatocytes and storing it in the form of glycogen. If blood glucose levels drop below normal, hepatocytes hydrolyze glycogen (**glycogenolysis**) into glucose and transport it out of the cells into the space of Disse (see Fig. 18.31), from which it enters the blood stream to elevate blood glucose to normal levels. Hepatocytes can also synthesize glucose from other sugars (such as fructose and galactose) or from noncarbohydrate sources (such as amino acids), a process known as ***gluconeogenesis***.

One of the most essential roles of the liver is the elimination of blood-borne ammonia by converting it into **urea**. There are two major sources of ammonia in the body, the deamination of amino acids by hepatocytes and the synthesis of ammonia by bacterial action in the alimentary canal.

Clinical Correlation

If the liver does not convert ammonia into urea, the individual's blood ammonia level rises to such an extent that the patient goes into hepatic coma, resulting in death.

Approximately 90% of the blood proteins are manufactured by the liver (see Fig. 18.31). These products include:

- Factors necessary for coagulation (such as fibrinogen, factor III, accelerator globulin, and prothrombin)
- Proteins required for the complement reactions
- Proteins that function in transport of metabolites
- Albumins

All of the globulins, except gamma (γ) globulins (antibodies), are also synthesized by the liver. Hepatocytes can also synthesize all of the nonessential amino acids that the body requires.

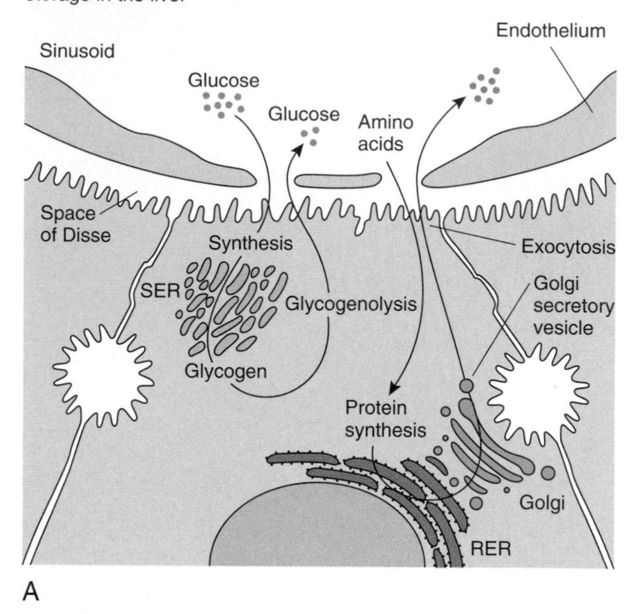

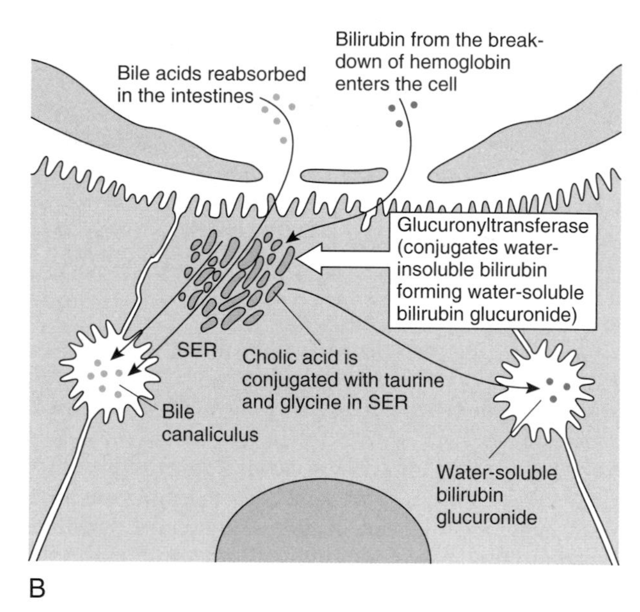

Fig. 18.31 Schematic diagram of a hepatocyte function. (A) Protein synthesis and carbohydrate storage. (B) Secretion of bile acids and bilirubin. SER, Smooth endoplasmic reticulum.

Vitamin Storage

Vitamin A is stored in the greatest amount in the liver, but vitamins K, D, and B_{12} are also present in substantial quantities. The liver contains enough vitamin storage to prevent deficiency of vitamin A for about 10 months, vitamin D for about 4 months, and vitamin B_{12} for more than 12 months.

Degradation of Hormones and Detoxification of Drugs and Toxins

The liver endocytoses and degrades hormones of the endocrine glands. The endocytosed hormones are either transported into the bile canaliculi in their native form to be digested in the lumen of the alimentary canal or delivered into late endosomes for degradation by lysosomal enzymes.

Drugs, such as barbiturates and antibiotics, and toxins are inactivated by hepatocytes in a two-step reaction. The **first phase** occurs in the cisterna of the SER, where drugs and toxins are inactivated by methylation or oxidation by **microsomal mixed-function oxidases**. The **second phase** occurs as the substrates formed in the first phase are conjugated with various intracellular cofactors, making the resultant substances water soluble so that they can be eliminated from the body.

Occasionally, as in the case of alcohol, detoxification occurs in peroxisomes rather than in the SER.

Clinical Correlations

Continued long-term use of certain drugs, such as barbiturates, decreases their effectiveness, requiring prescriptions of increased doses. This drug ***tolerance*** *is due to hypertrophy of the SER complement of hepatocytes and a concomitant increase in their mixed-function oxidases. The increase in organelle size and enzyme concentration is* ***induced*** *by the barbiturate, which is detoxified via oxidative demethylation. In addition, these hepatocytes concurrently become more efficient in detoxifying other drugs and toxins.*

Immune Function

Hepatocytes complex IgA with secretory component and release the secretory IgA into the bile canaliculi.

Most of the **IgA antibodies** formed by plasma cells in the mucosa of the alimentary canal enter the circulatory system and are transported to the liver. Hepatocytes complex the IgA with secretory component and release the complex into bile, which then enters the lumen of the duodenum. Thus, much of the luminal IgA enters the intestine in bile released via the common bile duct. The remainder of the luminal IgA is transported from the intestinal mucosa into the lumen by surface absorptive cells.

Kupffer cells, derived from monocyte precursors, are long-lived cells that are located within the lining of the hepatic sinusoids; some may also adhere to the luminal surface of endothelial cells. Kupffer cells have **Fc receptors**, as well as **receptors for complement**; thus, they can phagocytose foreign particulate matter. The importance of these cells is appreciable because blood from the portal vein contains a considerable number of microorganisms that enter the bloodstream from the lumen of the alimentary canal. These bacteria become opsonized in the lumen or mucosa of the gut or in the bloodstream. Kupffer cells recognize and endocytose at least 99% of these microorganisms. Kupffer cells also remove cellular debris and defunct erythrocytes from the blood.

Liver Regeneration

The liver has a great ability to regenerate after a hepatotoxic insult or even after three-quarters of the liver is excised.

Hepatocytes have a life span of approximately 150 days; thus, mitotic figures are only infrequently present. If hepatotoxic drugs are administered or a portion of the liver is excised, hepatocytes proliferate, and the liver regenerates its normal architecture and previous size.

The regenerative ability of the liver of rodents is so enormous that if 75% of the gland is excised, it regenerates to its normal size within 4 weeks. The human liver's regenerative capacity is much less than that of mice and rats. The mechanism of regeneration is controlled by hepatocyte growth factor, transforming growth factor-α, epidermal growth factor, and interleukin-6. Many of these factors are released by the hepatic stellate cells (Ito cells) located in the space of Disse, although hepatocyte growth factor is probably formed by mesenchymal cells of the liver and is bound to heparin in the liver's scant extracellular matrix. In most cases, the regeneration is due to the replicative capability of the remaining hepatocytes; however, if the hepatotoxic insult is too great, regeneration of the liver is performed by mitotic activity of the oval cells of the canals of Hering. Once the liver is regenerated to its normal size, the hepatocytes manufacture and release the cytokine **transforming growth factor-β**, which inhibits mitotic activity in the liver; thus, regeneration ceases.

GALLBLADDER

The **gallbladder** is a small, pear-shaped organ situated on the inferior aspect of the liver. It is about 10 cm in length and 4 cm in cross-section and can store about 70 mL of bile. This organ resembles a sack with a single opening. The bulk of the organ forms the **body**; the opening, which is continuous with the **cystic duct**, is called the ***neck***. The neck has an out pocketing, known as the **Hartmann pouch**, which is a region where gallstones frequently lodge. The gallbladder stores and concentrates bile and releases it into the duodenum as required.

Structure of the Gallbladder

The gallbladder is composed of four layers: epithelium, lamina propria, smooth muscle, and serosa/adventitia.

The mucosa of the empty gallbladder is highly folded into tall, parallel ridges (Figs. 18.32 and 18.33). As the gallbladder becomes distended with bile, the plication is reduced to a few short folds, and the mucosa becomes relatively smooth.

The lumen of the gallbladder is lined by a simple columnar epithelium, composed of two types of cells: the more common clear cells and the infrequent brush cells (Fig. 18.34). The oval nuclei of these cells are basally positioned, and the supranuclear cytoplasm displays occasional secretory granules containing mucinogen. In electron micrographs, their luminal surface displays short microvilli coated by a thin layer of glycocalyx. The basal region of the cytoplasm is particularly rich in mitochondria, providing abundant energy for the Na^+-K^+ ATPase pump present in the basolateral cell membrane.

The lamina propria is composed of a vascularized loose connective tissue that is well endowed with elastic and collagen fibers. In the neck of the gallbladder, the lamina propria houses simple tubuloacinar glands, which produce a small amount of mucus to lubricate the lumen of this constricted region. The thin, smooth muscle layer of the gallbladder is composed mostly of **obliquely** oriented fibers, whereas others are oriented longitudinally. Although the connective

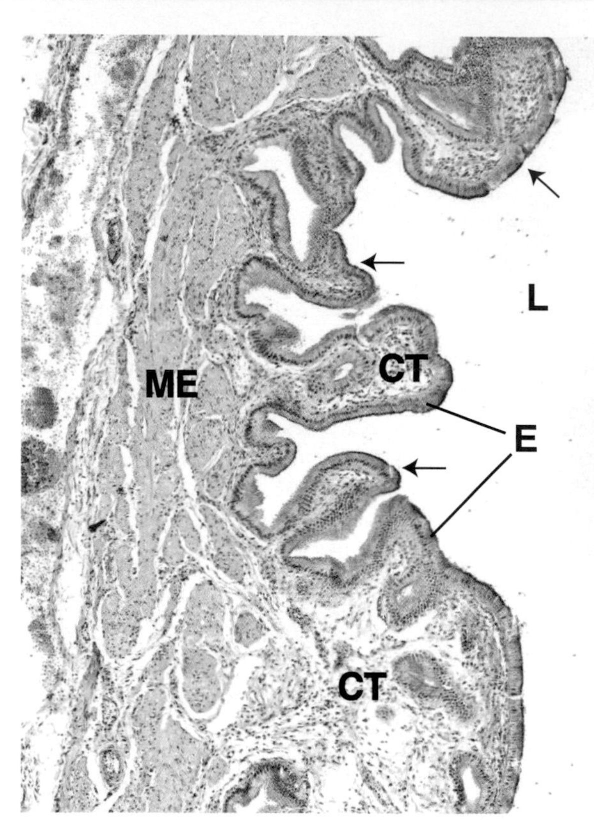

Fig. 18.32 This very-low-magnification photomicrograph of the empty gallbladder displays its muscularis externa (ME) as well as its folded mucosa *(arrows)*. A simple cuboidal epithelium (E) lines the lumen (L) of the gallbladder. The connective tissue (CT) of the lamina propria is unremarkable. (×56)

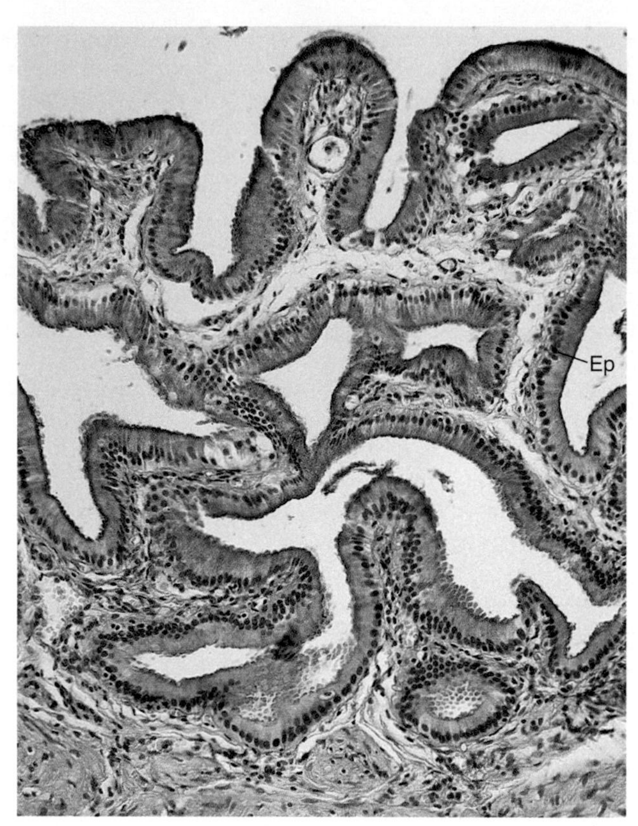

Fig. 18.33 Photomicrograph of an empty gallbladder. Observe that the mucosa of the gallbladder is highly folded, indicating that it is empty. Note that the lumen of the gallbladder is lined by a simple columnar epithelium (Ep). (×270)

tissue adventitia is attached to the Glisson capsule of the liver, it may be separated from it with relative ease. The nonattached surface of the gallbladder is invested by peritoneum, providing it with a smooth, simple squamous epithelial serosa.

Extrahepatic Ducts

The right and left **hepatic ducts** unite to form the **common hepatic duct**, which is joined by the **cystic duct**, arising from the gallbladder. The merger of these two ducts forms the **common bile duct**, 7 to 8 cm long, which fuses with the pancreatic duct to form the **ampulla of Vater**. The ampulla opens at the duodenal papilla into the lumen of the duodenum.

The opening of the common bile duct and of the pancreatic duct is controlled by a complex of four sphincter muscles, sphincter choledecus, sphincter pancreaticus, sphincter ampullae, and fasciculus longitudinalis, collectively called the ***sphincter of Oddi***. The locations and functions of these muscles are summarized in Table 18.5.

Histophysiology of the Gallbladder

The gallbladder stores, concentrates, and releases bile; bile release is triggered by CCK and vagal stimulation.

The primary functions of the gallbladder are to store, concentrate, and release bile. Bile is constantly manufactured by the liver and must make its way to the gallbladder. This activity requires that the sphincters choledecus, pancreaticus, and ampullae be maintained in a closed position so that the bile backs up the common bile duct and the cystic duct to enter the gallbladder.

Na^+ is actively transported from the basolateral region of the simple columnar epithelium of the gallbladder into the extracellular space and is passively followed by chloride (Cl^-) and water. To compensate for the loss of intracellular ions, apical ion channels permit Na^+ and Cl^- to enter the simple columnar cells, reducing the salt (NaCl) concentration of bile. The requirement for osmotic equilibrium drives water from the bile into the simple columnar cell, thus concentrating bile.

The signaling molecule **CCK** is released by I cells (DNES cells) of the duodenum in response to a fatty meal. This molecule comes in contact with CCK receptors on the smooth muscle cells of the gallbladder and causes them to contract intermittently. Concurrently, contact of CCK receptors with the smooth muscle cells of the sphincter of Oddi causes the sphincter muscles to relax. As a result, the rhythmic contractile forces of the gallbladder inject the bile into the lumen of the duodenum. In addition, **acetylcholine**, released by the vagal parasympathetic fibers, stimulates contraction of the gallbladder.

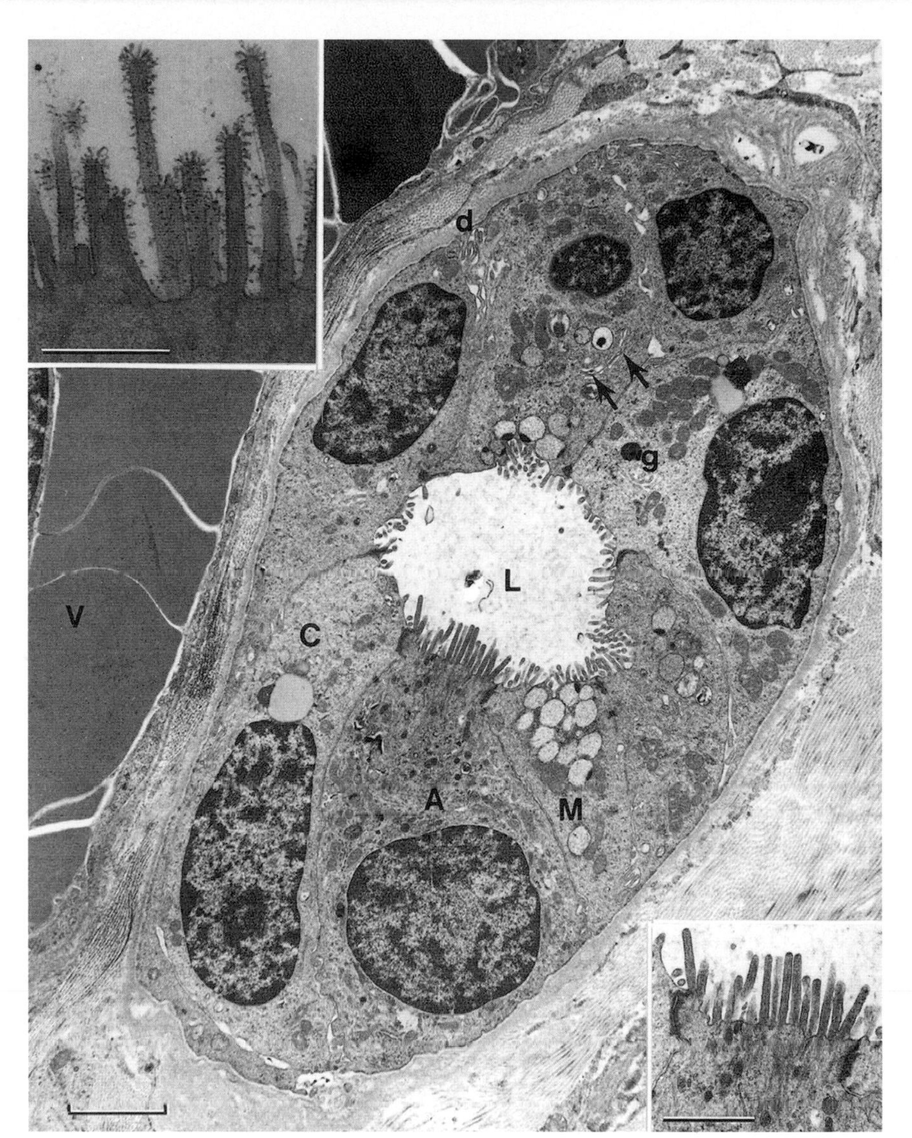

Fig. 18.34 Electron micrograph of the human gallbladder diverticulum displaying brush cells (A) and clear cells (C) of the epithelium. d, Interdigitations; g, granules; L, lumen; M, clear cells with mucoid granules. Bar = 2 µm. *Upper inset:* Clear cell microvilli. Bar = 0.5 µm. *Lower inset:* Brush cell microvilli. Bar = 1.0 µm. (From Gilloteaux J, Pomerants B, Kelly T. Human gallbladder mucosa ultrastructure: evidence of intraepithelial nerve structures. *Am J Anat.* 1989;184:321–333. Reprinted with permission from Wiley-Liss, Inc., a subsidiary of John Wiley & Sons, Inc.)

TABLE 18.5 The Sphincter of Oddi and Its Component Parts

Sphincter Muscle	Location and Function
Sphincter choledochus	Surrounds and controls terminal region of common bile duct to stop bile flow into duodenum
Sphincter pancreaticus	Surrounds and controls terminal portion of pancreatic duct to stop pancreatic juices from entering duodenum and prevents entry of bile into pancreatic duct
Sphincter ampullae	Surrounds and controls ampulla of Vater and prevents entry of bile and pancreatic juices into duodenum
Fasciculus longitudinalis	Located in triangular interval delineated by ampulla of Vater, pancreatic duct, and common bile duct; facilitates entry of bile into lumen of duodenum

Clinical Correlations

*Gallstones (cholelithiasis) are more common in women than in men and occur most frequently in the fourth decade of life. Approximately 20% of all women and 8% of all men have gallstones. Usually, people are unaware of their presence because gallstones are either small enough to be eliminated with normal bile flow or too large to leave the gallbladder. When they enter and become entrapped in the cystic or common hepatic ducts, gallstones obstruct bile flow and cause excruciating pain. Approximately 80% of gallstones are composed of cholesterol (**cholesterol stones**). Most of the remainder are formed from the calcium salt of bile, calcium bilirubinate (**pigment stones**), or a combination of cholesterol and calcified bilirubinate. Cholesterol stones are large (1–3 cm) and pale yellow, have numerous facets, and are few in number. Pigment stones are smaller (1 cm), black, and ovoid, and they occur in large numbers. Usually, both types of stones are radiolucent.*

Pathological Considerations

See Figs. 18.35 through 18.37.

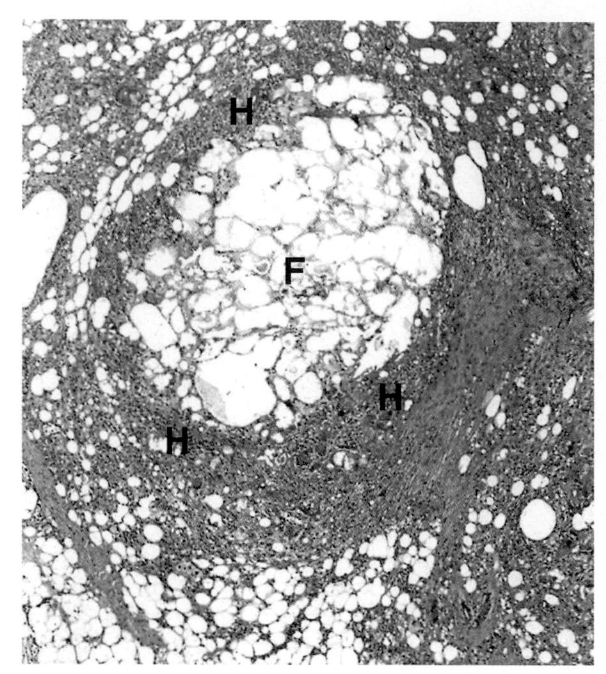

Fig. 18.35 Photomicrograph of the pancreas of a patient with acute pancreatitis. Observe the necrotic adipose tissue (F) that is enveloped by macrophages (H) whose cytoplasm is laden with phagocytosed lipid droplets. (Reprinted with permission from Young B, Stewart W, O'Dowd G. *Wheater's Basic Pathology: A Text, Atlas and Review of Histopathology*. 5th ed. Oxford: Churchill Livingstone/Elsevier Limited; 2011:174.)

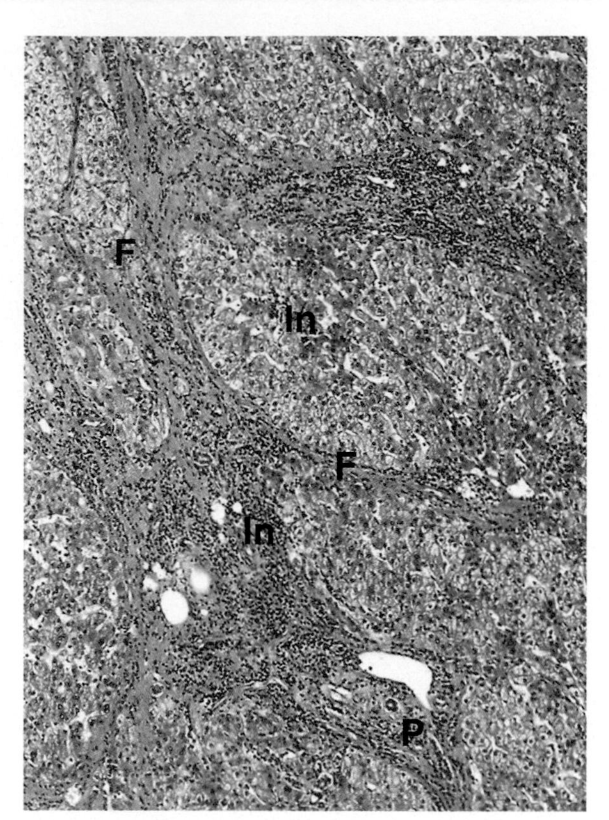

Fig. 18.36 Photomicrograph of a patient with progressive chronic hepatitis and consequent cirrhosis. Note that the portal areas (P) are invaded by inflammatory cells, resulting in areas of focal inflammation (In) and fibrosis (F) where portal areas are connected to each other by fibrous connective tissue. (Reprinted with permission from Young B, Stewart W, O'Dowd G. *Wheater's Basic Pathology: A Text, Atlas and Review of Histopathology*. 5th ed. Oxford: Churchill Livingstone/Elsevier Limited; 2011:170.)

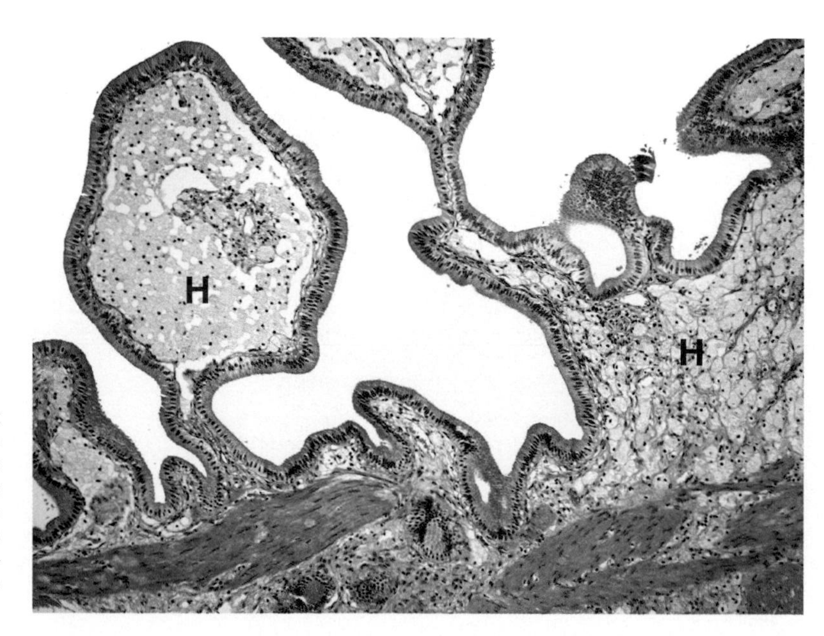

Fig. 18.37 Photomicrograph of the gallbladder of a patient with cholesterolosis, a condition that is frequently accompanied by cholesterol-based gallstone. Histological features include the deposition of lipids, including cholesterol, in the lamina propria of the gallbladder. Observe that the lamina propria is inundated by fat-laden macrophages (H). (Reprinted with permission from Young B, Stewart W, O'Dowd G. *Wheater's Basic Pathology: A Text, Atlas and Review of Histopathology*. 5th ed. Oxford: Churchill Livingstone/Elsevier Limited; 2011:174.)

Histology Laboratory Instructions: Digestive System—Glands

Major Salivary Glands

Parotid Gland

The parotid gland is a serous salivary gland whose connective tissue capsule sends connective tissue septa into the gland, subdividing it into lobules. Even at low magnification, the acini of this gland is noted to be composed of cells with round, basally located nuclei. The gland has numerous ducts, with a variable amount of connective tissue surrounding it (see Fig. 18.4, T, Ac, D). A medium magnification of a parotid gland lobule displays that a section of an acinus resembles a pepperoni pizza, where each triangular slice is the acinar cell and the single pepperoni is its round nucleus. The cross-sectional profiles of the striated duct is easily distinguishable from the acinus (see Fig. 18.5 Ac, SD).

Sublingual Gland

The sublingual gland produces a mixed secretion but is similar to the parotid gland in that its capsule forms connective tissue septa that subdivide the gland into lobules. Even at a low magnification, it is evident that the cells composing the mucous acini possess a froth-like cytoplasm with a thin, basally positioned nucleus, so that the section of the acinus resembles an anchovy pizza. Many of the mucous acini present with a serous demilune (see Fig. 18.6, CT, T, MA, *arrows*). At a medium magnification, the connective tissue septa appear better represented and the acinar cells of the mucous acini display the empty secretory vesicles that give the appearance of their frothy cytoplasm. Note also the cell membranes separating cells of the acinus from one another. The round nuclei and the homogeneous cytoplasm of the cells of the serous demilunes are clearly evident. The cross-sectional profiles of the striated ducts are easily distinguishable from the secretory elements (see Fig. 18.7, CT, T, MA, *arrowheads*, *arrows*, SD).

Submandibular Gland

The submandibular gland produces a mixed secretion and is similar to the sublingual gland in that its capsule forms connective tissue septa that subdivide the gland into lobules. A distinguishing feature of the submandibular gland is that it has many fewer mucous than serous acini. The most characteristic component of the submandibular gland is that it has a much larger number of striated duct profiles than do either the parotid or sublingual glands. Almost every mucous acinus is capped by a serous demilune (see Fig. 18.8, Se, SA, SD, M). At a medium magnification, the striated ducts still form a large percentage of the total area. Mucous acini capped with serous demilunes are well demonstrated. Additionally, there are many serous acini (see Fig. 18.9, SD, MA, SeD, SAc). At a high magnification, the flat nuclei of the cells composing the mucous acini and the round nuclei of the cells of serous acini are clearly evident. The serous components of the submandibular gland, either as serous acini or serous demilunes, far outnumber the mucous components of this gland. Note the cross-sectional profiles of a striated duct (see Fig. 18.10, *arrowheads*, *arrows*, SAc, SeD, MA, SD).

Pancreas

At low magnifications, it is easy to find areas of the pancreas that display both its exocrine components, the serous acini, and their excretory ducts, as well as its endocrine components, the islets of Langerhans (see Fig. 18.12, Ac, D, IL). At a high magnification, the centroacinar cells, pale cells in the center of the serous acinus, is sometimes very evident (see Fig. 18.13, CC, SA). Another high magnification photomicrograph of the pancreas was selected to display the intercalated ducts, formed by the centroacinar cells, which deliver the exocrine secretion of the acinar cells of the acinus to the intralobular ducts (see Fig. 18.14, arrows, Ac, ILD, *arrowheads*).

Liver

Because the pig liver possesses connective tissue elements that completely surround the classical lobule, it is a good way to begin learning the histology of the human liver. Note that in this very-low-magnification photomicrograph, the hexagonal morphology of the classical lobule is clearly outlined by connective tissue septa. The portal areas at the regions where three classical lobules contact each other and the central vein in the center of the classical lobule are clearly distinguishable (see Fig. 18.18, Se, PA, CV). At a medium magnification of a portal area, the portal vein, hepatic artery, bile duct, and lymph vessel are easily recognized. Hepatocytes and sinusoids are also clearly evident (see Fig. 18.19, PV, HA, BD, *arrow*, H, Si). Even at a low magnification of a classical lobule around its central vein, the sinusoids, situated between plates of liver cells, may easily be discerned. Because the dog from which this tissue was removed was injected with India ink prior to being sacrificed, its Kupffer cells are filled with phagocytosed ink particles, making these cells highly visible (see Fig. 18.20, CV, Si, LP, KC). At a medium magnification, the endothelial lining cells of the central vein are well illustrated, as are the sinusoids between plates of liver cells (see Fig. 18.21, *arrow*, CV, Si, H). Bile canaliculi are narrow channels created by the lateral domains of adjacent hepatocytes. These tiny continuous channels deliver their bile into canals of Hering, from which bile enters the bile ducts (see Fig. 18.23, *arrowheads*, *arrows*, BD). A low-magnification photomicrograph of the liver taken from a dog that was injected with India ink prior to being sacrificed displays sinusoids, located between adjacent plates of liver cells, emptying into the central vein. All of the dark blotches represent Kupffer cells that phagocytosed particles of the India ink. Observe a bile duct at the periphery of this classical liver lobule (see Fig. 18.24, Si, H, *arrows*, CV, KC, BD). A high magnification of a similar liver lobule displays the large nuclei of hepatocytes and liver sinusoids lined by endothelial lining cells, as well as Kupffer cells that phagocytosed particles of India ink (see Fig. 18.25, N, Si, K).

Gallbladder

A very-low-magnification photomicrograph of an empty gallbladder demonstrates that it has a highly folded mucosa that becomes flattened when its lumen is filled with bile. The mucosa is composed of a simple columnar epithelium and a loose connective tissue. The muscularis externa or, simply, the muscularis of the gallbladder, is arranged in an oblique fashion and is covered by an adventitia where it adheres to the liver and by a serosa on its free aspect (see Fig. 18.32, *arrows*, L, E, CT, ME). A medium magnification of the empty gallbladder displays its highly folded mucosa. The lumen of the gallbladder is lined by a simple columnar epithelium (see Fig 18.33, Ep).

19 Urinary System

The two kidneys not only remove toxic by-products of metabolism from the bloodstream by forming **urine** but they also **conserve** salts, glucose, amino acids, proteins, water, and additional materials required by the body. The kidneys also help regulate **blood pressure**, **hemodynamics**, and the body's **acid–base balance**. Urine is delivered from the kidneys into the two **ureters**, from which it passes to a storage organ, the **urinary bladder**. During voiding, the urinary bladder is emptied via the **urethra**, which delivers the urine to outside the body. The kidneys also have endocrine functions in that they produce **renin**, **erythropoietin**, and **prostaglandins**. Additionally, they convert a circulating not very active form of vitamin D_3 (**25-OH-vitamin D_3**) to the active vitamin, known as ***calcitriol*** (**1,25-[OH]$_2$ vitamin D_3**). The kidneys also have the ability to synthesize glucose from noncarbohydrate sources, the process known as ***gluconeogenesis***. Although it is the liver that is the usual site of gluconeogenesis, if necessary, the kidneys can match the liver's ability in glucose production.

The Body's Intake and Loss of Water

On a daily basis, an individual's intake of water is approximately 2.1 L, which is gained in the form of liquid plus the water content of food. An additional 200 mL of water is formed by cells of the body, due to carbohydrate oxidation.

Water is lost in the following manner: insensible loss, loss due to sweat, loss in the feces, and loss due to the kidneys.

- **Insensible water loss** occurs in two ways:
  - Via the process of breathing, an individual loses approximately 350 mL of water per day.
  - Via diffusion through the skin, an individual loses approximately 350 mL per day.
- **Water loss due to sweating** is only about 100 mL per day, but that can change according to weather conditions and physical activity. In fact, during very strenuous exercise, the loss may be as much as 10 L per day.
- **Water loss in feces** is approximately 100 mL per day.
- **Water loss through the kidneys** is approximately 1400 mL per day.

Therefore, the loss of water (2.3 L) equals the amount of water an individual takes in (2.3 L), and it is the responsibility of the kidneys to adjust the loss of water in urine to ensure this balanced water conservation. Because the kidneys play such an important role in the body's water balance, much of this chapter is dedicated to the discussion of the structure and functions of the kidneys.

Kidney

The kidneys have a concave region, known as the hilum, where the ureter, renal vein, renal artery, and lymph vessels pierce the kidney.

The kidneys are large, reddish, bean-shaped organs about 11 cm long, 4 to 5 cm wide, and 2 to 3 cm thick. They are embedded in perirenal fat positioned retroperitoneally on the posterior abdominal wall with their convex border situated laterally and their concave **hilum** facing medially. Because of the position of the liver, the right kidney is situated approximately 1 to 2 cm lower than the left. Branches of the renal artery and vein, lymph vessels, and ureter pierce each kidney at its hilum. The ureter is expanded at this region, forming the **renal pelvis**; a fat-filled extension of the hilum, the **renal sinus**, presses deeper into the kidney.

The kidney is invested by a thin, loosely adhering **capsule**, composed of an outer dense, irregular, collagenous, connective tissue with **fibroblasts** and occasional elastic fibers, and an inner layer composed mostly of **myoepithelial cells**.

OVERVIEW OF KIDNEY STRUCTURE

The kidney is subdivided into an outer cortex and an inner medulla.

A hemisected view of the kidney with the unaided eye displays the presence of a narrow outer **cortex** and a much wider inner **medulla** (Fig. 19.1). The cortical region appears dark brown and granular, whereas the medulla contains at least 8, but generally more than 12, discrete pyramid-shaped, pale, striated regions, the **renal pyramids**. The base of each pyramid is oriented toward the cortex, constituting the corticomedullary border, whereas its apex, known as the **renal papilla**, points toward the hilum. The apex is perforated by around 20 openings of the **ducts of Bellini**; this sieve-like region of the renal papilla is known as the **area cribrosa**. The renal papilla is surrounded by a cup-like space, the **minor calyx**, which joins two or three neighboring minor calyces to open into a **major calyx**. The three or four major calyces are larger spaces that empty into the **renal pelvis**, the expanded region of the proximal portion of the ureter. Neighboring pyramids are separated from each other by material resembling the cortex, the **cortical columns** (of Bertin).

The portion of the cortex overlying the base of each pyramid is known as a **cortical arch**. Macroscopically, three types of structures are present in the cortex: (1) red, dot-like granules, the **renal corpuscles**; (2) convoluted tubules, the **cortical labyrinth**; and (3) longitudinal striations, **medullary rays**, the cortical continuations of structures located in the renal pyramids.

Each renal pyramid, with its associated cortical arch and cortical columns, represents a **lobe** of the kidney. Hence, the human kidney is a multilobar organ. Each medullary ray, with part of the cortical labyrinth surrounding, it is considered a kidney **lobule** (bounded by **interlobular arteries**), which continues into the medulla as a cone-shaped structure, widest at the cortex and narrowest near the renal papilla.

Clinical Correlations

1. *During fetal development, the lobes of the kidney are accentuated by deep clefts, but this characteristic is normally obliterated in adults. When the lobation is retained after infancy, the condition is known as* **lobated kidney.**
2. *Another anomalous kidney development is known as* ***polycystic kidney disease*** *(PKD), which presents varied morphological features according to the severity of the affliction; it involves the appearance of thin-walled cysts on and in the kidneys. According to the National Kidney Foundation, approximately 600,000 people have PKD in the United States, distributed equally between men and women. In half the population diagnosed with PKD, the result is kidney failure by 60 years of age. By age 70 years, the incidence rises to 60%, for which the risk factors are gender (males are more at risk than are females); patients with hypertension; the presence of proteinurea or hematuria; and women with four or more pregnancies who also suffer from hypertension. There is no cure for PKD. Recently, however, the US Food and Drug Administration approved a new medication, tolvaptan, designed to decrease the rate of PKD in patients with the autosomal dominant form of PKD.*

URINIFEROUS TUBULES

The uriniferous tubule, the functional unit of the kidney, is composed of a nephron and collecting tubule.

The **uriniferous tubule**, a highly convoluted structure that modifies the fluid passing through it to form **urine** as its final output, is the functional unit of the kidney. It consists of two parts: the **nephron** and **collecting tubule** (see Fig. 19.1), each with a different embryological origin. Each kidney possesses approximately 1.3 million nephrons, several of which are drained by a single collecting tubule. Multiple collecting tubules join in the deeper aspect of the medulla to form increasingly larger ducts. The largest of these, the **ducts of Bellini**, perforate the renal papilla at the area cribrosa.

Uriniferous tubules are so densely packed that they leave only a little space for the connective tissue **stroma**, from which they are separated by an intervening **basal lamina**. Much of the stroma is occupied by the rich vascular supply of the kidney. The functional relationship between the vascular supply and uriniferous tubules is discussed later in the chapter.

Nephron

There are two types of nephrons, depending on the location of their renal corpuscles and the length of their Henle loop.

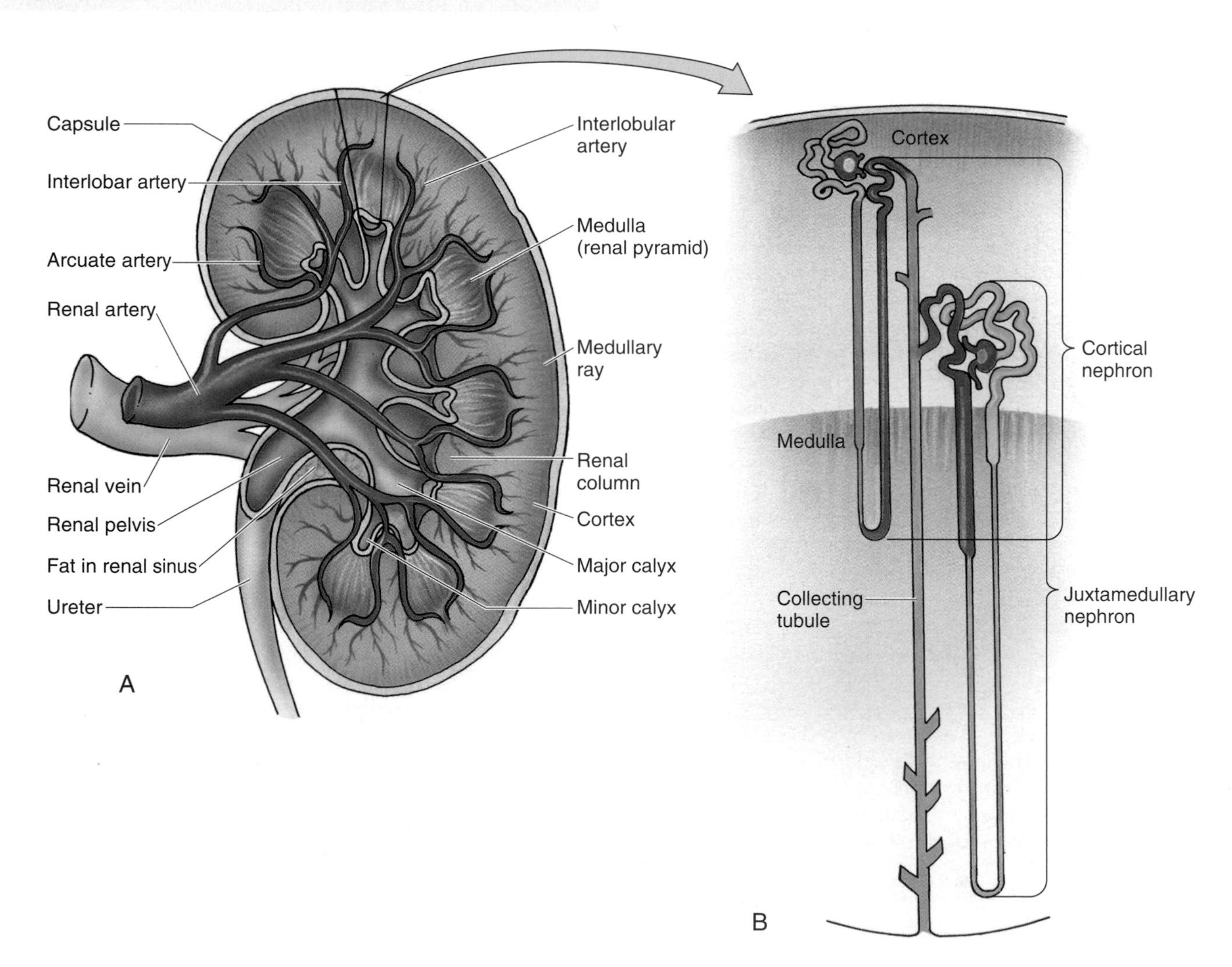

Fig. 19.1 The kidney. (A) Schematic diagram of a hemisected kidney illustrating its morphology and circulation. (B) Arrangement of cortical and juxtamedullary nephrons.

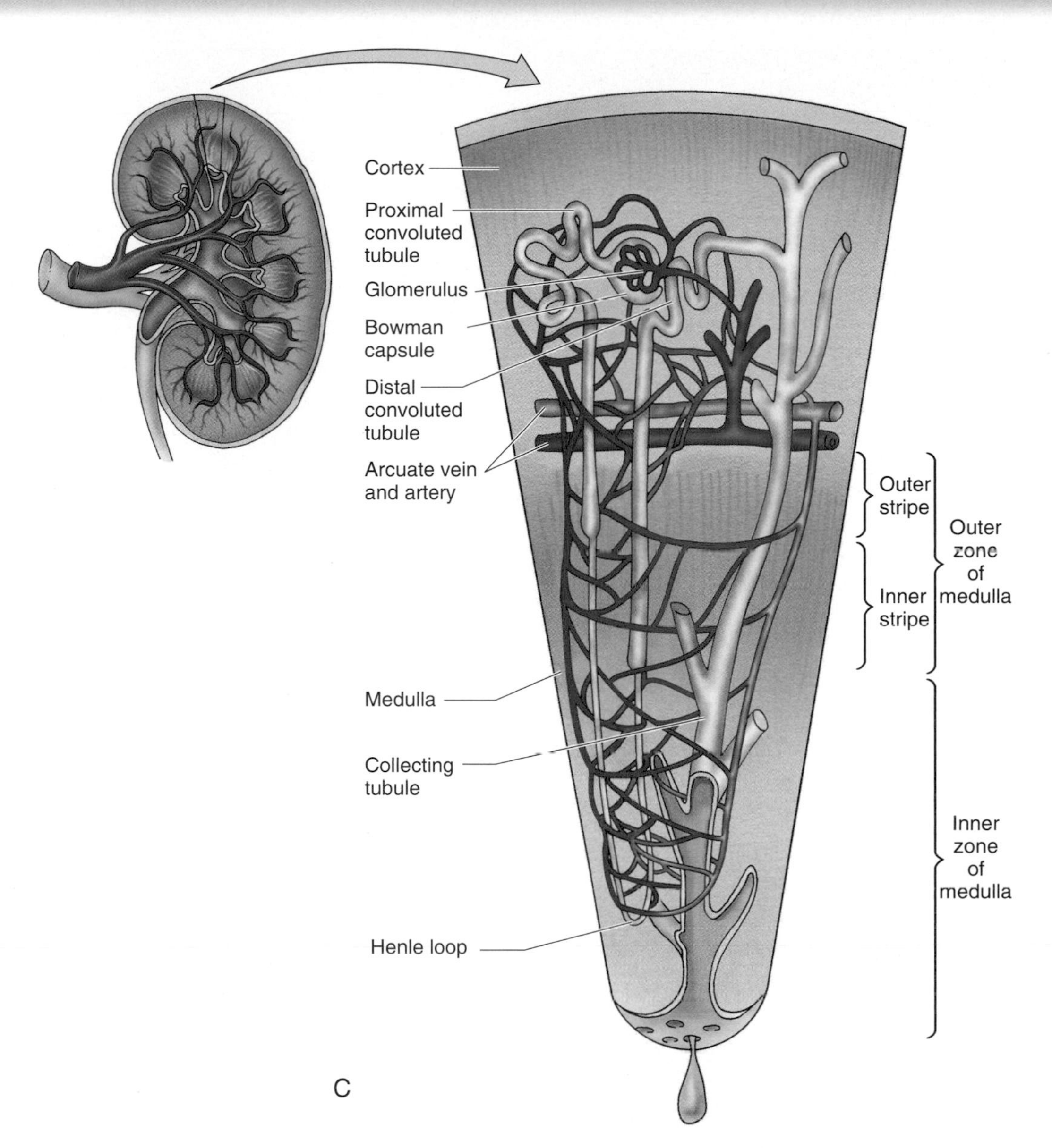

Fig. 19.1, cont'd (C) The uriniferous tubule and its vascular supply and drainage. The juxtamedullary nephron extends much deeper into the medulla than does the cortical nephron.

Two types of nephrons are found in the human kidney: (1) shorter **cortical nephrons**, subdivided into two groups, superficial and midcortical nephrons, neither of which extend deep into the medulla; and (2) the longer **juxtamedullary nephrons**, whose renal corpuscle is located in the cortex—at the corticomedullary junction—and whose tubular parts extend deep into the medulla (see Fig. 19.1). The specific locations of the two types of nephrons, the cellular composition of their various regions, and the specific alignments of these regions in register with one another permit the subdivision of the medulla into an **outer medulla** (**outer zone**) and an **inner medulla** (**inner zone**). The outer medulla is further subdivided into an **outer stripe** and an **inner stripe**. The regions of the medulla are illustrated in Fig. 19.1C (note that parts of the kidney have more than a single name; since that can be confusing, Table 19.1 lists the alternate names). Unless otherwise noted, all of the descriptions in this textbook refer to **juxtamedullary nephrons**, even though they constitute only 15% of all nephrons.

Each juxtamedullary nephron is about 40 mm long and its constituent parts are modified to perform specific physiological functions. The **Bowman capsule**, with its attendant glomerulus, filters the fluid expressed from the bloodstream. The subsequent tubular portions of the nephron (i.e., the **proximal tubule**, **thin limbs of Henle loop**, and **distal tubule**) modify the filtrate to form urine.

Clinical Correlations

Because nephrons cannot be regenerated as the individual ages, there is an age-related reduction in the number of nephrons. It has been reported that, after middle age (around 40 years of age), there is an annual 1% loss in the number of nephrons, so that 75-year-old individuals have 35% fewer nephrons than they did at age 40 years. Fortunately, the remaining nephrons compensate for the decrease by adapting to the deteriorated condition, and, provided that all other conditions remain normal, they are able to maintain normal physiological status.

TABLE 19.1 Alternate Names of Various Kidney Structures

Common Name	Alternate Names
Outer medulla	Outer zone
Inner medulla	Inner zone
Cortical column	Cortical column of Bertin
Bowman space	Urinary space
Primary process of podocyte	Major process of podocyte
Pedicel	Secondary process of podocyte
Ultrafiltrate	Glomerular ultrafiltrate
Proximal convoluted tubule	Pars convoluta of proximal tubule
Descending thick limb of Henle loop	Pars recta of proximal tubule
Ascending thick limb of Henle loop	Pars recta of distal tubule
Distal convoluted tubule	Pars convoluta of distal tubule
Extraglomerular mesangial cells	Polkissen; lacis cells; polar cushion
Cortical collecting tubules	Collecting tubules
Medullary collecting tubules	Collecting tubules
Ducts of Bellini	Papillary collecting tubules
Vasa recta	Arteriolae rectae and venae rectae

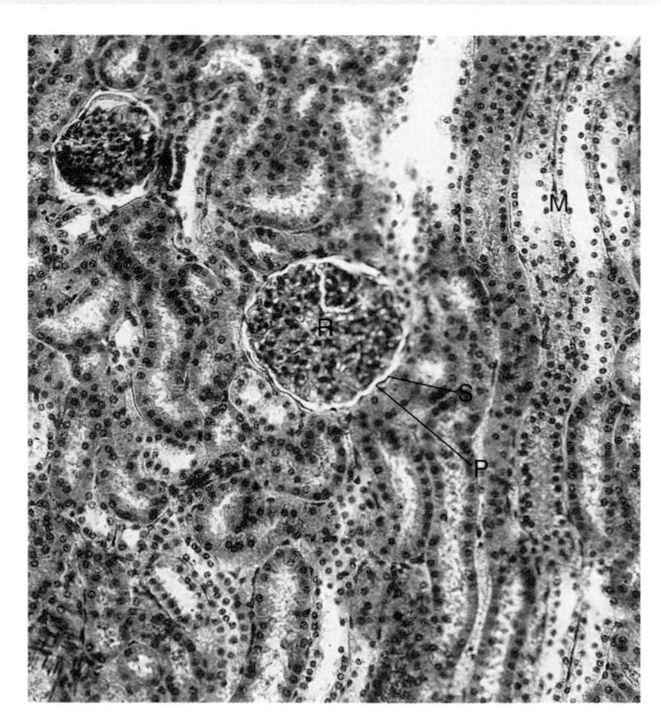

Fig. 19.2 Photomicrograph of the kidney cortex in a monkey illustrating renal corpuscles (R), medullary ray (M), and cross-sectional profiles of the uriniferous tubules. A portion of the urinary space (S) is clearly evident at the periphery of the renal corpuscle and is bounded by the simple squamous epithelium composing the parietal layer (P) of the Bowman capsule. (×132)

Renal Corpuscle

The renal corpuscle is composed of a tuft of capillaries, the glomerulus, surrounded by the Bowman capsule.

The **renal corpuscle**, an oval to round structure about 200 to 250 μm in diameter, is composed of a tuft of capillaries, the **glomerulus**, which is invaginated into the **Bowman capsule**, the dilated, blind, pouch-like, proximal end of the nephron (Figs. 19.2–19.5). During development, the capillaries become invested by the blind end of the tubular nephron, almost as if fingers of a hand were pushing into the end of an expanded balloon. Hence, the space inside the Bowman capsule, known as the **Bowman space** (**urinary space**), is decreased in volume. The glomerulus is in intimate contact with the **visceral layer of the Bowman capsule**, composed of modified epithelial

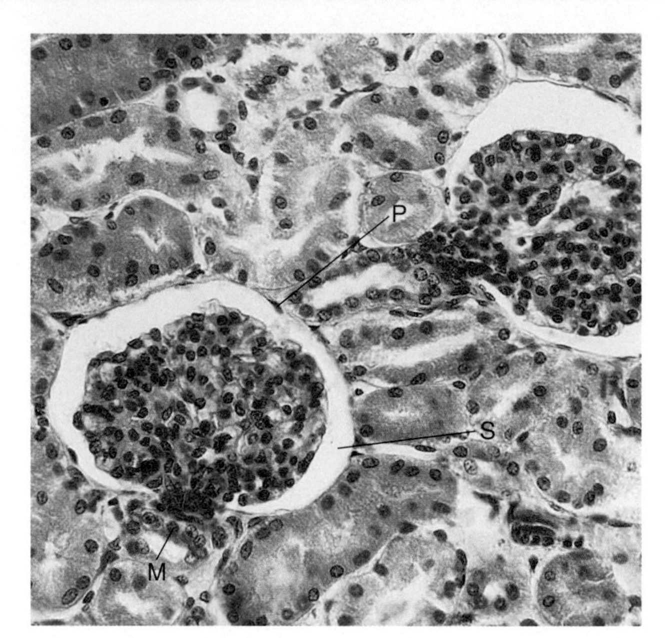

Fig. 19.3 Photomicrograph of the monkey renal corpuscle surrounded by cross-sectional profiles of proximal and distal tubules. The macula densa (M) and parietal layer of the Bowman capsule (P) are clearly evident as they enclose the clear space, a part of the urinary space (S). (×270)

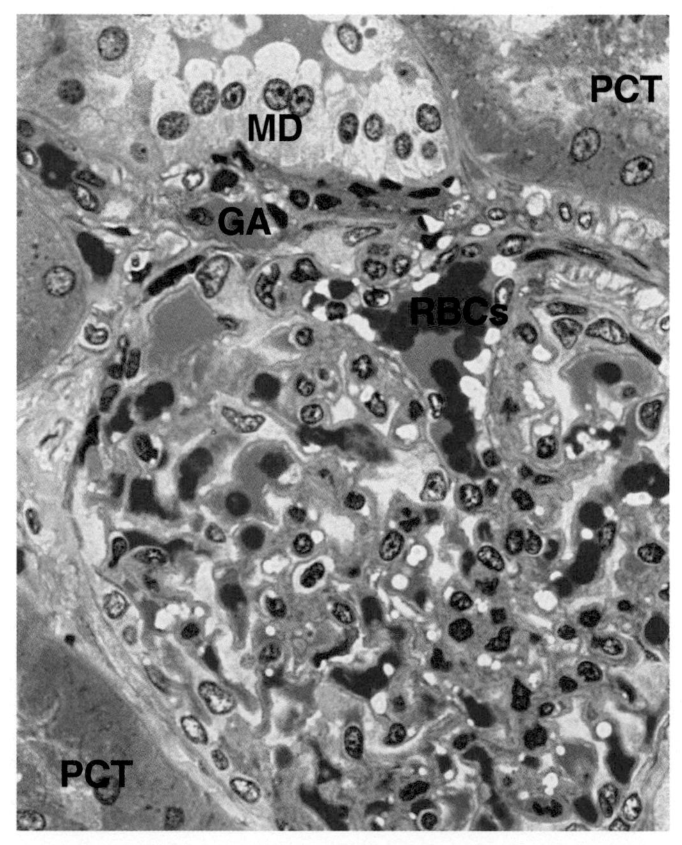

Fig. 19.4 This high-magnification photomicrograph of a renal corpuscle displays the red blood cells (RBCs) in the glomerulus. It also presents the afferent glomerular arteriole (GA) of the vascular pole in close association of the macula densa (MD) portion of the distal tubule. Cross-sectional profiles of the proximal convoluted tubule are also labeled. (×540)

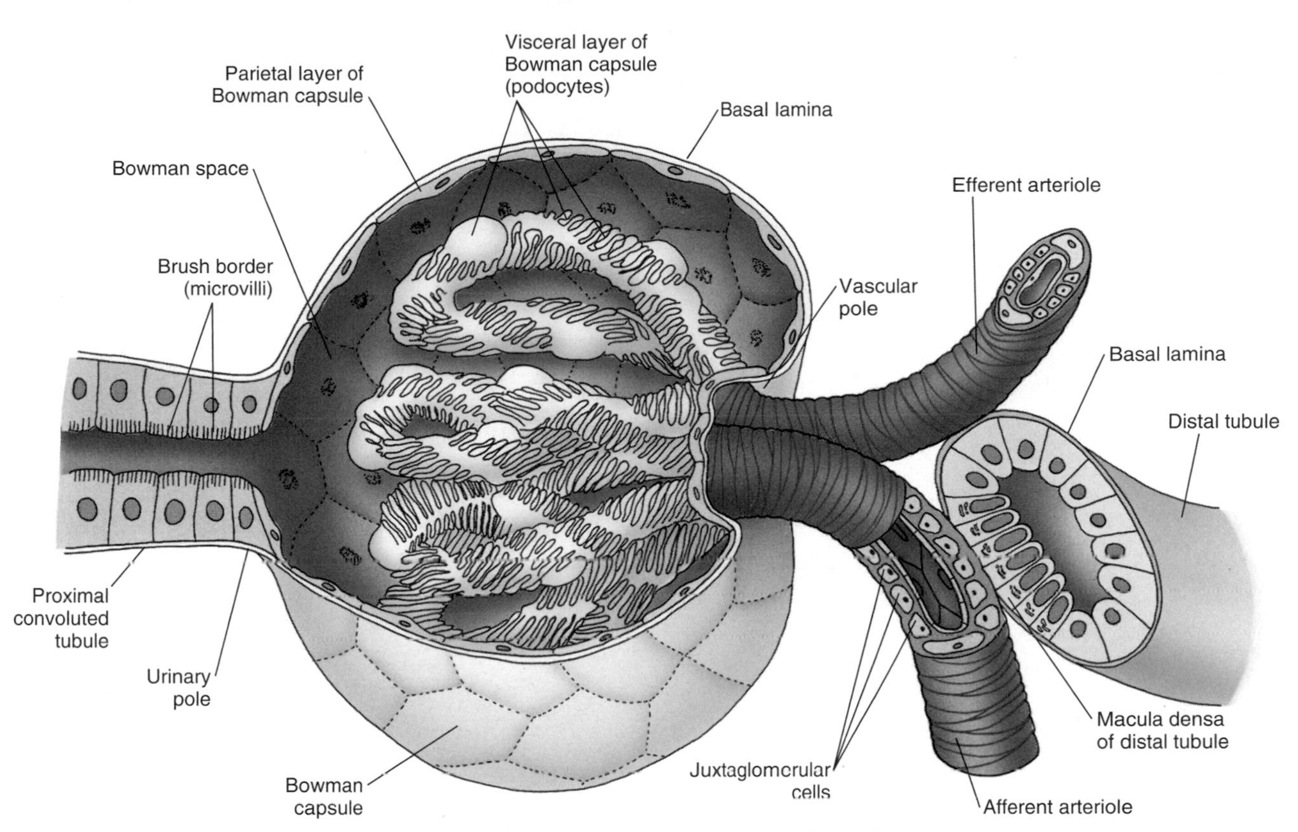

Fig. 19.5 Diagram of a renal corpuscle and its juxtaglomerular apparatus.

cells called **podocytes**. The outer wall surrounding the Bowman space, composed of simple squamous epithelial cells (surrounded by a thin basal lamina), is the **parietal layer of the Bowman capsule** (see Figs. 19.3–9.5).

The region where the vessels supplying and draining the glomerulus enter and exit the Bowman capsule is known as the **vascular pole**, whereas the region of continuation between the renal corpuscle and the proximal tubule, which drains the Bowman space, is called the **urinary pole**. The glomerulus is supplied by the short, straight **afferent glomerular arteriole**, a branch of the **interlobular artery**, and drained by the **efferent glomerular arteriole**. Although the outer diameter of the afferent arteriole is greater than that of the efferent arteriole, their luminal diameters are approximately equal. It is important to note that the glomerulus is a capillary bed that is supplied and drained by arterioles; the reader should bear in mind that most capillary beds are supplied by arterioles and drained by venules. The efferent glomerular arteriole presents greater resistance to blood flow than a venule would; therefore, blood pressure in the glomerulus is greater than in other capillary beds. Filtrate leaking out of the glomerulus enters the Bowman space through a complex **filtration barrier** composed of the endothelial wall of the glomerular capillary, the basal lamina, and the visceral layer of the Bowman capsule.

Glomerulus.

The glomerulus is composed of tufts of fenestrated capillaries supplied by the afferent glomerular arteriole and drained by the efferent glomerular arteriole.

The **glomerulus** is formed as several tufts of anastomosing capillaries that arise from branches of the afferent glomerular arteriole. The connective tissue component of the afferent arteriole does not enter the Bowman capsule, and the normal connective tissue cells are replaced by a specialized cell type of smooth muscle origin, known as **mesangial cells**. There are two groups of mesangial cells, both of which are of smooth muscle origin. **Extraglomerular mesangial cells** are located at the vascular pole, and pericyte-like **intraglomerular mesangial cells** are situated within the renal corpuscle (Figs. 19.6 and 19.7).

Intraglomerular mesangial cells are phagocytic and function in resorption of the basal lamina, but they demonstrate their smooth muscle origin because they are contractile and have receptors for vasoconstrictor agents such as **angiotensin II** and **atrial natriuretic peptide**. When these agents bind to their receptors, the mesangial cells reduce blood flow through the glomerulus. Both types of mesangial cells also synthesize various cytokines, such as interleukin-1, endothelins, platelet-derived growth factor, prostaglandin E_2 (PGE_2), and mesangial matrix. Moreover, they provide physical support to the capillaries of the glomerulus, along with podocytes and the glomerular basement membrane. The glomerulus is composed of fenestrated capillaries (Fig. 19.8; see Figs. 19.6 and 19.7) whose endothelial cells are highly attenuated, except for the region containing the nucleus; their fenestrae are *not covered by a diaphragm*. The pores are large, ranging between 70 and 90 nm in diameter; hence, these capillaries act as a barrier only to formed elements of the blood and to macromolecules whose effective diameter exceeds the size of the fenestrae (e.g., albumin, 69,000 daltons [Da]). These endothelial cells possess Aquaporin-1 channels in their cell membranes and manufacture cytokines, such as nitric oxide (NO) and PGE_2.

Basal Lamina. Investing the glomerulus is a glomerular basal lamina (~300 nm thick), consisting of three layers (see Figs. 19.7 and 19.8). The middle dense layer, the **lamina densa**, is about 100 nm in thickness and consists of type IV collagen. However, it does

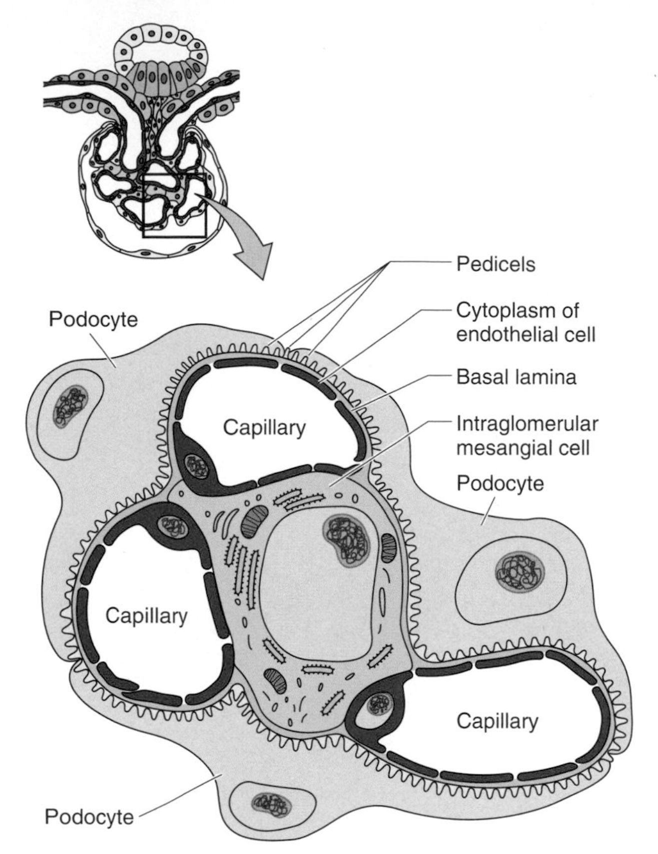

Fig. 19.6 Relationship between the intraglomerular mesangial cell, podocytes, and glomerulus.

not contain the usual type composed of α_1 and α_2 chains that are present in lamina densa of basal laminae in other regions of the body but rather the α_3, α_4, and α_5 chains. Less electron-dense layers—the **laminae rarae**, which contain **laminin**, **fibronectin**, and the highly hydrated polyanionic proteoglycans, perlacan and agrin, rich in **heparan sulfate**—are located on either side of the lamina densa. Some refer to a **lamina rara interna**, between the endothelial cells of the capillary and the lamina densa, and the **lamina rara externa**, between the lamina densa and the visceral layer of the Bowman capsule. Fibronectin and laminin assist the pedicels and endothelial cells to maintain their attachment to the lamina densa.

Clinical Correlations

*Mutations in the α_3 and α_4 chains of type IV collagen result in **Alport syndrome**, which is distinguished by loss of hearing, vision problems, and nephritis accompanied by microscopic hematuria. Patients with Alport syndrome frequently suffer from kidney failure and may, eventually, require a kidney transplant. The most common form of Alport syndrome is X-linked; therefore, males are more often affected than females, who tend to be carriers but still exhibit hematuria. Males usually die from kidney failure but females rarely do, unless they carry the mutations on both X chromosomes. The less common form of Alport syndrome is inherited as an autosomal recessive pattern (chromosome 2), which causes them to be carriers of the syndrome. If they have the same mutations on both copies of chromosome 2, then they exhibit Alport syndrome and males and females are affected equally.*

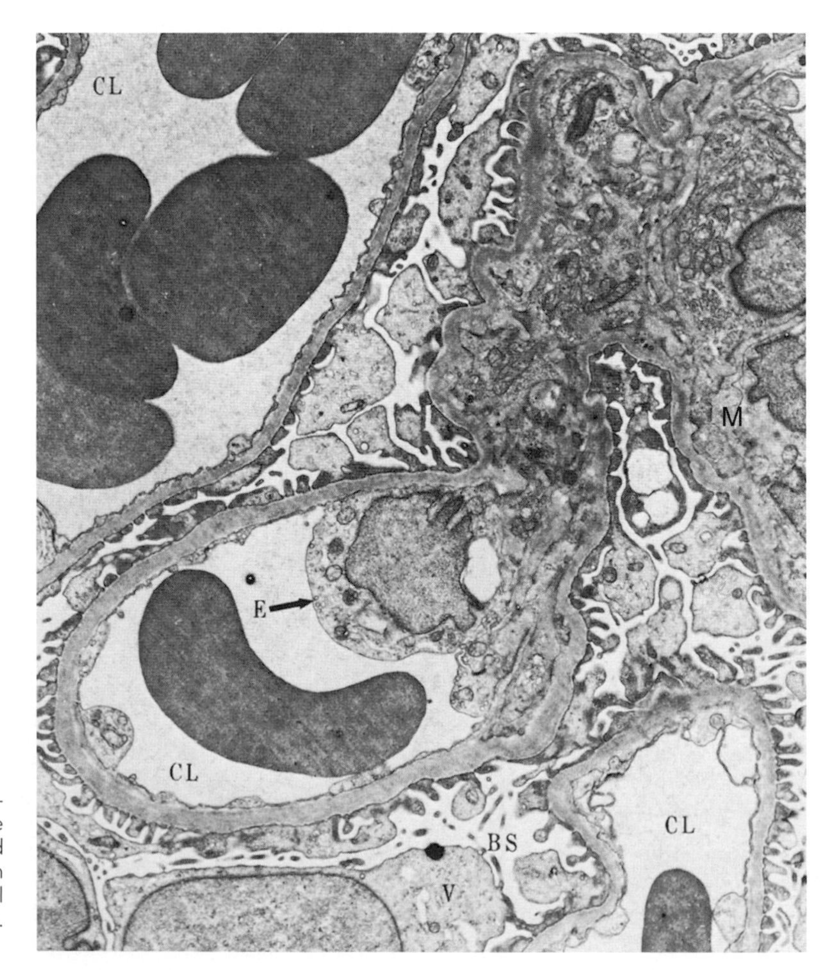

Fig. 19.7 Electron micrograph of a region of the human kidney glomerulus containing red blood cells (×4594). Note the association between the intraglomerular mesangial cell and the podocytes around the glomerular capillaries. BS, Bowman space; CL, capillary lumen; E, endothelial cell; M, mesangial cells; V, podocyte. (From Brenner BM, Rector FC. *The Kidney*. 4th ed. Vol 1. Philadelphia: WB Saunders; 1991.)

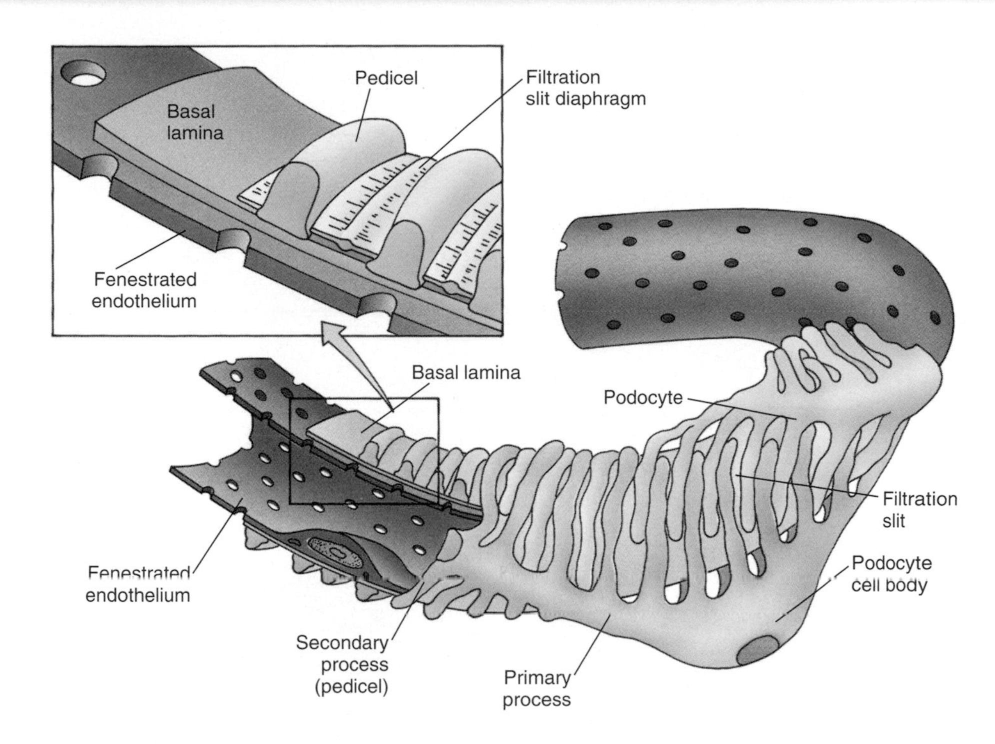

Fig. 19.8 Schematic diagram of the interrelationship of the glomerulus, podocytes, pedicels, and basal laminae.

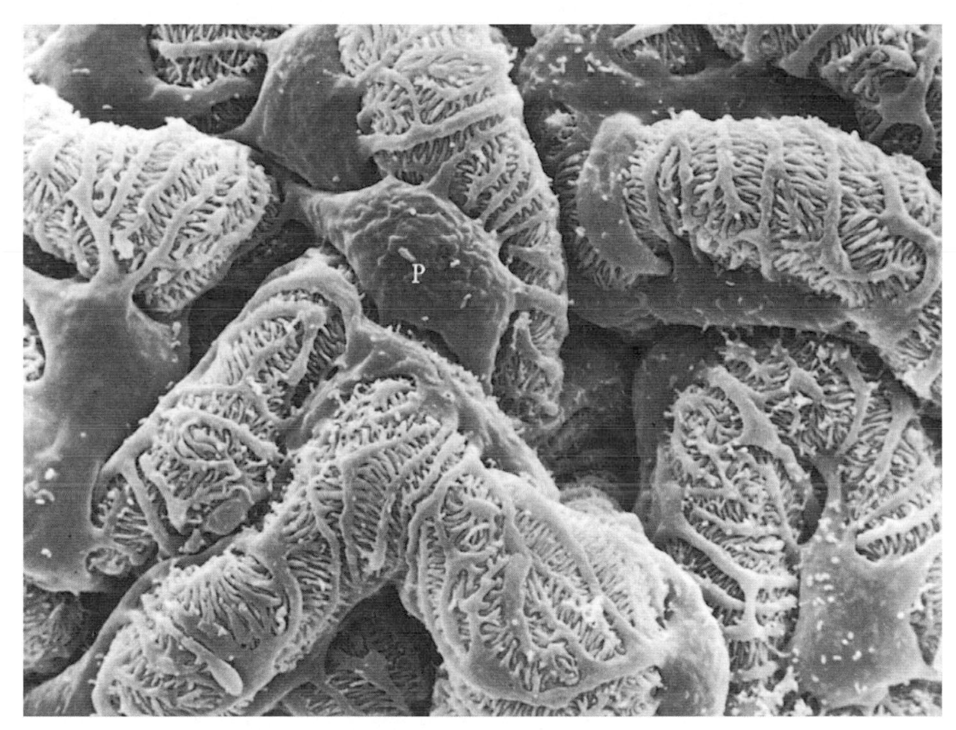

Fig. 19.9 Scanning electron micrograph of podocytes and their processes from the kidney of a rat (×4700). P, Podocytes. (From Brenner BM, Rector FC. *The Kidney*. 4th ed. Vol 1. Philadelphia: WB Saunders; 1991.)

Visceral Layer of the Bowman Capsule

The visceral layer of the Bowman capsule is composed of epithelial cells that become modified and are known as podocytes.

The visceral layer of the Bowman capsule is composed of epithelial cells that are highly modified to perform a filtering function. These large cells, called **podocytes**, bear numerous long, tentacle-like cytoplasmic extensions, **primary (major) processes**, which follow but usually do not come in close contact with the longitudinal axes of the glomerular capillaries. Each primary process bears many **secondary processes**, also known as **pedicels**, arranged in an orderly fashion. Pedicels completely envelop most of the glomerular capillaries by interdigitating with pedicels from neighboring major processes of different podocytes (Figs. 19.9–19.11). Podocytes also manufacture **glomerular endothelial growth factor** that functions not only in maintaining the integrity of the endothelial cells of the glomerulus but also prompts them, when the need arises, to enter the cell cycle.

Pedicels have a well-developed glycocalyx composed of the negatively charged sialoprotein **podocalyxin**, **podoplanin**, and **podoendin**. The negative charges are responsible for the electrostatic repulsion that contributes to the formation of the filtration barrier. Pedicels rest on the lamina rara externa of the basal lamina and possess $\alpha_3\beta_1$

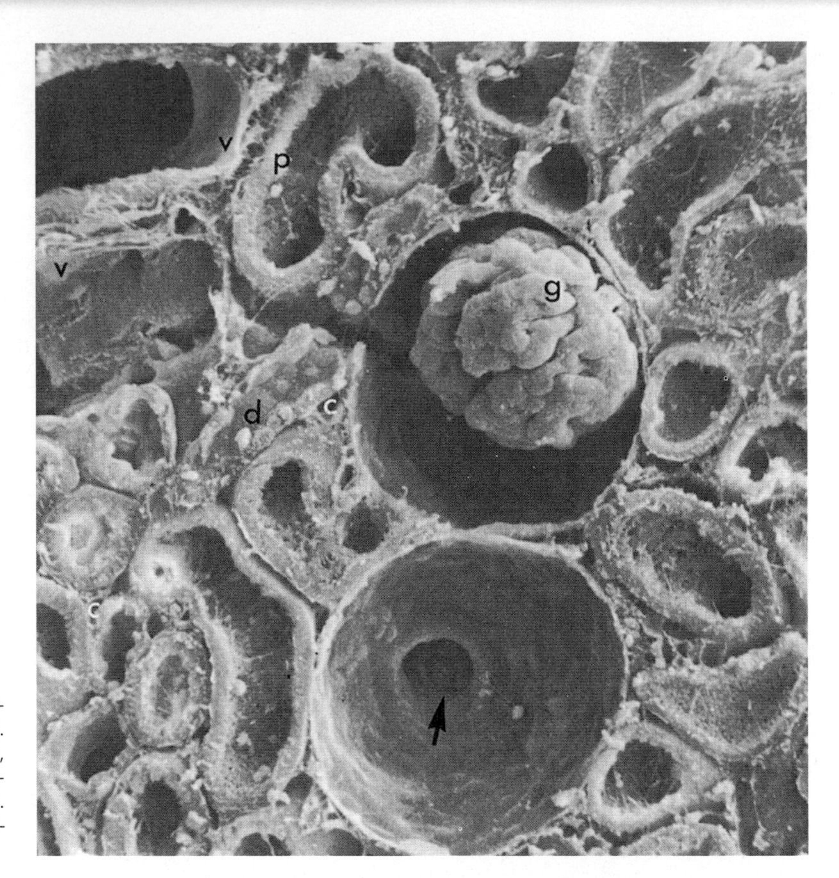

Fig. 19.10 Scanning electron micrograph of the rat renal cortex displaying a renal corpuscle with its glomerulus (g) (×543). The renal corpuscle below it does not have its glomerulus; thus, the urinary pole *(arrow)* is evident. C, Capillaries; d, distal convoluted tubule; P, proximal convoluted tubule; v, blood vessels. (From Leeson TS, Leeson CR, Paparo AA. *Text/Atlas of Histology*. Philadelphia: WB Saunders; 1988.)

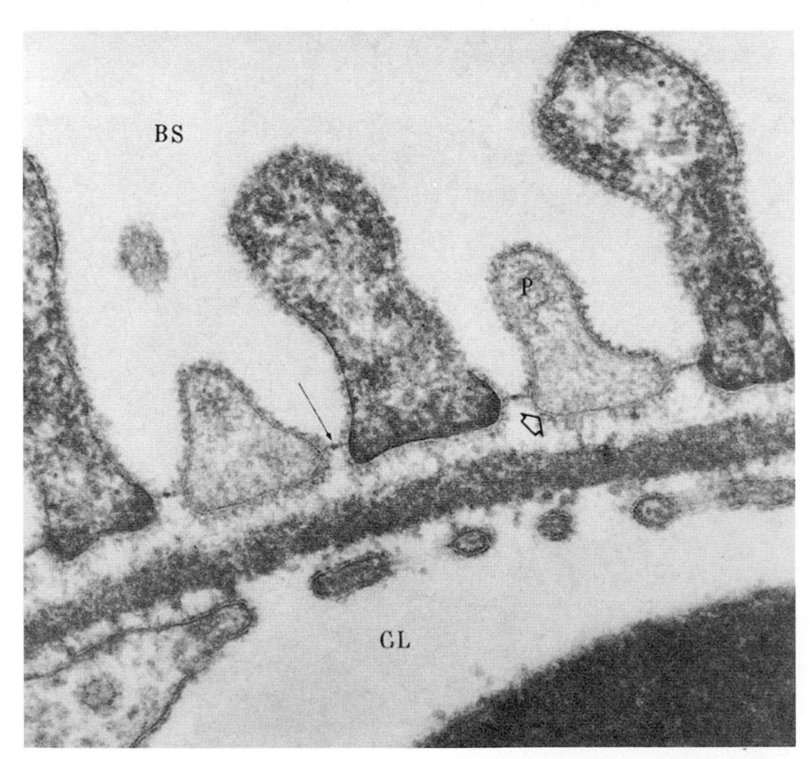

Fig. 19.11 Electron micrograph of pedicels and diaphragms bridging the filtration slits of a glomerulus in a rat (×86,700). BS, Bowman space; CL, capillary lumen. *Hollow arrow* indicates the laminae rara externa; the *arrow* indicates the filtration slit diaphragm. (From Brenner BM, Rector FC. *The Kidney*. 4th ed. Vol 1. Philadelphia: WB Saunders; 1991.)

integrins in their plasmalemma that assists them to adhere to the basal lamina. Their cytoplasm is devoid of organelles but does house microtubules and microfilaments. Interdigitation occurs in such a fashion that narrow clefts, 20 to 40 nm in width, known as ***filtration slits***, remain between adjacent pedicels. Filtration slits are not completely open; instead, they are covered by a thin **filtration slit diaphragm**, which extends between neighboring pedicels and acts as a part of the filtration barrier (see Figs. 19.8 and 19.11). The slit diaphragm of the two neighboring pedicels is composed of the extracytoplasmic moieties of the 40-nm-long transmembrane protein **nephrin** and the 20-nm-long **Neph1**. The intracytoplasmic component

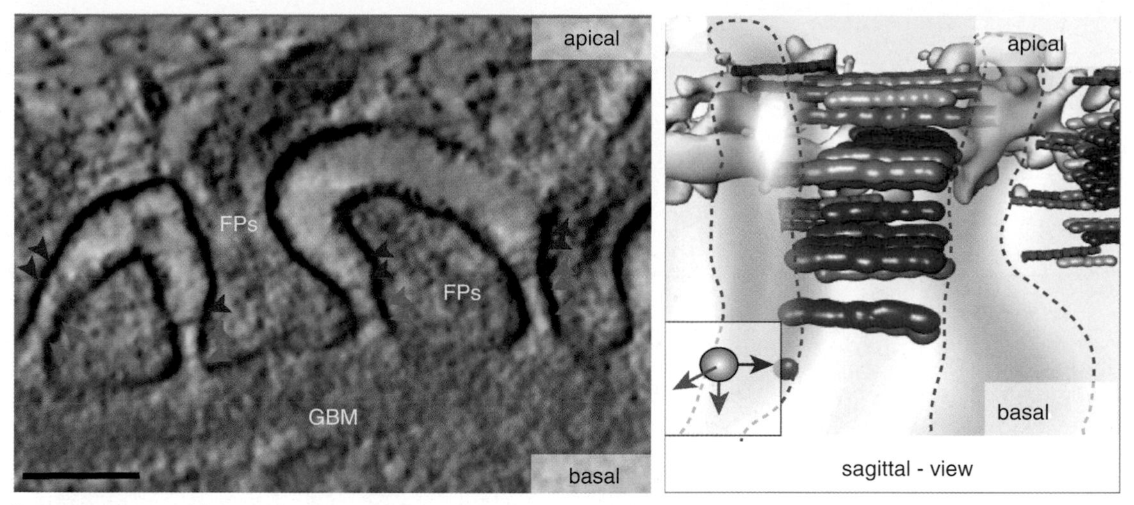

Fig. 19.12 *Left:* A sagittal view of four pedicels (FPs) sitting on the glomerular basal lamina (GBM) indicating the pedicels' basal and apical regions. Observe that the slit diaphragm is a multilayered structure, where the longer nephrin molecules *(red arrowheads)* form a single layer and are located apically, whereas the shorter Neph1 molecules are multilayered (blue arrowheads) and are located more basally. *Right:* A diagram illustrating the electron micrograph on the left. Note that the nephrin molecules *(red)* are longer and are located apically and the several layers of the shorter Neph1 molecules (blue) are located basally. (From Grahammer et al., "A flexible multilayered protein scaffold maintains the slit in between glomerular podocytes." https://doi.org/10.1172/jci.insight.86177)

of these two molecules are connected to actin filaments by two interlinking proteins, **CD2-associated protein** and **podocin**. It has been demonstrated that the slit diaphragm, unlike its simple image in conventional transmission electron microscopy (see Fig. 19.11) is a very complex, flexible, multilayered structure where Neph1 is located basally, forming several layers closer to the glomerular basal lamina, and nephrin is a single layer thick and is located more apically (Fig. 19.12). Because both nephrin and Neph1 are flexible, the distance between individual nephrin molecules and individual Neph1 molecules can be modulated as necessary, thereby making these spaces act as variable-sized pores. Therefore, the slit diaphragm is a barrier that can avoid being clogged by larger molecules by altering their pore size.

The cell body of the podocyte is not at all unusual in organelle content. It houses the irregularly shaped nucleus, as well as rough endoplasmic reticulum, Golgi apparatus, and numerous free ribosomes.

Filtration Process. Fluid leaving the glomerular capillaries is driven by the **blood pressure** in the glomerular capillary bed (60 mm Hg), but that is resisted by the **colloid osmotic pressure** of the blood in the glomerulus (32 mm Hg) and by the hydrostatic pressure of the fluid, known as the ***oncotic pressure***, in the urinary space (18 mm Hg). Therefore, there is a **net filtration pressure** of 10 mm Hg, which drives fluid into the urinary space. In order for the fluid to leave the glomerular capillaries, it has to pass through the fenestrae of the capillary endothelial cells. This fluid is then filtered by the glomerular basal lamina. The lamina densa traps larger molecules (> 69,000 Da), whereas the polyanions of the laminae rarae impede the passage of negatively charged molecules and molecules that are incapable of deformation. The fluid containing small molecules, ions, and macromolecules that penetrates the lamina densa must pass through the pores in the slit diaphragm of the filtration slits. If the macromolecules are uncharged and if they are 1.8 nm or less in diameter, they can pass without any hindrance through the slit diaphragm. If the uncharged macromolecules are greater than 4 nm in diameter, they cannot pass through the slit diaphragm and remain in the basal lamina. The fluid entering the Bowman space is called the **glomerular ultrafiltrate**. The rate at which the ultrafiltrate enters the urinary space per unit time (usually in mL/min) is referred to as the **glomerular filtration rate** (**GFR**).

Because the basal lamina traps larger macromolecules, it would become clogged were it not continuously phagocytosed by **intraglomerular mesangial cells** and replenished by both cells of the visceral layer of the Bowman capsule (podocytes) and glomerular endothelial cells.

Clinical Correlations

1. *The presence of albumin in the urine (albuminuria) is the result of increased permeability of the glomerular endothelium. Among the causes of this condition are vascular injury, hypertension, mercury poisoning, and exposure to bacterial toxins.*
2. *The basal lamina may also become impaired because of the deposition of antigen–antibody complexes that are filtered from the glomeruli or from the reaction of anti–basement membrane antibody with the basal lamina itself. Both of these instances produce types of glomerulonephritis.*
3. *In cases of lipoid nephrosis, the basal laminae are not congested with antibodies, but adjacent pedicels appear to fuse. This disease is one of the most prevalent kidney disorders in children.*
4. *Individuals with diabetic kidney disease present with proteinuria, which has been suggested to be a function of damaged or altered podocytes. Some of these problems may be due to apoptosis of podocytes, resulting in areas denuded of these cells where proteins can leak into the urinary space. Other problems may be due to alterations in the morphology of the slit diaphragms again permitting the escape of proteins into Bowman space; or some conditions result in podocyte hypertrophy, with a resultant detachment of the enlarged cells, again forming denuded regions where proteins can escape into the urinary space.*

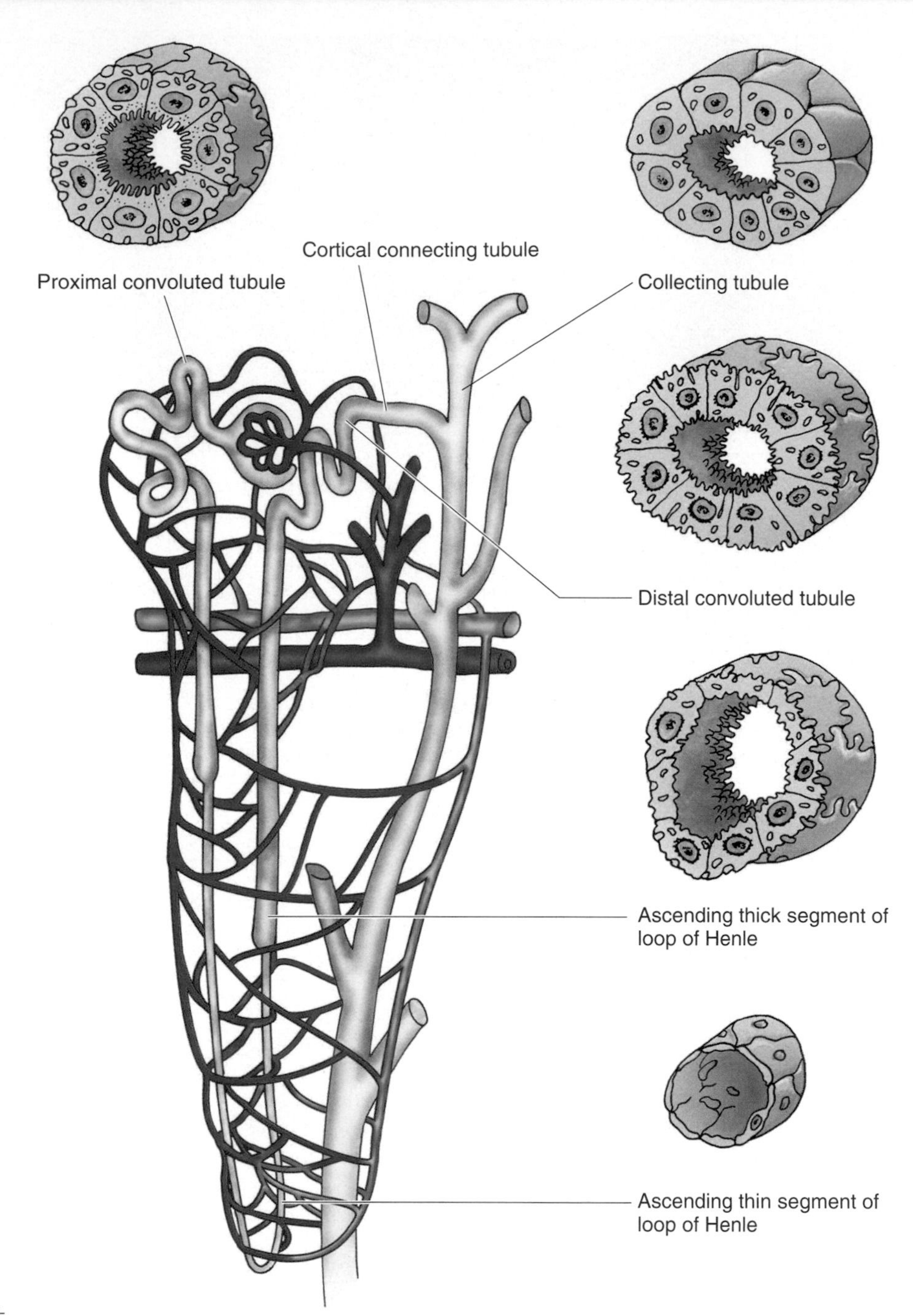

Fig. 19.13 Schematic diagram of the uriniferous tubule and its cross-sectional morphology as viewed with the light microscope.

Proximal Tubule

The proximal tubule has two regions: the proximal convoluted tubule and pars recta of the proximal tubule.

The **Bowman space** drains into the **proximal tubule** at the **urinary pole.** In this junctional region, sometimes called the *neck* of the proximal tubule (negligible in humans), the simple squamous epithelium of the parietal layer of the Bowman capsule joins the simple cuboidal epithelium of the proximal tubule (see Fig. 19.5). The proximal tubule, occupying much of the renal cortex, is approximately 60 μm in diameter and about 14 mm long. The tubule consists of a highly tortuous region, the **pars convoluta of the proximal tubule** (**proximal convoluted tubule**), located near renal corpuscles, and a straighter portion, the **pars recta of the proximal tubule** (**descending thick limb of Henle loop**), which descends in medullary rays within the cortex and then within the medulla to become continuous with the **descending thin limb of Henle loop** at the junction of the outer and inner stripes of the outer medulla.

Viewed with the light microscope, the convoluted portion of the proximal tubule is composed of a simple cuboidal type of epithelium with an eosinophilic, granular appearing cytoplasm (Figs. 19.13–19.15). These cells have an elaborate striated border and an intricate system of interlocking and interwoven lateral cell processes. Thus, the lateral cell membranes are usually

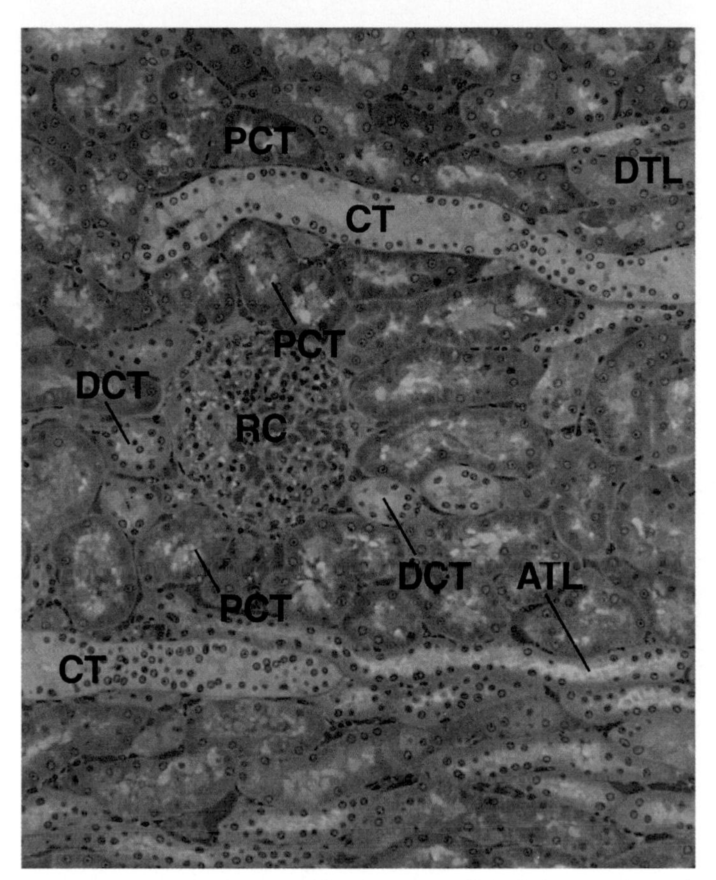

Fig. 19.14 The renal corpuscle in the cortex of the kidney is surrounded by profiles of both proximal convoluted tubule (PCT) and distal convoluted tubule (DCT). Note that the longer proximal convoluted tubule is represented by considerably more cross-sectional profiles than the shorter distal convoluted tubule. Observe the presence of cortical collecting tubules (CT) and ascending and descending thick limbs of Henle loop (ATL, DTL) that belong to the medullary rays, which form the center of a kidney lobule. (×132).

indistinguishable with the light microscope. The height of the cells varies with their functional state—from a low cuboidal to an almost high cuboidal epithelium.

The method and rapidity of fixation modify the microscopic morphology of the proximal convoluted tubule because its lumen is kept open by fluid pressure. Ideal fixation demonstrates wide open, empty lumina and no clumping of the striated border. However, paraffin sections usually display mostly occluded lumina; fluted and ragged-appearing striated borders; few, basally placed nuclei per cross-section of the tubule; and a lack of distinct lateral cell membranes. The cuboidal cells sit on a well-defined basement membrane, easily demonstrated by the periodic acid–Schiff reaction. Each cross-section is composed of approximately 10 to 20 cells, but because these cells are large, usually only six to eight nuclei are included in the plane of the section (see Figs. 19.14 and 19.15).

On the basis of the transmission electron microscopic features of its component cells, the proximal tubule can be subdivided into three regions: S_1, S_2, and S_3.

Cells of the **S_1 region**, the first two-thirds of the pars convoluta, have long (1.3–1.6 μm), closely packed microvilli and a system of intermicrovillar caveolae, known as ***apical canaliculi***, which extend into the apical cytoplasm (Fig. 19.16). The apical canaliculi are more extensive during active diuresis, suggesting that they function in resorption of proteins during tubular clearing of the **glomerular ultrafiltrate**. Mitochondria, Golgi apparatus, and other normal cellular components are also present in these cells. Elaborate lateral and basal processes may extend almost the entire height of the cell. These processes are long and narrow and usually accommodate elongated, tubular mitochondria.

Cells composing the **S_2 region**, the remainder of the pars convoluta, and much of the pars recta, are similar to those of the S_1 region, but they have fewer mitochondria and apical canaliculi, have less elaborate intercellular processes, and are lower in height.

Cells of the **S_3 region**, the remainder of the pars recta, are low cuboidal with few mitochondria. These cells have only infrequent intercellular processes and no apical canaliculi.

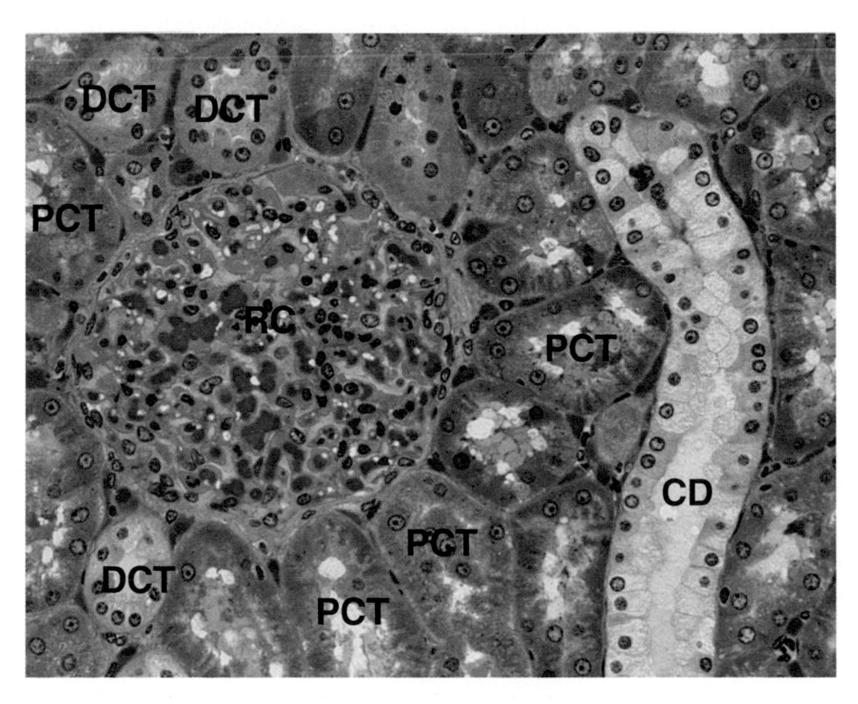

Fig. 19.15 This medium-magnification photomicrograph of a renal corpuscle (RC) displays the cross-sectional profiles of the proximal convoluted tubule (PCT) and of the distal convoluted tubule (DCT). Observe that in paraffin sections, the cells of the proximal convoluted tubule are larger and darker stained than the cells of the distal convoluted tubule. Note that the cells of the cortical collecting tubule (CD) resemble those of the distal convoluted tubule but their cell membranes are clearly discernible. (×270)

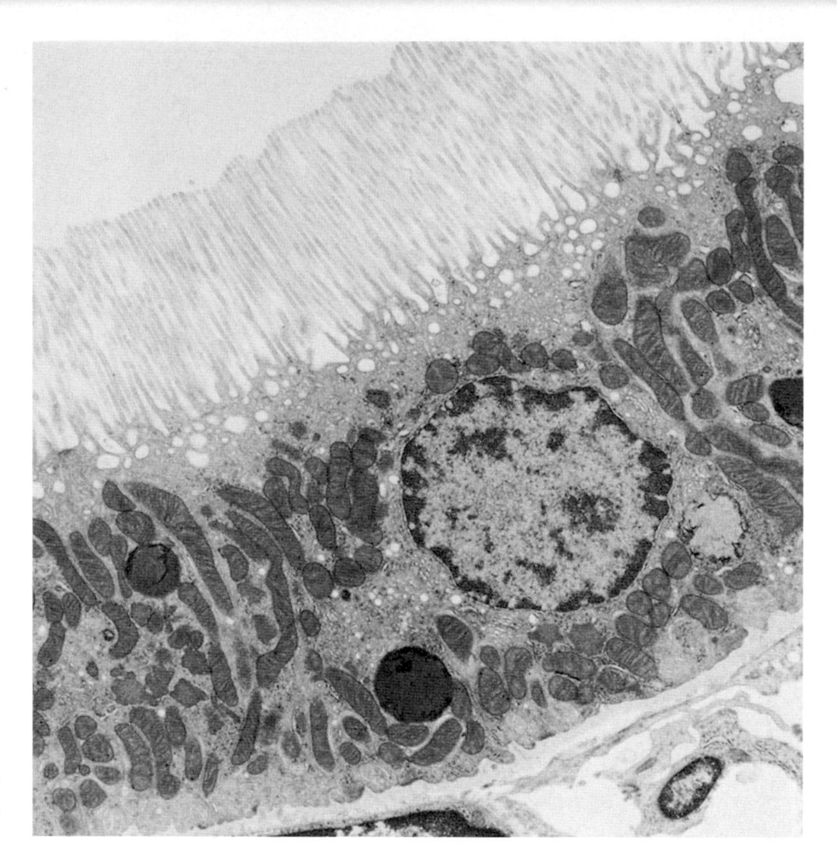

Fig. 19.16 Electron micrograph of the S_1 segment of the rat proximal tubule (×7128). (From Brenner BM, Rector FC. *The Kidney*. 4th ed. Vol 1. Philadelphia: WB Saunders; 1991.)

About 65% to perhaps as much as 80% of sodium (Na^+), chloride (Cl^-), and water is reabsorbed from the glomerular ultrafiltrate and transported into the connective tissue stroma by cells of the proximal tubule. Sodium is actively pumped out of the cell at the basolateral cell membranes by a **sodium pump** (Na^+-K^+ ATPase). The sodium is followed by chloride, not only through the tight junctions between cuboidal cells (i.e., via the **paracellular route**) but also via co-transport with sodium ions along the lateral cell membranes to maintain electrical neutrality and is also followed by water to maintain osmotic equilibrium. The water passes through tight junctions between the cuboidal cells, as well as through Aquaporin-1 channels located in the basolateral cell membrane. In addition, all of the glucose, amino acids, and protein in the glomerular ultrafiltrate are reabsorbed by the vacuolar endocytic apparatus of the cells of the proximal tubule. Moreover, the proximal tubule **excretes** a limited amount of H^+ ions into the ultrafiltrate (in exchange, Na^+ leaves the ultrafiltrate and enters the cell) and also **excretes** organic solutes (e.g., catecholamines, bile salts, and oxalate), drugs (e.g., penicillin), and toxins that must be rapidly removed from the body. Cells of the proximal tubules are able to monitor the ultrafiltrate by the presence of a single **primary cilium** on their luminal aspect.

Thin Limbs of Henle Loop.

The thin limbs of the loop of Henle have three regions: the descending thin limb, loop of Henle, and the ascending thin limb.

The pars recta of the proximal tubule continues as the **thin limb of Henle loop** (Fig. 19.17; see Fig. 19.13). This thin tubule, whose overall diameter is about 15 to 20 μm, is composed of squamous epithelial cells with an average height of 1.5 to 2.0 μm. The length of the thin segments varies with the location of the nephron (see Fig. 19.1). In cortical nephrons, the thin segment is only 1 to 2 mm long or may be completely absent. Juxtamedullary nephrons have much longer thin segments, 9 to 10 mm in length, forming a hairpin-like loop that extends deep into the medulla as far down as the renal papilla. The region of the loop continuous with the pars recta of the proximal tubule is called the **descending thin limb (of Henle** loop), the hairpin-like bend is **Henle loop**, and the region that connects Henle loop to the pars recta of the **distal tubule** is known as the **ascending thin limb (of Henle loop)**.

The nuclei of the cells composing the thin limbs bulge into the lumen of the tubule; hence, in paraffin section, these limbs resemble capillaries in cross-section (see Fig. 19.13). They may be distinguished from capillaries in that their epithelial cells are slightly thicker, their nuclei stain less densely, and their lumina contain no blood cells.

The fine structure of the epithelial cells constituting the thin segments is not unusual. They present a few short, stubby microvilli on their luminal surfaces and a few mitochondria in the cytoplasm surrounding the nucleus. Numerous processes project from the basal portion of the cell to interdigitate with those of neighboring cells.

It is possible to differentiate among four types of epithelial cells composing different regions of Henle loop according to their structural features in transmission electron micrographs but cannot be differentiated in light micrographs. The locations and fine structural features of the four cell types are listed in Table 19.2.

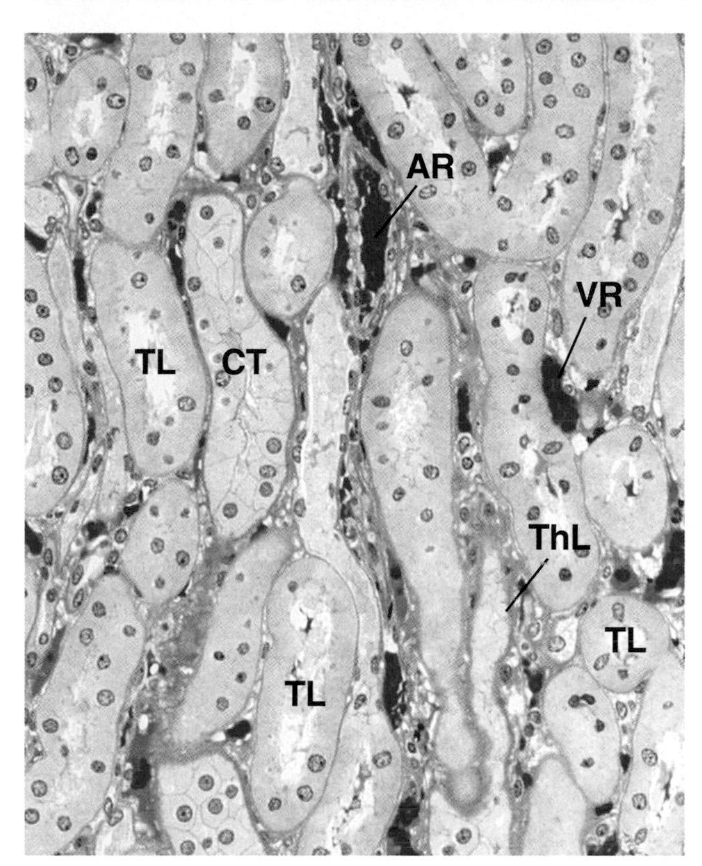

Fig. 19.17 The renal medulla displays the collecting tubules (CT), thick (TL) and thin (ThL) limbs of Henle loop as well as the arteria (AR) and vena (VR) recta. Observe the scant connective tissue elements of the medulla, much of which is occupied by the vasa recta. (×270)

The descending thin limb is highly permeable to water owing to the presence of numerous Aquaporin-1 water channels; it is moderately permeable to urea, and slightly permeable to sodium, chloride, and other ions. The major difference between the ascending and descending thin limbs is that the ascending thin limb is only slightly permeable (almost impermeable) to water and is highly permeable to sodium and chloride. The significance of this difference in water permeability is discussed later.

Distal Tubule

The distal tubule has three regions: the pars recta (the ascending thick limb of Henle loop), the macula densa, and the pars convoluta (the distal convoluted tubule).

The **distal tubule** is subdivided into the **pars recta**, which, as the continuation of the ascending thin limb of Henle loop, is also known as the **ascending thick limb of Henle loop** (**pars recta of the distal tubule**), and the **distal convoluted tubule** (**pars convoluta of the distal tubule**). The ascending thick limb, just before it continues as the distal convoluted tubule, has a modified region called the **macula densa**.

The ascending thick limb of Henle loop, 9 to 10 mm in length and 30 to 40 µm in diameter, ascends straight up through the medulla to reach the cortex. The low cuboidal epithelial cells composing the ascending thick limb have centrally placed, round to slightly oval nuclei and a few club-shaped, short microvilli. Although the lateral aspects of these cells interdigitate, the interrelationships between neighboring cells are not nearly as elaborate as in the proximal convoluted tubules. Basal interdigitations are much more extensive, however, and the number of mitochondria is greater in these cells than in those of the proximal convoluted tubules. Moreover, these cells form highly efficient zonulae occludentes with their neighboring cells.

TABLE 19.2 Cell Types Composing the Thin Limbs of Henle Loop

Cell Type	Location	Fine Structural Features
I	Cortical nephrons	Squamous cells with no lateral processes and no interdigitations
II	Juxtamedullary nephrons; descending thin limb of the outer zone of the medulla	Squamous cells with numerous, long, radiating processes that interdigitate with those of neighboring cells; fascia occludentes between cells; infoldings of the basal plasmalemma
III	Juxtamedullary nephrons; descending thin limb of the inner zone of the medulla	Squamous cells with fewer processes and interdigitations than those of type II
IV	Juxtamedullary nephrons; ascending thin limb	Squamous cells with numerous, long, radiating processes that interdigitate with those of neighboring cells as in type II cells; no infoldings of the basal plasmalemma

The thick ascending limb is almost impermeable to water or urea. Its cells have **1-sodium**, **1-potassium**, **2-chloride co-transporters** that function in the active transport chloride, sodium, and potassium from the lumen of the tubule into the cell of the thick ascending limb (thus, every two chloride ions are accompanied by a single sodium and single potassium ion). At the same time, sodium-potassium ATPase pumps of the basal cell membrane (contacting the basal lamina) deliver equimolar quantities of K^+ ions into the cell and Na^+ ions out of the cell. Additionally, Na^+-H^+ co-transporters at the luminal surface deliver a limited amount of hydrogen ions into the lumen (mildly acidifying the ultrafiltrate) and reabsorb sodium ions from the lumen into the cell. Thus, as the filtrate reaches the cortex of the kidney within the lumen of the distal tubule, its salt concentration is low and its urea concentration remains high. Cells of the thick ascending limb also manufacture **Tamm-Horsfall protein** (**uromodulin**), which they release into the lumen. Uromodulin impedes the formation of kidney stones and decreases the chances of urinary tract infection.

As the ascending thick limb of the Henle loop passes near its own renal corpuscle, it lies between the afferent and efferent glomerular arterioles. This region of the pars recta of the distal tubule houses the **macula densa**, a component of the **juxtaglomerular apparatus** (described in the next section). Because the cells of the macula densa are tall and narrow, the nuclei of these cells are much closer together than those of the remainder of the distal tubule, appearing dark and dense—hence the name *macula densa*.

Distal convoluted tubules are short (4–5 mm) with an overall diameter of 25 to 45 µm. In paraffin sections, the lumina of these tubules are wide open, the granular cytoplasm of the low cuboidal lining epithelium is paler than those of proximal convoluted tubules, and, because the cells are narrower, more nuclei

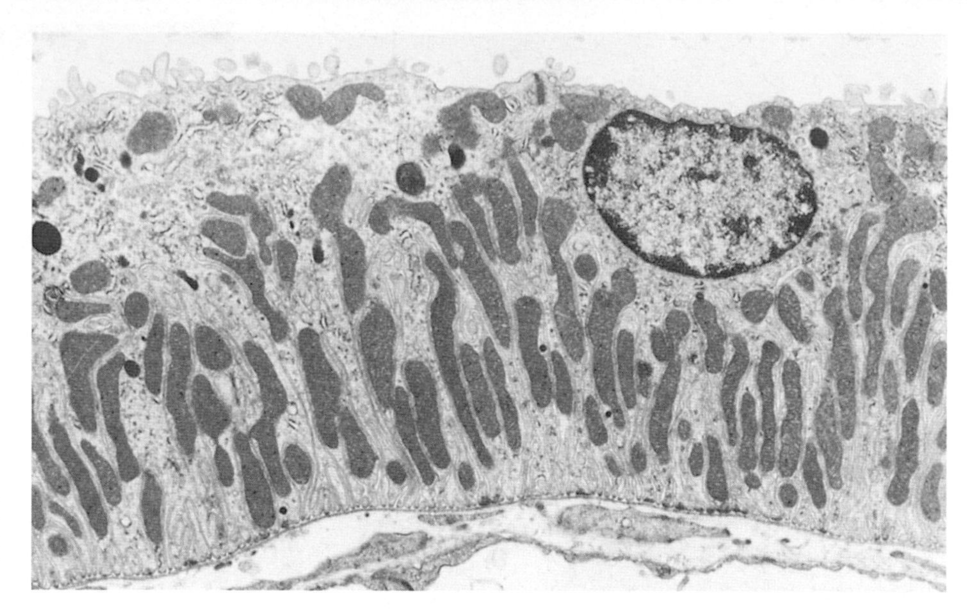

Fig. 19.18 Electron micrograph of the distal convoluted tubule (×8100). (From Brenner BM, Rector FC. *The Kidney*. 4th ed. Vol 1. Philadelphia: WB Saunders; 1991.)

are apparent in tubular cross-section. The ultrastructure of these cells demonstrates a clear, pale cytoplasm with a few blunt apical microvilli (Fig. 19.18). Nuclei are more or less round and apically located, having one or two dense nucleoli. Mitochondria are not as numerous, and the basal interdigitations are not as extensive as those of the ascending thick limb of Henle loop.

Because distal convoluted tubules are much shorter than proximal convoluted tubules, any section of the kidney cortex presents many more cross-sections of proximal convoluted tubules than cross-sections of distal convoluted tubules. Indeed, as indicated earlier, the ratio of cross-sections of proximal to distal convoluted tubules surrounding any renal corpuscle is usually 7 : 1.

Distal convoluted tubules usually ascend slightly above their own renal corpuscles and drain into the arched portion of the collecting tubules.

Similar to the thick ascending limbs, the distal convoluted tubule is almost impermeable to water and urea. However, in the basolateral plasmalemma of its cells, high Na^{+}-K^{+} ATPase activity powers sodium-potassium exchange pumps. Thus, in response to the hormone **aldosterone**, these cells can actively reabsorb almost all of the remaining sodium (and, passively, chloride) from the lumen of the tubule into the renal interstitium. In addition, potassium and hydrogen ions are actively secreted *into* the lumen, contributing to the control of the body's extracellular fluid potassium level and the acidity of urine, respectively.

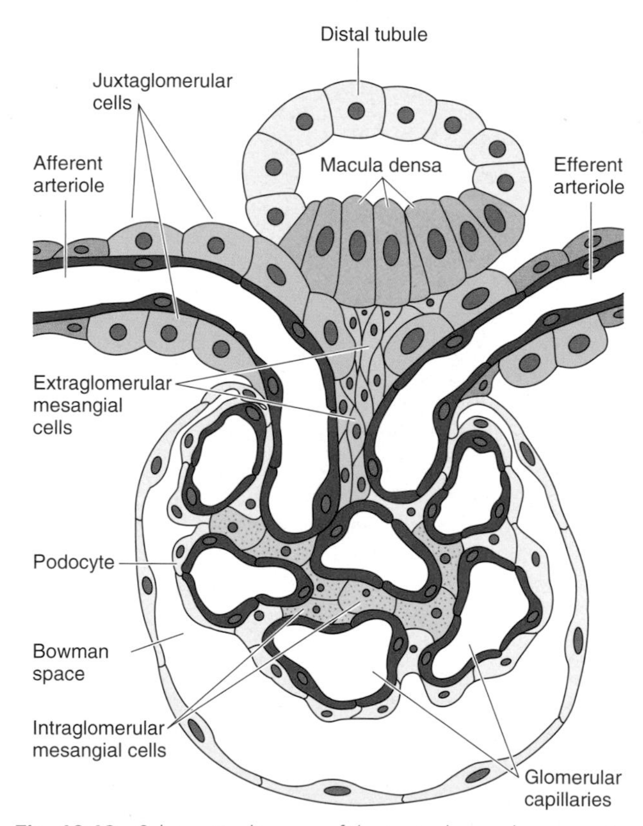

Fig. 19.19 Schematic diagram of the juxtaglomerular apparatus.

Juxtaglomerular Apparatus

The juxtaglomerular apparatus has three components: the macula densa of the distal tubule, juxtaglomerular cells of the afferent glomerular arteriole, and extraglomerular mesangial cells. It activates the renin-angiotensin-aldosterone system to regulate blood pressure.

The **juxtaglomerular apparatus** consists of the **macula densa** of the distal tubule, **juxtaglomerular cells** of the adjacent afferent (and, occasionally, efferent) glomerular arteriole, and the **extraglomerular mesangial cells** (also known as polkissen, lacis cells, and polar cushions). These structures are illustrated schematically in Fig. 19.19. By monitoring the forming urine as it enters the distal convoluted tubule, the macula densa activates, when necessary, the **renin-angiotensin-aldosterone system** to regulate blood pressure and the body's fluid balance.

The cells of the **macula densa** are tall, narrow, pale cells with centrally to apically placed nuclei (Figs. 19.19 and 19.20). They appear to function as chemo- and mechanoreceptors that, when conditions require, release paracrine factors that act on the juxtaglomerular cells and on extraglomerular

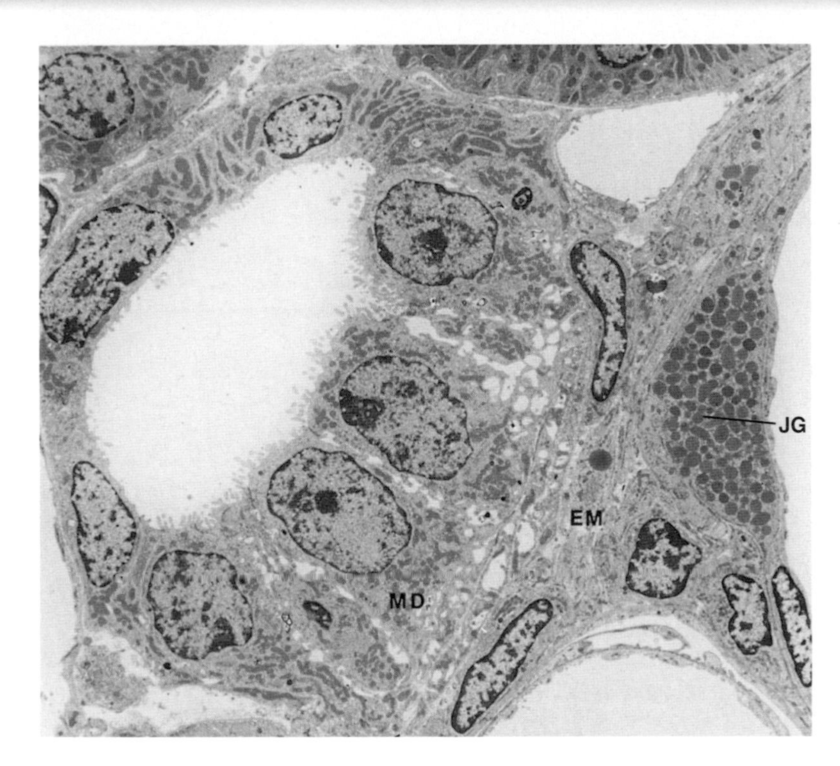

Fig. 19.20 Electron micrograph of the juxtaglomerular apparatus from the kidney of a rabbit. The macula densa (MD), juxtaglomerular cell (JG; containing electron-dense granules), and extraglomerular mesangial (EM) cells are displayed (×2552). (From Brenner BM, Rector FC. *The Kidney*. 4th ed. Vol 1. Philadelphia: WB Saunders; 1991.)

mesangial cells. With the electron microscope, macula densa cells demonstrate numerous microvilli; a primary cilium that monitors the conditions of the ultrafiltrate; small mitochondria; an infranuclearly located Golgi apparatus; and basally located small, membrane-bound dense granules, 60 to 130 nm in diameter (see Fig. 19.20). The basal membranes of macula densa cells display dense granule-containing cytoplasmic projections that contact extraglomerular mesangial cells whose basal lamina fused with the basal lamina of the macula densa cells.

The **juxtaglomerular cells**, modified smooth muscle cells located in the tunica media of afferent (and, occasionally, efferent) glomerular arterioles, are richly innervated by sympathetic nerve fibers. The nuclei of these cells are round instead of the spindle shape seen in smooth muscle cells. Juxtaglomerular cells contain specific granules demonstrated to be the proteolytic enzyme **renin** (see Fig. 19.20). Small quantities of **angiotensin-converting enzyme (ACE)**, **angiotensin I**, and **angiotensin II** are also present in these cells.

Juxtaglomerular cells and the cells of the macula densa have a special spatial relationship because the basal lamina, normally present between epithelium and other tissues, is absent at this point, permitting intimate contact between cells of the macula densa and the juxtaglomerular cells.

The extraglomerular mesangial cells, the third member of the juxtaglomerular apparatus, occupy the space bounded by the afferent arteriole, macula densa, efferent arteriole, and vascular pole of the renal corpuscle. These cells may contain occasional granules and are probably contiguous with the intraglomerular mesangial cells. The functional significance of the juxtaglomerular apparatus is discussed later in the chapter.

Collecting Tubules

Collecting tubules, composed of a simple cuboidal epithelium, convey and modify the ultrafiltrate from the nephron to the minor calyces of the kidney.

Collecting tubules are not part of the nephron. They have different embryological origins, and it is only later in development that they meet the nephron and join it to form the continuous uriniferous tubule. The distal convoluted tubules of several nephrons join to form a short **cortical connecting tubule** that leads into the **cortical collecting tubule**. The glomerular ultrafiltrate that enters the cortical collecting tubule is modified as it passes through the various regions of the collecting tubules to be delivered to the medullary papillae. Collecting tubules are about 20 mm long and have three recognized regions:

- Cortical
- Medullary
- Papillary

Cortical collecting tubules (see Figs. 19.14 and 19.15) are located in the medullary rays and are composed of two types of cuboidal cells:

- **Principal cells** (**light cells**) have oval, centrally located nuclei; a few small mitochondria; and short, sparse microvilli. The basal membranes of these cells display numerous infoldings. Because the lateral cell membranes are not plicated, they are clearly evident with the light microscope. These cells possess numerous Aquaporin-2 channels that are very sensitive to **antidiuretic hormone** (**ADH**) and become completely permeable to water, permitting these cells to reabsorb water from the ultrafiltrate, thus ***concentrating*** urine.
- **Intercalated cells** (**dark cells**) display numerous apical vesicles 50 to 200 nm in diameter, microplicae on their apical plasmalemma, and an abundance of mitochondria. The nuclei of these cells are round and centrally located. There are two types of intercalated cells: (1) **type α cells**, whose luminal membrane possesses H^+-ATPase that functions in transporting H^+, even against high-concentration gradients, into the lumen of the tubule, thus acidifying urine; and (2) **type β cells**, whose basolateral membrane possesses H^+-ATPase and functions in reabsorbing H^+ and secreting HCO_3^-, thus making the urine less acidic.

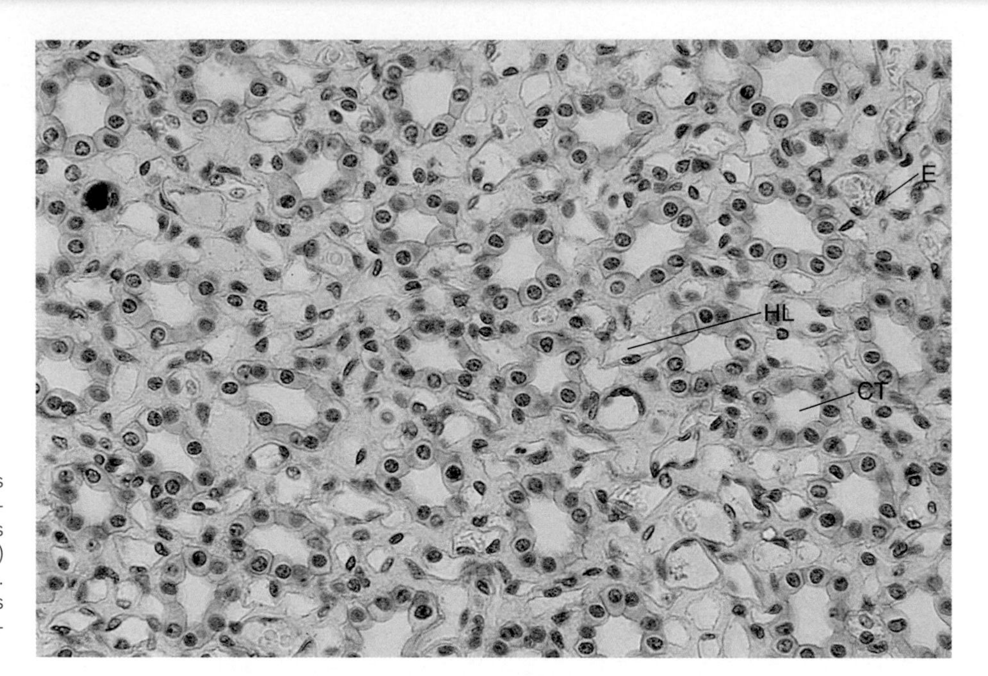

Fig. 19.21 The medulla of the kidney displays the simple cuboidal epithelium of the collecting tubules (CT) as well as the simple squamous epithelium of the thin limbs of Henle loop (HL) and the endothelial cells (E) of the vasa recta. Note that the connective tissue components are sparse and consist mostly of vascular elements. (×270)

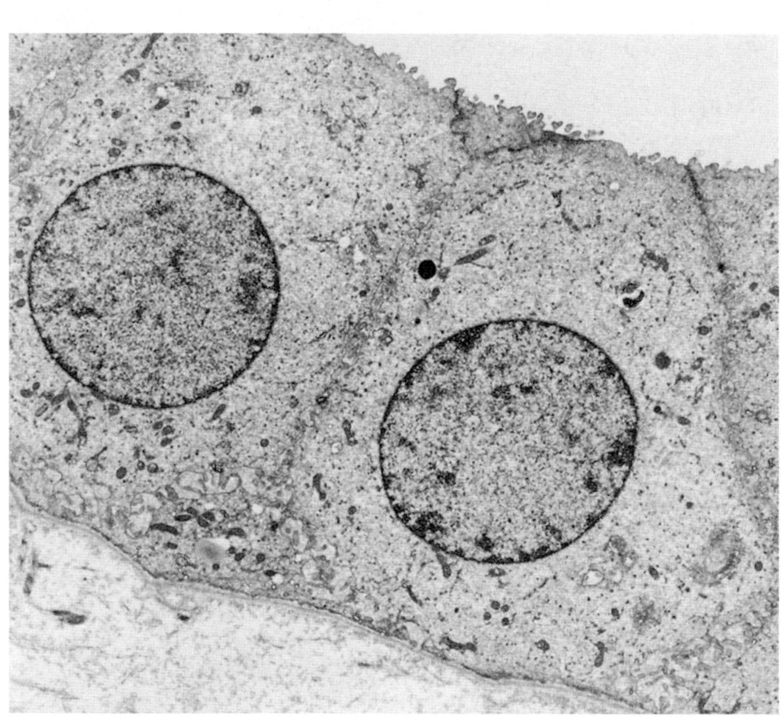

Fig. 19.22 Electron micrograph of a collecting tubule from a rabbit kidney (×4790). (From Brenner BM, Rector FC. *The Kidney*. 4th ed. Vol 1. Philadelphia: WB Saunders; 1991.)

Medullary collecting tubules (Figs. 19.17, 19.21, and 19.22) are of larger caliber because they are formed by the union of several cortical collecting tubules. Those in the **outer zone** of the medulla are similar to the cortical collecting tubules in that they display both principal and intercalated cells, whereas tubules of the **inner zone** of the medulla have principal cells only. The cells of these ducts are also able to excrete hydrogen ions into the lumen of the duct, thereby acidifying urine.

Papillary collecting tubules (**ducts of Bellini**; Fig. 19.23) are each formed by the confluence of several medullary collecting tubules. These are large ducts, 200 to 300 μm in diameter, which open at the area cribrosa of the renal papilla to deliver the urine that they convey into the minor calyx of the kidney. Each duct of Bellini collects urine from as many as 5000 nephrons. These ducts are lined by tall columnar principal cells only; each cell possesses a primary cilium that probably is responsible for monitoring the urine in its lumen.

Collecting tubules are impermeable to water. However, in the presence of **ADH**, they become permeable to water (and in the medullary collecting tubules to urea). Thus, in the absence of ADH, urine is copious and hypotonic; in the presence of ADH, the volume of urine is low and concentrated.

Renal Interstitium

The renal interstitium is a very flimsy, scant amount of loose connective tissue housing three types of cells: fibroblasts, macrophages, and interstitial cells.

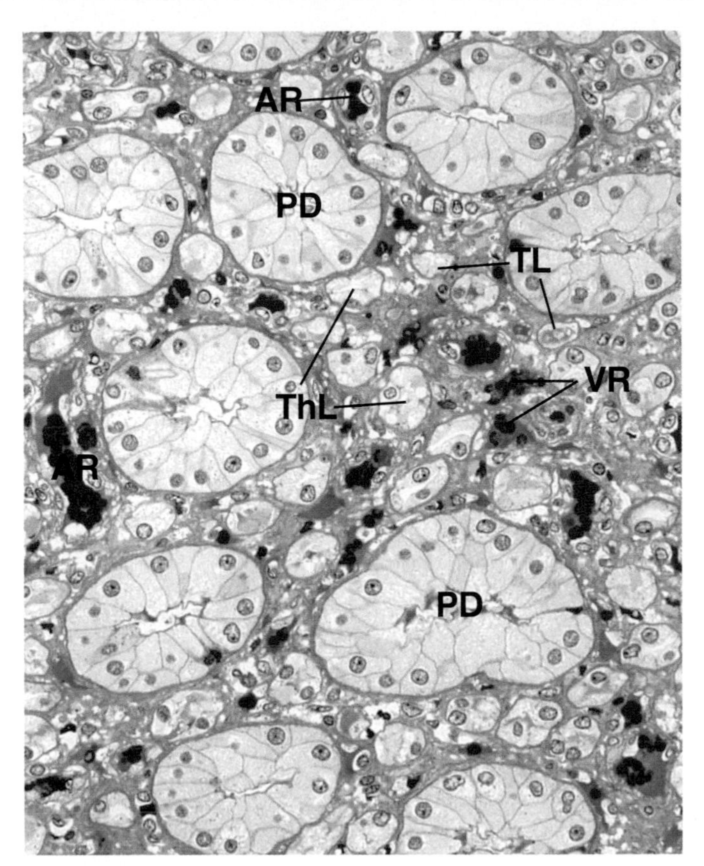

Fig. 19.23 This medium-magnification photomicrograph of the renal papilla displays the circular profiles of numerous papillary ducts (PD) near the area cribrosa, accompanied by cross-sections of the thin (TL) and thick limbs (ThL) of Henle loop. Note also the thick-walled arteria recta (AR) housing many erythrocytes; VR is vena recta. (×270)

The kidney is invested by a dense, irregular, collagenous type of connective tissue, with some elastic fibers interspersed among the bundles of collagen. This capsule is not attached firmly to the underlying cortex. As blood vessels enter the hilum, they travel in a thin connective tissue cover, most of which is derived from the capsule. The cortical region has only delicate connective tissue elements that constitute less than 10% of the cortical volume and is associated mostly with the basement membranes investing the uriniferous tubules and their vascular supply. The two cellular components of the cortical connective tissue are **fibroblasts** and cells that are believed to be macrophages, known as **interstitial dendritic cells**.

The medullary interstitial connective tissue component is more extensive than that found in the cortex; in fact, it occupies more than 20% of the volume of the medulla. Embedded in this connective tissue are the various components of the uriniferous tubules, as well as the extensive vascular network located in the medulla. The cell population of medullary interstitium consists of fibroblasts, macrophages (interstitial dendritic cells), pericytes, and interstitial cells. The first three have been described in Chapter 6; therefore, only interstitial cells are discussed here. **Interstitial cells** appear to be situated like the rungs of a ladder, one on top of the other, and are most numerous between straight collecting tubules and the ducts of Bellini. They have elongated nuclei and numerous cytoplasmic lipid droplets. It is believed that interstitial cells synthesize **medullipin I**, a substance that is converted in the liver to **medullipin II**, a potent vasodilator that lowers blood pressure.

Renal Circulation: Arterial Supply

The two kidneys receive 20% of the total blood volume (1200 mL) per minute via the large branches of the abdominal aorta known as the renal arteries.

The two kidneys receive an extensive blood supply (1200 mL every minute) via the large **renal arteries**, direct branches of the abdominal aorta (see Fig. 19.1). Before entering the hilum of the kidney, the renal artery bifurcates into an anterior and posterior division, which, in turn, subdivide to form a total of five **segmental arteries**. The branches of any one segmental artery do not form anastomoses with the branches of other segmental arteries. Hence, if blood flow through one of these arteries is blocked, circulation to the region of the kidney supplied by the affected vessel is interrupted. Therefore, the kidney is said to be subdivided into vascular segments, with each segment supplied by a specific artery.

The first subdivisions of the segmental arteries are called **lobar arteries**, one for each lobe of the kidney. These, in turn, branch to form two or three **interlobar arteries**, which travel between the renal pyramids to the corticomedullary junction. At the corticomedullary junction, these arteries form a series of vessels (perpendicular to the parent vessel) that, to a large extent, remain at that junction, occupying the same curved plane. Because these arteries describe a slight arc over the base of the renal pyramid, they are called **arcuate arteries**.

Although arcuate arteries once were believed to anastomose, more recent studies suggest that terminal branches of these arteries do not join each other. Instead, terminal branches, as all other branches of the arcuate arteries, ascend into the cortex, forming interlobular arteries.

Interlobular arteries ascend within the cortical labyrinth approximately halfway between neighboring medullary rays. Hence, they travel in the interstices between any two lobules. Many branches arise from the interlobular arteries. These branches supply the glomeruli of renal corpuscles and are known as **afferent glomerular arterioles**. Some of the interlobular arteries ascend through the cortex to reach the kidney capsule. Here, they contribute to the formation of the capsular plexus. Most of the interlobular arteries, however, terminate as afferent glomerular arterioles.

Each glomerulus is drained by another arteriole, the **efferent glomerular arteriole**. There are two fates for efferent glomerular arterioles, those draining glomeruli of cortical nephrons and those draining glomeruli of juxtamedullary nephrons.

Efferent glomerular arterioles from *cortical nephrons* are short and branch to form a system of capillaries, the **peritubular capillary network**. This capillary bed supplies the entire cortical labyrinth, with the obvious exception of the glomeruli. Thus, the kidney possesses a dual capillary bed, one responsible for the formation of the ultrafiltrate, the glomerulus with a high hydrostatic pressure of about 60 mm Hg, and the second, the peritubular capillary bed with a low hydrostatic pressure of about 12 mm Hg. This hydrostatic pressure differential permits the exceptionally efficient reabsorption of the fluid conserved by the uriniferous tubules.

The endothelial cells of the peritubular capillary network manufacture and release 90% of the body's hormone **erythropoietin**; the remaining 10% is formed by hepatocytes.

The efferent glomerular arterioles, derived from glomeruli of juxtamedullary nephrons, as well as from glomeruli located in the lower quadrant of the cortex, each give rise to 10 to 25 long, hairpin-like capillaries that dip deep into the medulla (Figs. 19.13, 19.24, and 19.25). Their descending limbs have a narrow bore and are called **arteriolae rectae**; their ascending limbs are much greater in diameter and are called **venae rectae**. Frequently, these vessels are simply called **vasa recta**. The hairpin-like shape of the vasa recta, which closely follows and wraps around the two limbs of Henle loop and the collecting tubule, is essential in the physiology of urine concentration (see later discussion).

Renal Circulation: Venous Drainage

The arcuate veins receive blood from the cortex via the stellate veins and interlobular veins and from the medulla via the venae rectae; arcuate veins are drained by the interlobar veins that deliver their blood into the renal vein.

Venae rectae drain blood from the medulla and deliver their blood to **arcuate veins**, vessels that follow the paths of the same-named arteries. Blood from the superficial aspect of the cortex is collected into a star-shaped system of subcapsular veins called **stellate veins**; blood from the peritubular capillary bed is drained by the **deep cortical veins.** The stellate veins and deep cortical veins deliver their blood into the **interlobular veins**, which—paralleling the same-named arteries—deliver their blood to the **arcuate veins**. Hence, arcuate veins drain blood both from the medulla and the cortex. Arcuate veins empty into **interlobar veins** that unite, near the hilum, to form the **renal vein**, which delivers its blood into the **inferior vena cava**. Note the absence of lobar and segmental veins, in contrast to the presence of such named arteries in the arterial system of the kidney.

Lymphatic Supply of the Kidney

Lymph vessels of the kidney probably follow the larger arteries.

The **lymphatic supply** of the kidney is not completely understood. It is believed that most lymphatic vessels follow the larger arteries. According to most authors, the lymphatic supply of the kidney may be subdivided into superficial and deep aspects located in the subcapsular region and medulla, respectively. The two systems may or may not join near the hilum, where they form several large lymphatic trunks. Lymph nodes in the vicinity of the vena cava and abdominal aorta receive lymph from the kidneys. There are lymph vessels in the cortex that do not follow

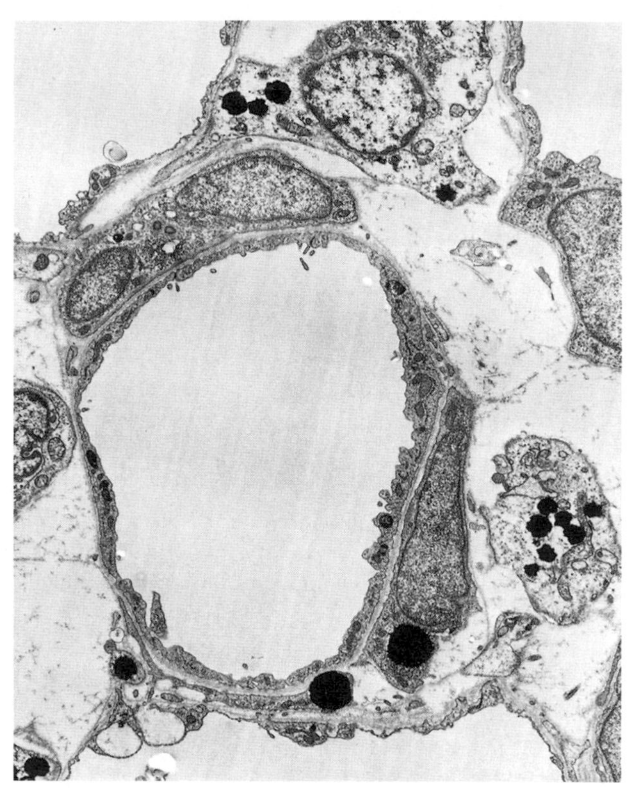

Fig. 19.24 Electron micrograph of the arteria recta of a rat kidney. (From Takahashi-Iwanaga H. The three-dimensional cytoarchitecture of the interstitial tissue in the rat kidney. *Cell Tissue Res.* 1991;264:269–281.)

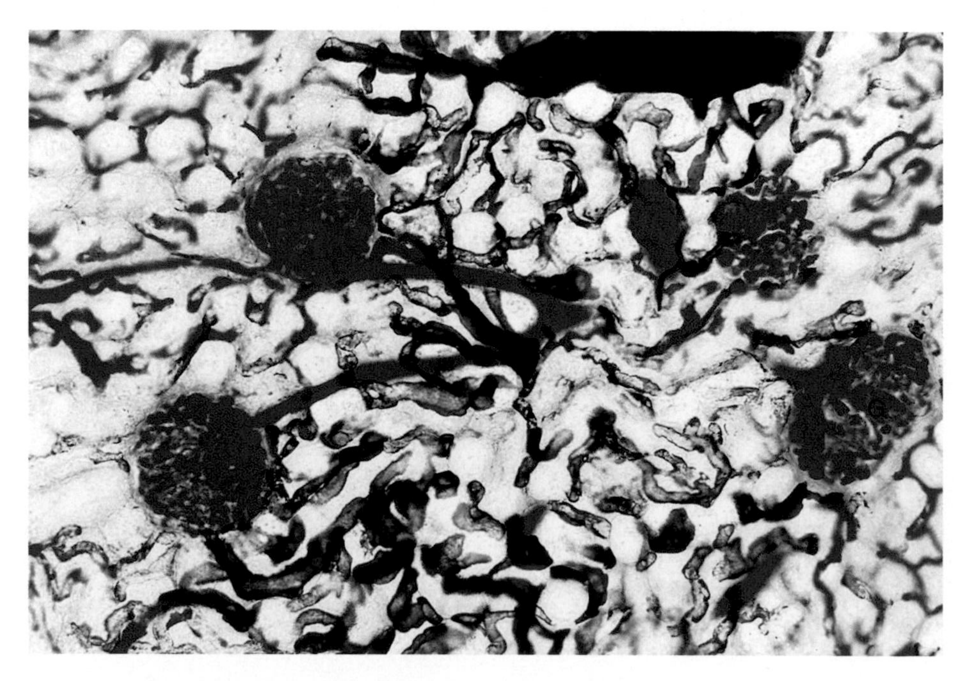

Fig. 19.25 Injected kidney displaying the rich vascular supply of the kidney cortex. Note that the glomeruli are clearly evident. (×132)

the larger arteries, but they do drain their lymph into a plexus of lymph vessels at the hilum.

RENAL INNERVATION

Most nerve fibers that reach the kidney are unmyelinated, sympathetic fibers that form the renal plexus, traveling along the renal artery. The cell bodies of these fibers are probably located in the aortic and celiac plexuses. Sympathetic fibers are distributed by branches of the renal arterial tree, and these vessels are modulated by some of these fibers. Additional sympathetic fibers reach the epithelium of the renal tubules, the juxtaglomerular and interstitial cells, and the capsule of the kidney. Sensory fibers and parasympathetic fibers (probably from the vagus nerve) have also been described in the kidney.

Recapitulation of Kidney Functions

The kidneys regulate blood pressure. They also play a role in excretion, as well as controlling body fluid composition and volume. Specifically, they regulate solute components (e.g., sodium, potassium, chloride, glucose, and amino acids) and acid–base balance. Thus, during the summer, when a great deal of fluid is lost through perspiration, the urinary output is reduced in volume and increased in osmolarity. During the winter months, when fluid loss through perspiration is minimal, the urinary output is increased in volume, and the urine is dilute. Moreover, the kidneys excrete detoxified end products; regulate the osmolality of urine; and secrete substances such as medullipin I, renin, prostaglandins, and erythropoietin. They can also function in gluconeogenesis.

Also, in the presence of parathyroid hormone, the kidneys facilitate the conversion of a less active form of vitamin D_3 (25-OH-vitamin D_3) to **calcitriol (1,25-[OH]$_2$-vitamin D_3)**, its most active form, which is responsible for the increased absorption of calcium and phosphate ions by the digestive system and their transport into the extracellular fluid compartment of the body. Although all of these functions are important aspects of kidney histophysiology, only the mechanism of urine formation is discussed in this chapter.

Recapitulation of the Mechanism of Urine Formation

The two kidneys receive about one-fifth the total blood volume (1200 mL) per minute, and they manufacture about 1 to 2 mL of urine per minute.

The two kidneys receive a large volume of circulating blood because the renal arteries are large and are direct branches of the abdominal aorta. Inulin, a fructose polymer, can be used to measure the glomerular filtration rate (GFR) Such studies have shown that the entire blood supply circulates through the two kidneys every 5 minutes, which means that approximately 1200 mL of blood enters the two kidneys each minute, of which 125 mL/min of glomerular filtrate, the typical GFR for an adult human, is formed in the average male. Thus, 180 L of glomerular filtrate is formed each day, of which only 1.5 to 2.0 L is excreted as urine. Therefore, every day, at least 178 L of the glomerular filtrate is reabsorbed by the two kidneys, and only about 1% of the total glomerular filtrate is excreted.

The structure and function of the various regions of the uriniferous tubule are presented in Table 19.3.

TABLE 19.3 Structure and Function of the Uriniferous Tubule

Region of Uriniferous Tubule	Major Functions	Miscellaneous Comments
Renal corpuscle: Simple squamous epithelium, fused basal laminae, podocytes	Filtration	Filtration barrier: endothelial cell, fused basal laminae, filtration diaphragm
Proximal tubule: Simple cuboidal epithelium	Resorption of 65%–80% of water, sodium, and chloride (reducing volume of ultrafiltrate); resorption of 100% of protein, amino acids, glucose, and bicarbonate	Sodium pump in basolateral membrane; ultrafiltrate is isotonic with blood
Descending thin limb of Henle loop: Simple squamous epithelium	Completely permeable to water and slightly permeable to salts (reducing volume of ultrafiltrate)	Ultrafiltrate is hypertonic with respect to blood; urea enters lumen of tubule
Ascending thin limb of Henle loop: Simple squamous epithelium	Impermeable to water, permeable to salts; sodium and chloride leave tubule to enter renal interstitium	Ultrafiltrate is hypertonic with respect to blood; urea leaves renal interstitium and enters the lumen of tubule
Ascending thick limb of Henle loop: Simple cuboidal epithelium	Impermeable to water; chloride and sodium leave tubule to enter renal interstitium	Ultrafiltrate becomes hypotonic with respect to blood; sodium-chloride pump in basolateral cell membrane is responsible for establishment of osmotic gradient in interstitium of outer medulla
Macula densa: Simple columnar cells	Monitors sodium level and volume of ultrafiltrate in lumen of distal tubule	Contacts and communicates with juxtaglomerular cells
Juxtaglomerular cells: Modified smooth muscle cells	Synthesize and release renin into bloodstream	Renin initiates the reaction for the eventual formation of angiotensin II (see Table 19.4)
Distal convoluted tubule: Simple cuboidal epithelium	Responds to aldosterone by reabsorbing sodium and chloride for lumen	Ultrafiltrate becomes more hypotonic (in the presence of aldosterone); sodium pump in basolateral membrane; potassium is secreted into the lumen
Collecting tubule: Simple cuboidal epithelium	In the presence of ADH, water and urea leave the lumen to enter the renal interstitium	Urine becomes hypertonic in the presence of ADH; urea in interstitium is responsible for gradient of concentration in interstitium of the inner medulla

ADH, Antidiuretic hormone.

Filtration in the Renal Corpuscle

Fluid component from the blood passes through the filtration barrier to become the ultrafiltrate.

As blood passes from the afferent glomerular arteriole into the glomerulus, it encounters a region of differential pressure, where the intracapillary blood pressure (60 mm Hg) is greater than the two opposing forces: the colloid osmotic pressure of the blood (32 mm Hg) and the oncotic pressure (i.e., the fluid pressure) in the Bowman space (18 mm Hg), forcing fluid from the capillary into that space. Therefore, the net effect, the **filtration force**, is 10 mm Hg. The fluid entering the Bowman space is called the (**glomerular**) **ultrafiltrate**.

Because of the tripartite **filtration barrier** (endothelial cell, basal lamina, filtration slit diaphragm), cellular material and large macromolecules cannot leave the glomerulus; thus, the ultrafiltrate is similar to plasma (without its constituent macromolecules). Molecules greater than 69,000 Da (e.g., albumin) are trapped by the basal lamina. In addition to molecular weight, the molecular shape and charge of a molecule and the functional state of the filtration barrier all influence the ability of a molecule to traverse the filtration barrier. Because the filtration barrier has negatively charged components, macromolecules that are negatively charged are less able to cross the filtration barrier, compared with positively charged or neutral macromolecules.

Resorption in the Proximal Tubule

The proximal tubule is the site of mass movement, where a tremendous amount of electrolytes, glucose, amino acids, protein, and water is conserved.

The **ultrafiltrate** leaves the Bowman space via the urinary pole to enter the proximal convoluted tubule, where modification of this fluid begins. Materials reabsorbed from the lumen of the proximal tubule enter the tubular epithelial cells, from which they are exocytosed into the interstitial connective tissue. Here, the reabsorbed substances enter the peritubular capillary network and are returned to the body via the bloodstream.

Most resorption of materials from the ultrafiltrate occurs in the proximal tubule. Normally, the following amounts are absorbed in the proximal tubule: 100% of proteins, glucose, amino acids; almost 100% of bicarbonate ions; 65% to 80% of sodium and chloride ions; and 65% to 80% of the water.

Na^+-K^+ ATPase, the active transport **sodium pump** in the basolateral plasma membrane of the proximal tubule cell, pumps sodium out of the cell and into the renal interstitium. This movement of sodium ions out of the cell at the basolateral membrane causes sodium in the lumen of the tubule to leave the ultrafiltrate and enter the cell through its apical cell membrane via various **carrier-mediated transports**. In this fashion, the net sodium movement is from the ultrafiltrate into the renal connective tissue. To maintain electrical neutrality, chloride ions passively follow sodium, also via carrier-mediated transports and chloride channels. Further, to maintain osmotic equilibrium, water passively follows sodium (by osmosis) through Aquaporin-1 channels.

Additionally, energy-requiring pumps, located in the apical plasmalemma of proximal tubule cells, co-transport amino acids and glucose with sodium into the cell to be released into the renal interstitium. Proteins, brought into the cell by pinocytotic vesicles, are degraded by hydrolytic enzymes within late endosomes.

Each day, as much as 140 g of glucose, 430 g of sodium, 500 g of chloride, 300 g of bicarbonate, 18 g of potassium ions, 54 g of protein, and approximately 142 L of water are conserved by the **proximal tubules** of the kidney.

The proximal tubule also releases certain substances into the tubular lumen. These include hydrogen ions (H^+), ammonia, phenol red, hippuric acid, uric acid, organic bases, ethylenediaminetetraacetate, and certain drugs, such as penicillin.

Henle Loop and the Countercurrent Multiplier System

The long Henle loop of the juxtamedullary nephron is responsible for the establishment of the countercurrent multiplier system.

The osmolarity of the glomerular ultrafiltrate is the same as that of circulating blood. This osmolarity is not altered by the proximal tubule because water has left its lumen in response to the movement of ions. However, the osmotic pressure of *formed urine* is different from that of blood. The osmotic pressure differential is established by the remaining regions of the uriniferous tubule. As indicated earlier, the osmolarity and volume of urine vary, demonstrating that the kidneys can and do modulate these factors.

A gradient of osmolarity, increasing from the corticomedullary junction to deep into the medulla, is maintained in the renal medullary interstitium. The long loops of Henle of **juxtamedullary nephrons** aid not only in the creation but also in the maintenance of this osmotic gradient via a **countercurrent multiplier system** (Fig. 19.26). The cells of the descending thin limb of Henle loop are freely permeable to water (via Aquaporin-1 channels) and moderately permeable to urea but only slightly permeable to salts (including sodium and chloride). Therefore, the movement of water reacts to the osmotic forces in its microenvironment. The ascending thin limb is almost completely impermeable to water but is very permeable to salts. It is important to understand at this point (to be explained later) that *urea enters* the lumina of both the descending and ascending thin limbs of Henle loop.

The thick ascending limb of Henle loop is completely impermeable to water; however, **1-sodium, 1-potassium, 2-chloride co-transporters** (**pumps**) actively remove, in proportion, 2 chloride ions and 1 sodium and 1 potassium ion from the lumen of the tubules; these enter the cells of the ascending thick limb of Henle loop. At the same time, sodium-potassium ATPase pumps of the basolateral cell membrane (contacting the basal lamina) deliver equimolar quantities of K^+ ions into the cell (from the renal interstitium) and Na^+ ion (along with chloride ions via an energy-requiring system) out of the cells (into the renal interstitium). Additionally, Na^+-H^+ co-transporters at the luminal surface deliver a limited amount of hydrogen ions into the lumen, mildly acidifying the ultrafiltrate and reabsorbing sodium ions from the lumen into the cell. However, urea cannot enter or leave the lumen of the ascending thick limb. As the filtrate ascends, it contains increasingly fewer sodium and chloride ions but the same amount of water; hence, the amount of salts that may be transferred out into the interstitium decreases. Thus, a gradient of salt concentration is established in the renal interstitium so that the highest interstitial osmolarity is deep in

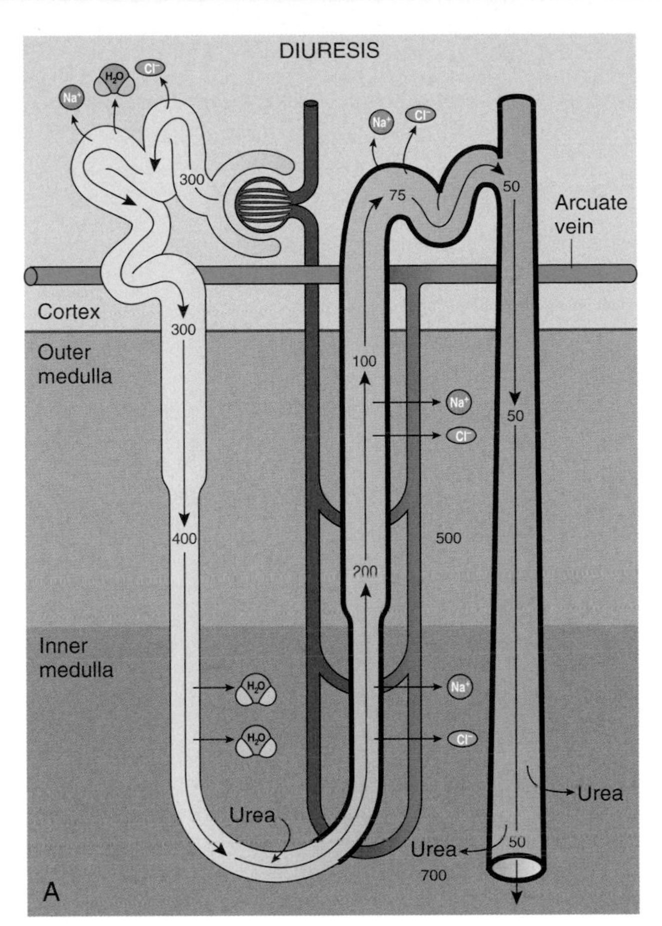

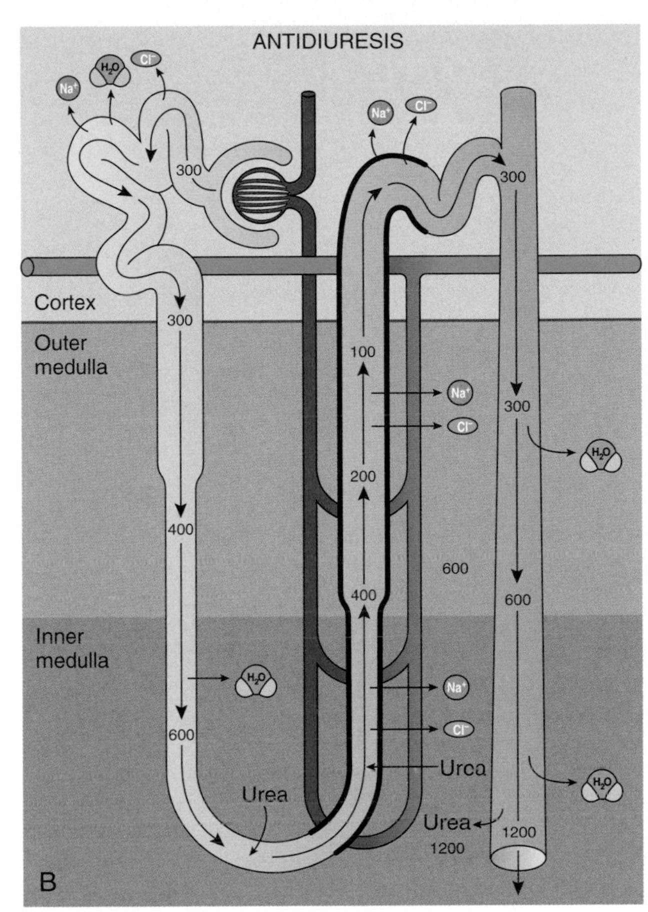

Fig. 19.26 Histophysiology of the uriniferous tubule. (A) In the absence of antidiuretic hormone (ADH; diuresis). (B) In the presence of ADH (antidiuresis). Numbers indicate milliosmoles per liter. Areas outlined by a *thick line* indicate that the tubule is impermeable to water. In the presence of ADH, the collecting tubule changes so that it becomes permeable to water, and the concentration in the interstitium of the inner medulla increases. The vasa recta is simplified in this drawing because it encompasses the entire uriniferous tubule (see Fig. 19.1).

the medulla, and the osmolarity of the interstitium decreases toward the cortex.

Because the medulla is tightly packed with thick and thin (ascending and descending) limbs of Henle loop and collecting tubules, the gradient of osmolarity that is established is pervasive and affects all of the tubules equally (see Fig. 19.26).

Therefore, keeping the foregoing in mind, we can recap the movement of ions and water, once again starting as the ultrafiltrate, which, as the reader should recall, is isotonic with blood as it leaves the pars recta of the proximal tubule. As the ultrafiltrate descends in the thin descending limb of Henle loop, it loses water (*reducing volume and increasing osmolarity*), reacting to the osmotic gradient of the interstitium so that the intraluminal filtrate more or less becomes equilibrated with that of the surrounding connective tissue. This fluid of high osmolarity now ascends in the thin ascending limb of Henle loop, which is mostly impermeable to water but not to salts. Thus, the volume of the ultrafiltrate does not change (i.e., the volume is the same when the ultrafiltrate leaves the ascending thin limb as when it entered it), but the osmolarity of the ultrafiltrate inside the tubule adjusts to the osmolarity of the interstitium.

The fluid entering the ascending thick limb of Henle loop passes a region that is impermeable to water but has **1-sodium, 1-potassium, 2-chloride co-transporters** (**pumps**), which removes chloride, sodium, and potassium ions from the lumen. Because water cannot leave the lumen, the ultrafiltrate becomes *hypotonic, but its volume remains constant* as it ascends to the cortex in the ascending thick limb. The chloride and sodium that were transferred from the lumen of the ascending thick limb into the connective tissue are responsible for the establishment of a concentration gradient in the renal interstitium of the outer medulla.

Monitoring the Filtrate in the Juxtaglomerular Apparatus

When cells of the macula densa detect a low sodium concentration in the ultrafiltrate, they cause juxtaglomerular cells to release the enzyme renin, which converts angiotensinogen circulating in the blood to angiotensin I.

The cells of the macula densa monitor the filtrate volume and sodium concentration. If sodium concentration is below a specific threshold, macula densa cells do two things:

- They cause dilation of the afferent glomerular arterioles, increasing blood flow into the glomerulus.
- When necessary, they activate the **renin-angiotensin-aldosterone system** to regulate blood pressure and the body's fluid balance by instructing juxtaglomerular cells to release the enzyme **renin** into circulation.

Renin cleaves from **angiotensinogen**, a large protein manufactured by hepatocytes and released into the bloodstream, a decapeptide known as **angiotensin I**, a mild vasoconstrictor. In the capillaries of the lungs, but also to a lesser extent in those of the kidneys and other organs of the body,

TABLE 19.4 Effects of Angiotensin II

Function	Result
Acts as a potent vasoconstrictor	Increased blood pressure
Facilitates synthesis and release of aldosterone	Resorption of sodium and chloride from lumen of distal convoluted tubule
Facilitates release of ADH	Resorption of water from lumen of collecting tubule
Increases thirst	Increased tissue fluid volume
Inhibits renin release	Feedback inhibition
Facilitates release of prostaglandins	Vasodilation of afferent glomerular arteriole, thus maintaining glomerular filtration rate

ADH, Antidiuretic hormone.

angiotensin-converting enzyme (**ACE**) converts angiotensin I to **angiotensin II**, a hormone with numerous biological effects (Table 19.4).

As a potent vasoconstrictor, angiotensin II reduces the luminal diameter of blood vessels, constricting the *efferent glomerular arterioles*, further increasing pressure within the glomerulus. The increased intraglomerular pressure, along with the increased volume of blood flow, results in the increased GFR of a larger volume of blood. Angiotensin II also influences the adrenal cortex to release **aldosterone**, a hormone that acts primarily on cells of the distal convoluted tubules, increasing their reabsorption of sodium and chloride ions. Additionally, angiotensin II facilitates the release of **ADH** from the posterior pituitary (neurohypophysis), which causes the collecting tubules to become permeable to water, thereby reabsorbing water from the lumen and releasing it into the renal interstitium (see following section on the loss of water and urea from filtrate in collecting tubules).

Clinical Correlations

One of the causes contributing to ***chronic essential hypertension*** *is the presence of elevated levels of angiotensin II. Elevated blood levels of angiotensin II were once believed to be due to the excessive release of renin from the juxtaglomerular cells of the juxtaglomerular apparatus. It is now understood that the increased activity of angiotensin-converting enzyme, rather than the renal release of renin, is directly responsible for elevating the concentration of angiotensin II.*

Loss of Water and Urea from Filtrate in Collecting Tubules

Antidiuretic hormone (vasopressin) causes the conservation of water and the excretion of concentrated urine.

The filtrate that leaves the distal convoluted tubule to enter the connecting tubule is hypotonic. As the collecting tubule passes through the renal medulla to reach the area cribrosa, it is also subject to the same osmotic gradients as the ascending and descending limbs of Henle loop. In the absence of **ADH**, the cells of the collecting tubule and, to a lesser extent, of the distal convoluted tubule are completely impermeable to water (see Fig. 19.26). Therefore, the filtrate, or urine, is not modified in the collecting tubule, and the urine remains dilute (hypotonic).

Under the influence of ADH, however, the cells of the collecting tubule (and, in animals other than humans and monkeys, also the distal convoluted tubules) become freely permeable to water and the medullary collecting tubules also to urea. As the filtrate descends through the renal medulla in the collecting tubule, it is subject to the osmotic pressure gradients established by loops of Henle and water leaves the lumina of the collecting tubules to enter the interstitium. Hence, the urine, *in the presence of ADH*, becomes **concentrated** (**hypertonic**).

In addition, the concentration of urea becomes extremely high in the lumen of the collecting tubule, and, in the presence of ADH, it passively enters the interstitium of the inner medulla. **Thus, much of the concentration gradient of the renal interstitium in the *inner medulla* is due to the presence of *urea*, whereas, in the *outer medulla*, the presence of *sodium* and *chloride* are responsible for the establishment of the concentration gradient.**

TABLE 19.5 Types of Aquaporins and Their Locations in the Uriniferous Tubule

Aquaporins	Location	Function
Aquaporin-1 (AQP1)	Proximal tubule and thin descending limb of Henle loop	These segments are always permeable to water.
Aquaporin-2 (AQP2)	In the presence of ADH, they are in the luminal surface of principal cells of the collecting tubules. In the absence of ADH, they are stored in apically located vesicles of principal cells of collecting tubules.	In the presence of ADH, AQP2 channels are inserted into the luminal membranes of principal cells, and water can traverse the cell to enter the renal interstitium.
Aquaporin-3 and Aquaporin-4 (AQP3 and AQP4)	Always present in the basolateral cell membranes of the principal cells of tubules; in the presence of ADH they are inserted into the luminal plasmalemma.	The basolateral cell membranes of the principal cells of collecting ducts are always permeable to water.

ADH, Antidiuretic hormone.

The action of ADH is believed to be dependent on V_2 receptors (vasopressin receptor) located in the basolateral plasma membranes of **principal cells** of the collecting tubules. Once ADH binds to a V_2 receptor,

- Gs proteins are activated.
- Adenylate cyclase generates cyclic adenosine monophosphate (cAMP).
- Aquaporin-2 channels (AQP2), as well as AQP3 and AQP4, are inserted into the luminal plasma membrane (Table 19.5)
- Water, from the lumen of the collecting tubule, enters the cell.
- Water leaves the cell via Aquaporin-3 (AQP3) and Aquaporin-4 (AQP4) channels (that are always present in the basolateral cell membranes) to enter the renal interstitium.
- The increase in the interstitial fluid volume causes an increase in blood pressure, thereby increasing GFR.

Clinical Correlations

Congenital nephrogenic diabetes insipidus is an X-linked disorder evidenced clinically in male infants only, although it may also have a certain degree of clinical penetrance in female infants. This condition, in affected males, manifests itself in the formation of a copious quantity of dilute urine due to the malformation of the V_2 receptor. Additional symptoms include fever, vomiting, hypernatremia, and extreme dehydration. The blood level of antidiuretic hormone (ADH) is normal or somewhat elevated; however, the aberrant ADH receptor cannot activate Gs proteins. Consequently, aquaporins are not inserted into the luminal plasma membranes of collecting tubule, resulting in the inability to concentrate urine.

Vasa Recta and Countercurrent Exchange System

The lumen of the arterial limb of the vasa recta has a smaller diameter than that of the venous limb, both limbs are freely permeable to electrolytes and water.

The vasa recta helps maintain the osmotic gradient in the medulla because both arterial and venous limbs are freely permeable to water and salts (Fig. 19.27). Therefore, as the blood courses down the arterial limb, it loses water and gains salts, and as it returns via the venous limb, it loses salts and gains water, thus acting as a **countercurrent exchange system**.

This mechanism ensures that the system of osmotic gradients remains undisturbed because the osmolarity of the blood in the vessels is more or less equilibrated with that of the interstitium. However, as indicated earlier, the luminal diameter of the venous limb is larger than that of the arterial limb. Therefore, the volume of salts and fluid being returned from the medulla into the venous system by the venous limb is greater than that being brought into the medulla by the arterial limb.

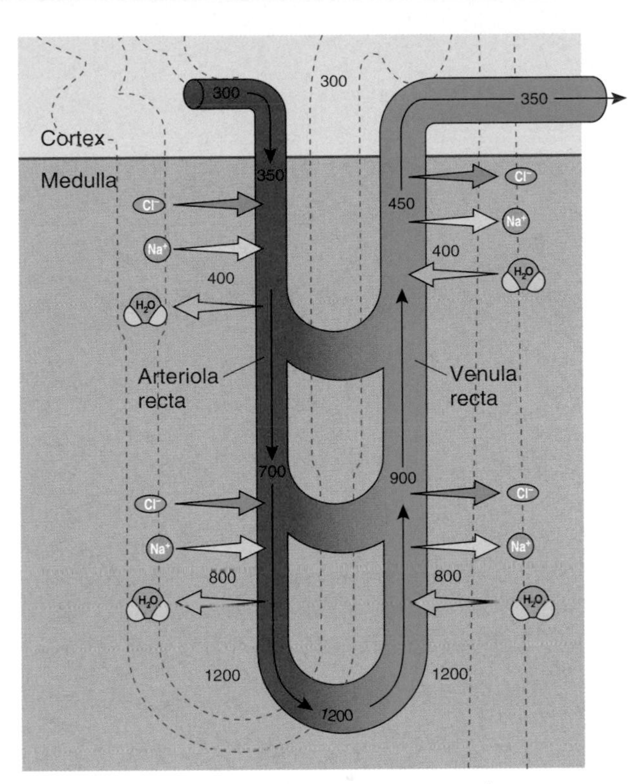

Fig. 19.27 Histophysiology of the vasa recta. Numbers represent milliosmoles per liter. The arteriola recta is smaller in diameter than the venula recta.

Excretory Passages

The excretory passages of the urinary system consist of the minor and major calyces, pelvis of the kidney, ureter, single urinary bladder, and single urethra.

CALYCES

Each minor calyx accepts urine from the renal papilla of a renal pyramid; as many as four minor calyces may deliver their urine to a major calyx.

The renal papilla of each renal pyramid fits into a **minor calyx**, a funnel-shaped chamber that accepts urine leaving the ducts of Bellini at the area cribrosa (Fig. 19.28). The portion of the apex of the pyramid that projects into the minor calyx is covered by **transitional epithelium**, which acts as a barrier, separating the urine from the underlying interstitial connective tissue. Deep to the lamina propria is a thin muscular coat composed entirely of smooth muscle. This muscular layer propels the urine into a **major calyx**, one of three or four larger funnel-shaped chambers, each of which collects urine from two to four **minor calyces**. The major calyces are similar in structure to the minor calyces, as well as to the expanded proximal region of

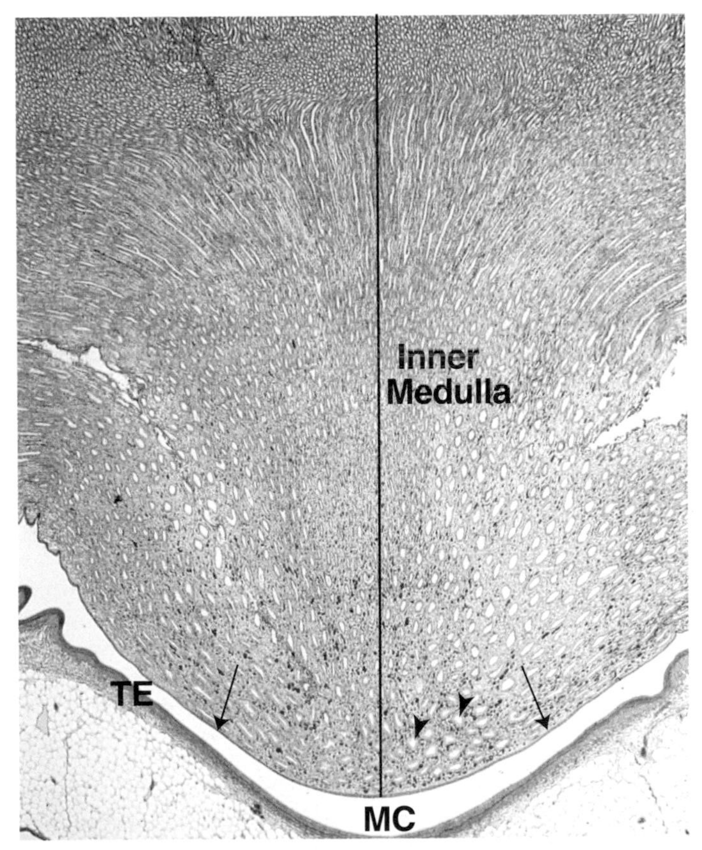

Fig. 19.28 Note that the minor calyx (MC) receives urine from the papillary ducts of Bellini *(arrowheads)* that leave the medulla of the pyramids at the area cribrosa *(between the two arrows)*. The minor calyx is lined by transitional epithelium. (×56)

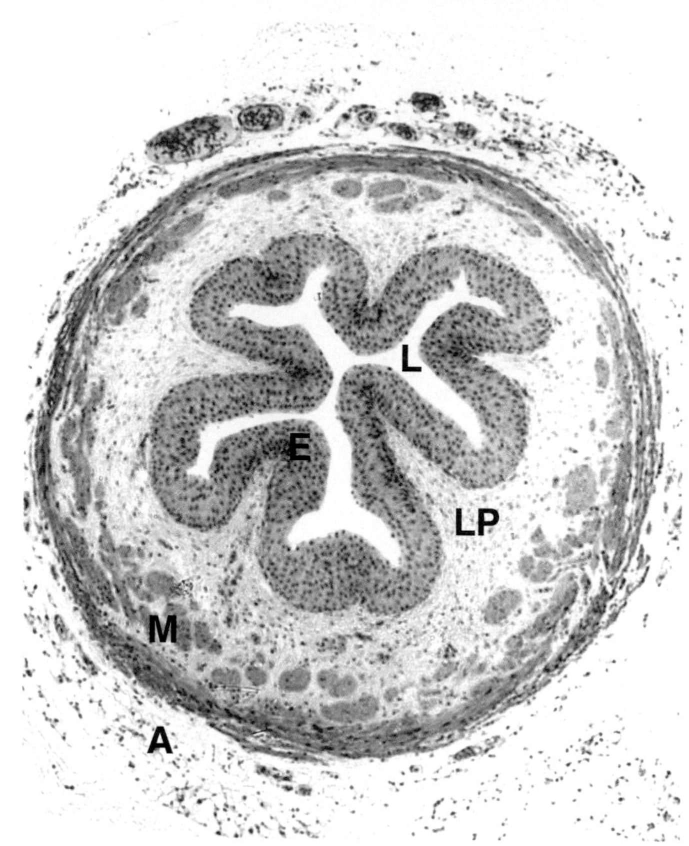

Fig. 19.29 This very-low-magnification photomicrograph of a cross-section of a ureter displays the transitional epithelium (E) lining the lumen (L). The lamina propria (LP) is a dense, irregular, collagenous connective tissue surrounded by an inner longitudinal and outer circular layer of smooth muscle fibers (M). Observe that the muscle coat is surrounded by a fibrous connective tissue (A). (×56)

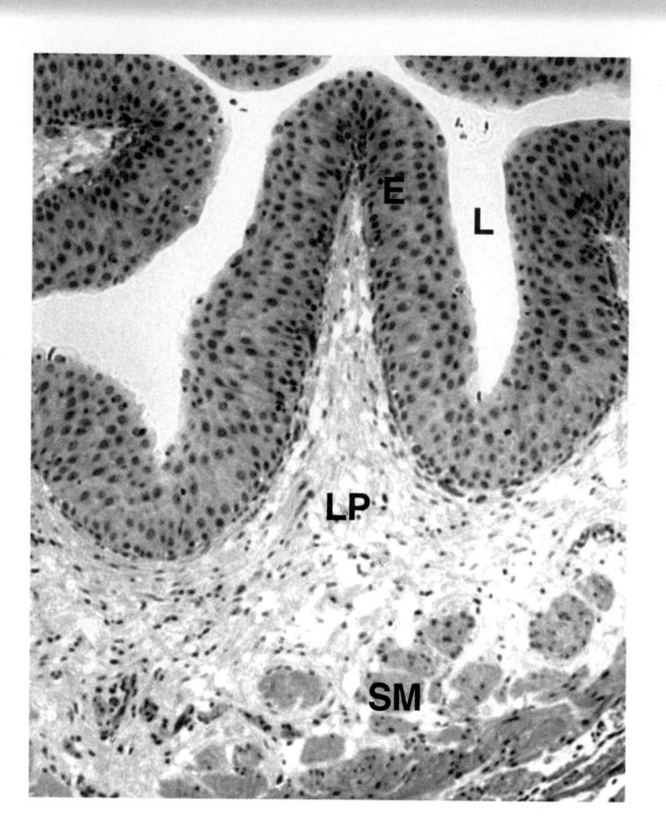

Fig. 19.30 This low-magnification photomicrograph of a cross-section of the ureter displays the transitional epithelial (E) lining of the lumen (L). The lamina propria (LP) is composed of a dense, irregular, collagenous connective tissue surrounded by the inner longitudinal and outer circular layers of smooth muscle fibers (SM). (×132)

the ureters, the **renal pelvis**. The walls of the excretory passages thicken from the minor calyces to the urinary bladder.

URETER

The ureters deliver urine from the kidneys to the urinary bladder.

Each **ureter** is about 3 to 4 mm in diameter, is approximately 25 to 30 cm long, and pierces the base of the urinary bladder. The ureters are hollow tubes consisting of a mucosa, which lines the lumen, a muscular coat (muscularis), and a fibrous, connective tissue covering (Figs. 19.29 and 19.30).

The **mucosa** of the ureter presents several folds, which project into the lumen when the ureter is empty but are absent when the ureter is distended. The **transitional epithelial lining**, three to five cell layers in thickness, overlies a layer of dense, irregular fibroelastic connective tissue, which constitutes the **lamina propria**. As always, the epithelium is separated from the underlying lamina propria by a basal lamina.

The **muscularis** of the ureter is composed of two predominantly inseparable layers of smooth muscle cells. The arrangement of the layers is opposite that found in the digestive tract because the outer layer is arranged circularly and the inner layer is longitudinally disposed. This arrangement is true for the proximal two-thirds of the ureter, but in the lower third, near the urinary bladder, a third muscle layer, whose fibers are oriented longitudinally, is added onto the existing surface of the existing muscle coat. Hence, the muscular fiber orientation in the lower third of the ureter is **outer longitudinal**, **middle circular**, and **inner longitudinal**. However, it should be noted that, just as in the digestive tract, these muscle layers are arranged in a helical configuration, where the pitch of the helices varies from short to long, giving the appearance of circular or longitudinal orientations.

The **fibrous outer coat** of the ureter is unremarkable. At its proximal and distal terminals, it blends with the capsule of the kidney and the connective tissue of the bladder wall, respectively. Contrary to expectation, urine does not pass down the ureter because of gravitational forces; instead, muscular contraction of the ureteric wall establishes peristalsis-like waves that convey urine to the urinary bladder. As the ureters pierce the posterior aspect of the base of the bladder, they pass obliquely for about 2 to 3 cm through the muscular wall of the urinary bladder. Because the muscular wall of the urinary bladder is under constant tonus, the portions of the ureters that pass through this muscular wall become compressed, preventing the reflux of urine back into the ureters. As the ureters open into the bladder lumen, a valve-like flap of mucosa hangs over each ureteric orifice, also contributing to the prevention of regurgitation of urine from the bladder back into the ureters.

URINARY BLADDER

The urinary bladder stores urine until it is ready to be voided.

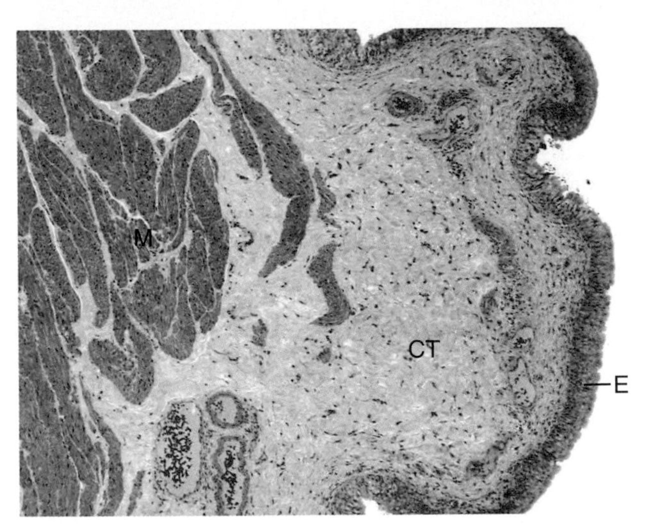

Fig. 19.31 Low-power photomicrograph of a monkey urinary bladder. Observe the epithelium (E), subepithelial connective tissue (CT), and muscular coat (M) of the bladder. (×58)

The **urinary bladder** is essentially an organ for storing urine until the pressure becomes sufficient to induce the urge for micturition (emptying the bladder). It has major anatomical regions, the larger **body** that expands to store the urine and the much smaller **neck**, which connects the bladder to the urethra. Histologically, the bladder has a **mucosa** composed of a **transitional epithelium** (**urothelium**) and an underlying dense irregular collagenous connective tissue layer, the **lamina propria**, surrounded by a thick **smooth muscle coat**. The outermost coat of the bladder is a **serosa** on its posterior aspect, whereas its anterior aspect has an **adventitia** that causes the bladder to adhere to the anterior abdominal wall (Figs. 19.31–19.33). The triangular region of the interior surface of the bladder, whose apices are the orifices of the two ureters and the urethra, is known as the ***trigone***. The mucosa of the trigone is always smooth. The embryonic origin of the trigone differs from that of the remainder of the bladder.

The mucosa of the empty bladder, with the exception of the trigone region, is arranged in numerous folds, which disappear when the bladder becomes distended with urine. During distention, the large, round, **dome-shaped cells** of the transitional epithelium become stretched and change their morphology to become flattened.

The accommodation of the dome-shaped cell shape is performed by a unique feature of the **transitional epithelial cell plasmalemma**, which is composed of a mosaic of specialized, rigid, thickened regions, **plaques**, interspersed by normal cell membrane, known as the **interplaque regions**. When the bladder is empty, the plaque regions are folded into irregular, angular contours, which disappear when the cell becomes stretched. These rigid plaque regions, anchored to intracytoplasmic filaments, resemble gap junctions, but this similarity is superficial only. Plaques appear to be impermeable to water and salts; thus, these cells act as osmotic barriers between the urine and the underlying lamina propria. The superficial cells of the transitional epithelium are held together by desmosomes and, possibly, by tight junctions, which also aid the establishment of the osmotic barrier by preventing the passage of fluid between the cells.

The **lamina propria** of the bladder has two layers, a more *superficial* (just deep to the epithelium) dense, irregular,

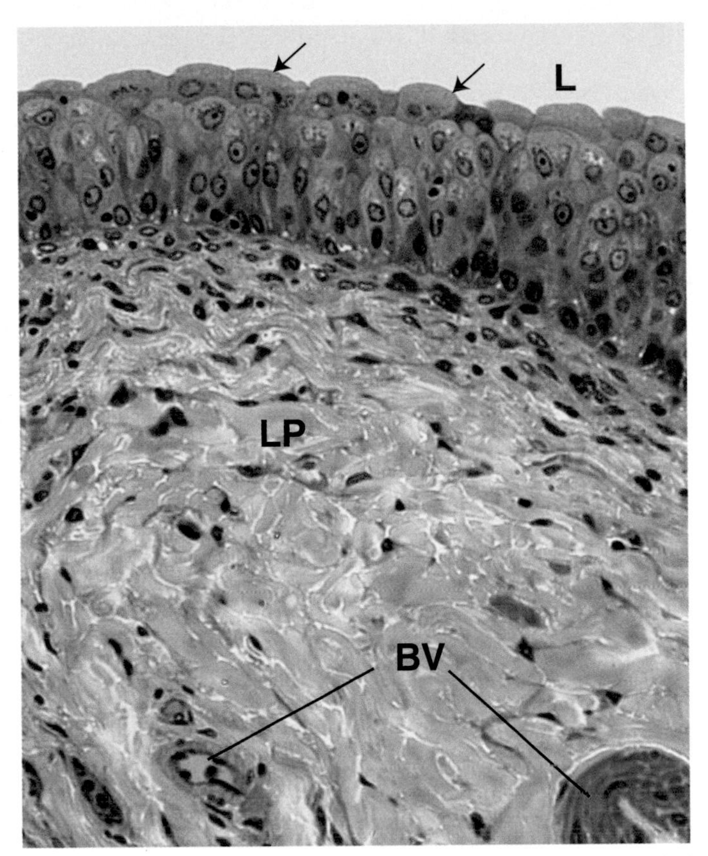

Fig. 19.32 This medium-magnification photomicrograph of the bladder displays the dome-shaped cells *(arrows)* of the transitional epithelium (E). The cellular lamina propria (LP) is well vascularized (BV). (×270)

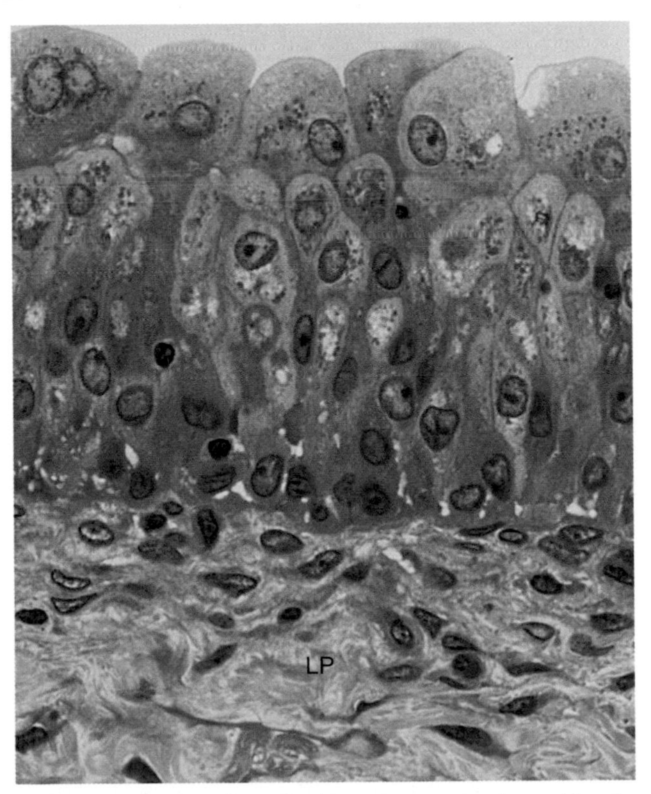

Fig. 19.33 High magnification photomicrograph of transitional epithelium from the bladder of a monkey. Observe the very large dome-shaped cells abutting the lumen. (×540)

collagenous connective tissue and a *deeper*, looser layer of connective tissue composed of a mixture of collagen and elastic fibers. The lamina propria contains no glands, except at the region surrounding the urethral orifice, where **mucous glands** may be found. Usually, these glands extend only into the superficial layer of the lamina propria. They secrete a clear viscous fluid that apparently lubricates the urethral orifice.

The entire muscular coat of the urinary bladder, known as the **detrusor muscle**, is composed of three interlaced layers of smooth muscle fibers that are evident only in the region of the neck of the bladder. Here, they are arranged as a thin inner longitudinal layer, a thick middle circular layer, and a thin outer longitudinal layer. The middle circular layer is interwoven with elastic fibers and forms the **internal sphincter muscle** around the internal orifice of the neck of the bladder just before it joins the urethra. The constant tonus of this muscle averts the emptying of the bladder until the fluid pressure becomes strong enough to relax the internal sphincter and initiate voiding. Fortunately, in humans and many domesticated animals, emptying can be controlled by the voluntary nervous system because of the presence of a second sphincter muscle. As the urethra passes through the floor of the pelvis, a region known as the *urogenital diaphragm*, **skeletal muscle fibers** form the **external sphincter of the bladder**, which is, in reality, a sphincter of the **membranous urethra**. This sphincter muscle is under voluntary control; even though the detrusor muscle contracts and the internal sphincter muscle of the bladder relaxes to attempt to empty the bladder, voluntary contraction of the external sphincter prevents urine from entering the urethra. (The innervation of the bladder and the control of micturition is described in the next section.)

The **adventitia** of the bladder is composed of a dense, irregular collagenous type of connective tissue containing a generous amount of elastic fibers. On the posterior aspect, the adventitia is covered by a peritoneal reflection onto the wall of the bladder, forming a **serosa**.

Clinical Correlations

Cancer of the bladder is one of the most common cancers. Fully 50% of the cases involve individuals who smoke, although, in 30% of the cases, it is attributed to exposure to carcinogens such as naphthylamine and benzidine in the workplace. Bladder cancer may occur in younger individuals, but it is more frequent in older males (66%) than in older females (33%) and almost always begins in the transitional epithelium of the bladder. Symptoms of bladder cancer are blood in the urine, with or without pain, followed by painful and frequent urination later. Bladder cancer is usually diagnosed early enough to be cured, but remission does occur. Thus, patients should be monitored for the rest of their lives. Almost 200,000 people die annually worldwide from bladder cancer.

MICTURITION

Micturition (**urination**; **emptying of the urinary bladder**) is a process that is controlled by both the autonomic nervous system and voluntary nervous system. The autonomic control of the urinary bladder has two components, sensory and motor. The **sensory fibers** originate in stretch receptors and monitor how much the bladder wall is stretched by the accumulated urine. The **motor component** is under the control of **parasympathetic nerves** whose preganglionic fibers, originating from preganglionic parasympathetic neurons located in spinal cord segments S2 and S3, synapse on postganglionic parasympathetic neurons located in small parasympathetic ganglia residing in the wall of the urinary bladder. **Postganglionic fibers** from these ganglia innervate the detrusor muscle and the internal sphincter of the bladder. When the bladder is stretched to a certain extent, the signals from the stretch receptors initiate *contraction of the detrusor muscle and relaxation of the internal urinary sphincter* so that the bladder can expel the urine. However, for actual urination to occur, the **somatic motor fibers** carried by the pudendal nerve must permit the *relaxation of the external sphincter of the bladder*, thus opening the lumen of the membranous portion of the urethra. The average individual voids about 1.5 to 2.0 L of urine per day.

URETHRA

The urethra conveys urine from the urinary bladder to outside the body.

The urinary bladder is drained by a single tubular structure, the **urethra**, which communicates with the outside, permitting elimination of urine from the body. As the urethra pierces the **perineum** (**urogenital diaphragm**; **floor of the pelvis**), skeletal muscle fibers from that perineum form the **external sphincter muscle** surrounding the urethra. This muscle permits voluntary control of micturition (see previous section). The urethra of the male is longer than that of the female and has a dual function, acting as a route for urine as well as for semen.

Clinical Correlations

Loss of voluntary control over the ***external sphincter muscle*** *of the urethra causes* ***urinary incontinence****, a condition affecting primarily older women.*

Female Urethra

The female urethra is about 4 to 5 cm in length and 5 to 6 mm in diameter. It extends from the urinary bladder to the external urethral orifice just above and anterior to the opening of the vagina. Normally, the lumen is collapsed, except during micturition. It is lined by a **transitional epithelium** near the bladder and by a **stratified squamous nonkeratinized epithelium** along the remainder of its length. Interspersed in the epithelium are patches of pseudostratified columnar epithelium. The mucosa is arranged in elongated folds because of the organization of the fibroelastic **lamina propria**. Along the entire length of the urethra are numerous clear, mucus-secreting **glands of Littre**.

A thin, vascular, erectile coat surrounds the mucosa, resembling the corpus spongiosum of the male. The muscular layer of the urethra is continuous with that of the bladder but is composed of two layers only, an inner longitudinal and outer circular smooth muscle layer. As discussed earlier, as the urethra pierces the perineum, a skeletal muscle sphincter surrounds it and permits voluntary control of micturition.

Male Urethra

The male urethra is about 20 cm long, and its three regions are named according to the structures through which they pass.

- **Prostatic urethra.** Three to 4 cm long, it lies entirely in the prostate gland. It is lined by a transitional epithelium and receives the openings of many tiny ducts of the prostate, the prostatic utricle (a rudimentary homologue of the uterus), and the paired ejaculatory ducts.
- **Membranous urethra.** One to 2 cm long. This segment is so named because it passes through the perineum. It is lined by stratified columnar epithelium interspersed with patches of pseudostratified columnar epithelium. As indicated earlier, skeletal muscle fibers from the perineum form a sphincter around this portion of the urethra, which provides voluntary control over micturition.
- **Spongy urethra (penile urethra).** The longest portion of the urethra (15 cm long), it passes through the length of the penis, terminating at the tip of the glans penis as the external urethral orifice. This segment is so named because it is located in the corpus spongiosum. It is lined by stratified columnar epithelium interspersed with patches of pseudostratified columnar and stratified squamous, nonkeratinized epithelia. The enlarged terminal portion of the urethra in the glans penis (the **navicular fossa**) is lined by stratified squamous, nonkeratinized epithelium.

The **lamina propria** of all three regions is composed of a loose fibroelastic connective tissue with a rich vascular supply. It houses numerous **glands of Littre**, whose mucous secretion lubricates the epithelial lining of the urethra.

Clinical Correlations

Urinary tract infections (UTIs) usually affect the urinary bladder (acute cystitis); however, in some cases, the infection may travel up the ureters and involve the kidneys (pyelonephritis). In the case of acute cystitis, the symptoms are frequent urination and painful or burning sensations during voiding. However, if these conditions are accompanied by fever and pain in the lower back and, occasionally, vomiting, all of which developed in a short period of time, the physician should suspect pyelonephritis. In most cases, the infection is caused by the invasion of the urinary tract by the microorganism Escherichia coli *(*E. coli*). Because the most common source of* E. coli *is the anus, UTIs are more frequent in females than in males because the proximity of the urethra to the anus. Additionally, in women who have undergone hysterectomy, the connection of the bladder to the anterior abdominal wall is weakened, and the bladder tends to prolapse, thus making emptying the bladder more difficult. The trapped urine has the tendency to permit the proliferation of* E. coli *in the bladder, thereby increasing the chances of acute cystitis. In most cases, antibiotic treatment eliminates acute cystitis. Pyelonephritis is a very serious disease that should be treated with antibiotics and, at times, even by surgical intervention.*

Pathological Considerations

See Figs. 19.34 through 19.36.

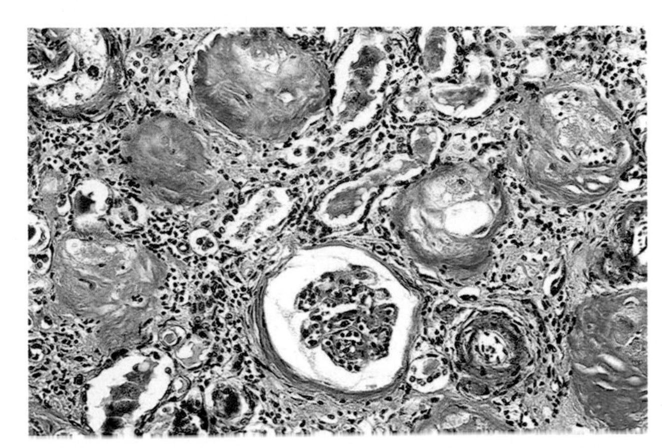

Fig. 19.34 Photomicrograph of the kidney of a patient with chronic glomerulonephritis. Observe in this Masson trichrome–stained tissue that most of the glomeruli have been replaced by blue-stained collagen fibers. (Reprinted with permission from Kumar V, Abbas AK, Aster JC. *Robbins and Cotran Pathologic Basis of Disease*. 9th ed. Philadelphia: Elsevier; 2015:925.)

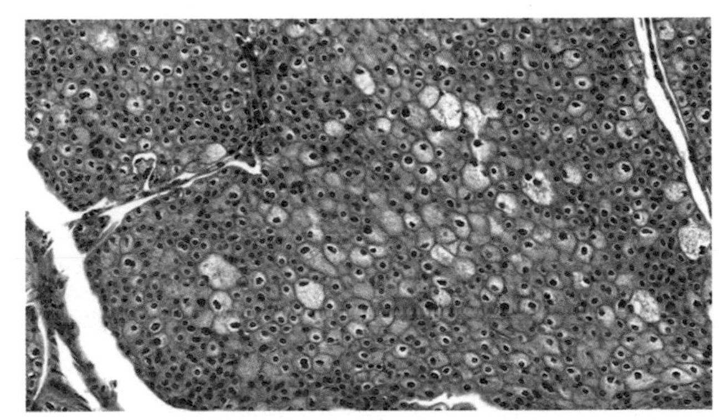

Fig. 19.35 Photomicrograph of the kidney of a patient with chromophobe-type renal cell carcinoma as evidenced by the presence of pale chromophobe-like cells that display a perinuclear halo. (Reprinted with permission from Kumar V, Abbas AK, Aster JC. *Robbins and Cotran Pathologic Basis of Disease*. 9th ed. Philadelphia: Elsevier; 2015:955.)

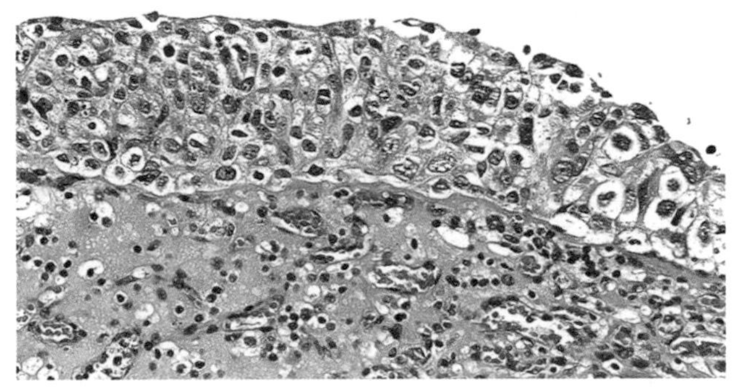

Fig. 19.36 Photomicrograph of the urinary bladder of a patient with flat carcinoma in situ. Observe the characteristic enlarged, pleomorphic nuclei of the transitional epithelial cells. (Reprinted with permission from Kumar V, Abbas AK, Aster JC. *Robbins and Cotran Pathologic Basis of Disease*. 9th ed. Philadelphia: Elsevier; 2015:967.)

Histology Laboratory Instructions: Urinary System

Kidney

Cortex

The kidney cortex is characterized by the renal corpuscles that are surrounded by the proximal and distal convoluted tubules of the cortical labyrinth and medullary rays composed of cortical collecting tubules and pars recta of the proximal and distal tubules. Note that even at low magnification, the parietal layer of the Bowman capsule and urinary space are clearly evident (see Fig. 19.2, R, M, P, S). At medium magnification, the parietal layer of the Bowman capsule is seen to be composed of a simple squamous epithelium that surrounds the urinary space. The macula densa portion of the distal tubule's pars recta is clearly evident due to the closely packed nuclei of the macula densa cells. The proximal convoluted tubules are distinguishable by the darker stain of their large cells in comparison with the smaller, lighter staining cells of the distal convoluted tubule (see Fig. 19.3, P, S, M). At high magnification, the glomerular capillaries of the renal corpuscle can be seen to be filled with blood, and the relationship between the afferent glomerular arteriole and the macula densa is apparent. Observe that the large, dark-staining cells of the proximal convoluted tubule are well represented (see Fig. 19.4, RBCs, GA, MD, PCT).

Another low-magnification photomicrograph of the kidney cortex displays the renal corpuscle surrounded by cross-sectional profiles of a proximal convoluted tubule (PCT) and a distal convoluted tubule (DCT). Because the proximal convoluted tubule is much longer than the distal convoluted tubule, the ratio of PCT to DCT profiles is about 7:1. Proximal convoluted tubules have larger, darker-staining cells when compared with distal convoluted tubule cells. Medullary rays, housing cortical collecting tubules and ascending thick limbs and descending thick limbs of Henle loop are clearly evident. Note that the cell membranes of collecting tubules are clearly evident, permitting them to be recognized with ease. Cells of the descending thick limbs resemble those of the proximal convoluted tubules, whereas the cells of the ascending thick limbs resemble those of the distal convoluted tubules (see Fig. 19.14, RC, PCT, DCT, CT, ATL, DTL). A medium-magnification photomicrograph of the kidney cortex presents a renal corpuscle surrounded by profiles of proximal and distal convoluted tubules displaying numerical and histological differences, demonstrating an approximately 7:1 ratio of proximal to distal convoluted profiles, as well as the darker, larger cells of the proximal versus smaller, lighter cells of the distal convoluted tubule. The cortical collecting duct exhibits the lightly stained cells with obvious cell membranes (see Fig. 19.15, RC, PCT, DCT, CD).

Medulla

A longitudinal section of the outer zone of the renal medulla at medium magnification displays the thin and thick limbs of Henle loop. Observe that the cells composing the thin limb are squamous, whereas those of the thick limb are low cuboidal to cuboidal in shape. The medullary collecting tubules are not any different from their cortical portions, displaying their characteristically obvious cell membranes. The difference between the arteria recta and vena recta are obvious in that the arteria recta has a thicker wall than the vena recta (see Fig. 19.17, TL, ThL, CT, AR, VR). A cross-section of a similar region of the outer zone of the renal medulla displays the cuboidal cells of the medullary collecting tubules, as well as thin limbs of Henle loop and the endothelial cells of the vasa recta (see Fig. 19.21, CT, HL, E).

A cross-section of the renal papilla displays the large papillary ducts of Bellini that resemble the collecting tubules in that their cells are lightly stained and present obvious cell membranes between adjoining cells. However, these cells are columnar rather than cuboidal in shape. Also, observe the difference between the cuboidal-shaped cells of the thick limbs of Henle loop and the squamous cells of the thin limbs of Henle loop. Observe also the thick walls of the arteria recta (see Fig. 19.23, PD, ThL, TL, AR).

Calyces (Minor Calyx)

The inner medulla of the kidney ends at the renal papilla, where the papillary ducts of Bellini open at the area cribrosa to deliver the urine into the minor calyx, a funnel-shaped structure that is lined by transitional epithelium and opens into a major calyx (see Fig. 19.28, *arrowheads, area between the two arrows*, MC, TE).

Ureter

A very-low-magnification photomicrograph of a cross-section of a ureter displays the transitional epithelium lining its lumen. Note that the dense, irregular, collagenous connective tissue of the lamina propria is surrounded by two layers of smooth muscle fibers, an inner longitudinal and an outer circular (the opposite of the digestive tract). The muscle coat is surrounded by a fibrous connective tissue, known as the adventitia (see Fig. 19.29, E, L, LP, M, A). A higher magnification of the ureter displays the transitional epithelial lining of the lumen. It demonstrates the cellularity of the lamina propria and the two smooth muscle layers of the muscle coat (see Fig. 19.30, E, L, LP, SM).

Urinary Bladder

A very low magnification of the urinary bladder displays its thick transitional epithelium and a thick connective tissue layer, the lamina propria, which is thrown into folds when the bladder is empty. The thick muscle coat is also evident (see Fig. 19.31, E, CT, M). A medium magnification of the urinary bladder displays the transitional epithelial lining of the lumen. Observe that the surface-most cells of the transitional epithelium are large, dome-shaped cells. The lamina propria is well endowed by cellular and vascular elements (see Fig. 19.32, E, L, *arrows*, LP, BV). At high magnification, the dome-shaped cells are well defined and it is obvious that some of the cells have two nuclei. Observe the cellularity of the lamina propria (see Fig. 19.33, LP).

20 Female Reproductive System

The **female reproductive system** consists of the internal reproductive organs (the two ovaries, two oviducts, uterus, and vagina; Fig. 20.1) and the external genitalia (the clitoris, labia majora, and labia minora).

Prior to puberty, the female reproductive organs are incompletely developed. They remain so until **gonadotropic hormones** secreted by the pituitary gland signal the initiation of puberty. Thereafter, further differentiation of the reproductive organs occurs, culminating in **menarche**, the first menstrual flow. The average age at which menarche takes place is 12.7 years, but varies between 9 to 15 years of age. After the first menstrual flow, the menstrual cycle, which involves many hormonal, histological, and psychological changes, is repeated approximately each month (28 days) throughout the entire reproductive years, unless it is interrupted by pregnancy. As a woman nears the end of her reproductive years, her menstrual cycles become less regular, as hormonal and neurological signals begin to change. This culminates in complete cessation of menstruation, known as **menopause**, after which, limited involution of the reproductive organs occurs. On average, menopause in women in the United States occurs at 51 years of age but generally ranges between 48 and 55 years of age. However, it may begin even in the early 40s.

Although the mammary glands are not considered to belong to the female reproductive system, their physiology and function are so closely associated with the reproductive system that they are discussed in this chapter.

Ovaries

Each ovary, covered by the germinal epithelium, is indistinctly divided into a cortex and medulla.

Each **ovary** is approximately 3 cm long, 1.5 to 2 cm wide, and 1 cm thick, each weighing approximately 14 g. The ovaries are located in the pelvis and are suspended in the **broad ligament of the uterus** by an attachment called the ***mesovarium***, a special fold of the peritoneum through which blood vessels reach the ovaries (see Fig. 20.1).

EMBRYONIC DEVELOPMENT OF THE OVARIES

The Y chromosome is responsible for the development of the male gonads; in its absence, the default formation of **ovaries** will occur. Prior to the fourth week of development, epithelially covered **gonadal ridges** form on the posterior aspects of the abdominal wall. About 1 week later, cells derived from the epithelial cover pass through the substance of the gonadal ridges to form a group of cells known as the **primitive sex cords**. By the sixth week of development, these gonadal ridges form structures known as **indifferent gonads**—indifferent because they do not as yet exhibit male or female characteristics. Within a few days of the formation of the primitive sex cords, cells from the yolk sac, known as **primordial germ cells**, invade the gonadal ridges and rapidly proliferate, thus enlarging the gonadal ridges. These primordial germ cells differentiate into **oogonia,** which proliferate by mitosis. However, some of these cells begin their first **meiotic division**, entering the **prophase of meiosis I**, and become known as **primary oocytes**. During the seventh week of development, another group of cells from the epithelial cover, called the **germinal epithelium**, burrows into the *cortical aspect* of the gonadal ridges to establish **cortical sex cords**. After their formation, these **cortical sex cords** dissociate into individual flat cells that migrate to each primary oocyte and form a single layer of cells, now known as **follicular cells,** around it. The primary oocyte and its surrounding flat follicular cells are collectively known as a **primordial follicle**. The follicular cells release the signaling molecule **oocyte maturation inhibitor**, preventing meiosis from continuing, forcing the primary oocyte to remain in the **dictyate** (**prolonged diplotene**) **phase** of **prophase I** of **meiosis I** until just before it is ovulated.

By the fifth month of development, there are as many as 7 million oogonia and primary oocytes present in the developing ovary. Then, suddenly, many of these oogonia and primary oocytes undergo **atresia** and die, so that, at birth, there are only 1 to 2 million primordial follicles present in the two ovaries. Most of these become atretic over the next decade or so of life, and at menarche a young woman has less than 200,000 primordial follicles in the two ovaries. Generally, ovulation will occur every 28 days for the next 30 to 40 years, with one oocyte released each month, for a total of about 450 oocytes released over the reproductive period. The remaining follicles degenerate and die over the same period of time.

Clinical Correlation

The development of a female is the default condition that requires the absence of a Y chromosome. If a Y chromosome is present, two of its genes, SRY (sex-determining region of the Y chromosome) *and* SOX9 *(a gene that codes for a transcription factor known by the same name) become activated. The former expresses the protein known as* testis-determining factor*, which inhibits the regions of the X chromosome that code for the development of a female. The protein SOX9 has several functions, including the prompting of* Sertoli cells *to form* antimullerian hormone (AMH)*. AMH prevents the formation of the female reproductive tract (see Chapter 21 on the male reproductive system) and activates* fibroblast growth factor-9*, which encourages Sertoli cell proliferation and thereby the continued synthesis and release of the protein SOX9. This prompts a continuous supply of AMH and development of an embryo of the male gender.*

GENERAL DESCRIPTION OF THE OVARIES

The ovaries are covered by a low cuboidal, mesothelial derivative known as the **germinal epithelium**, which was originally believed to give rise to the germ cells. Although this is now

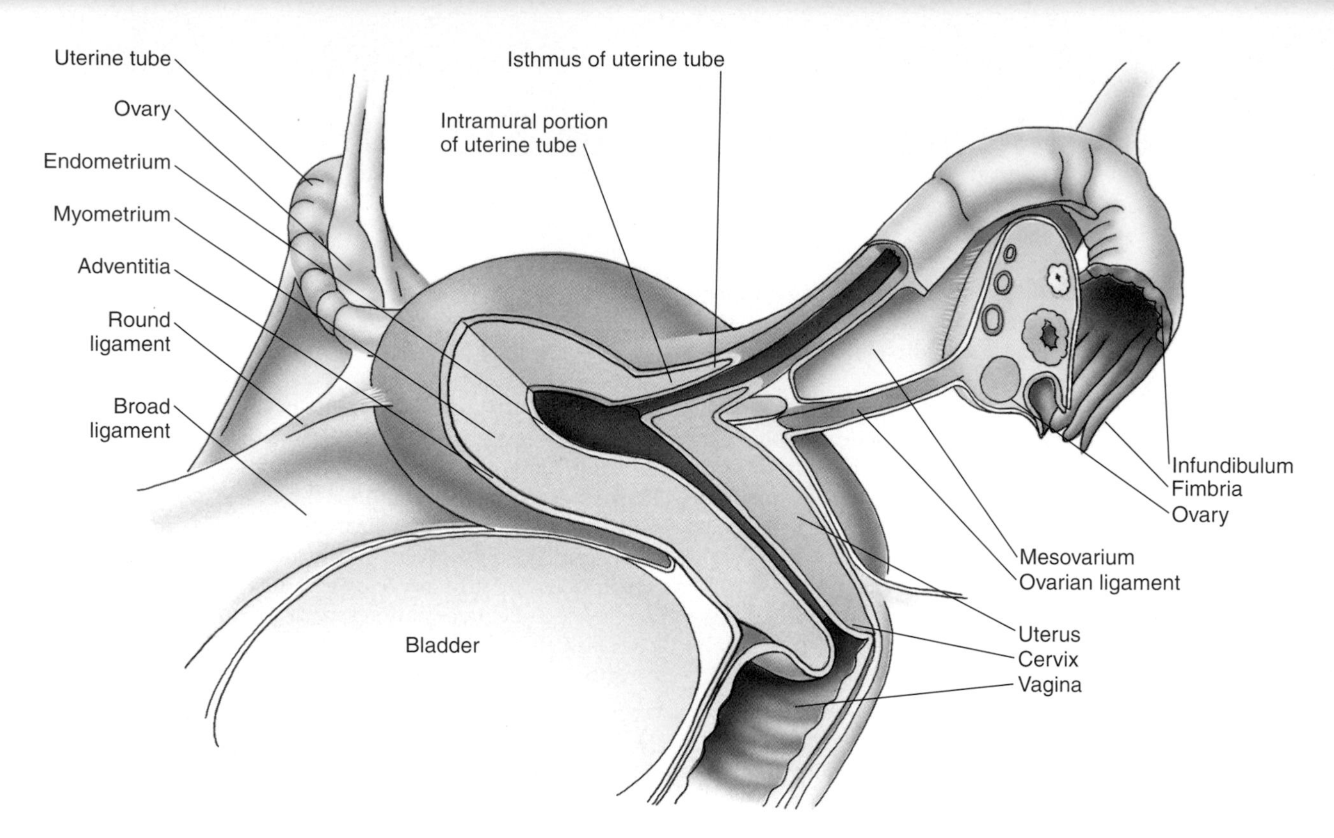

Fig. 20.1 Schematic diagram of the female reproductive tract. Note that the ovary is sectioned to show the developing follicles and that the uterus and fallopian tube are both opened to display their respective lumina.

known to be incorrect the name persists. Deep to the germinal epithelium is a poorly vascularized, dense, irregular collagenous connective tissue capsule, the **tunica albuginea**, whose type I collagen fibers are oriented approximately parallel to the surface of the ovary. Each ovary is subdivided into the highly cellular **cortex** and a richly vascularized loose connective tissue **medulla** whose blood vessels are derived from the ovarian arteries. Histologically, however, the division between the cortex and the medulla is indistinct.

OVARIAN CORTEX

The ovarian cortex is composed of the connective tissue stroma that houses ovarian follicles in various stages of development.

The **ovarian cortex** of a sexually mature female is composed of a connective tissue framework, the **stroma** (**interstitial compartment**), housing fibroblast-like **stromal cells** (**interstitial cells**) and **ovarian follicles** in various stages of development (Fig. 20.2A).

The Ovarian Cortex at Onset of Puberty

The pulsatile release of gonadotropin-releasing hormone has the major responsibility for the initiation of puberty.

Prior to reaching puberty, all of the follicles of the ovarian cortex are in the **primordial follicle** stage. **Gonadotropin-releasing hormone (GnRH**, also known as **luteinizing hormone-releasing hormone**, **LHRH)**, a polypeptide composed of 10 amino acids and produced by the neurosecretory neurons of the arcuate nucleus and preoptic area of the hypothalamus, has a major role in initiating puberty. The release of LHRH is pulsatile, occurring approximately every 90 minutes, and its half-life in the bloodstream is only about 2 to 4 minutes. The pulsatility of LHRH release is a prerequisite not only for the onset of menarche but also for the maintenance of the normal ovulatory and menstrual cycles throughout the reproductive life of the female.

The pulsatile release of **GnRH** (and the nonpulsatile release of the hormone **leptin**) results in a parallel, pulsatile, release of gonadotropins (**follicle-stimulating hormone** [**FSH**] and **luteinizing hormone** [**LH**]) by basophils of the anterior pituitary, culminating in the commencement of follicular development and the onset of the ovulatory cycle (Table 20.1). The ovulatory cycle, follicular development, and hormonal interrelationships are described next.

Ovarian Follicles

Ovarian follicles mature through four developmental stages: primordial, primary, secondary, and graafian.

Ovarian follicles are surrounded by stromal connective tissue and consist of a **primary oocyte** and its associated **follicular cells** (**granulosa cells**) arranged in a single spherical layer or several concentric layers around the primary oocyte. Follicular cells, similar to the germinal epithelium, are derived from the **mesothelial epithelium** and possibly also from a second source, the primitive sex cords of the **mesonephros,** a precursor of the kidney.

There are two stages of follicular development based on the growth of the follicle that are also categorized by the development of the oocyte and follicular cells (Table 20.2; see Fig. 20.2B): **nongrowing follicles**, namely, **primordial follicles**; and **growing follicles** that are of three types—**primary follicles** (both *unilaminar* and *multilaminar*), **secondary** (**antral**) **follicles**, and **graafian** (**mature**) **follicles**.

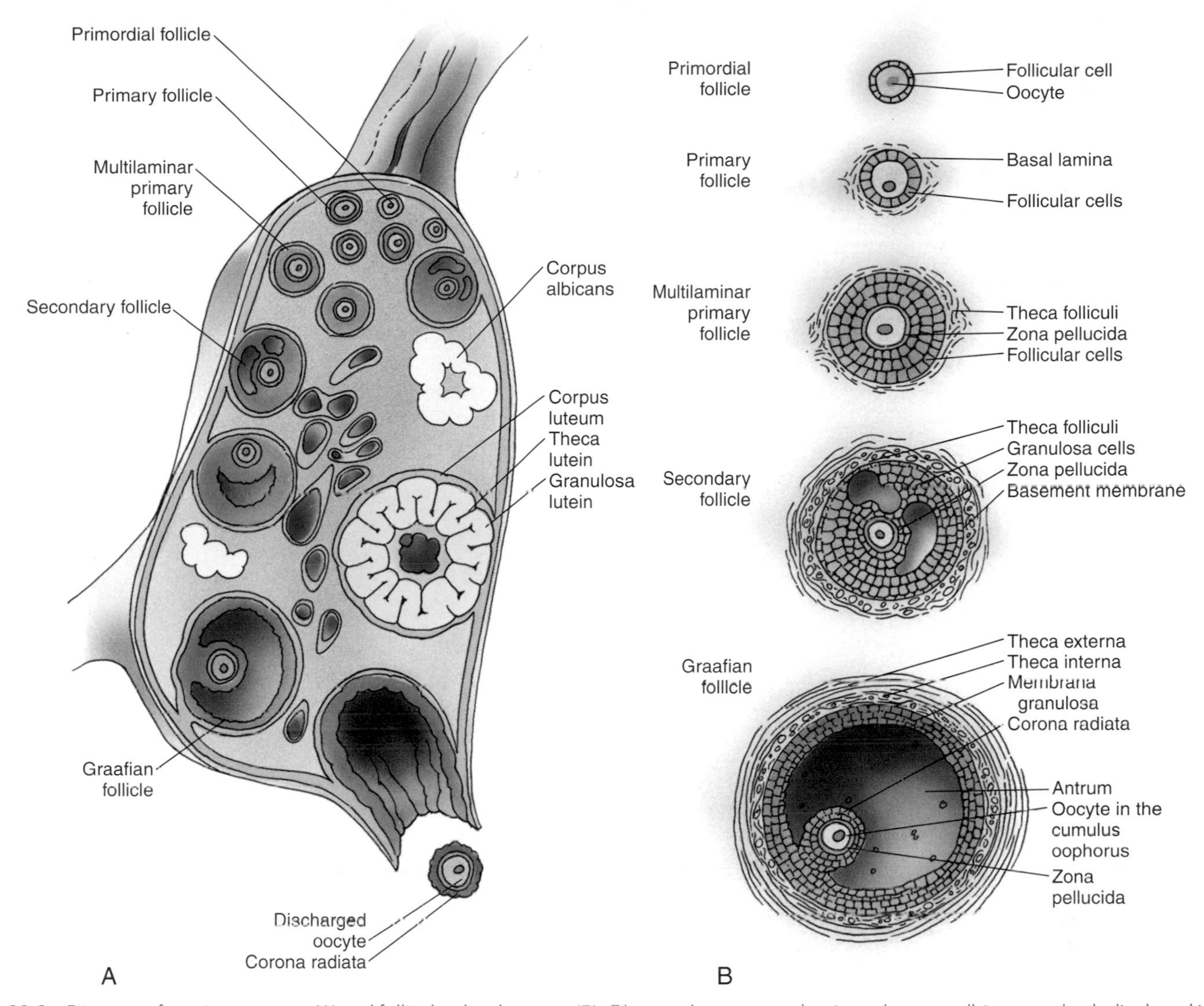

Fig. 20.2 Diagram of ovarian structure (A) and follicular development (B). Observe that a corpus lutein and corpus albicans are both displayed in the ovary. Note that all of the stages of follicular development, from the primordial follicle stage to the graafian follicle stage, are presented.

TABLE 20.1 Pulsatility Rate of LHRH Release

Rate of Release	Direct Results	Effects of Direct Results
Less than 60 minutes	Downregulates LHRH receptor formation	Anovulation due to lack of gonadotropin responsivity
Greater than 90 minutes	Inadequate stimulation of basophils	Anovulation and amenorrhea
Between 60 and 90 minutes	Adequate number of LHRH receptors on basophils	Normal ovulatory cycle

LHRH, Luteinizing hormone–releasing hormone.

Recruitment of the primordial follicle to become a primary follicle and *activation* of primary follicles to become secondary follicles are *independent* of FSH. Secondary and later follicles, however, are under the influence of FSH. Follicular development usually culminates in the release of a single oocyte (ovulation).

Primordial Follicles

Primordial follicles, composed of a single layer of flattened follicular cells that surround the primary oocyte, are separated from the ovarian stroma by a basement membrane; they are considered to be the basic reproductive units of the ovary.

Primordial follicles are abundant before birth, after which they become fewer in number; they are considered to be the basic reproductive units of the ovary. The primordial follicle is composed of a **primary oocyte** surrounded by a single layer of flattened **follicular cells** (Figs. 20.3 and 20.4).

The **primary oocyte**, a spherical cell about 25 μm in diameter, has a large, acentric nucleus with a single nucleolus. The nucleoplasm appears vesicular because of its uncoiled chromosomes. The cytoplasm possesses numerous mitochondria, abundant Golgi complexes, rough endoplasmic reticulum (RER) with a sparse amount of ribosomes, and annulate lamellae. Moreover, primary oocytes house vesicles

TABLE 20.2 Stages of Ovarian Follicular Development

Stage	FSH Dependent	Oocyte	Zona Pellucida	Follicular Cells or Granulosa	Liquor Folliculi	Theca Interna	Theca Externa
Primordial follicle	No	Primary oocyte	None	Single layer of flat cells	None	None	None
Unilaminar primary follicle	No	Primary oocyte	Present	Single layer of cuboidal cells	None	None	None
Multilaminar primary follicle	No	Primary oocyte	Present and microvilli of primary oocyte form gap junctions with filopodia of corona radiata cells	Several layers of follicular cells (now called *granulosa cells*)	None	Present	Present
Secondary follicle	Yes	Primary oocyte	Present with gap junctions	Spaces develop between granulosa cells	Accumulate in spaces between granulosa cells	Present	Present
Graafian follicle	Yes, until it becomes the dominant follicle	Primary oocyte surrounded by corona radiata in cumulus oophorus	Present with gap junctions	Form membrana granulosa and cumulus oophorus	Fills the antrum	Present	Present

FSH, Follicle-stimulating hormone.

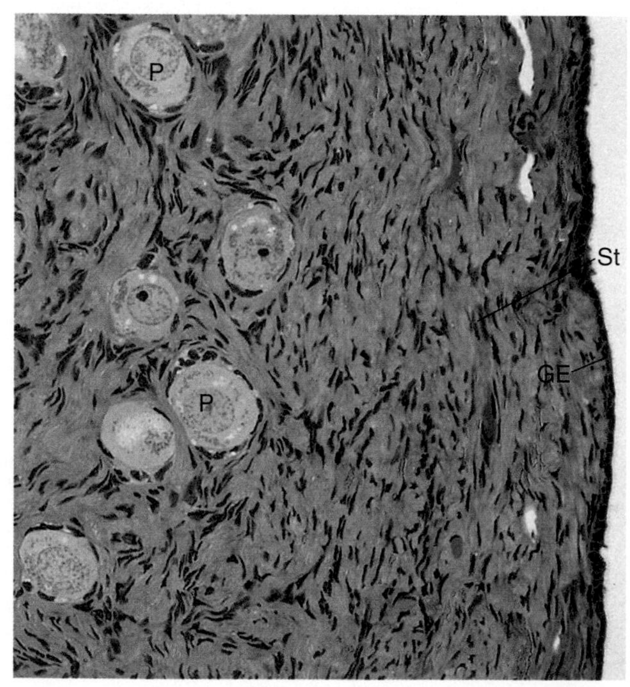

Fig. 20.3 Light micrograph of the ovarian cortex demonstrating mostly primordial follicles (P), which are primary oocytes surrounded by follicular cells. The germinal epithelium (GE) as well as the ovarian stroma (St) of the cortex are also evident in this photomicrograph. (×270)

that occupy the cortical region of the cell, just beneath the plasmalemma. These vesicles are known as ***cortical granules***, which house proteolytic enzymes that will function during the process of fertilization (see the section on fertilization). Primary oocytes remain in the **dictyate stage of prophase** of **meiosis I** until ovulation even if that occurs 30 to 40 years later.

The primary oocyte is completely surrounded by squamous **follicular cells** attached to each other by desmosomes and separated from the connective tissue stroma by a basement membrane.

Clinical Correlations

During the dictyate stage, mRNAs are transcribed in the nucleus of the primary oocyte; however, they are not translated until after meiosis I resumes. It appears that regulatory proteins must polyadenylate the 3′ end of the mRNA, but this site is blocked and the mRNA remains dormant. Once the site is freed, proteins such as eukaryotic translation initiation factor 4E (eIF4E) and cytoplasmic polyadenylation element binding protein (CPEB) can stimulate polyadenylation of the dormant mRNA, permitting it to be translated.

Primary Follicles

There are two types of primary follicles, unilaminar and multilaminar, depending on the number of layers of follicular cells that surround the primary oocyte.

Primordial follicles develop into **primary follicles** distinguished as a result of changes in the primary oocyte, follicular cells, and surrounding stromal tissue (Fig. 20.5).

The **primary oocyte** grows to about 100 to 150 μm in diameter, with an enlarged nucleus (these nuclei are sometimes called ***germinal vesicles***). Several Golgi complexes are scattered throughout the cell, the RER becomes rich with ribosomes, free ribosomes are abundant, and mitochondria are numerous and dispersed throughout the cell.

Follicular cells become cuboidal in shape. As long as only a single layer of follicular cells encircles the oocyte, the follicle is called a ***unilaminar primary follicle***. Once a primordial follicle

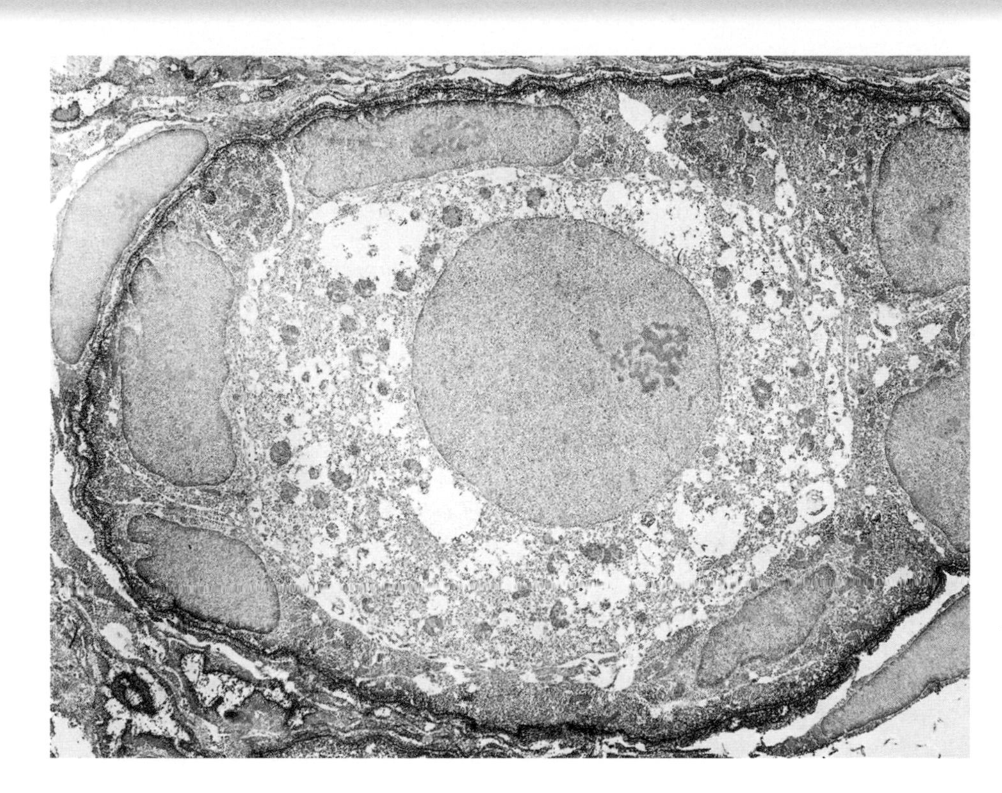

Fig. 20.4 Electron micrograph of a primordial ovarian follicle of a rat ovary (×6200). Observe the oocyte surrounded by follicular cells. (From Leardkamolkarn V, Abrahamson DR. Immunoelectron microscopic localization of laminin in rat ovarian follicles. *Anat Rec.* 1992;233:41–52. Reprinted with permission from Wiley-Liss, Inc., a subsidiary of John Wiley & Sons, Inc.)

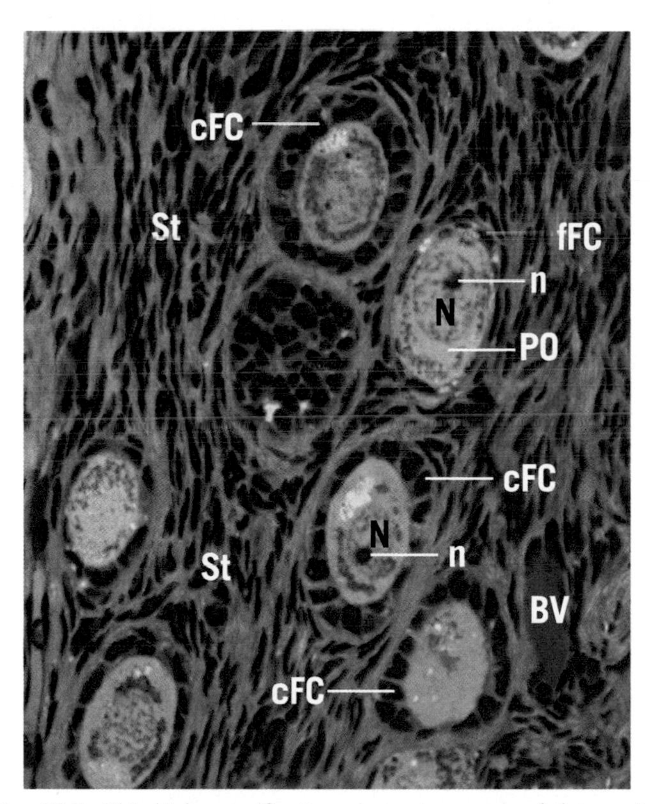

Fig. 20.5 This high-magnification photomicrograph of the ovarian cortex displays the highly cellular stroma (St) and several primordial and unilaminar primary follicles. The primordial follicle has a single layer of flat follicular cells (fFC) surrounding the primary oocyte (PO), whereas the unilaminar primary follicle has a single layer of cuboidal follicular cells (cFC) surrounding the primary oocyte. Note the large, vesicular-appearing nuclei (N) and the single dense nucleoli (n) of the primary oocytes. The stroma has a rich vascular supply (BV). (×540)

is *recruited*, both the follicular cells and the primary oocyte participate in the *transformation* of the primordial follicle into the primary follicle by expressing transcription factors such as **newborn oogenesis homeobox**, **spermatogenesis and oogenesis helix-loop-helix 1 and 2**, and **forkhead box L2**. All of these factors plus other signaling molecules—such as **activin**, **epidermal growth factor**, **insulin-like growth factor**, and **calcium ions**—act at the level of the microenvironment of a particular developing primary follicle, so that other neighboring primordial follicles are not prompted into becoming primary follicles. In fact, other local factors—such as phosphorylated **forkhead box O3**, manufactured by the primary oocyte, and **anti-Mullerian hormone,** secreted by follicular cells (granulosa cells) of neighboring growing follicles—inhibit the transformation of most primordial follicles in their vicinity into a primary follicle.

Multilaminar Primary Follicle. When the follicular cells proliferate and stratify, forming several layers of cells around the primary oocyte, the follicle is called a ***multilaminar primary follicle***, and the follicular cells are more commonly referred to as ***granulosa cells***. The proliferative activity of the granulosa cells is due to the growth factors **activin**, **bone morphogenic protein-15**, and **growth differentiation factor-9** produced by the primary oocyte. As the multilaminar primary follicle continues to develop, its granulosa cells begin to express some FSH receptors on their cell membranes.

During this stage, an amorphous substance (the **zona pellucida**) appears, separating the oocyte from the surrounding follicular cells. The zonula pellucida is composed of four different glycoproteins—ZP_1, ZP_2, ZP_3, and ZP_4—secreted by the oocyte (see later section on fertilization for the functions of these glycoproteins). Filopodia of the follicular cells invade the zonula pellucida and come in contact with the oocyte plasmalemma, forming gap junctions with each other (composed of **connexin 43**), as well as gap junctions with the microvilli of the primary oocyte (using **connexin 37**). It is through these connexin

37–based gap junctions that follicular cells communicate with the primary oocyte throughout follicular development, and it is through connexin 43–based gap junctions that they communicate with each other.

Stromal cells begin to be organized around the multilaminar primary follicle, forming an inner **theca interna** composed mostly of a richly vascularized cellular layer and an outer **theca externa** composed mostly of fibrous connective tissue. This process of reorganization of the stromal cells, as well as the growth of the primary oocyte in diameter, are due to the secretion of **kit ligand** (**stem cell factor**) by the granulosa cells. As kit ligand is being released, both the primary oocyte and granulosa cells in the immediate vicinity of the primary oocyte express **kit ligand receptors**; the binding of kit ligand to its receptors effects changes in the primary oocyte and stromal cells. The cells composing the theca interna also possess **LH receptors** on their plasmalemma. These cells assume the ultrastructural characteristics of steroid-producing cells. Their cytoplasm accumulates numerous lipid droplets and has abundant smooth endoplasmic reticulum (SER), and the cristae of their mitochondria are tubular. These theca interna cells produce the male sex hormone **androstenedione**, which enters the granulosa cells, whose enzyme **aromatase** converts it into the estrogen **estradiol** (female sex hormone). The granulosa cells are separated from the theca interna by a thickened basal lamina.

Secondary (Antral) Follicles

Secondary follicles are similar to multilaminar primary follicles except for the presence of accumulations of liquor folliculi among the granulosa cells.

The multilaminar primary follicle continues to develop and increase in size, reaching up to 200 μm in diameter. A large spherical follicle is formed with numerous layers of granulosa cells around the primary oocyte (whose size from this point on remains constant, owing to the continued release of **oocyte maturation inhibitor** by the theca interna cells). Several intercellular spaces develop within the mass of granulosa cells and become filled with a fluid known as ***liquor folliculi***. Once the multilaminar primary follicle displays the presence of liquor folliculi, it is known as a ***secondary follicle*** (although some refer to this phase as a **tertiary follicle** or **antral follicle**). These follicular cells continue to express an increasing amount of FSH receptors on their cell membranes (Figs. 20.6 and 20.7).

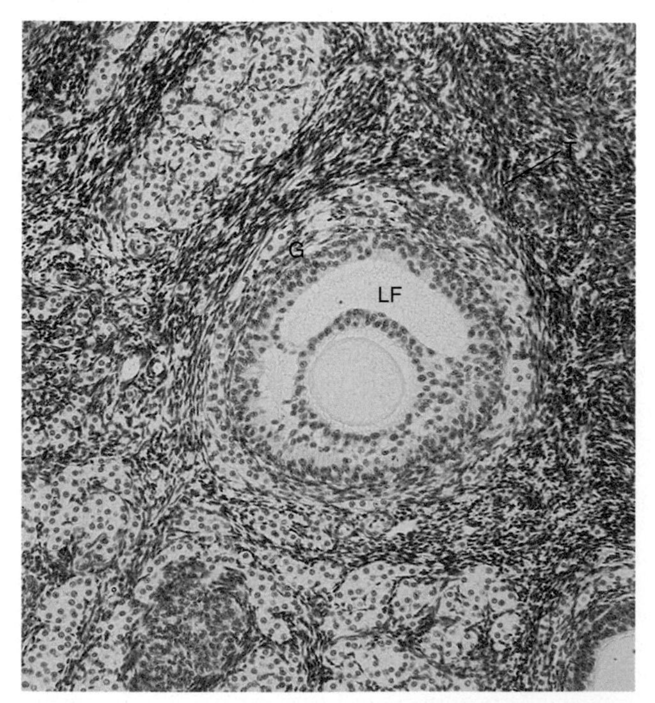

Fig. 20.6 Light micrograph of a secondary follicle. Observe the primary oocyte and the follicular fluid surrounded by membrana granulosa. Note also the presence of the basement membrane between the granulosa cells (G) and the theca interna (T). LF, Liquor folliculi. (×132)

Continued proliferation of the granulosa cells of the secondary follicle depends on **FSH** released by basophil cells of the anterior pituitary. Under the influence of FSH, the number of layers of the granulosa cells increases, as does the number of liquor folliculi–containing extracellular spaces. This fluid, an exudate of plasma, contains glycosaminoglycans, proteoglycans, and steroid-binding proteins produced by the granulosa cells. Moreover, it contains the hormones **progesterone**, **estradiol**, **inhibin**, **follistatin** (**folliculostatin**) and **activin**, which regulate the release of LH and FSH. In addition, FSH (along with estrogen) induces the granulosa cells to manufacture receptors for LH, which become incorporated into their plasmalemma.

Clinical Correlations

Granulosa cell tumors are of two types, juvenile and adult, mostly depending on the age of the affected individual. These are mostly benign, constituting approximately 5% of ovarian tumors. They resemble the membrana granulosa of ovarian follicles; occasionally, they display the presence of small, gland-like structures containing acidophilic extracellular fluids, known as Call-Exner bodies. The granulosa cells frequently manufacture estrogens, which, in prepubertal females, may cause early menarche. In adult females, the excess estrogen can cause hyperplasia, and even cancer, of the endometrium and proliferative breast disease. At times, these tumors may produce male sex hormones, causing masculinization of the patient. Granulosa tumors often produce elevated levels of serum inhibin. Recent investigations revealed the presence of mutations in the FOXL2 *genes that function in the maturation of adult granulosa cells. However, the same mutation is seldom present in the juvenile form of the tumor, indicating a lack of genetic similarity between the two forms of this condition.*

Graafian (Mature) Follicles

Graafian follicles, also known as mature follicles, may be as large as the entire ovary; it is these follicles that undergo ovulation.

Continued proliferation of the granulosa cells and continued formation of liquor folliculi result in the formation of a **graafian (mature) follicle** whose diameter reaches 2.5 cm by the time of ovulation. The graafian follicle may be observed as a transparent bulge on the surface of the ovary, nearly as large as the ovary itself.

As more fluid is produced, individual droplets of **liquor folliculi** coalesce to form a single fluid-filled chamber, the **antrum**. The granulosa cells become rearranged so that the primary oocyte is now surrounded by a small group of granulosa cells

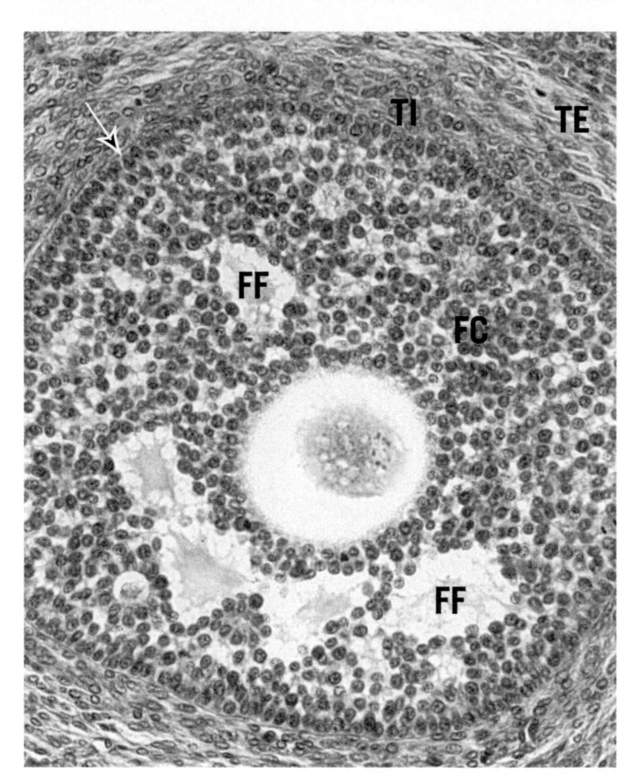

Fig. 20.7 This medium magnification of a secondary follicle displays the multiple layers of the granulosa cells (FC) and the accumulation of extracellular droplets of follicular fluid (FF). Note the presence of a basement membrane *(arrow)* between the granulosa cells and the tunica intima (TI) whose cellular nature differentiates it from the fibrous nature of the tunica externa (TE). (×270)

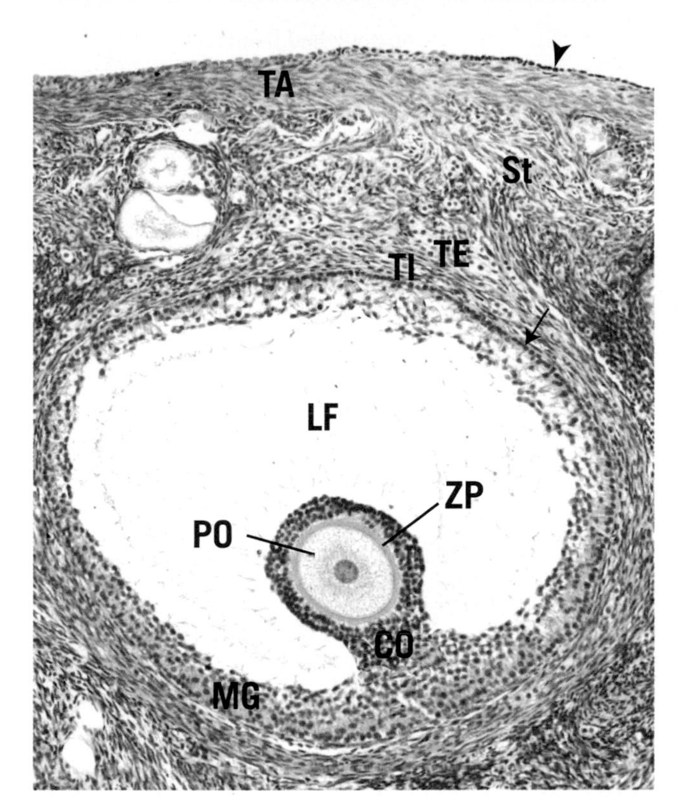

Fig. 20.8 This small, developing graafian follicle is in the cortex of the ovary, as is evidenced by its germinal epithelium *(arrowhead)* covering the tunica albuginea (TA). Observe the large liquor folliculi (LF)–filled antrum surrounded by the membrana granulosa. Note that the cumulus oophorus (CO) juts into the antrum and contains the primary oocyte (PO) that is separated from the corona radiata portion of the cumulus granulosa cells by the zona pellucida (ZP). The mural granulosa cells (MG) surround the antrum and are separated from the theca interna (TI) by a basement membrane *(arrow)*. The periphery of the theca externa (TE) blends into the cortical stroma (St). (×132)

TABLE 20.3 Types of Granulosa Cells

Cells	Characteristics of the Cells
Membrana granulosa cells	• About the basement membrane • Have LH and FSH receptors • Function in steroidogenesis due to the presence of the enzyme aromatase (estradiol, progesterone) • Produces the regulatory hormones activin, inhibin, folliculostatin, and insulin-like growth factor I. • Form the bulk of the corpus luteum • Line the antrum
Cumulus oophorus granulosa cells	• Are not active in steroidogenesis • Surround the oocyte • Contact the oocyte plasmalemmae by their filopodia • Do not possess many LH receptors • Divide to form cells of the membrana granulosa • Are ovulated along with the oocyte

FSH, Follicle-stimulating hormone; *LH*, luteinizing hormone.

that project out from the wall into the fluid-filled antrum. This structure is called the **cumulus oophorus**. The loosely arranged low cuboidal granulosa cells immediately adjacent to the zona pellucida move slightly away from the oocyte, but their filopodia remain within the zona pellucida, maintaining contact with the primary oocyte. This single layer of granulosa cells that immediately surrounds the primary oocyte is called the **corona radiata**. At this time, two different types of granulosa cells may be distinguished, **cumulus granulosa cells** and the **membrana (mural) granulosa cells** (Table 20.3), where the membrana granulosa cells form the wall of the antrum and the cumulus granulosa cells function in directing the development of the primary oocyte (Figs. 20.8 and 20.9).

Toward the end of this stage, stromal cells become enlarged, and the theca interna is invaded by capillaries that nourish them, as well as the avascular granulosa cells. Most of the developing follicles that reach this stage of development undergo atresia, but some of the granulosa cells associated with the atretic follicles do not degenerate. Instead, they form **interstitial glands**, which secrete small amounts of androgens until menopause is concluded. A few secondary follicles continue to develop into mature follicles.

The theca interna cells continue to display **LH receptors** and under the influence of LH synthesize **androstenedione** (**androgen**), the male sex hormone. The androgens cross the basement membrane and enter the cells of the membrana granulosa, where the androgens are transformed by the enzyme **aromatase** into **estradiol** (**estrogen**).

The theca externa is a dense, irregular, collagenous connective tissue that possesses smooth muscle cells and a rich vascular supply that provides oxygen and nutrients for the theca interna, granulosa cells, and primary oocyte.

The fluid pressure, owing to the continued formation of liquor folliculi, causes the cumulus oophorus—composed of the primary oocyte, corona radiata, and associated cumulus granulosa cells—to become detached from its base to float freely within the liquor folliculi (see Fig. 20.2B).

Ovulation

The process of releasing the secondary oocyte from the graafian follicle is known as ovulation.

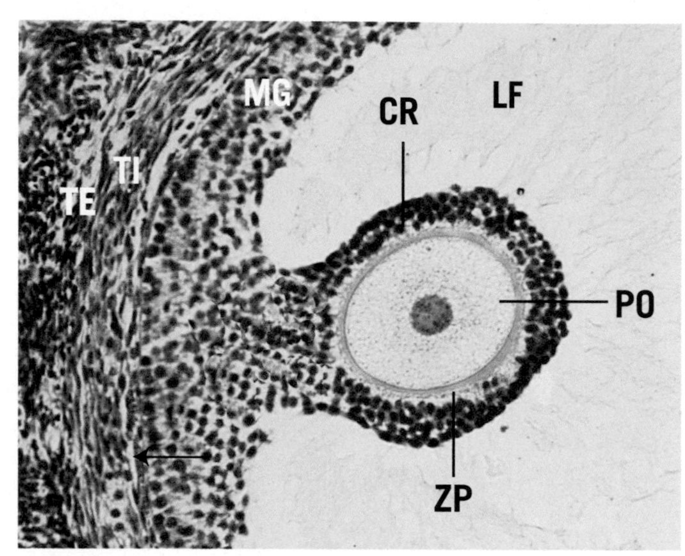

Fig. 20.9 This photomicrograph is a higher magnification of the cumulus oophorus region of Fig. 20.8. Observe that the primary oocyte (PO) is surrounded by the zona pellucida (ZP) and that the innermost layer of the cumulus granulosa cells, known as the corona radiata (CR) and whose filopodia penetrate the zona pellucida. Note that the membrana granulosa (MG) is separated from the theca interna (TI) by a well-developed basement membrane *(arrow)*. The outermost region of the theca externa (TE) blends in with the connective tissue stroma of the ovarian cortex. (×270)

By the 14th day of the menstrual cycle, estrogen produced mostly by the developing graafian follicle, but also by the remaining secondary follicles, causes elevation of blood estrogen to levels high enough to have the following effects:

- Negative feedback inhibition shuts off FSH release by the anterior pituitary.
- A sudden surge of LH is released by basophils of the anterior pituitary.

The surge in LH levels results in increased blood flow to the ovaries, and capillaries within the theca externa begin leaking plasma, resulting in edema. Concomitant with edema formation, histamine, prostaglandins, and collagenase are released in the vicinity of the graafian follicle. Additionally, plasminogen activator levels, the enzyme that catalyzes the conversion of plasminogen to plasmin, increase in the follicle, and the newly formed plasmin facilitates the proteolysis of the membrana granulosa, permitting ovulation to occur (Fig. 20.10 and Table 20.4).

In addition, the LH surge is responsible for the following events:

1. A local factor, maturation-promoting factor, is released by the primary oocyte.
2. Under the influence of **maturation-promoting factor**, composed of **cyclin B** and **cyclin-dependent kinase**, the primary oocyte of the graafian follicle resumes and completes its first meiotic division, resulting in the formation of two daughter cells, the **secondary oocyte** and the **first polar body.** Because of the uneven distribution of the cytoplasm, the first polar body is composed of a nucleus surrounded by only a narrow rim of cytoplasm; it will degenerate and die within a few days.
3. The newly formed secondary oocyte enters the **second meiotic division** but is arrested in **metaphase** and remains at that stage until fertilization.

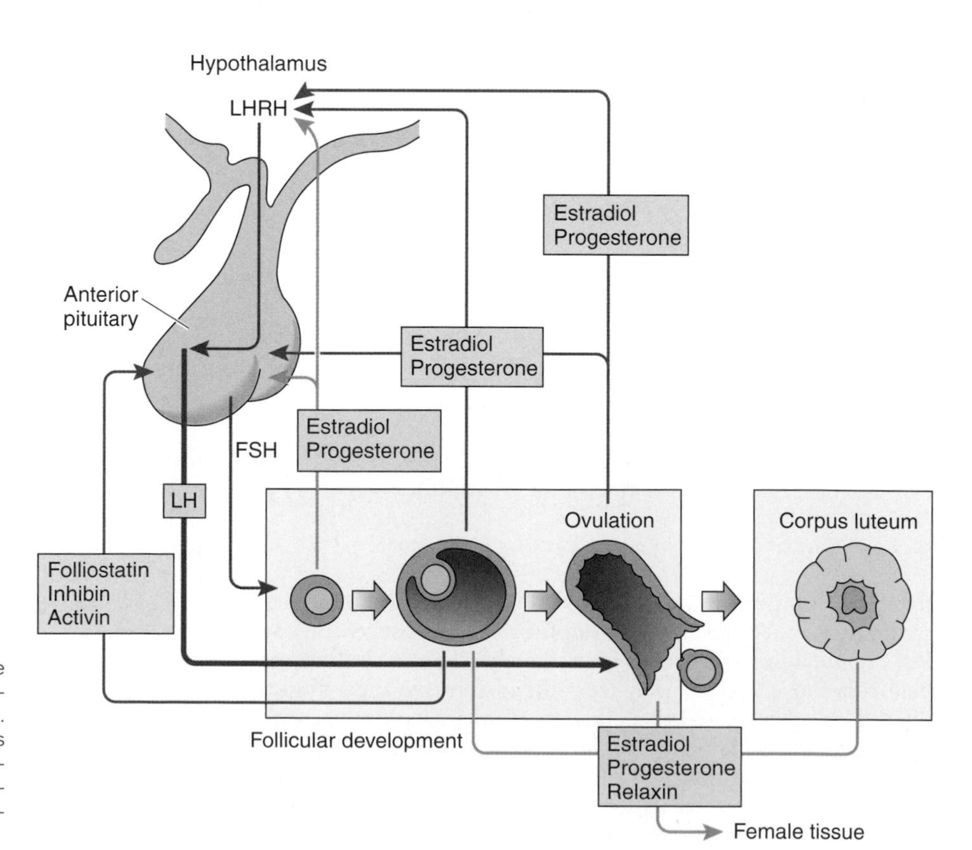

Fig. 20.10 Schematic diagram illustrating the hormonal interactions between the hypothalamo-pituitary axis and the female reproductive system. Note that folliostatin and inhibin both suppress follicle-stimulating hormone (FSH) release, whereas activin facilitates the release of FSH. LHRH, Luteinizing hormone-releasing hormone; LH, luteinizing hormone.

TABLE 20.4 Major Hormones Involved in the Female Reproductive System

Hormone	Source	Function
Gonadotropin-releasing hormone (LHRH)	Hypothalamus	Stimulates release of FSH and LH from anterior pituitary gland
Prolactin-inhibiting factor	Hypothalamus	Inhibits release of prolactin by acidophils of anterior pituitary gland
Follicle-stimulating hormone (FSH)	Basophils of anterior pituitary gland	Stimulates secretion of estrogen and development of ovarian follicles (from secondary follicle onward)
Luteinizing hormone (LH)	Basophils of anterior pituitary gland	Stimulates formation of estrogen and progesterone; promotes ovulation and formation of corpus luteum
Estradiol	Granulosa cells of ovary; granulosa-lutein cells of corpus luteum; and the placenta	Inhibits release of FSH and LHRH; triggers surge of LH; causes proliferation and hypertrophy of myometrium of uterus; causes development of female sexual characteristics, including breasts and body fat; stimulates milk production before and at parturition
Progesterone	Granulosa cells of the ovary; theca-lutein and granulosa-lutein cells of the corpus luteum; placenta	Inhibits the release of LHRH from the hypothalamus and LH from the basophils of the anterior pituitary; causes the development of the uterine endometrium and regulates the viscosity of the mucus produced by the glands of the uterine cervix; causes the development of female sexual characteristics, including breasts; suppresses T cell–mediated rejection of the fetus
Inhibin	Granulosa cells of the ovary; granulosa-lutein cells of the corpus luteum	Inhibits FSH secretion by basophils of the anterior pituitary
Activin	Oocyte	Promotes granulosa cell proliferation
Human chorionic gonadotropin (hCG)	Placenta	Assists in the maintenance of the corpus luteum; promotes the release of progesterone
Human placental lactogen (human chorionic somatomammotropin)	Placenta	Promotes mammary gland development during pregnancy; promotes lactogenesis
Chorionic thyrotropin	Placenta	Stimulates thyroid hormone release
Insulin-like growth factors I and II	Placenta	Stimulates cytotrophoblast growth and development
Endothelial growth factor	Placenta	Supports trophoblast development and function
Fibroblast growth factor	Placenta	Induces cytotrophoblast proliferation
Colony-stimulating factor	Placenta	Induces cytotrophoblast proliferation
Tumor necrosis factor	Placenta	Inhibits cytotrophoblast proliferation
Leptin	Placenta	Assists in transplacental transport of nutrients; maintains maternal nutrient status
Relaxin	Placenta	Facilitates parturition by softening the fibrocartilage of the pubic symphysis; softens the cervix and facilitates its dilation in preparation for parturition
Oxytocin	Hypothalamus via the posterior pituitary	Stimulates smooth muscle contraction of the uterus during orgasm and during parturition; stimulates contraction of myoepithelial cells of the mammary gland, assisting in milk ejection

4. The presence and continued formation of proteoglycans and hyaluronic acid by the granulosa cells attract water, causing an even greater increase not only in the size of the graafian follicle but also in the loosening of the membrana granulosa.
5. Just before ovulation, the surface of the ovary, where the graafian follicle is pressing against the tunica albuginea, loses its blood supply.
6. This thinned, avascular region becomes blanched and is known as the ***stigma.*** The connective tissue at the stigma degenerates, as does the wall of the graafian follicle in contact with the stigma, forming an opening between the peritoneal cavity and the antrum of the graafian follicle.
7. Through this opening, the secondary oocyte and its attendant follicular cells and some of the liquor folliculi are gently released from the ovary, resulting in **ovulation.** Although the average menstrual cycle is 28 days long, some cycles are longer, and others are shorter. However, ovulation is always on the 14th day before the beginning of the next menstruation.
8. The remnants of the graafian follicle are converted into the corpus hemorrhagicum and then the corpus luteum.

It would appear from the previous description that the entire process of the recruitment of the primordial follicle into a graafian follicle and ovulation of the secondary oocyte occurs in approximately 14 days; however, that is not so. Instead, the time period required is much greater, for it takes almost 10 months for the primordial follicle to become a secondary follicle and a subsequent 2 months for ovulation to occur. Not all follicles are in the same stage of development; therefore, usually one dominant follicle will be ready to release its secondary oocyte every 28 days or so. All of the oocyte and granulosa cells of follicles that have reached the secondary follicle stage (but are not going to ovulate) undergo atresia and degenerate, but their theca cells do not undergo apoptosis; instead, they dedifferentiate into stromal cells. Usually, only one of the follicles that reaches the graafian follicle stage will ovulate, which is known as the ***dominant follicle***. All of the follicles that have reached the graafian follicle stage are FSH dependent except for the dominant follicle that begins to produce large quantities of the hormone **inhibin** that shuts off FSH release by the pituitary gland (but does not act on GnRH release by the hypothalamus). Once FSH is no longer produced, those follicles that are FSH dependent undergo atresia. However, the primordial, unilaminar primary, multilaminar primary follicles, as well as the dominant follicle do not undergo atresia because they are FSH independent. Therefore, the dominant follicle is able to progress to ovulation.

The distal, fimbriated end of the oviduct, which presses against the ovary, captures the ovulated secondary oocyte and its attendant follicular cells. They enter the **infundibulum** of the **oviduct** and begin their journey into the ampulla, where the secondary oocyte may be fertilized (see Fig. 20.1). If fertilization does not occur within approximately 24 hours, the secondary oocyte degenerates and its remnants become phagocytosed. The process of fertilization is discussed later in the chapter.

Corpus Luteum

The corpus luteum, formed from the remnants of the graafian follicle, is a temporary endocrine gland that manufactures and releases hormones that support the uterine endometrium.

After the secondary oocyte and its associated follicular cells are ovulated, the remainder of the graafian follicle collapses and becomes folded. Some of the ruptured blood vessels leak blood into the follicular cavity, forming a central clot, resulting in a structure known as the ***corpus hemorrhagicum***. As the clot is removed by phagocytes, continued high levels of **LH**, in conjunction with the hormones estradiol, insulin-like growth factors I and II, human chorionic gonadotrophin, and prolactin convert the corpus hemorrhagicum into a temporary structure known as the ***corpus luteum***, which functions as a *temporary endocrine gland* (Figs. 20.11 and 20.12). This highly vascularized structure is composed of granulosa-lutein cells (modified granulosa cells) and theca-lutein cells (modified theca interna cells). The basement membrane between the former theca interna and membrana granulosa disintegrates and the blood vessels of the theca interna, in response to the **angiogenic factors**, **fibroblast growth factor**, and **vascular endothelial growth factor**, invade the membrane granulosa. The maintenance of the corpus luteum is **LH dependent**.

Granulosa Lutein Cells

Granulosa cells of the graafian follicle differentiate into granulosa-lutein cells that manufacture progesterone and convert androgen to estrogen.

The granulosa cells remaining in the central region of the follicle become modified into large, pale-staining cells (30–50 μm in diameter) called **granulosa lutein cells**, which account for about 80% of the parenchymal cell population of the corpus luteum. These cells display many long microvilli and all of the organelles necessary for steroid production, including abundant SER and RER, abundant mitochondria, several well-developed Golgi complexes, and some lipid droplets scattered throughout the cytoplasm (Figs. 20.11–20.13). Granulosa lutein cells produce **progesterone** and convert androgens produced by the theca lutein cells into **estrogens**.

- Progesterone production is dependent on the presence of **low-density lipoprotein** (**LDL**) **cholesterol receptors** on the basal plasmalemmae of these cells, as well as on the presence of **steroidogenic acute regulatory (StAR) proteins.** LDL cholesterol receptors transfer LDL cholesterol into the granulosa-lutein cells and StAR proteins transfer the LDL cholesterol into the mitochondria of these cells. Within the mitochondria, the LDL cholesterol is transformed into **pregnenolone**, which, in the cytoplasm, is converted into **progesterone.**
- The conversion of androgens—synthesized in the theca-lutein cells and transferred into the granulosa-lutein cells—into estrogens is dependent on the enzyme **aromatase.**

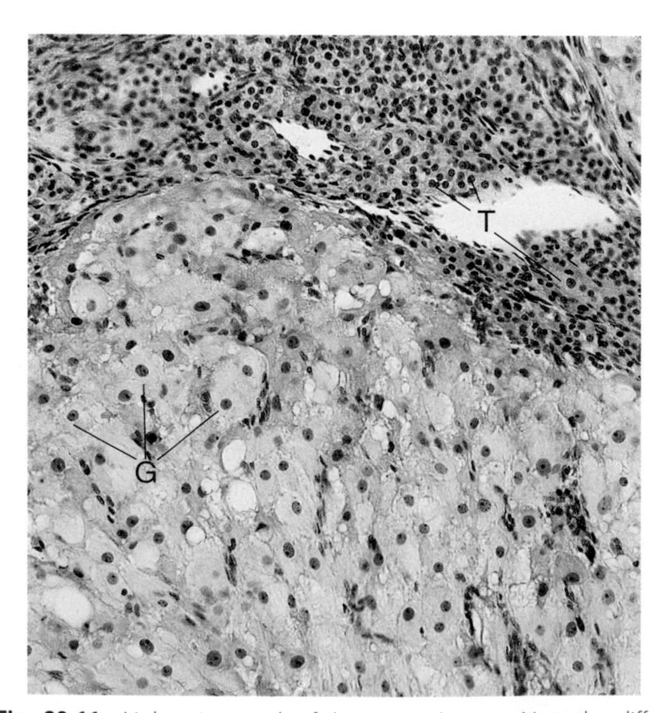

Fig. 20.11 Light micrograph of the corpus luteum. Note the difference between the large granulosa-lutein (G) and small theca-lutein (T) cells. (×132)

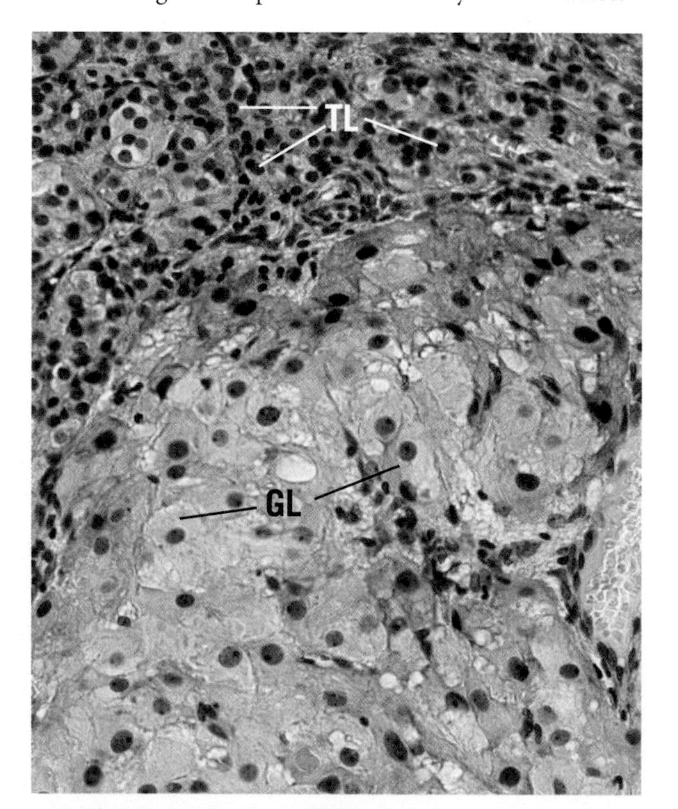

Fig. 20.12 This medium-magnification photomicrograph of the corpus luteum displays the large, lightly staining granulosa-lutein cells (GL) and the smaller, darker-staining theca lutein cells (TL). (×270)

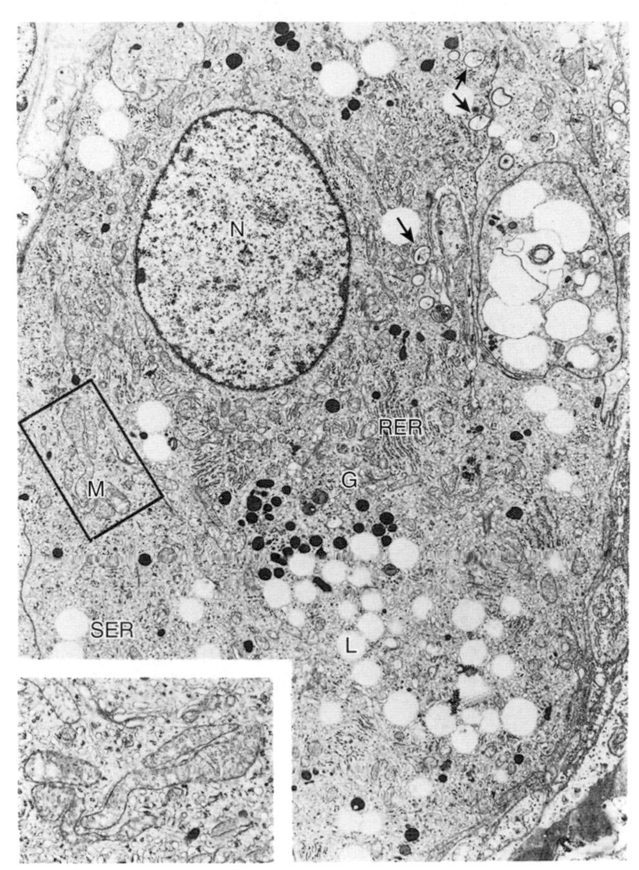

Fig. 20.13 Electron micrograph of a rhesus monkey granulosa lutein cell with its large acentric nucleus and numerous organelles. G, Golgi apparatus; L, lipid droplet; M, mitochondria (displayed at a higher magnification in *inset, lower left*); N, nucleus; RER, rough endoplasmic reticulum; SER, smooth endoplasmic reticulum (×6800). (From Booher C, Enders AC, Hendrick X, Hess DL. Structural characteristics of the corpus luteum during implantation in the rhesus monkey [*Macaca mulatta*]. *Am J Anat.* 1981;160:1736. Reprinted with permission from Wiley-Liss, Inc., a subsidiary of John Wiley & Sons, Inc.)

Theca Lutein Cells

Theca lutein cells, derived from the cells of the theca interna, secrete progesterone, androgens, and some estrogens.

The **theca interna cells** become modified into hormone-secreting cells known as **theca lutein cells**, dark-staining small cells (approximately 15 µm in diameter) that are located at the periphery of the corpus luteum and account for about 20% of the corpus luteum's parenchymal cell population. They specialize in the production of **androgens**, as well as some **progesterone** and estrogens.

Progesterone and estrogens secreted by granulosa lutein and theca lutein cells continue to inhibit the secretion of LH and FSH, respectively. The absence of FSH continues to prevent the development of new follicles, thus preventing a second ovulation. If pregnancy does not occur, the absence of LH leads to degeneration of the corpus luteum, forming the **corpus luteum of menstruation**. If pregnancy does occur, **human chorionic gonadotropin** (**hCG**), secreted by the placenta, maintains the corpus luteum for about 3 months. Now called the **corpus luteum of pregnancy**, it grows to a diameter of 5 cm and continues to secrete hormones necessary for the maintenance of pregnancy. Although the placenta becomes the main site of production of the various hormones involved in maintaining pregnancy 2 to 3 months after its formation, the corpus luteum of pregnancy continues to manufacture these hormones for several months.

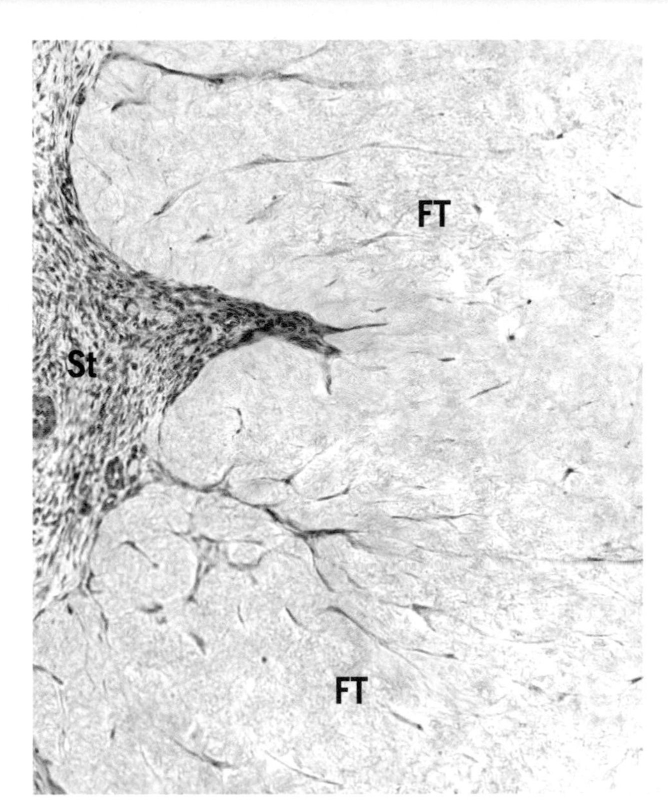

Fig. 20.14 This low-magnification photomicrograph displays the highly cellular stroma (St) of the ovary and the lack of cellularity of the fibrous tissue (FT) component of the corpus albicans. (×132)

Corpus Albicans

As the corpus luteum degenerates and is being phagocytosed by macrophages, fibroblasts enter, manufacture type I collagen, and form a fibrous structure known as the corpus albicans.

The corpus luteum of menstruation (or of pregnancy) is invaded by fibroblasts, becomes fibrotic, recruits **T cells**, and ceases to function. Its remnants undergo autolysis, a process known as **luteolysis**, because the T cells release the cytokines **interferon-γ** that recruits macrophages. The newly recruited macrophages release **tumor necrosis factor α** (**TNF-α**), which induces granulosa lutein and theca lutein cells to undergo apoptosis, and the macrophages phagocytose the remnants of the apoptotic cells. The fibrous connective tissue that forms in the place of the corpus luteum is known as the **corpus albicans** (Fig. 20.14) and remains for some time before being reabsorbed. The remnants of the corpus albicans persist as a scar on the surface of the ovary.

Atretic Follicles

Follicles that undergo degeneration are known as atretic follicles.

The ovaries contain many follicles in various stages of development. Many of the follicles degenerate before reaching the mature stage, but multiple graafian follicles develop during each menstrual cycle. Nevertheless, once a dominant follicle forms, the remaining FSH-dependent follicles undergo atresia. The resulting **atretic follicles** are eventually phagocytosed by macrophages. Thus, normally, only the single dominant follicle ovulates during each menstrual cycle. Occasionally, two separate follicles develop to maturity and ovulate, leading to fraternal twins if both oocytes are fertilized, although only about 2% of all follicles reach the mature stage and are primed to undergo ovulation. Of all follicles present in the ovaries at menarche, just 0.1% to 0.2% develop to maturity and undergo ovulation.

OVARIAN MEDULLA

The ovarian medulla is a richly vascularized fibroelastic connective tissue housing connective tissue cells, interstitial cells, and hilar cells.

The central region of the ovary, the **medulla**, is composed of fibroblasts loosely embedded in a collagen-rich meshwork containing elastic fibers (see Fig. 20.2A). The medulla also contains large blood vessels, lymph vessels, and nerve fibers. The premenstrual human ovarian medulla has a few clusters of epithelioid **interstitial cells** that secrete estrogens. In mammals having large litters, the ovaries contain many clusters of these interstitial cells, which collectively are called the **interstitial gland**. In humans, most of these interstitial cells involute during the first menstrual cycle and have little, if any, function.

Hilar cells constitute another group of epithelioid cells in the ovarian medulla. These cells have a similar configuration of organelles and contain the same substances in their cytoplasm as Leydig cells of the testes. These cells secrete androgens.

OVIDUCTS (FALLOPIAN TUBES)

The oviducts act as a conduit for spermatozoa to reach the secondary oocyte and to convey the fertilized egg to the uterus.

The **oviducts** (**fallopian tubes**) are paired, muscular-walled tubular structures approximately 12 cm long, each with an open free end and an open attached end (see Fig. 20.1). Each oviduct becomes continuous with the wall of the uterus at its attached end, where it traverses the uterine wall to open into its lumen. The free end of the oviduct opens into the peritoneal cavity close to the ovaries.

Each oviduct is said to have four anatomical regions:

- Beginning at the free end is the **infundibulum**, whose open end is fringed with projections called **fimbriae** that help capture the ovulated secondary oocyte and its adherent follicular cells.
- The longest region is the expanded **ampulla**, where fertilization usually takes place.
- The **isthmus** is the narrowed portion between the ampulla and the uterus.
- The attached end is known as the **intramural region** because it pierces and passes through the uterine wall to open into the lumen of the uterus.

The wall of each oviduct is composed of three layers (Fig. 20.15), the mucosa, muscularis, and serosa.

The **mucosa** is characterized by many longitudinal folds that are present in all four regions of the oviduct but are most pronounced in the ampulla, where they branch. In the other regions, the mucosal folds are reduced to low elevations (Figs. 20.16 and 20.17). The **simple columnar epithelium** that lines the lumen is tallest in the infundibulum and shortens as the oviduct approaches the uterus. Simple columnar epithelium is composed of two types of cells: nonciliated peg cells and ciliated columnar cells.

Peg cells have no cilia. They have a secretory function, providing a nutritive and protective environment for maintaining spermatozoa on their migration route to reach the secondary oocyte. Products within the secretions of the peg cells facilitate

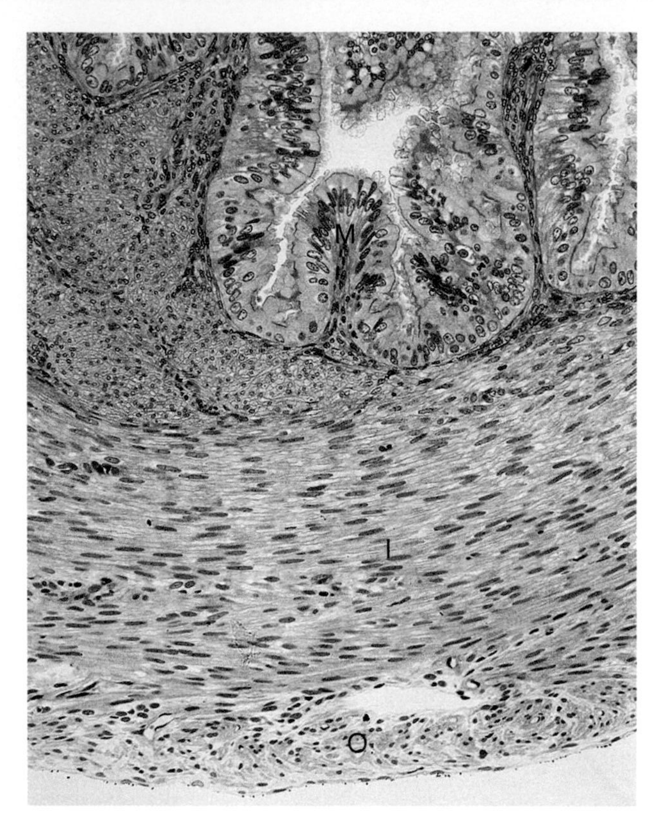

Fig. 20.15 Light micrograph of the oviduct in cross-section. Observe the outer longitudinal (O) and inner circular (I) muscle layers and the mucosa (M). Note that the mucosa is thrown into folds that reduce the size of the lumen (×132).

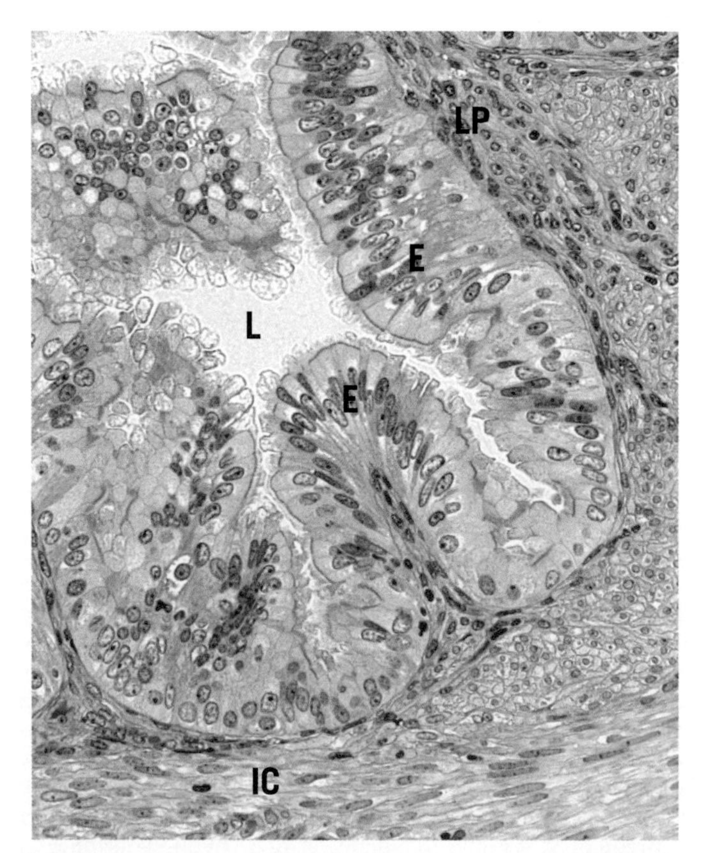

Fig. 20.16 This medium-magnification photomicrograph displays that the lining of the lumen (L) is composed of a simple columnar epithelium (E), which is surrounded by a highly cellular and richly vascularized lamina propria (LP). The inner circular (IC) smooth muscle layer is clearly evident. (×270)

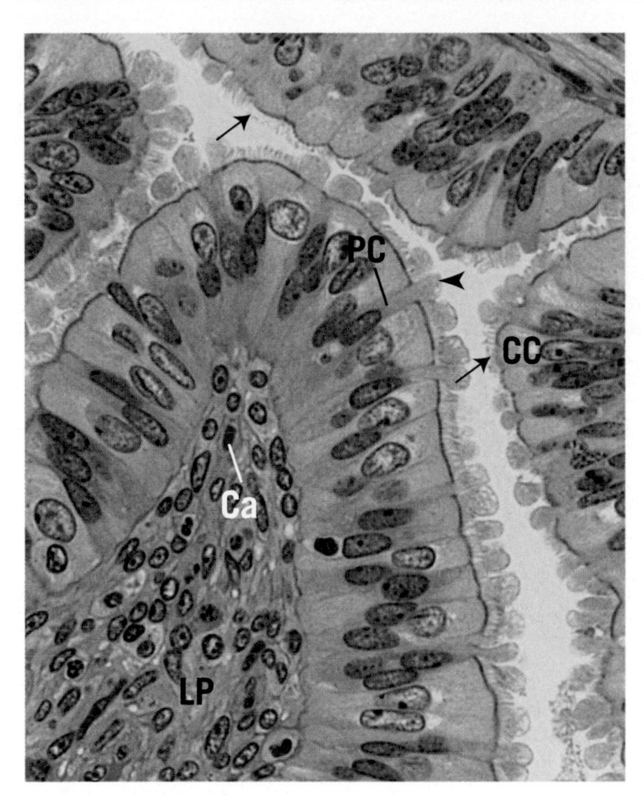

Fig. 20.17 A high magnification of the epithelium and lamina propria (LP) presents the two types of cells constituting the epithelium of the oviduct: the ciliated cells (CC), whose cilia are indicated by *arrows*, and the peg cells (PC) that have no cilia, but present cytoplasmic extensions that bulge into the lumen *(arrowhead)*. Note that the lamina propria is highly cellular and possesses a rich vascular supply (Ca). (×540)

capacitation of spermatozoa, a process whereby spermatozoa become fully mature and capable of fertilizing the ovum. It is not known whether human spermatozoa require capacitation because they are capable of in vitro fertilization of the ovum without being exposed to the female reproductive tract. If there is such a requirement, the sojourn in the female reproductive tract necessitates only a minimal amount of time. Secretory products also provide nutrition and protection to the ovum; if the ovum is fertilized, the same secretions provide nutrients to the embryo during the initial phases of its development. The secretions of peg cells coupled with the movement of the fluid toward the uterus inhibit microorganisms from the uterus moving to the oviduct and into the peritoneal cavity. The number of peg cells is progesterone dependent in that they increase in number if progesterone is present.

The **cilia** of **ciliated cells** beat in unison toward the uterus. As a result, the fertilized ovum, spermatozoa, and viscous liquid produced by the peg cells are all propelled toward the uterus (Fig. 20.18). The number of ciliated cells is also estrogen dependent in that they, too, increase in number if estrogen is present.

The **lamina propria** of the oviduct mucosa is unremarkable because it is composed of loose connective tissue containing fibroblasts, mast cells, lymphoid cells, collagen, and reticular fibers. The **muscularis** consists of poorly defined inner circular and outer longitudinal layers of smooth muscle. Loose connective tissue also fills spaces between the bundles of muscle. A simple squamous epithelium provides the **serosal covering** of the oviduct. The loose connective tissue between the serosa and the muscularis contains many blood vessels and autonomic nerve fibers.

Because the oviducts are so richly vascularized with mostly large veins, contractions of the muscularis during ovulation constrict the engorged veins. This constriction causes distention of the entire oviduct and brings the fimbriae into contact with the ovary, aiding the capture of the released secondary oocyte. Continued rhythmic contractions of the layers of the muscularis, coupled with the beating of the cilia within, help propel the captured oocyte to the uterus.

UTERUS

The uterus is a muscular organ consisting of a fundus, body, and cervix.

The uterus, a single, thick, pear-shaped structure located in the midline of the pelvis, receives at its broad, closed end the terminals of the paired oviducts. The uterus is a robust muscular organ about 7 cm long, 4 cm wide, and 2.5 cm thick. The lumen of the nongravid uterus is only about 10 mL in volume; by the time of parturition, it has increased to more than 5 L. The uterus is divided into three regions (see Fig. 20.1): the **body**, which is the broad portion into which the oviducts open; the **fundus**, the rounded base of the uterus, which is located superior to the entry ports of the oviducts; and the **cervix**, which is the narrow, circular portion of the uterus that protrudes and opens into the vagina.

Body and Fundus

The uterine wall of the body and the fundus is composed of an **endometrium**, **myometrium**, and either an **adventitia** or **serosa**.

Endometrium

The endometrium is the mucosal lining of the uterus, consisting of two layers: the superficial functionalis and the deeper located basalis.

The endometrium, or mucosal lining of the uterus, is composed of a simple columnar epithelium consisting of **nonciliated secretory columnar cells** and **ciliated cells**, and a lamina propria that houses simple branched **tubular glands** extending as far as the myometrium (Fig. 20.19). Although the secretory cells of the glands resemble cells of the surface epithelium, they possess no cilia. The dense, irregular, collagenous connective tissue of the **lamina propria** is highly cellular and contains star-shaped cells, macrophages, leukocytes, and an abundance of reticular fibers.

The endometrium consists of two layers (see Fig. 20.19):

- **Functionalis.** A thick, superficial layer whose thickness ranges between 1 and 7 mm depending on the stage of the menstrual cycle. It is this layer that is sloughed at menstruation.
- **Basalis.** A much thinner, deep layer, approximately 1 mm in thickness, which is not sloughed during menstruation. The glands and connective tissue elements of the basalis proliferate and thereby regenerate the functionalis during each menstrual cycle.

The **functionalis** is vascularized by numerous coiled **helical arteries**, which originate from the **arcuate arteries** of the stratum vasculare, located in the middle layer of the myometrium. The coiled arteries give rise to a rich capillary network that supplies the glands and connective tissue of the functionalis. It is the helical arteries that permit the development of the **hemochorioendothelial type of placenta**, as well as the process of

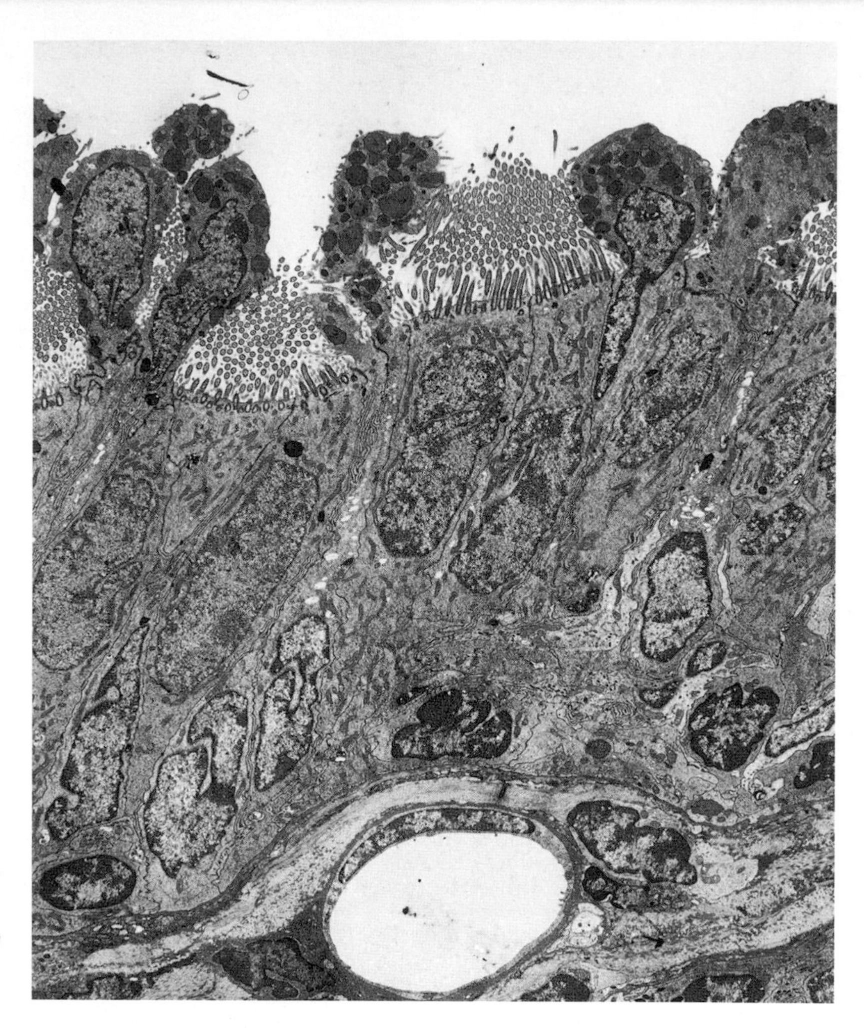

Fig. 20.18 Electron micrograph of the oviduct epithelium. Note the bulbous apices of the peg cells as well as the cilia of the ciliated cells (×40,000). (From Hollis DE, Frith PA, Vaughan JD, et al. Ultrastructural changes in the oviductal epithelium of Merino ewes during the estrous cycle. *Am J Anat.* 1984;171:441–456. Reprinted with permission from Wiley-Liss, Inc., a subsidiary of John Wiley & Sons, Inc.)

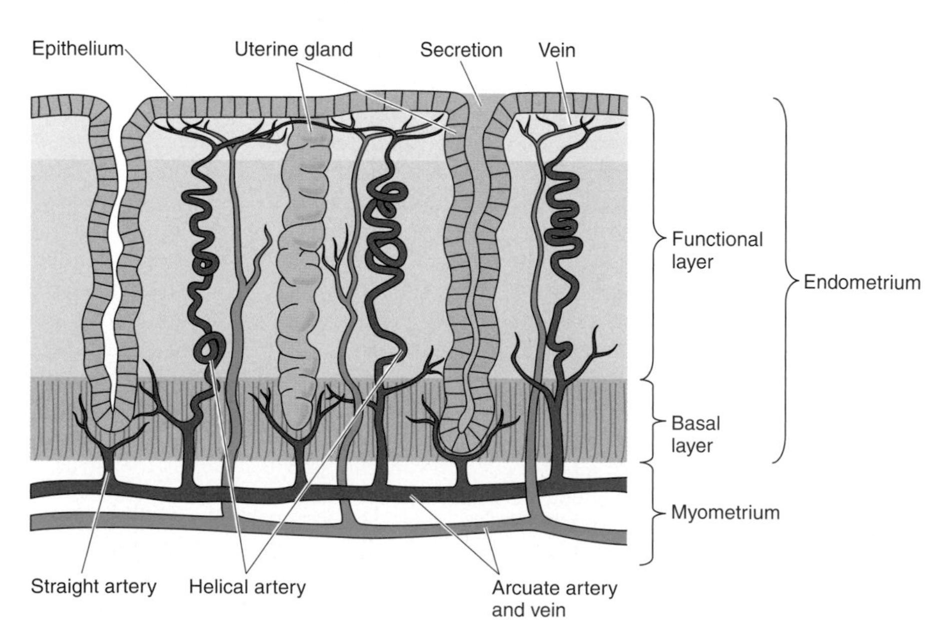

Fig. 20.19 Diagram of the uterine endometrium characterized by the basal and functional layers. Observe that the basal layer is supplied by the straight arteries, whereas the functionalis layer is served by the coiled vessels known as the *helical arteries.*

menstruation, the hormone-dependent casting off of the functional layer of the endometrium. Another set of arteries, the **straight arteries**, also originate from the arcuate arteries but are much shorter and supply only the basalis; they are responsible for maintaining the basalis during the process of menstruation.

Myometrium

The myometrium is composed of inner longitudinal, middle circular, and outer longitudinal layers of smooth muscle.

The thick muscular wall of the uterus, the **myometrium**, is composed of *three layers* of smooth muscle. **Longitudinal muscle** makes up the *inner* and *outer layers*, whereas the richly *vascularized middle layer* contains mostly **circularly** arranged smooth muscle bundles. Because this houses the **arcuate arteries**, it is called the **stratum vasculare**. As the uterus narrows toward the cervix, the smooth muscle layers are replaced mostly by fibrous connective tissue. At the cervix, the former smooth muscle layer is composed of dense, irregular, collagenous connective tissue containing elastic fibers and only a small number of scattered smooth muscle cells.

The size and number of the myometrial muscle cells are related to estrogen levels. The muscle cells are largest and most numerous during pregnancy, when estrogen levels are very high. They are smallest after the conclusion of menstruation, when estrogen levels are low. When estrogen is absent, the myometrial muscle atrophies, with some cells succumbing to **apoptosis**. Although most of the increase in uterine size during pregnancy is related to **hypertrophy** of the smooth muscle cells, the number of smooth muscle cells also increases, suggesting that **hyperplasia** also occurs. However, it is as yet unclear whether the increase in cell number results only from division of smooth muscle cells or also from differentiation of undifferentiated cells into smooth muscle fibers.

Clinical Correlations

Uterine smooth muscle cells undergo contraction due to various causes. Moderate contraction may occur during sexual stimulation. During menstruation, in some women, the smooth muscle cells of the uterus may constrict powerfully enough to cause considerable pain. Contractions of the pregnant uterus during delivery are very painful and powerful enough to expel the fetus, and later the placenta, from the uterus. Contractions during parturition are due to the actions of the paracrine hormone ***prostaglandin****, manufactured and released by the myometrium and fetal membranes, and by the hormone* ***oxytocin****, released from the pars nervosa of the pituitary gland. After delivery, oxytocin continues to stimulate uterine contractions, which inhibit excessive blood loss from the detachment site of the placenta.*

Uterine Serosa or Adventitia

Much of the anterior portion of the uterus, as it lies against the urinary bladder, is covered by **adventitia**, making that area **retroperitoneal**. The fundus and posterior portion of the body are covered by a **serosa**; therefore, this area is **intraperitoneal**.

Clinical Correlations

The presence of endometrial tissue in the pelvis or peritoneal cavity is known as ***endometriosis****. This often painful condition may cause dysmenorrhea and even infertility. It has been recently reported that women with endometriosis who are infertile had a decreased level of the enzyme* ***histone deacetylase 3*** *(HDAC3) in their uterine lining; in fact, as many as half of infertile women have been shown to have endometriosis. Mice engineered with low HDAC3 levels in their uterine epithelium were sterile; apparently, the embryos of these HDAC3-deficient mice were unable to adhere to the uterine lining and, therefore, could not implant into the uterine wall. Additionally, these mice had a much greater amount of fibrosis in their uterus than mice with normal levels of HDAC3.*

The origin of endometrial tissue outside the uterus is not known, but three theories have been suggested. The ***regurgitation theory*** *proposes that menstrual flow escapes from the uterus via the fallopian tubes to enter the peritoneal cavity and some of the endometrial cells become established there. The* ***metaplastic theory*** *supposes that the epithelial cells of the peritoneum differentiate into endometrial cells and launch a population of endometrial cells. The* ***vascular (lymphatic) dissemination theory*** *proposes that endometrial cells enter vascular (or lymphatic) channels during menstruation and are distributed by the blood (or lymph) vascular system and initiate the formation of an endometrial cell population. The risk of developing endometriosis increases with early menarche (10 years of age or younger), having close relatives with endometriosis, having been exposed to diethylstilbestrol while in utero, and having been born underweight.*

These extrauterine endometrial tissues also undergo cyclic changes. Hemorrhaging of this tissue may cause adhesions and extreme pain. If endometriosis is not corrected, the pelvic viscera may be embroiled in a fibrotic mass, possibly resulting in sterility.

Cervix

The terminal end of the uterus (the cervix) extends into the vagina.

The **cervix** is the terminal end of the uterus that protrudes into the vagina (see Fig. 20.1). Its wall consists mostly of dense, collagenous connective tissue containing many elastic fibers and only a few smooth muscle fibers. The lumen of the cervix is lined by a **mucus-secreting simple columnar epithelium**. However, its external surface, where the cervix protrudes into the vagina, is covered by a **stratified squamous nonkeratinized epithelium** similar to that of the vagina. Cervical mucosa contains branched **cervical glands**. Although the cervical mucosa changes during the menstrual cycle, it does not slough during menstruation.

At the midpoint in the menstrual cycle, around the time of ovulation, the cervical glands secrete a serous fluid that facilitates entry of the spermatozoa into the uterus. At other times, especially during pregnancy, the secretions of the cervical glands become more viscous, forming a plug of thickened mucus in the orifice of the cervix, thwarting the entry of sperm and microorganisms into the uterus. The hormone **progesterone** regulates the changes in the viscosity of the cervical gland secretions.

At the time of parturition, another luteal hormone, **relaxin**, induces lysis of collagen in the cervical walls. This results in a softening of the cervix, facilitating cervical dilation, and makes it easier for the fetus to enter the birth canal.

Clinical Correlations

*The **Papanicolaou (Pap smear) technique** is a diagnostic tool for detecting cervical cancer. It is performed by aspirating cervical fluid from the vagina or taking scrapings directly from the cervix. The tissue or fluid is prepared and stained on a microscope slide and then examined for variations in the cell populations to detect anaplasia, dysplasia, and carcinoma. Recently, the United States Preventive Services Task Force suggested that instead of Pap smear testing, women between 30 and 65 years old should be tested for **human papilloma virus (HPV)** every 5 years because the HPV test is a better indicator of cervical carcinoma. It has been reported that women receiving negative HPV results are significantly less likely to be diagnosed with cervical cancer than women with negative Pap smears.*

***Cervical carcinoma** is one of the most common cancers in women, although it is rare in virgins and in nulliparous women (women who have not given birth). The incidence increases in women with multiple sex partners and herpes infections. It develops from the stratified squamous nonkeratinized epithelium of the cervix, where it is called **carcinoma in situ**. If detected by Pap smear in this stage, it can usually be successfully treated with surgery. If not detected early, however, it may invade other areas and metastasize, changing to **invasive carcinoma**, which carries a poor prognosis.*

MENSTRUAL CYCLE

The menstrual cycle is divided into the menstrual, proliferative (follicular), and secretory (luteal) phases.

Ideally, the average menstrual cycle is 28 days. Although the successive events constituting the cycle occur continuously, they can be described in three phases: **menstrual phase**, **proliferative (follicular) phase**, and **secretory (luteal) phase** (Fig. 20.20). These histologically recognizable phases depend on the levels of estradiol and progesterone.

Menstrual Phase (Day 1 to Day 3 or 4)

The menstrual phase is characterized by the desquamation of the functionalis layer of the endometrium.

Menstruation, which begins on the day that bleeding from the uterus starts, occurs if fertilization does not take place and serum **FSH** and **LH** levels are still very low. The corpus luteum becomes nonfunctional about 14 days after ovulation, thus reducing the levels of **progesterone** and **estradiol**.

A couple of days before bleeding begins, the functionalis layer of the endometrium becomes deprived of blood as the coiled **helical arteries** become intermittently constricted and dilated. After 2 days or so, the coiled arteries become permanently constricted, reducing oxygen to the functionalis layer, leading to a shutdown of the glands, invasion by leukocytes, ischemia, and eventual **necrosis** of the **functionalis**. Shortly thereafter, the coiled arteries dilate again; however, because these coiled arteries have been weakened by the previous events, they rupture. The disgorged blood removes patches of the functionalis to be

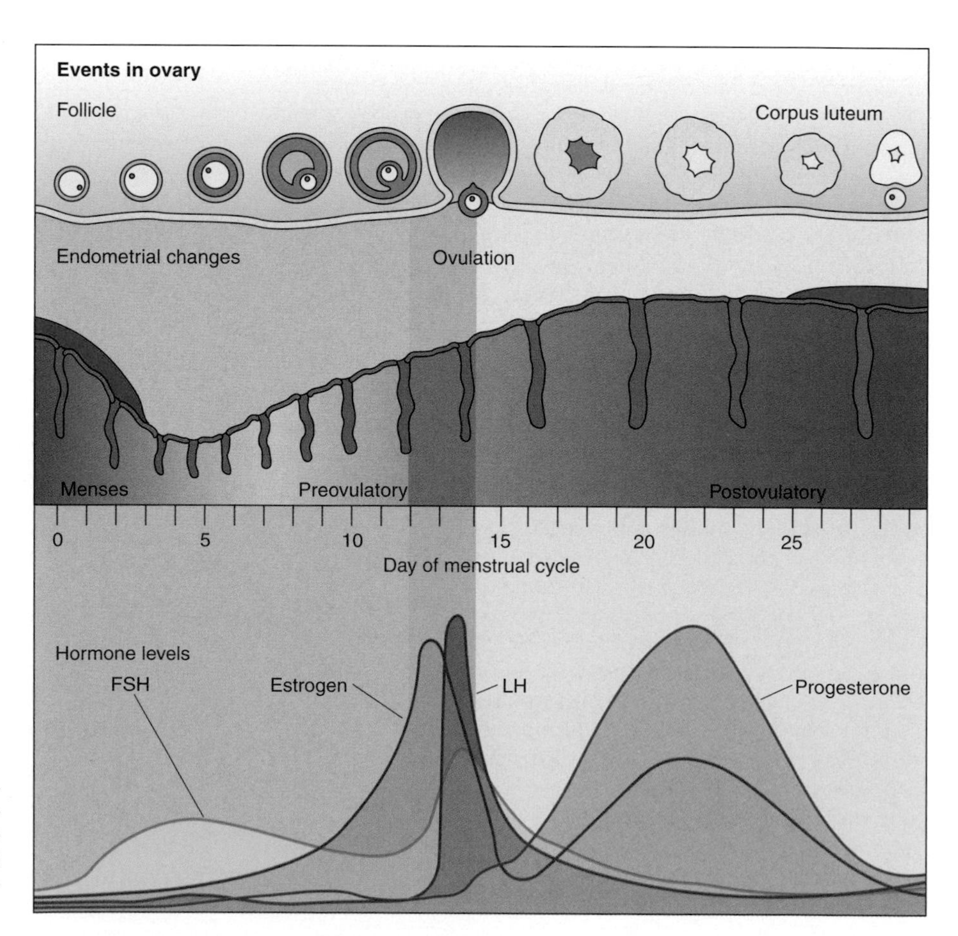

Fig. 20.20 Diagram correlating the events in follicular development, ovulation, hormonal interrelationships, and the menstrual cycle. Note that the levels of estrogen and luteinizing hormone (LH) are highest at the time of ovulation. FSH, Follicle-stimulating hormone.

eliminated as a **hemorrhagic discharge** (**menses**), initiating menstruation on day 1 (Fig. 20.21).

Although the entire functionalis layer of the endometrium is sloughed, it is not completely released from the wall immediately; rather, this process continues for 3 to 4 days. During a normal menstrual period, the approximate blood loss is only 35 mL, although in some women it may be greater. It is important to note that during the menstrual phase, there is an *inhibition* of the blood clotting mechanism.

Before and during the menstrual phase, the basalis layer of the endometrium continues to be vascularized by its own **straight arteries** and, thus, remains viable. The basal cells of the glands of the basalis begin to proliferate, and the newly formed cells migrate to the surface to begin reepithelialization of the connective tissue wound of the uterine lumen. These events commence the proliferative phase.

Proliferative (Follicular) Phase (Day 4 or 5 to Day 14)

The proliferative phase is characterized by a reepithelialization of the lining of the endometrium and renewal of the functionalis.

The proliferative phase (also called the ***follicular phase*** because it occurs at the same time as the development of the ovarian follicles) begins when menstrual flow ceases, on about day 4 or 5, and continues through day 14. The proliferative phase is characterized by reepithelialization of the lining of the endometrium; reconstruction of the glands, connective tissue, and coiled arteries of the lamina propria; and renewal of the entire functionalis (Fig. 20.22). The process of proliferation is driven by the increasing levels of the hormone **estradiol** produced by the granulosa cells of the developing follicles but especially by the **dominant follicle** of the ovary. Estradiol binds to **estradiol receptors** in the stromal cells, forming **estradiol-estradiol receptor complexes** that act as transcriptional factors that activate dozens of genes. These genes code for paracrine type **growth factors** that, in turn, act on epithelial and endothelial cells, inducing their proliferation.

During this phase, the functional layer becomes much thicker (up to 2–3 mm) because of the proliferation of the cells in the base of the glands, whose blood supply remained intact, which were unaffected during the menstrual phase. As stated earlier, it is these cells that are responsible for the formation of the epithelial lining of the uterus and for the establishment of new glands in the functionalis. These tubular glands are straight, not yet coiled, but their cells begin to accumulate glycogen, as do the cells of the stroma that proliferated to renew the stroma of the functionalis. The coiled arteries that were lost in the menstrual phase are replaced but are not tightly coiled and reach only two-thirds of the way into the functionalis.

By the 14th day of the menstrual cycle (ovulation), the functionalis layer of the endometrium has been fully restored to its

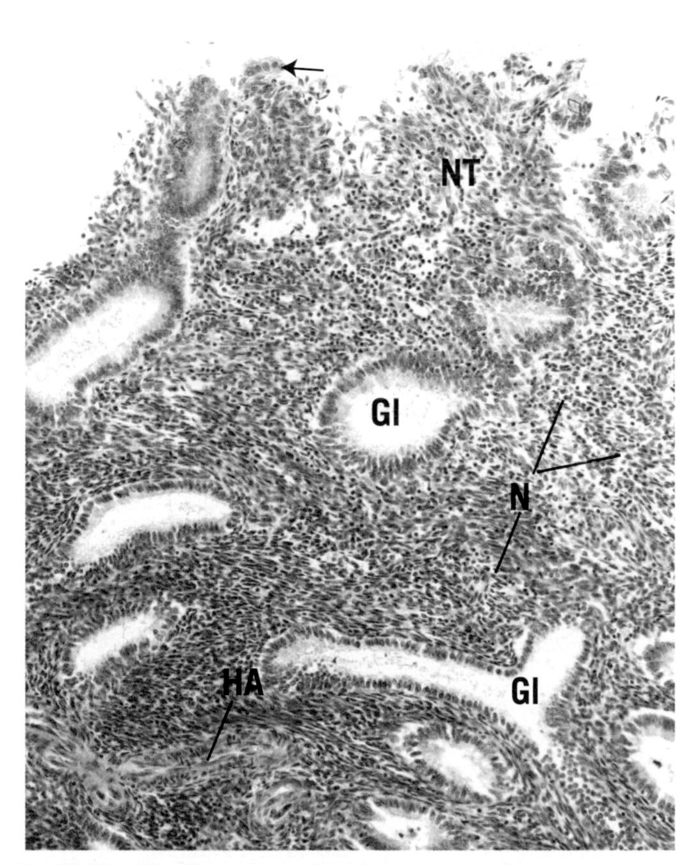

Fig. 20.21 This photomicrograph of the uterus in the menstrual phase displays the disrupted epithelial lining *(arrow)* of the simple columnar epithelial lining of the endometrium. Observe the nuclei (N) of free leukocytes in the necrotic tissue (NT) that will be discharged. Some of the uterine glands (Gl) still appear healthy and a segment of a helical artery (HA) still appears intact. (×132)

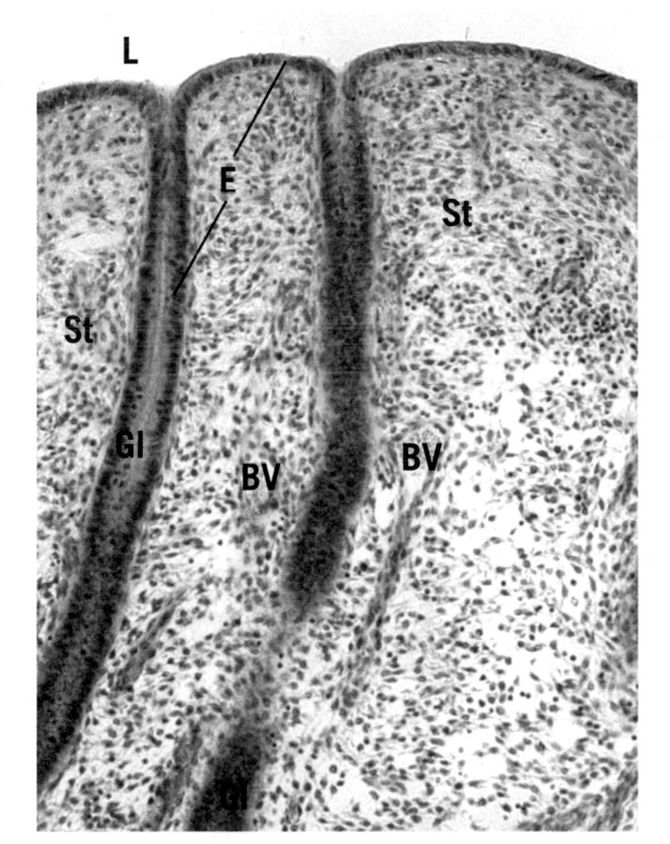

Fig. 20.22 The proliferative phase of the uterus displays the reestablished simple columnar epithelium (E) lining the lumen (L) of the uterus as well as the uterine glands (Gl). Note that the functionalis layer looks healthy with a stroma (St) that has very few invading lymphocytes. Note the helical arteries (BV) that supply the functionalis layer of the endometrium. The uterine glands are well represented but have not as yet started to produce their secretory products. (×132)

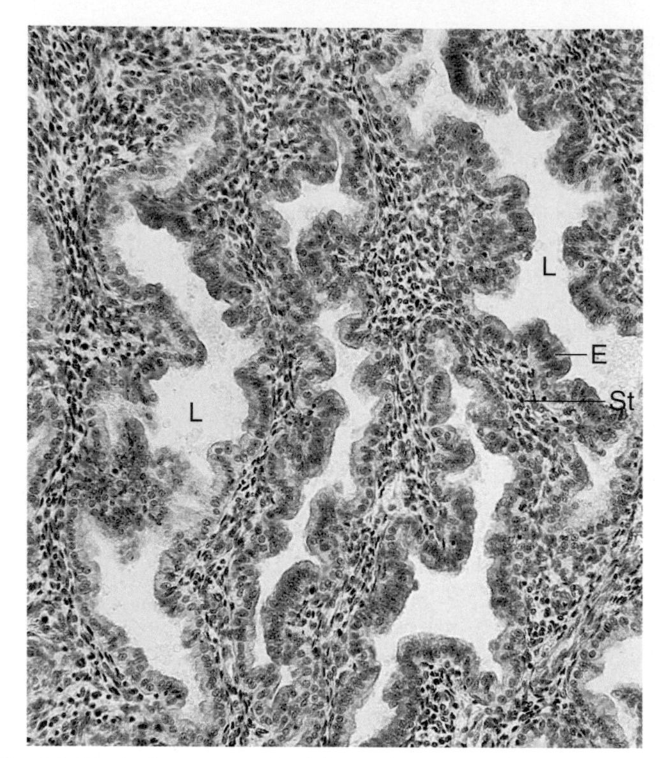

Fig. 20.23 Light micrograph of the endometrium of the uterus in the luteal phase. Note the simple columnar epithelial lining (E) of the lumina (L) of the glands surrounded by stromal cells (St). (×132)

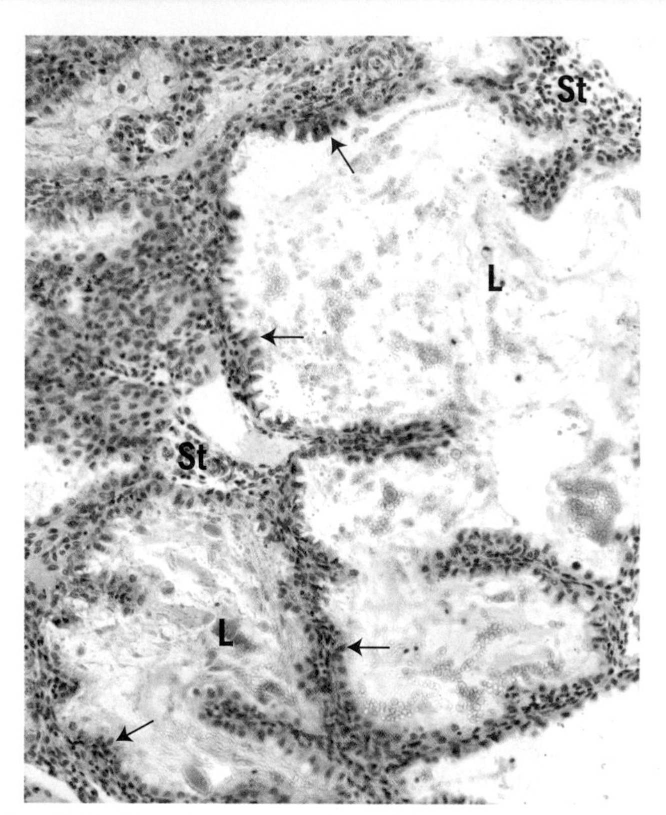

Fig. 20.24 This photomicrograph is of the endometrial glands in the late luteal phase, displaying their coiled characteristics, as well as the large amount of secretory product housed in the lumina (L) of the glands. Some of the cells lining the gland are taller and plumper than their neighbors; thus, the lining has a "sawtoothed" appearance *(arrows)*. The stroma (St) appears compressed among the many dilated glands. (×132)

previous status, with a full complement of epithelium, glands, stroma, and coiled arteries.

Secretory (Luteal) Phase (Days 15–28)

The secretory phase is characterized by thickening of the endometrium as a result of edema and accumulated glycogen secretions of the highly coiled endometrial glands.

The secretory phase (or **luteal phase**) commences after ovulation and is driven by the hormone **progesterone** released by the **granulosa lutein cells** of the **corpus luteum** and to a limited extent by **estradiol** produced by the theca lutein cells of the corpus luteum. Stromal cells possess **progesterone receptors**, and the **progesterone–progesterone receptor complexes** (**P-PR complexes**) not only act as transcription factors but also decrease the expression of estradiol receptors. Additionally, P-PR complexes activate genes that code for enzymes that inactivate estradiols. Moreover, P-PR complexes activate other genes responsible for differentiation of the endometrium, making it receptive for the arrival of the early embryo.

During this phase, the endometrium continues to thicken as a result of edema and accumulated glycogen secretions of the endometrial glands, which become *highly convoluted* and *branched*. The secretory products first accumulate in the basal region of the cytoplasm of the cells constituting the endometrial glands. As more secretory product is manufactured, the secretory granules move apically and are released into the lumen of the gland. This **glycogen-rich material** will nourish the conceptus before the formation of the placenta.

Most of the changes that result in the thickening of the endometrium are attributed to the functionalis, although the lumina of the glands located in the basalis are also filled with secretory product (Figs. 20.23 and 20.24).

The coiled arteries of the functionalis attain full development, becoming more coiled and extending fully into the functional layer, by the 22nd day. Thus, at this point in the secretory phase, the endometrium is about 6 to 7 mm thick.

The secretory phase completes the cycle as the 28th day approaches, presaging the menstrual phase of a new menstrual cycle. The menstrual phase is driven by the *reduction* in the hormones that promote the growth and development of the functionalis layer of the endometrium.

FERTILIZATION, IMPLANTATION, AND PLACENTAL DEVELOPMENT

Fertilization

Fertilization, the fusion of the sperm and the oocyte, occurs in the ampulla of the oviduct.

As the secondary oocyte and its attendant follicular cells are transported down the oviduct to the uterus by the cilia of the ciliated cells and by rhythmic contractions of the smooth muscle of the oviduct (Fig. 20.25), they are nourished by the nutrient-rich fluid produced by peg cells of the mucosal epithelium.

Spermatozoa, introduced into the vagina during sexual intercourse, pass through the cervix, the uterine lumen, and up the oviduct to the ampulla to encounter the secondary oocyte. In order to have the ability to fertilize a secondary oocyte, the spermatozoon has to progress through three stages: maturation, capacitation, and hyperactivity.

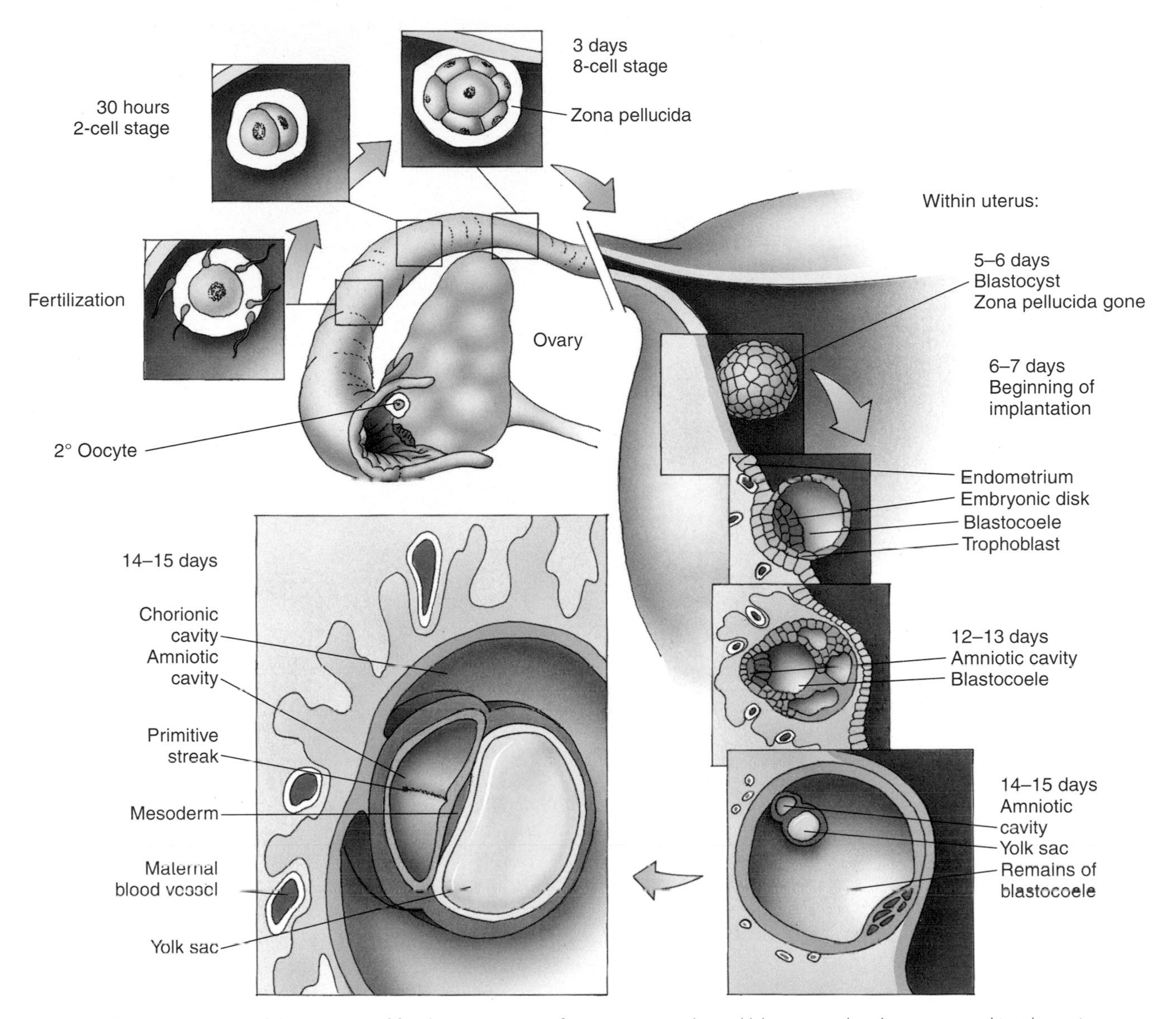

Fig. 20.25 Diagram of the process of fertilization, zygote formation, morula and blastocyst development, and implantation.

- The process of **maturation** occurs in the male reproductive tract. Prior to maturation, the spermatozoon can travel only in a circular direction, whereas after maturation, it can travel in a forward direction. While in the male reproductive tract, the spermatozoon is subject to a high concentration of the prostate manufactured **fertilization-promoting peptide** (**FPP**) that prevents the spermatozoon from undergoing capacitation.
- Once the spermatozoon is deposited in the female reproductive tract, the level of FPP is diluted by the vaginal secretions and the reduced level of FPP prompts the spermatozoon to begin **capacitation.** The process of capacitation entails a modification of the acrosomal membrane in that cholesterol and certain glycoproteins, known as **decapacitation factors**, are removed from the membrane, making it more flexible and able to bind to zona pellucida receptors. Additionally, calcium ion channels, known as **CatSpers** (**cation channels of spermatozoa**) in the flagellar membrane open, allowing the influx of calcium ions.
- The increased entry of calcium ions into the spermatozoon elevates **cAMP** levels within the spermatozoon, inducing it to be more vigorous and a stronger swimmer, a condition known as **hyperactivity.** Due to its enhanced swimming abilities, the spermatozoon has an increased capability to pass through the zona pellucida to reach and fertilize the secondary oocyte.

Fertilization usually occurs in the ampulla (Fig. 20.26). At this time, the cells of the corona radiata still surround the **zona pellucida**, a gel-like substance consisting of four related glycoproteins named *ZP1, ZP2, ZP3,* and *ZP4.* These glycoproteins act to prevent polyspermy; that is, they ensure that only a single spermatozoon is able to bind to and penetrate the secondary oocyte. **ZP3** binds to the first spermatozoon to reach the zona pellucida and triggers the spermatozoon to initiate the acrosome reaction (see upcoming discussion). **ZP2** assists ZP3 in binding the spermatozoon to the zona pellucida. **ZP1** acts to cross-link ZP2 with ZP3 so that they are no longer able to bind to spermatozoa, thus taking further steps to prevent polyspermy. The role of ZP4 is not yet understood.

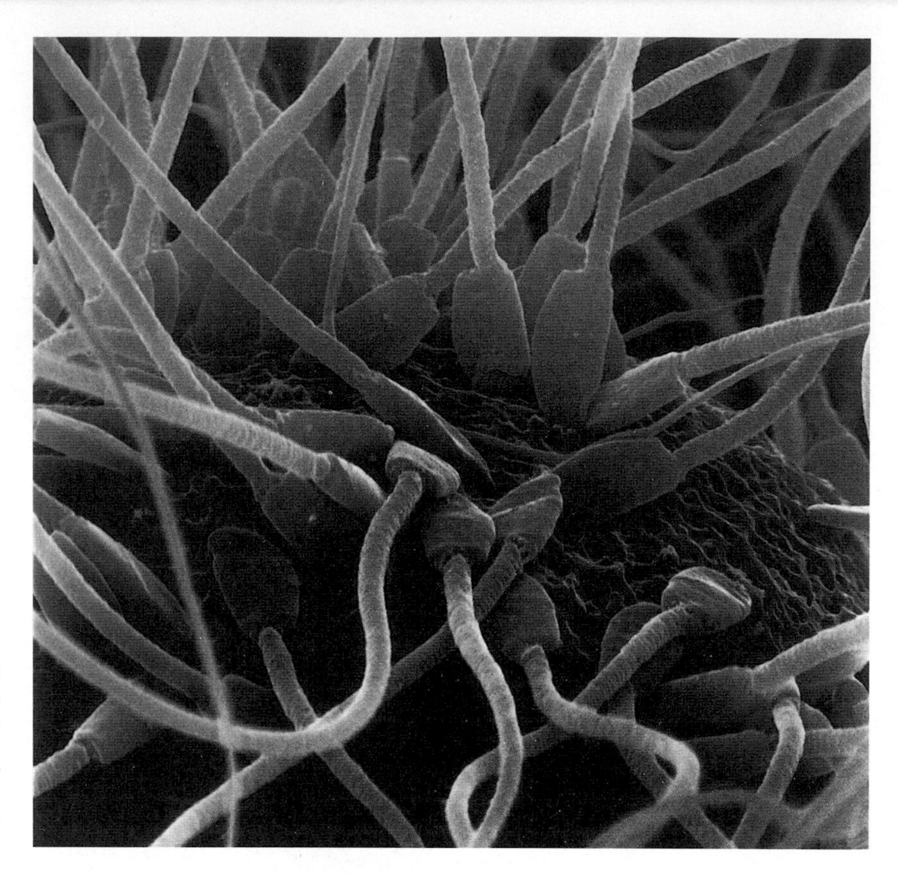

Fig. 20.26 Scanning electron micrograph of fertilization. Observe that the large number of spermatozoa are trying to make their way through the cells of the corona radiata, but only a single spermatozoon will be able to fertilize the egg (×5700). (From Phillips DM, Shalgi R, Dekel N. Mammalian fertilization as seen with the scanning electron microscope. *Am J Anat.* 1985;174:357–372. Reprinted with permission from Wiley-Liss, Inc., a subsidiary of John Wiley & Sons, Inc.)

The **acrosome reaction** results in the release of the acrosomal enzymes into the zona pellucida. The liberated enzymes, especially the inner acrosomal membrane-bound enzyme **acrosin**, decrease the viscosity of the zona pellucida, facilitating the flagellar movement of the spermatozoa to propel the sperm toward the oocyte. Once the spermatozoon penetrates the entire width of the zona pellucida, it enters the **perivitelline space**, located between the zona pellucida and the oocyte cell membrane, and can reach the oocyte.

When the spermatozoon contacts the secondary oocyte membrane, the spermatozoon membrane's integral protein molecules, known as **fertilin**, bind with the oocyte membrane's **integrin** and **CD9 molecules**, ensuring a strong attachment between them. This contact between the sperm and the oocyte is responsible for the **cortical reaction**, which is an additional process that prevents **polyspermy**. The cortical reaction has a fast and a slow component.

- The **fast component** involves a change in the resting membrane potential of the oocyte plasma membrane that prevents contact between the oocyte and another sperm. This alteration of the membrane potential lasts only a few minutes.
- The **slow component** involves the release of the contents of numerous cortical granules located in the oocyte's cytoplasm into the **perivitelline space.** Enzymes, such as **ovastacin**, within the cortical granules act to hydrolyze ZP2 and ZP3 molecules, the sperm receptors, in the zona pellucida, preventing additional spermatozoa from reaching the oocyte. The alteration in the ZP proteins causes the zona pellucida to become a firmer, thicker, more viscous gel that prevents other spermatozoa from penetrating it. The cortical granules also release polysaccharides in to the perivitelline space. As these polysaccharides become hydrated, they swell, pressing the zona pellucida away from the secondary oocyte, enlarging the perivitelline space and making it even more difficult for a second spermatozoon to contact the oocyte.

At this time, the spermatozoon's **centrosome** and its nucleus, called the **male pronucleus,** enter the cytoplasm of the secondary oocyte, triggering it to resume and complete its second meiotic division. This results in an unequal division of the oocyte cytoplasm, forming two haploid cells—the large **ovum** and the very small second polar body, which, similar to the first polar body, is composed of a nucleus surrounded by only a narrow rim of cytoplasm. It will degenerate and die within a few days.

The resultant haploid nucleus of the ovum, known as the **female pronucleus**, and the haploid male pronucleus both lose their nuclear envelopes as they travel toward each other and their chromosomes mingle, forming a new cell known as the **zygote**, with the diploid number of chromosomes. Thus, the event of fertilization is completed. The zygote enters its first *mitotic division*, forming two identical daughter cells, a process that initiates the development of an embryo. It should be recognized that the mitotic spindle apparatus of the embryo is derived from the spermatozoon, whereas the mitochondria and much of the cytoplasm is derived from the ovum.

The window of time between ovulation and fertilization is about 24 hours. If fertilization does not occur during this period, the secondary oocyte degenerates and is phagocytosed by macrophages.

Implantation

Implantation is the process that occurs as the blastocyst becomes embedded in the uterine endometrium.

As the zygote continues its journey through the oviduct on its way to the uterus, it undergoes numerous mitotic divisions, becoming the spherical cluster of cells known as the **morula** (see Fig. 20.25). With further divisions and modifications, the morula is transformed into the **blastocyst**, composed of a hollow ball of cells, whose lumen contains a somewhat viscous fluid and a few cells at one pole. The peripheral cells are known as **trophoblasts**, and the cells trapped inside the blastocyst are the **embryoblasts**. The blastocyst enters the uterine cavity about 4 to 6 days after fertilization; on the sixth or seventh day, it begins to embed itself into the uterine wall, a process known as **implantation**. The trophoblasts of the blastocyst stimulate the transformation of the **stromal cells** of the uterine endometrium into pale-staining **decidual cells**, whose stored glycogen probably provides nourishment for the developing embryo.

The **embryoblast cells** develop into the embryo, whereas **trophoblast cells** give rise to the embryonic portion of the placenta. Trophoblast cells proliferate rapidly, forming an inner conglomeration of individual cells, which are mitotically active and are known as **cytotrophoblasts**, and a thicker outer syncytium of cells that do not undergo mitosis, called **syncytiotrophoblasts**.

As the **cytotrophoblasts** proliferate, the newly formed cells join the syncytiotrophoblasts, enlarging the syncytium enough so that by the ninth day after fertilization, vascular spaces can form within the substance of the syncytium. As these spaces increase in number, they coalesce into larger, labyrinthine spaces known as **lacunae** (**trophoblastic lacunae**). As the syncytium continues to grow in size, it erodes the lining of the endometrium, permitting deep penetration of the blastocyst into the wall of the endometrium. By the 11th day of gestation, implantation is complete and the endometrial epithelium seals over the implantation site.

Placenta

The placenta is a vascular tissue derived from the uterine endometrium, as well as from the developing embryo.

At parturition, or birth, the placenta is a highly vascularized disk-shaped structure, about 18 cm in diameter and 2.5 cm thick in its middle, weighing about 600 g.

Development of the Placenta

Maternal blood vessels form blood sinusoids in the uterine endometrium. Blood from these sinusoids empties into the trophoblastic lacunae that surround the developing embryo, providing nourishment for it. With further growth and development, the **placenta**, more accurately known as the **hemochorioendothelial placenta**, begins to be formed, with the resultant separation between the blood of the developing embryo and that of the mother (maternal blood). The reason that it is referred to as a *hemochorioendothelial placenta* is because only three layers—the fetal endothelial vessels of the placenta, embryonic connective tissue, and a layer of trophoblasts—are interposed between the maternal blood and the fetal blood.

Cells of the trophoblast give rise to the **chorion**, which evolves into the **chorionic plate**, which gives rise to the **chorionic villi** (Fig. 20.27).

The developing trophoblasts induce changes in the endometrium in their vicinity, altering it to begin the formation of the maternal portion of the placenta. This altered maternal tissue, called the **decidua**, is subdivided into three regions:

- The **decidua capsularis** is interposed between the uterine lumen and the developing embryo.
- The **decidua basalis** is interposed between the developing embryo and the myometrium.
- The **decidua parietalis** composes the balance of the decidua.

Initially, the entire embryo is surrounded by decidua in order to nourish it. The region of the chorion in contact with the decidua capsularis forms short, insubstantial villi, thus remaining mostly smooth surfaced. That smooth-surfaced region of the chorion is known as the **chorion laeve**. The region of the decidua basalis, however, becomes highly vascularized by maternal blood vessels; it is in this region that the placenta develops. The region of the chorionic plate in contact with the decidua basalis forms extensive chorionic villi, known as **primary chorionic villi**; thus, this region of the chorion is known as the **chorion frondosum**.

The primary villi are composed of both syncytiotrophoblasts and cytotrophoblasts. With further development, extraembryonic mesenchymal cells enter the core of the primary villi, converting them into **secondary chorionic villi**. The connective tissue of the secondary villi becomes vascularized by extensive **capillary beds**, which are linked to the developing vascular supply of the embryo, at which point they are known as **tertiary villi**.

As development continues, the cytotrophoblast population decreases because these cells join the syncytium and contribute to its growth. The decidua basalis forms large vascular spaces, known as **lacunae**, which are compartmentalized into smaller regions by extensions of the decidua called **placental septa**. Secondary villi project into these vascular spaces and are surrounded by maternal blood that is delivered to and drained from the lacunae by maternal blood vessels of the decidua basalis.

Most of the villi are not anchored to the decidua basalis but are suspended in maternal blood of the lacunae similar to roots of vegetables grown in hydroponic environments; these are known as **free villi** (**terminal villi**). The villi anchored to the decidua basalis are called **anchoring villi** (Figs. 20.28 and 20.29). Capillaries of free and anchoring villi are near the surface of the villi and are separated from the maternal blood by a slight amount of connective tissue and the syncytiotrophoblasts (and occasional cytotrophoblasts) covering the secondary villus. Thus, as indicated earlier in the definition of the hemochorioendothelial placenta, maternal blood and fetal blood do not intermix. Instead, nutrients and oxygen from the maternal blood diffuse through the syncytiotrophoblasts and cytotrophoblasts (and their basal laminae), connective tissue, and endothelial cells (and their basal lamina) of the capillaries of the villi to reach the fetal blood. These structures form the **placental barrier**. Certain substances, such as water, oxygen, carbon dioxide, small molecules, some proteins, lipids, hormones, drugs, and some antibodies (especially immunoglobulin G) can penetrate the placental barrier, whereas most macromolecules cannot. Some of these substances, such as IgG, are able to penetrate the placental barrier via specific carrier-mediated transport.

In addition to being the site where nutritious substances, waste, and gases are exchanged between maternal and fetal blood, the placenta, specifically the syncytiotrophoblasts, serves as an endocrine organ, secreting **human chorionic gonadotropin** (**hCG**), **chorionic thyrotropin**, **progesterone**, **estrogen**, **human chorionic somatomammotropin** hormone (also known as lactogenic hormone), endothelial growth factor, platelet-derived growth factor, fibroblast growth factor, TNF-α, transforming growth factor, insulin-like growth factor I, insulin-like growth factor II, colony-stimulating factor, as well as interleukin 1, interleukin 3, leptin, and relaxin. Also, stromal connective tissue cells of the decidua form the **decidual cells**, which enlarge and synthesize **prolactin** and **prostaglandins** (see Table 20.4).

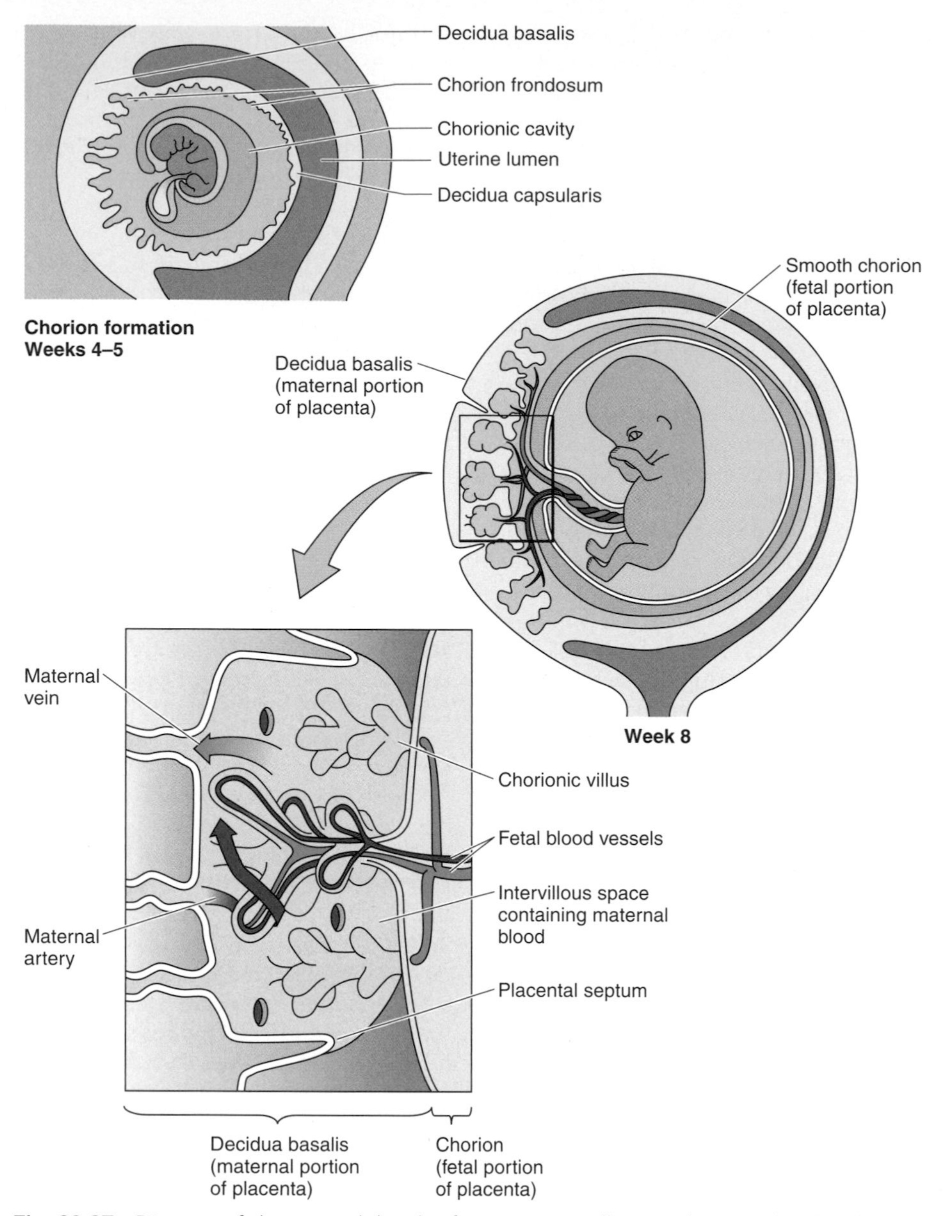

Fig. 20.27 Diagram of chorion and decidua formation as well as circulation within the placenta.

Clinical Correlations

1. *The blastocyst usually implants into the upper third of the anterior or posterior wall of the uterus; it is in that location that the placenta will begin to develop. Occasionally, in 1 of 200 pregnancies, implantation occurs lower down in the uterus, near the cervix, where the endometrium is much thinner and the connective tissue stroma is much denser. As the placenta begins to develop and enlarge, it covers partially or completely the opening of the cervix, making normal, vaginal delivery an untenable option. This condition is referred to as* ***placenta previa****, usually necessitating the delivery of the baby via a cesarean section.*
2. ***Placenta accreta*** *is a condition in which the placenta, instead of attaching to the basalis layer of the endometrium, grows deeper into the wall of the uterus and attaches to the myometrium. This condition can be exceptionally dangerous because after delivery of the baby, the delivery of the placenta may cause complications, including heavy bleeding. In fact, as many as 7% of women experiencing placenta accrete may die owing to blood loss. The chances of placenta accreta occurring is greatly increased if the previous pregnancy was complicated by placenta previa or if the previous delivery was performed by a caesarean section. It has been noted that the incidence of placenta accreta has increased from 1 in 30,000 deliveries in the 1950s to 1 in 2500 deliveries in 2018.*
3. *The* ***placenta*** *was believed to be a sterile organ; however, recent reports indicate that it harbors nonpathogenic microbes. Interestingly, the* ***placental microbiota*** *does not resemble that of the vagina; instead, it resembles the microbiota of the oral cavity. The phyla represented included Proteobacteria, Fusobacteria, Firmicutes, Bacteroidetes, and Tenericutes. It has been suggested that this is the first exposure of the newborn to his or her microbiome because the newborn possesses many of the bacteria present in the placenta. Additionally, the newborn also receives vaginal microbiota during normal delivery, as well as microorganisms from individuals who come in physical contact with the neonate.*

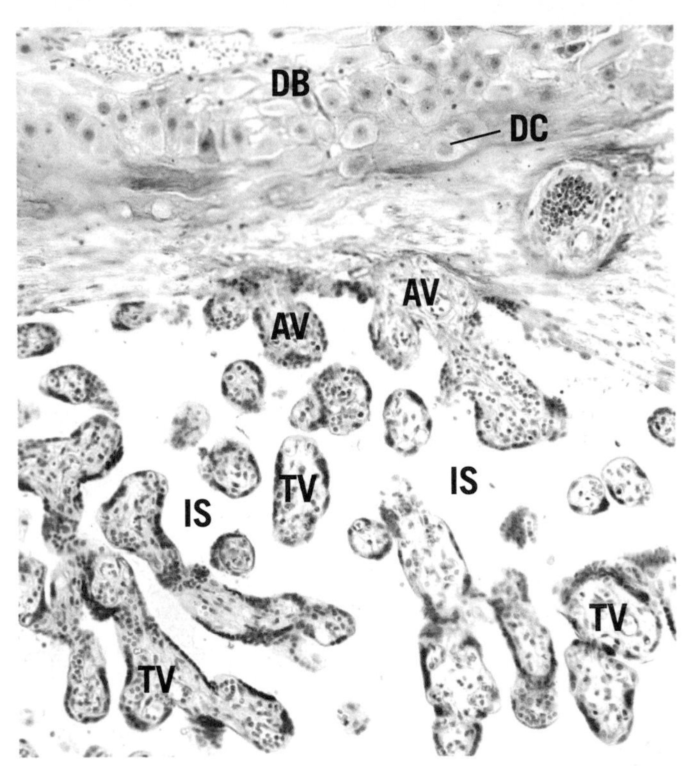

Fig. 20.28 This low-magnification light micrograph of the developing placenta. Note that the decidua basalis (DB) possesses numerous decidual cells and that the anchoring chorionic villi (AV) are attached to it. The blindly ending terminal villi (TV) end in the intervillous spaces; in the living person, these are filled with maternal blood. (×132)

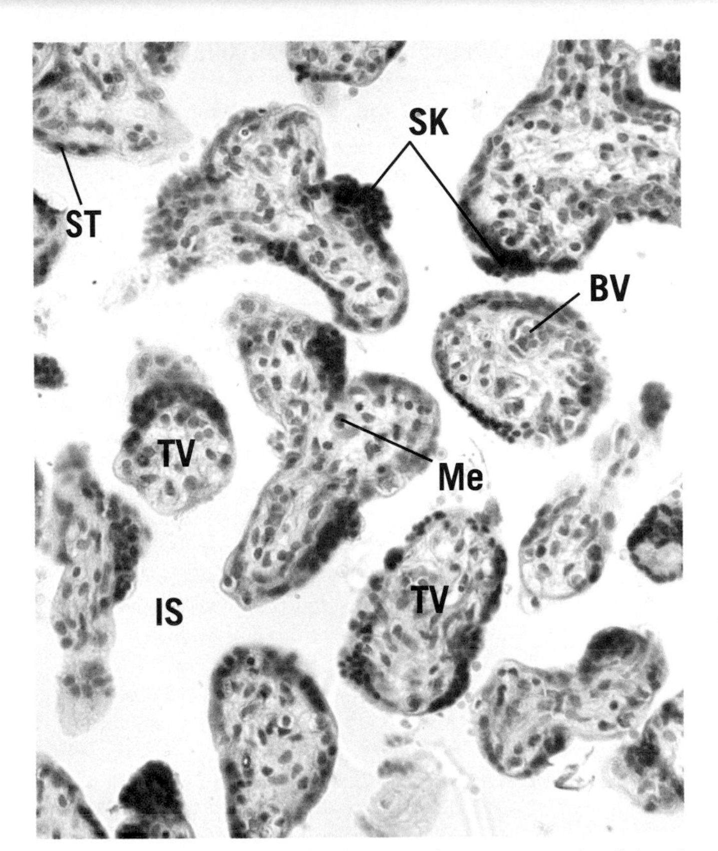

Fig. 20.29 This medium magnification photomicrograph of the developing placenta displays the intervillous spaces that are occupied by cross and oblique sections of terminal villi (TV) with their small blood vessels of the embryo (BV) surrounded by mesoderm (Me). The terminal villi are finger-shaped processes whose external aspect is covered by syncytiotrophoblasts (ST) whose nuclei frequently form clusters, known as syncytial knots (SK). (x270)

MATERNAL CHANGES DURING PREGNANCY

On the average, at full term, the mother gains approximately 12.5 kg (Table 20.5), has gastroesophageal reflux, has bouts of constipation, experiences reduction in bile delivery to the duodenum with a resultant formation of gallstones, has an increased glomerular filtration rate and urine production, has an increased blood volume, increased heart rate, and reduced diastolic blood pressure. Additionally, because the diaphragm is displaced, the mother's expiratory reserve volume is reduced by almost half.

TABLE 20.5 Sources of Weight Gain in the Gravid Mother at Term

Source of Weight Gain	Weight (kg)
Fetus	3.5
Placenta	0.6
Amniotic fluid	0.8
Uterus	1.0
Breasts	0.4
Blood	1.5
Extravascular fluid	1.5
Maternal fat gained (as fat reserve)	3.2
Total	12.5

VAGINA

The vagina, a fibromuscular sheath, is composed of three layers: mucosa, muscularis, and adventitia.

The vagina is a fibromuscular tubular structure 8 to 9 cm in length connected to the uterus proximally and the vestibule of the external genitalia distally. The vagina consists of three layers: **mucosa, muscularis**, and **adventitia**.

The lumen of the vagina is lined by a thick, **stratified squamous nonkeratinized epithelium** (150–200 μm thick), although some of the superficial cells may contain some keratohyalin (Figs. 20.30 and 20.31). Langerhans cells in the epithelium function in antigen presentation to T lymphocytes housed in the inguinal lymph nodes. The epithelial cells are stimulated by estrogen to synthesize and store large deposits of **glycogen**, which is released into the lumen as the vaginal epithelial cells are sloughed. Naturally occurring vaginal bacterial flora metabolize the glycogen, forming **lactic acid**, which is responsible for the low pH in the lumen of the vagina, especially at the midpoint of the menstrual cycle. The lowered pH also helps restrict pathogenic invasion.

The **lamina propria** of the vagina is composed of a loose fibroelastic connective tissue containing a rich vascular supply in its deeper regions, which is occasionally referred to as the submucosa. The lamina propria also contains numerous lymphocytes and neutrophils that reach the lumen by passing through extracellular spaces during certain periods in the menstrual cycle, where they participate in immune responses. Although the vagina does not contain glands, there is an increase in vaginal fluid during sexual stimulation, arousal, and intercourse that serves to lubricate its lining. The fluid is derived from the transudate present in the lamina propria combined with secretions from glands of the cervix.

The **muscularis** layer of the vagina is composed of smooth muscle cells arranged so that the mostly longitudinal bundles of the external aspect intermingle with the more circularly arranged bundles nearer the lumen. A sphincter muscle, composed of skeletal muscle fibers, encircles the vagina at its external opening.

Dense, fibroelastic connective tissue constitutes the **adventitia** of the vagina, attaching it to surrounding structures. Contained within the adventitia is a rich vascular supply, with a vast venous plexus and nerve bundles derived from the pelvic splanchnic nerves.

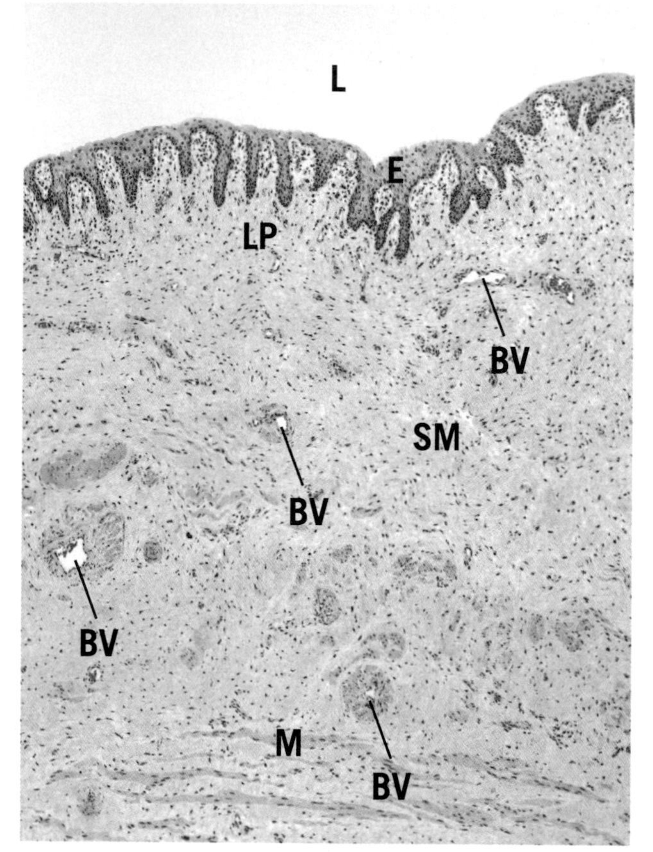

Fig. 20.30 The vagina, a fibromuscular tubular structure, is composed of three layers, the mucosa, muscularis, and an adventitia. The lumen (L) is usually collapsed and is lined by a stratified squamous epithelium (E). The lamina propria (LP) is composed of a loose fibroelastic connective tissue with a rich vascular supply in its deeper region; some refer to this deeper area as the submucosa (SM). The deepest region of the vaginal wall is the muscular layer (M), which possesses poorly differentiated inner circular and outer longitudinal smooth muscle fibers. The outermost adventitia is out of the view of this photomicrograph. (×56)

Clinical Correlations

The most common forms of ***sexually transmitted diseases (STDs)*** *are HPV infections, chlamydia, gonorrhea, syphilis, herpes, trichomoniasis, and human immunodeficiency virus (HIV). Another STD that has been known since the early 1980s is* Mycoplasma genitalium *infection (Mgen). Even though it is more common than gonorrhea in that it infects up to 3% of the US population, it was only in 2015 that the Center for Disease Control and Prevention (CDC) recognized it as an STD that should be monitored. The concern is that people with Mgen frequently have no symptoms and, when they do, they are similar to those of gonorrhea and chlamydia—pelvic pain, vaginal discharge, postcoital pain, and, at times, postcoital bleeding. Because the symptoms are similar and because not much attention has been brought to Mgen, the patients are not treated with antibiotics against* M. genitalium*. This leads to worsening of the infection, with possibly very serious consequences, such as infertility, pelvic inflammatory disease, inflammation of the urethra, and other related problems.*

EXTERNAL GENITALIA

The external genitalia (vulva) are composed of the labia majora, labia minora, vestibule, and clitoris.

The **labia majora** are two folds of skin heavily endowed with adipose tissue and a thin layer of smooth muscle. The homologue of these structures in the male is the scrotum, with the smooth muscle layer corresponding to the dartos muscle of the scrotum. The labia majora are covered with coarse hair on their external surface but are devoid of hair on their smooth inner surface. Numerous sweat glands and sebaceous glands open on both surfaces.

The **labia minora**, located medial and slightly deep to the labia majora, are the homologues of the urethral surface of the penis in the male. The labia minora are two smaller folds of skin devoid of hair follicles and adipose tissue. Their core is composed of a spongy connective tissue containing elastic fibers arranged in networks. They contain numerous sebaceous glands and are richly supplied with blood vessels and nerve endings.

The cleft situated between the right and left labia minora is the **vestibule**, a space that receives secretions of the **glands of Bartholin**, paired mucus-secreting glands, and many small **minor vestibular glands**. Also located in the vestibule are the orifices of the urethra and the vagina. In virgins, the orifice of the vagina is narrowed by a thin fold of epithelially enclosed fibrovascular tissue called the ***hymen***.

The **clitoris**, the female homologue of the penis, is located between the folds of the labia minora superiorly, where the two labia minora unite to form the prepuce over the top of the **glans clitoridis**. The clitoris is covered by stratified squamous epithelium and is composed of two **erectile bodies** containing numerous blood vessels and sensory nerves, including Meissner and Pacinian corpuscles, which are sensitive during sexual arousal.

MAMMARY GLANDS

The mammary glands, modified sweat glands, are compound tubuloalveolar glands that consist of 15 to 20 lobes radiating out from the nipple and are separated by adipose and collagenous connective tissue.

Mammary glands are modified sweat glands that secrete milk, a fluid that contains proteins, lipids, and lactose, as well as lymphocytes and monocytes, antibodies, minerals, and fat-soluble vitamins, to provide the proper nourishment for the newborn.

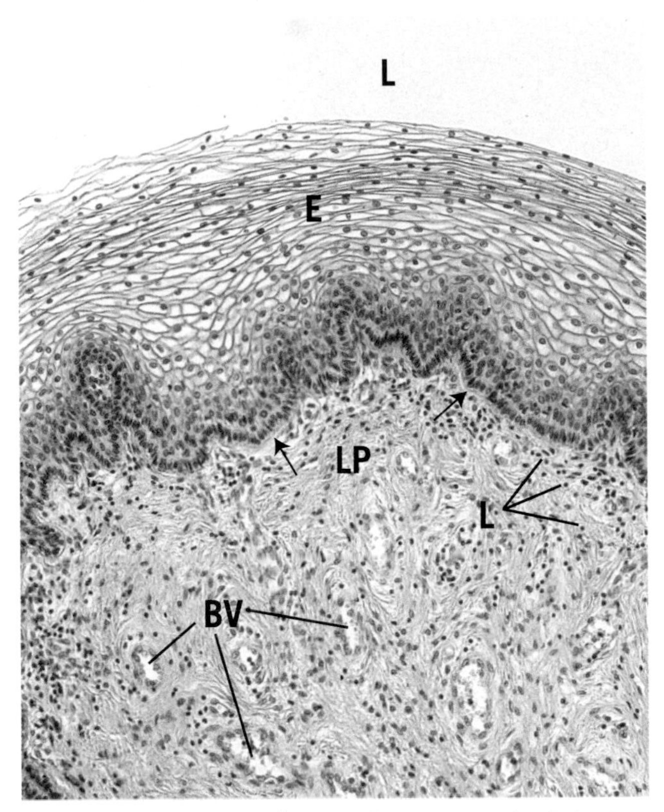

Fig. 20.31 This low-magnification photomicrograph of the human vagina displays a lumen (L) lined by a thick stratified squamous nonkeratinized epithelium (E) whose deeper cells are denser appearing, whereas the epithelial cells in its more superficial regions are filled with glycogen. The epithelium is separated from the lamina propria (LP) by a well-defined basement membrane *(arrows)*. Observe that the lamina propria is infiltrated by lymphoid cells (L) and note the rich vascular supply (BV) of the lamina propria. (×132)

The mammary glands develop in the same manner and are of the same structure in both sexes until puberty, when changes in the hormonal secretions in females cause further development and structural changes within the glands. Secretions of **estradiol** and **progesterone** from the ovary (as well as from the placenta) and **prolactin** from the acidophils of the anterior pituitary gland and human somatomammotropin from the placenta initiate development of **lobules** and **terminal ductules**. Full development of the ductal portion of the breast requires **glucocorticoids** and further activation by anterior pituitary **somatotropin**.

Concomitant with these events is an increase in connective tissue and adipose tissue within the stroma, causing the gland to enlarge. Full development occurs at about 20 years of age, with minor cyclic changes during each menstrual period, whereas major changes occur during pregnancy and in lactation. After age 40 years or so, the secretory portions, as well as some of the ducts and connective tissue elements of the breasts begin to atrophy, and they continue this process through menopause.

The glands within the breasts are classified as **compound tubuloacinar glands**, consisting of 15 to 20 lobes radiating out from the nipple and separated from each other by adipose tissue and collagenous connective tissue. Each lobe is drained by its own **lactiferous duct**, leading directly to the **nipple**, where it opens onto the surface. Before reaching the nipple, each of the ducts is dilated to form a **lactiferous sinus** for milk storage and then narrows before passing through the nipple (Fig. 20.32).

Resting Mammary Glands

Acini are not developed in the resting mammary gland.

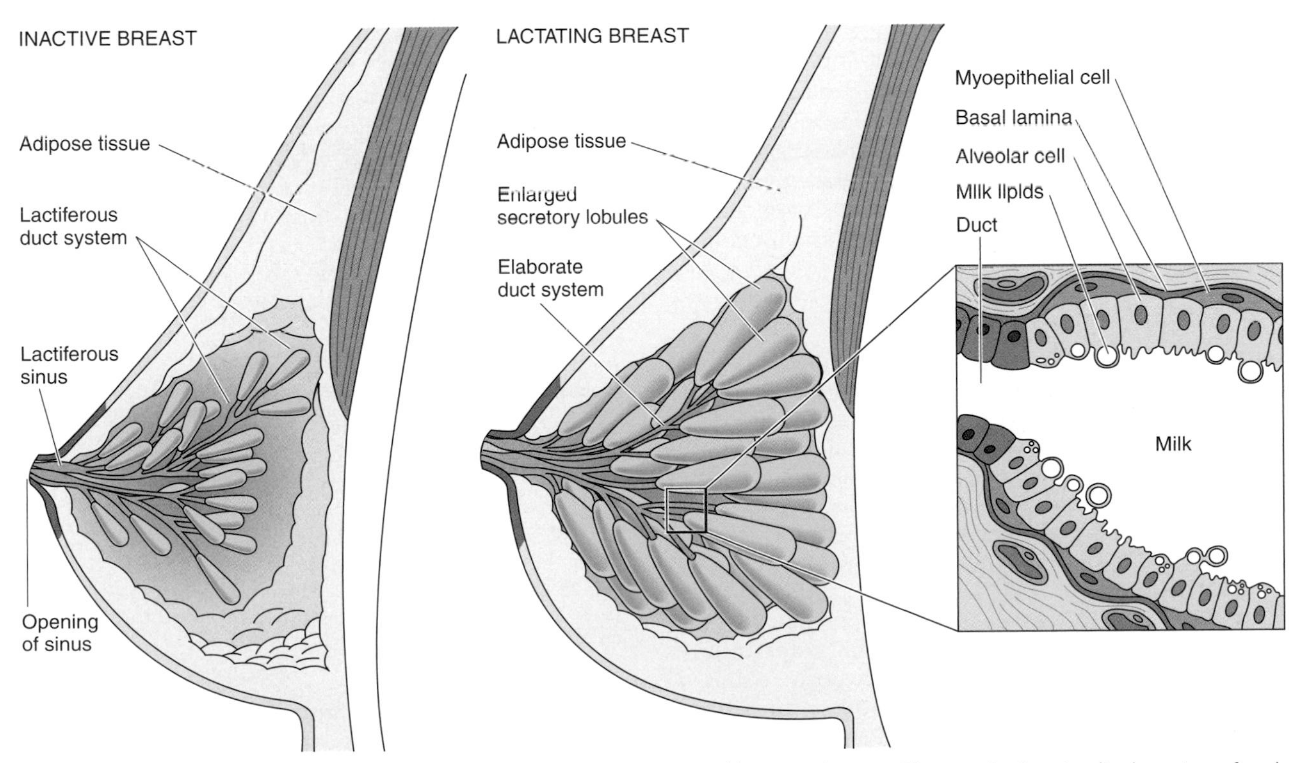

Fig. 20.32 Diagram comparing the glandular differences between a resting and lactating breast. Observe the longitudinal section of a gland and duct of the active mammary gland.

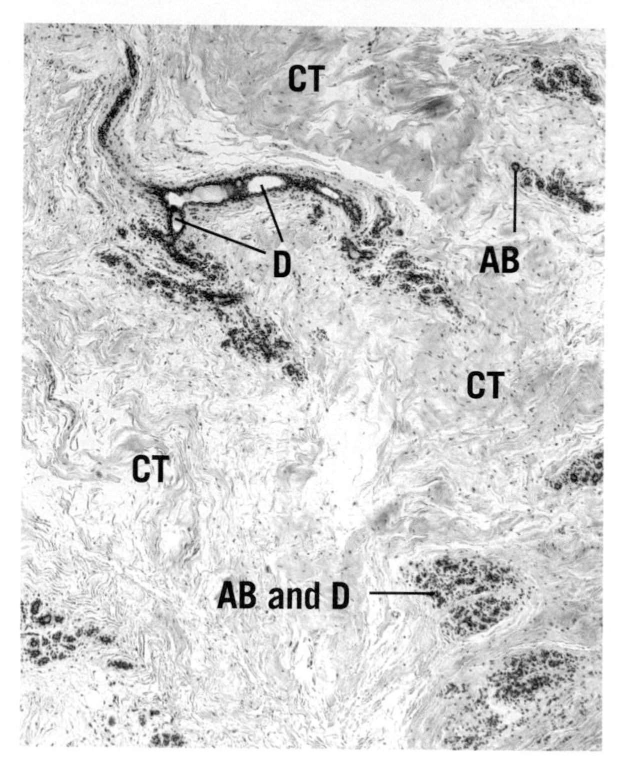

Fig. 20.33 This very-low-magnification photomicrograph of a resting (inactive) mammary gland displays the small alveolar buds (AB) and ducts (D) surrounded by a dense collagenous type of connective tissue (CT). (×56)

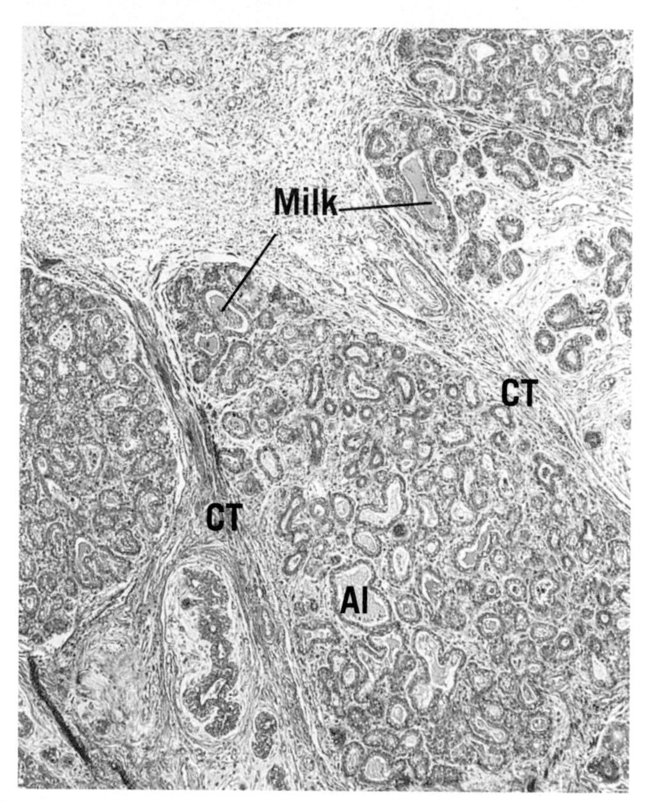

Fig. 20.34 This very-low-magnification photomicrograph of a lactating mammary gland displays lobules of alveoli (Al) where some of the alveoli contain milk. Note that the lobules are separated by compressed collagenous connective tissue (CT) elements. (×56)

Resting (nonsecreting or **nonlactating)** mammary glands of nonpregnant women have the same basic architecture as the lactating (active) mammary glands, except that they are smaller and without developed acini (Fig. 20.33); acini development occurs during pregnancy only. Near the opening at the nipple, lactiferous ducts are lined by a stratified squamous (keratinized) epithelium. The lactiferous sinus and the lactiferous duct leading to it are lined by stratified cuboidal epithelium, whereas the smaller ducts leading to the lactiferous duct are lined by a simple columnar epithelium. Stellate myoepithelial cells located between the epithelium and the basal lamina also wrap around the developing acini and become functional during pregnancy.

Lactating (Active) Mammary Glands

During pregnancy, the terminal portions of the ducts branch and grow and develop secretory units known as acini.

Mammary glands are activated by elevated surges of **estrogen** and **progesterone** (as well as human somatomammotropin from the placenta) during pregnancy to become lactating glands to provide milk for the newborn. At this time, the terminal portions of the ducts branch and grow and the acini develop and mature (Figs. 20.34–20.36). As pregnancy progresses, the breasts enlarge as a result of hypertrophy of the glandular parenchyma and engorgement with **colostrum**, a protein-rich fluid, in preparation for the newborn. Within a few days after birth, when estrogen and progesterone secretions have subsided, **prolactin**, secreted by acidophils of the anterior pituitary gland, activates the secretion of milk, which replaces the colostrum.

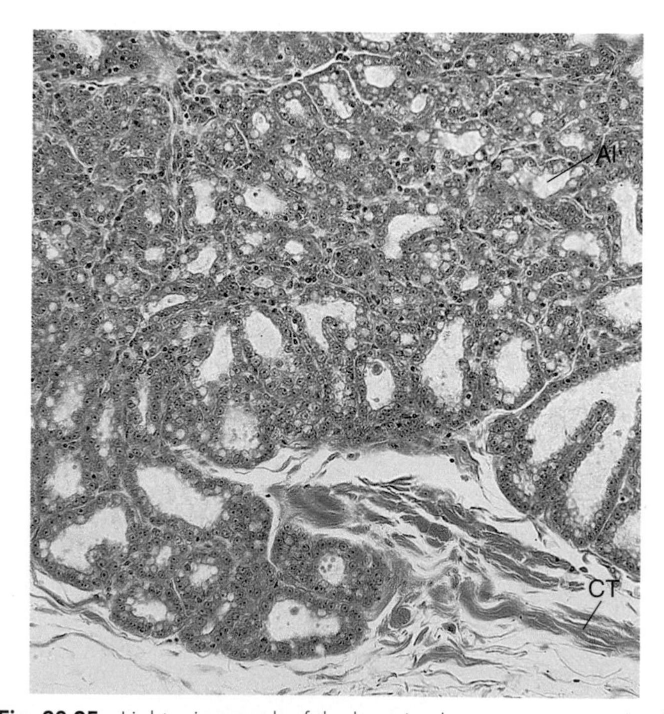

Fig. 20.35 Light micrograph of the lactating human mammary gland. Observe the crowded alveoli and note that various regions of the gland are in different stages of the secretory process (×132).

The **alveoli** of the lactating (active) mammary glands are composed of cuboidal cells partially surrounded by a meshwork of myoepithelial cells. These secretory cells possess abundant RER and mitochondria, several Golgi complexes, many lipid droplets, and numerous vesicles containing caseins (milk proteins) and lactose (Fig. 20.37). However, not all regions of the alveolus are in the same stage of production because different alveoli display various degrees of preparation for synthesis of milk substances (see Fig. 20.35).

The secretions of the alveolar cells are of two kinds: lipids and proteins.

Lipids are stored as droplets within the cytoplasm. They are released from the secretory cells, most probably by the **apocrine** mode of exocytosis, whereby small droplets coalesce to form increasingly larger droplets that move to the periphery of the cell. Once there, they project as cytoplasmic blebs into the lumen; eventually, these lipid droplets containing blebs are pinched off and become part of the secretory product. Each bleb then consists of a central lipid droplet surrounded by a very narrow rim of cytoplasm and enclosed by a plasmalemma.

Proteins synthesized within these secretory cells are liberated from the cells by the **merocrine** mode of exocytosis in much the same manner as would be expected of other cells that synthesize and release proteins into the extracellular space.

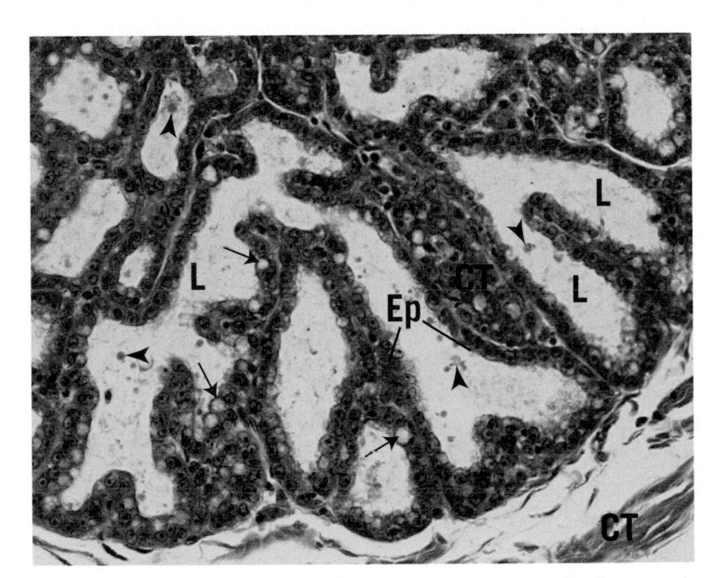

Fig. 20.36 This medium-magnification photomicrograph of a part of a lobule of a lactating mammary gland presents the branching tubuloacinar units. Note that their lumina (L) contain milk solids *(arrowheads)* and the cuboidal epithelial cells (Ep) have large droplets of milk lipids *(arrows)* and lactose at the apical region of the cells ready to be released, probably via apocrine mode of exocytosis into the lumen. (×270)

Areola and Nipple

The circular, heavily pigmented skin in the center of the breast is the **areola**. It contains sweat glands and sebaceous glands at its margin, as well as **areolar glands (of Montgomery)** that resemble both sweat and mammary glands. In the center of the areola is the **nipple**, a protuberance covered by stratified squamous keratinized epithelium containing the terminal openings of the lactiferous ducts (Fig. 20.38). In fair-skinned individuals, a pinkish color is imparted to the nipple as a result of the color of blood in the rich vascular supply within the long dermal papillae that extend near its surface. During pregnancy, the color becomes darker because of increased pigmentation of the areola and the nipple.

The core of the nipple is composed of dense, irregular collagenous connective tissue with abundant elastic fibers connected to the surrounding skin or interlaced within the connective tissue and a rich component of smooth muscle cells. The wrinkling of the skin on the nipple results from the attachments of the elastic fibers. The abundant smooth muscle fibers are arranged in two ways: circularly around the nipple and radiating longitudinally along the long axis of the nipple. The contraction of these muscle fibers is responsible for erection of the nipple.

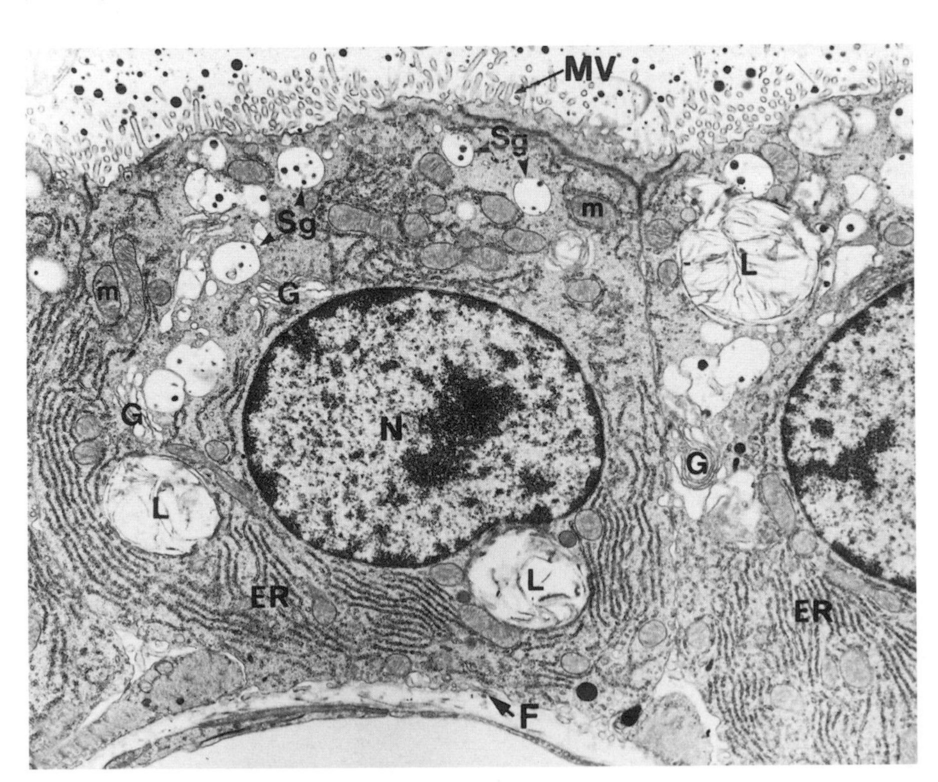

Fig. 20.37 Electron micrograph of an acinar cell from the lactating mammary gland of the rat. Note the large lipid droplets (L), abundant rough endoplasmic reticulum (ER), and the Golgi apparatus (G). F, Folds of the basal plasmalemma; m, mitochondria; MV, microvilli; Sg, secretory granules (×9000). (From Clermont Y, Xia I, Rambourg A, et al. Structure of the Golgi apparatus in stimulated and nonstimulated acinar cells of mammary glands of the rat. *Anat Rec.* 1993;237:308–317. Reprinted with permission from Wiley-Liss, Inc., a subsidiary of John Wiley & Sons, Inc.)

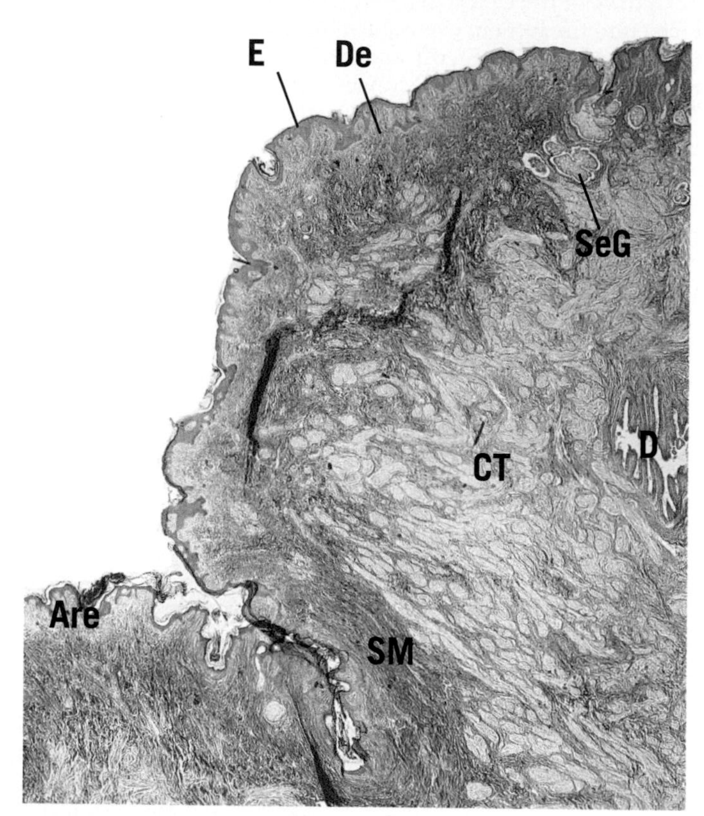

Fig. 20.38 Light micrograph of a human nipple shows a small part of the areola (Are). A lactiferous duct (D) is seen on its way to the surface. Note that the nipple is covered by skin, with a thin epidermis (E) and a thicker dermis (De) housing sebaceous glands (SeG). The dense collagenous connective tissue core (CT) is interwoven with elastic fibers and smooth muscle bundles (SM). (×14)

Most of the sebaceous glands located around the lactiferous ducts open onto the surface or sides of the nipple, although some open into the lactiferous ducts just before those ducts open onto the surface.

Mammary Gland Secretions

Prolactin is responsible for the production of milk by the mammary glands; oxytocin is responsible for the milk ejection reflex.

Although the expectant mother's mammary gland is prepared to secrete milk even before parturition, certain hormones prohibit this from occurring. However, when the placenta is detached after the baby is born, **prolactin** from the anterior pituitary stimulates the production of milk, which reaches full capacity in a few days. Before that, for the first 2 or 3 days after birth, a protein-rich thick fluid called ***colostrum*** is secreted. This high-protein secretion, rich in vitamin A, sodium, and chloride, also contains lymphocytes and monocytes, minerals, lactalbumin, and antibodies (immunoglobulin A) to nourish and protect the newborn.

Milk, usually produced by the fourth day after parturition, is a fluid that contains minerals, electrolytes, carbohydrates (including lactose), immunoglobulins (mostly immunoglobulin A), proteins (including caseins), and lipids. Production of milk results from the stimuli of sight, touch, handling of the newborn, and anticipation of nursing, events that create a surge in **prolactin** release. Once initiated, milk production is continuous, with the milk being stored within the duct system.

Concomitant with the production of prolactin, **oxytocin** is released from the posterior lobe of the pituitary. Oxytocin initiates the **milk ejection reflex** by inducing contractions of the myoepithelial cells around the alveoli and the ducts, thus expelling the milk.

Clinical Correlations

1. *Mothers who cannot* ***breastfeed*** *their infants on a regular feeding schedule are inclined to experience poor lactation. This may motivate a decision to discontinue nursing altogether, with the result that the infant is deprived of the passive immunity conferred by ingesting antibodies from the mother.*
2. ***Breast cancer****, second only to lung cancer as one of the major causes of cancer-related death in women, may be of two different types:* ***ductal carcinoma*** *of the ductal cells and* ***lobular carcinoma*** *of the terminal ductules. Detection must be early or the prognosis is poor because the carcinoma may* ***metastasize*** *to the axillary lymph nodes and from there to the lungs, bone, and brain. At the recommendation of the medical profession, early detection through self-examination and mammography has helped to reduce breast cancer mortality rates. In the year 2005, approximately 270,000 women and 1700 men were diagnosed with breast cancer in the United States, and approximately 40,000 women and 500 men died of breast cancer. There is an inverse relationship between the age of the woman and her risk of contracting the disease in that, in 2005, one out of 2200 women younger than the age of 30 years contracted breast cancer, whereas 1 of 54 and 1 of 23 women contracted breast cancer under 50 and 60 years of age, respectively. Although breast cancer is more likely to occur at an older age, younger women tend to have more aggressive breast cancers. In younger women, a family history of breast cancer should prompt genetic analysis for the presence of mutations or deficiencies in the BRCA1 and BRCA2 genes (on chromosomes 17 and 11, respectively). If either gene is mutated, the patient should go for genetic counseling, as well as for regular screening for the evidence of tumors. If focal calcifications, premalignant, or malignant lesions are suspected on the basis of mammography, needle biopsies should be performed to determine whether the lesion is suspicious.*
3. *In 2017, the Food and Drug Administration modified its earlier counsel concerning* ***breast implant–associated anaplastic large cell lymphoma (BIA-ALCL)****, a cancer of the lymphatic system. It appears that women with breast implants have a slightly greater risk of having* ***anaplastic large cell lymphoma (ALCL)*** *than women without an implant. Although the incidence of ALCL is approximately 2 per million women, it is a little greater in women who had a textured implant rather than a smooth implant. In fact, of the 231 cases of BIA-ALCL for which the implant type was reported, 28 were smooth and 203 were textured implants. Women diagnosed with BIA-ALCL developed the condition several years after the implant was placed.*

Stem Cells

There are special cells, known as **stem cells**, which possess the ability to divide and form daughter cells that are identical to themselves (**symmetrical division**) and to form daughter cells that differentiate into somatic cells with specific characteristics (asymmetrical division). There are two basic types of stem cells: those that are present in the early embryo only, specifically the cells of the **morula** and the **inner cell mass** (**embryoblasts**) of the blastocyst, known as **embryonic stem cells** (**ESCs**); and those that remain in most adult tissues, known as **adult stem cells** (**ASCs**). These two categories are different because ESCs are **pluripotent**, that is, they can differentiate into any cell of the three germ layers (ectoderm, mesoderm, and endoderm), whereas adult stem cells have a limited differentiation capability. Examples of adult stem cells have been discussed in most chapters of this textbook, as in cells of the stratum basale of the epidermis, regenerative cells of the lining of the digestive tract, osteoprogenitor cells of bone, and hematopoietic stem cells of the bone marrow, among many others.

Embryonic stem cells, therefore, may be harvested from blastocysts of in vitro fertilization, and, if cultured appropriately, these cells can divide symmetrically an untold number of times without losing their undifferentiated state and without undergoing the senescence to which other types of cultured cells eventually succumb. This ability is attributed to the high concentration of the enzyme **telomerase** in these cells that protects them from losing the ability to divide. Given the proper signals, these cells can then undergo asymmetrical division and form any particular cell derivative of any of the three germ layers. These ESCs can be used in **stem cell therapy** to replace defective cells of the adult; for instance, they can be coaxed into forming beta cells of the islets of Langerhans, which can produce insulin in individuals with type I diabetes. However, ethical considerations prevent their use in human beings.

Adult stem cells function in replacing injured tissue (as pericytes of blood vessels) and also to replenish discarded cells, such as those of the blood. In the first decade of the 21st century, a major accomplishment was reported—that fully differentiated adult somatic cells can be reprogrammed to become pluripotential cells, which were named **induced pluripotent stem cells (iPSCs)**. These cells behave just as if they were embryonic stem cells, that is, morphologically, they are identical to ESCs, possess the same high levels of telomerase, display the same surface markers as ESCs, and have the ability to be induced to differentiate into cells of all three germ layers. The major benefit of these cells is that the somatic cells can be harvested from the individual patient and reprogrammed to become iPSCs, and the patient's immune system will not mount an immune response against them. Unfortunately, currently, it is difficult to control iPSCs because only some of the reprogrammed cells form the requisite differentiated cell, and others can form teratomas and other tumors. It is hoped that continued research into stem cells will ameliorate these problems.

Pathological Considerations

See Figs. 20.39 through 20.42.

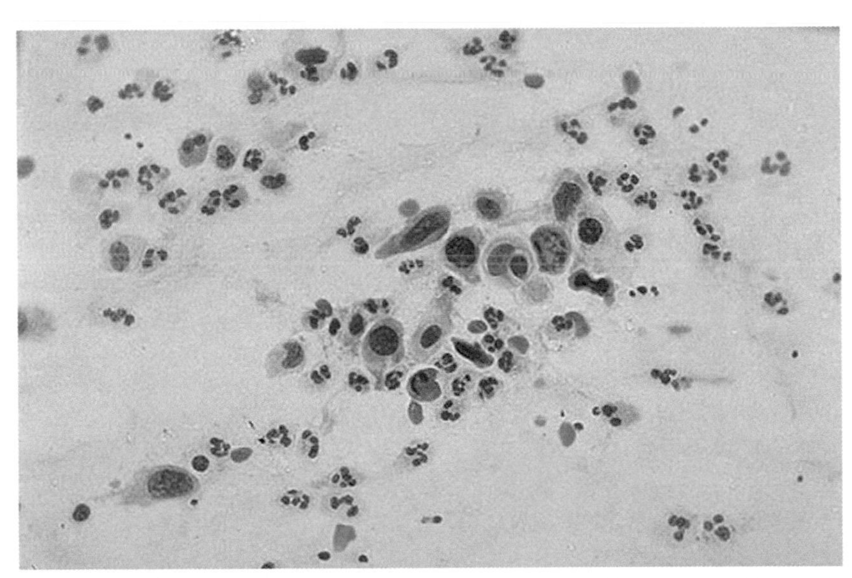

Fig. 20.39 Photomicrograph of cervical squamous carcinoma present in a Pap smear. Note the presence of large, pleomorphic cells in the center of the field. The large number of inflammatory cells and erythrocytes indicate an aggressive, ulcerative, and invasive lesion. (Reprinted with permission from Klatt EC. *Robbins and Cotran: Atlas of Pathology*. 2nd ed. Philadelphia: Elsevier; 2010:324.)

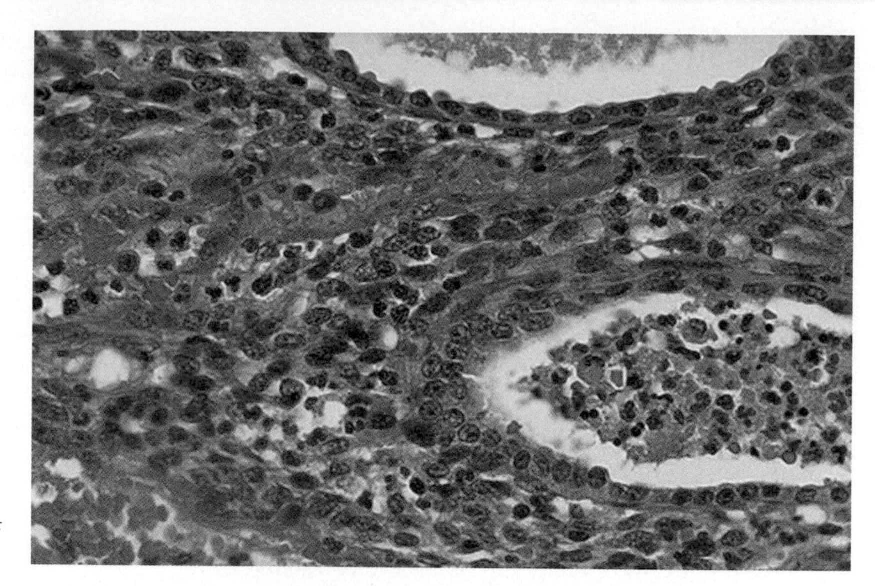

Fig. 20.40 Photomicrograph of the uterus of a patient with acute endometriosis. This condition is evidenced by the presence of neutrophils scattered throughout the stroma and glands of the endometrium. (Reprinted with permission from Klatt EC. *Robbins and Cotran: Atlas of Pathology*. 2nd ed. Philadelphia: Elsevier; 2010:333.)

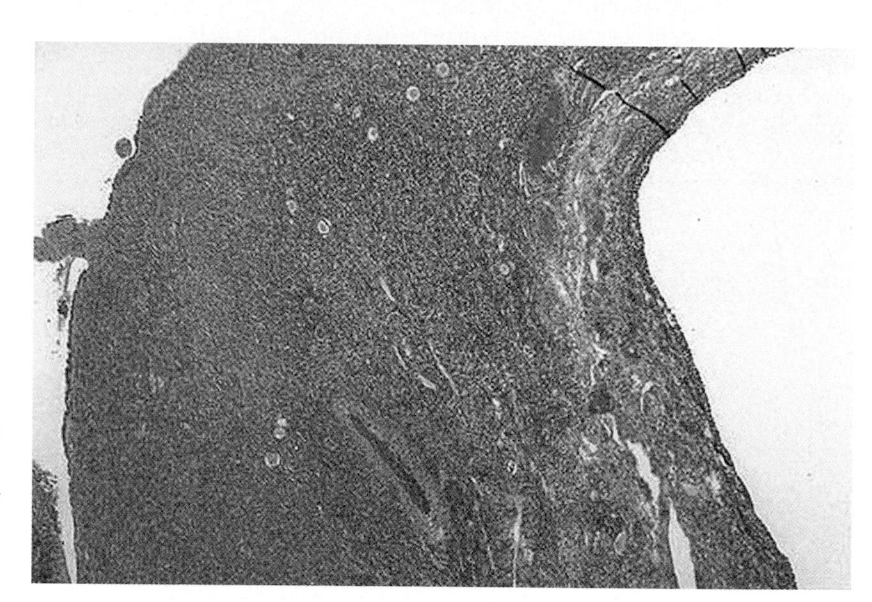

Fig. 20.41 Photomicrograph of the ovary of a patient with polycystic ovarian disease. This condition is characterized by a very thick ovarian cortex *(left side of the field)*, as well as the presence of numerous follicle cysts (one of which is displayed on the *right side of the field*). (Reprinted with permission from Klatt EC. *Robbins and Cotran: Atlas of Pathology*. 2nd ed. Philadelphia: Elsevier; 2010:341.)

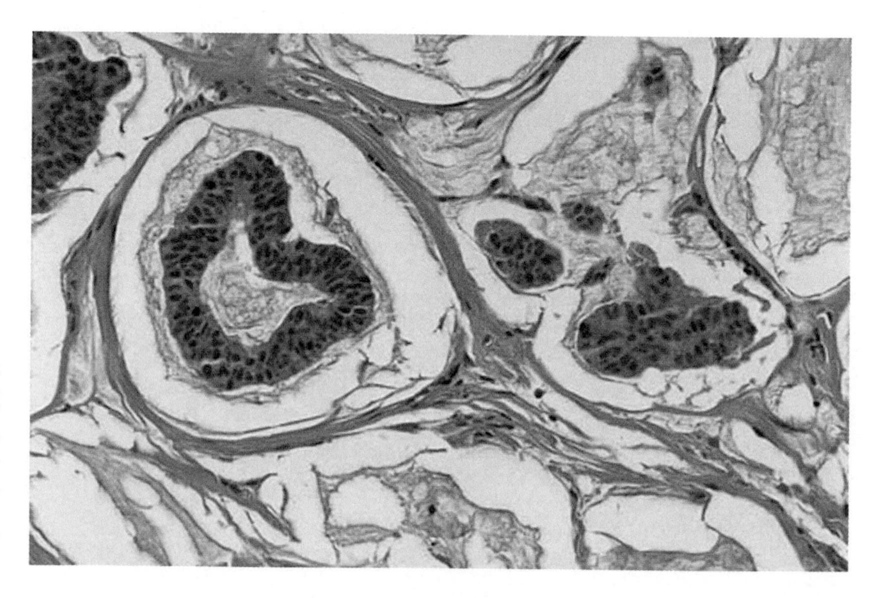

Fig. 20.42 Photomicrograph of the breast of a patient with mucinous carcinoma of the breast (also known as *colloid carcinoma of the breast*). This condition is a form of ductal carcinoma, an invasive breast cancer, in which the malignant cells are surrounded by a large amount of mucin that they manufacture. Frequently, this type of tumor is associated with mutations in the *BRCA* gene. (Reprinted with permission from Klatt EC. *Robbins and Cotran: Atlas of Pathology*. 2nd ed. Philadelphia: Elsevier; 2010:377.)

Histology Laboratory Instructions: Female Reproductive System

Ovary

Primordial Follicle

The cortex of the ovary houses a plethora of ovarian follicles in various stages of development. The most numerous of these are the primordial follicles, which consist of a single layer of flat follicular cells that surround a primary oocyte. In this photomicrograph, the simple cuboidal germinal epithelium and the very cellular ovarian stroma are well represented (see Fig. 20.3, P, GE, St).

Primary Follicle

As the primordial follicles begin the maturation process to become unilaminar primary follicles, the follicular cells differentiate into a single layer of cuboidal cells that surround the primary oocyte whose large, vesicular appearing nucleus houses a single, large nucleolus. As the unilaminar primary follicle continues to develop, its follicular cells undergo mitosis to form two or more follicular cell layers around the primary oocyte, differentiating into multilaminar primary follicles. The ovarian stroma is a highly cellular connective tissue with a well-developed vascular supply. Note the primordial follicle with its flat follicular cells surrounding the primary oocyte (see Fig. 20.5, cFC, N, n, St, BV, fFC).

Secondary Follicle

Secondary, antral, follicles resemble multilaminar primary follicles in that they have several layers of follicular cells (granulosa cells) surrounding the primary oocyte except that there are accumulations of liquor folliculi in the extracellular spaces of the granulosa cells. Note that the granulosa cells are surrounded by the theca interna (see Fig. 20.6, G, LF, T). At a higher magnification, the follicular cells are clearly seen to be cuboidal and the follicular fluid occupies several, possibly interconnected, extracellular spaces. Note that the granulosa cells are separated from the theca interna by a well-defined basement membrane. Observe that the theca interna is more cellular than is the theca externa (see Fig. 20.7, FC, FF, TI, *arrow*, TE).

Graafian (Mature) Follicle

Graafian (mature) follicles are very large structures that bulge off the ovaries and may be as large as the ovary itself. This mature follicle is still in the process of development even though the liquor folliculi has collected into a single chamber, known as the antrum, which is surrounded by mural granulosa cells (membrana granulosa), follicular cells several cell layers thick. The cumulus oophorus is composed of the cumulus granulosa cells, whose innermost layer, the corona radiata, contacts the zona pellucida, which surrounds the primary oocyte. The theca interna is separated from the membrana granulosa by the well-developed basement membrane. The theca externa surrounds the theca interna and its peripheral aspect blends in with the stroma of the ovarian cortex. The capsule of the ovary, the tunica albuginea, is covered by a simple cuboidal (at times simple squamous) epithelium, known as the germinal epithelium, a region of the peritoneum (see Fig. 20.8, LF, MG, CO, ZP, PO, TI, *arrow*, TE, St, TA, *arrowhead*). A higher magnification of the region of the cumulus oophorus displays the theca externa and the theca interna, as well as the basement membrane that separates the theca interna from the membrana granulosa. The liquor folliculi surrounds the cumulus oophorus, which houses the primary oocyte, which is surrounded by the zona pellucida. Observe that filopodia of the cells of the corona radiata penetrate the zona pellucida to contact the cell membrane of the primary oocyte (see Fig. 20.9, TE, TI, *arrow*, MG, LF, PO, CR, ZP).

Corpus Luteum

After ovulation, the remnant of the dominant follicle becomes reorganized and forms the corpus hemorrhagicum, which becomes transformed into the corpus luteum, a highly vascularized temporary endocrine gland, composed basically of two cell types: the large, lightly stained, vesicular-appearing derivatives of the granulosa cells of the dominant follicle, known as granulosa-lutein cells, and the smaller, theca interna cell derivatives, the theca-lutein cells (see Fig. 20.11, G, T). At higher magnification, the morphology of the granulosa-lutein cells and the theca-lutein cells are more evident (see Fig. 20.12, GL, TL).

Corpus Albicans

As the corpus luteum finishes its function, it becomes invaded by fibroblasts, T cells, and macrophages and undergoes luteolysis. The fibroblasts manufacture collagen fibers; as the corpus luteum becomes fibrotic, it becomes known as the corpus albicans, which is surrounded by the ovarian stroma. The difference between the highly cellular stroma and the fibrous tissue of the corpus albicans is self-evident (see Fig. 20.14, St, FT).

Oviduct

The oviduct (fallopian tube) acts as a conduit for spermatozoa to reach the secondary oocyte and as a conduit conveying the fertilized egg to the uterus. In order to be able to do that, the oviduct possesses a thick muscularis composed of an inner circular and an outer longitudinal smooth muscle layer. The outer smooth muscle layer is covered by a subserous connective tissue and a simple squamous epithelium, the serosa. The lumen of the oviduct is lined by a highly folded mucosa that, owing to its complex longitudinal folds, reduces the size of the lumen. The mucosa consists of a richly vascularized lamina propria and an epithelium composed of two types of cells: (1) peg cells that possess no cilia but manufacture a nutrient-rich substance that provides nutrition for the spermatozoa as well as for the fertilized ovum; and (2) ciliated cells whose cilia assist in the movement of the fertilized egg as well as for the movement of spermatozoa to reach the secondary oocyte (see Fig. 20.15, I, O, M). A higher magnification of the mucosa and inner circular smooth muscle layer demonstrates the folded nature of the mucosa. Note that the lumen is lined by a simple columnar epithelium deep to which is the lamina propria (see Fig. 20.16, IC, E, LP). At high magnification, the two types of cells that constitute the oviduct simple columnar epithelium are clearly distinguishable. Note the presence of cilia of the wider ciliated cells and the apical bulging of the cytoplasm of the narrow peg cells. Observe the capillaries in the cell-rich lamina propria (see Fig. 20.17, *arrow*, CC, *arrowhead*, PC, Ca, LP).

Phases of the Uterine Endometrium

Menstrual Phase (Day 1 to Day 3 or 4)

The menstrual phase of the uterine endometrium lasts 3 to 4 days. The simple columnar epithelial lining is disrupted and the underlying necrotic tissue houses free leukocytes whose nuclei are clearly evident. During the first day or so of the menstrual phase, many of the uterine glands and helical arteries appear to be healthy (see Fig. 20.21, *arrow*, NT, N, Gl, HA).

Proliferative (Follicular) Phase (Day 4 or 5 to Day 14)

The menstrual phase is followed by the proliferative (follicular) phase when the endometrium begins the healing and restorative process. The simple columnar epithelial lining of the lumen is reestablished and the uterine glands begin to be formed but do not as yet produce secretions. The stroma of the functionalis layer appears healthy, with almost an absence of the invading leukocytes noted in the menstrual phase. The helical arteries are also penetrating the functionalis layer (see Fig. 20.22, E, L, Gl St, BV).

Secretory (Luteal) Phase (Day 15 to 28)

The early secretory (luteal) phase of the endometrium presents with glands that are beginning to be coiled and whose lumina are lined by a columnar epithelium that is beginning to manufacture the secretory product that will nourish the developing embryo prior to the formation of the placenta. The stroma becomes more condensed and reduced in volume (see Fig. 20.23, L, E, St). The late luteal phase displays endometrial glands that are more branched and more coiled and whose lumina are filled with secretory material. The epithelial lining of the glands have a sawtooth appearance because some of the columnar cells of this simple columnar epithelium are taller and plumper than their neighbors. The stroma is even more compressed than it was in the early luteal phase (see Fig. 20.24 L, *arrows*, St).

Placenta

Viewing the placenta at a low magnification displays the decidual cells of the decidua basalis, as well as the anchoring chorionic villi that are attached to the decidua basalis. The blindly ending terminal villi are bathed in the maternal blood that fills the intervillous spaces (see Fig. 20.28, DC, DB, AV, TV, IS). A medium magnification of the placenta displays the fetal blood vessels surrounded by the mesoderm of the terminal villi that are cut in cross-sections and oblique sections as they are bathed in the maternal blood located in the intervillous spaces. Observe that the terminal villi are covered by syncytiotrophoblasts whose nuclei frequently form clusters, known as syncytial knots (see Fig. 20.29, BV, Me, TV, IS, ST, SK).

Vagina

The vagina is a fibromuscular sheath whose lumen is lined by a stratified squamous nonkeratinized epithelium. The lamina propria is a loose type of fibroelastic connective tissue whose deeper region is richly vascularized and is occasionally referred to as the submucosa. The deepest region of the vaginal wall is the muscular layer, possessing poorly differentiated inner circular and outer longitudinal smooth muscle fibers. The outermost layer of the wall of the vagina is composed of fibroelastic connective tissue, known as the adventitia, which aids the vagina in adhering to the surrounding structures (see Fig. 20.30, L, E, LP, BV, SM, M). The deeper layers of the stratified squamous nonkeratinized epithelium lining the lumen of the vagina are composed of denser-appearing cells, whereas the more superficial layers are filled with glycogen and, consequently, are larger and lighter staining. A well-defined basement membrane separates the epithelium from the vascular lamina propria, which is often infiltrated by lymphoid cells (Fig. 20.31, E, L, *arrows*, BV, LP).

Mammary Gland

When the mammary gland is not producing milk, it is said to be resting (inactive). When it is actively producing milk to supply nourishment to the infant, it is said to be lactating (active).

Resting (Inactive) Mammary Gland

The resting (inactive) mammary gland displays numerous ducts and alveolar buds surrounded by dense, irregular, collagenous connective tissue, as well as lobules of adipose tissue (see Fig. 20.33, D, AB, CT).

Lactating (Active) Mammary Gland

The lactating (active) mammary gland has lobules of alveoli, many of whose lumina house milk. The lobules are separated from each other by compressed dense collagenous connective tissue elements (see Fig. 20.34, Al, Milk, CT). At a higher magnification, the alveoli are noted to be branched, and connective tissue elements are noted to separate lobules of alveoli from each other (Fig. 20.35 AI, CT). At medium magnification, the branching of the alveoli is clearly evident and their lumina display the presence of milk solids. Note that the glandular epithelial cells of the alveoli have large droplets of milk lipids at their apical region that will be released via the apocrine mode of secretion (see Fig. 20.36 L, *arrowheads*, Ep, *arrows*).

Nipple

The nipple is a skin-covered protuberance in the middle of the areola that contains the terminal openings of the lactiferous ducts. The thin epidermis of the nipple overlies the equally thin dermis that houses numerous sebaceous glands. The core of the nipple is composed of a dense, irregular fibroelastic connective tissue interwoven with smooth muscle fiber bundles that causes the nipple to become erect during sexual stimulation and when exposed to cold temperature (see Fig. 20.38, Are, D, E, De, SeG, CT, SM).

21 Male Reproductive System

The two testes suspended in the scrotum, a system of intratesticular and extratesticular genital ducts, associated glands, and the male copulatory organ (the penis), constitute the male reproductive system (Fig. 21.1). **Spermatozoa** formation—as well as the synthesis, storage, and release of the male sex hormone testosterone—are performed by the two testes.

The glands associated with the male reproductive tract are the paired **seminal vesicles**, the single **prostate gland**, and the two **bulbourethral glands (of Cowper)**, which form the noncellular portion of **semen** (spermatozoa suspended in the secretions of the accessory glands), which not only nourishes the spermatozoa but also provides a fluid vehicle for their delivery into the female reproductive tract. The **penis** has a dual function: it serves as the conduit of urine from the urinary bladder to outside of the body and delivers semen to the female reproductive tract during copulation.

Testes

The testes, located in the scrotum, are paired organs that produce spermatozoa and testosterone.

Each testis of a mature male is an oval organ approximately 4 cm long, 2 to 3 cm wide, and 3 cm thick. In approximately 60% of males, the left testis is suspended 1 to 2 cm lower in the scrotum than the right testis. The testes develop on the posterior wall of the abdominal cavity behind the peritoneum and carry with them a sack of peritoneum as they descend into the scrotum. This peritoneal pouch, the **tunica vaginalis**, forms a serous cavity encompassing the anterolateral aspect of each testis, permitting it some degree of mobility within its scrotal compartment.

The wall of the scrotum houses smooth muscle fibers, the **dartos muscle**, which contributes to the regulation of the temperature within the scrotum. In cold temperature, the dartos muscle contracts, not only releasing heat of contraction but also bringing the testes closer to the body wall. The paired **cremaster muscles**, skeletal muscles located in the inguinal canal also bring the testes closer to the body wall as they contract. The main function of the cremaster muscles is protection of the testes by moving them out of harm's way during copulation, as well as when the individual is experiencing fear. Even though they are skeletal muscles, they act in an involuntary fashion most of the time, although they may be activated voluntarily when the abdominal muscles are contracted.

GENERAL STRUCTURE AND VASCULAR SUPPLY OF THE TESTES

Connective tissue septa divide the testis into lobuli testis, each of which houses one to four seminiferous tubules.

The testis has a two-layered capsule, the outer dense, irregular, collagenous connective tissue, the **tunica albuginea**. Immediately deep to it is the highly vascularized loose connective tissue, the **tunica vasculosa.** The posterior aspect of the tunica albuginea is somewhat thickened, forming the **mediastinum testis**, from which connective tissue septa radiate to subdivide each testis into approximately 250 pyramid-shaped intercommunicating compartments known as the **lobuli testis** (Fig. 21.2).

Each lobule contains one to four blindly ending **seminiferous tubules**, which are surrounded by a richly innervated and highly vascularized loose connective tissue derived from the tunica vasculosa. Dispersed throughout this connective tissue are small clusters of endocrine cells, the **interstitial cells (of Leydig)**, responsible for the synthesis of testosterone.

Spermatozoa are produced by the **seminiferous epithelium** of the seminiferous tubules. Spermatozoa enter short straight ducts, **tubuli recti**, which connect the open end of each seminiferous tubule to the **rete testis,** a system of labyrinthine spaces housed within the mediastinum testis. The spermatozoa leave the rete testis through 10 to 20 short tubules, the **ductuli efferentes**, which eventually fuse with the **ductus epididymis**, the first part of the extratesticular genital ducts. From the epididymis spermatozoa enter the ductus deferens (vas deferens). From there they reach the ejaculatory ducts, which lead the spermatozoa to the urethra, where the secretions of the accessory genital glands join the spermatozoa. The spermatozoa, suspended in these secretions, form the semen, which leaves the male reproductive system at the tip of the penis, through the external urethral orifice.

Blood to each testis is supplied by the **testicular artery** (a branch of the abdominal aorta) which, during embryogenesis, descends with the testis into the scrotum, accompanied by the **ductus deferens (vas deferens)**. The testicular artery forms several branches that pierce the capsule of the testis to supply the testicular capillary beds, whose blood is drained into several intertwining veins, the **pampiniform plexus of veins,** which are wrapped around the testicular artery. The artery, veins, lymph vessels, nerve fibers, and ductus deferens together form the **spermatic cord**, which passes through the inguinal canal, the passageway from the abdominal cavity to the scrotum.

Blood in the pampiniform plexus of veins is cooler than that in the testicular artery and, therefore, acts to reduce the temperature of the arterial blood, forming a **countercurrent heat exchange system.** In this fashion, it helps keep the temperature of the testes about 2°C lower than that of the remainder of the body. At this cooler temperature (35°C), spermatozoa develop normally. If they developed at body temperature (36.7°C–37.1°C), spermatozoa would be sterile. Also, because the testes, unlike the ovaries, are not located in the body cavity but rather in the scrotum, they are exposed to a lower temperature. This enhances the cooling effect of the pampiniform plexus of veins.

Lymphatic drainage of the testes is accomplished by lymph vessels that accompany the testicular arteries to drain into the periaortic lymph nodes.

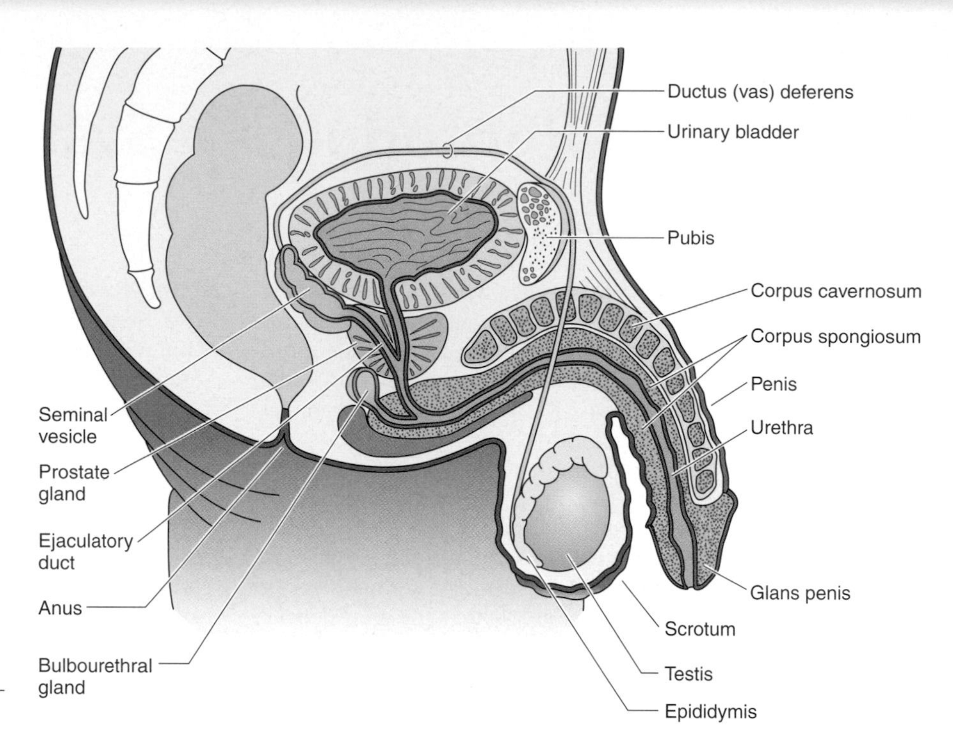

Fig. 21.1 Schematic diagram of the male reproductive system.

> ***Clinical Correlations***
>
> 1. *Because hyperthermia has been identified as a factor in male infertility, it has been reported that males who work with laptop computers held on their laps for 1 hour of continuous use exhibited an increase in scrotal temperatures by as much as 2.8°C. Although these studies are not conclusive, it is suggested that boys and young men may wish to limit the use of computers on their laps.*
> 2. *The temperature of the testes also varies with the type of underwear that male subjects wear. It has been demonstrated that men wearing boxer shorts have about 17% higher sperm count, 25% higher sperm concentration, and 33% more motile spermatozoa than men wearing tight briefs that bring the testes closer to the abdominal wall, increasing the testicular temperature. However, in spite of these differences, in both groups of individuals tested the sperm counts, sperm concentration, and sperm motility were within normal limits. A problem may occur in men who are having difficulties in impregnating their partners; the reduction in sperm count, concentration, and motility in these individuals may be sufficient to interfere with the fertility of their spermatozoa.*
> 3. *Metastatic testicular cancers spread via the lymphatic drainage into the periaortic lymph nodes and from there to their various final destinations.*

SEMINIFEROUS TUBULES

Seminiferous tubules are composed of a thick seminiferous epithelium surrounded by a thin connective tissue, the tunica propria.

Seminiferous tubules are highly convoluted hollow tubules, 30 to 70 cm long and 150 to 250 μm in diameter; they are surrounded by extensive capillary beds. About 1000 seminiferous

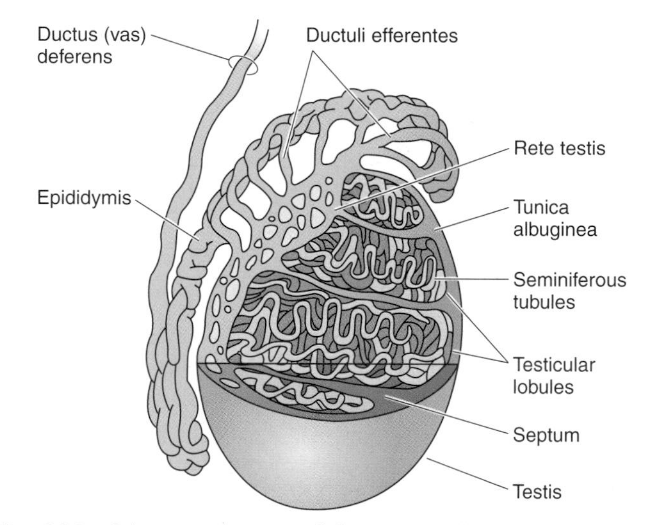

Fig. 21.2 Schematic diagram of the testis and epididymis. Lobules and their contents are not drawn to scale.

tubules are present in the two testes, for a total length of nearly 0.5 km (0.3 mile), dedicated to the production of spermatozoa. Approximately 85% to 90% of the volume of each testis is occupied by the seminiferous tubules.

The wall of the seminiferous tubule is composed of a slender connective tissue layer, the **tunica propria,** and a thick seminiferous epithelium. The tunica propria and the seminiferous epithelium are separated from each other by a well-developed **basal lamina**. The connective tissue comprises mostly interlaced, slender, type I collagen fiber bundles housing several layers of fibroblasts. **Myoid cells**, similar to smooth muscle, are also present, which impart contractility to the seminiferous tubules.

The seminiferous epithelium (or **germinal epithelium**) is several cell layers thick (Figs. 21.3–21.6) and is composed of two types of cells: Sertoli cells and spermatogenic cells (Figs. 21.6 and Fig. 21.7). The latter cells are in various stages of maturation.

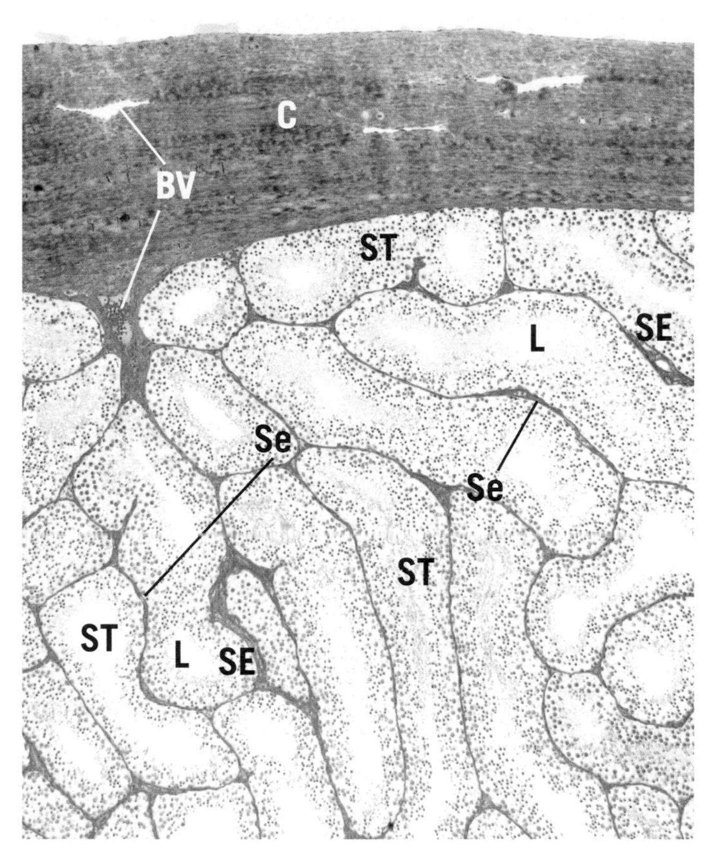

Fig. 21.3 At a very low magnification, the vascular supply (BV) of the testicular capsule (C) is well illustrated. Observe that the walls (Se) are closely applied to each other and that the thick seminiferous epithelium (SE) of the seminiferous tubules (ST) are pale in comparison. The lumina (L) of the seminiferous tubules are clearly visible. (×56)

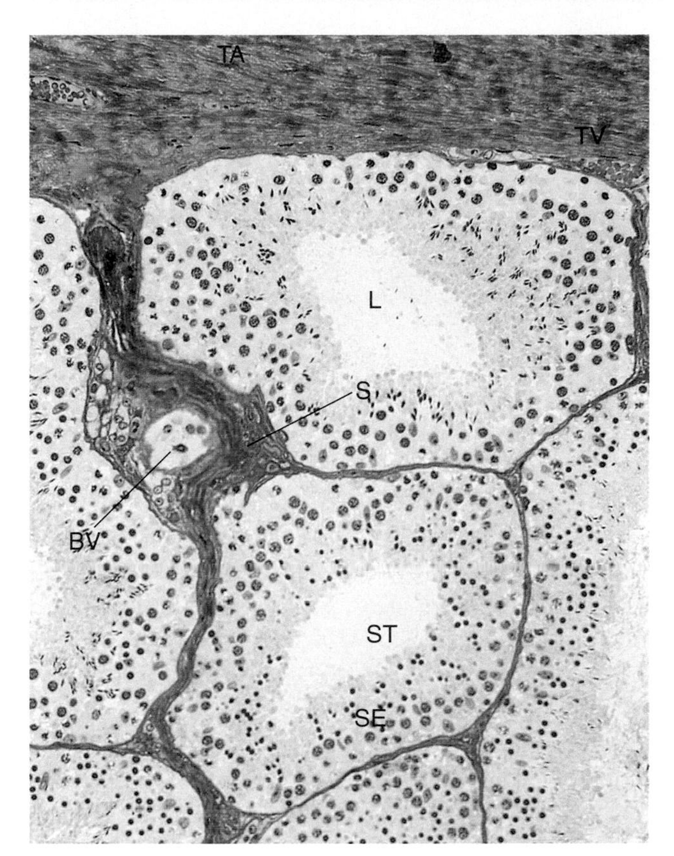

Fig. 21.4 Photomicrograph of the capsule of a monkey testis and cross-sectional profiles of seminiferous tubules (ST), blood vessel (BV), tunica albuginea (TA), tunica vasculosa (TV), lumen (L), seminiferous epithelium (SE), and septa (Se). (×132)

Sertoli Cells

Sertoli cells support, protect, and nourish spermatogenic cells; phagocytose cytoplasmic remnants of spermatids; secrete androgen-binding protein, hormones, and a nutritive medium; and establish the blood–testis barrier.

Sertoli cells are tall, columnar cells whose basolateral infoldings envelop groups of spermatogenic cells and their highly folded apical cell membranes project into the lumina of the seminiferous tubules, where they couch developing spermatozoa. These cells have a basally located, clear, oval nucleus with a large, centrally positioned nucleolus (see Figs. 21.6 and 21.7). Their cytoplasm has been shown to house inclusion products known as ***crystalloids of Charcot-Böttcher***, the composition and function of which are not known. The basal cell membrane of Sertoli cells possesses receptors for follicle-stimulating hormone (FSH) and for androgens.

Electron micrographs reveal that the cytoplasm of Sertoli cells is replete with profiles of smooth endoplasmic reticulum (SER), but only a limited amount of rough endoplasmic reticulum (RER). Sertoli cells possess numerous mitochondria, a well-developed Golgi apparatus, and numerous vesicles that belong to the endolysosomal complex. The cytoskeletal elements of these cells are also abundant, indicating that one of their functions is to provide structural support for the developing gametes.

The lateral cell membranes of adjacent Sertoli cells form occluding junctions, thus subdividing the lumen of the seminiferous tubule into two isolated, concentric compartments (see Figs. 21.7 and 21.8). The **basal compartment** is narrower, located basal to the zonulae occludentes, and surrounds the wider **adluminal compartment**. Thus, the zonulae occludentes of the Sertoli cells establish a blood–testis barrier that isolates the adluminal compartment from connective tissue influences, protecting the developing gametes from the immune system. Because spermatogenesis begins after puberty, the newly differentiating germ cells, which have a different chromosome number, as well as express different surface membrane receptors and molecules, would be considered "foreign cells" by the immune system. Were it not for the isolation of germ cells from the connective tissue compartments by the zonulae occludentes of the Sertoli cells, an immune response would be mounted against them.

Sertoli cells perform the following functions:

- Physical and nutritional support of the developing germ cells
- Phagocytosis of cytoplasm eliminated during spermiogenesis
- Establishment of a blood–testis barrier by the formation of zonulae occludentes between adjacent Sertoli cells
- Synthesis and release of **androgen-binding protein (ABP)**, a macromolecule that facilitates an increase in the concentration of testosterone in the seminiferous tubule by binding to it and preventing it from leaving the tubule
- Synthesis and release (during embryogenesis) of **antimullerian hormone,** which suppresses the formation of the mullerian duct (precursor of the female reproductive system) and, thus, establishes the "maleness" of the developing embryo

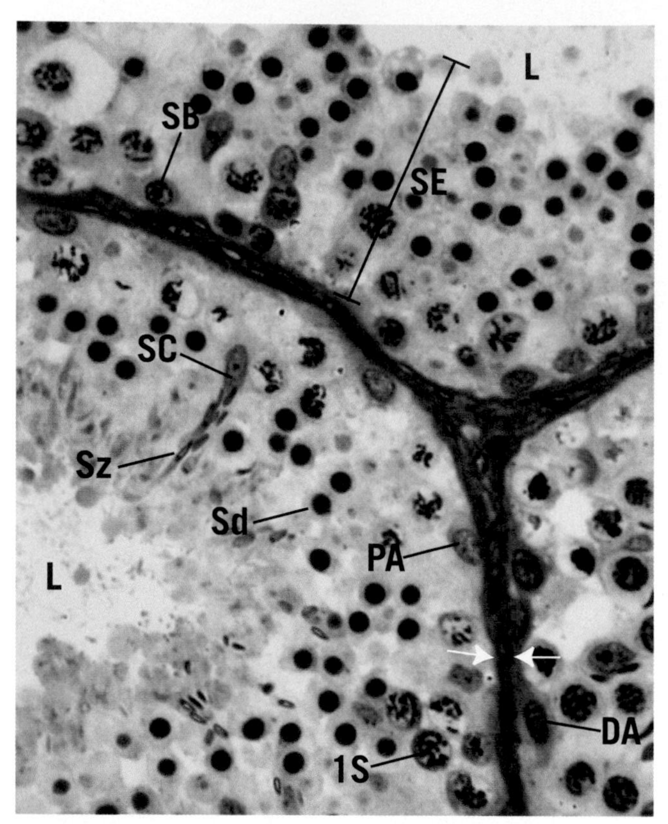

Fig. 21.5 In this high-magnification photomicrograph of the testis, as three seminiferous tubules contact each other their narrow tunicae propriae appear to fuse with each other *(between the white arrows)*. Observe that the thick seminiferous epithelia (SE) are composed of supportive Sertoli cells (SC) and spermatogenic cells in various stages of development—dark A type spermatogonia (DA), pale A type spermatogonia (PA) and type B spermatogonia (SB) —all lying against the basement membrane separating them from the tunica propria. Primary spermatocytes (1S), spermatids (Sd), and spermatozoa (Sz) are also easily recognized. Secondary spermatocytes are elusive because they quickly transition into spermatids, with a very short life span of about 10 hours. The lumina of the seminiferous tubules are divided into an adluminal and basal compartment. (×540)

- Synthesis and secretion of **inhibin**, a hormone that inhibits the release of FSH by the anterior pituitary
- Synthesis of **activin**, a hormone that facilitates the release of FSH from the anterior pituitary
- Secretion of a fructose-rich medium that nourishes and facilitates the transport of spermatozoa to the genital ducts
- Synthesis and secretion of **Ets-related molecule (ERM) transmission factor**, which sustains the stem cell lines necessary for spermatogonia formation
- Synthesis and secretion of **testicular transferrin**, an apoprotein that accepts iron from serum transferrin and conveys it to maturing gametes
- Synthesis and secretion of molecules, such as **Fas ligand** (**Fas-L**) that forces cells expressing Fas receptors into apoptosis; therefore if cytotoxic T cells enter the adluminal compartment, Fas-L would force them into apoptosis, protecting the forming germ cells against an immune response.

Spermatogenic Cells

The process of spermatogenesis, whereby spermatogonia give rise to spermatozoa, is divided into three phases: spermatocytogenesis, meiosis, and spermiogenesis.

Most of the cells composing the thick seminiferous epithelium are **spermatogenic cells** in various stages of maturation (see Figs. 21.5–21.7). Some of these cells, **spermatogonia**, are located in the basal compartment, whereas most of the developing cells—**primary spermatocytes**, **secondary spermatocytes**, **spermatids**, and **spermatozoa**—occupy the adluminal compartment. Spermatogonia are diploid cells that undergo mitotic division to form more spermatogonia and primary spermatocytes, which migrate from the basal into the adluminal compartment. Primary spermatocytes enter the **first meiotic division** to form secondary spermatocytes, which undergo the **second meiotic division** to form **haploid** cells known as ***spermatids***. These haploid cells are transformed into spermatozoa (mature sperm) through shedding of much of their cytoplasm, rearrangement of their organelles, and formation of flagella.

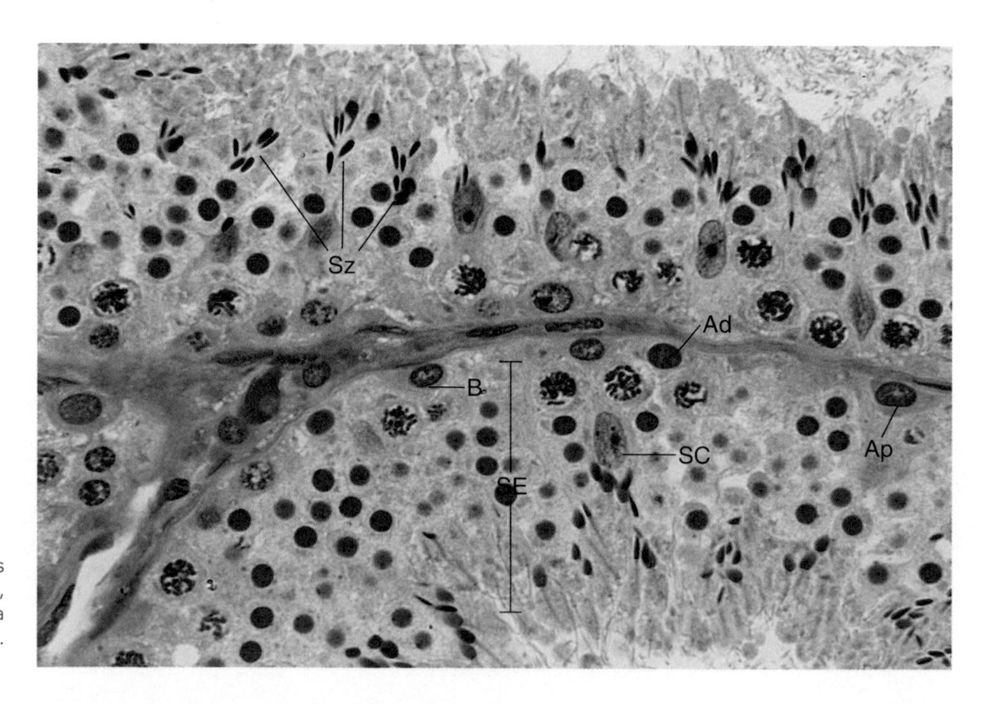

Fig. 21.6 Seminiferous tubule. Seminiferous epithelium (SE), pale spermatogonia A (Ap), dark spermatogonia A (Ad), spermatogonia B (B), Sertoli cell (SC), and spermatozoa (Sz). (×540)

The various cell types that result from this process of cell maturation, called ***spermatogenesis***, are diagrammed in Fig. 21.9. The maturation process is divided into three phases:

- **Spermatocytogenesis**—Differentiation of spermatogonia into primary spermatocytes
- **Meiosis**—Reduction division whereby diploid primary spermatocytes reduce their chromosome complement, forming haploid spermatids
- **Spermiogenesis**—Transformation of spermatids into spermatozoa (sperm)

Differentiation of Spermatogonia

Spermatogonia are diploid (2n) and are influenced by testosterone at puberty to enter the cell cycle.

Spermatogonia, small, diploid germ cells located in the basal compartment of the seminiferous tubules (see Figs. 21.7 and 21.9), lie on the basement membrane and, subsequent to puberty, become influenced by testosterone to enter the cell cycle. There are three categories of spermatogonia:

- **Dark type A spermatogonia** are small (12 µm in diameter), dome-shaped cells that have flattened, oval nuclei with abundant heterochromatin, imparting a dense appearance to the nucleus. They are **reserve cells** that have *not* entered the cell cycle but may do so. Their mitotic rate is slow and they are quite resistant to insults such as low levels of ionizing radiation. Once they undergo mitosis, they form additional dark type A spermatogonia and pale type A spermatogonia.
- **Pale type A spermatogonia** are identical to the dark type A cells, but their nuclei have abundant euchromatin, giving them a pale appearance. These cells have only a few organelles, including mitochondria, a limited Golgi complex, some RER, and numerous free ribosomes. They are induced by testosterone to *proliferate* by undergoing mitosis, giving rise to additional pale type A spermatogonia and to type B spermatogonia.
- **Type B spermatogonia** resemble pale type A spermatogonia, but usually their nuclei are round rather than flattened. They are the most sensitive of the spermatogenic cells to the deleterious effects of ionizing radiation. These cells also divide mitotically to give rise to primary spermatocytes.

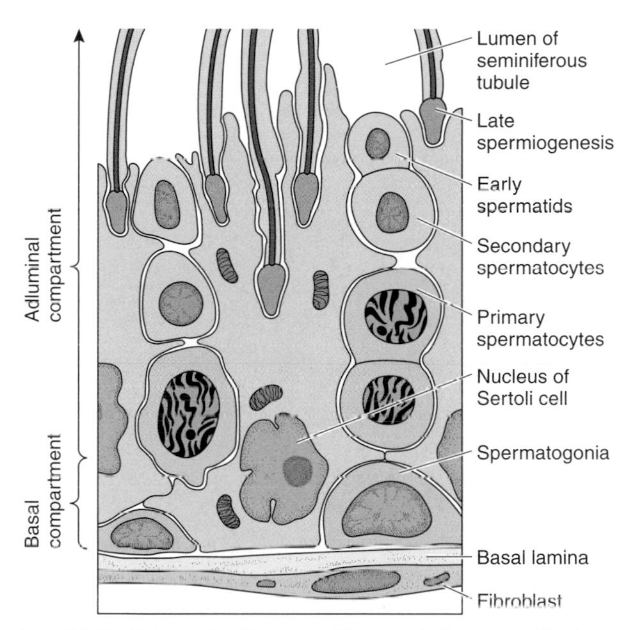

Fig. 21.7 Schematic diagram of the seminiferous epithelium.

Meiotic Division of Spermatocytes

The first meiotic division of the primary spermatocyte, followed by the second meiotic division of the secondary spermatocyte, reduces the chromosome number and deoxyribonucleic acid (DNA) content to the haploid (n) state in the spermatids.

As soon as **primary spermatocytes** are formed, they migrate from the basal compartment into the adluminal compartment. As these cells migrate between adjacent Sertoli cells, they form zonulae occludentes with the Sertoli cells, helping maintain the integrity of the blood–testis barrier. Primary spermatocytes are the largest cells of the seminiferous epithelium (see Fig. 21.7), possessing large, vesicular-appearing nuclei whose chromosomes are in various stages of condensation. Shortly after their

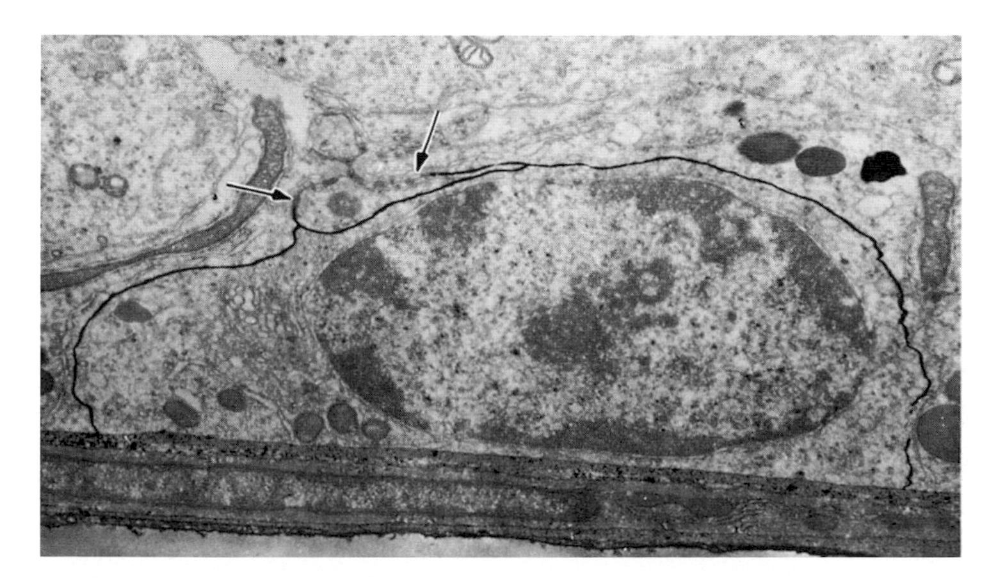

Fig. 21.8 Electron micrograph of the basal compartment of the seminiferous epithelium (×15,000). The testis has been perfused with an electron-dense tracer (lanthanum nitrate) to demonstrate that the occluding junctions *(arrows)* between adjacent Sertoli cells prevent the tracer from entering the adluminal compartment. (From Leeson TS, Leeson CR, Papparo AA. *Text/Atlas of Histology*. Philadelphia: WB Saunders; 1988.)

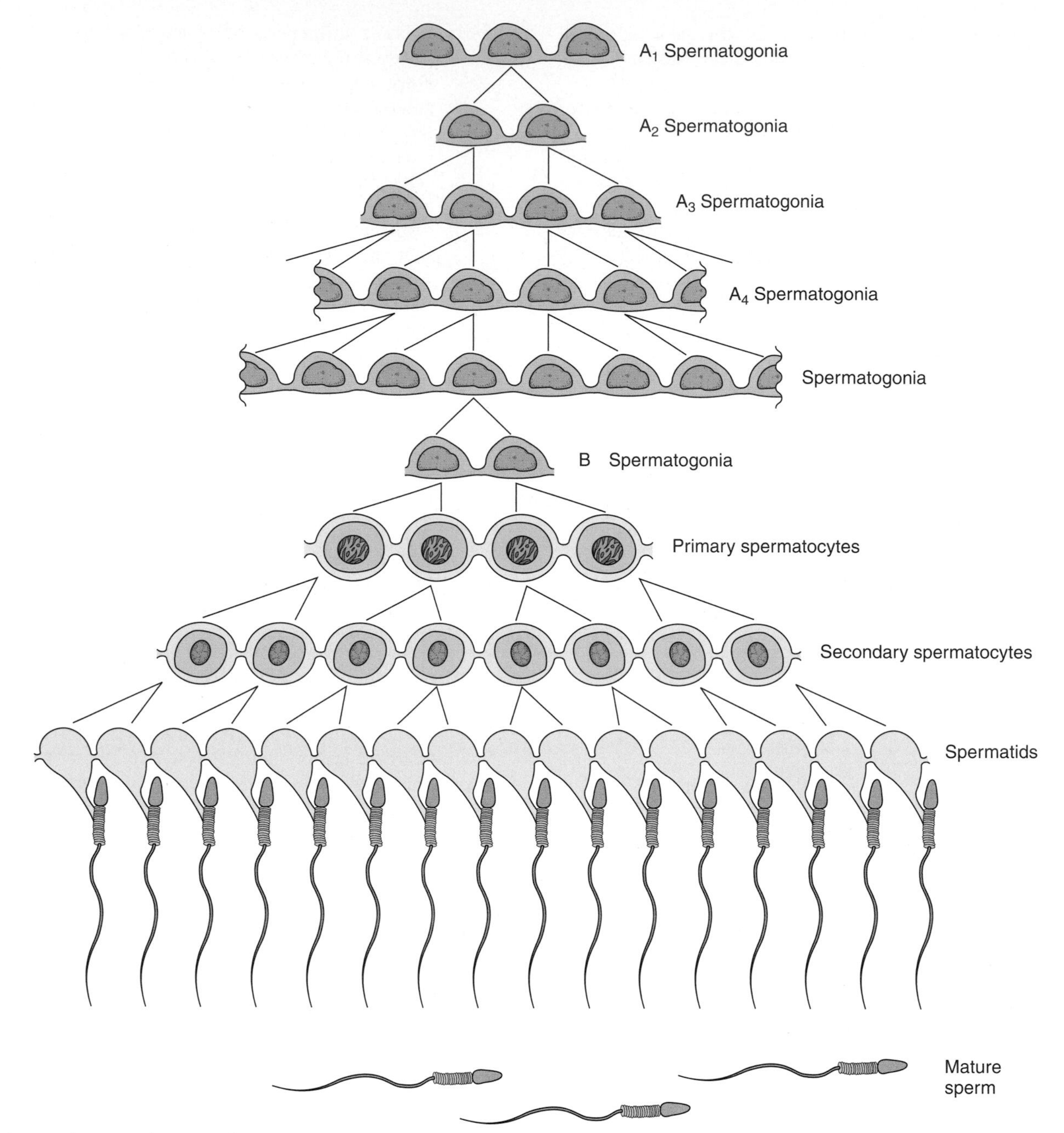

Fig. 21.9 A schematic diagram of spermatogenesis, displaying the intercellular bridges that maintain the syncytium during differentiation and maturation. (Modified from Ren X-D, Russell L. Clonal development of interconnected germ cells in the rat and its relationship to the segmental and subsegmental organization of spermatogenesis. *Am J Anat*. 1991;192:127. Reprinted with permission from Wiley-Liss, Inc., a subsidiary of John Wiley & Sons, Inc.)

formation, primary spermatocytes duplicate their DNA to obtain a 4n DNA content; however, the chromosome number remains diploid (2n).

During the **first meiotic division**, the DNA content is halved (to 2n DNA) in each daughter cell and the chromosome number is reduced to haploid (n). During the **second meiotic division,** the DNA content of each new daughter cell is reduced to haploid (1n DNA), whereas the chromosome number remains unaltered (haploid).

Prophase I of the first meiotic division lasts for as long as 22 days and involves four stages:

- Leptotene
- Zygotene
- Pachytene
- Diakinesis

The chromosomes of a primary spermatocyte begin to condense, forming long threads during **leptotene** and pairing with their homologues during **zygotene**. Further condensation yields short, thick chromosomes, recognizable as **tetrads**, during **pachytene.** The exchange of segments (**crossing over**) of homologous chromosomes occurs during **diakinesis**; this random genetic recombination results in the unique genome of each gamete and contributes to the variation of the gene pool.

During **metaphase I**, the paired homologous chromosomes line up at the equatorial plate. The members of each pair pull apart and then migrate to opposite poles of the cell in **anaphase**

I; the daughter cells separate (although a cytoplasmic bridge remains), forming two secondary spermatocytes during **telophase I**.

Because the homologous chromosomes are segregated during anaphase, the X and Y chromosomes are sorted into separate secondary spermatocytes, eventually forming spermatozoa that carry either an X or a Y chromosome. Thus, it is the spermatozoon that determines the chromosomal (genetic) sex of the future embryo.

Secondary spermatocytes are relatively small cells; because they are present for less than 10 hours, they are not readily seen in the seminiferous epithelium. These cells, which contain 2n DNA, do not replicate their chromosomes; they quickly enter the second meiotic division, forming two haploid (1n DNA) **spermatids**.

During mitosis of spermatogonia and meiosis of spermatocytes, nuclear division (**karyokinesis**) is accompanied by a **modified cytokinesis**. As each cell divides to form two cells, a **cytoplasmic bridge** remains between them, holding the newly formed cells tethered to each other (see Fig. 21.9). Because this incomplete division occurs over a number of mitotic and meiotic events, it results in the formation of a **syncytium** of cells, a large number of spermatids that are connected to one another. This connection enables the spermatogenic cells to communicate with each other and, thus, to synchronize their activities.

Clinical Correlations

The most common abnormality due to nondisjunction of the XX homologues is known as Klinefelter syndrome. *Individuals with this syndrome usually have XXY chromosomes (an extra X chromosome). They are typically infertile, tall and thin, exhibit various degrees of masculine characteristics (including small testes), and are somewhat challenged mentally. Approximately equal numbers of the individuals with Klinefelter syndrome are due to nondisjunction of paternally and maternally derived chromosomes.*

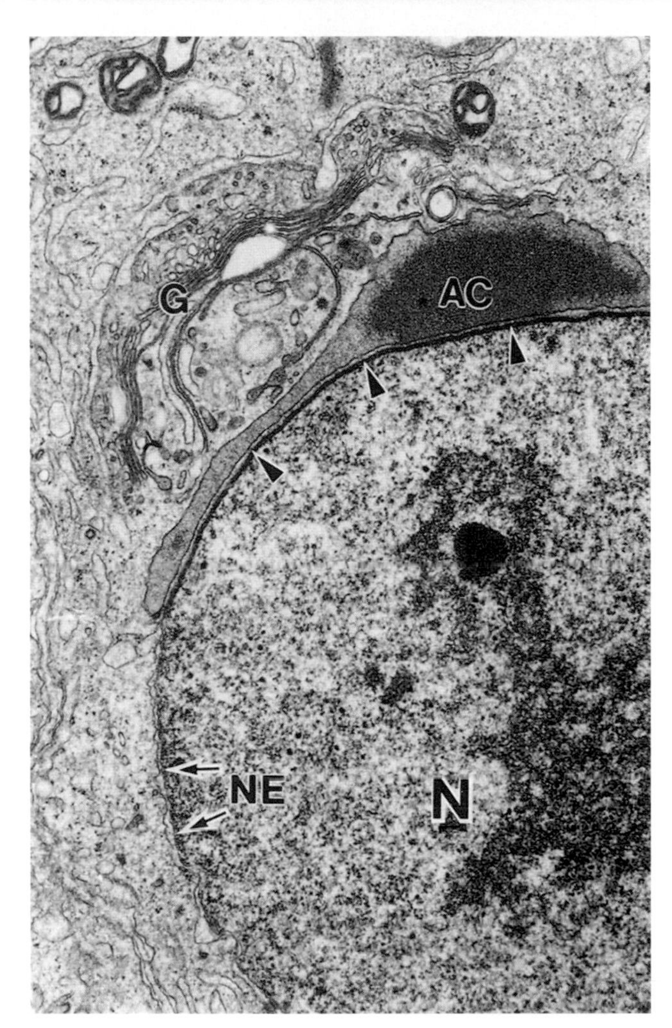

Fig. 21.10 Electron micrograph of the cap stage of a rodent spermatid (×18,000). AC, Acrosome; G, Golgi apparatus; N, nucleus; NE, nuclear envelope. (From Oshako S, Bunick D, Hess RA, et al. Characterization of a testis specific protein localized in the endoplasmic reticulum of spermatogenic cells. *Anat Rec.* 1994;238:335-348. Reprinted with permission from Wiley-Liss, Inc., a subsidiary of John Wiley & Sons.)

Transformation of Spermatids (Spermiogenesis)

Spermatids discard much of their cytoplasm, rearrange their organelles, and form a flagellum to become transformed into spermatozoa. This process of transformation is known as spermiogenesis.

Spermatids are small, round haploid cells (8 µm in diameter). All of the spermatids that are the progeny of a single pale type A spermatogonium are connected to one another by cytoplasmic bridges. They form small clusters and occupy a position near the lumen of the seminiferous tubule. These cells have abundant RER, numerous mitochondria, and a well-developed Golgi complex. During their transformation into spermatozoa, they accumulate hydrolytic enzymes, rearrange and reduce the number of their organelles, form flagella and associated cytoskeletal apparatus, and shed some of their cytoplasm. This process of **spermiogenesis** is subdivided into four phases (Figs. 21.10 and 21.11).

- Golgi phase
- Cap phase
- Acrosomal phase
- Maturation phase

Golgi Phase. During the **Golgi phase** of spermiogenesis, hydrolytic enzymes are formed on the RER, modified in the Golgi apparatus, and packaged by the ***trans*-Golgi network** as small, membrane-bound **preacrosomal granules**. These small vesicles fuse, forming an **acrosomal vesicle**. Viewed with transmission electron microscopy, the hydrolytic enzymes in the acrosomal vesicle are noted as an electron-dense material known as the ***acrosomal granule***. The acrosomal vesicle comes into contact with and becomes bound to the nuclear envelope, establishing the anterior pole of the developing spermatozoon.

As the acrosomal vesicle is being formed, the centrioles leave the vicinity of the nucleus, one of which participates in the formation of the **flagellar axoneme**. After the generation of the microtubules is initiated, the centrioles return to the vicinity of the nucleus to assist in the formation of the **connecting piece**, a structure that will surround the centrioles (see later description of the spermatozoon).

Cap Phase. During the **cap phase**, the acrosomal vesicle increases in size, and its membrane partially surrounds the nucleus (see Fig. 21.10). As this vesicle enlarges to its final size, it becomes known as the ***acrosome*** (***acrosomal cap***).

Acrosomal Phase. The **acrosomal phase** is characterized by several alterations in the morphology of the spermatid.

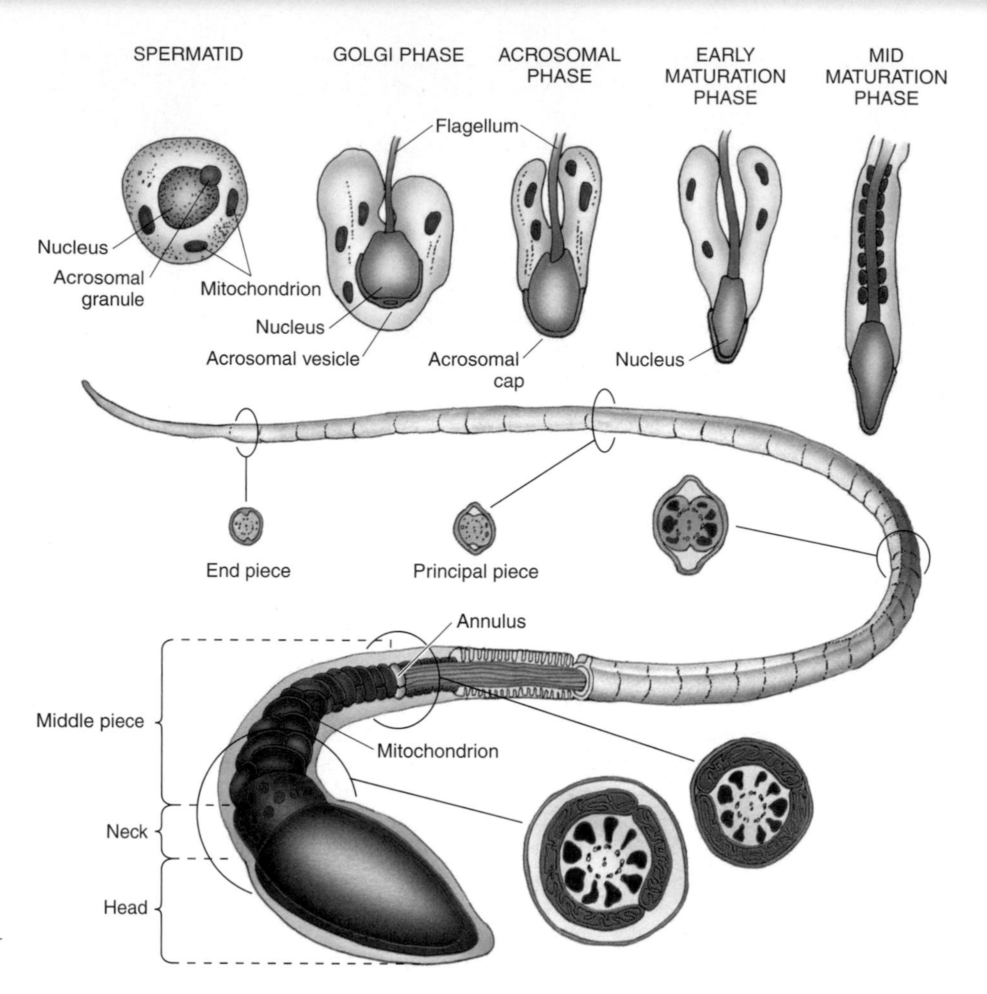

Fig. 21.11 Schematic diagram of spermiogenesis and of a mature spermatozoon.

The nucleus becomes condensed, the cell elongates, and the mitochondria shift location.

The chromosomes become tightly condensed and tightly packaged. As the chromosomal volume decreases, the volume of the entire nucleus is also reduced. Additionally, the nucleus becomes flattened and assumes its specific morphology.

Microtubules assemble to form a cylindrical structure, the **manchette**, which aids in the elongation of the spermatid. As the elongating cytoplasm reaches the microtubules of the flagellar axoneme, the manchette microtubules disassemble. Their place is assumed by the **annulus,** an electron-dense, ring-like structure that delineates the junction of the spermatozoon's **middle piece** with its **principal piece** (see Fig. 21.11). A mitochondrial sheath forms around the axoneme of the middle piece of the tail of the spermatozoon.

During formation of the mitochondrial sheath and elongation of the spermatid, nine columns of **outer dense fibers** form around the axoneme. These dense fibers are attached to the connecting piece formed during the Golgi phase. After their establishment, the dense fibers become surrounded by ribs, a series of ring-like, dense structures known as the ***fibrous sheath***.

Maturation Phase. The **maturation phase** is characterized by the shedding of spermatid cytoplasm. As the excess cytoplasm is released, the syncytium is disrupted and individual spermatozoa are liberated from the large cellular mass. The cytoplasmic remnants are phagocytosed by Sertoli cells, and the disengaged spermatozoa are released into the lumen of the seminiferous tubule (**spermiation**).

Note that the newly formed spermatozoa are **immotile** and cannot fertilize an oocyte. Spermatozoa gain motility while passing through the epididymis. Only after they enter the female reproductive system do spermatozoa become **capacitated** (i.e., become capable of fertilization).

Structure of Spermatozoa

Spermatozoa are composed of a head, housing the nucleus, and a tail that is divided into four regions: neck, middle piece, principal piece, and end piece.

The **spermatozoa** (**sperm**), produced by spermatogenesis, are long cells (~ 65 μm). Each spermatozoon is composed of a head, housing the nucleus, and a tail, which accounts for most of its length (Fig. 21.12).

Head of the Spermatozoon. The flattened head of the spermatozoon is about 5 μm long and is surrounded by plasmalemma (see Figs. 21.11 and 21.12). It is occupied by the condensed electron-dense nucleus, containing only 1 member of the 23 pairs of chromosomes (22 autosomes + the Y chromosome—or 22 autosomes + the X chromosome), and the **acrosome**, which partially surrounds the anterior aspect of the nucleus and contacts the cell membrane of the spermatozoon anteriorly. It houses various enzymes, including neuraminidase,

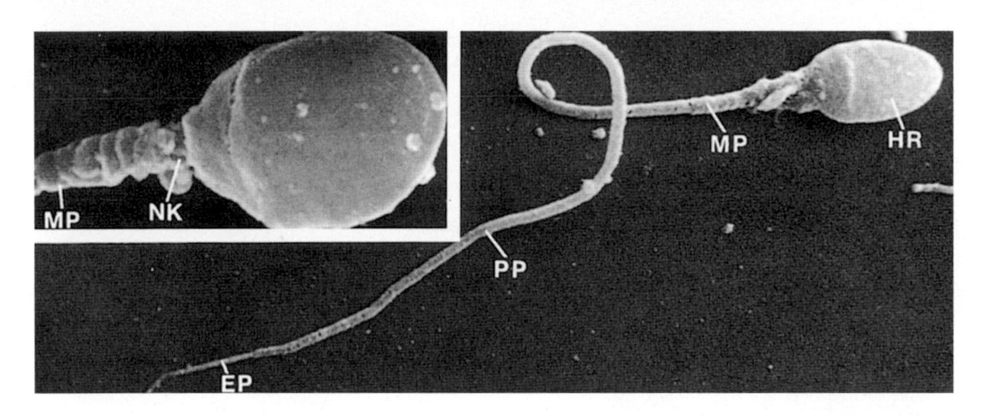

Fig. 21.12 Scanning electron micrograph of human spermatozoa. The entire spermatozoon is shown: head region (HR), middle piece (MP), principal piece (PP), and end piece (EP) (×650). *Inset,* Head, neck (NK), and middle piece (MP) (×15,130). (From Kessel RG. *Tissue and Organs: A Text Atlas of Scanning Electron Microscopy.* San Francisco: W. H. Freeman; 1979.)

hyaluronidase, acid phosphatase, aryl sulfatase, and a trypsin-like protease known as ***acrosin***.

Binding of a spermatozoon to the ZP3 molecule of the zona pellucida triggers the **acrosomal reaction**, the release of the acrosomal enzymes that digest a path for the sperm to reach the oocyte, facilitating the process of fertilization. The acrosomal reaction and process of fertilization are described in Chapter 20.

Tail of the Spermatozoon. The tail of the spermatozoon is subdivided into four regions: neck, middle piece, principal piece, and end piece (see Figs. 21.11 and 21.12). The plasmalemma of the spermatozoon's head is continuous with the plasma membrane of the spermatozoon's tail.

The **neck** (~ 5 μm long), which connects the head to the remainder of the tail, is composed of the cylindrical arrangement of the nine columns of the **connecting piece** that encircles the two centrioles, one of which is usually fragmented. The posterior aspects of the columnar densities are continuous with the nine **outer dense fibers**.

The **middle piece** (~ 5 μm long), located between the neck and the principal piece, is characterized by the presence of the mitochondrial sheath, which encircles the **outer dense fibers** and the central-most **axoneme**. The middle piece stops at the **annulus**, a ring-like, dense structure to which the plasmalemma adheres, preventing the mitochondrial sheath from moving caudally into the tail. Also, two of the nine outer dense fibers terminate at the annulus and the remaining seven continue into the principal piece.

The **principal piece** (~ 45 μm long), the longest segment of the tail, extends from the annulus to the end piece. The axoneme of the principal piece is continuous with that of the middle piece. Surrounding the axoneme are the seven outer dense fibers that are continuous with those of the middle piece and are surrounded, in turn, by the **fibrous sheath**. The principal piece tapers near its caudal extent, where both the outer dense fibers and the fibrous sheath terminate, and is continuous with the end piece.

The **end piece** (~ 5 μm long) is composed of the central axoneme surrounded by plasmalemma. The axoneme is disorganized in the last 0.5 to 1.0 μm, so that instead of the nine doublets and two singlets, 20 haphazardly arranged, individual microtubules are evident. Recent studies using cryo-electron tomography demonstrated that, within the hollow region of these microtubule singlets, a left-handed interrupted helical protein, **tail axoneme intraluminal spiral** (**TAILS**), binds to the internal aspects of the microtubule wall. It is suggested that this newly noted structure may assist in microtubule stabilization, determine the direction of spermatozoa motility, or facilitate rapid forward acceleration of the spermatozoon.

Clinical Correlations

Mutations in the gene that codes for the protein ***beta defensin 126 (DEFB126)*** *has been demonstrated to reduce male fertility. Apparently, DEFB126 is necessary for the sperm to be able to navigate freely through the female genital tract because spermatozoa with mutated forms of this protein often are trapped in the mucous secretions lining the uterus and oviducts.*

Cycle of the Seminiferous Epithelium

The seminiferous epithelium displays 16-day cycles; four cycles are required to complete spermatogenesis.

Because germ cells that arise from a single pale type A spermatogonium are connected by cytoplasmic bridges, they constitute a syncytium and can readily communicate with each other and synchronize their development. Careful examination of the human seminiferous epithelium reveals six possible characteristic associations of developing cell types, known as the **six stages of spermatogenesis**, because they are undergoing synchronized transformations to form spermatozoa (Fig. 21.13). Each cross-sectional profile of a seminiferous tubule may be subdivided into three or more wedge-shaped areas, where each area displays cells in the same stage of spermatogenesis but different from the cells in the other two or more areas.

Clinical Correlations

Studies following the fate of tritium-labeled thymidine (^{3}H-thymidine) injected into the testes of human volunteers have demonstrated that radioactivity appears at 16-day intervals in the same stage of spermatogenesis. Each 16-day interval is known as a ***cycle of the seminiferous epithelium****, and the process of spermatogenesis requires the passage of 4 cycles, or 64 days. Examination of serial cross-sections of a single seminiferous tubule reveals that the same stage of the seminiferous epithelium continues to reappear at specific distances along the length of the tubule. The distance between two identical stages of the seminiferous epithelium is called the* ***wave of the seminiferous epithelium****. Thus, in humans, there are six repeating waves of the seminiferous epithelium, corresponding to the six stages.*

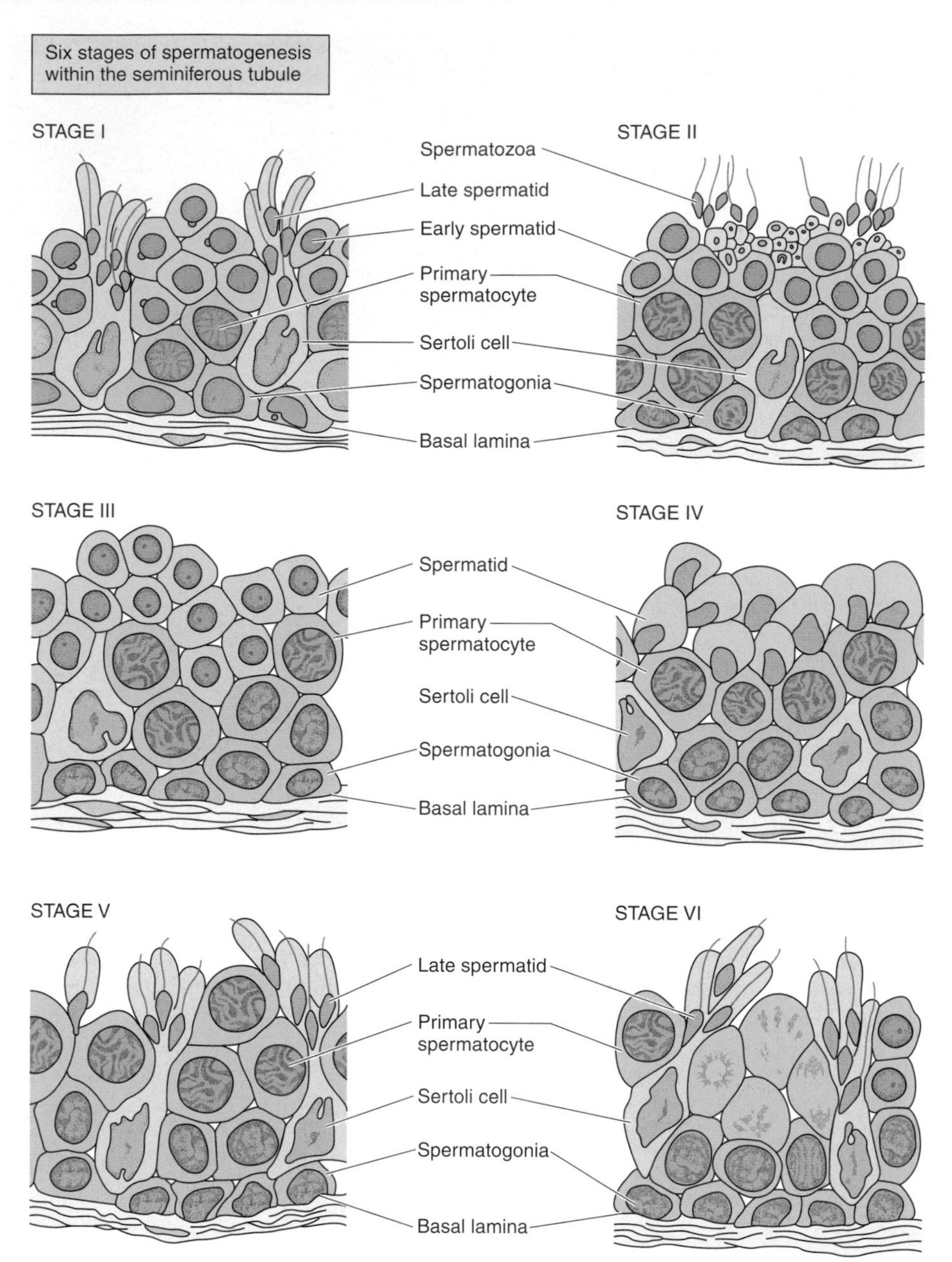

Fig. 21.13 Schematic diagram of the six stages of spermatogenesis in the human seminiferous tubule. (From Clermont Y. The cycle of the seminiferous epithelium in man. *Am J Anat.* 1963;112:35-52. Reprinted with permission from Wiley-Liss, Inc., a subsidiary of John Wiley & Sons, Inc.)

INTERSTITIAL CELLS OF LEYDIG

The interstitial cells of Leydig, scattered among connective tissue elements of the tunica vasculosa, secrete testosterone.

The seminiferous tubules are embedded in the tunica vasculosa, a richly vascularized, loose connective tissue housing scattered fibroblasts, mast cells, and other cellular constituents normally present in loose connective tissue. Also dispersed throughout the tunica vasculosa are small collections of endocrine cells, the **interstitial cells (of Leydig)**, which produce the hormones **testosterone** and **insulin-like factor 3 (INSL 3)**. The former facilitates spermatogenesis, and the latter facilitates the descent of the testes into the scrotum in fetal life. During puberty and in the adult, INSL 3 enhances the release of testosterone by Leydig cells and maintains the health of spermatogenic cells.

Interstitial cells of Leydig are polyhedral and approximately 15 μm in diameter (Figs. 21.14 and 21.15). They have a single nucleus; occasionally, they may be binucleate. Viewed with transmission electron microscopy, Leydig cells are typical steroid-producing cells that have mitochondria with tubular cristae, a large accumulation of SER, and a well-developed Golgi apparatus (Fig. 21.16). These cells also house some RER and numerous lipid droplets, but they contain no secretory vesicles because testosterone is probably released as soon as its synthesis is complete. Lysosomes and peroxisomes are also evident, as are lipochrome pigments (especially in older men). The cytoplasm also contains crystallized proteins, the **crystals of Reinke**, a characteristic of human interstitial cells.

HISTOPHYSIOLOGY OF THE TESTES

The principal functions of the testes are the production of spermatozoa and the synthesis and release of testosterone.

The two testes form about 120 million spermatozoa per day by a process that may be considered a holocrine type of secretion.

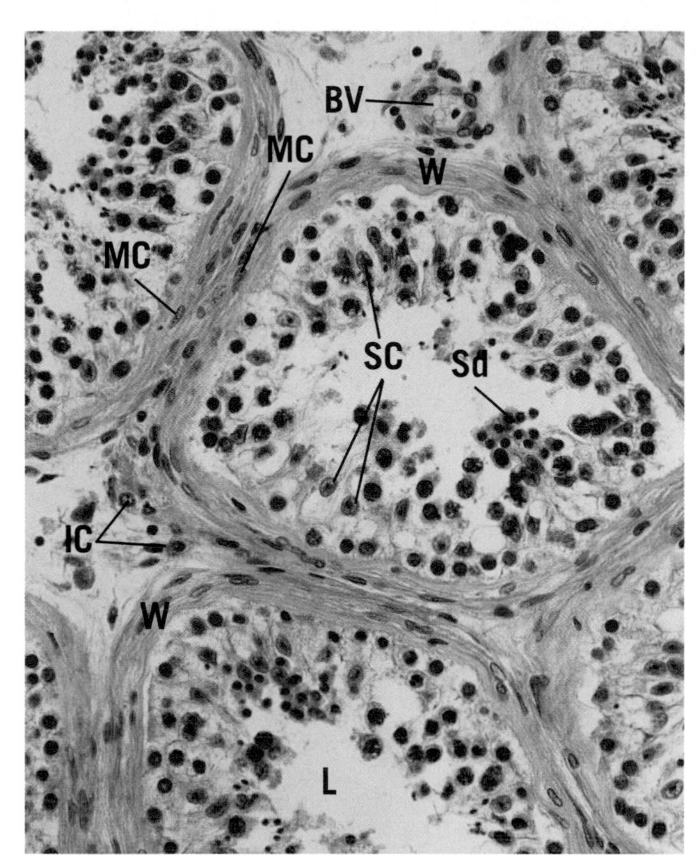

Fig. 21.14 This medium magnification of the seminiferous tubules displays interstitial cells of Leydig (IC) located in the vascular (BV) tunica vasculosa surrounding the seminiferous tubules whose walls (W) possess myoid cells (MC) along with fibroblasts. The lumina (L) of the seminiferous tubules present the cytoplasmic debris discarded by spermatids (Sd) undergoing spermiogenesis and the cytoplasmic remnants are phagocytosed by Sertoli cells (SC). (×270)

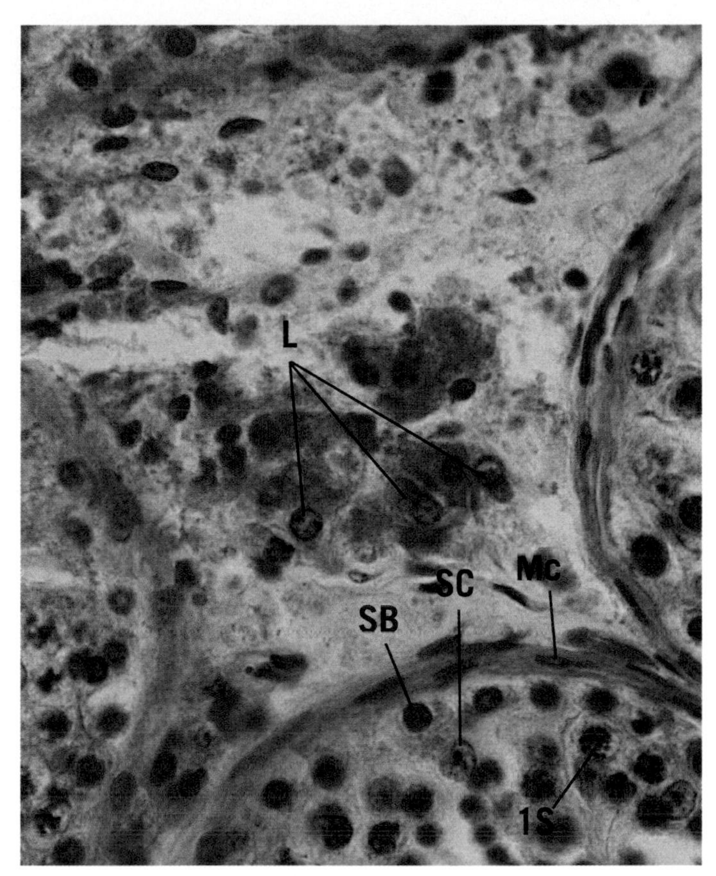

Fig. 21.15 This high-magnification light micrograph of the tunica vasculosa displays a cluster of interstitial cells of Leydig (L). Observe the three cross-sections of a seminiferous tubule whose wall houses fibroblasts as well as myoid cells (Mc). Note the presence of a spermatogonia B in the basal compartment and the primary spermatocytes (1S) in the adluminal compartment. The nucleus of the Sertoli cell is also in the adluminal compartment, although these cells span both compartments. (×540)

Sertoli cells of the seminiferous epithelium also produce a fructose-rich fluid that acts to nourish and transport the newly formed spermatozoa from the lumen of the seminiferous tubule to the extratesticular genital ducts.

Luteinizing hormone (LH), a gonadotropin released from the anterior pituitary gland, binds to LH receptors on the Leydig cells, activating adenylate cyclase of these cells to form cyclic adenosine monophosphate (cAMP). Activation of protein kinases of the Leydig cells by cAMP induces inactive **cholesterol esterases** to become active and cleave free cholesterol from intracellular lipid droplets. The first step in the pathway of testosterone synthesis is also LH-sensitive because LH activates **cholesterol desmolase**, the enzyme that converts free cholesterol into pregnelonone. The various products of the synthetic pathway are shuttled between the SER and mitochondria until **testosterone**, the male sex hormone, is formed and is ultimately released by these cells (Fig. 21.17).

Because blood testosterone levels are not sufficient to initiate and maintain spermatogenesis, FSH—another anterior pituitary gonadotropin—induces Sertoli cells to synthesize and release **androgen-binding protein** (**ABP**; Fig. 21.18). As its name implies, ABP binds testosterone, preventing the hormone from leaving the region of the seminiferous tubule, thus, elevating the testosterone levels in the local environment sufficiently to sustain spermatogenesis.

Release of LH is inhibited by increased levels of testosterone and dihydrotestosterone, whereas release of FSH is inhibited by the hormone **inhibin** and enhanced by the hormone **activin**. Both are produced by Sertoli cells (see Fig. 21.18). It is interesting to note that estrogens, female sex hormones, are also bound by ABP and, thus, can reduce the levels of spermatogenesis.

Germ cell loss due mostly to apoptosis during the meiosis phase of spermatogenesis can be as high as 40%; this number is increased after the individual reaches 40 years of age. It is presumed that this loss would be much greater were it not for the hormone **INSL 3**, produced by the interstitial cells of Leydig, which protects spermatogenic cells from apoptosis.

Clinical Correlations

The hormone ***insulin-like 3*** *is a product of the* ISNL3 *gene. In males, it appears to function not only in preventing spermatogenic cells from entering the apoptotic pathway but also in embryonic development during the descent of the testes, where* INSL3 *controls enlargement and development of the gubernacula aiding in the positioning of the testes into the scrotal sac. It has been demonstrated that, in certain cases, mutations in the* ISNL3 *gene result in cryptorchidism.*

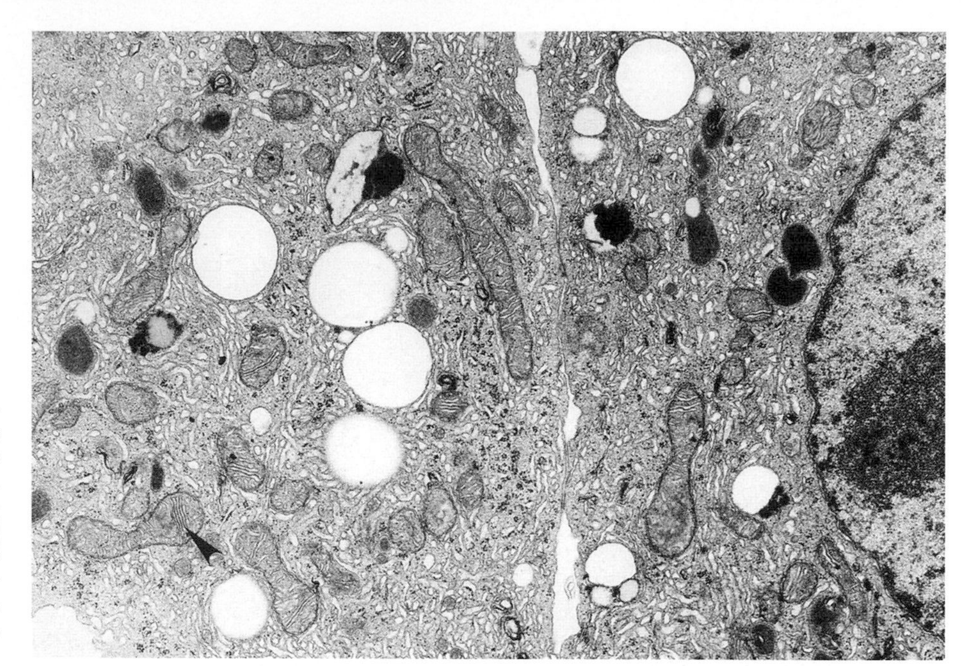

Fig. 21.16 Low-magnification electron micrograph exhibits areas of two human Leydig cells (×18150). Mitochondria are relatively uniform in diameter and, even at low magnification, stacked lamellae are an evident form of the cristae *(arrowhead)*. (From Prince FP. Mitochondrial cristae diversity in human Leydig cells: a revised look at cristae morphology in these steroid-producing cells. *Anat Rec.* 1999;254:534-541. Reprinted with permission from Wiley-Liss, Inc., a subsidiary of John Wiley & Sons, Inc.)

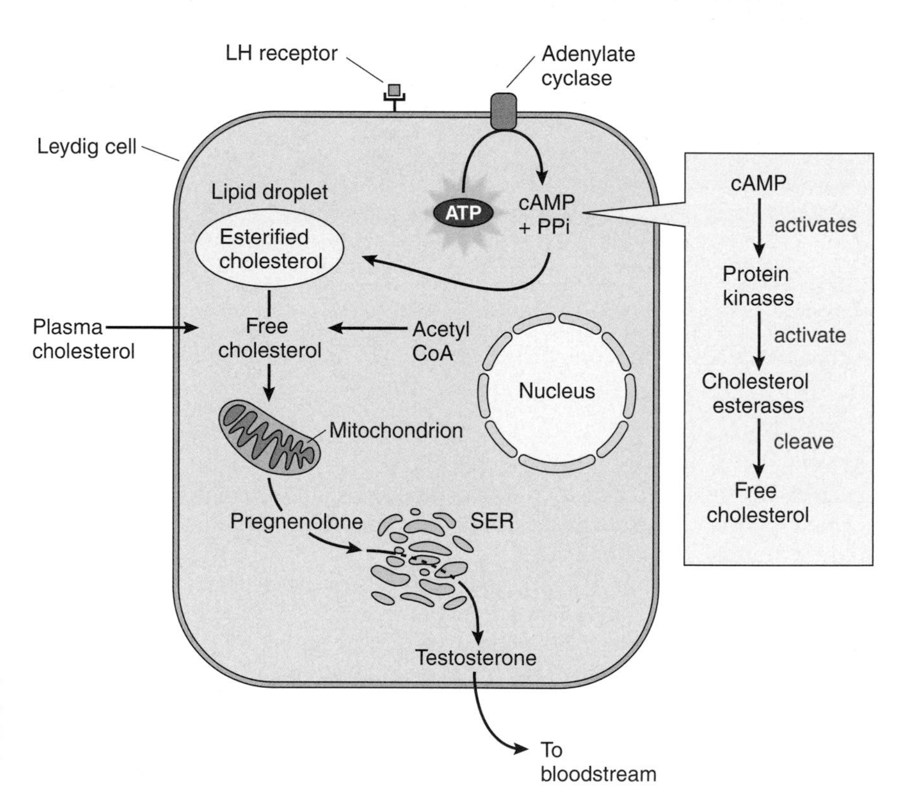

Fig. 21.17 Schematic diagram of testosterone synthesis by the interstitial cells of Leydig. ATP, Adenosine triphosphate; cAMP, cyclic adenosine monophosphate; CoA, coenzyme A; LH, luteinizing hormone; SER, smooth endoplasmic reticulum.

Testosterone is also required for the appearance and maintenance of the male secondary sexual characteristics, as well as for the normal functioning of the seminal vesicles, prostate, and bulbourethral glands. The cells that require testosterone possess **5α-reductase**, the enzyme that converts testosterone to its more active form, **dihydrotestosterone**.

Genital Ducts

There are two categories of genital ducts, those located within the testes (**intratesticular**) and those located external to the testes (**extratesticular;** Table 21.1).

INTRATESTICULAR GENITAL DUCTS

The genital ducts located within the testis connect the seminiferous tubules to the epididymis. These intratesticular ducts are the tubuli recti and the rete testis (see Fig. 21.2).

Tubuli Recti

The tubuli recti deliver spermatozoa from the seminiferous tubules into the rete testis.

The **tubuli recti** are short, straight tubules lined by Sertoli cells in their first half, near the seminiferous tubule, and by a

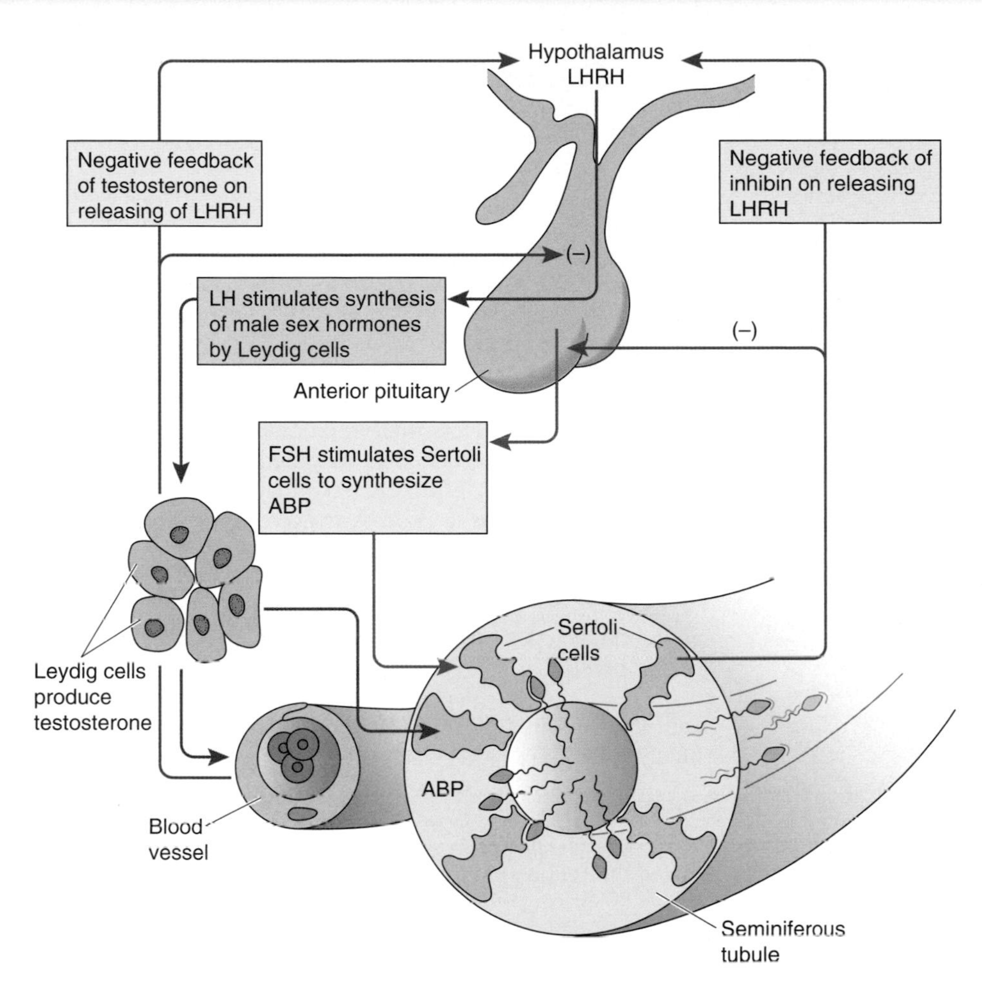

Fig. 21.18 Schematic diagram of the hormonal control of spermatogenesis. ABP, Androgen-binding protein; FSH, follicle-stimulating hormone; LH, luteinizing hormone; LHRH, luteinizing hormone–releasing hormone. (From Fawcett DW. *Bloom and Fawcett's A Textbook of Histology*. 10th ed. Philadelphia: WB Saunders; 1975.)

TABLE 21.1 Histological Features and Functions of Male Genital Ducts

Duct	Epithelial Lining	Supporting Tissues	Function
Tubuli recti	Sertoli cells in proximal half; simple cuboidal epithelium in distal half	Loose connective tissue	Convey spermatozoa from the seminiferous tubules to the rete testis
Rete testis	Simple cuboidal epithelium	Vascular connective tissue	Conveys spermatozoa from the tubuli recti to the ductuli efferentes
Ductuli efferentes	Patches of nonciliated cuboidal cells alternating with ciliated columnar cells	Thin, loose connective tissue surrounded by a thin layer of circularly arranged smooth muscle cells	Convey spermatozoa from the rete testis to the ductus epididymis
Ductus epididymis	Pseudostratified epithelium composed of short basal cells and tall principal cells (with stereocilia)	Thin, loose connective tissue surrounded by a layer of circularly arranged smooth muscle cells	Conveys spermatozoa from the ductuli efferentes to the ductus deferens
Ductus (vas) deferens	Stereociliated pseudostratified columnar epithelium	Loose fibroelastic connective tissue; thick three-layered smooth muscle coats; *inner* and *outer* longitudinal, *middle* circular	Delivers spermatozoa from tail of epididymis to ejaculatory duct
Ejaculatory duct	Simple columnar epithelium	Folded subepithelial connective tissue, giving lumen irregular appearance; no smooth muscle	Delivers spermatozoa and seminal fluid to prostatic urethra at colliculus seminalis

simple cuboidal epithelium in their second half, near the rete testis. The cuboidal cells have short, stubby microvilli, and most possess a single flagellum. The tubuli recti are continuous with the seminiferous tubules and deliver the spermatozoa to the rete testis.

Rete Testis

Immature spermatozoa pass from the tubuli recti into the rete testis, labyrinthine spaces lined by cuboidal epithelium.

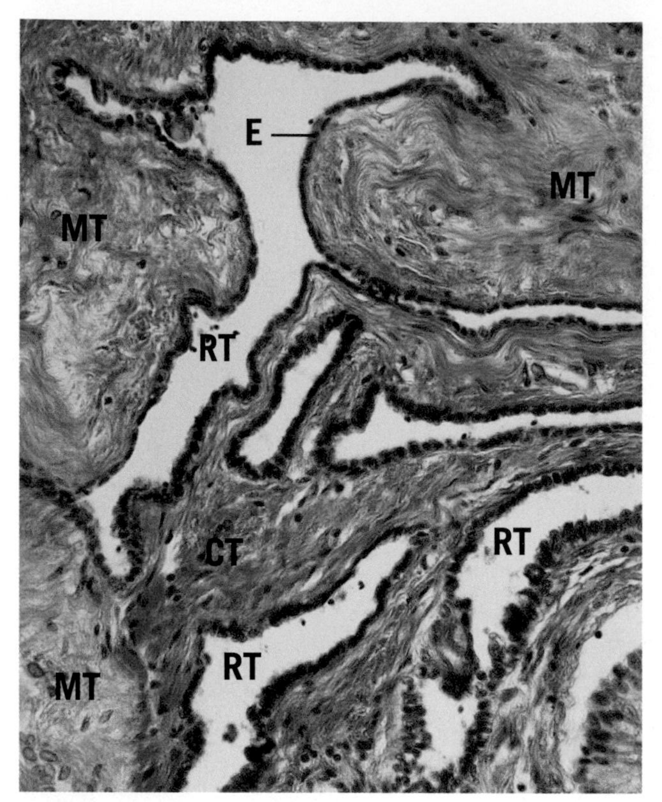

Fig. 21.19 The rete testis (RT) is composed of labyrinthine spaces lined by a simple cuboidal ciliated epithelium within the mediastinum testis (MT). (×270)

The **rete testis** consists of labyrinthine spaces, lined by a simple cuboidal epithelium, within the mediastinum testis. These cuboidal cells, which resemble those of the tubuli recti, have numerous short microvilli with a single flagellum (Figs. 21.19 and 21.20).

EXTRATESTICULAR GENITAL DUCTS

The extratesticular genital ducts are the ductuli efferentes, ductus epididymis, ductus deferens, and ejaculatory duct.

The **extratesticular genital ducts** associated with each testis are the ductuli efferentes, ductus epididymis, the ductus (vas) deferens, and the ejaculatory duct (see Fig. 21.1). The epididymis secretes numerous factors that, in an unknown manner, facilitate maturation of spermatozoa. As noted previously, however, spermatozoa cannot fertilize a secondary oocyte until they undergo **capacitation**, a process triggered by secretions produced in the female genital tract (see Chapter 20).

Epididymis

The ductuli efferentes and the ductus epididymis form the epididymis.

Each **epididymis** is formed by the ductuli efferentes and the ductus epididymis.

Ductuli Efferentes

The ductuli efferentes are interposed between the rete testis and the ductus epididymis.

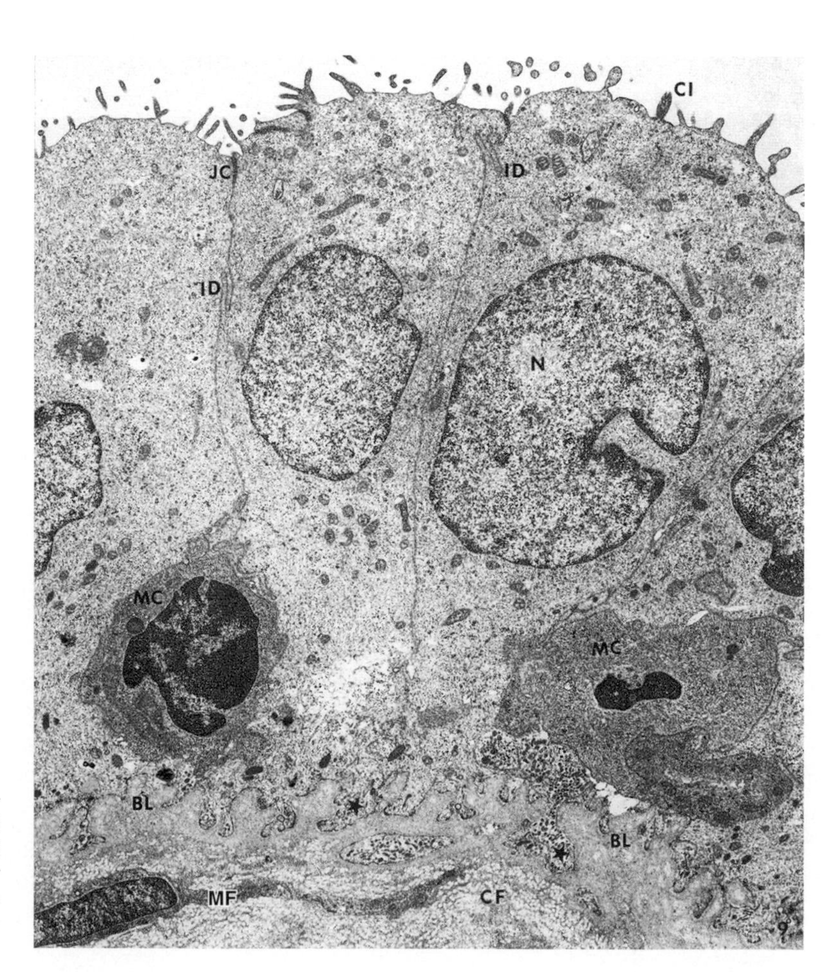

Fig. 21.20 Electron micrograph of the epithelium of the bovine rete testis (×19,900). BL, Basal lamina; CF, collagen fibers; CI, cilium; ID, interdigitation of the lateral plasmalemmae; JC, junctional complexes; MC, monocellular cell; MF, myofibroblast; N, nucleus. (From Hees H, Wrobel KH, Elmagd AA, Hees I. The mediastinum of the bovine testis. *Cell Tissue Res.* 1989;255:29-39.)

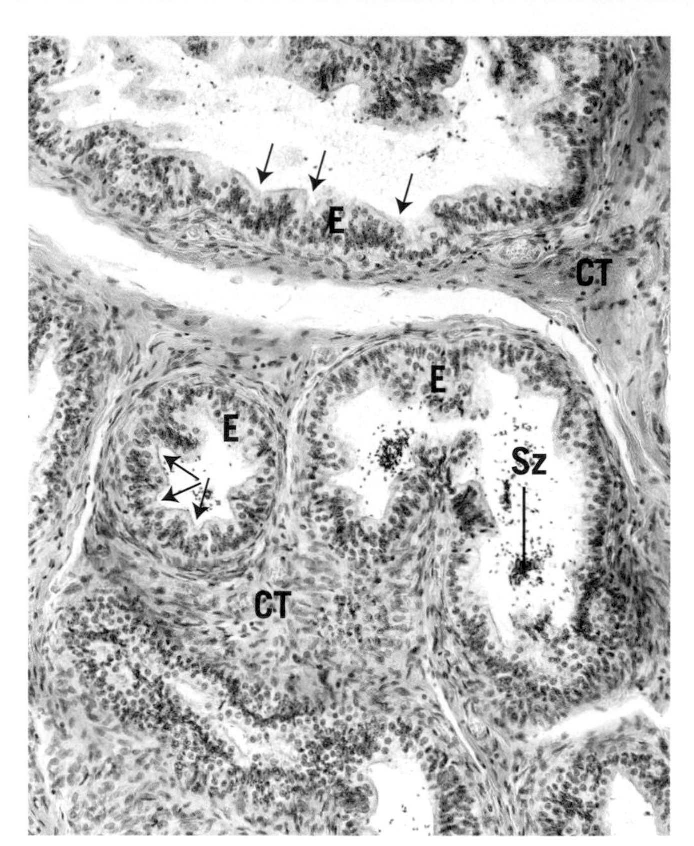

Fig. 21.21 The ductuli efferentes are lined by a simple epithelium (E) composed mostly of two types of cells, patches of ciliated columnar cells alternating with patches of nonciliated cuboidal cells, with the occasional presence of stem cells. This alteration of cell shapes is responsible for the scalloped appearance *(arrows)* of the epithelium. The lumina of the ductuli efferentes are occupied by spermatozoa suspended in the fluid matrix manufactured and released by Sertoli cells of the seminiferous tubule. The connective tissue (CT) walls of the ductuli efferentes possess smooth muscle fibers that, along with the cilia of the columnar cells, propel the spermatozoa toward the ductus epididymis. (×132)

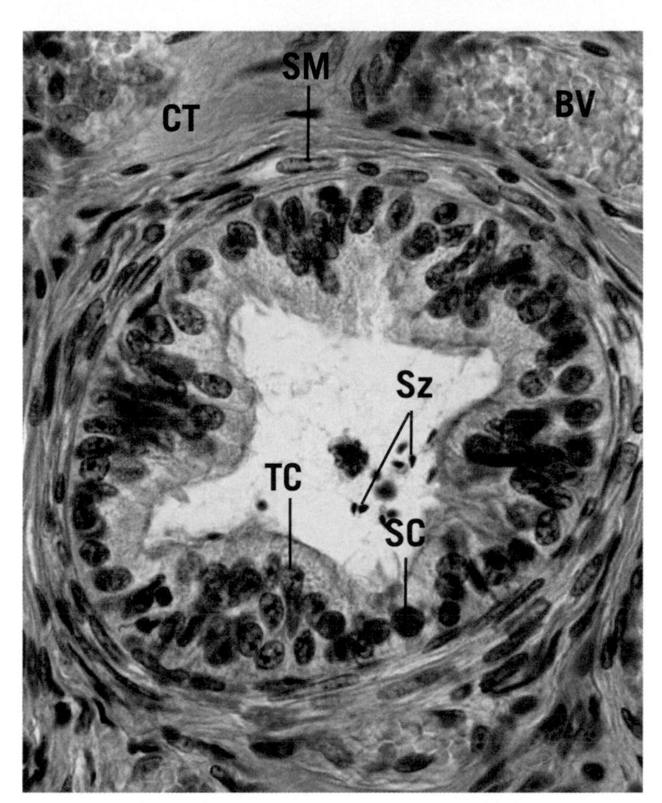

Fig. 21.22 A medium-magnification photomicrograph of a cross-section of a ductuli efferentes displays the vascular (BV) connective tissue (CT) surrounding the ductules, as well as the smooth muscle cells (SM) of the wall of the ductuli efferentes. The tall columnar cells (TC) of the epithelium of the ductuli efferentes possess elongated nuclei, whereas the short cuboidal cells (SC) have round nuclei. Note the presence of spermatozoa in the lumen of the ductule. (×270)

The 10 to 20 **ductuli efferentes** are short tubules that drain spermatozoa from the rete testis and pierce the tunica albuginea of the testis to conduct the sperm to the ductus epididymis (see Fig. 21.2). Thus, the ductuli efferentes become confluent with the ductus epididymis at this point.

The simple epithelial lining of the lumen of each ductule consists of patches of **nonciliated cuboidal cells** alternating with regions of **ciliated columnar cells.** The successive clusters of short and tall epithelial cells impart a scalloped appearance to the lumina of the ductuli efferentes, a notable characteristic of these ductules (Figs. 21.21 and 21.22). The cuboidal cells are richly endowed with lysosomes, and their apical plasmalemmae display numerous invaginations indicative of endocytosis. These cells are believed to **resorb** most of the luminal fluid elaborated by the Sertoli cells of the seminiferous tubule. The cilia of the columnar cells probably move the spermatozoa toward the epididymis. Occasional stem cells are also present scattered among the cuboidal and columnar cells. These stem cells are responsible for giving rise to new cuboidal and columnar cells to maintain a constant epithelial population.

The simple epithelium sits on a basal lamina that separates it from the thin, loose connective tissue wall of each ductule. The connective tissue is surrounded by a thin layer of smooth muscle cells that are circularly arrayed and, by undergoing rhythmic contractions, assist in propelling their luminal contents into the epididymis.

Ductus Epididymis

The ductus epididymis is a thin, long, highly convoluted tubule composed of three regions: the head, body, and tail.

The **ductus epididymis** is a thin, long (4–6 m in length), highly convoluted tubule that is folded into a space only 5 cm long on the posterior aspect of the testis (see Fig. 21.2). The epididymis may be subdivided into three regions: head, body, and tail. The head, formed by the union of the 10 to 20 ductuli efferentes, becomes highly coiled and continues as the equally highly coiled body. The distal portion of the tail, which stores spermatozoa for a short time, loses its convolutions as it becomes continuous with the ductus deferens.

The lumen of the epididymis is lined by a **pseudostratified epithelium** composed of two cell types (Figs. 21.23–21.25):

- **Short basal cells**—Pyramidal to polyhedral. They have round nuclei in which large accumulations of heterochromatin impart a dense appearance to this structure. The sparse cytoplasm of these cells is relatively clear, with a scarcity of organelles. It is believed that the basal cells function as stem cells, regenerating themselves and the principal cells as the need arises.
- **Tall principal cells**—They have irregular, oval nuclei with one or two large nucleoli. These nuclei are much paler than those of the basal cells and are located basally within the cell.

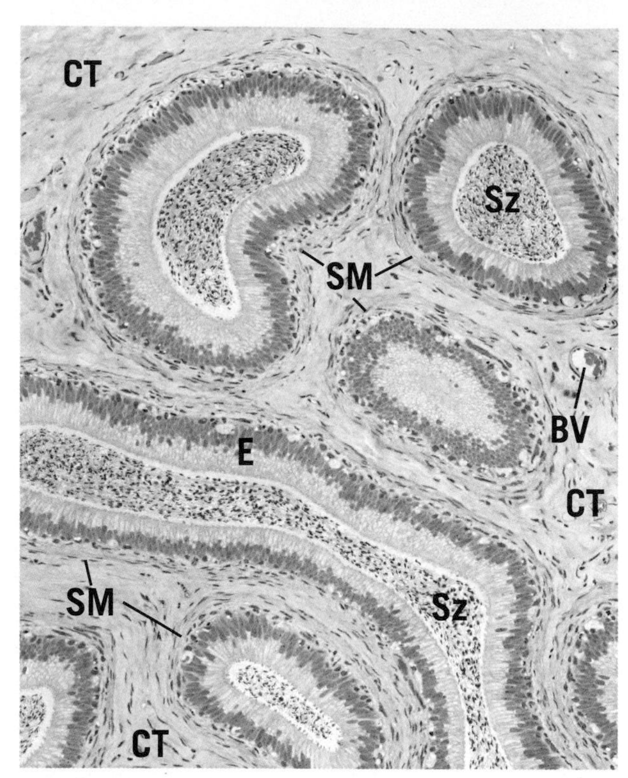

Fig. 21.23 The pseudostratified epithelium (E) of the epididymis lines its spermatozoa-filled (Sz) lumen, and the wall of the epididymis possesses a well-developed smooth muscle layer (SM) that blends with the connective tissue (CT), which attaches this very long, thin tube to the tunica albuginea of the testis. (×132)

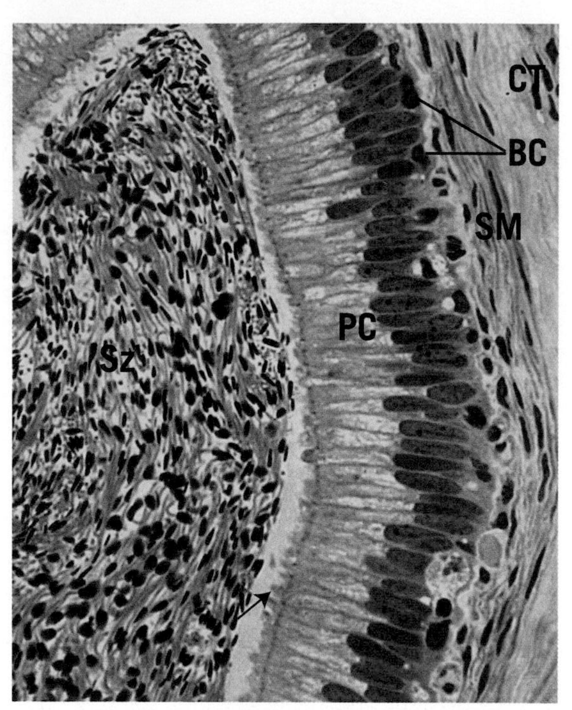

Fig. 21.25 This high-magnification photomicrograph of the epididymis displays the two cell types of the pseudostratified epithelium, the short basal cells (BC) and the tall, stereociliated *(arrow)* principal cells (PC). Note the spermatozoa-filled lumen, as well as the smooth muscle cells (SM) located in the wall of the epididymis just deep to a very thin, lamina propria–like connective tissue. Thicker connective tissue (CT) elements attach the epididymis to the tunica albuginea of the testis. (×540)

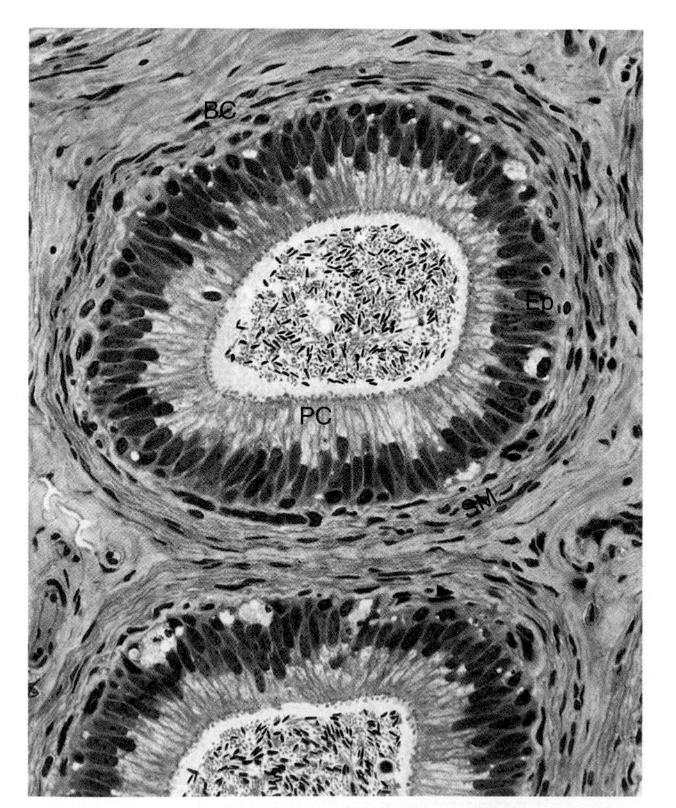

Fig. 21.24 Photomicrograph of the epididymis in a monkey, showing smooth muscle (SM), principal cells (PC), epithelium (Ep), and basal cells (BC). (×270)

The cytoplasm of the principal cell houses abundant RER located between the nucleus and the basal plasmalemma. The cytoplasm also has a large, supranuclearly positioned Golgi complex, numerous profiles of apically located SER, endolysosomes, and multivesicular bodies. The apical cell membranes of the principal cells display a profusion of pinocytotic and coated vesicles at the bases of the many **stereocilia** that project into the lumen of the epididymis. These long, branched, cellular extensions are clusters of nonmotile microvilli that appear to form clumps as they adhere to one another.

The principal cells resorb the luminal fluid, which is endocytosed by pinocytotic vesicles and delivered to the endolysosomes for disposal. Additionally, these cells phagocytose remnants of spermatid cytoplasm that were not removed by Sertoli cells. Principal cells also manufacture **glycerophosphocholine**, a glycoprotein that inhibits spermatozoon capacitation, preventing the spermatozoon from fertilizing a secondary oocyte until the sperm enters the female genital tract. The high level of **fertilization promoting peptide** (**FPP**) also prevents the spermatozoon from undergoing capacitation until it reaches the female reproductive tract, where FPP levels become diluted.

The epithelium of the epididymis is separated by a basement membrane from the underlying circularly arranged smooth muscle cells whose **peristaltic contractions** help conduct the spermatozoa to the ductus deferens. The smooth muscle layer increases in thickness from the head of the epididymis to the body, where a second layer of smooth muscle cells, arranged more or less longitudinally, is added between the basement membrane and the circular smooth muscle layer. This second smooth muscle cell layer becomes more distinct in the beginning of the tail of the ductus epididymis. In the distal portion of the tail of the ductus epididymis, a third longitudinally arranged smooth muscle layer is added so that there is an inner and an outer longitudinally oriented and an intervening, middle circular smooth muscle layer. These smooth muscle layers will match those of the ductus deferens.

A connective tissue layer peripheral to the smooth muscle cells maintains the epididymis in a folded state and attaches it to the tunica albuginea of the testis.

Ductus Deferens (Vas Deferens)

The ductus deferens (also known as the vas deferens) is a muscular tube that conveys spermatozoa from the tail of the epididymis to the ejaculatory duct.

Each **ductus deferens** (also known as the ***vas deferens***) is a thick-walled muscular tube with a small, irregular lumen that conveys spermatozoa from the tail of the epididymis to the ejaculatory duct (see Figs. 21.1 and 21.2). As indicated earlier, the ductus deferens is accompanied by the spermatic artery, spermatic plexus of nerves, lymphatic vessels, and the pampiniform plexus of veins to form the **spermatic cord**. The cremaster muscle, skeletal muscle fibers derived from the internal oblique muscle, originate from the inguinal ligament. They form long, fibrous loops that surround the spermatic cord, are entwined with a fascial layer known as the cremasteric sheath, and extend as far down as and attach to the tunica vaginalis of the testis. This muscle acts to draw the testis toward the body wall when the person is cold or is experiencing fear.

The stereociliated **pseudostratified columnar epithelium** of the ductus deferens is similar to that of the epididymis, although the principal cells are shorter. A basal lamina separates the epithelium from the underlying loose fibroelastic connective tissue, which has numerous folds, making the lumen appear irregular. The thick smooth muscle coat surrounding the connective tissue is composed of three layers, inner and outer longitudinal layers with an intervening middle circular layer. The smooth muscle coat is invested by a thin layer of loose fibroelastic connective tissue (Figs. 21.26 and 21.27).

Clinical Correlations

Because the ductus deferens has a muscular wall 1 mm thick, it is easily perceptible through the skin of the scrotum as a dense, rolling tubule. Vasectomy (surgical removal of part of the ductus deferens) is performed via a small slit through the scrotal sac, sterilizing the person.

The dilated terminus of each ductus deferens, known as the **ampulla**, has a highly folded, thickened epithelium. As the ampulla approaches the prostate gland, it is joined by the

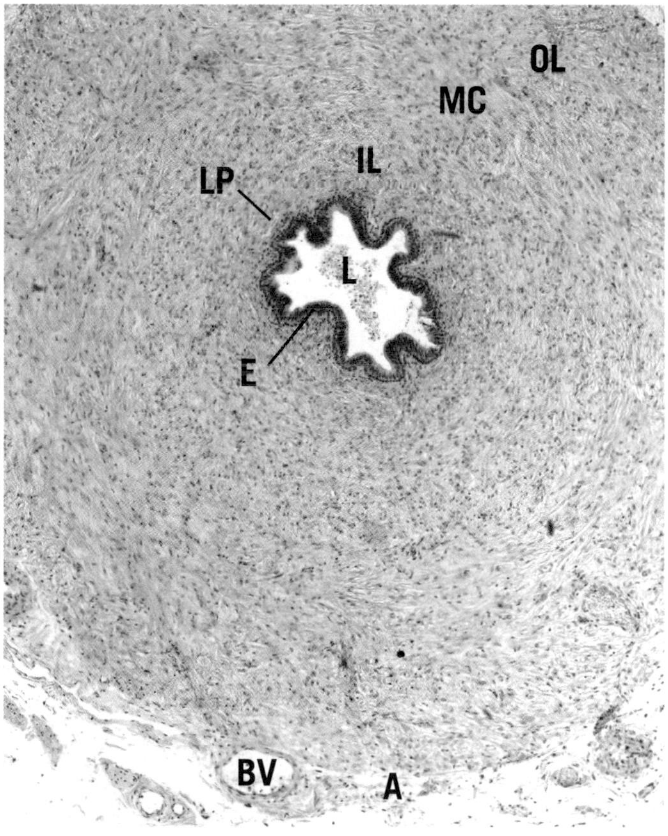

Fig. 21.26 The lumen (L) of the human ductus deferens is lined by a pseudostratified columnar epithelium (E) surrounded by a thin lamina propria (LP) that is thrown into folds. The thick muscular coat of the ductus deferens is composed of three layers of smooth muscle: inner longitudinal (IL), middle circular (MC), and outer longitudinal (OL). The adventitia (A) surrounding the outer longitudinal layer of smooth muscle conveys the vascular supply (BV) of the ductus deferens. (×56)

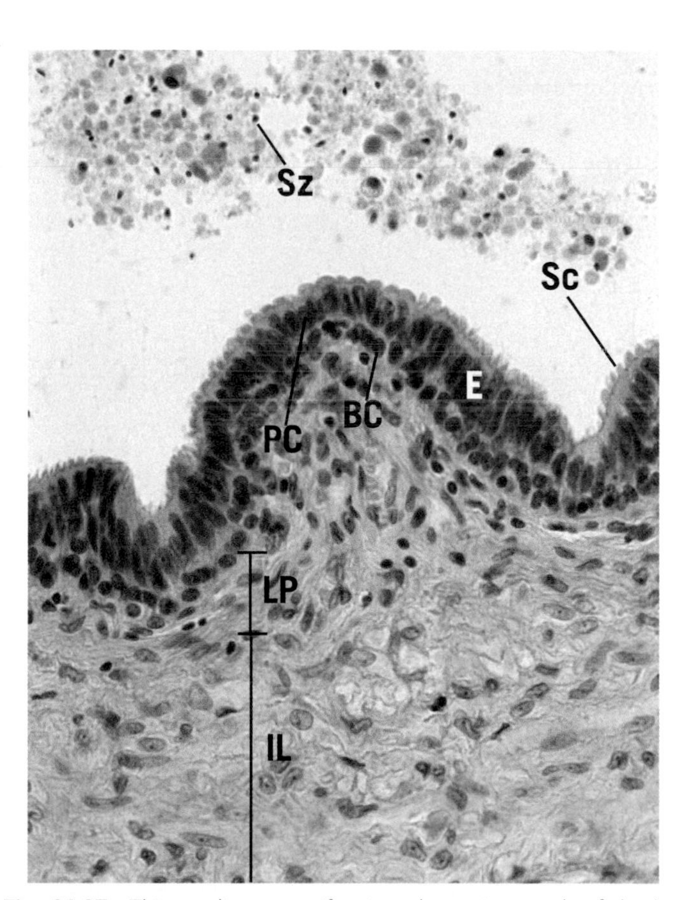

Fig. 21.27 This medium-magnification photomicrograph of the human ductus deferens displays the presence of spermatozoa (Sz) in its lumen and the two cell types of its epithelial (E) lining: the stereociliated (Sc) tall principal cells (PC) and the short basal cells (BC). Note the loose connective tissue constituting the lamina propria (LP) and the inner longitudinal layer (IL) of the smooth muscle coat. (×270)

seminal vesicle. The continuation of the junction of the ampulla with the seminal vesicle is called the **ejaculatory duct**.

Ejaculatory Duct

The ampulla of the ductus deferens joins the seminal vesicle to form the ejaculatory duct, which then enters the prostate gland and opens in the prostatic urethra.

Each **ejaculatory duct** is a short, straight tubule that enters the substance of and is surrounded by the prostate gland (see Fig. 21.1). The ejaculatory duct ends as it pierces the posterior aspect of the prostatic urethra at the **colliculus seminalis**. The lumen of the ejaculatory duct is lined by a simple columnar epithelium. The subepithelial connective tissue is folded, a feature responsible for the irregular appearance of its lumen. The ejaculatory duct has no smooth muscle in its wall.

Accessory Genital Glands

The male reproductive system has five **accessory glands**: the paired seminal vesicles, the single prostate gland, and the paired bulbourethral glands (see Fig. 21.1).

SEMINAL VESICLES

The paired seminal vesicles, located adjacent to the posterior wall of the prostate gland, secrete a viscous fluid that constitutes about 70% of the ejaculate.

The paired **seminal vesicles** are highly coiled tubular structures about 15 cm long. They are located between the posterior aspect of the neck of the bladder and the prostate gland and join the ampulla of the ductus deferens just above the prostate gland.

The mucosa of the seminal vesicles is highly convoluted, forming labyrinth-like cul-de-sacs that, in three dimensions, are observed to open into a central lumen. The lumen is lined by a **pseudostratified columnar epithelium** composed of short basal cells and low columnar cells (Figs. 21.28 and 21.29)

Each short **columnar cell** has numerous short microvilli and a single flagellum projecting into the lumen of the gland. The cytoplasm of these cells displays RER, Golgi apparatus, numerous mitochondria, some lipid and **lipochrome pigment** droplets, and abundant secretory granules. The height of the cells varies directly with blood testosterone levels. The subepithelial connective tissue is **fibroelastic** and surrounded by smooth muscle cells, arranged as an inner circular layer and outer longitudinal layer. The **smooth muscle coat** is, in turn, surrounded by a flimsy layer of fibroelastic connective tissue.

The seminal vesicles once were believed to store spermatozoa, some of which are always present in the lumen of this gland. It is now known that these glands produce a yellow, viscous, **fructose-rich seminal fluid** that constitutes 60% of the volume of semen. Although seminal fluid also contains amino acids, citrates, prostaglandins, and proteins, fructose is its principal constituent because it is the source of energy for spermatozoa. The characteristic pale-yellow color of semen is due to the lipochrome pigment released by the seminal vesicles.

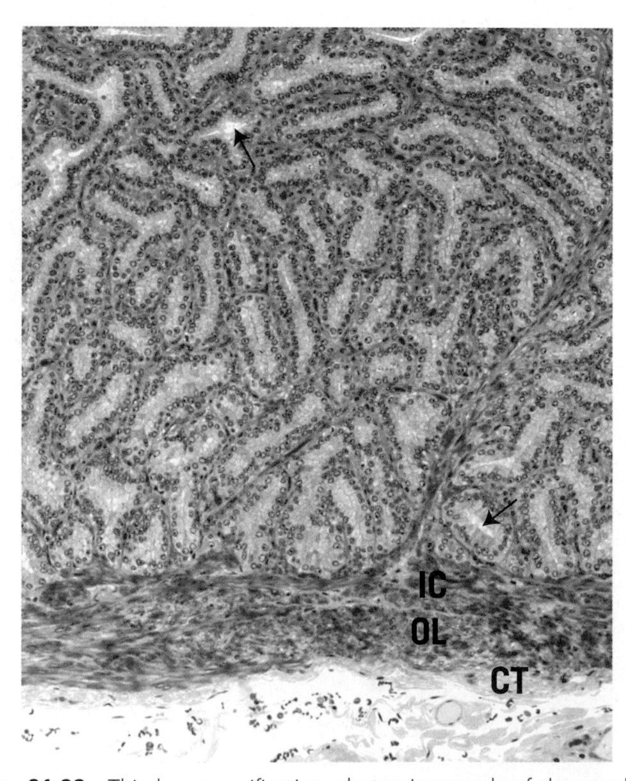

Fig. 21.28 This low-magnification photomicrograph of the monkey seminal vesicle presents various oblique and cross-sections *(arrows)* of this highly convoluted gland. Note the inner circular (IC) and outer longitudinal (OL) smooth muscle layers surrounded by a loose fibroelastic connective tissue (CT). (×132)

PROSTATE GLAND

The prostate gland, surrounding a portion of the urethra, secretes acid phosphatase, fibrinolysin, and citric acid directly into the lumen of the urethra.

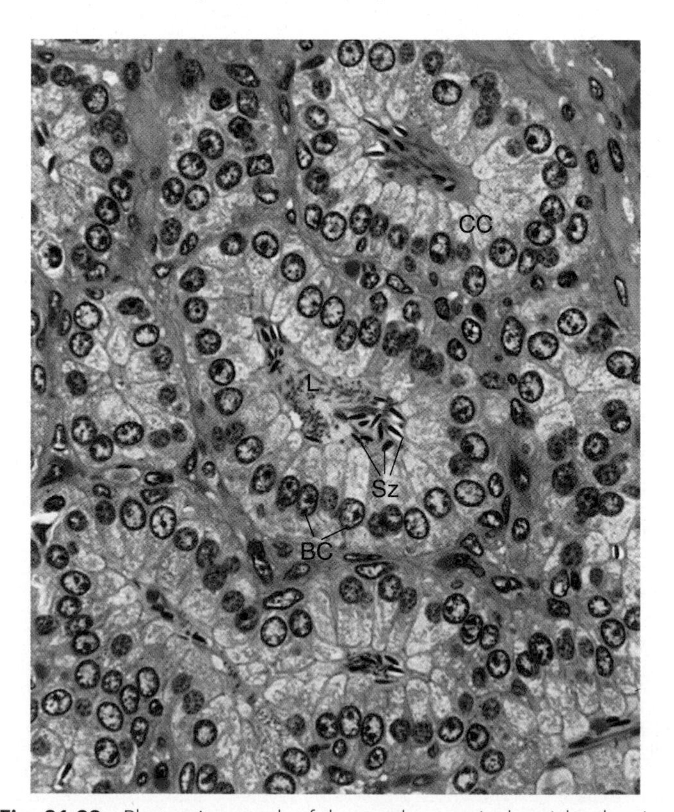

Fig. 21.29 Photomicrograph of the monkey seminal vesicle, showing spermatozoa (Sz), lumen (L), basal cells (BC), and columnar cells (CC). (×270)

The **prostate gland**, the largest of the accessory glands, is pierced by the urethra and the ejaculatory ducts (Figs. 21.30–21.32). The slender **capsule** of the gland is composed of a richly vascularized, dense, irregular collagenous connective tissue interspersed with **smooth muscle cells**. The connective tissue **stroma** of the gland is derived from the capsule; therefore, it is also enriched by smooth muscle fibers in addition to their normal connective tissue cells.

The prostate gland, a conglomeration of 30 to 50 individual **compound tubuloacinar glands**, is arranged in three discrete, concentric layers:

- Mucosal
- Submucosal
- Main

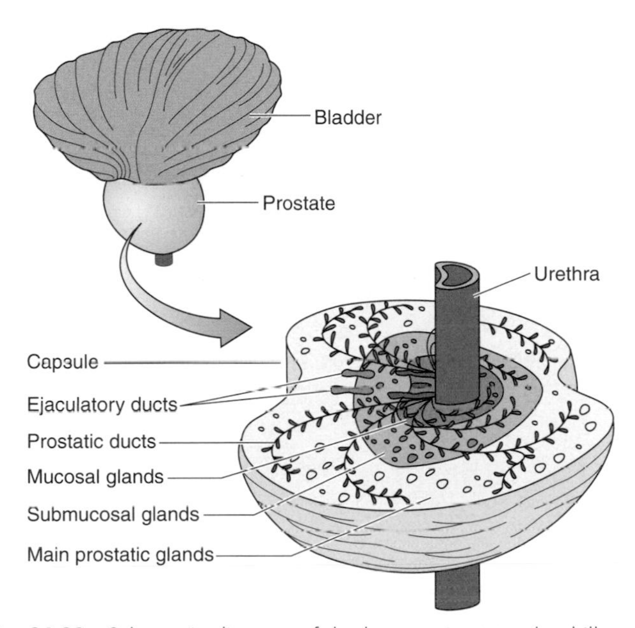

Fig. 21.30 Schematic diagram of the human prostate gland illustrating the mucosal, submucosal, and main prostatic glands.

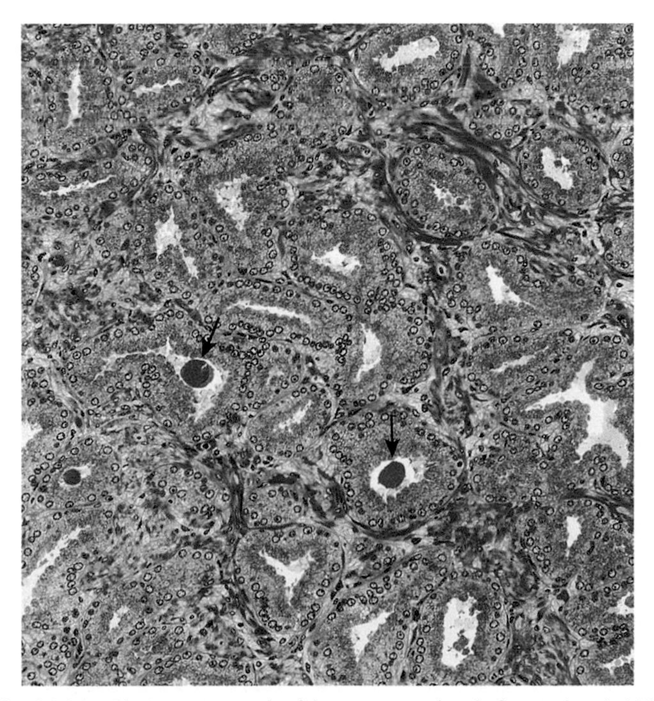

Fig. 21.31 Photomicrograph of the prostate gland of a monkey (×132). *Arrows* represent prostatic concretion.

Each tubuloacinar gland has its own duct that delivers its secretory product into the prostatic urethra.

The **mucosal glands** are closest to the urethra and, thus, are the smallest of the glands. The **submucosal glands** are peripheral to the mucosal glands; consequently, they are larger than the mucosal glands. The largest and most numerous of the glands are the peripheral-most **main glands**, which compose the bulk of the prostate.

The components of the prostate gland are lined by a **simple** to **pseudostratified columnar epithelium** (see Figs. 21.31 and 21.32), the cells of which are well endowed with organelles responsible for the synthesis and packaging of proteins. Hence, these cells have an abundant RER, a large Golgi apparatus, numerous secretory granules (Fig. 21.33), and many lysosomes.

The lumina of the tubuloacinar glands frequently house round to oval calcified glycoproteins, known as **prostatic concretions** (**corpora amylacea**), whose numbers increase with a person's age (see Figs. 21.31 and 21.32) but whose significance is not understood.

The **prostatic secretion** constitutes approximately 30% of the semen. It is a serous, white fluid rich in lipids, proteolytic enzymes, acid phosphatase, fibrinolysin, and citric acid. The formation, synthesis, and release of the prostatic secretions are regulated by **dihydrotestosterone**, the active form of testosterone.

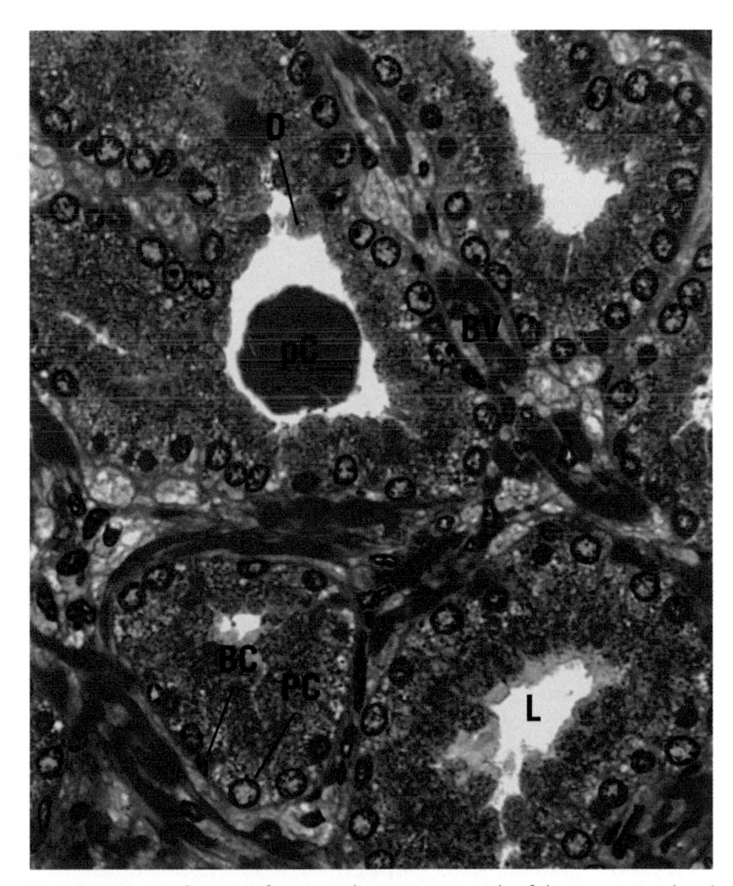

Fig. 21.32 High-magnification photomicrograph of the prostate gland displaying the presence of prostatic concretions (pC) in the lumen (L) of the gland. The epithelium is composed of a simple to pseudostratified epithelium composed of two cell types: basal cells (BC) and principal cells (PC). Note that some of the principal cells possess dome-shaped (D) protrusions that bulge into the lumen. (×540)

Clinical Correlations

As men age, the prostatic stroma and mucosal and submucosal glands begin to enlarge, a condition known as ***benign prostatic hypertrophy (BPH)****. The enlarged prostate partially strangulates the urethra, resulting in difficulties with urination. Approximately 40% of men older than 50 years of age are afflicted with this condition; the percentage increases to 95% by the 80th year. It has been suggested, based on some clinical studies of patients with BPH who ate 5 to 15 g of pumpkin seeds every day, that the oil in these seeds improved their symptoms by reducing both the frequency of nocturnal urination and urinary leaking.*

The second most common form of cancer in males is ***adenocarcinoma of the prostate****, affecting approximately 30% of men over 75 years of age. Frequently, the cancer cells enter the circulatory system and metastasize to bone. A simple blood test to detect* ***prostatic-specific antigen*** *has been developed that permits early detection of prostatic adenocarcinoma. Although tumor growth can be detected by digital palpation through the rectum, a biopsy is required for confirmation. Surgery or radiotherapy are the usual treatments, but they are not without possible side effects, such as impotence and incontinence.*

BULBOURETHRAL GLANDS

The paired bulbourethral glands, located at the root of the penis, secrete a slippery lubricating solution directly into the urethra.

The **bulbourethral glands** (**Cowper glands**) are small (3-5 mm in diameter) and are located at the root of the penis, just at the beginning of the membranous urethra (see Fig. 21.1). Their fibroelastic capsule contains not only fibroblasts and smooth muscle cells but also skeletal muscle fibers derived from the muscles of the urogenital diaphragm. Septa derived from the capsule divide each gland into several lobules. The epithelium of these compound tubuloacinar glands varies from **simple cuboidal** to **simple columnar**.

The secretion produced by the bulbourethral glands is a thick, slippery fluid containing galactose and sialic acid that probably plays a role in lubricating the lumen of the urethra. During the process of ejaculation, this viscous fluid precedes the remainder of the semen.

HISTOPHYSIOLOGY OF THE ACCESSORY GENITAL GLANDS

The bulbourethral glands produce a viscous, slippery fluid that lubricates the lining of the urethra. It is the first of the glandular secretions to be released subsequent to erection of the penis. Just before ejaculation, secretions from the prostate are discharged into the urethra, as are the spermatozoa from the ampulla of the ductus deferens. The prostatic secretions apparently help the spermatozoa achieve motility. The final secretions arise from the seminal vesicles, which are responsible for a significant increase in the volume of the semen. Their fructose-rich fluid is used by the spermatozoa for energy.

The ejaculate, known as ***semen***, consists of secretions from the accessory glands and 200 to 400 million spermatozoa. It is about 3.5 mL in volume in humans, with a pH of about 7.5 due to the buffering action of the prostatic secretions.

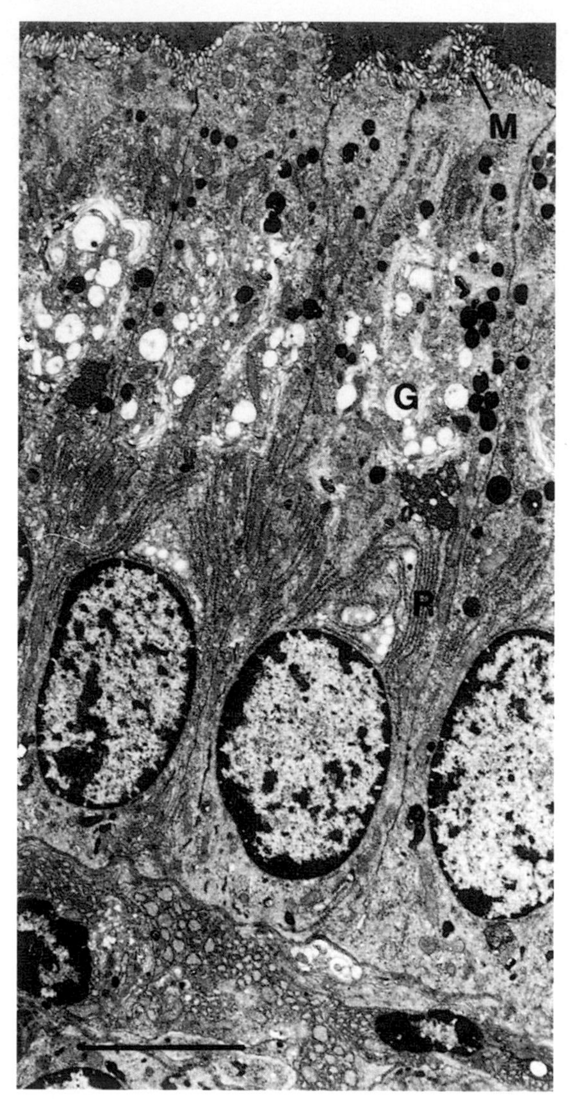

Fig. 21.33 Electron micrograph of the prostate gland in the hamster. G, Golgi apparatus; M, microvilli; R, rough endoplasmic reticulum. Bar = 5 μm. (From Toma JG, Buzzell GR. Fine structure of the ventral and dorsal lobes of the prostate in a young adult Syrian hamster, *Mesocritetus auratus*. *Am J Anat.* 1988;181:132-140. Reprinted with permission from Wiley-Liss, Inc., a subsidiary of John Wiley & Sons, Inc.)

Penis

The penis functions as an excretory organ for urine and as the male copulatory organ for the deposition of spermatozoa into the female reproductive tract.

The **penis** is composed of three columns of **erectile tissue**, each enclosed by its own dense, fibrous connective tissue capsule, the **tunica albuginea** (Fig. 21.34).

Two of the columns of erectile tissue, the **corpora cavernosa,** are positioned dorsally; their tunicae albugineae are discontinuous in places, permitting communication between their erectile tissues. The third column of erectile tissue, the **corpus spongiosum,** is positioned ventrally. Because the corpus spongiosum houses the penile portion of the urethra (see Chapter 19), it is also called the **corpus cavernosum urethrae.** The corpus spongiosum ends distally in an enlarged, bulbous portion, the **glans penis** (head of the penis). The tip of the glans penis is pierced by the end of the urethra as a vertical slit.

The three corpora are surrounded by a common loose connective tissue sheath, but no hypodermis, and are covered by thin skin. The skin of the proximal portion of the penis has coarse pubic hairs and numerous sweat and sebaceous glands. The distal portion of the penis is hairless and has only a few sweat glands. Skin continues distal to the glans penis to form a retractable sheath, the **prepuce**, which is lined by a mucous membrane, a moist, stratified squamous nonkeratinized epithelium. When an individual is circumcised, it is the prepuce that is removed.

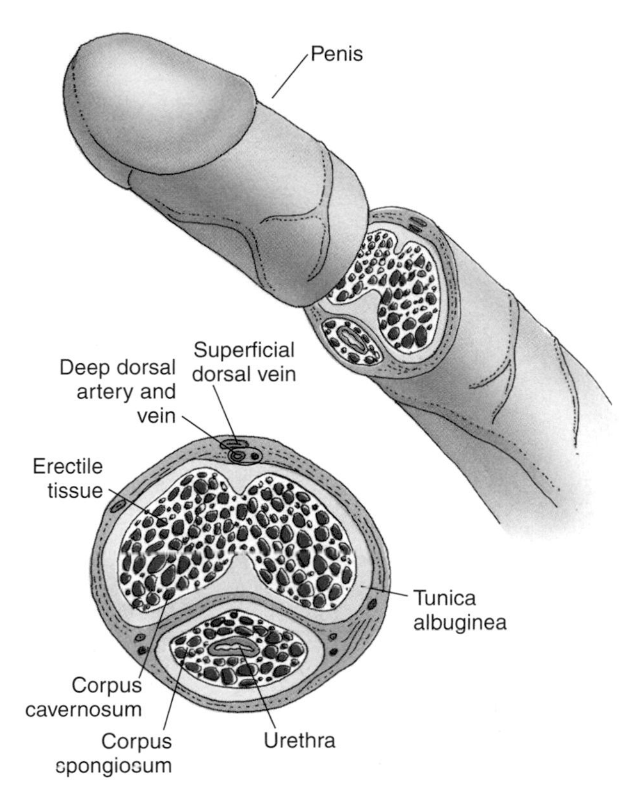

Fig. 21.34 Schematic illustration of the penis in cross-section.

Clinical Correlations

1. *It has been reported that circumcision of adults alters the microbiome at the glans penis by decreasing the resident anaerobic population and replacing it with aerobic organisms because removal of the prepuce eliminates the moist, warm, anaerobic environment that was present beneath the prepuce. Whether this factor accounts for the 50% to 60% reduction in HIV occurrence in newly circumcised males is not known.*
2. *Occasionally, in uncircumcised males, the distal end of the prepuce may become constricted, a condition known as phimosis, so that during an erection the glans penis cannot fit through the opening of the prepuce, causing considerable pain and even a tearing of the tissue. It is possible to relieve the condition by the application of topical steroid creams. However, if that does not result in stretching of the prepuce, then the treatment of choice is circumcision, whereby the prepuce is surgically removed so that it no longer interferes with erection.*
3. *Paraphimosis is a very rare occurrence in which the constricted prepuce is trapped so that it cannot be pulled over the glans penis. If this condition is not relieved and the constricted foreskin begins to strangulate circulation to the glans, it can have extremely serious consequences, including gangrene. Therefore, an individual suffering from paraphimosis should be treated by a physician as soon as possible, within 1 to 2 hours, so that the constriction can be alleviated.*

STRUCTURE OF ERECTILE TISSUE

Vascular spaces within the erectile tissues become engorged with blood, causing erection of the penis.

Erectile tissue of the penis contains numerous variably shaped, endothelially lined spaces that are separated from one another by trabeculae of connective tissue and smooth muscle cells (Figs. 21.35 and 21.36). The vascular spaces of the corpora cavernosa are larger centrally and smaller peripherally near the tunica albuginea. However, the vascular spaces of the corpus spongiosum are similar in size throughout its extent. The trabeculae of the corpus spongiosum contain more elastic fibers and fewer smooth muscle cells than those of the corpora cavernosa.

The erectile tissues of the corpora cavernosa receive blood from branches of the **deep** and **dorsal arteries of the penis** (see Fig. 21.36). These branches penetrate the walls of the trabeculae of the erectile tissue and form either capillary plexuses, which supply some blood flow into the vascular spaces, or coiled arteries (**helical arteries**), which are important sources of blood to the vascular spaces during erection of the penis.

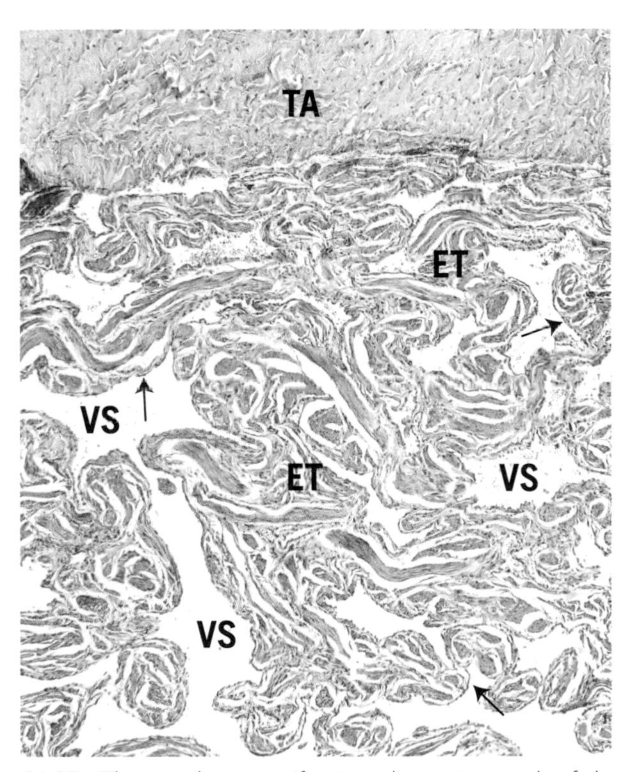

Fig. 21.35 This very-low-magnification photomicrograph of the human corpus cavernosum displays the endothelial lining *(arrows)* of the vascular spaces (VS) of the erectile tissue (ET) surrounded by the dense, irregular connective tissue that forms the tunica albuginea (TA). (×56)

Venous drainage occurs via three groups of veins, which are drained by the **deep dorsal vein** (see Fig. 21.36).

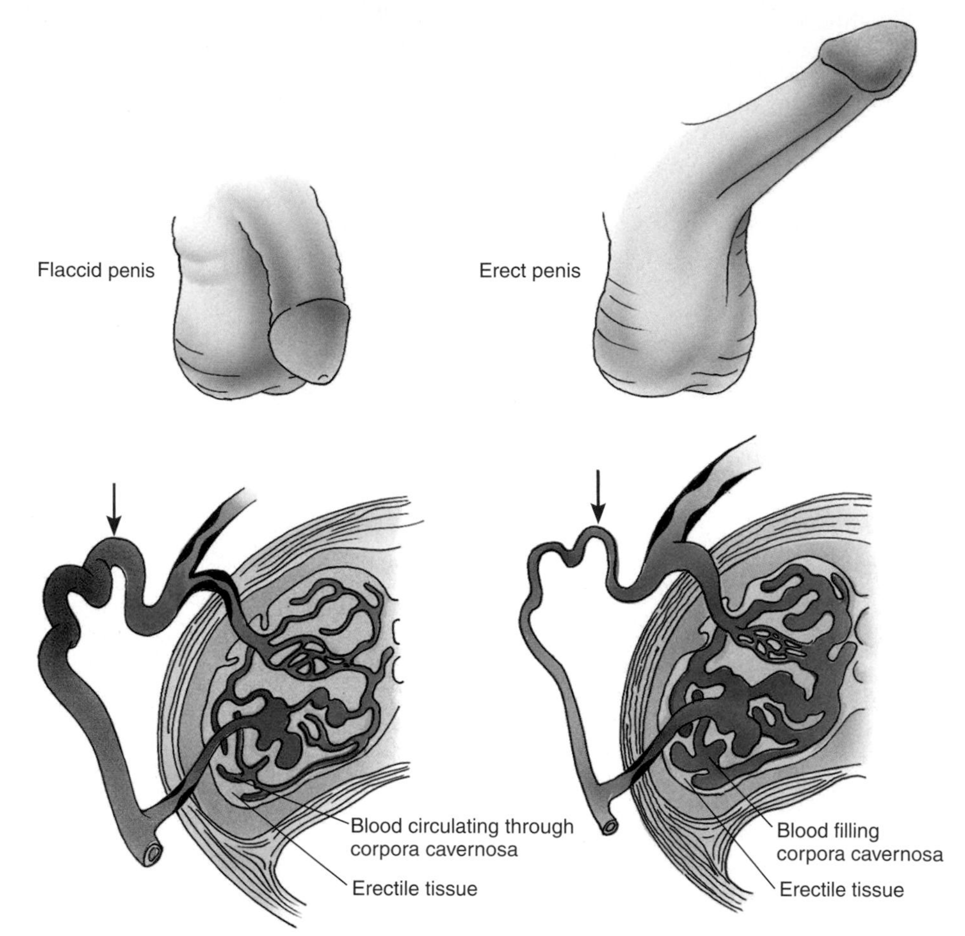

Fig. 21.36 Schematic illustration of circulation in the flaccid and erect penis. The arteriovenous anastomosis *(arrow)* in the flaccid penis is wide, diverting blood flow into the venous drainage. In the erect penis, the arteriovenous anastomosis is constricted, and blood flow into the vascular spaces of the erectile tissue is increased, causing the penis to become turgid with blood. (From Conti G. *Acta Anat.* The erection of the human penis and its morphologic vascular basis. 1952; 14:217–262.)

The three groups of veins arise from the base of the glans penis, dorsal aspect of the corpora cavernosa, and ventral aspect of the corpora cavernosa and corpus spongiosum. Additionally, some of the veins leave the erectile tissue at the root of the penis and drain into the plexus of veins that drain the prostate gland.

MECHANISMS OF ERECTION, EJACULATION, AND DETUMESCENCE

Erection is controlled by the parasympathetic nervous system. It is a result of sexual, tactile, olfactory, visual, auditory, and/or psychological stimulation. Ejaculation is controlled by the sympathetic nervous system.

When the penis is flaccid, the vascular spaces of the erectile tissue contain little blood. In this condition, much of the arterial blood flow is diverted into arteriovenous anastomoses that connect the branches of the deep and dorsal arteries of the penis to veins that deliver their blood into the deep dorsal vein (see Fig. 21.36). Thus, the majority of the blood flow bypasses the vascular spaces of the erectile tissue.

Erection occurs when blood flow is shifted to the vascular spaces of the erectile tissues (the corpora cavernosa and, to a more limited extent, the corpus spongiosum), causing the penis to enlarge and become turgid (see Fig. 21.36). During erection, the tunica albuginea surrounding the erectile tissues is stretched and decreases in thickness from 2 mm to 0.5 mm.

The shift in blood flow that leads to erection is controlled by the **parasympathetic nervous system** following sexual stimulation (e.g., pleasurable tactile, olfactory, visual, auditory, and/or psychological stimuli). The parasympathetic impulses trigger local release of **nitric oxide**, which causes relaxation of smooth muscles of the branches of the deep and dorsal arteries of the penis, increasing the flow of blood into the organ. Simultaneously, the arteriovenous anastomoses undergo constriction, diverting the flow of blood into the helical arteries of the erectile tissue. As these spaces become engorged with blood, the penis enlarges and becomes turgid, leading to erection. The veins of the penis become compressed, and the blood is trapped in the vascular spaces of the erectile tissue, maintaining the penis in an erect state (see Fig. 21.36).

Clinical Correlations

Penile fracture, the rupturing of the tunica albuginea of one or both corpora cavernosa, is a very rare condition resulting from vigorous masturbation or vaginal intercourse that places great bending force on the erect penis. The most common cause of penile fracture is vaginal intercourse in which the person penetrated assumes the top position and does not realize that the penis is in a misaligned position and is being bent to such an extent that the movement causes considerable pain. Penile fracture is a very serious condition, especially if the lesion affects the urethra, dorsal veins, arteries, or nerves; a surgeon should treat the patient as soon as possible.

Continued stimulation of the glans penis results in **ejaculation**, the forceful expulsion of **semen** from the male genital ducts. Each ejaculate, which has a volume of about 3.5 mL in humans, consists of secretions from the accessory genital glands and 200 to 400 million spermatozoa. Subsequent to erection, the bulbourethral glands release a viscous fluid that lubricates the lining of the urethra. Just before ejaculation, the prostate gland discharges its secretion into the urethra, and spermatozoa from the ampullae of the two ductus deferentes are released into the ejaculatory ducts. The prostatic secretion apparently helps the spermatozoa achieve motility. The final secretion added to semen is a fructose-rich fluid, released from the seminal vesicles, that provides energy to the spermatozoa. This secretion forms much of the volume of the ejaculate.

Clinical Correlations

1. *A single ejaculate normally contains approximately 60 to 100 million spermatozoa per milliliter. A male whose sperm count is less than 20 million spermatozoa per milliliter of ejaculate is considered* ***sterile.*** *Interestingly, men who watch more than 20 hours of television per week have a 45% lower sperm count than men who do not watch television. Additionally, men who are more active and exercise have a 75% greater sperm count than do men who do not exercise. The reason for these findings is not known.*
2. *The inability to achieve erection is known as* ***impotence.*** *Temporary erectile dysfunction can result from psychological factors or drugs (e.g., alcohol), whereas permanent impotence can be caused by many factors, including lesions in certain regions of the brain and hypothalamus, as well as spinal cord injuries, autonomic innervation malfunction, stroke, Parkinson disease, diabetes, multiple sclerosis, and even psychological disorders.*

Ejaculation, unlike erection, is regulated by the **sympathetic nervous system.** These impulses trigger the following sequence of events:

- Contraction of the smooth muscles of the genital ducts and accessory genital glands forces the semen into the urethra.
- The sphincter muscle of the urinary bladder contracts, preventing the release of urine (or the entry of semen into the bladder).
- The bulbospongiosus muscle, which surrounds the proximal end of the corpus spongiosum (bulb of the penis), undergoes powerful, rhythmic contractions, resulting in forceful expulsion of semen from the urethra.

Ejaculation is followed by the cessation of parasympathetic impulses to the vascular supply of the penis. As a result, the arteriovenous shunt is reopened, blood flow through the deep and dorsal arteries of the penis is diminished, and the vascular spaces of the erectile tissues are slowly emptied of blood by the venous drainage. As the blood leaves these vascular spaces, the penis undergoes **detumescence** and becomes flaccid.

Clinical Correlations

The neurotransmitter ***nitric oxide (NO)*** *released by the endothelial cells of the sinusoids (i.e., vascular spaces of the erectile tissues) activate guanylate cyclase of smooth muscle cells to produce cyclic guanosine monophosphate (cGMP) from guanosine triphosphate (GTP), thus relaxing the smooth muscle cells. Relaxation of the smooth muscle cells permits the accumulation of blood in the sinusoids; these enlarged vessels compress the small return venous channels that drain the sinusoids, resulting in the erection of the penis.*

After ejaculation or when the parasympathetic impulses cease and cGMP levels dwindle, another enzyme, ***phosphodiesterase,*** *destroys the cGMP, permitting smooth muscle contraction to occur again, the sinusoids begin to be drained of blood, and the erection is terminated.*

Although ***sildenafil (Viagra)*** *was originally developed as a treatment for heart failure, it was found to produce erections in many patients. Further study showed that the medication blocked phosphodiesterase from inhibiting cGMP degradation, thus leading to erection.*

Pathological Considerations

See Figs. 21.37 through 21.40.

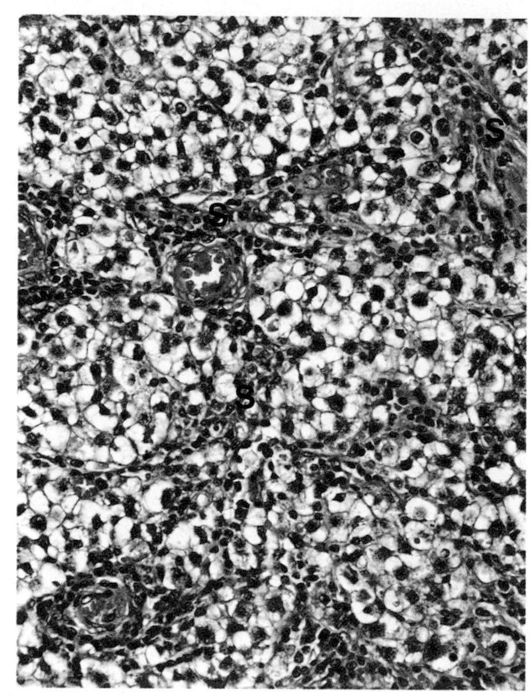

Fig. 21.37 Photomicrograph of a patient with classical seminoma, the most common testicular tumor. Note the presence of clusters of numerous polygonal-shaped cells with clear cytoplasm. The clusters are separated by slender connective tissue septa (S). (Reprinted with permission from Young B, Stewart W, O'Dowd G. *Wheater's Basic Pathology: A Text, Atlas and Review of Histopathology.* 5th ed. Oxford: Churchill Livingstone/Elsevier Limited; 2011:248.)

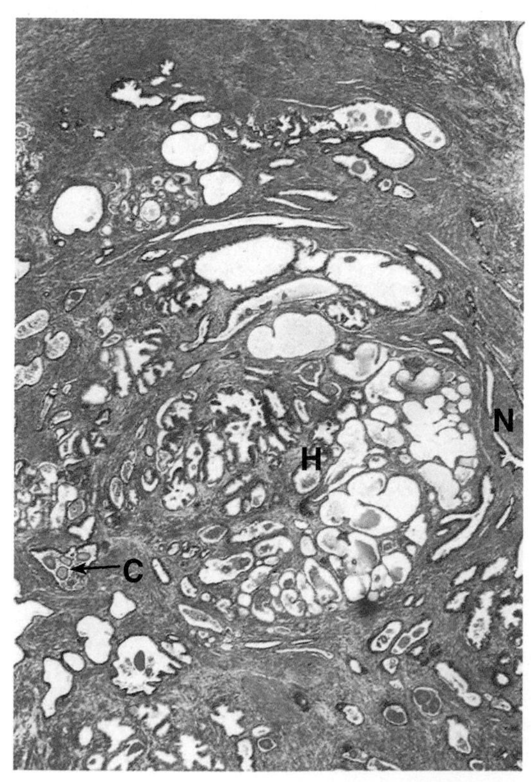

Fig. 21.38 Photomicrograph of a patient with benign prostatic hyperplasia. Observe the hyperplastic prostatic tissue (H) compressing the normal tissue (N) at the periphery. Note the presence of corpora amylacea (C) throughout the tissue. (Reprinted with permission from Young B, Stewart W, O'Dowd G. *Wheater's Basic Pathology: A Text, Atlas and Review of Histopathology.* 5th ed. Oxford: Churchill Livingstone/Elsevier Limited; 2011:251.)

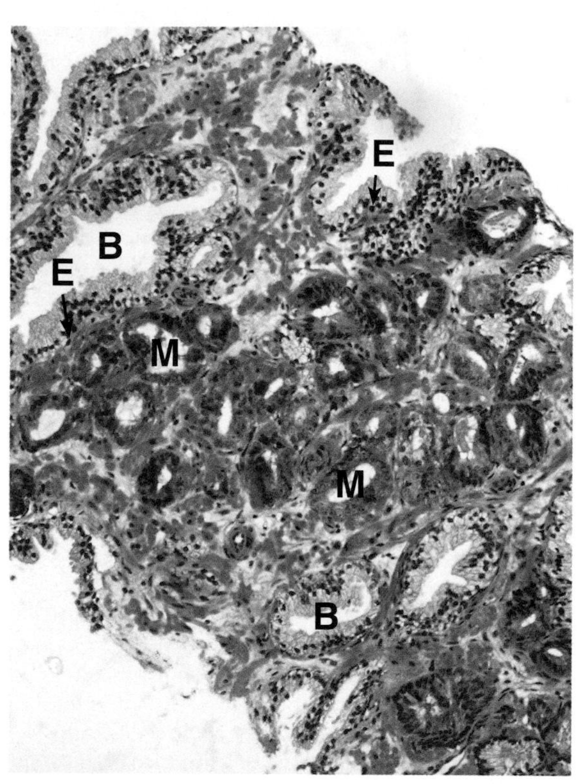

Fig. 21.39 Photomicrograph of a patient with prostatic adenocarcinoma. This is a higher-grade cancer and is characterized by the presence of malignant glandular tissue (M) interspersed among the benign glandular tissue (B). Note that the prominent basal cell layer (E) present in the benign glands is absent in the malignant tissue. (Reprinted with permission from Young B, Stewart W, O'Dowd G. *Wheater's Basic Pathology: A Text, Atlas and Review of Histopathology.* 5th ed. Oxford: Churchill Livingstone/Elsevier Limited; 2011:252.)

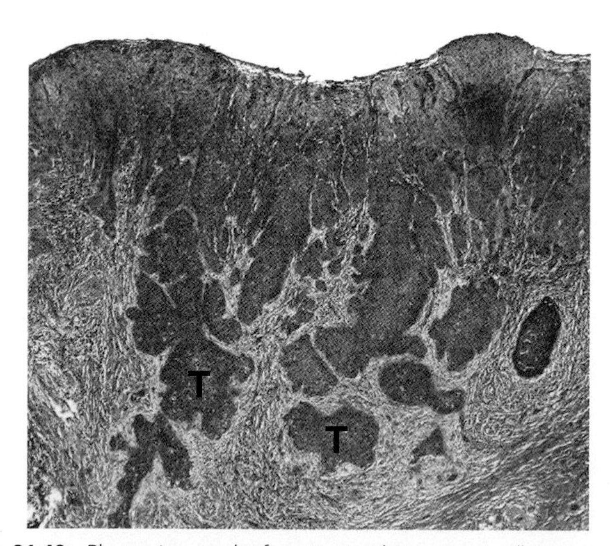

Fig. 21.40 Photomicrograph of a patient with squamous cell carcinoma of the glans penis. Note that this keratinizing squamous cell carcinoma invaded the underlying connective tissue, presenting with islands of tumor cells (T) deep in the glans penis. (Reprinted with permission from Young B, Stewart W, O'Dowd G. *Wheater's Basic Pathology: A Text, Atlas and Review of Histopathology.* 5th ed. Oxford: Churchill Livingstone/Elsevier Limited; 2011:253.)

Histology Laboratory Instructions: Male Reproductive System

Testes

Seminiferous Tubules

Each testis has a thick, vascularized, connective tissue capsule that becomes thickened at the mediastinum testis. Septa derived from the mediastinum subdivides the testis into 250 compartments, where each compartment has one to four highly coiled seminiferous tubules whose lumen is lined by seminiferous epithelium (see Fig. 21.3, C, BV, ST, L, SE). Viewed with a low magnification, the capsule of the testis is seen to be subdivided into an outer, thick, collagenous connective tissue layer, the tunica albuginea, and a deeper layer composed of a loose, vascular connective tissue, the tunica vasculosa. The septa that subdivide the testis into compartments have a good vascular supply. The lumen of the seminiferous tubule is lined by a seminiferous epithelium (see Fig. 21.4, TA, TV, S, BV, L, ST, SE). Viewed at a high magnification, the thin wall, the tunica propria, of the seminiferous tubule is apparent where three cross-sectional profiles contact each other. The lumen of the seminiferous tubule is lined by a seminiferous epithelium composed of Sertoli cells and spermatogenic cells in various stages of development, dark A, pale A, and type B spermatogonia, all lying on the basement membrane within the basal compartment. The adluminal compartment houses the apical portion of Sertoli cells along with primary and secondary spermatocytes, spermatids, and spermatozoa. Note that secondary spermatocytes have a very short lifespan. Therefore, they are very seldom visible (see Figs. 21.5 and 21.6, between *white arrows*, L, SE, SC, PA, DA, 1S, Sd, Sz).

Interstitial Cells of Leydig

As its name implies, the tunica vasculosa that surrounds the seminiferous tubules is richly endowed by blood vessels. Embedded in this vascular loose connective tissue are clusters of interstitial cells of Leydig that manufacture and release the male sex hormone, testosterone. Observe that the wall of the seminiferous tubule houses myoid cells and that the lumen of the seminiferous tubule is lined by the seminiferous epithelium, whose Sertoli cells and spermatids are easily distinguishable (see Fig. 21.14, BV, IC, W, MC, L, SC, Sd). Observe in this high-magnification photomicrograph the cluster of interstitial cells of Leydig surrounded by the tunica vasculosa. Note the presence of myoid cells in the wall of the seminiferous tubule, as well as the spermatogonia B, Sertoli cells, and primary spermatocytes of the seminiferous epithelium (see Fig. 21.15, L, Mc, SB, SC, 1S).

Rete Testis

The labyrinthine spaces located in the mediastinum testis, known as the rete testis, conveys spermatozoa from the tubuli recti to the ductuli efferentes. The rete testis is lined by a ciliated simple cuboidal epithelium (see Fig. 21.19, MT, RT, E).

Epididymis

Ductuli Efferentes

The 10 to 20 ductuli efferentes that drain spermatozoa from the rete testis are lined by a simple epithelium composed of patches of nonciliated cuboidal cells alternating with patches of ciliated columnar cells, which give the lumina a festooned appearance. The connective tissue walls of the ductuli efferentes possess numerous smooth muscle fibers (see Fig. 21.21, Sz, E, *arrows*, CT). A medium magnification of a cross-section of a ductulus efferens displays the spermatozoa in its lumen, as well as the simple epithelium composed of tall ciliated columnar cells and short cuboidal cells. Observe the smooth muscle cells interspersed with the connective tissue elements in its wall and the blood vessels in its immediate vicinity (see Fig. 21.22, Sz, TC, SC, BV).

Ductus Epididymis

A low magnification of the ductus epididymis demonstrates that the lumen of the ductus epididymis, lined by a pseudostratified stereociliated epithelium, is filled with spermatozoa. A basement membrane separates the epithelium from the circular layer of smooth muscle fibers. Connective tissue elements hold the folded regions of the ductus epididymis to each other and to the tunica albuginea of the testis (see Fig. 21.23, E, Sz, SM, CT). At a medium magnification, the short basal cells and the tall principal cells are easily demonstrated. Note also the circularly arranged smooth muscle cells surrounding the epithelium of the ductus epididymis (see Fig. 21.24, BC, PC, SM, Ep). A high magnification of the ductus epididymis, the connective tissue of the epididymis, is evident as it surrounds the circular smooth muscle cell layer. Note that the short basal cells and the tall principal cells with their stereocilia constitute the epithelium of the ductus epididymis and that its lumen is filled with spermatozoa (see Fig. 21.25, CT, SM, BC, PC, *arrow*, Sz).

Ductus Deferens (Vas Dferens)

At a very low magnification, the lumen of the thick, muscular ductus deferens is seen to be thrown into folds lined by a pseudostratified epithelium due to the folding of the thin connective tissue layer, the lamina propria. Observe that the thick muscle layer is grouped into an inner and outer longitudinal smooth muscle layer and an intervening circularly arranged smooth muscle layer. The loose connective tissue adventitia is well supplied by blood vessels (see Fig. 21.26, L, E, LP, IL, OL, MC, A, BV). A medium magnification of the epithelium lining the spermatozoa-filled lumen is clearly noted to be pseudostratified columnar, with basal cells and stereociliated, taller columnar cells. The thin lamina propria is surrounded by the inner longitudinal layer of smooth muscle cells (see Fig. 21.27, E, Sz, BC, PC, Sc, LP, IL).

Accessory Genital Glands

Seminal Vesicles

At a low magnification, the seminal vesicle is a highly coiled tubular structure, as evidenced by the numerous oblique and cross-sections of the gland. Observe the inner circular and outer longitudinal smooth muscle fibers surrounded by a fibroelastic connective tissue (see Fig. 21.28, *arrows*, IC, OL, CT). At a medium magnification, the epithelium is noted to be pseudostratified columnar, composed of short basal cells and low columnar cells. The lumen of the seminal vesicles contains spermatozoa (see Fig. 21.29, BC, CC, L, Sz).

Prostate Gland

This low-magnification photomicrograph displays the presence of prostatic concretions in the lumina of the gland (see Fig. 21.31, *arrows*). At a high magnification, the basal cells and principal cells of the epithelium are evident, as well as the dome-shaped protuberance of the apical aspect of some principal cells. Note that some of the lumina of the gland exhibits the presence of prostatic concretions (see Fig. 21.32, BC, PC, D, L, pC).

Penis

Corpus Cavernosum

The tunica albuginea of the corpus cavernosum is a thick, dense, irregular, collagenous connective tissue that surrounds the erectile tissue. Observe that the vascular spaces are lined by the endothelium, a simple squamous epithelium (see Fig. 21.35, TA, ET, VS, *arrows*).

22 Special Senses

There are five special senses—smell, taste, feeling, vision, and hearing—each of which is perceived by receptors specific to that particular sense. The sense of smell and its receptors were described in Chapter 15; the sense of taste was described in Chapter 16; the sense of feeling (pressure, touch, pain, temperature, and proprioception) was partially described in Chapter 14 but will be elaborated on here; and the other two special senses, vision and hearing, will be described in detail to follow. Special sense receptors, when stimulated by environmental stimuli, transduce this sensory input into electrical signals and convey them to the central nervous system (CNS). These sensory receptors are classified into three types, depending on the source of the stimulus: exteroceptors, proprioceptors, and interoceptors.

Exteroceptors, located near the body surface, are specialized to perceive stimuli from the external environment. These receptors—sensitive to temperature, touch, pressure, and pain—are components of the **general somatic afferent** pathways and are described in the first part of this chapter. Other exteroceptors, specialized for perceiving light (sense of vision) and sound (sense of hearing), are components of the **special somatic afferent** pathways (discussed later).

Proprioceptors are specialized receptors located in joint capsules, tendons, and intrafusal fibers within muscles (see Chapter 8). These **general somatic afferent** receptors transmit sensory input to the CNS, which is translated into information that relates to an awareness of the body in space and movement. Certain receptors of the **vestibular (balance) mechanism** (see later discussion), located within the inner ear, are specialized for receiving stimuli related to motion vectors within the head. This input is transmitted to the brain for processing into awareness of motion for corrective balancing.

Interoceptors are specialized receptors that perceive sensory information from within organs of the body; therefore, the modality serving this function is **general visceral afferent**.

Specialized Peripheral Receptors

Certain peripheral receptors specialized to receive particular stimuli include mechanoreceptors, thermoreceptors, and nociceptors.

The dendritic endings of certain sensory receptors located in various regions of the body—including muscles, tendons, skin, fascia, and joint capsules—are specialized to receive particular stimuli. These adaptations help the dendrite respond to a particular stimulus. Thus, these receptors are classified into three types:

- Mechanoreceptors, which respond to touch (Figs. 22.1–22.4)
- Thermoreceptors, which respond to cold and warmth
- Nociceptors (pain receptors) and pruriceptors (itch receptors)—the former respond to pain due to mechanical stress, extremes of temperature differences, and chemical substances; the latter respond to itch sensations

Although these specialized receptors generally are triggered only by a particular stimulus, any stimulus that is intense enough can trigger any receptor.

MECHANORECEPTORS

Mechanoreceptors respond to mechanical stimuli that may in some fashion alter the morphology either of the receptor or the tissues surrounding the receptor. Stimuli that trigger the mechanoreceptors are touch, stretch, vibrations, and pressure.

Nonencapsulated Mechanoreceptors

Nonencapsulated mechanoreceptors are simple unmyelinated receptors present in the skin, connective tissues, and surrounding hair follicles.

Peritrichial nerve endings, the simplest form of mechanoreceptors, are unmyelinated, lack Schwann cells, and are not covered by a connective tissue capsule. Such nerve endings are located in the epidermis of skin, especially in regions of great sensitivity, such as the face and the cornea, where they respond to stimuli related to touch and pressure (see Fig. 22.1D). Additionally, peritrichial nerve endings are wrapped around the base and shaft of hair follicles and function in touch perception related to the deformation of the hairs. Moreover, some naked nerve endings function as nociceptors or as thermoreceptors.

Merkel disks are slightly more complex mechanoreceptors (see Fig. 22.1A). Specialized for perceiving discriminatory touch, these receptors are composed of an expanded unmyelinated nerve terminal associated with **Merkel cells**, specialized epithelial cells interspersed with keratinocytes in the stratum basale of the skin (see Fig. 14.1). These receptors are located mostly in glabrous (nonhairy) skin and regions of the body more sensitive to touch.

Encapsulated Mechanoreceptors

Encapsulated mechanoreceptors exhibit characteristic structures and are present in specific locations.

Pacinian corpuscles, another example of the encapsulated mechanoreceptors, are located in the dermis and hypodermis in the digits of the hands and in the breasts, as well as in connective tissue of the joints, periosteum, and mesentery. These mechanoreceptors are specialized to perceive **pressure**, **touch**, and **vibration**. Pacinian corpuscles are large, ovoid receptors 1 to 2 mm long by 0.1 to 0.7 mm in diameter (see Figs. 22.1C, 22.2, and 22.3). Each large Pacinian corpuscle is composed of a single myelinated fiber that, almost as soon as it enters the corpuscle, loses its myelin sheath and courses the entire length of the corpuscle as an unmyelinated nerve fiber. The **inner core** of the corpuscle contains the nonmyelinated nerve terminal and its Schwann cells, surrounded by approximately 60 layers of modified fibroblasts, each layer separated from the next by a small fluid-filled space. An additional group of 30 less dense modified fibroblasts, the **outer core**, surrounds the inner core.

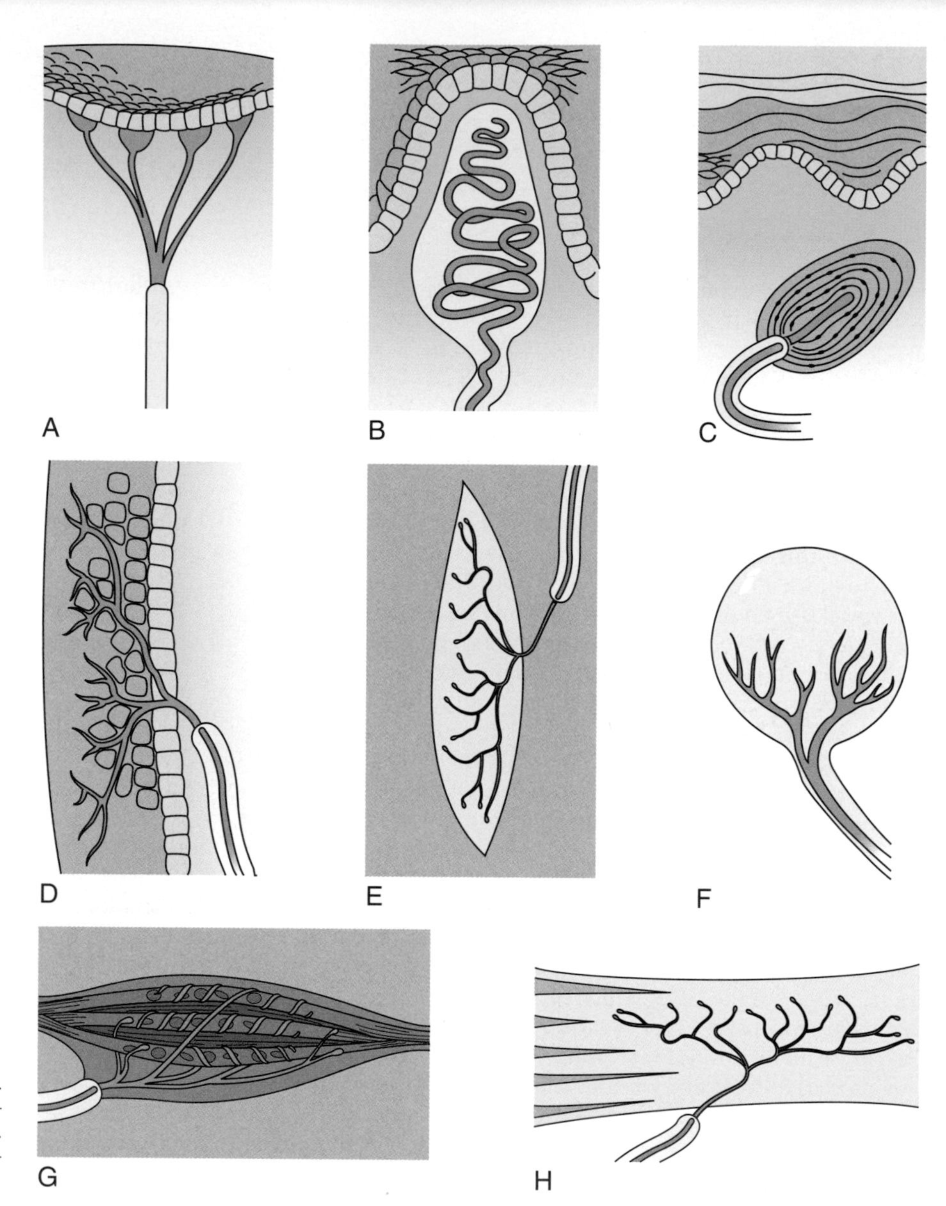

Fig. 22.1 Diagram of various sensory receptors. (A) Merkel disk. (B) Meissner corpuscle. (C) Pacinian corpuscle. (D) Peritricial (naked) nerve endings. (E) Ruffini corpuscle. (F) Krause end bulb. (G) Muscle spindle. (H) Golgi tendon organ.

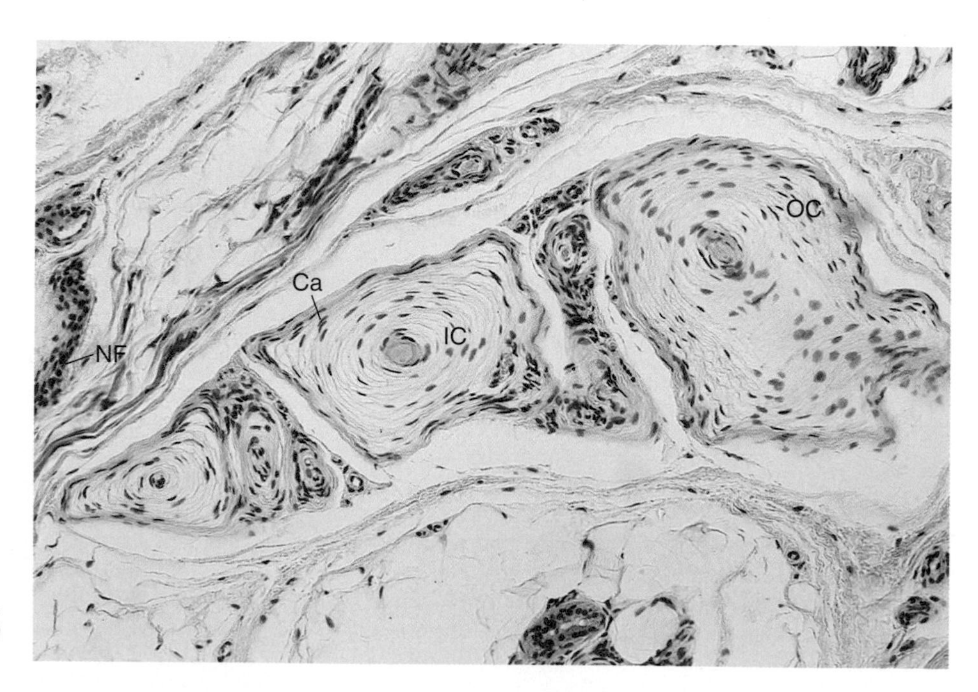

Fig. 22.2 Pacinian corpuscles. Inner core (IC), outer core (OC), nerve fiber (NF), capsule (Ca) (×132).

The entire structure has a collagenous connective tissue **capsule** that surrounds the outer core. The arrangement of the cells in the lamellae makes the histological section of a Pacinian corpuscle resemble an onion sliced in half.

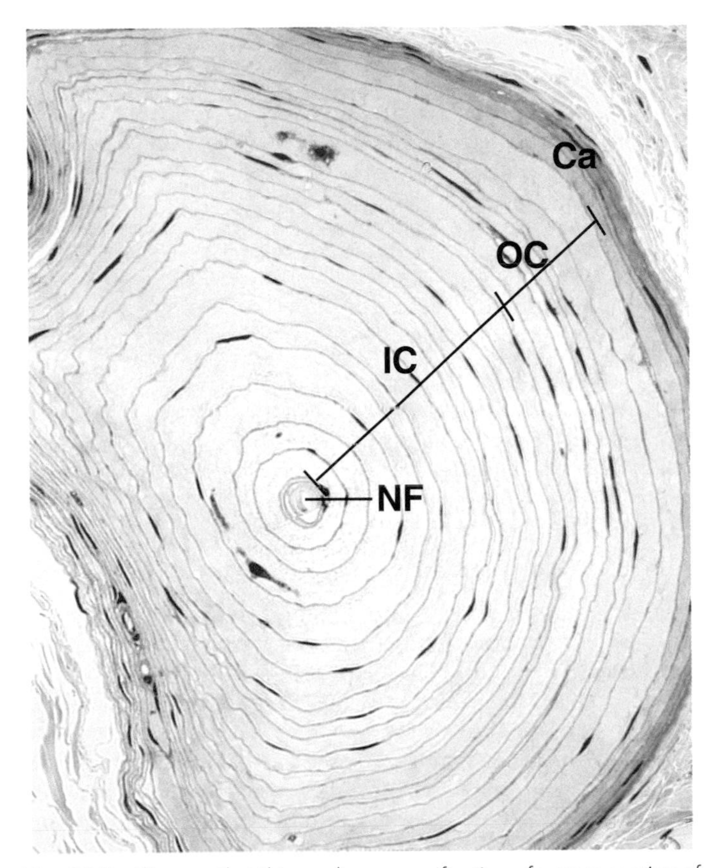

Fig. 22.3 Observe that this medium magnification of a cross-section of a small Pacinian corpuscle resembles an onion sliced in half. The nerve fiber (NF) has already lost its myelin sheath and is surrounded by several layers of fibroblast-like cells with fluid-filled spaces between the layers that form the inner core (IC). The outer core (OC) surrounds the inner core, which is, in turn, surrounded by a collagenous capsule (Ca). (×270)

Meissner corpuscles (see Fig. 22.4) are encapsulated mechanoreceptors specialized for **tactile discrimination**. These receptors are located in the dermal papillae of the glabrous portion of the fingers and palms of the hands, where they account for about half of the tactile receptors. They also are located in the eyelids, lips, tongue, nipples, skin of the feet, and skin of the forearms. Meissner corpuscles, located in the dermal papillae, measure 80 to 150 μm × 20 to 40 μm with their long axes oriented perpendicular to the skin surface (see Fig. 22.1B). Each Meissner corpuscle is formed by three or seven nerve terminals and their associated Schwann cells, all of which are encapsulated by connective tissue. A single myelinated nerve fiber branches to innervate several corpuscles; however, just after entering the corpuscle, the nerve fiber branch loses its myelin sheath. Contained within the capsule are stacks of epithelioid cells, possibly modified Schwann cells or fibroblasts, which serve to separate the branching nerve terminals. Meissner corpuscles respond to **fine touch** and are especially sensitive to **edges** and **points** and to **movements** of these objects, and they respond to slipping of the skin against an object so that the individuals can adjust the strength of their grip. These corpuscles have a receptive field of approximately 4 mm in diameter and respond to a pressure that depresses the skin of their receptive fields by less than 10 μm.

Ruffini endings (**corpuscles**) are encapsulated endings located in the dermis of the skin, nail beds, periodontal ligaments, and joint capsules. These large receptors, 1 mm long by 0.2 mm in diameter (see Fig. 22.1E), are composed of **branched nonmyelinated** terminals interspersed with collagen fibers and surrounded by four to five layers of modified fibroblasts. The connective tissue capsule surrounding each of these receptors is anchored at each end, increasing their sensibility to **stretching**, **touch**, and **pressure** in the skin and joint capsules.

Krause end bulbs are spherical, encapsulated nerve endings located in the papillary region of the dermis, joints, conjunctiva, peritoneum, genital regions, and subendothelial connective tissues of the oral and nasal cavities (see Fig. 22.1F). Originally,

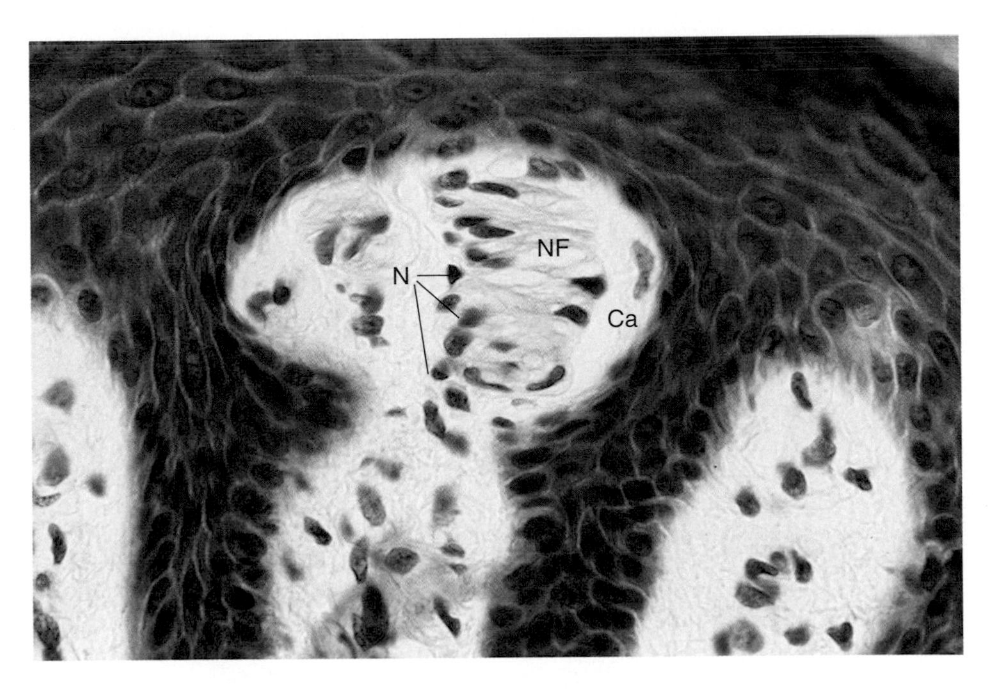

Fig. 22.4 Meissner corpuscle. Nuclei (N), capsule (Ca), nerve fibers (NF). (×540)

they were thought to be receptors sensitive to cold, but present evidence does not support this concept. Their function is unknown.

Both **muscle spindles** and **Golgi tendon organs** are encapsulated mechanoreceptors involved in proprioception. **Muscle spindles** (see Fig. 22.1G) provide feedback concerning the changes in muscle length, as well as the rate of alteration in the length of the muscle; **Golgi tendon organs** (see Fig. 22.1H) monitor the tension, as well as the rate at which the tension is being produced, during movement. Information from these two sensory structures is processed mostly at the unconscious levels within the spinal cord. However, the information also reaches the cerebellum, and even the cerebral cortex, so that the individual may sense muscle position. Golgi tendon organs and muscle spindles are discussed in Chapter 8.

THERMORECEPTORS

Thermoreceptors, which respond to temperature differences of about 2°C, are of three types: warmth receptors, cold receptors, and temperature-sensitive nociceptors.

Although specific receptors have not been identified for warmth, it is assumed that these receptors are naked endings of small nonmyelinated nerve fibers that respond to temperature increases (greater than 40°C to 42°C). It has been reported recently that ion channels, known as ***transient receptor V1 channels*** (also known as ***capsaicin receptors***) open when the temperature of the tissue in their immediate vicinity rises to higher than 43°C or when substances such as capsaicin or acids are encountered and Na^+ ions can enter the cell, depolarizing it. The information relayed to the CNS is interpreted as burning pain. Cold receptors are derived from naked nerve endings of myelinated fibers that branch and penetrate the epidermis and respond to temperatures lower than 25°C to 30°C. Because thermoreceptors are not activated by physical stimulation, they are believed to respond to differing rates of temperature-dependent biochemical reactions.

NOCICEPTORS AND PRURICEPTORS

Nociceptors are receptors sensitive to pain; pruriceptors respond to itching sensations.

Nociceptors are responsible for pain perception. These receptors are naked endings of myelinated nerve fibers that branch freely in the dermis before entering the epidermis. Nociceptors are divided into three groups: (1) those that respond to mechanical stress or damage; (2) those that respond to extremes in heat or cold; and (3) those that respond to chemical compounds such as bradykinin, serotonin, and histamine.

Nociception is dependent on opening of voltage-gated Na^+ ion channels. There are nine types of known voltage-gated Na^+ ion channels; each type opens at slightly different voltages. Three of the nine channels react to painful stimuli. These are known as *Na_V1.7*, *Na_V1.8*, and *Na_V1.9*, where Na_V = voltage-gated sodium ion channel and 1.7 is the seventh, 1.8 is the eighth, and 1.9 is the ninth voltage-gated sodium ion channel.

Itching (**pruriception**) is a somatic sensation that may be due to local causes, such as a tiny insect walking on one's arm or to generalized and systemic causes such as a form of dermatitis or even to cancer and organ failure. The mechanism of an itch is better known in mice than in humans, but it is assumed that there may be a close correlation in the two species. It has been demonstrated in mice that itching sensation is conveyed by C fibers to the murine spinal cord, where secondary neurons reside that are capable of expressing gastrin-releasing peptide receptors (GRPR). Apparently, there are a number of GRPR types of neurons and they are activated by various types of G protein–coupled receptors that respond to a particular cause of the itching sensation. Moreover, there seems to be a relationship between pain and itching sensations because they share similar but not identical pathways, but they both involve receptors in the skin, spinal cord, and brain.

Clinical Correlations

Chronic neuropathic pain (usually in the hands and feet) is one of the most common illnesses in the world, affecting a large segment of the U.S. population. Many individuals with this condition present with mutations in the nociceptor ion channels (especially NaV1.7) so that these ion channels are hyperactive and open even during conditions that would not be painful under normal circumstances. Normally, the resulting information is transmitted to the central nervous system (CNS), where interneurons intercept the information and inhibit its transmission (postsynaptic inhibition). The inhibition is due to the presence of a ***chloride transporter*** *in the interneuron plasmalemma (also present in other neuron plasma membranes), known as* ***potassium/chloride co-transporter 2 (KCC2)****. In a normal individual, when pain is detected,* ***microglia*** *of the spinal cord release a signaling molecule that acts on interneurons to reduce their KCC2 transporters, and the interneuron can no longer inhibit the pain signal from being transmitted to higher levels in the CNS. In patients with neuropathic pain, what normally would be a nonpainful stimulus will cause the diminution of KCC2 levels in the interneurons and the stimulus, instead of being blocked by the interneuron, is permitted to be transmitted, erroneously, resulting in pain sensations.*

Eye

The bulb of the eye is composed of three tunics: fibrous, vascular, and neural.

The **eyes** (**eyeballs**), the **photosensory organs** of the body, are approximately 24 mm in diameter and are located within the bony orbits of the skull. Light passing through the cornea and several refractory structures of the eyeballs is focused by the lens on the light-sensitive portion of the neural tunic of the eye, the **retina**, which contains the photosensitive **rods** and **cones**. Through a series of several layers of nerve cells and supporting cells, the partially assembled visual information is transmitted by the optic nerve to the brain for final processing.

About the fourth week of embryogenesis, the eyes begin to develop from three different sources. The future retina and optic nerve, the outgrowths of the forebrain, are the first to be observed. The continued growth of this outgrowth induces the surface ectoderm to develop into the lens and some of the accessory structures of the anterior portion of the eye. Later in development, adjacent mesenchyme condenses to form the tunics and associated structures of the eyeballs.

The eye is composed of three tunics (coats; Fig. 22.5): the **tunica fibrosa** (**fibrous tunic**), which forms the tough outer coat

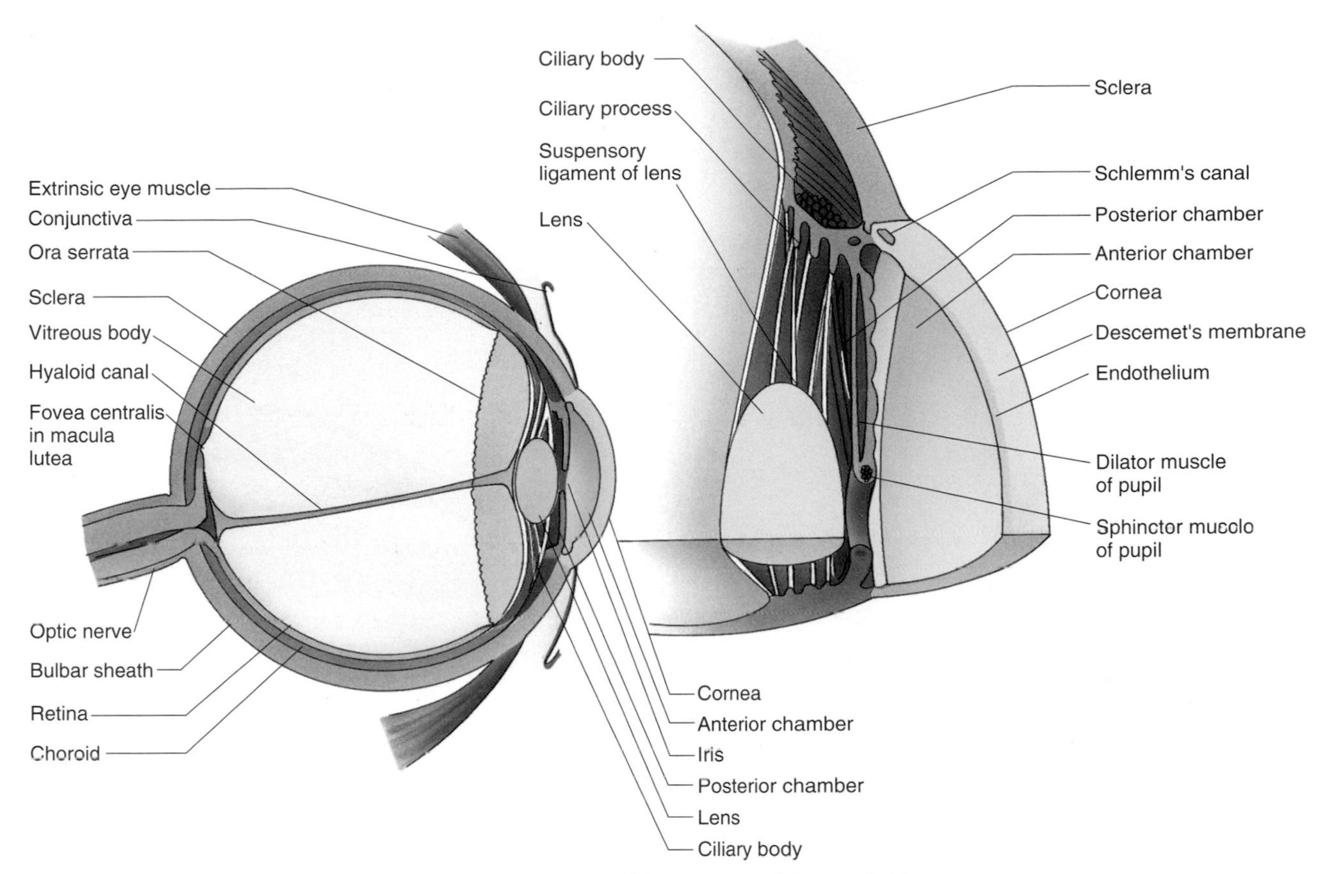

Fig. 22.5 Diagram of the anatomy of the eye (orb).

of the eye; the **tunica vasculosa** (**vascular tunic; uvea**), which is composed of the pigmented and vascular middle coats; and the **retina** (**neural tunic**), which constitutes the innermost coat of the eyeball.

The **extrinsic muscles** of the eye, which are responsible for coordinated movements of the eyes to gain access to various visual fields, insert into the fibrous tunic. Smooth muscles located within the eyeball accommodate focusing of the lens and function to control the aperture of the pupil. Located outside the eyeball, but still within the orbit, is the **lacrimal gland** (tear gland), which secretes **lacrimal fluid** (tears) that moistens the anterior surface of the eye and the inner surface of the eyelids by passing through the **conjunctiva**, a transparent membrane that covers and protects the anterior surface of the eye.

TUNICA FIBROSA

The tunica fibrosa is composed of the sclera and cornea.

The external fibrous tunic of the eye, the **tunica fibrosa**, is divided into the **sclera** and **cornea** (see Fig. 22.5). The white, opaque **sclera** covers the posterior five-sixths of the eyeball, whereas the colorless, transparent **cornea** covers the anterior one-sixth of the eyeball.

Sclera

The white opaque sclera is composed of type I collagen fibers interlaced with elastic fibers.

The **sclera**, a tough fibrous connective tissue layer that covers approximately 85% of the eyeball, is about 1 mm thick posteriorly, thinning at the equator and then thickening again near its junction with the cornea. It is covered by the conjunctiva, composed of a stratified squamous nonkeratinized to a stratified cuboidal epithelium with occasional goblet cells. Blood vessels visible on the surface of the sclera pierce the sclera to reach the tunica vasculosa, where they distribute to various components of the eye.

The sclera has three indistinctly recognizable layers. Just deep to the conjunctiva is the first layer, a thin, looser type of collagenous connective tissue layer, the **episclera**. The second and thickest layer, composed of a dense, collagenous connective tissue, is known as the **stroma** (**Tenon capsule, sclera proper**), whose interlacing type I collagen fiber bundles alternating with networks of elastic fibers provide the architectural support for the shape of the eyeball, which is maintained by intraocular pressure from the aqueous humor (located anterior to the lens) and the vitreous body (located posterior to the lens). The third layer, the **suprachoroid lamina**, is a thin, connective tissue layer that houses elongated, flat fibroblasts throughout its substance and **melanocytes** in its deeper aspect. At the sclera-corneal junction, the deep surface of the suprachoroid lamina is covered by a simple squamous epithelium, known as the **scleral endothelium**.

Tendons of the **extraocular muscles** insert into the **stroma**. The eyeball, along with its various parts and attached extraocular muscles, moves in unison within the periorbital fat–filled bony orbit (Fig. 22.6).

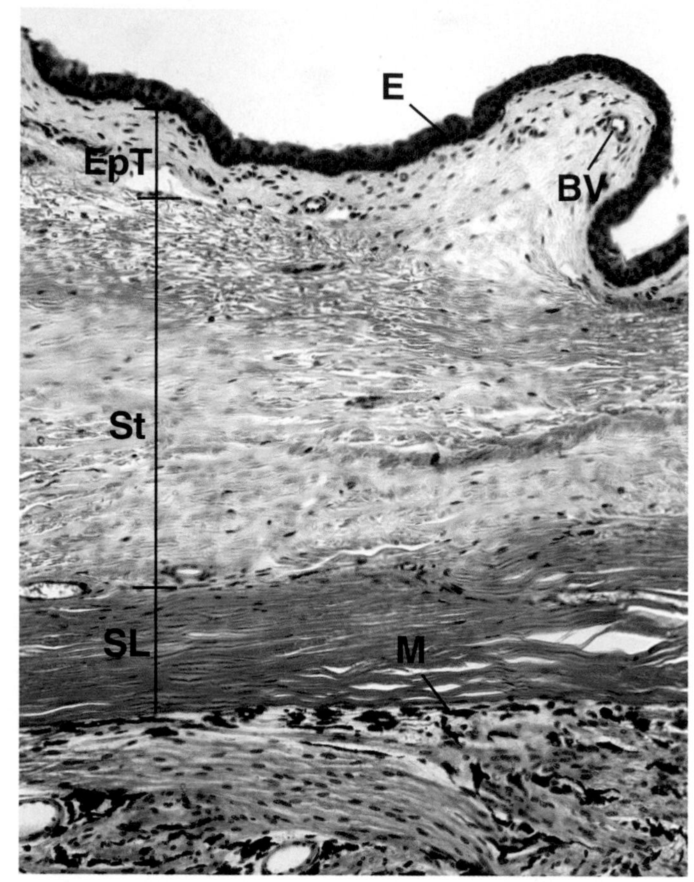

Fig. 22.6 The sclera, white of the eye, is nearly avascular, although it has some blood vessels (BV) associated with it. Its external surface is covered by the epithelium of the conjunctiva, a stratified squamous nonkeratinized to a stratified cuboidal epithelium (E). The episclera (EpT), stroma (St), and the melanocytes (M) of the suprachoroid lamina (SL) are well displayed. (×132)

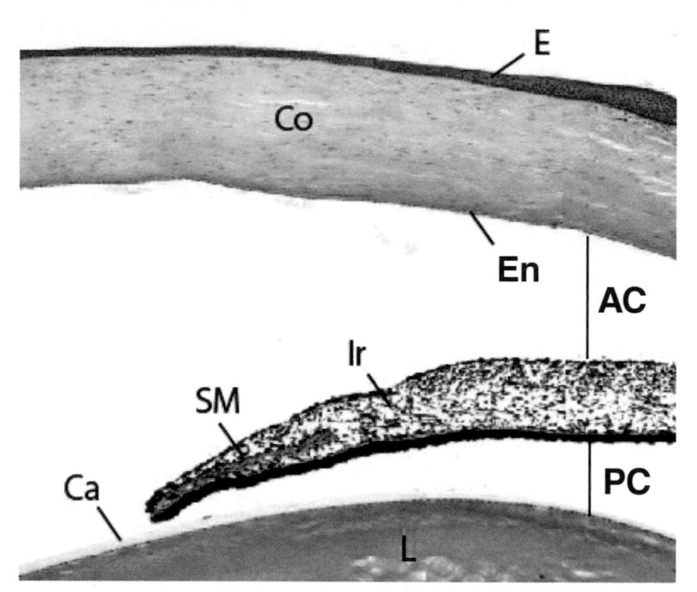

Fig. 22.7 This very-low-magnification photomicrograph of the anterior region of the eyeball presents the cornea (Co) with its corneal epithelium (E) and corneal endothelium (En), which abuts the anterior chamber (AC). Observe the iris (Ir) with its smooth muscle fibers, and the posterior chamber (PC) between the iris and the thin capsule (Ca) of the lens (L). (×56)

Cornea

The cornea is the transparent bulging anterior one-sixth of the eyeball.

The **cornea** is the transparent, avascular, and highly innervated anterior portion of the fibrous tunic that bulges out anteriorly from the eyeball (Figs. 22.7 and 22.8) It is slightly thicker than the sclera and is composed of six histologically distinct layers:

- Corneal epithelium
- Bowman membrane
- Stroma
- Pre-Descemet layer (Dua layer)
- Descemet membrane
- Corneal endothelium

The **corneal epithelium**, the continuation of the conjunctiva (a mucous membrane covering the anterior sclera and lining the internal surface of the eyelids), is a stratified, squamous, nonkeratinized epithelium composed of five to seven layers of cells that covers the anterior surface of the cornea. The larger superficial cells have microvilli and exhibit zonulae occludentes, whereas the remaining cells of the corneal epithelium interdigitate with and form desmosomal contacts with one another, and their cytoplasm contains the usual array of organelles, along with intermediate filaments. The corneal epithelium is highly innervated by pain fibers with numerous free nerve endings. Mitotic figures are observed mostly near the periphery of the cornea, with a turnover rate of approximately 7 days, and damage to the cornea is repaired rapidly as cells migrate to the defect to cover the injured region. Subsequently, mitotic activity replaces

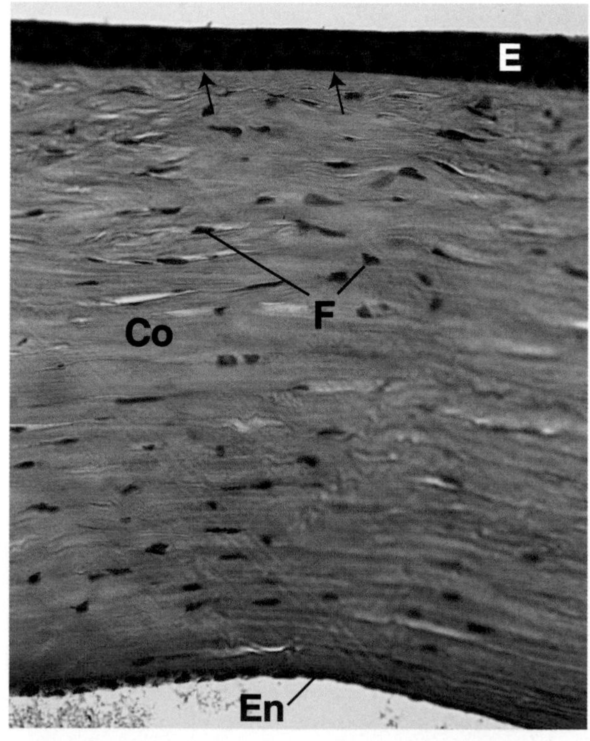

Fig. 22.8 At medium magnification, the stratified squamous epithelium (E) of the cornea is well demonstrated, as is the thin acellular Bowman membrane *(arrows)* that separates the epithelium from the transparent stroma with its collagen fibers (Co) and thin fibroblasts (F). Note the thin simple squamous to cuboidal endothelium (En) that separates the cornea from the aqueous humor of the anterior chamber. (×270)

the cells that migrated to the wound. The corneal epithelium also functions in transferring water and ions from the stroma into the conjunctival sac.

The **Bowman membrane**, a fibrillar lamina 6 to 30 µm thick composed of type I collagen fibers arranged in an apparently random fashion, lies immediately deep to the corneal epithelium. It is believed that this membrane is synthesized by both the corneal epithelium and cells of the underlying stroma. The sensory nerve fibers pass through this structure to enter and terminate in the epithelium.

The transparent **stroma** is composed of collagenous connective tissue consisting mostly of type I collagen fibers that are arranged in 200 to 250 lamellae, each about 2 µm thick. The collagen fibers within each lamella are arranged parallel to one another, but fiber orientation shifts in adjacent lamellae. The collagen fibers are interspersed with thin elastic fibers embedded in ground substance containing mostly chondroitin sulfate and keratan sulfate. Long, slender fibroblasts are also present among the collagen fiber bundles. The stroma constitutes approximately 90% of the cornea, making it the cornea's thickest layer; during inflammation, lymphocytes and neutrophils infiltrate it. At the **limbus** (sclera-corneal junction) is a **scleral sulcus** whose inner aspect at the stroma is depressed and houses endothelium-lined spaces known as the **trabecular meshwork** that lead to the **canal of Schlemm**, the site of outflow of the aqueous humor from the anterior chamber of the eye into the venous system.

Clinical Correlations

The sclera, the white of the eye, is nontransparent because of its high degree of hydration. However, if one dries a small area of the scleral surface by blowing dry air on it, that dried region becomes transparent. The cornea, however, is transparent because extracellular fluid is constantly being resorbed from its surfaces, partially dehydrating the substance of this transparent layer of the eyeball. Tears keep the modified conjunctival covering the cornea moist without adding water to the stroma of the cornea.

The pre-Descemet layer (**Dua layer**) is a 15-µm, thin, tough collagenous membrane that is probably manufactured by the fibroblasts of the stroma. It has been suggested that the durability of this recently discovered layer protects the cornea from damage, whereas physical injury that breaches the integrity of the pre-Descemet layer may result in **corneal hydrops** (infiltration of an aqueous fluid into the corneal stroma).

The **Descemet membrane** is a thick basement membrane interposed between the stroma and the underlying endothelium. Although this membrane is thin, only 5 µm at birth and homogeneous in younger persons, in older adults it becomes thicker (17 µm), presenting with cross-striations and hexagonal fiber patterns.

The **corneal endothelium**, which lines the internal (posterior) surface of the cornea, is a **simple squamous** to **simple cuboidal epithelium**, whose cells exhibit numerous pinocytotic vesicles, and their membranes have sodium pumps that transport sodium ions (Na^+) into the anterior chamber; these ions are passively followed by chloride ions (Cl^-) and water. Thus, excess fluid within the stroma is resorbed by the endothelium, keeping the stroma relatively dehydrated, a condition necessary for the maintenance of the refractive quality of the cornea. The corneal endothelium is responsible for synthesis of proteins that form the Descemet membrane.

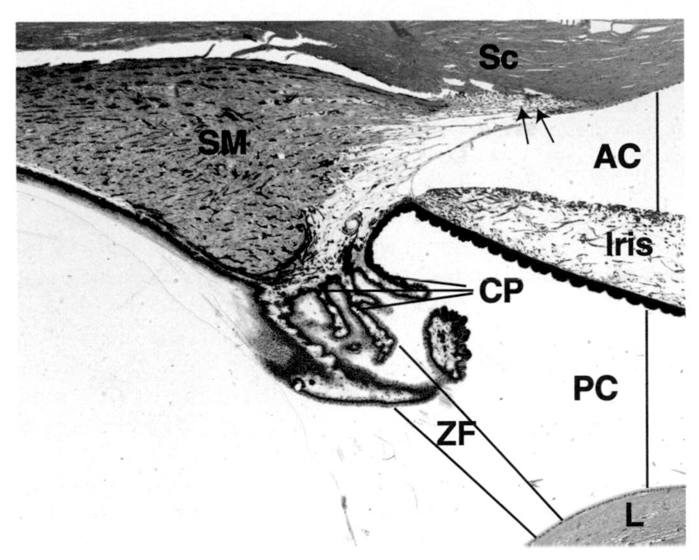

Fig. 22.9 This low-magnification photomicrograph presents the smooth muscle (SM) of the ciliary body and the ciliary processes (CP), as well as the proximal portion of the iris that separates the anterior chamber (AC) from the posterior chamber (PC) located between the iris and the lens (L). The lines drawn from the ciliary processes to the lens represent the zonular fibers (ZF). Observe the canal of Schlemm *(arrows)* at the junction of the sclera–corneal junction (Sc). (×132)

Clinical Correlations

H-Y antigens, products of genes located on the Y chromosome, are expressed on the cell membranes of almost every cell in the male body. If a female has not been exposed to these antigens prior to birth, then the unexposed female will react to the antigens as nonself and will mount an immune response against them. This is an important consideration in corneal transplants because in a major study, it was shown that approximately 22% of females receiving a male cornea rejected it, whereas in female-to-female corneal transplant the failure rate was 18%.

TUNICA VASCULOSA

The vascular middle tunic of the eye, the tunica vasculosa (also known as the uvea), is composed of three parts: (1) the choroid, (2) ciliary body, and (3) iris (Fig. 22.9; see Fig. 22.5).

Choroid

The choroid, the pigmented posterior portion of the middle vascular tunic, is loosely attached to the sclera and separated from the retina by the Bruch membrane.

The **choroid**, the well-vascularized, pigmented layer of the posterior wall of the eyeball, is loosely attached to the tunica fibrosa. It is composed of loose connective tissue containing numerous fibroblasts and other connective tissue cells and has a rich vascular supply. The black color of the choroid is due to the myriad of melanocytes present in it. The inner surface of the choroid, because of its abundance of small blood vessels, is known as the **choriocapillary layer** and is responsible for providing nutrients to the retina. The choroid is separated from the retina by the 1- to 4-µm-thick **Bruch membrane**, which is composed of a network of elastic fibers located in the central region and sandwiched on both sides by collagen fiber layers. The outer aspect of each collagen fiber layer is covered by a basal lamina that belongs to capillaries on one side and the **pigment epithelium** of the retina on the other side.

Ciliary Body

The ciliary body is a wedge-shaped portion of the choroid located in the lumen of the orb between the iris and vitreous body and projecting toward the lens.

The **ciliary body** is the wedge-shaped extension of the choroid that rings the inner wall of the eye at the level of the lens, occupies the space between the **ora serrata** (the serrated junction where the retina ends) and the attached portion of the iris. One surface of the ciliary body abuts the sclera at the sclera–corneal junction; another surface abuts the vitreous body. The medial surface projects toward the lens, forming short, finger-like projections known as the **ciliary processes** (see Fig. 22.9).

The ciliary body is composed of loose connective tissue containing numerous elastic fibers, blood vessels, and melanocytes. Its inner surface is lined by the **pars ciliaris of the retina**, a pigmented layer of the retina that is composed of two cell layers. The outer cell layer, which faces the lumen of the eyeball, is a nonpigmented columnar epithelium (**nonpigmented ciliary epithelium**). The inner cell layer is composed of a pigmented simple columnar epithelium (**pigmented ciliary epithelium**), which is rich in melanin pigments.

The anterior third of the ciliary body has about 70 **ciliary processes**, which radiate out from a central core of connective tissue containing abundant fenestrated capillaries. **Zonular fibers**, composed of fibrillin, radiate from the ciliary processes to insert into the lens capsule, forming the **suspensory ligaments of the lens**, which suspend the lens in place.

The ciliary processes are covered by the same two layers of epithelia that cover the ciliary body. The inner nonpigmented layer has many interdigitations and infoldings; its cells transport a protein-poor plasma filtrate, the **aqueous humor**, into the posterior chamber of the eye. The aqueous humor flows from the posterior chamber into the anterior chamber by passing through the **pupillary aperture** between the iris and the lens. The aqueous humor exits the anterior chamber by passing into the trabecular meshwork near the limbus and, finally, as stated earlier, into the canal of Schlemm, which leads directly into the venous system. The aqueous humor provides nutrients and oxygen for the lens and cornea.

The bulk of the ciliary body is composed of three bundles of smooth muscle cells called the ciliary muscle. One bundle, because of its orientation, stretches the choroid, altering the opening of the canal of Schlemm for drainage of the aqueous humor. The remaining two muscle bundles, attached at the scleral spur (the junction point of the sclera, cornea, and ciliary body, just peripheral to the attachment of the iris), function in reducing tension on the zonulae. Contractions of this muscle, mediated by parasympathetic fibers of the oculomotor nerve (Cranial Nerve [CN] III), stretch the ciliary body, thereby releasing tension on the suspensory ligaments of the lens. As a result, the lens becomes thicker and more convex. This action permits focusing on nearby objects, a process called accommodation. Relaxation of all three muscle bundles increases tension on the zonule, which flattens the lens, enabling the eye to focus on distant objects. Constant adjustments between various degrees of contraction and relaxation are required to permit focusing on objects that are distant, intermediate, and close up.

Clinical Correlations

Glaucoma is a constellation of conditions resulting from prolonged increased intraocular pressure caused by the failure of drainage of the aqueous humor from the anterior chamber of the eye. It is the world's leading cause of blindness, second only to cataracts. In ***chronic glaucoma,*** *the most common condition, the continued increase of intraocular pressure causes progressive damage to the eye, specifically, the optic nerve. The gradual loss of vision, if left untreated, results in blindness. Fortunately, a simple daily application of a variety of prescription eyedrops alleviates the condition. However, patient compliance (at least in the United States) is a major problem—approximately 50% to 75% of the patients fail to renew their prescription. Surgical treatments, such as canaloplasty, in which the canal of Schlemm is enlarged via microcatheterization, or trabeculectomy, in which a partial scleral flap is made and loosely sutured in position, provide a space for the fluid to drain from the eye. Additionally, in third-world countries, the access to ophthalmologists, as well as the availability and price of prescription drugs are major obstacles to proper glaucoma treatment. Currently, it is estimated that there are almost 60 million people affected worldwide and almost 3.5 million people with glaucoma in the United States.*

Iris

The iris, the colored anterior extension of the choroid, is a contractile diaphragm that controls the diameter of the pupillary aperture.

The **iris** is a circular colored disc with a centrally located round hole known as the **pupil** (**pupillary aperture**). It is the anteriormost extension of the choroid, situated between the posterior and anterior chambers of the eye so that it completely covers the lens except at the pupil. The iris is thickest in the middle, becoming thinner both toward its attachment to the ciliary body and at the rim of the pupil (see Figs. 22.7 and 22.9).

The *anterior surface* of the iris displays two concentric rings: the **pupillary zone**, lying nearest the pupil, and the wider **ciliary zone**; the two are separated by the **collarette**, the thickest part of the iris. This surface of the iris is irregular, with trenches extending into it; it also contains contraction furrows, which are easily distinguished when the pupil is dilated. An incomplete layer of pigmented cells and fibroblasts covers the anterior surface of the iris. Deep to this layer is the **stroma**, a poorly vascularized connective tissue containing numerous fibroblasts and melanocytes, which gives way to a well-vascularized, loose connective tissue zone.

The *posterior surface* of the iris is smooth and covered by the continuation of the two layers of retinal epithelium that cover the ciliary body. The surface facing the lens is composed of heavily pigmented cells, which block the light from passing through the iris except at the pupil. The epithelial cells facing the stroma of the iris have extensions that form the **dilator pupillae muscle**, consisting of myoepithelial cells. Another muscle, the **sphincter pupillae muscle**, is located in a concentric ring around the pupil. Contractions of these smooth muscles alter the diameter of the pupil, which changes inversely with the amount of light impinging on the iris. Thus, bright light causes constriction of the pupillary diameter, whereas dim light dilates it. As their names imply, the dilator pupillae muscle, innervated by the **sympathetic nervous system**, dilates the pupil; whereas the sphincter pupillae muscle, innervated by **parasympathetic fibers** of the oculomotor nerve (CN III), constricts the pupil.

The abundant population of melanocytes in the epithelium and stroma of the iris not only blocks the passage of light into the eye (except at the pupil) but also imparts color to the eyes.

Clinical Correlations

The eyes are dark when the number of melanocytes is high, and they are blue when the number of melanocytes is low. Approximately 6000 to 10,000 years ago, every person had brown eyes, but a mutation in the HERC2 gene that appeared in a single female was transmitted down the generations. The mutation in this gene affects a neighboring gene, known as OCA2, which is responsible for the formation of melanin in the iris. The final result is that the pigment cells of the iris produce less melanin than in irises without the mutation and the stroma of the iris contains much less melanin than individuals with brown eyes. Consequently, the irises of these individuals are blue.

Lens

The lens, the transparent biconvex disk located directly behind the pupil, focuses light rays on the retina.

The lens of the eye is a flexible, biconvex, transparent disk composed of epithelial cells and their secretory products. The lens consists of three parts: lens capsule, subcapsular epithelium, and lens fibers (see Fig. 22.5).

The **lens capsule** is a basal lamina, 10 to 20 μm thick, containing mostly type IV collagen and glycoprotein that covers the epithelial cells and envelops the entire lens. This elastic, transparent, homogeneous structure, which refracts light, is thickest anteriorly.

The **subcapsular epithelium** is located only on the anterior and lateral surfaces of the lens, immediately deep to the lens capsule (Figs. 22.10 and 22.11). It is composed of a single layer of cuboidal cells, which communicate with each other via gap junctions. The apices of these cells are directed toward the lens fibers and interdigitate with them, especially in the vicinity of the equator, where they are elongated and columnar in shape.

The substance of the lens is composed of approximately 2000 long cells, known as **lens fibers**, that lie immediately deep to the subcapsular epithelium (see Figs. 22.10–22.12). These highly differentiated cells in the shape of hexagonal solids arise from cells of the subcapsular epithelium, which lose their nuclei and organelles and continue elongating until they reach a length of 7 to 10 μm. This process of elongation, known as **maturation**, continues throughout the life of the individual. Eventually, these cells become filled with special lens proteins, known as **crystallins**, that increase the refractory index of the lens fibers.

As indicated earlier, the lens is suspended in its location in the eyeball by the presence of zonular fibers (suspensory ligaments of the lens) that are attached to the ciliary processes. When the smooth muscles of the ciliary body are in the contracted state, there is little tension on the ligaments, and the lens is more convex so that near vision is sharper. During the relaxation of the ciliary muscles, the tension on the ligaments is increased, making the lens flatter and sharpening distant vision.

Clinical Correlations

Presbyopia *is the inability of the eye to focus on near objects (accommodation) and is caused by an age-related decrease in the elasticity of the lens. As a result, the lens cannot become spherical for exact focusing. This condition can be corrected with eyeglasses, contact lenses, or LASIK (laser-assisted in situ keratomileusis) eye surgery.*

Cataract *formation is usually also an age-related condition in which the lens becomes opaque, impairing vision. This condition may be due to an accumulation of pigment or other substances, as well as to excessive exposure to ultraviolet radiation. Although cataracts do not usually respond to medication and eventually lead to blindness, the opaque lens may be excised and replaced with a corrective artificial lens.*

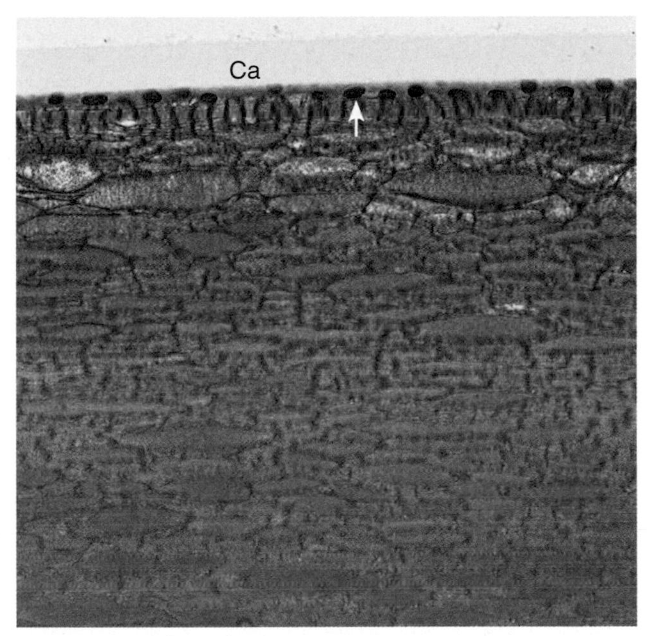

Fig. 22.10 Light micrograph of the lens (×132). Note the simple cuboidal epithelium *(arrow)* on the anterior surface and the capsule (Ca) covering the epithelium.

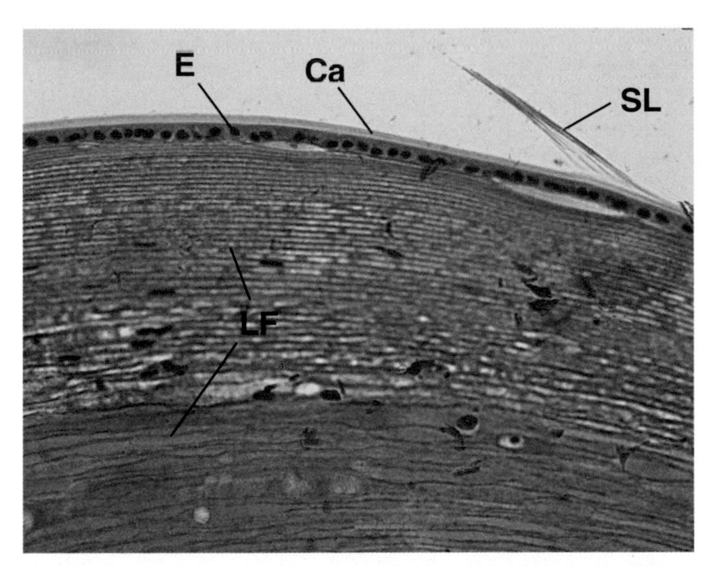

Fig. 22.11 This medium-magnification photomicrograph of the lens displays the zonular fibers that form the suspensory ligaments of the lens (SL) as they insert into the capsule (Ca) of the lens. Deep to the capsule is the simple cuboidal subcapsular epithelium (E) that covers the bulk of the lens, composed of elongated cells known as lens fibers (LF). (×270)

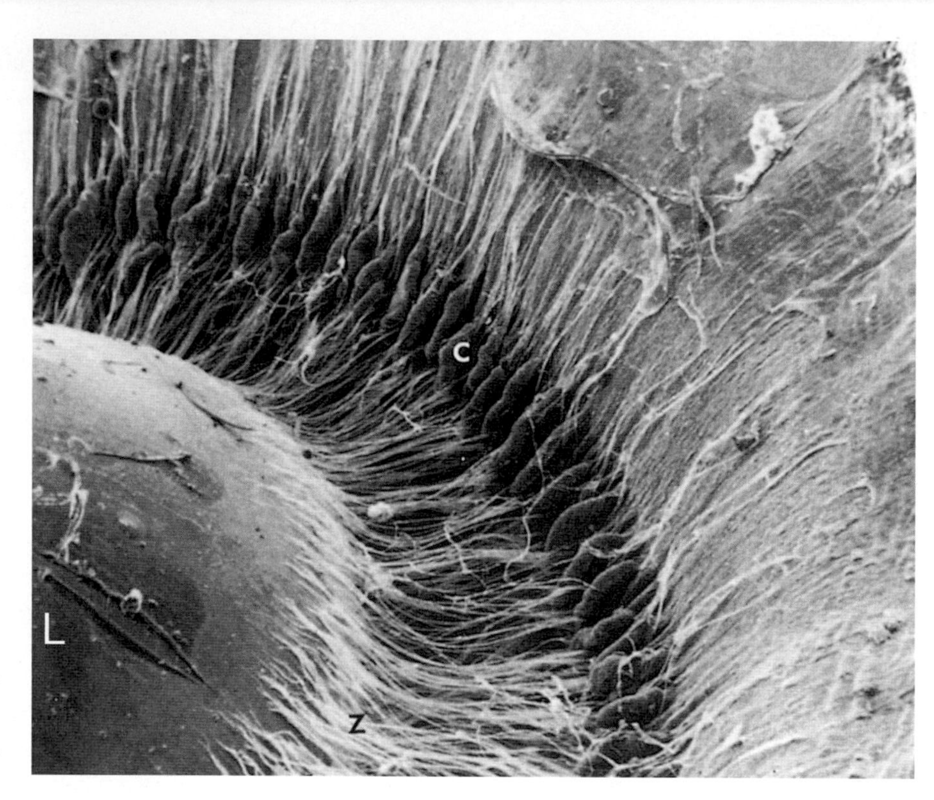

Fig. 22.12 Scanning electron micrograph of the posterior surface of the lens (×28). C, Ciliary body; L, lens; Z, zonula fibers. (From Leeson TS, Leeson CR, Paparo AA. *Text/Atlas of Histology*. Philadelphia: WB Saunders; 1988.)

Vitreous Body

The **vitreous body**, a transparent refractile gel that fills the **vitreous cavity** (cavity of the eye behind the lens), is composed mostly (99%) of water containing a minute amount of electrolytes, collagen fibers, and hyaluronic acid. It adheres to the retina over its entire surface, especially at the ora serrata. Occasional macrophages and small cells called **hyalocytes** are observed at the periphery of the vitreous body; these are believed to synthesize the collagen and the hyaluronic acid. The fluid-filled **hyaloid canal**, a narrow channel that was occupied by the hyaloid artery in the fetus, extends through the entire vitreous body from the posterior aspect of the lens to the optic disk.

Clinical Correlations

Eye floaters (vitreous opacities) specks, clouds, cobwebs and the like that individuals appear to see out in front of their eyes represent small debris that is floating in the vitreous body caused by its dehydration. These objects cast shadows on the retina that are translated by the brain as images in front of the eyes. Although most of the time these floaters will naturally resolve, some persons find that their lives are disrupted with the presence of floaters, especially when they are reading or driving. Specialized laser treatments can obliterate the floaters.

RETINA (NEURAL TUNIC)

The retina, composed of 10 layers, possesses specialized receptor cells, called rods and cones, which are responsible for photoreception.

The **retina**, the third and innermost tunic of the eye, develops from the optic cup, an evagination of the diencephalon, which gives rise to the primary optic vesicle. Later in development, this structure invaginates to form a bilaminar secondary optic vesicle from which the retina develops, whereas the stalk of the optic cup becomes the optic nerve. The retina contains the photoreceptor cells, known as **rods** and **cones**.

The retina is formed of an outer **pigmented layer** that develops from the outer wall of the optic cup, whereas the neural portion of the retina develops from the inner layer of the optic cup and is called the **retina proper**. The pigmented layer of the retina covers the entire internal surface of the eyeball, reflecting over the ciliary body and posterior wall of the iris, whereas the retina proper stops at the ora serrata. The cells composing the retina proper constitute a highly differentiated extension of the brain.

The **optic disk**, located on the posterior wall of the eyeball, is approximately 1.75 mm in diameter and is the exit site of the optic nerve. Because it contains no photoreceptor cells, it is insensitive to light and is therefore called the **blind spot** of the retina (Figs. 22.13 and 22.14). About 0.7 mm lateral to the **optic disk** is a yellow-pigmented zone, called the **macula lutea** (**yellow spot**), approximately 5.5 mm in diameter. At its center is a depression, 1.5 mm in diameter, known as the **fovea** (**fovea centralis**). Its central portion, the **foveola**, is where visual acuity is the greatest.

The retina has a dual blood supply. Much of the internal layers of the retina, from the internal segments of the rods and cones through the optic nerve fiber layer, is supplied by the **central retinal artery**, which gains access to the eyeball via the center of the optic nerve and forms numerous branches on the surface of the internal aspect of the retina. The external layers of the retina that constitute the outer segments of the rods and cones and the pigment epithelium are served by the vascular supply of the **choroid**.

The portion of the retina that functions in photoreception faces the inner surface of the choroid layer from the optic disk to the ora serrata and is composed of 10 distinct layers (Figs. 22.15 and 22.16). The retina has 10 named layers; by convention, the numbering starts from adjacent to the choroid to where

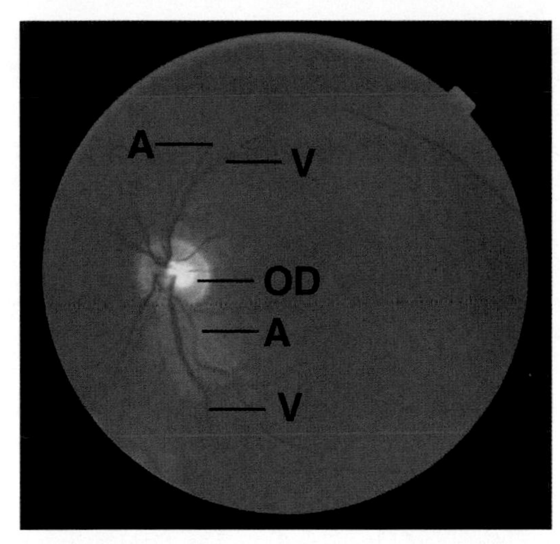

Fig. 22.13 This fundus photograph of the retina displays the optic disc (OD) and arteries (A) and veins (V) of the retina. Note that the veins are wider and darker than the arteries. (Courtesy Dr. Edward C. Watters III, MD)

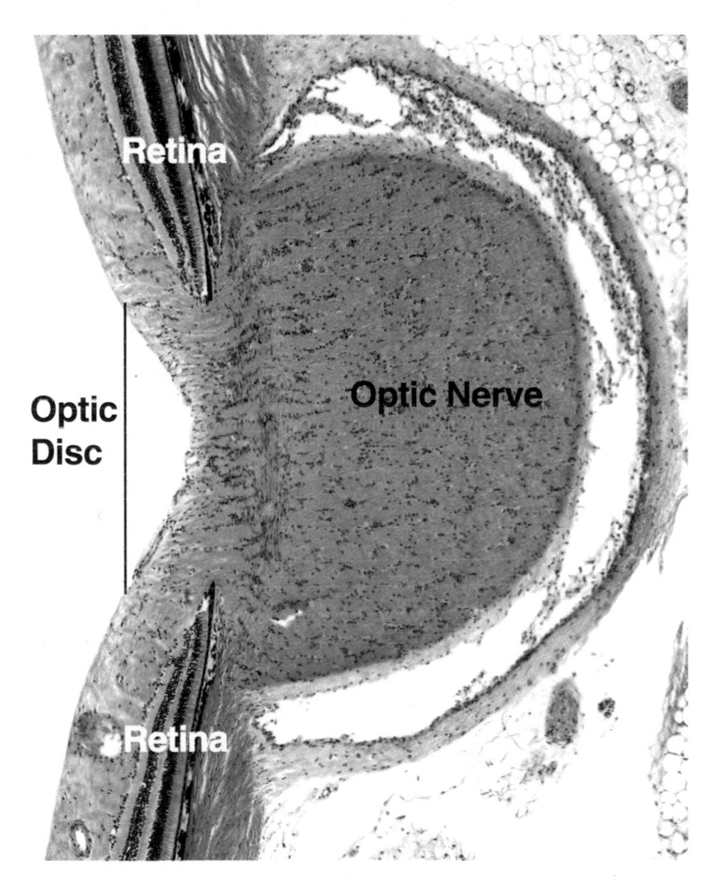

Fig. 22.14 This very-low-magnification photomicrograph of the optic disc demonstrates that the retinal layers stop at the periphery of the optic disc, the blind spot of the retina. The axons of the various nerve cells of the retina are gathered to form the optic nerve at the optic disc. (×56)

the vitreous humor abuts the retina. It should be noted that the light entering the eyeball reaches the tenth layer (inner limiting membrane) first and the first layer (pigment epithelium) last. These 10 layers are as follows (see also Table 22.1):

1. Pigment epithelium
2. Layer of rods and cones
3. Outer limiting membrane
4. Outer nuclear layer

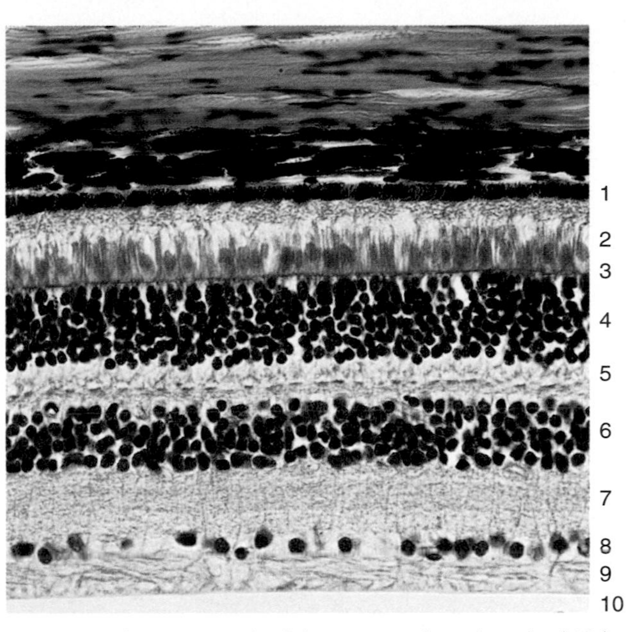

Fig. 22.15 Light micrograph of the retina with its described 10 layers (×270). (1) Pigment epithelium, (2) lamina of rods and cones, (3) external limiting membrane, (4) outer nuclear layer, (5) outer plexiform layer, (6) inner nuclear layer, (7) inner plexiform layer, (8) ganglion cell layer, (9) optic nerve fiber layer, and (10) inner limiting membrane.

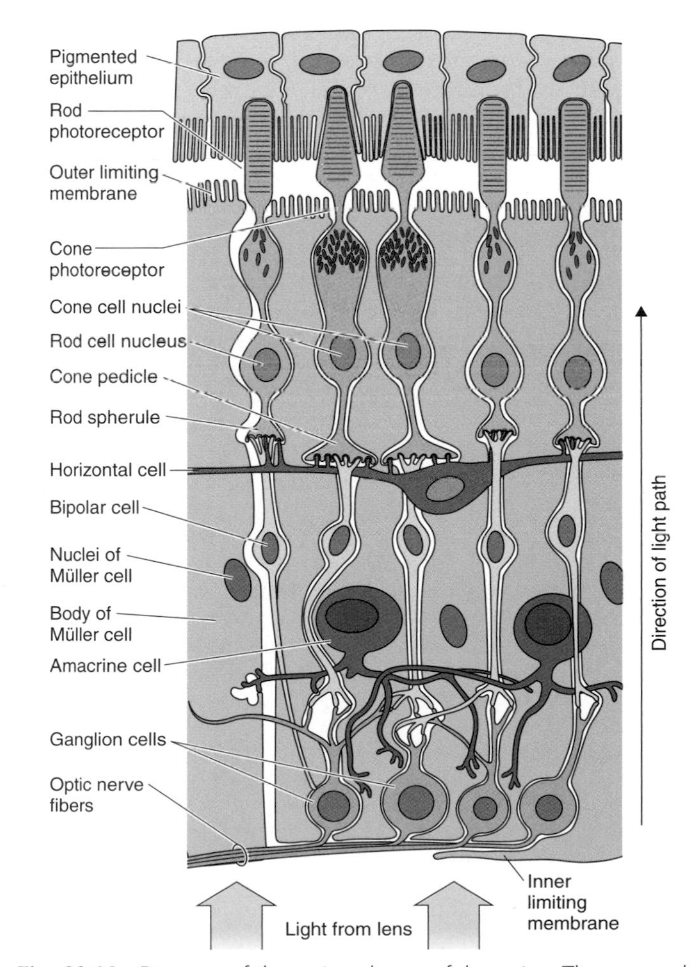

Fig. 22.16 Diagram of the various layers of the retina. The space observed between the pigmented layer and remainder of the retina is an artifact of development and does not exist in the adult, except during detachment of the retina.

TABLE 22.1 Cells of the Retina and Their Functions

Cell	Function
Pigment cells	Absorption of light, preventing light reflection; phagocytosis of spent membranous disks from rods and cones; esterifying and storing vitamin A to release it to rods and cones when needed.
Rods	Photosensitive cells responsible for monochromatic vision during low light conditions.
Cones	Photosensitive cells responsible for color vision during bright light conditions.
Bipolar neurons	Synapse with rods and cones and transmit information from these photoreceptor cells to dendrites of ganglion cells.
Horizontal cells	Transmit information from rods and cones to bipolar cells and regulate the transmission of this information by bipolar cells via lateral inhibition.
Amacrine cells	Act as interneurons controlling whether visual information should be transmitted to the visual center of the brain.
Müller cells	Support the cells of the retina physically and physiologically; act as if they were fiber-optic cables by guiding various wavelengths of light to the correct photoreceptor cells.
Ganglion cells	Relay information from rods and cones to the visual center of the brain; a small fraction of ganglion cells responsible for providing information concerning daylight and night to the regions of the brain responsible for establishing the body's circadian rhythm; some of these cells are also control the pupillary reflex.

5. Outer plexiform layer
6. Inner nuclear layer
7. Inner plexiform layer
8. Ganglion cell layer
9. Optic nerve fiber layer
10. Inner limiting membrane

Only three of the ten layers are composed of neurons that receive, integrate, and relay or transmit impulses to the brain for processing. These three layers are the photoreceptor cells (rods and cones), bipolar cells, and the ganglion cells; all of the other layers have supporting functions. The following sections describe the 10 layers of the retina starting with layer 1, which is adjacent to the choroid, and ending with layer 10, which contacts the vitreous humor.

Pigment Epithelium (Layer 1)

The **pigment epithelium**, originating from the outer layer of the optic cup, is composed of cuboidal to columnar cells (14 μm wide and 10 to 14 μm tall) that are attached to the Bruch membrane, which separates these cells from the choroid. The nuclei of these cells are basally located, as are their mitochondria, which are especially abundant in the numerous cytoplasmic invaginations with the Bruch membrane. Desmosomes, zonulae occludentes, and zonulae adherentes are present on the lateral cell membranes, forming the **blood–retina barrier**. Moreover, gap junctions on the lateral cell membranes permit intercellular communication. The cell apices exhibit microvilli and sleeve-like structures that surround and isolate, but are not attached to, the tips of individual rods and cones.

The most distinctive feature of the pigment cells is their abundance of melanin granules, which these cells synthesize and store in their apical regions. Additionally, smooth endoplasmic reticulum, rough endoplasmic reticulum (RER), and Golgi apparatus are abundant in the cytoplasm.

Pigmented epithelial cells have a number of functions. They absorb light after it has passed through and stimulated the photoreceptors, preventing reflections from the tunics, which would impair focus; continually phagocytose spent membranous disks from the tips of the photoreceptor rods and cones; play an active role in vision by esterifying vitamin A derivatives in their smooth endoplasmic reticulum; and store vitamin A in their cytoplasm, which they release to rods and cones as needed.

Clinical Correlations

1. *Individuals with albinism are unable to produce melanin pigment; therefore, the light that enters the eyeball is not absorbed by the pigment epithelium. Instead, the light is reflected throughout the eyeball. Consequently, the impinging light excites many more rods and cones than in a nonalbino individual, reducing the ability of those with albinism to see clearly. Usually, these individuals, instead of having 20/20 vision, have 20/100 to 20/200 vision.*
2. *Because the sleeve-like extensions of the pigment epithelial cells merely surround the photoreceptor rod and cone tips, sudden hard jolts may disengage them, resulting in* **detachment of the retina***, a common cause of partial blindness. The condition can be corrected surgically by "spot welding" the two structures back together. However, if this condition is left unattended, the rods and cones die because they will have lost the metabolic support normally provided by the pigment epithelium. Their death leaves a blind spot in the visual field corresponding to the area where the photoreceptors were lost.*
3. **Age-related macular degeneration** *(*AMD*) is a condition that appears usually in individuals who are at least 50 years old. The region of the macula of these patients begins to undergo degenerative changes resulting initially in blurred vision and eventually central blindness but peripheral vision is virtually unaffected. Unfortunately, the region of the macula provides the greatest visual acuity. Therefore, patients suffering from the late stages of macular degeneration are mostly blind.* **Early to intermediate AMD** *presents very little if any symptoms. However, ophthalmologic examination discloses the presence of medium (90–100 μm in diameter) to large (> 180 μm) drusen (yellow deposits of lipids and lipoproteins between the retina and the choroid) and even bundles of melanin pigments derived from cells of layer 1 (pigment epithelium).* **Late AMD** *has two distinct forms: neovascular AMD (wet AMD) and geographic atrophy (dry AMD). Of the 6 million people worldwide who have AMD, 80% have dry and 20% have wet AMD. Usually,* **neovascular AMD** *develops rapidly; blood vessels invade the region deep to the retina and, when they reach the region of the macula, foveal vision becomes compromised.*

Clinical Correlations—cont'd

Usually, these new blood vessels are fragile; as they break, they release blood that accumulates deep to the macula, further complicating the condition. If untreated, the damage to the retina will cause loss of retinal cells. ***Geographic atrophy*** *is a much slower process that involves destruction of layers 1 and 2 (layer of pigment epithelium and layer of rods and cones, respectively) resulting in an irreversible loss of vision. There are treatment possibilities for neovascular AMD that involve the use of vascular endothelial growth factor (VEGF) inhibitors and lasers to coagulate the aberrant blood vessels (this procedure is not recommended in the region of the macula, however). At this writing, there were no treatment modalities for geographic atrophy; however, in 2017, two separate studies reported that injected stem cells programmed to differentiate into retinal pigment epithelial cells survived for more than 3 years and caused some improvement in patients' vision. Further studies are needed to confirm these early results.*

Layer of Rods and Cones (Layer 2)

Rods and **cones** are polarized photoreceptor cells whose apical portions, known as the **outer segments**, are specialized dendrites. The outer segments of both rods and cones are surrounded by pigmented epithelial cells (see Fig. 22.16) and their basal regions form synapses with the underlying cells of the bipolar layer. There are approximately 100 to 120 million rods and only 3 million cones in each retina. *Rods are specialized receptors for perceiving objects in dim light; cones are specialized receptors for perceiving objects in bright light.* Cones are further adapted for color vision; rods perceive only light and cannot differentiate colors. Rods and cones are unevenly distributed in the retina in that cones are highly concentrated in the fovea; thus, this is the area of the retina where high-acuity vision occurs.

Rods

Rods are the photoreceptors of the retina specialized for perceiving dim light.

Rods are elongated cells (50 μm long by 2–5 μm in diameter) oriented parallel to one another but perpendicular to the retina. These cells are composed of an **outer segment**, **inner segment**, **nuclear region**, and **synaptic region** (Fig. 22.17).

The **outer segment of the rod**, its dendritic end, presents close to 1000 flattened membranous lamellae oriented perpendicular to the rod's long axis (Fig. 22.18; see Fig. 22.17). Each lamella represents an invagination of the plasmalemma, which is detached from the cell surface, thus forming a disk. Each disk is composed of two membranes separated by an 8-nm space. The membranes contain a specific form of the light-sensitive pigments **opsins**, known as **rhodopsin** (**visual purple**). Because the outer segment is longer in rods than in cones, rods contain more rhodopsin, respond more slowly than cones, and have the capacity to collectively summate the reception. The cell membrane of the outer segment houses **cyclic guanosine monophosphate (cGMP)–gated Na^+ ion channels** that are kept open by the cGMP that are bound to the gates if there are no photons impinging on the rod, that is, if it is dark. Therefore, in the dark, Na^+ ions may enter the outer segment of the rod.

The **inner segment of the rod** is separated from the outer segment by a constriction called the **connecting stalk**. Passing through the connecting stalk and into the outer segment of the rod is a modified cilium (lacking the central singlet microtubules) that arises from a basal body located at the apical end of the inner segment. Congregated near the interface with the connecting stalk are abundant mitochondria and cytoplasmic glycogen granules, both necessary for the production of energy for the visual process. The cytoplasm basal to the mitochondria is rich in microtubules, polysomes, smooth endoplasmic reticulum, RER, and Golgi complexes. Proteins produced in the inner segment migrate to the outer segment, where they become incorporated into the disks. The disks gradually migrate to the apical end of the outer segment and are eventually shed into the sheaths of the pigment cells, where they will be phagocytosed. The length of time from protein incorporation through migration and finally to shedding is less than 2 weeks. The lateral cell membrane of the inner segment has adenosine triphosphate (ATP)–driven sodium-potassium pumps that deliver potassium into the rod and drive sodium out of the rod. The lateral cell membrane of the inner segment also houses

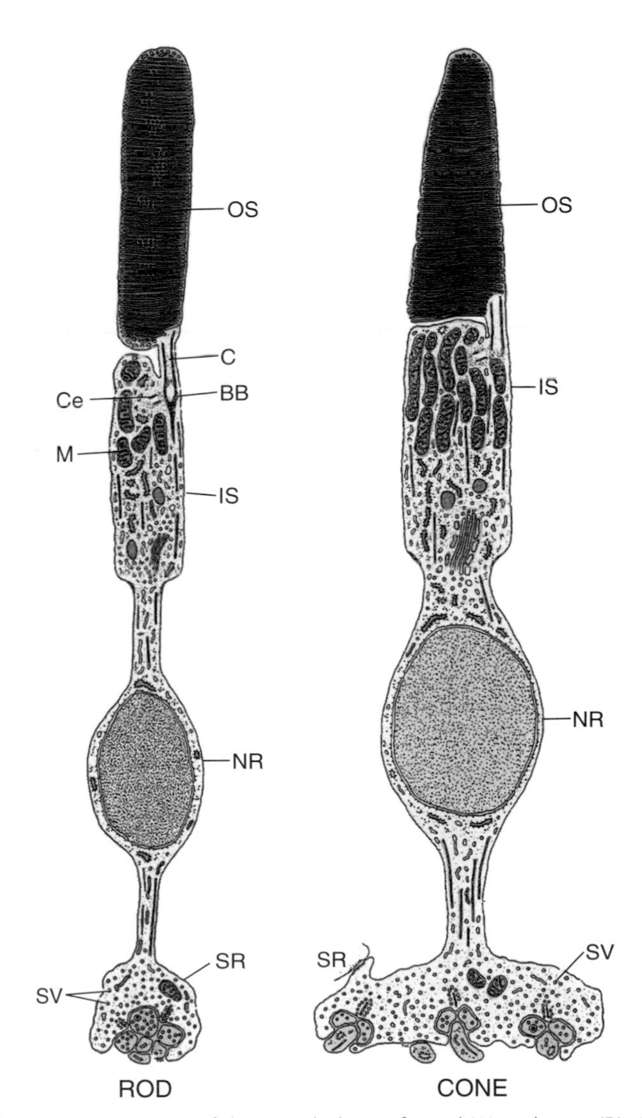

Fig. 22.17 Diagram of the morphology of a rod (A) and cone (B). OS, Outer segment; BB, basal body; C, connecting stalk; Ce, centriole; IS, inner segment; M, mitochondria; NR, nuclear region; SR, synaptic region; SV, synaptic vesicles. (From Lentz TL. *Cell Fine Structure: An Atlas of Drawings of Whole-Cell Structure*. Philadelphia: WB Saunders; 1971.)

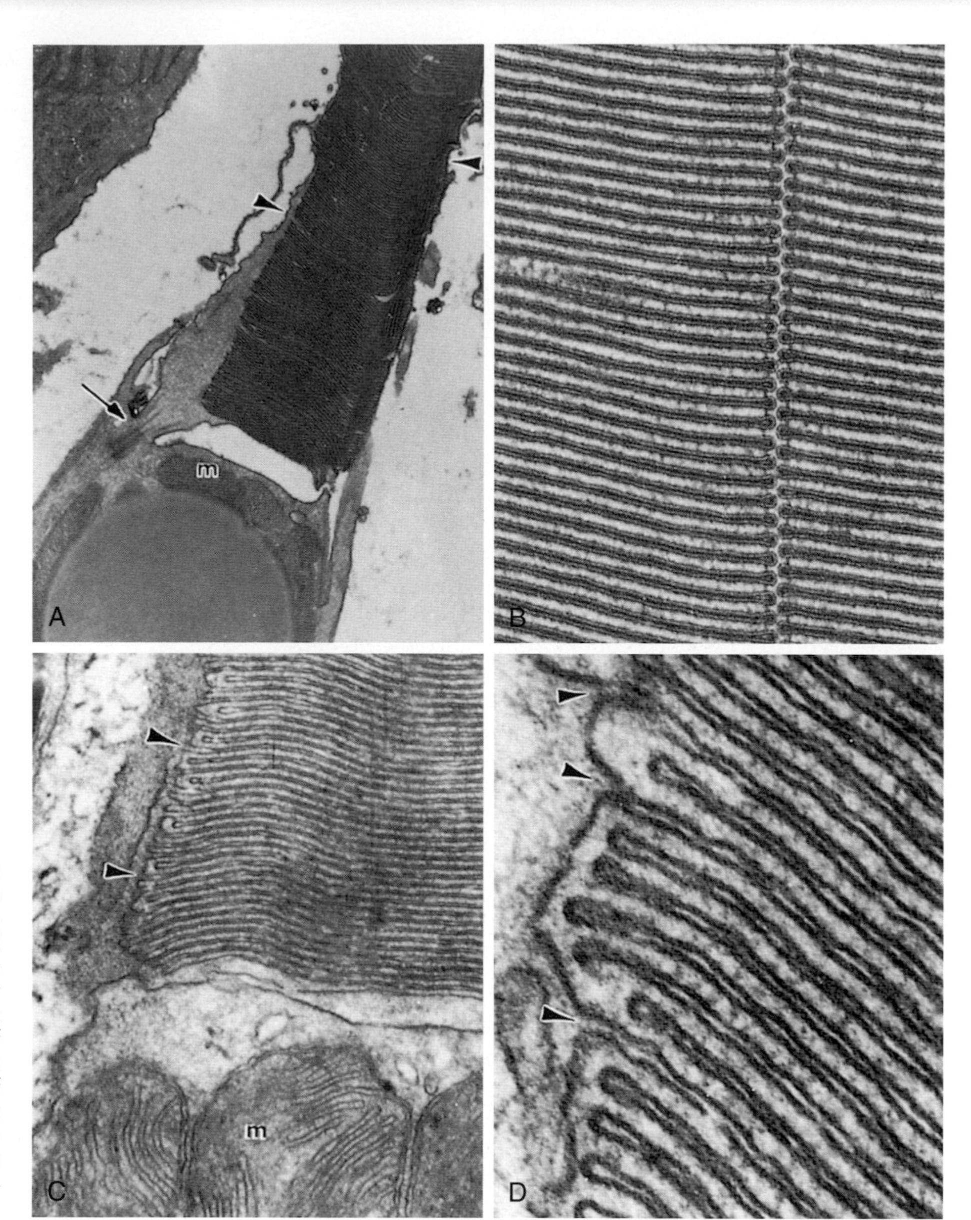

Fig. 22.18 Electron micrographs of rods from the eye of a frog and cones from the eye of a squirrel. (A) Disks in the outer segment and mitochondria (m) in the inner segment of the rod of a frog; *arrow* points to a cilium connecting the inner and outer segments (×16,200). (B) Higher magnification of the disks of the outer segment of the rod of a frog (×76,500). (C) Junction of the outer and inner segments of the cone of a squirrel (×28,800). (D) Higher magnification of the disks of the outer segment of a squirrel eye showing continuity of the lamellae with the plasmalemma *(arrowheads)* (×82,800). (From Leeson TS, Leeson CR, Paparo AA. *Text/Atlas of Histology*. Philadelphia: WB Saunders; 1988.)

nongated K^+ channels through which K^+ ions can leave the rod. These ion channels operate the same way whether light is impinging on the rod or not and maintain the cell membrane potential at −40 mV. When light impinges on a rod, the cGMP-gated Na^+ ion channels of the outer segment become closed. Thus, sodium cannot enter the rod and cause the cytoplasmic face of the rod cell membrane to become more negative (−70 to −80 mV) compared with its outer face, causing the rod to become **hyperpolarized**. *Therefore, it is the hyperpolarization of the rod plasmalemma rather than depolarization that causes the rod to fire.*

It was stated earlier that the rod membrane contains a light-sensitive pigment known as **rhodopsin**, a light-sensitive molecule composed of a carotene-like pigment **11-*cis* retinal** and the protein **scotopsin**. When photons impinge on rhodopsin, within picoseconds the *cis*-retinal is transformed into **all-*trans* retinal**, changing its molecular conformation from a bent structure to a straight structure. This conformational alteration disrupts the bond between the retinal and scotopsin; within milliseconds, the rhodopsin molecule is transformed into **activated rhodopsin**, the molecule responsible for the electrical alterations within the rod. Activated rhodopsin is stable for 1 or 2 seconds and then is digested by the enzyme **rhodopsin kinase** into all-*trans* retinal and scotopsin. In order to replenish rhodopsin, the energy-requiring reaction occurs in which the enzyme **retinal isomerase** converts all-*trans* retinal to 11-*cis* retinal. Once converted, it immediately binds to scotopsin to form rhodopsin. Interestingly, the same enzyme can convert **vitamin A (11-*cis* retinol)** to 11-*cis* retinal, ensuring an abundant supply of rhodopsin.

Activated rhodopsin acts on **transducin**, a G protein, by inducing it to activate the enzyme cGMP phosphodiesterase to convert cGMP to 5′-cGMP. The decrease in cGMP levels causes the sodium channels of the outer segment to close because cGMP is no longer bound to the gates, preventing the entry of Na^+ ions into the rod, thus causing the rod cell membrane to become hyperpolarized. It should be noted that the impingement of even a single photon on a rod has a tremendous effect by being able to influence the movements of millions of sodium ions in that rod (Fig. 22.19).

As indicated earlier, the signal from rods is not induced by depolarization, as it is in most cells; rather, light-induced hyperpolarization causes the signal to be transmitted through the various cell layers to the ganglion cells, where the signal generates an action potential along the axons to the brain.

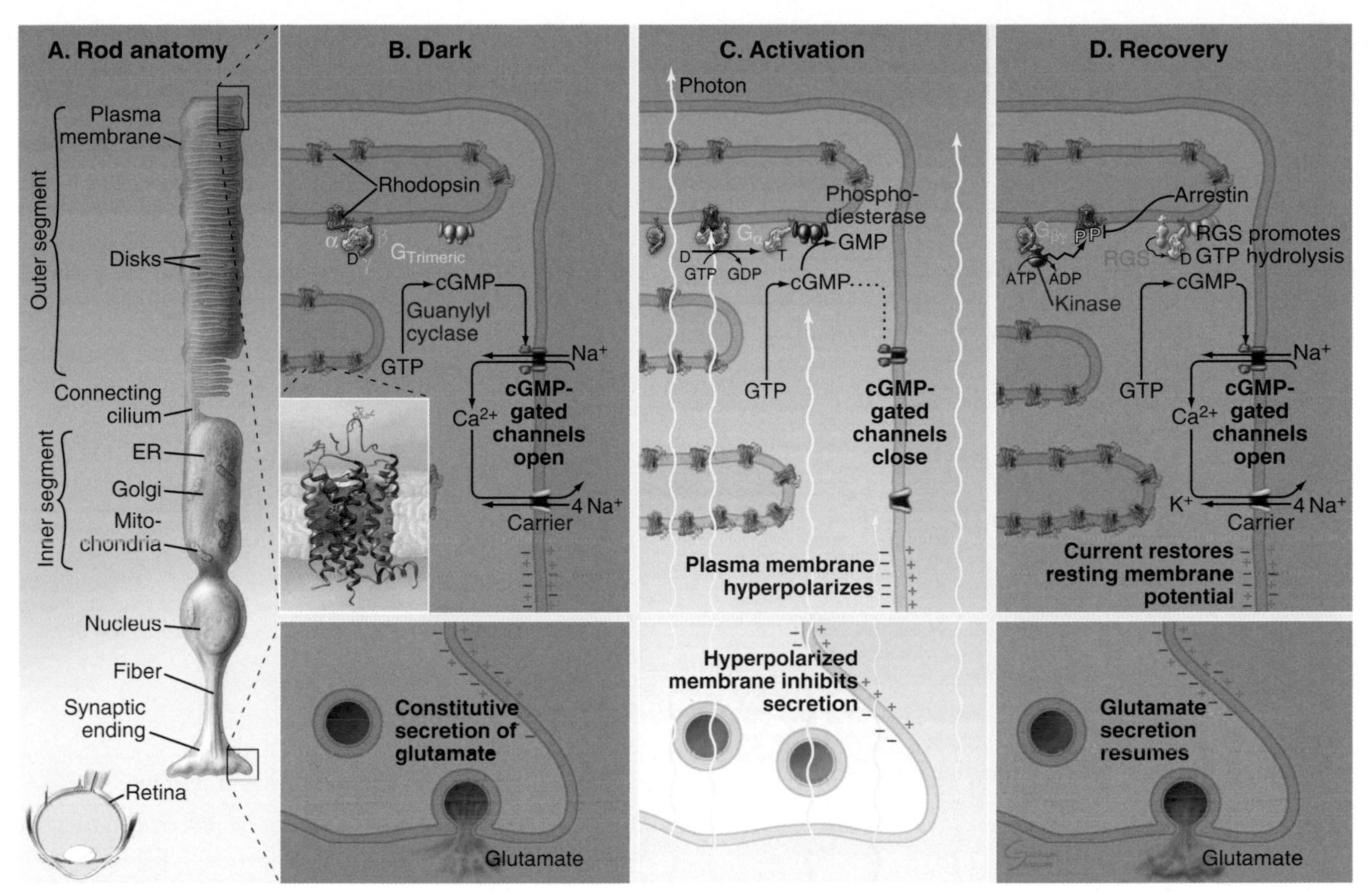

Fig. 22.19 Vertebrate visual transduction. (A) Drawing of a rod cell. Disks in the outer segment are rich in rhodopsin. ER, endoplasmic reticulum. (B–D) Drawings of small portions of an outer segment *(upper panels)* and the synaptic terminal of a rod cell *(lower panels)* in three physiological states. Active components are highlighted by bright colors. (B) Resting cell in the dark. Constitutive production of cyclic guanosine monophosphate (cGMP) keeps a subset of the plasma membrane cGMP-gated channels open most of the time, allowing an influx of Na+ and Ca2+. At this membrane potential, the synaptic terminal constitutively secretes the neurotransmitter glutamate. Ca2+ leaves the outer segment via a sodium/calcium exchange carrier in the outer segment; Na+ leaves the cell via a sodium pump in the plasma membrane of the inner segment. (C) Absorption of a photon activates one rhodopsin, allowing it to catalyze the exchange of GTP for GDP bound on many molecules of transducin (GT). This dissociates GTα from Gβγ. Each GTα-GTP binds and activates one molecule of phosphodiesterase (attached to the disk membrane by N-terminal isoprenyl groups), which rapidly converts cGMP to guanosine monophosphate (GMP). As the concentration of free cGMP declines, the cGMP-gated channels close, leading to hyperpolarization of the plasma membrane and inhibition of glutamate secretion at the synaptic body. (D) Recovery is initiated when rhodopsin kinase phosphorylates activated rhodopsin. Binding of arrestin to phosphorylated rhodopsin prevents further activation of GT. Phosphodiesterase and an RGS protein cooperate to stimulate hydrolysis of GTP bound to GT, returning GT to the inactive GTα-GDP state. Synthesis of cGMP by guanylyl cyclase returns the cytoplasmic concentration of cGMP to resting levels and opens the cGMP-gated channels. Constitutive secretion of glutamate resumes. ADP, adenosine diphosphate; ATP, adenosine triphosphate. (From Pollard T. D., and, Earnshaw, W. C. *Cell Biology*. 3rd ed. Philadelphia: Elsevier; 2017. Fig. 27.2)

The **nuclear region** of rods houses the nucleus and many of the organelles of the cell. The **synaptic region** displays short cytoplasmic processes that form synapses with bipolar and horizontal cells. The synaptic vesicles housed in the synaptic region contain the neurotransmitter substance **glutamate**, which they continuously release into the synaptic cleft when the rods **are not** hyperpolarized.

Rods are most sensitive to greenish-blue light whose wavelength is about 505 nm and completely insensitive to red light and beyond (640 nm).

Clinical Correlations

A severe lack of vitamin A causes ***night blindness*** *because the amount of available rhodopsin is greatly reduced. Because vitamin A is stored in great supply by the liver, it takes as long as 1 year of vitamin A deficiency in the individual's diet before night blindness becomes evident. Fortunately, night blindness caused by a vitamin A deficiency can be reversed rapidly by a vitamin A injection.*

Cones

Cones are specialized photoreceptors of the retina for perceiving bright light and color.

Although the morphology and mode of function of the cones is similar to that of rods, cones are activated in bright light and produce greater visual acuity compared with rods. There are three types of cones, L cones (long wavelength), M cones (medium wavelength), and S cones (short wavelength), each containing a different variety of the photopigment **opsin**, known as **photopsin** and responding to different wavelengths of light. Thus, each variety of photopsin has a maximum sensitivity to one of three colors of the spectrum—red, green, and blue. The difference resides in the opsins rather than in the 11-*cis* retinal (see Tables 22.1 and Table 22.2).

Cones are elongated cells (60 μm long × 5 to 8 μm in diameter), being longer and narrower at the fovea centralis (70 μm long × 1.5 μm in diameter). Their structure is similar to that

TABLE 22.2 Peak Light Absorption by Opsins in Rods and Cones

Rod/Cones	Wavelength of Light (nm)
Rods	505
Blue-sensitive pigment in cones (S cones)	445
Green-sensitive pigment in cones (M cones)	535
Red-sensitive pigment in cones (L cones)	570

L, Long wavelength; M, medium wavelength; S, short wavelength.

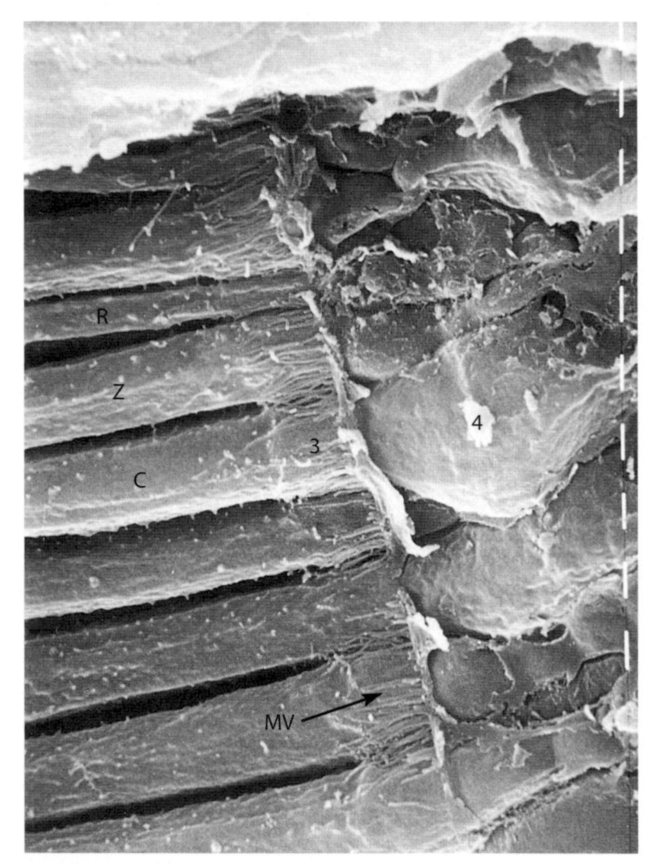

Fig. 22.20 Scanning electron micrograph of the retina in a monkey in a displaying cone (C) and a few rods (R) (×5800). 3, External limiting membrane; 4, outer nuclear layer; MV, microvilli belonging to the Müller cells; Z, inner segments. (From Borwein B, Borwein D, Medeiros J, McGowan J. The ultrastructure of monkey foveal photoreceptors, with special reference to the structure, shape, size, and spacing of the foveal cones. *Am J Anat.* 1980;159:125–146. Reprinted with permission from John Wiley & Sons, Inc.)

of rods, with the following few exceptions (Fig. 22.20; see Figs. 22.17B and 22.18):

- Their apical terminal (outer segment) is shaped more like a cone than a cylinder.
- The disks of cones, although composed of lamellae of the plasmalemma, are attached to the plasma membrane, unlike the lamellae of the rods, which are separated from the plasma membrane.
- Protein produced in the inner segment of cones is inserted into the disks throughout the entire outer segment. In the rods, it is concentrated in the most distal region of the outer segment.
- Unlike rods, cones are sensitive to color and provide greater visual acuity.
- Recycling of the cone photopigment does not require the retina pigment cells for the processing.
- Cones are not nearly as sensitive (as much as 100 times less sensitive) to light as rods, but they are still able to discriminate color in relatively poorly lit conditions.
- The synaptic vesicles housed in the synaptic region of cones, just as in rods, contain the neurotransmitter substance **glutamate**, which they **stop releasing** into the synaptic cleft when they become hyperpolarized.

The mechanism of photoreception in cones is very similar to that in rods, but cones react to different wavelengths than do rods (see Table 22.2).

Clinical Correlations

Each type of cone can distinguish approximately 100 shades of color. Most mammals have two types of cones and are said to be **dichromatic***; therefore, they distinguish 10,000 different colors. Because humans have three types of cones, people are said to be trichromatic and are able to distinguish 1 million different colors. It has been reported that some people possess four types of cones, tetrachromats, who can distinguish 100 million different colors.*

External (Outer) Limiting Membrane (Layer 3)

Although the term ***external limiting membrane*** is still used in descriptions of the layers of the retina, this structure is not a membrane. Instead, electron micrographs have revealed this "layer" to be a region of zonulae adherentes between Müller cells (modified neuroglial cells) and the photoreceptors. Distal to this, microvilli of the Müller cells project into the interstices between the inner segments of the rods and cones.

Outer Nuclear Layer (Layer 4)

The **outer nuclear layer** consists of a zone occupied mainly by the nuclei of the rods and cones. In histological sections, the nuclei of rods are smaller, more rounded, and more darkly stained than the nuclei of cones.

Outer Plexiform Layer (Layer 5)

Axodendritic synapses between the photoreceptor cells and dendrites of bipolar and horizontal cells are located in the **outer plexiform layer**. There are two types of synapses in this layer: (1) *flat synapses*, which display the usual synaptic histology; and (2) *invaginated synapses*. Invaginated synapses are unique in that they consist of a dendrite of a single bipolar cell and a dendrite from each of two horizontal cells, thus making a **triad**. Located within this invaginated synaptic region is a ribbon-like lamella (**synaptic ribbon**) containing a neurotransmitter substance. It is believed that this structure captures and assists in distributing the neurotransmitter glutamate.

Inner Nuclear Layer (Layer 6)

The nuclei of bipolar, horizontal, amacrine, and Müller cells compose the **inner nuclear layer**.

Bipolar neurons are interposed between photoreceptor cells and ganglion cells. These neurons may be contacted by many rods (10 near the macula to as many as 100 contacts near the ora serrata), permitting summation of the signals, which is especially useful in low light intensity. Cones, however, do not converge, at least not those near the fovea. Instead, each cone synapses with several bipolar cells, further enhancing visual acuity. Axons of the bipolar cells synapse with dendrites of the ganglion cells. There are two types of bipolar neurons: those that become **depolarized** upon being stimulated by the glutamine released by rods or cones and those that become **hyperpolarized** when stimulated by glutamine released by rods or cones. It is believed that the two types of cells assist in enhancing visual contrast (see the following discussion).

Horizontal cells located in this layer synapse with the synaptic junctions between the photoreceptor cells and the bipolar cells. As their name implies, these cells transmit information in a horizontal plane only (i.e., in the outer plexiform layer) from rods and cones to bipolar cells. These cells enhance visual contrast by permitting the transmission of impulses from bipolar cells that have been excited in the immediate vicinity of cones and rods that are hyperpolarized but inhibit the transmission of impulses by bipolar cells peripheral to the area of light impingement. This mechanism is known as ***lateral inhibition***.

Amacrine cells are located at the inner limits of this layer. Their dendrites all exit from one area of the cell and terminate on synaptic complexes between bipolar cells and ganglion cells. They also synapse on **interproximal cells** that are interspersed with bipolar cell bodies. There are many different types of amacrine cells—some synapse with bipolar cells and ganglion cells, some with bipolar cells and other amacrine cells. Some amacrine cells respond when a visual signal begins and others when a visual signal ends. Therefore, they respond to changes in light intensity, whereas still other amacrine cells respond to an object moving across the visual field. Basically, amacrine cells appear to function as interneurons that control whether specific visual information should be transmitted to the visual center of the brain.

Müller cells are neuroglial cells that extend between the vitreous body and inner segments of the rods and cones. It is here that Müller cells end by forming zonulae adherentes with the photoreceptor cells represented by the external limiting membrane. Microvilli extend from their apical surface. Thus, Müller cells function as supporting cells for the neural retina. This support is twofold: physical/physiological and as light conducting.

- **Physical/physiological support.** Involves maintaining the proper relationships among the cells of the retina, regulating the extracellular ion levels, neurotransmitter levels, and insulating the various cellular components of the retina.
- **Light-conducting support.** Involves the separation of the various wavelengths of light and guiding of the impinging photons of correct wavelength to the rods and cones that are designed for their maximal reception. Therefore, Müller cells appear to act as if they were wavelength-specific fiber-optic cables.

Inner Plexiform Layer (Layer 7)

The processes of amacrine, bipolar, and ganglion cells are intermingled in the inner plexiform layer. **Axodendritic synapses** between the axons of bipolar cells and dendrites of ganglion cells and amacrine cells also are located here. As in the outer plexiform layer, there are two types of synapses in this layer: *flat* and *invaginated*. Invaginated synapses consist of an axon of a single bipolar cell and two dendrites of either amacrine cells or ganglion cells or one dendrite from each of the two different cells, thus making a **dyad**. Also located within this synapse is a shortened version of the **synaptic ribbon**, which contains neurotransmitter substances.

Ganglion Cell Layer (Layer 8)

Cell bodies of large multipolar neurons of the ganglion cells, up to 30 μm in diameter, are located in the **ganglion cell layer**. The axons of these neurons pass to the brain. Hyperpolarization of the rods and cones indirectly activates these ganglion cells, which then generate an action potential that is passed by their axons to the brain via the visual relay system. There are four types of ganglion cells: W cells, X cells, Y cells, all three dedicated to vision, and the **photosensitive retinal glial cells** (**PSRGCs**) dedicated to relaying information to the pineal gland, informing that structure as to whether it is day or night and to regulating the pupillary reflex.

- **W ganglion cells.** These are the smallest, with a cell body that is approximately 10 μm in diameter, and the slowest, with a conduction velocity of 8 m/sec. The amacrine and bipolar cells that synapse with W cells convey information mostly from rods and are responsible for much of the night vision.
- **X ganglion cells.** They comprise most of the ganglion cells and are 10 to 15 μm in diameter, with a conduction velocity of 15 m/sec. These cells are responsible for most of the color vision because they receive information from amacrine and bipolar cells that synapse with cones. Each X cell receives information from a small region of the retina; therefore, they provide information that is specific for location of the visual event.
- **Y ganglion cells.** They are larger than and relay information faster than W or X cells, reaching 30 μm in diameter and a conduction velocity of at least 50 m/sec. They receive information from bipolar and amacrine cells from large areas of the visual field. Y ganglion cells are responsible for monitoring changes in the entire visual field but do not provide precise information concerning the location of the visual event.
- **Photosensitive retinal glial cells. PSRGCs** constitute a very small fraction, approximately 2% to 3%, of the ganglion cells of the retina. These cells possess a photopigment, similar to the opsins of the rods and cones, known as **melanopsin.** They project to the suprachiasmatic nucleus and indirectly to the pineal gland, regions responsible for the establishment of the body's circadian rhythm. When PSRGCs are exposed to light, they send information to these regions, indicating that presence of light. When they do not send information, it indicates that it is dark. Interestingly, PSRGCs also receive input from amacrine cells and bipolar cells that synapse with rods and cones, providing a redundancy, thus ensuring that regions of the brain that establish the circadian rhythm receive pertinent information about daylight and dark (see the section concerning the pineal gland in Chapter 13). These cells are also responsible for the pupillary reflex whereby the pupil opens or closes depending on the amount of light impinging on the retina.

Optic Nerve Fiber Layer (Layer 9)

Nerve fibers are formed of unmyelinated axons of the ganglion cells in the **optic nerve fiber layer**. These axons become myelinated as the nerve pierces the sclera.

Inner Limiting Membrane (Layer 10)

Basal laminae of the Müller cells compose the **inner limiting membrane**.

Fovea Centralis and Foveola

The **fovea centralis** is a specialized, avascular area of the retina about 1.5 mm in diameter. It is the central region of the macula

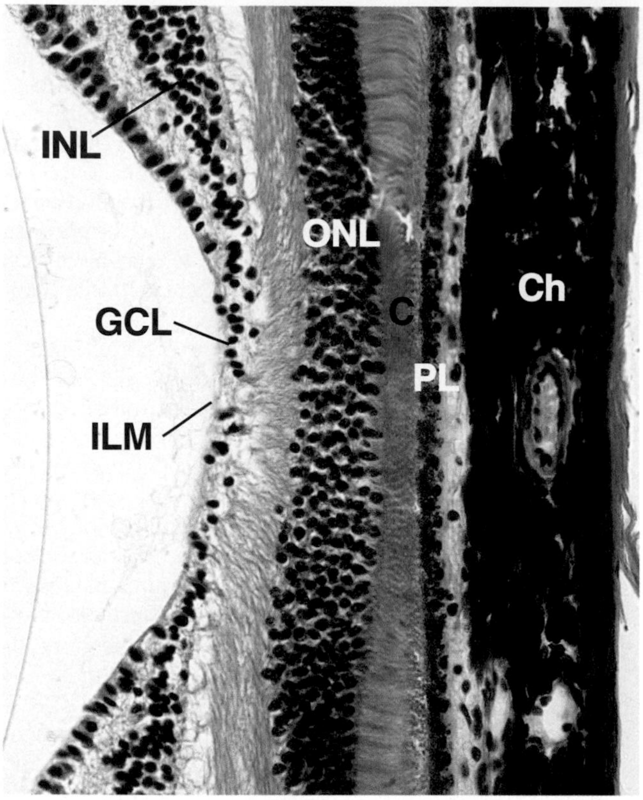

Fig. 22.21 The retina at the foveola, the center of the fovea centralis, is much thinner than anywhere else. Note that, as expected, the inner limiting membrane (ILM) lies against the ganglion cell layer (GCL) but the optic nerve fiber layer and the inner nuclear layer are absent. The outer plexiform layer, the outer nuclear layer (ONL), the external limiting membrane, and the layer of cones (C) are all present; however, rods are absent. The pigment epithelium (PL) adheres tightly to the choroid. (×132)

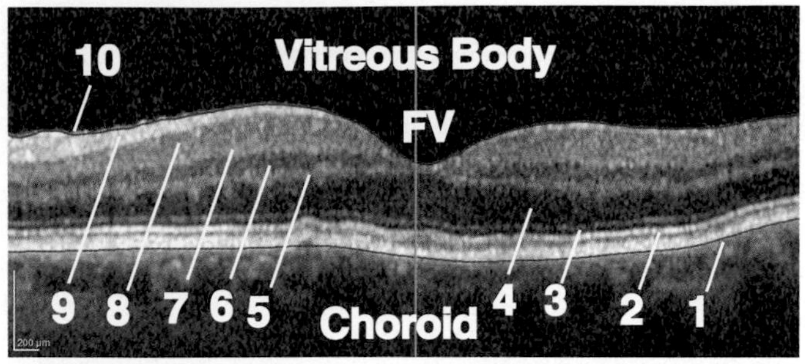

Fig. 22.22 This optical coherence tomography of the retina of the left eye displays the foveola (FV, *green vertical line going through it*) demonstrating that a number of the retinal layers disappear at the foveola. As described earlier in the text, the retinal layers, starting at the choroid, are numbered 1 through 10. Pigment epithelium of the retina (1); lamina of rods and cones (2); external limiting membrane (3); outer nuclear layer (4); outer plexiform layer (5); inner nuclear layer (6); inner plexiform layer (7); ganglion cell layer (8); optic nerve fiber layer (9); and inner limiting membrane (10). (Courtesy Dr. Roma Desai, O.D.)

lutea, which is about 5.5 mm in diameter. The central portion of the fovea centralis is the **foveola**, which has the greatest visual acuity and is approximately 0.35 mm in diameter. The foveola has no rods; its layer 2, the layer of rods and cones, consists almost entirely of cones, which are packed tightly as a number of the other layers of the retina are pushed aside. These cones are somewhat different from other cones of the retina because they are narrower, only about 1.5 μm in diameter. Therefore, more cones can fit in per unit area here than elsewhere in the retina. One may think of the configuration of cones in the foveola as a region of high definition because there are more "pixels" per unit area. As distance from the foveola increases, the number of cones decreases and the number of rods increases (Figs. 22.21 and 22.22).

IMAGE PROCESSING IN THE RETINA

For a considerable period of time, it was believed that photoreceptor cells (rods and cones) of the retina convey raw data to the brain for processing. In that concept, the retina was believed to act as a digital camera sending pixels to the brain and the neurons of the visual cortex interpreted the pixels as visual images that are associated with pictures of the outside world. In the past decade, this view has been greatly modified, demonstrating that a considerable amount of preprocessing of these pixels occurs in the retina and the information that is conveyed to the visual cortex is a much more elaborate representation of the external world than previously thought. It appears that the retina builds a series of primitive "videos" that it sends to the visual cortex. Some of these videos consist only of the periphery of the images focused on the retina, whereas other videos provide data concerning silhouettes and essential features; still others tract focus on the direction and duration of motion across the visual field. It is these videos that are provided to the visual cortex, whose neurons "compile" and "edit" the information to construct a comprehensive image of the actual scene that the individual perceives.

ACCESSORY STRUCTURES OF THE EYE

Conjunctiva

The conjunctiva is the mucous membrane lining the eyelids and reflecting onto the sclera of the anterior surface of the eye.

A transparent mucous membrane, known as the **conjunctiva**, lines the inner surface of the eyelids (**palpebral conjunctiva**) and covers the sclera of the anterior portion of the eye (**bulbar conjunctiva**). The conjunctiva is composed of a stratified columnar epithelium that contains goblet cells overlying a basal lamina and a lamina propria composed of loose connective tissue. Secretions of the goblet cells become a part of the **tear film**, which aids in lubricating and protecting the epithelium of the anterior aspect of the eye. At the corneoscleral junction, where the cornea begins, the conjunctiva continues as the stratified squamous **corneal epithelium** and is devoid of goblet cells.

Clinical Correlations

Conjunctivitis is an inflammation of the conjunctiva, usually associated with hyperemia (excessive blood flow) and a discharge. It may be caused by a number of bacterial agents, viruses, allergens, and parasitic organisms. Some forms of conjunctivitis are extremely contagious, are damaging to the eye, and may cause blindness if untreated.

Eyelids

Eyelids, covered externally by skin and internally by the conjunctiva, provide a protective barrier for the anterior surface of the eye.

The eyelids are formed as folds of skin that cover the anterior surface of the developing eye. Accordingly, stratified squamous epithelium of skin covers their external surface; at the **palpebral fissure**, palpebral conjunctiva covers their inner surface. The eyelids are supported by a framework of **tarsal plates** composed of dense, fibrous connective tissue. Sweat glands are located in the skin of the eyelids, as are fine hairs and sebaceous glands. The dermis of the eyelids is generally thinner than in most skin, contains numerous elastic fibers, and is without fat. The margins of the eyelids contain **eyelashes** arranged in rows of three or four, but they are without arrector pili muscles.

Modified sweat glands, called ***glands of Moll***, form a simple spiral before opening into the eyelash follicles. **Meibomian glands**, modified sebaceous glands located in the tarsus of each lid, open on the free edge of the lids. The oily substance secreted by these glands becomes incorporated into the tear film and impedes evaporation of the tears. Other smaller modified sebaceous glands, the **glands of Zeis**, are associated with the eyelashes and secrete their product into the eyelash follicles.

Lacrimal Apparatus

The lacrimal apparatus keeps the anterior surface of the eye lubricated with tears, preventing dehydration of the cornea.

The lacrimal apparatus of each eye consists of

- The **lacrimal gland**, which secretes the **lacrimal fluid** (tears)
- The **lacrimal canaliculi**, which carry the lacrimal fluid away from the surface of the eye
- The **lacrimal sac**, a dilated portion of the duct system
- The **nasolacrimal duct**, which delivers the lacrimal fluid to the nasal cavity

The **lacrimal gland** has two unequal parts. The larger, almond-shaped part lies in the lacrimal fossa located in the superolateral aspect of the orbit; the smaller, palpebral part is attached to the fornix of the conjunctiva just outside the conjunctival sac. The two parts are attached on their lateral aspects. Their 6 to 12 ducts open into the conjunctival sac at the lateral portion of the superior conjunctival fornix. The gland is a serous, compound tubuloacinar gland that resembles the parotid gland. Myoepithelial cells completely surround its secretory acini (Figs. 22.23 and 22.24).

Lacrimal fluid (**tears**) is composed mostly of water. This sterile fluid, containing the antibacterial agent **lysozyme**, passes through the secretory ducts to enter the conjunctival sac. The upper eyelids, by blinking, wash the tears over the anterior portion of the sclera and cornea, keeping them moist and protected from dehydration. The lacrimal fluid is wiped in a medial direction and enters the **lacrimal punctum**, an aperture located in each of the medial margins of the upper and lower eyelids. The punctum of each eyelid leads directly to **lacrimal canaliculi**, which join into a common conduit that leads to the lacrimal sac. The walls of the lacrimal canaliculi are lined by stratified squamous epithelium.

The **lacrimal sac** is the dilated superior portion of the nasolacrimal duct. It is lined by pseudostratified ciliated columnar epithelium.

The inferior continuation of the lacrimal sac, the **nasolacrimal duct**, is also lined by pseudostratified ciliated columnar epithelium. This duct carries the lacrimal fluid into the inferior meatus located in the floor of the nasal cavity.

Clinical Correlations

Dry eye syndrome (DES), a condition in which the eye does not have enough moisture to keep it comfortable, is the most common eye disease, affecting approximately 6% of the population, but it may affect fully one-third of older individuals. The eyes of these individuals feel tired, scratchy, and uncomfortable. The three principal causes of DES are not enough tear production, as in Sjögren syndrome, or other diseases, postmenopausal conditions in women, certain prescription drugs, and the production of tears that evaporate too quickly. Recently, a fifth possible cause has been added: spending long periods of time staring at computer monitors, tablets, or smartphone screens. It has been noted that individuals who stare at these devices blink less frequently than when not occupied in those endeavors. Their tears dry up before the blinking of the eyelids can spread the tears across the cornea. If untreated, dry eyes can cause corneal ulcerations, corneal scarring, and, occasionally, perforation of the cornea, leading to possible loss of vision.

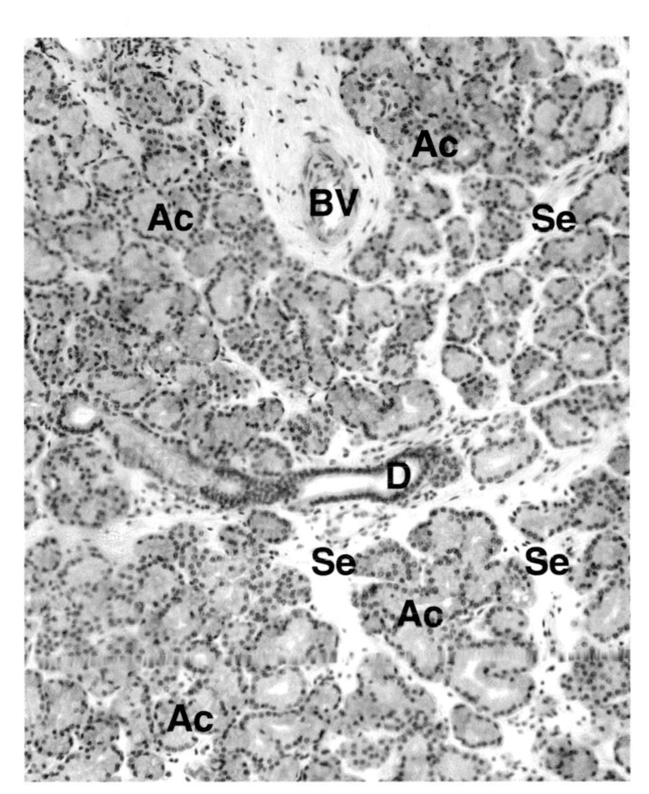

Fig. 22.23 This low-magnification photomicrograph demonstrates that the lacrimal gland is subdivided into lobules by connective tissue septa (Se), which also conveys blood vessels (BV) in and out of the gland and ducts (D), which receive tears from the acini (Ac) and deliver the tears to the surface of the eyeball. (×132)

Ear (Vestibulocochlear Apparatus)

The ear, the organ of hearing and balance, is composed of three regions: the outer ear, middle ear, and inner ear.

The ear, the organ of hearing, as well as the organ of equilibrium or balance, is divisible into three parts: (1) the external ear, (2) middle ear (tympanic cavity), and (3) inner ear (Fig. 22.25).

Sound waves received by the **external ear** are translated into mechanical vibrations by the tympanic membrane (eardrum). These vibrations then are amplified by the bony ossicles in the **middle ear** (**tympanic cavity**) and transferred to the fluid medium of the **inner ear** at the oval window. The inner ear, a perilymph-filled bony labyrinth in which is suspended a membranous labyrinth, regulates hearing (the cochlear portion) and maintains balance (the vestibular portion). Sensory input into the entire vestibulocochlear apparatus is transmitted to the brain by the two divisions of the vestibulocochlear nerve (CN VIII).

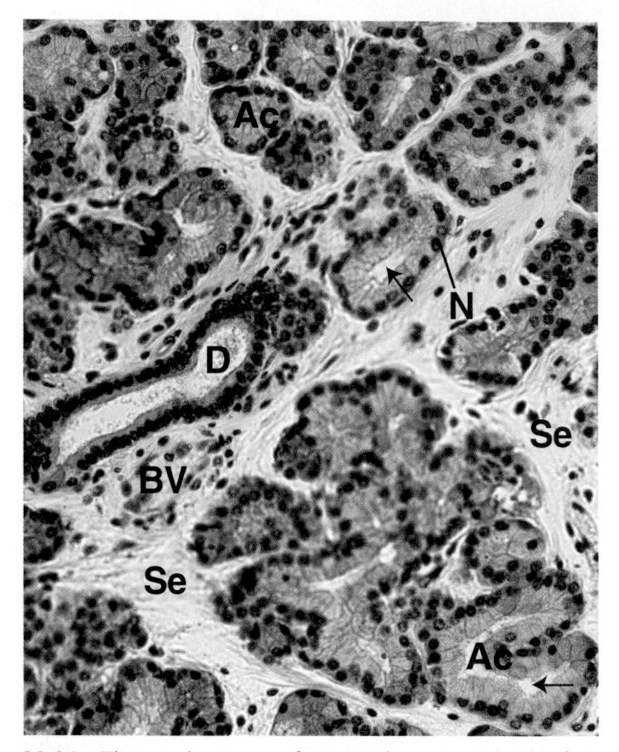

Fig. 22.24 This medium-magnification photomicrograph of the lacrimal gland displays the connective tissue septa (Se) as well as blood vessels (BV) and ducts (D). Observe the lumina *(arrows)* of the acini (Ac), as well as the nuclei (N) of the acinar cells. (×270)

EXTERNAL EAR

The external ear is composed of the auricle, external auditory meatus, and tympanic membrane.

The **external ear** is composed of the auricle (pinna), external auditory meatus, and tympanic membrane (see Fig. 22.25). The **auricle** develops from parts of the first and second branchial arches. Its general shape, size, and specific contours are usually distinctive for each person, with familial similarities. The pinna is composed of an irregularly shaped plate of elastic cartilage covered by thin skin that adheres tightly to the cartilage. The cartilage of the pinna is continuous with the cartilage lining the cartilaginous portion of the external auditory meatus.

The **external auditory meatus** is the canal that extends from the pinna into the temporal bone to the external surface of the tympanic membrane. Its superficial portion is composed of elastic cartilage, which is continuous with the cartilage of the pinna. Temporal bone replaces the cartilage as support within the inner two-thirds of the canal. The external auditory meatus is covered with skin containing hair follicles, sebaceous glands, and modified sweat glands known as ***ceruminous glands***, which produce a waxy material called ***cerumen*** (earwax). Hair and the sticky wax help prevent objects from penetrating deep into the meatus.

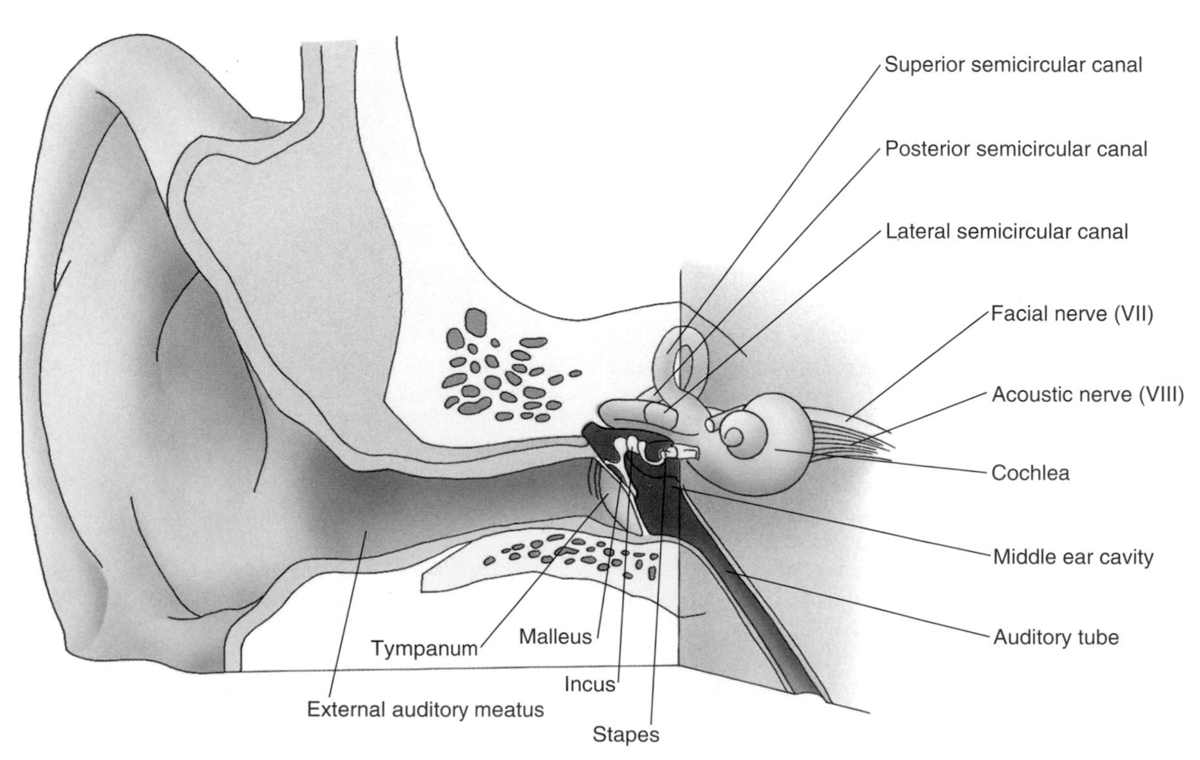

Fig. 22.25 Diagram of the anatomy of the ear.

Clinical Correlations

1. *Earwax, produced by the ceruminous glands of most of the world's population, has a sticky consistency. However, a large percent of individuals of East Asian descent have a desiccated, crumbling earwax that does not form a self-sticking substance. The formation of the dry variety of earwax is due to a mutation that occurred approximately 25,000 to 30,000 years ago in the ABCC11 gene (ATP-binding cassette subfamily C member 11). Interestingly, people with this mutation also have less odorous armpits than the rest of the human population (See also Chapter 14).*
2. *Impaction by earwax, that is, complete blocking of the external auditory meatus, occurs in 10% of young children, 20% in adults, and 30% in seniors, but in approximately 60% of seniors living in nursing homes. This easily remedied condition can result in loss of hearing, tinnitus, and vertigo. In patients who are already suffering with dementia, it can exacerbate mental deterioration. Removal of the earwax should be performed by physicians who specialize in ear, nose, and throat treatment or audiologists trained in the proper technique. Self-cleaning by the use of Q-tips or other devices is not recommended because the device used usually pushes the earwax farther into the ear canal, aggravating the deleterious effects of the earwax.*

The **tympanic membrane** covers the deepest end of the external auditory meatus. It represents the closing plate between the first pharyngeal groove and the first pharyngeal pouch, where ectoderm, mesoderm, and endoderm are in close proximity. The external surface of the tympanic membrane is covered by a thin epidermis derived from ectoderm, whereas its internal surface is composed of a simple squamous to cuboidal epithelium derived from endoderm. Sensory nerve fibers and a thin layer of mesodermal elements—including collagen fibers, elastic fibers, and fibroblasts—is interposed between the two epithelial layers of the tympanic membrane. This membrane receives sound waves transmitted to it by air through the external auditory meatus, which cause it to vibrate. In this fashion, the sound waves are converted into mechanical energy that is transmitted to the bony ossicles in the middle ear.

Clinical Correlations

Occasionally, individuals suffering from infections of the middle ear experience a sudden relief of the pain that they have endured and feel fluid draining from the opening of their external ear canal. This is due to a rupture of the eardrum, where a small perforation formed as a result of the fluid pressure impinging on the middle-ear side of the tympanic membrane. In most cases, the rupture heals in less than a month. In small children who suffer from recurrent middle-ear infection, a tympanostomy tube (a small tube) is positioned in the tympanic membrane for a few months to allow the infection to subside and to stop the continued buildup of fluid or pus in the middle ear.

MIDDLE EAR

The middle ear (tympanic cavity) houses the three bony ossicles: the malleus, incus, and stapes.

The **middle ear**, or **tympanic cavity**, is an air-filled space located in the petrous portion of the temporal bone. This space communicates posteriorly with the mastoid air cells and anteriorly, via the **auditory tube** (**eustachian tube**), with the pharynx (see Fig. 22.25). The three bony ossicles are housed in this space, spanning the distance between the tympanic membrane and the membrane at the oval window.

The superior portion of the tympanic cavity is lined by simple squamous epithelium, whereas the remainder of the cavity is lined by a pseudostratified ciliated columnar epithelium that is continuous with the internal lining of the tympanic membrane and with the epithelium in the vicinity of the auditory tube.

Clinical Correlations

The tympanic cavity is lined by two different epithelia. According to recent investigations, the pseudostratified ciliated epithelium is derived from endoderm, whereas the simple squamous epithelium is of neural crest origin. This region of the tympanic cavity is less resistant to microbial infections than is the region near the auditory tube and near the internal lining of the eardrum.

The lamina propria over the bony wall adheres to it tightly and does not contain glands, but the lamina propria overlying the cartilaginous portion contains many mucous glands whose ducts open into the lumen of the tympanic cavity. Additionally, goblet cells and lymphoid tissue are present in the vicinity of the pharyngeal opening. In its deepest two-thirds, the bony housing of the tympanic cavity gives way to cartilage as it approaches the auditory tube.

During swallowing, blowing the nose, and yawning, the pharyngeal orifice of the auditory tube opens, permitting an equalization of air pressure in the tympanic cavity with that in the external auditory meatus, which is located on the opposite side of the tympanic membrane. This is why swallowing, blowing one's nose, or yawning relieves the "ear pressure" during rapid ascent or descent when one is flying in an airplane or riding in a fast-moving elevator of a very tall building.

Located within the medial wall of the tympanic cavity are two openings, the **oval window** and **round window**, which connect the middle ear cavity to the inner ear. These two windows are formed by membrane-covered voids in the **bony wall**. The three bony ossicles—the **malleus**, **incus**, and **stapes**—are articulated in series by synovial joints lined with simple squamous epithelium. The malleus is attached to the tympanic membrane, with the incus interposed between it and the stapes, which, in turn, is attached to the oval window. Two small skeletal muscles, the **tensor tympani** and **stapedius**, modulate movements of the tympanic membrane and bony ossicles to prevent damage from very loud sounds. Vibrations of the tympanic membrane set the ossicles into motion. Because of their lever action, the oscillations are magnified to vibrate the membrane of the oval window, setting the fluid medium of the cochlear division of the inner ear into motion. Essentially, the force of movement due to the lever action is increased by a factor of about 1.3. The surface area of the tympanic membrane (55 mm^2) is 17 times greater than the footprint of the stapes (3.2 mm^2); these two factors (17 times 1.3) provide a 22-fold increase between the force that impinges on the tympanic membrane versus the force acting on the fluid on the other side of the oval window, amplifying by a factor of 22 the energy of the original sound waves entering the external auditory meatus (the external ear canal).

INNER EAR

The **inner ear** is composed of the **bony labyrinth**, an irregular, hollowed-out cavity located within the petrous portion of the temporal bone, and the **membranous labyrinth**, which is suspended within the bony labyrinth (Fig. 22.26).

Semicircular canals:
Superior
Posterior
Lateral
Ampulla
Recess for utricle
Recess for saccule
Vestibule
Oval window
Round window
Cochlea
A
BONY

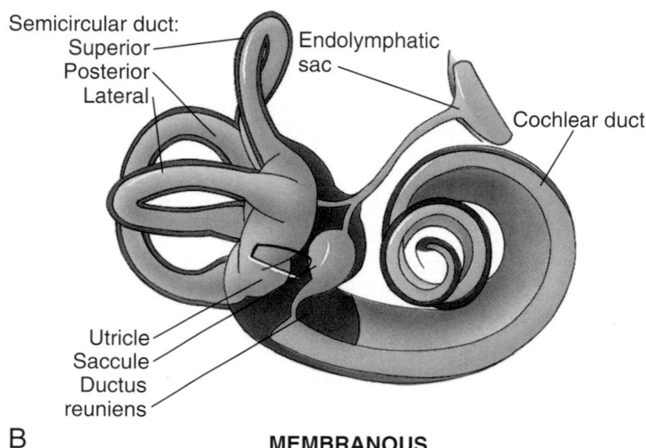

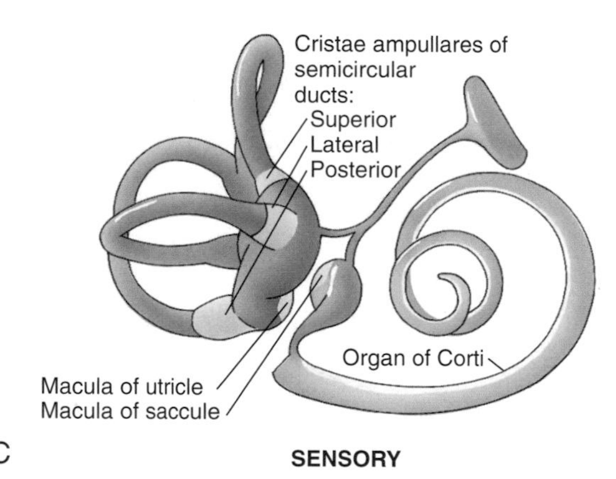

Fig. 22.26 Diagram of the cochlea of the inner ear. (A) Anatomy of bony labyrinth. (B) Anatomy of the membranous labyrinth. (C) Sensory labyrinth.

Bony Labyrinth

The bony labyrinth has three components: the semicircular canals, vestibule, and cochlea.

The **bony labyrinth**—composed of the semicircular canals, vestibule, and cochlea—is lined with endosteum and is separated from the membranous labyrinth by the **perilymphatic space**. This space is filled with a clear fluid similar in composition to the extracellular fluid, called the **perilymph** (Table 22.3), within which the membranous labyrinth is suspended.

TABLE 22.3 Sodium and Potassium Concentrations of Perilymph, Endolymph, Extracellular Fluid, and Cytosol

Fluid	Sodium (mmol/L)	Potassium (mmol/L)
Perilymph	140.0	7
Endolymph	1.3	157
Extracellular fluid	140.0	5
Cytosol	12.0	140

The three **semicircular canals** (**superior**, **posterior**, and **lateral**) are oriented at 90 degrees to one another (see Fig. 22.26). One end of each canal is enlarged; this expanded region is called the **ampulla**. All three semicircular canals arise from and return to the vestibule, but one end of each of two of the canals shares an opening to the vestibule. Consequently, there are only five, rather than six, orifices to the vestibule. Suspended within the canals are the **semicircular ducts**, which are regionally named continuations of the membranous labyrinth.

The **vestibule** is the central portion of the bony labyrinth located between the anteriorly placed cochlea and the posteriorly placed semicircular canals. Its lateral wall contains the **oval window** (**fenestra vestibuli**), covered by a membrane to which the footplate of the stapes is attached, and the **round window** (**fenestra cochleae**), covered only by a membrane. The vestibule also houses specialized regions of the membranous labyrinth (the **utricle** and the **saccule**).

The **cochlea** arises as a hollow bony spiral that turns upon itself, like a snail shell, two and one-half times around a central bony column, the **modiolus**. The modiolus projects into the spiraled cochlea with a shelf of bone called the **osseous spiral lamina** through which traverse blood vessels and the **spiral ganglion**, the cochlear division of the vestibulocochlear nerve.

Membranous Labyrinth

The membranous labyrinth is filled with endolymph and possesses the following specialized areas: the saccule and utricle, semicircular ducts, and cochlear duct.

The **membranous labyrinth** is composed of an epithelium derived from the embryonic ectoderm, which invades the developing temporal bone and gives rise to two small sacs, the **saccule** and **utricle**, as well as to the **semicircular ducts** and the **cochlear duct** (see Fig. 22.26). Circulating through the entire membranous labyrinth is **endolymph**, a viscous fluid that resembles the cytosol (intracellular fluid) in its ionic composition (i.e., it is sodium poor but potassium rich; see Table 22.3).

Thin strands of connective tissue arising from the endosteum of the bony labyrinth pass through the perilymph to be inserted into the membranous labyrinth. In addition to anchoring the membranous labyrinth to the bony labyrinth, these connective tissue strands carry blood vessels that nourish the epithelia of the membranous labyrinth.

Saccule and Utricle

The saccule and utricle, sac-like structures lying in the vestibule, contain neuroepithelial hair cells that are specialized to sense position of the head and linear movement.

The **saccule** and **utricle** are connected by a small duct, the **ductus utriculosaccularis**. Small ducts from each join to form

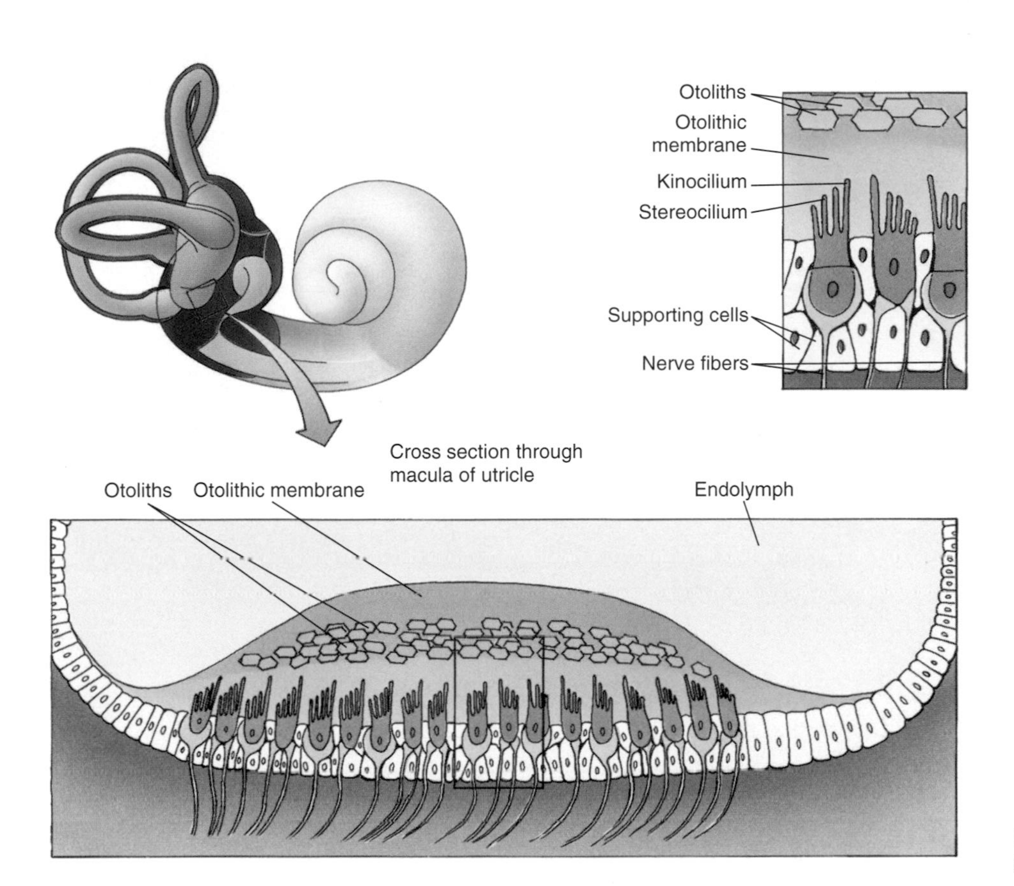

Fig. 22.27 Diagram of hair cells and supporting cells in the macula of the utricle.

the **endolymphatic duct**, whose dilated blind end is known as the **endolymphatic sac**. Another small duct, the **ductus reuniens**, joins the saccule with the duct of the cochlea (see Fig. 22.26).

The walls of the saccule and utricle are composed of a thin outer vascular layer of connective tissue and an inner layer of simple squamous to low cuboidal epithelium. Specialized regions of the saccule and utricle act as receptors for sensing the orientation of the head relative to gravity and acceleration, respectively. These receptors are called the **macula of the saccule** and the **macula of the utricle**.

The maculae of the saccule and utricle are located so that they are perpendicular (i.e., the macula of the saccule is located predominantly in the wall, thus detecting linear vertical acceleration, whereas the macula of the utricle is located mostly in the floor, thus detecting linear horizontal acceleration). The epithelium of the nonreceptor regions of the saccule and utricle is composed of light and dark cells. **Light cells** have a few microvilli, and their cytoplasm contains a few pinocytotic vesicles, ribosomes, and only a small number of mitochondria. The cytoplasm of the **dark cells**, however, contains an abundance of coated vesicles, smooth vesicles, and lipid droplets, as well as numerous elongated mitochondria located in compartments formed by infoldings of the basal plasma membrane. Nuclei of the dark cells are irregular in shape and are often located apically. It is believed that light cells play a role in absorption and that dark cells control endolymph composition by transporting K^+ ions into the endolymph using potassium ion channels in the apical plasmalemmae of the dark cells.

Clinical Correlations

The potassium ion channels of dark cells that transfer K^+ ions from the dark cell into the endolymph are composed of a regulatory protein (KCNE1) and a channel protein (KCNQ1). The potassium channel ancillary regulatory protein (KCNE1) modulates the channel proteins (KCNQ1). Certain mutations in the gene coding for the protein KCNE1 disturb the flow of K^+ ions into the endolymph, altering its ionic composition. Consequently, the entire epithelial lining of superior aspect of the ampullae, utricle, and saccule become damaged, resulting in the breakdown of the vestibular apparatus.

The maculae are thickened areas of the epithelium, 2 to 3 mm in diameter. They are composed of two types of **neuroepithelial hair cells**, called **type I hair cells** and **type II hair cells**, and supporting cells that sit on a basal lamina (Figs. 22.27 and 22.28). Nerve fibers from the vestibular division of the vestibulocochlear nerve supply the neuroepithelial cells.

Each type I or type II hair cell has a single kinocilium and 50 to 100 stereocilia arranged in rows according to length, with the longest (10 μm) being nearest the kinocilium.

Type I hair cells are plump cells with a rounded base that narrows toward the neck (see Fig. 22.28). Their cytoplasm contains occasional RER, a supranuclear Golgi complex, and numerous small vesicles. Each stereocilium, which is anchored in a dense terminal web, is a long microvillus with a core of many actin filaments cross-linked by **fimbrin**. The filamentous core imparts rigidity to the stereocilia so that bending can occur only in the neck region, near their site of origin from the apical plasma membrane. The

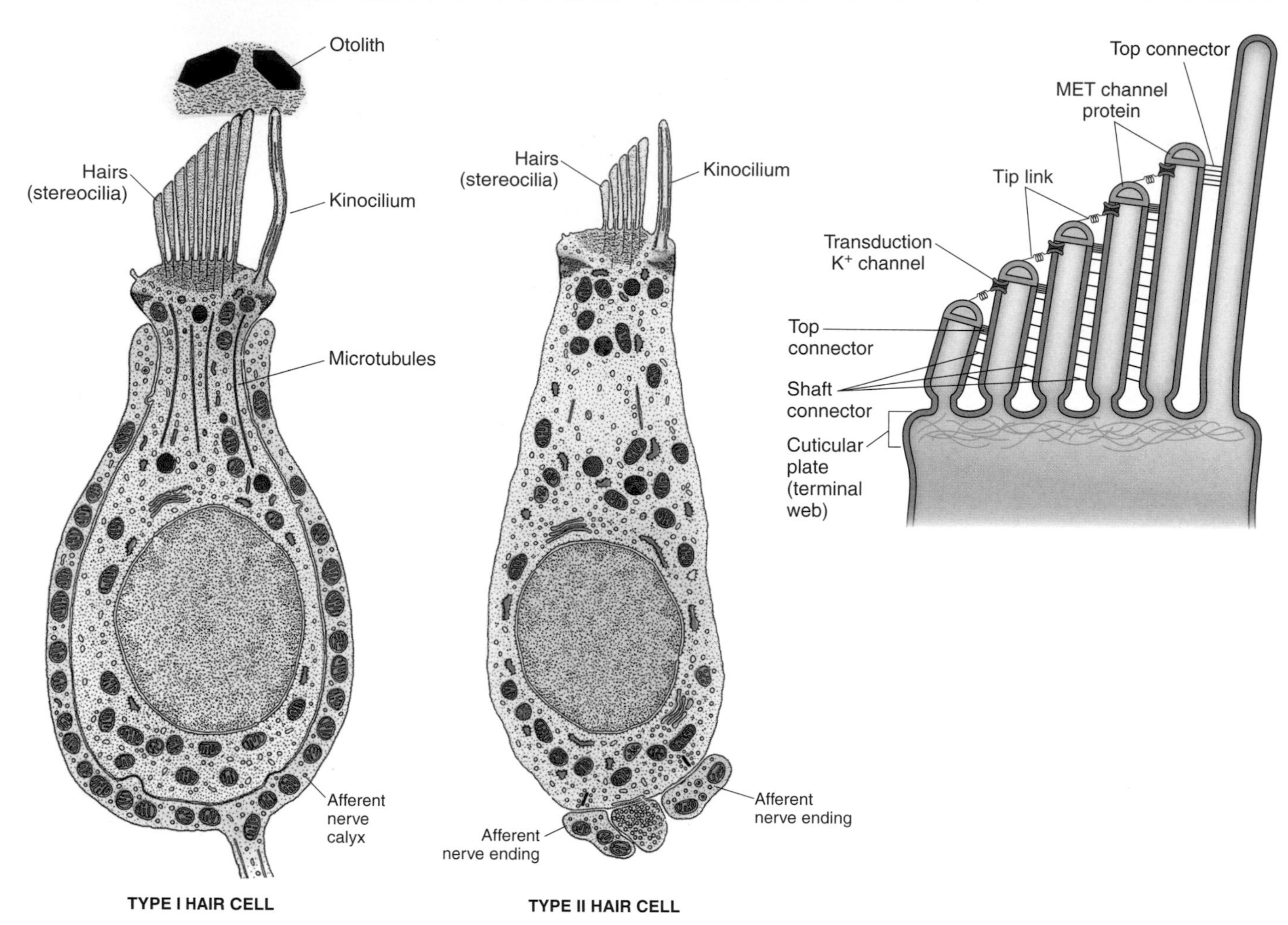

Fig. 22.28 Diagram demonstrating the morphology of type I and type II neuroepithelial (hair) cells of the maculae of the saccule and utricle. The otolithic membrane is not shown with the type II hair cell. The relationship of stereocilia with each other and with the kinocilium is illustrated on the right side of this figure. The skeletons of the stereocilia and kinocilia (not illustrated) are anchored into the cuticular plate (terminal web) of the hair cells. Note that the stereocilia are attached by tip links, top connectors, and shaft connectors. The locations of the mechanoelectric transducer channel proteins (MET channel proteins) and transduction K+ channels are also illustrated. The stereocilium adjacent to the kinocilium is connected to it by a top connector. When the stereocilia bend toward the kinocilium (as illustrated here), the K+ channels of the stereocilia open, the hair cell becomes depolarized, and the neurotransmitter substance is released. When the stereocilia bend in the opposite direction (away from the kinocilium), the K+ channels of the stereocilia close, the cell becomes hyperpolarized, and the neurotransmitter substance is not released. (Modified from Lentz TL. Cell Fine Structure: An Atlas of Drawings of Whole-Cell Structure. Philadelphia: WB Saunders; 1971.)

top of each stereocilium possesses **mechanoelectrical transduction channels** (**MET channels**) that are responsible for transducing mechanical events into electrical signals. As the person's head moves, the stereocilia bend *toward* the kinocilium, which opens the MET channels, permitting the movement of K^+ ions into the stereocilia, **depolarizing** the hair cell. When the person's head stops moving, the stereocilia bend *away from* the kinocilium, closing the MET channels, preventing K^+ ions from entering the stereocilia, thus **hyperpolarizing** the hair cell. To ensure that the stereocilia move in the same direction and open/close the MET channels simultaneously, they are connected by unusually long cadherin molecules, known as **tip links,** which are responsible for the opening or closing of the neighboring MET channels. The movement of K^+ ions into the stereocilia and, of course, into the cytoplasm of the hair cells depolarizes the hair cells, causing the opening of basally located **voltage-gated calcium channels**. The entry of calcium into the hair cells drives the neurotransmitter-containing vesicle to fuse with the presynaptic regions of the basal hair cell plasma membrane, releasing the neurotransmitter into the synaptic cleft. The released neurotransmitter substance contacts its receptor on the postsynaptic membrane of the afferent nerve fiber, causing it to transmit the signal to the CNS from processing. In addition to the opening of the voltage-gated calcium channels, **basally located voltage gated potassium channels** also open and the K+ ions that entered at the MET channels will leave the hair cell basally. To ensure that the stereocilia maintain contact with each other, additional links hold them together by various links along their length. The side links near their top are known as **top connectors**, the ones along the side are known as **side connectors**, and the ones at the bottom of the stereocilia are known as **foot connectors**.

Type II hair cells are similar to type I hair cells with regard to the stereocilia and kinocilium, but their shape is more columnar and their cytoplasm contains a larger Golgi complex and more vesicles (see Fig. 22.28).

Supporting cells of the maculae, which are interposed between both types of hair cells, have a few microvilli. Thick junctional complexes bind these cells to each other and to the hair cells. They exhibit a well-developed Golgi complex and secretory granules, suggesting that they may help maintain the hair cells and that they may contribute to the production of endolymph.

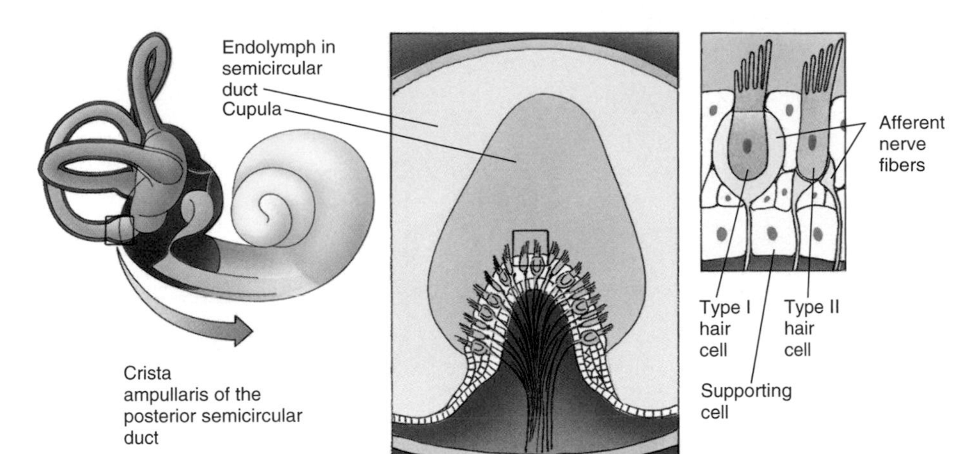

Fig. 22.29 Diagram of the hair cells and supporting cells in one of the cristae ampullares of the semicircular canals.

Innervation of the hair cells is derived from the vestibular division of the vestibulocochlear nerve. The rounded bases of the type I hair cells are almost entirely surrounded by a cup-shaped afferent nerve fiber. Type II hair cells exhibit many afferent fibers synapsing on the basal area of the cell. Structures resembling **synaptic ribbons** are present near the bases of type I and type II hair cells. The synaptic ribbons of the type II hair cells probably function in synapses with efferent nerves, which are thought to be responsible for increasing the efficiency of synaptic release.

The stereocilia of the neuroepithelial hair cells are covered by and embedded in a thick, gelatinous, glycoprotein mass, the **otolithic membrane**. The surface region of this membrane contains small calcium carbonate crystals known as **otoliths** or **otoconia** (see Figs. 22.27 and 22.28).

Semicircular Ducts

Each of the three semicircular ducts contains an expanded region, the ampulla, where specialized receptors (neuroepithelial hair cells) sense linear and angular movement.

Each **semicircular duct**, a continuation of the membranous labyrinth arising from the utricle, is housed within its semicircular canal and thus conforms to its shape. Each of the three ducts is dilated at its lateral end (near the utricle). These expanded regions, called the **ampullae**, contain the **cristae ampullares**, which are specialized receptor areas. Each crista ampullaris is composed of a ridge whose free surface is covered by sensory epithelium consisting of **neuroepithelial hair cells** and **supporting cells** (Fig. 22.29). The supporting cells sit on the basal lamina, whereas the hair cells do not; rather, the hair cells are cradled between the supporting cells. The neuroepithelial hair cells, also known as **type I hair cells** and **type II hair cells**, exhibit the same morphology as the hair cells of the maculae. The **cupula**, a gelatinous glycoprotein mass overlying the crista ampullaris, is similar to the otolithic membrane in structure and function, but it is cone shaped and does not contain otoliths. The functional mechanism of the vestibular apparatus is described in the section titled Vestibular Functions.

Cochlear Duct (Scala Media) and Organ of Corti

The cochlear duct (scala media) and its organ of Corti are responsible for the mechanism of hearing.

The **endolymph**-filled **cochlear duct** (**scala media**), a diverticulum of the saccule, is another regionally named portion of the membranous labyrinth. It is a wedge-shaped receptor organ housed in the bony cochlea and is surrounded by perilymph containing compartments that are separated from it by two membranes (Figs. 22.30–22.33). The roof of the **cochlear duct** is the **vestibular membrane** (**Reissner membrane**); the floor of the cochlear duct is the **basilar membrane**. The perilymph-filled compartment lying above the vestibular membrane is called the **scala vestibuli**; the perilymph-filled compartment lying below the basilar membrane is the **scala tympani**. These two perilymph-containing compartments communicate with each other at the **helicotrema**, near the apex of the cochlea.

The **vestibular membrane** is composed of two layers of squamous epithelial cells separated by a basal lamina. The inner layer is the lining cells of the scala media, and the outer layer is the lining cells of the scala vestibuli. Numerous tight junctions seal both layers of cells, ensuring a high ionic gradient across the membrane. The **basilar membrane**, extending from the spiral lamina at the modiolus to the lateral wall, supports the organ of Corti and is composed of two zones: the zona arcuata and the zona pectinata. The **zona arcuata** is thinner, lies more medial, and supports the organ of Corti. The **zona pectinata** is similar to a fibrous meshwork containing a few fibroblasts.

The lateral wall of the cochlear duct, extending between the vestibular membrane and the spiral prominence, is covered by a pseudostratified epithelium called the **stria vascularis**. Unlike most epithelia, it contains an *intraepithelial plexus of capillaries*. The stria vascularis is composed of three cell types: marginal, basal, and intermediate. All three cell types have different embryonic origins. Marginal cells originate from the otic epithelium; basal cells arise from the otic mesenchyme; and intermediate cells are melanocyte-like cells, originating from neural crest cells.

Light-staining **basal cells** and **intermediate cells** have a less dense cytoplasm, containing only a few mitochondria. Both have cytoplasmic processes that radiate out from the cell surfaces to interdigitate with the cell processes of the marginal cells and with other intermediate cells. Moreover, intermediate cells possess pigment granules in their cytoplasm. Basal cells also have cellular processes that ascend around the bases of the marginal cells, forming cup-like structures that isolate and support the marginal cells. Dark-staining **marginal cells** have abundant microvilli on their free surfaces. Their dense cytoplasm contains numerous mitochondria and small vesicles. Labyrinthine,

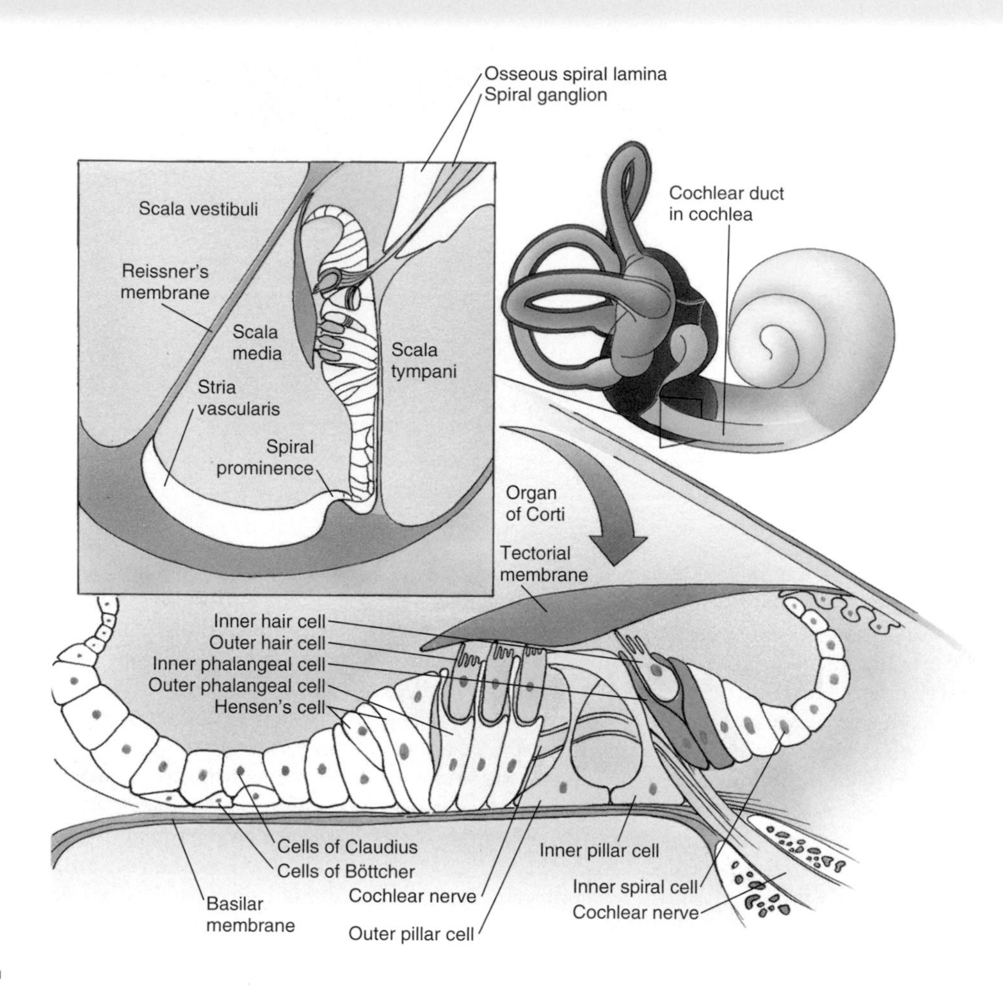

Fig. 22.30 Diagram of the organ of Corti.

narrow cell processes containing elongated mitochondria are abundant on the basilar portion of the cells.

Intraepithelial capillaries, derived from mesoderm, are positioned in such a fashion that they are surrounded by basal processes of the marginal cells and the ascending processes of the basal and intermediate cells.

The stria vascularis manufactures endolymph and delivers it into the scala media; its **marginal cells** are responsible for delivering K^+ ions into the endolymph. The basal cells line the basal aspect of the stria vascularis and form a cellular membrane between the stria vascularis and the spiral ligament. The function of the intermediate cells is not known, but the absence of these cells in atrophied stria vascularis results in sensorineural deafness.

The **spiral prominence** is also located on the inferior portion of the lateral wall of the cochlear duct. It is a small protuberance that juts out from the periosteum of the cochlea into the cochlear duct throughout its entire length. The basal cells of the stria vascularis are continuous with the vascular layer of cells covering the spiral prominence. Inferiorly, these cells of the spiral prominence are reflected into the spiral sulcus, where they become cuboidal. Other cells of this layer continue onto the basilar lamina as the **cells of Claudius**, which overlie the smaller **cells of Böttcher** (see Fig. 22.30). The latter cells are located only in the basilar turns of the cochlea. Cells of Claudius are believed to be supporting cells, whereas cells of Böttcher have been shown to possess high levels of **calmodulin** and **nitric oxide synthase**, suggesting that they function in the processes of secretion and absorption, as well as in the control of calcium ion levels in the endolymph.

At the narrowest portion of the cochlear duct, the periosteum covering the spiral lamina bulges out into the scala media, forming the **limbus of the spiral lamina** (**spiral limbus; limbus**). Part of the limbus projects over the **internal spiral sulcus** (**internal spiral tunnel**). The upper portion of the limbus is the **vestibular lip**, and the lower portion is called the **tympanic lip** of the limbus, a continuation of the basilar membrane. Numerous perforations in the tympanic lip accommodate branches of the cochlear division of the vestibulocochlear nerve (acoustic nerve). **Interdental cells** located within the body of the spiral limbus secrete the **tectorial membrane**, a proteoglycan-rich gelatinous mass containing numerous fine keratin-like filaments, that overlies the organ of Corti. Stereocilia of specialized receptor hair cells of the organ of Corti are embedded in the tectorial membrane (see Fig. 22.30).

Organ of Corti. The **organ of Corti**, the specialized receptor organ for hearing, lies on the basilar membrane and is composed of **neuroepithelial hair cells** and several types of **supporting cells**. Although the supporting cells of the organ of Corti have different characteristics, they all originate on the basilar membrane and contain bundles of microtubules and microfilaments, and their apical surfaces are all interconnected at the free surface of the organ of Corti. Supporting cells include **pillar cells**, **phalangeal cells** (also known as **Dieter cells**), **border cells**, and **cells of Hensen** (see Figs. 22.30–22.33).

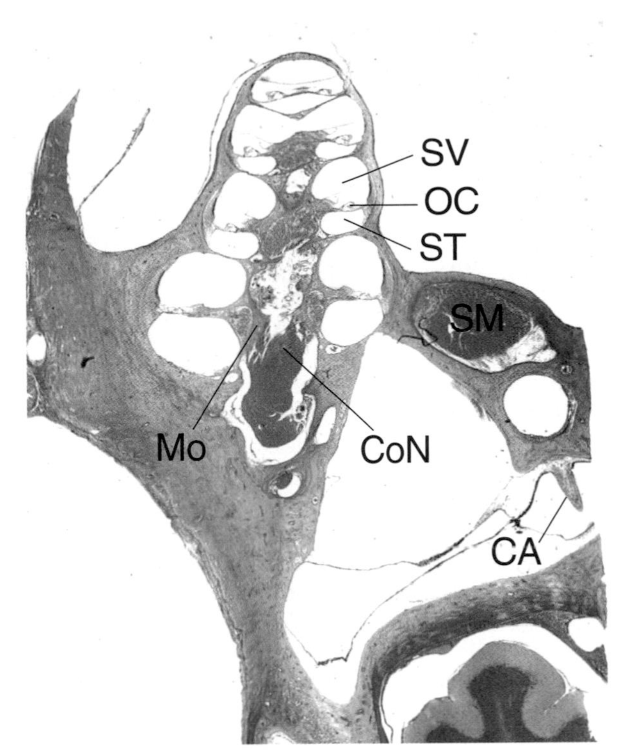

Fig. 22.31 This very-low-magnification photomicrograph of the cochlea displays the bony modiolus (Mo), the cochlear nerve (CoN), and the osseous spiral laminae supporting the organ of Corti (OC) with the scala vestibuli (SV) and the scala tympani (ST) positioned below the basilar membrane of the organ of Corti. Observe the crista ampullaris (CA), recognizable by its cone-shaped cupula overlying it. Observe the cross-section of the stapedius muscle (SM). (×14)

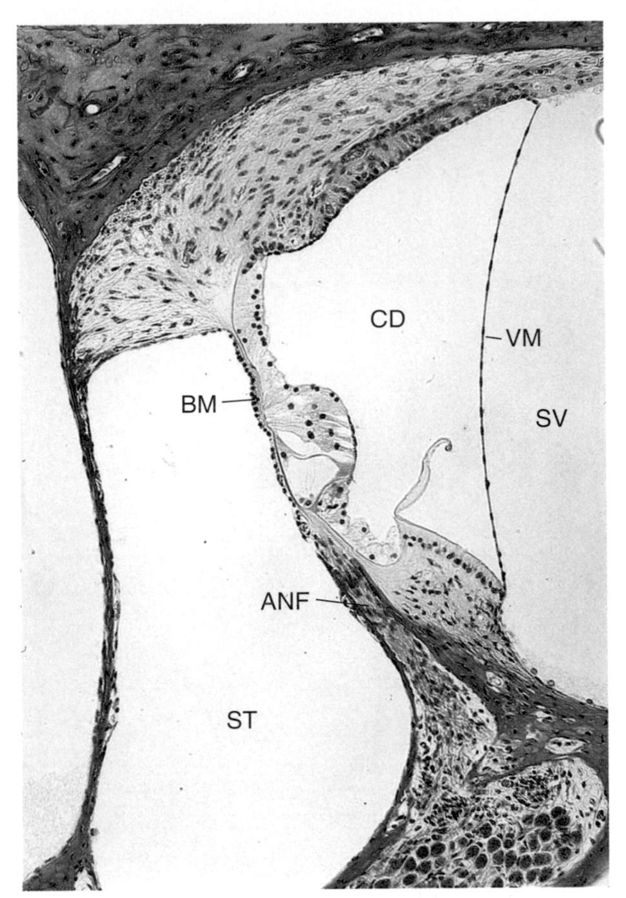

Fig. 22.32 Light micrograph of the organ of Corti sitting on the basilar membrane (BM) within the cochlea (×180). The cochlear duct (CD), containing endolymph, is limited by the vestibular membrane (VM) and the basilar membrane (BM). The scala vestibuli (SV) and the scala tympani (ST) contain perilymph. Observe the spiral ganglion and the vestibulocochlear (acoustic) nerve fibers (ANF) coming from the hair cells of the organ of Corti.

Supporting Cells of the Organ of Corti.

The supporting cells of the organ of Corti are the inner and outer pillar cells, inner and outer phalangeal cells, border cells, cells of Hensen, and cells of Böttcher.

Inner and **outer pillar cells** (Table 22.4) are tall cells with wide bases and apical ends; thus, they are shaped like an elongated "I." They are attached to the basilar membrane, and each one arises from a broad base. The central portions of both inner and outer pillar cells are deflected away from each other, becoming the walls of the **inner tunnel**, where the inner pillar cells form the medial wall of the inner tunnel and the outer pillar cells form the lateral wall of the inner tunnel. At their apices, both inner and outer pillar cells are again in contact with each other. Their cytoplasm contains bundles of microfilaments and microtubules. Inner pillar cells outnumber outer pillar cells, with three inner pillar cells usually abutting two outer pillar cells. The pillar cells support not only the hair cells of the organ of Corti but also the tectorial and basilar membranes.

Outer phalangeal cells (**outer Dieter cells**) are tall columnar cells that are attached to the basilar membrane. Their apical aspects are cup shaped to support not only the basilar portions of the outer hair cells but also the bundles of efferent and afferent nerve fibers, which pass between them on their way to the hair cells. Because their cup-shaped apices cradle the hair cells, the outer phalangeal cells do not reach the free surface of the organ of Corti. However, originating from the lateral aspect of each of these outer phalangeal cells is a small **phalangeal process** whose microtubules and microfilaments confer a degree of firmness and rigidity to it. This rigid phalangeal process extends to the outer hair cells, forming a flattened distal cuticular plate that forms a solid contact with its cradled outer hair cell and an adjacent outer hair cell. These cuticular plates form a stiff membranous sheet, known as the **reticular membrane**, that extends from the outer hair cells to the cells of Hensen. The reticular membrane isolates the bodies of the outer hair cells from the endolymph, creating a micro-compartment surrounding the outer hair cells and outer phalangeal cells. This is known as the **space of Nuel**, which communicates with the **outer tunnel** that is bound by the cells of Hensen. Therefore, the reticular membrane forms a cover over the space of Nuel and the outer tunnel. The extracellular fluid in these two isolated micro-compartments is known as **cortilymph**, which resembles perilymph of the scala vestibuli and the scala tympani rather than the endolymph of the cochlear duct.

Inner phalangeal cells (**inner Dieter cells**) are located deep to the inner pillar cells. Unlike the outer phalangeal cells, they completely surround the inner hair cells that they support.

Border cells delineate the inner border of the organ of Corti. They are slender cells that support the inner aspects of the organ of Corti.

Cells of Hensen define the outer border of the organ of Corti. These tall cells are located between the outer phalangeal cells and the shorter cells of Claudius, which rest on the underlying **cells of Böttcher**.

All of these cells support the outer aspects of the organ of Corti (see Fig. 22.30).

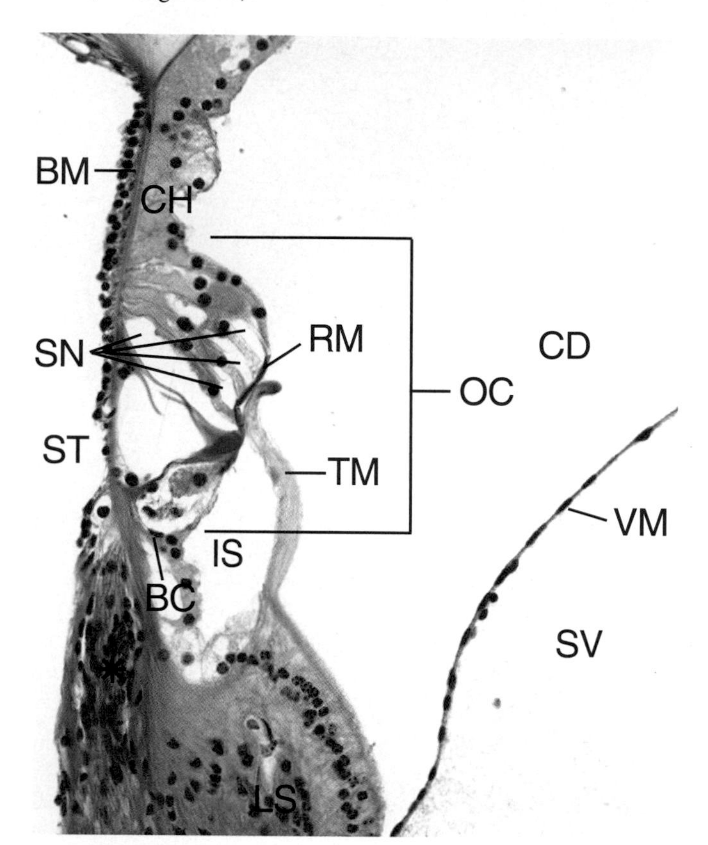

Fig. 22.33 This medium magnification of the organ of Corti (OC) displays the vestibular membrane (VM) separating the scala vestibuli (SV) from the cochlear duct (CD), which extends from the border cell (BC) to the cells of Hensen (CH). Observe the limbus spiralis (LS) and the cochlear nerve fibers *(asterisk)*. Note that the internal spiral sulcus (IS) is overlain by the tectorial membrane (TM), which rests on the inner and outer hair cells. Note that the organ of Corti rests on the basilar membrane (BM), which separates the organ of Corti from the scala tympani (ST). Note also the internal spiral sulcus (IS) covered by the tectorial membrane and that the reticular membrane (RM) isolates the outer and inner hair cells and the space of Nuel (SN) from the endolymph present in the cochlear duct. (×270)

TABLE 22.4 Supporting Cells of the Organ of Corti

Cell	Function
Inner and outer pillar cells	Form the inner tunnel; support hair cells; support tectorial and basilar membranes.
Outer phalangeal cells (outer Dieter cells)	Support the basilar portion of outer hair cells; support bundles of nerve fibers; form the space of Nuel.
Inner phalangeal cells (inner Dieter cells)	Support and completely surround hair cells.
Border cells	Support and define the inner aspect of the organ of Corti.
Cells of Hensen	Support and define the outer aspect of the organ of Corti.
Cells of Claudius	Support cells of Hensen and the outer aspect of the organ of Corti.
Cells of Böttcher	Possess high levels of **calmodulin** and **nitric oxide synthase**, suggesting that these cells function in the control of calcium ion levels and in the processes of secretion and absorption.

Neuroepithelial Cells (Hair Cells) of the Organ of Corti.

There are two types of neuroepithelial cells in the organ of Corti: inner hair cells and outer hair cells.

Neuroepithelial hair cells are specialized for transducing impulses for the organ of hearing. Depending on their locations, these cells are called **inner hair cells** and **outer hair cells.**

Inner hair cells, a single row of approximately 3500 cells, each about 12 μm in diameter, are supported by inner phalangeal cells. These inner hair cells extend the inner limit of the entire length of the organ of Corti. Inner hair cells are short and exhibit a centrally located nucleus, numerous mitochondria (especially beneath the terminal web), RER and smooth endoplasmic reticulum, and small vesicles. The basal aspect of these cells also contains microtubules. Their apical surface contains 50 to 60 stereocilia arranged in a "V" shape. The core of the stereocilia contains microfilaments, cross-linked with fimbrin, as in the type I hair cells of the vestibular labyrinth. The microfilaments of the stereocilia merge with those of the terminal web. Although a kinocilium is not present in inner hair cells, a basal body and centriole are both evident in the apical region of these cells. The basal aspects of these cells synapse with afferent fibers of the cochlear division of the vestibulocochlear nerve.

Outer hair cells, supported by outer phalangeal cells, are located near the outer limit of the organ of Corti and are arranged in rows of three (or four) along the entire length of this organ (see Fig. 22.30). There are approximately 12,000 outer hair cells, each about 8 μm in diameter. They are elongated cylindrical cells whose nuclei are located near their bases. Their cytoplasm contains abundant RER, and their mitochondria are located basally. The cytoplasm of those cells just beneath the lateral walls contains a **cortical lattice** composed of 5- to 7-nm filaments cross-linked by thinner filaments, which appears to support the cell and resist deformation.

Cochlear nerve fibers synapse on the lateral and basilar portion of the hair cells, with a large preponderance terminating on the *inner* and only about 5% to 10% terminating on the *outer* hair cells. Extending from the apical surface of the outer hair cells are as many as 100 stereocilia organized in the shape of the letter "W." These stereocilia vary in length and are arranged in ordered gradation. Like inner hair cells, outer hair cells do not have a kinocilium but do have a basal body.

Vestibular Functions

The vestibular function is the sense of position in space and during movement.

The sense of position in space and during movement is essential to activate and deactivate certain muscles that function in accommodating the body for balance. The sensory mechanism for this function is the **vestibular apparatus**, which is located in the inner ear. This apparatus comprises the utricle, saccule, and semicircular ducts.

Stereocilia of neuroepithelial hair cells located in the ampullae of the utricle and saccule are embedded in the otolithic membrane. **Linear movements** of the head cause displacement of the endolymph, which disturbs the positioning of the otoliths within the otolithic membrane and, consequently, the membrane itself, thereby bending the stereocilia of the hair cells. Movements of the stereocilia are transduced into action potentials, which are conducted by synapses to the vestibular division of the vestibulocochlear nerve for transmittal to the brain.

Circular movements of the head are sensed by receptor sites in the semicircular ducts housed within the semicircular canals. Stereocilia of the neuroepithelial hair cells of the cristae ampullares are embedded in the cupula. Movements of the endolymph within the semicircular ducts disturb the orientation of the cupula, which subsequently distorts the stereocilia of the hair cells. This mechanical stimulus is transduced to an electrical impulse, which is transferred by synapse to branches of the vestibular division of the vestibulocochlear nerve for transmission to the brain.

Information concerning the linear and circular movements of the head, recognized by receptors of the inner ear, is transmitted to the brain via the vestibular division of the vestibulocochlear nerve. There, it is interpreted and adjustments to the balance are initiated by activation of specific muscle masses responsible for posture.

Cochlear Functions

The cochhlea functions in the perception of sound.

Clinical Correlations

***Ménière disease** is a disorder with hearing loss resulting from excess fluid accumulation in the endolymphatic duct. Other symptoms include vertigo, tinnitus, nausea, and vomiting. Some drugs can relieve vertigo and nausea. There are three stages—early, middle, and late—in the progression of this disease. The **early stage** is exemplified by sudden onset of vertigo, dizziness, nausea, and vomiting. Tinnitus, a sense of blocked ears, and hearing loss are present temporarily, but once the vertigo subsides, its side-effects resolve themselves. Most patients experience these attacks 6 to 12 times a year. The **middle stage** is distinguished by milder attacks of vertigo but tinnitus and hearing loss become more severe. During remission, the symptoms are relieved for as long as 4 months. The **late stage** is characterized by very infrequent or even no attacks of vertigo, but the sense of balance, especially when in a dark place, is very poor. Hearing loss becomes increasingly severe. Moreover, tinnitus becomes a constant—and at times unbearable—problem, so much so that the vestibular division of the vestibulocochlear nerve may have to be severed. In extreme cases, the semicircular canals and cochlea may have to be surgically removed. Most people with Ménière disease have only one affected ear, but almost half of the affected individuals will eventually suffer with the condition in both ears.*

***Tinnitus** has affected people even in ancient times, as indicated by information noted on clay tablets preserved from the Assyrian empire and from papyrus scrolls from ancient Egypt.*

Sound waves collected by the external ear pass into the external auditory meatus and are received by the tympanic membrane, which is set into motion. The tympanic membrane converts sound waves into mechanical energy. Vibrations of the tympanic membrane set the malleus—and, consequently, the remaining two ossicles—into motion.

As indicated earlier, because of a mechanical advantage rendered by the articulations of the three bony ossicles and the difference between the surface area of the tympanic membrane and the foot of the stapes, the mechanical energy is amplified about 22 times when it reaches the membrane of the fenestra vestibuli (oval window). Movements of the oval window membrane initiate pressure waves in the perilymph within the scala vestibuli. Because fluid (in this instance, perilymph) is incompressible, the wave is passed through the scala vestibuli, through the helicotrema, and into the scala tympani and is dissipated via the membrane covering the round window. The pressure wave in the perilymph of the scala tympani causes the basilar membrane to vibrate.

Because the **organ of Corti** is firmly attached to the **basilar membrane**, a rocking motion within the basilar membrane is translated into a shearing motion on the stereocilia of the hair cells that are embedded in the overlying rigid tectorial membrane. When the shearing force produces a deflection of the stereocilia toward the taller stereocilia, the cell becomes depolarized, generating an impulse that is transmitted via the afferent nerve fibers of the cochlear division of the vestibulocochlear nerve (Fig. 22.34).

The differences in sound frequency or pitch are distinguished because regions of the basilar membrane, which becomes longer with each turn of the cochlea, vibrate at different frequencies relative to its width. Therefore, *low-frequency sounds* are near the apex of the cochlea (in the vicinity of the helicotrema), whereas *high-frequency sounds* are near the base of the cochlea (in the region of the oval window). Evidence suggests that outer hair cells contain the necessary machinery to react rapidly to efferent input, causing them to vary the length of their stereocilia, which alters the shear force between the tectorial membrane and basilar membrane, thus "tuning" the basilar membrane. This action then alters the response of the sound-detecting inner hair cells, affecting their reaction to different frequencies.

Clinical Correlations

1. **Conductive deafness** may be caused by any condition that impedes the conduction of sound waves from the external ear through the middle ear and into the organ of Corti of the inner ear. Conditions that can lead to conductive deafness include the presence of foreign bodies, **otitis media**, and **otosclerosis** (fixation of the footplate of the stapes in the oval window).
2. **Otitis media** is a common infection of the middle ear cavity in young children. It usually develops from a respiratory infection that involves the auditory tube. Fluid buildup in the middle ear cavity dampens the tympanic membrane, constricting the movements of the bony ossicles. Antibiotics are the usual treatment.
3. **Nerve deafness** usually results from a disease process that interrupts transmission of the nerve impulse. The interruption may be located anywhere in the cochlear division of the acoustic nerve, from the organ of Corti to the brain. Disease processes that can lead to nerve deafness include rubella, tumors of the nerve, and nerve degeneration.
4. Neuroepithelial hair cells of the organ of Corti possess **nicotinic acetylcholine receptors (nAChRs)** that decrease the sensitivity of hair cells to the volume of sound. At high decibels, as is apparent during certain music concerts and at many clubs, nAChRs cause hair cells to be desensitized and thus protect the individual from becoming deaf after long-term exposure to music at high volume. Interestingly, people living in exceptionally quiet areas of the world, such as the Mabaan people of South Sudan (near Ethiopia), have remarkably good hearing even into old age.
5. **Age-related hearing loss (ARHL)** has historically been attributed to damage to the inner hair cells. However, recent studies have demonstrated that the synaptic contact between the hair cells and the auditory nerve is the apparent causative factor. During exposure to very loud noise, the hair cells remain stable but the end feet (terminals) of the auditory nerve may be severely injured, a situation that also occurs in ARHL, where the end feet degenerate due to the aging process. These synaptic losses were not considered because the soma of the affected neurons did not show signs of degeneration for years after synaptic contact with the inner hair cells was terminated and because only high-threshold auditory nerve fibers were affected. Investigations are progressing in the use of neurotrophins to induce neurite regeneration from the neurons whose end feet were destroyed. Other research groups are using vitamins A, C, and E as well as magnesium to reverse ARHL in rats. Magnesium is a cochlear vasodilator and the three vitamins listed are free-radical scavengers; the combination of these four substances were shown to ameliorate ARHL in these rats. Further studies must be performed before they can be applied to humans.

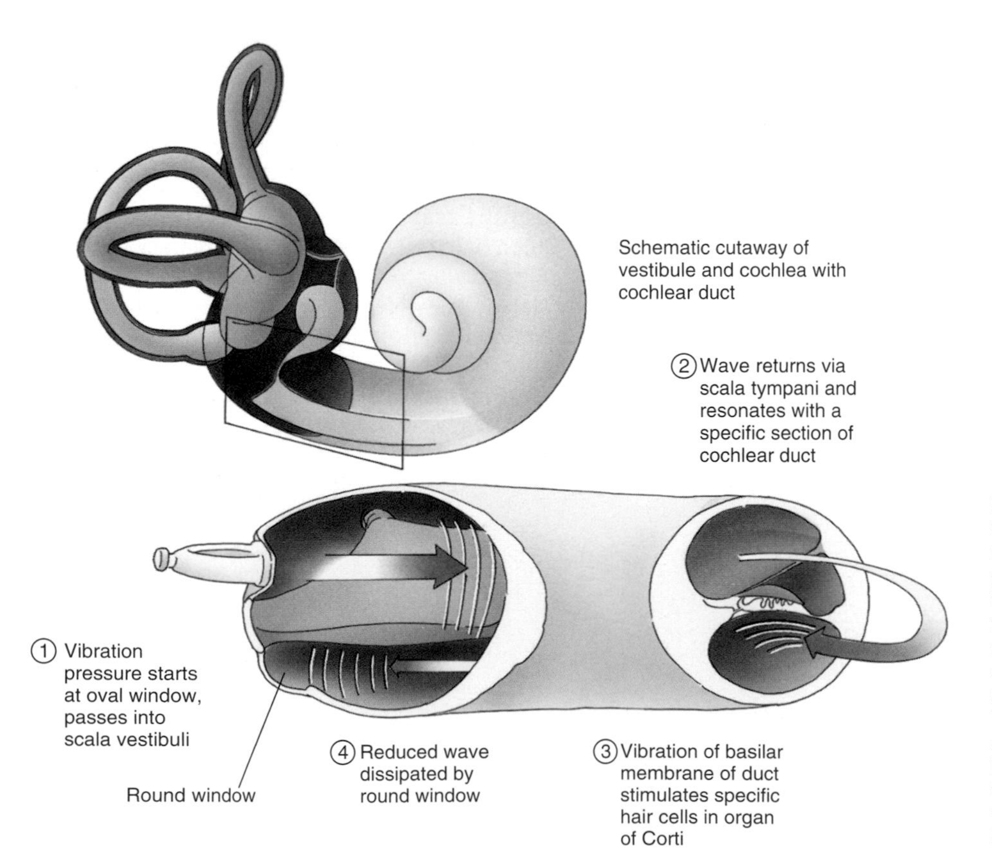

Fig. 22.34 Schematic diagram of how vibrations of the footplate of the stapes move the membrane on the oval window. This action produces pressure in the perilymph, located in the scala vestibuli. At the helicotrema, where the scala vestibuli and scala tympani communicate, the pressure wave within the perilymph of the scala tympani sets the basilar membrane and organ of Corti sitting on it into motion. This causes a shearing motion on the hair cells of the basilar membrane, which is transduced into an electric current and, in turn, is transmitted by a synapse to the cochlear division of the vestibulocochlear nerve for conduction to the brain for processing.

Pathological Considerations

See Figs. 22.35 through 22.37.

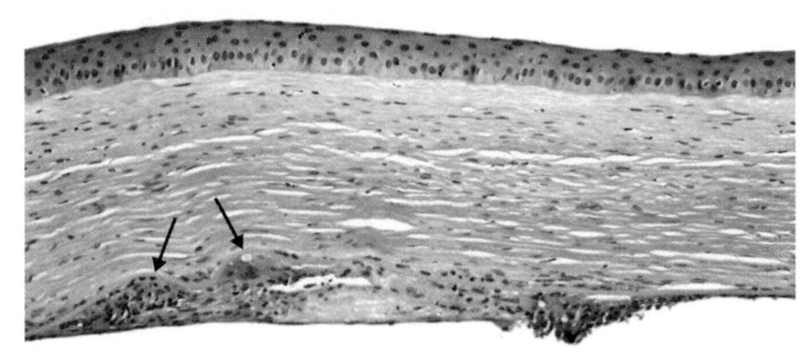

Fig. 22.35 Photomicrograph of the cornea of a patient with chronic herpes simplex keratitis. Observe that the number of fibroblasts is greatly increased when compared with a healthy cornea; also note the presence of the granulomatous reaction in the Descemet membrane *(arrows)*, a characteristic of this condition. (Reprinted with permission from Kumar V, Abbas AK, Aster JC. *Robbins and Cotran Pathologic Basis of Disease*. 9th ed. Philadelphia: Elsevier; 2015:1325.)

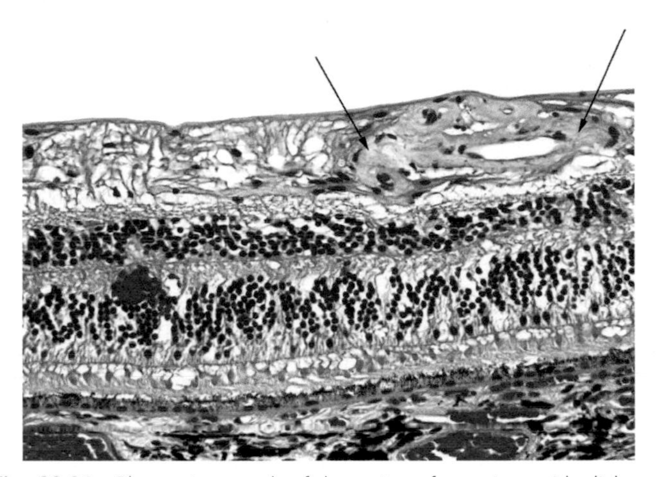

Fig. 22.36 Photomicrograph of the retina of a patient with diabetes mellitus. Observe the presence of tangled vascular elements deep to the internal limiting membrane *(between the two arrows)*, a characteristic of intraretinal angiogenesis. Note also the hemorrhage within the outer plexiform layer of the retina. (Reprinted with permission from Kumar V, Abbas AK, Aster JC. *Robbins and Cotran Pathologic Basis of Disease*. 9th ed. Philadelphia: Elsevier; 2015:1337.)

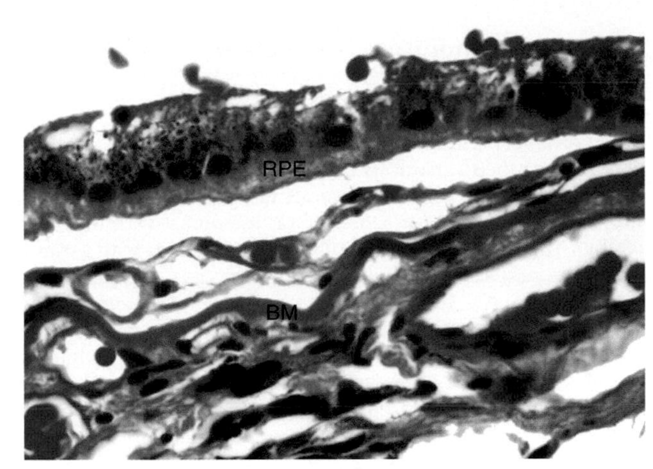

Fig. 22.37 Photomicrograph of the choroid of a patient with "wet" age-related macular degeneration. Observe the presence of a vascular membrane interposed between the retinal pigment epithelium (RPE) and Bruch membrane (BM). Observe the dense color of BM to the right of the label, indicative of local calcification. (Reprinted with permission from Kumar V, Abbas AK, Aster JC. *Robbins and Cotran Pathologic Basis of Disease*. 9th ed. Philadelphia: Elsevier; 2015:1338.)

Histology Laboratory Instructions: Special Senses

Peripheral Receptors

Pacinian Corpuscles

At a low magnification, Pacinian corpuscles resemble an onion; in histological sections, they resemble the cut surface of an onion sliced in half. Each Pacinian corpuscle has a myelinated fiber that almost as soon as it enters the corpuscle loses its myelin sheath. The inner core of the corpuscle contains the nonmyelinated nerve terminal and its Schwann cells, surrounded by approximately 60 layers of modified fibroblasts, each layer separated from the next by a small fluid-filled space. An additional group of 30 less dense modified fibroblasts, the outer core, surrounds the inner core. The entire structure has a collagenous connective tissue capsule that surrounds the outer core (see Fig. 22.2, NF, IC, OC, Ca). At a medium magnification, the central nerve fiber and its surrounding layers of modified fibroblasts, forming the inner core and the less dense modified fibroblasts, forming the outer core, are easily recognizable. The outer core, also composed of modified fibroblasts, is surrounded by the collagenous connective tissue capsule (see Fig. 22.3 NF, IC, OC, Ca).

Meissner Corpuscles

Meissner corpuscles, usually located in the dermal papillae of the nonhairy skin, are formed by a few nerve terminals and their associated Schwann cells that are completely surrounded by a collagenous connective tissue capsule. Each branching nerve terminal within a Meissner corpuscle is surrounded by stacks of epithelial cells whose nuclei are well stained with hematoxylin and eosin (H&E) stain (see Fig. 22.4, NF, Ca, N).

Eye

Sclera

The sclera, the white of the eye, is nearly avascular covered by the conjunctiva, a stratified squamous nonkeratinized to a stratified cuboidal epithelium with occasional goblet cells. Deep to the conjunctiva, the sclera has three layers: the thin collagenous connective tissue, known as the episclera; the thick collagenous connective tissue layer, called the stroma; and another thin connective tissue layer, the suprachoroid lamina, which possesses melanocytes in its deeper layer. Observe the blood vessel passing through the sclera (see Fig. 22.6, E, EpT, St, SL, M, BV).

continued

Histology Laboratory Instructions: Special Senses—cont'd

Cornea

Viewed at a very low magnification, the transparent cornea is seen to have a stratified squamous nonkeratinized epithelium on its external surface and a simple squamous to cuboidal corneal endothelium lining its internal surface, which is in contact with the anterior chamber. This photomicrograph also presents the iris with its smooth muscle, the posterior chamber, as well as the capsule of the lens (see Fig. 22.7, Co, E, AC, Ir, SM, PC, Ca, L). At medium magnification of the cornea, the stratified squamous anterior epithelial cover, Bowman membrane, and simple squamous to cuboidal corneal endothelium are well demonstrated. Between these two epithelia, the stroma of the cornea is seen to be composed of collagen fiber bundles that are manufactured by the numerous fibroblasts whose nuclei are quite evident (see Fig. 22.8, E, *arrows*, Co, F).

Ciliary Body

The ciliary body seen at low magnification displays its prominent smooth muscle, as well as the ciliary processes. In the vicinity of the corneal–scleral junction, the canal of Schlemm is visible, as is the root of the iris that separates the anterior chamber from the posterior chamber. These two chambers communicate with each other at the pupil. The lens is suspended in its location by the zonular fibers (suspensory ligaments), which are represented in this photomicrograph by two black lines drawn from the ciliary processes to the lens (see Fig. 22.9, SM, CP, Sc, *arrows*, Iris, AC, PC, L, ZF).

Lens

The lens, viewed at even a low magnification, displays its capsule, which is simply a very thick basal lamina. Deep to the capsule is the simple cuboidal subcapsular epithelium, present only on the anterior and lateral surfaces of the lens. The bulk of the lens is composed of approximately 2000 elongated, hexagonal solid-shaped cells, known as lens fibers, which are derived from the subcapsular epithelium (see Fig. 22.10, *arrow*, Ca). At medium magnification, the lens capsule, subcapsular epithelium, and suspensory ligaments of the lens are well displayed. The elongated cells, known as lens fibers, are also evident (see Fig. 22.11, Ca, E, SL, LF).

Retina

The retina is the innermost tunic of the eye containing the photoreceptor cells that transmit their information to neurons of the retina, which then collect and partially construct the visual information to convey it to the brain via the optic nerve. The exit site of the optic nerve is known as the optic disc, located in the posterior wall of the retina. Note that all of the retinal layers stop at the optic disc, the blind spot of the retina (see Fig. 22.14, Retina, Optic Nerve, Optic Disc). There are ten named layers of the retina, starting at the choroid and ending at the vitreous humor. Each named layer is represented by a number 1 to 10; these layers are presented at a medium magnification in this photomicrograph. The choroid is not part of the retina but the internal-most aspect of the choroid is richly endowed with melanocytes, making it appear black. Layer 1 of the retina, the pigment epithelium, is in direct contact with the choroid; 2 = layer of rods and cones; 3 = outer limiting membrane; 4 = outer nuclear layer; 5 = outer plexiform layer; 6 = inner nuclear layer; 7 = inner plexiform layer; 8 = ganglion cell layer; 9 = optic nerve fiber layer; and 10 = inner limiting membrane. The inner limiting membrane is composed of the basal lamina of the Müller cells; it is in direct contact with the vitreous body (see Fig. 22.15, 1, 2, 3, 4, 5, 6, 7, 8, 9, 10). The region of the retina that provides the most acute vision is the foveola, located in the center of the fovea centralis. At the edge of the fovea centralis, the layers of the retina begin to become thinner; at the foveola, the retina is very thin. Observe that the inner limiting membrane and the ganglion cell layer are present at the foveola but the optic nerve fiber layer and inner nuclear layer are both absent. The outer plexiform layer, outer nuclear layer, external limiting membrane, and layer of cones are all present; however, rods are absent. The pigment epithelium adheres tightly to the choroid (see Fig. 22.21, ILM, GCL, INL, ONL, C, PL, Ch).

Lacrimal Gland

The lacrimal gland is a serous, compound tubuloacinar gland whose ducts open into the conjunctival sac. It is subdivided into a number of lobules by connective tissue septa that convey vascular elements to and from the gland. The acini of the gland display the round nuclei of their acinar cells (see Fig. 22.23, D, Se, BV, Ac). At a medium magnification, the lumina and the round nuclei of the acinar cells composing the acini are well demonstrated. Observe that the ducts and blood vessels are located in the connective tissue septa (see Fig. 22.24, *arrow*, N, Ac, D, BV, Se).

Ear

Inner Ear: Cochlea and Crista Ampullaris

In this very-low-magnification photomicrograph, the cochlea is seen to be a hollow bony spiral that turns on itself, like a snail shell, two and one-half times around a central bony column, the modiolus. The modiolus projects into the spiraled cochlea with a shelf of bone called the osseous spiral lamina, through which traverse blood vessels, the spiral ganglion, and the cochlear nerve, a division of the vestibulocochlear nerve. Observe that the spiraling cochlea supports the organ of Corti, below which is the scala tympani. The space above the organ of Corti is divided by the vestibular membrane into two compartments: the cochlear duct (scala media) and scala vestibuli. The scalae tympani and vestibuli contain the extracellular fluid–like perilymph and the two scalae communicate with each other at the helicotrema; the cochlear duct houses the intracellular fluid–like endolymph. Observe the crista ampullaris of the semicircular canal, recognizable by the overlying cone-shaped cupula. The cross-section of the stapedius muscle is also evident (see Fig. 22.31, Mo, OC, ST, SV, CA, SM).

Inner Ear: Organ of Corti

The organ of Corti sits on the basilar membrane, which separates the perilymph-containing scala tympani from the endolymph-containing cochlear duct (scala media). The vestibular membrane separates the cochlear duct from the perilymph-containing scala vestibuli (see Fig. 22.32, BM, ST, CD, VM, SV). At a medium magnification, the organ of Corti, which sits on the basilar membrane, is seen to extend from the border cells to the cells of Hensen. Below the basilar membrane is the scala tympani. The vestibular membrane separates the cochlear duct (scala media) from the scala vestibuli. Observe that the tectorial membrane overlies the organ of Corti and the internal spiral sulcus. Note that the reticular membrane isolates the outer and inner hair cells and the space of Nuel from the endolymph present in the cochlear duct (see Fig. 22.33, OC, BM, BC, CH, ST, VM, CD, SV, TM, IS, RM, SN).

INDEX

Note: Page numbers followed by "f" indicate figures, "t" indicate tables, and "b" indicate boxes.

E

F

O

P

T